D1583598

DIAGNOSTIC IMAGING

OF THE JAWS

DIAGNOSTIC IMAGING OF THE JAWS

Robert P. Langlais, D.D.S., M.S., F.A.C.D.
Professor, University of Texas Health Science Center at San Antonio
School of Dentistry
San Antonio, Texas

Olaf E. Langland, D.D.S., M.S., F.A.C.D.
Professor, University of Texas Health Science Center at San Antonio
School of Dentistry
San Antonio, Texas

Christoffel J. Nortjé, B. Ch.D., Ph.D.
Professor of Maxillofacial Radiology
University of Stellenbosch
School of Dentistry
Tygerberg, Republic of South Africa

A Lea & Febiger Book

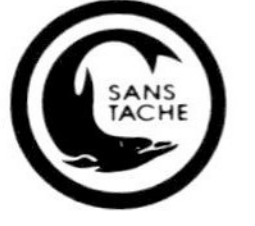

Williams & Wilkins
BALTIMORE • PHILADELPHIA • HONG KONG
LONDON • MUNICH • SYDNEY • TOKYO
A WAVERLY COMPANY

1995

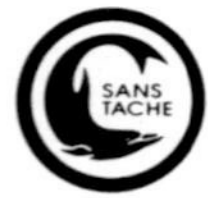

Executive Editor—D. Cooke
Development Editor—S. Zinner
Project Editor—D. DiRienzi
Production Manager—Mary Clare Beaulieu

Williams & Wilkins
200 Chester Field Parkway
Malvern, PA 19355 USA

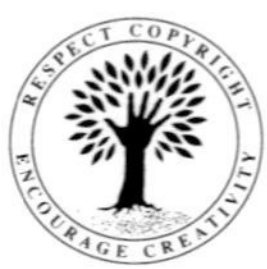

Accurate indications, adverse reactions, and dosage schedules for drugs are provided in this book, but it is possible they may change. The reader is urged to review the package information data of the manufacturers of the medications mentioned.

Printed in the United States of America

Library of Congress Cataloging-in-Publication Data

Diagnostic imaging of the jaws / [edited by] Robert P. Langlais, Olaf E. Langland, Christoffel J. Nortjé.—1st ed.
p. cm.
Includes index.
ISBN 0-683-04809-0
1. Jaws—Radiography. 2. Teeth—Radiography. 3. Jaws—Radiography—Atlases. 4. Teeth—Radiography—Atlases. I. Langlais, Robert P. II. Langland, Olaf E. III. Nortjé, Christoffel J.
[DNLM: 1. Jaw Diseases—diagnosis—atlases. 2. Radiography, Dental—atlases. 3. Jaw—pathology—atlases. WU 17 D536 1994]
RK309.D53 1994
617.5′22—dc20
DNLM/DLC
for Library of Congress 94-7878
CIP

94 95 96 97 98
1 2 3 4 5 6 7 8 9 10

This Book is Dedicated to:

Denyse
Gwen
Marie

Preface

This is a textbook of oral and maxillofacial radiologic interpretation intended for dental students, dentists, dental specialists, and medical radiologists. An attempt has been made to include all the more common abnormalities that may produce radiographic changes in the jaws and most of the rare ones; therefore, it can be used as a general source of reference.

The text contained in this book was written by the primary authors, and much of the illustrative material was supplied by the contributing authors. Because radiology is a pictorial science, many high-quality illustrations must be included to learn it. An analysis of 11 of the chapters shows a ratio of 1.6 pages of text to 1 page of illustrations. We searched wide and far to find the best possible group of contributing authors to supply this material. We made enormous efforts to find excellent examples of cases illustrating the typical radiologic features and the most common variations. Our special contributors have also aided by helping us with our literature reviews, case selections, and other tasks relative to the production of the final manuscript.

We have tried to produce a textbook of oral and maxillofacial radiographic interpretation that includes radiographs of high quality. We have been dismayed in the past by the number of poor-quality radiographs reproduced in textbooks and articles on pathology and radiology. To rectify this deficiency, almost all our radiographs have been reproduced by the Log E-Tronic process. We are sure you will notice the difference in clarity and definition of these illustrations.

Several of the goals that evolved as we wrote this book include the introduction of the regular usage of the descriptive terminology developed by medical radiologists; the provision of complete descriptions of each entity; observations on the nature and behavior of the lesion; and expansion of the number of histologically accurate radiologic diagnoses. With all the information available to us, we were dumbfounded to find the paucity of really accurate and detailed information on the radiology of the jaws. Typically, the radiologic description would range from a single descriptive term such as "multilocular" to varying degrees of added information such as size, margin characteristics, or location. In developing some of the unique descriptions in this text, we have attempted first to determine whether a lesion develops through several phases and relate the radiologic changes to these stages with the use of appropriate radiologic terms. For example, the ameloblastoma is generally described as an expansile multilocular radiolucency. In actual fact, the lesion begins as an unilocular cyst-like radiolucency, without expansion; multilocularity and expansion are later features. Thus, as some conditions develop, they evolve through stages that are radiologically distinct. This is important because the radiograph can supply information on the nature and behavior of an individual lesion. For example, questions relating to active versus dormant, aggressive versus nonaggressive, tendency for recurrence or not, rapidity of growth, and signs of regression, healing, or recurrence may all be answered with some accuracy by studying the radiographs of a given lesion. Because some of our findings have never been described elsewhere, we have been careful to indicate that these interpretations have originated with us. As some of our unique descriptions are based on a limited number of cases, we hope they will withstand the test of time or stimulate others to add to our observations.

As we have done on other occasions, we have classified the various conditions on the basis of their radiologic appearance. Thus, the list of diseases in a given chapter represents a differential diagnosis for the disorders contained herein. Our classification is based on the classic, most common, or mature radiologic presentation of an entity, and other variations are described in the same place. Thus, if the reader wants to learn about a disease, all the information will be found within a single description. In addition, the entities contained in any given chapter are in a similar order, beginning with developmental or hereditary problems, followed by reactive, traumatic, or inflammatory disorders, then cystic conditions, tumors and fibro-osseous maladies, first benign then malignant, and finally, systemic or metabolic disease. As it turns out, most of these categories of disorders can be found in one or several chapters. For example, most cysts are in the chapter on interradicular radiolucencies; most odontogenic and vascular lesions are in the pericoronal and multilocular chapters; fibro-osseous conditions are under periapical and generalized radiopacities; systemic-metabolic diseases are under generalized rarefactions; bone tumors fall into the category of solitary radiopacities; and finally, inflammatory and malignant problems fall into the chapter on poorly defined lesions. The text has been organized with multiple headings such as pathology, clinical features, treatment and prognosis, and radiology; within the radiology section, many subheadings can be found including location, general radiologic features, specific subheadings for the jaws, skull, and other parts of the skeleton if pertinent. Because the science of accurate radiologic interpretation is a deductive process that occurs before the histologic diagnosis is made, all ancillary information about the patients, such as age, sex, and symptoms, should be known; understanding the basic pathogenesis is also invaluable in learning and explaining the radiologic changes produced by a lesion.

Moreover, in almost all textbooks of dental radiographic interpretation, the very subjects that need the most extensive coverage, for instance caries, periodontal disease, and periapical disease, are covered only superficially or not at all. In this textbook, the reader will be pleased to discover comprehensive coverage of the dental diseases as well as the developmental conditions of the jaws and teeth.

We believe, as many other radiologists believe, that radiologic interpretation is "true detective" work. The radiograph is like a single page in a "whodunit" novel. The finished radiograph provides the dentist with a window into the many pathologic changes occurring within the patient as a result of disease. The radiograph does not provide the diagnosis, however. It provides only one piece of evidence in the diagnostic puzzle. If the student has a knowledge of anatomy, especially of the head and neck, and can observe the changes that the disease produces on the radiograph, it will be possible to identify the pathologic process(es) produced by those radiographic changes. It is our goal, as it is for many other teachers of radiology, to teach students to recognize radiographic patterns and, in turn, to define the pathophysiologic process producing that pattern.

No field of dentistry has made such dramatic changes as oral and maxillofacial radiology in the past two decades. The revolution in radiology began in the early 1970s with the development of ultrasound and computed tomography (CT); then in the early 1980s, magnetic resonance (MR) was perfected. Radiology is constantly changing. Improvements in computer technology have resulted in three-dimensional imaging and digital imaging. Digital processing of data will carry radiology into the twenty-first century. The days of film/screen imaging are numbered. The technique of picture archiving and computer storage (PACS) is now a reality and will become more generally available in the next few years. We hope that future editions of this textbook will be able to keep us up to date with the new changes in the use of diagnostic imaging in dentistry.

San Antonio, Texas — ***Robert P. Langlais***

San Antonio, Texas — ***Olaf E. Langland***

Tygerberg, South Africa — ***Christoffel J. Nortjé***

Acknowledgments

We express our appreciation to our many colleagues, contributors, and Eastman Kodak Company, who generously and willingly gave permission to use illustrative material and diagrams from their published works. We acknowledge with gratitude those many individuals throughout the world who have contributed radiographs of their cases. Without their kind assistance this book would not have been completed.

We acknowledge Dieter Karkut and April Cox, photographers, for their excellent quality of Log E-Tronic prints of most all the radiographs in this book. The illustrations and diagrams were skillfully prepared by Chuck Whitehead, medical illustrator.

We thank our secretaries, Peggy Campbell, Jerry Franklin, and Patricia Gonzales, who contributed unselfishly of their time, skillfully typing each chapter many times and carefully collecting illustrative material in the preparation of this manuscript.

Another source of great pleasure and inspiration has been, and still remains, the association we have with dental students. A special sense of gratitude is felt for the dental students for they have added pleasure and fullness to our lives as teachers of radiology.

R.P.L.
O.E.L.
C.J.N.

Contributing Authors

Masao Araki, D.D.S., Ph.D.
Instructor of Radiology
Nihon University School of Dentistry
Tokyo, Japan

Luis Ronaldo Archila, D.D.S.
Research Assistant Professor
University of Texas Health Science Center at San Antonio
School of Dentistry
San Antonio, Texas
Private Practice in Oral and Maxillofacial Radiology
Guatemala City, Guatemala

Roman Carlos, D.D.S., M.S.
Private Practice of Oral Pathology
Guatemala City, Guatemala

Alvaro Castro Delgado, D.D.S.
Professor and Chief of Radiology Clinic
Faculty of Odontology
Pontificia Universidad Javeriana
Santa Fé de Bogotá, Colombia

Gabriel Castro Delgado, D.D.S.
Professor and Chief of Radiology Clinic
Faculty of Odontology
Pontificia Universidad Javeriana
Santa Fé de Bogotá, Colombia

Israel Chilvarguer, D.D.S., M.S., Ph.D.
Assistant Professor of Radiology
University of São Paulo Dental School
São Paulo, Brazil

Pairat Dhiravarangkura, D.D.S.
Professor of Radiology
Chulalonghorn University
Bangkok, Thailand

Fernando Erales, D.D.S., M.S.
Private Practice of Oral and Maxillofacial Radiology
Guatemala City, Guatemala

Hajime Fuchihata, D.D.S., Ph.D.
Professor and Chairman of Oral and Maxillofacial Radiology
Faculty of Dentistry
Osaka University
Osaka, Japan

Yoshishige Fujiki, D.D.S., D. Med. Sci.
Honorary Professor
Asahi University School of Dentistry
Gifu, Japan

Koji Hashimoto, D.D.S., Ph.D.
Assistant Professor of Radiology
Nihon University School of Dentistry
Tokyo, Japan

Kazuya Honda, D.D.S., Ph.D.
Instructor of Radiology
Nihon University
Tokyo, Japan

Takinmori Noikura, Ph.D., D.D.S.
Professor of Dental Radiology
Dental School
Kagoshima University
Kagoshima, Japan

Takeshi Ohba, D.D.S., D. M. Sc.
Professor and Chairman of Dental Radiology
Kyushu Dental College
Kitakyushu, Japan

Chang Seo Park, D.D.S., M.S., Ph.D.
Associate Professor and Chairman of Dental Radiology
College of Dentistry
Yonsei University
Seoul, Korea

M.E. Parker, B. Ch. D. (U.W.C.), M. Dent. Rad. (Lond.)
Professor and Head of Diagnosis and Radiology
Faculty of Dentistry
University of the Western Cape
Stellenbosch, Republic of South Africa

Elias Romero, D.D.S., M.S.
Universidad Autonoma de Nuevo León
Monterrey, Mexico

Eiko Sairenji, D.D.S., D. Med. Sci., F.R.S.H. (Engld.)
Professor of Radiology
Nihon University
Tokyo, Japan

Harry C. Schwartz, D.M.D., M.D., F.A.C.S.
Chief of Maxillofacial Surgery
Southern California Permanente Medical Group
Associate Professor of Oral and Maxillofacial Surgery
University of California, Los Angeles
Los Angeles, California

Gunilla Tronje, D.D.S., Ph.D.
Docent in Oral Radiology
Karolinska Institutet
Stockholm, Sweden

Special Contributors

Marden Alder, D.D.S., M.S.
University of Texas Health Science Center
San Antonio, Texas

Lilian Chilvarquer, D.D.S., M.S.
Instituto de Documentaçao Ortodontica e Radiodiagnostico
São Paulo, Brazil

S. Brent Dove, D.D.S., M.S.
University of Texas Health Science Center
San Antonio, Texas

Denise Kassebaum, D.D.S., M.S.
University of Colorado
Denver, Colorado

Craig S. Miller, D.D.S., M.S.
University of Kentucky
Lexington, Kentucky

Richard Monahan, D.D.S., M.S.
Northwestern University
Chicago, Illinois

Thomas Schiff, D.M.D., F.I.C.D., F.A.C.D.
University of the Pacific
San Francisco, California

Contents

Chapter 1

Decision Making in Dental Radiology

Although a variety of oral health care workers can provide a multitude of diagnostic and therapeutic services, only the dentist is permitted to diagnose disease and to prescribe treatment. Because no recognized specialty of radiology exists in the dental profession in the United States, the practitioner assumes the responsibility of ordering the appropriate radiologic studies and accurately interpreting the radiography in light of current knowledge with respect to diagnostic quality, recognition of abnormality, and assessment of any changes discernible in the image.

DIAGNOSTIC SEQUENCE

The diagnostic sequence consists of the following information as it relates to the patient in question:

1. Demographic information with respect to age, sex, and race.
2. Chief complaint and its history.
3. Social, medical, and dental history.
4. Laboratory values.
5. Radiologic findings.
6. Additional examinations, tests, or consultations as required.

Throughout this text, we refer to specific information with respect to each condition that relates to the information needed to perform an accurate diagnostic sequence. For this reason, each condition is outlined as follows:

Overview.
Pathology.
Clinical features.
Treatment and prognosis.
Radiology.

Within the radiology section, applicable subdivisions include:

General or skeletal radiologic features if applicable.
Radiology of the skull and facial bones if applicable.
Radiology of the jaws including location, radiologic features, and relation to teeth.
Features on other imaging methods including linear and multidirectional tomography, computed tomography (CT), magnetic resonance (MR), scintigraphy, and other less common adjunctive imaging techniques including arthroscopy, arthrography, sialography, angiography, and others as needed.

VIEWING THE RADIOGRAPH

To obtain the maximum amount of information when viewing radiographs, the following principles should be observed:

1. Interpret only from properly exposed and processed radiographs.
2. Use multiple views and imaging methods when these are required to demonstrate all the radiographic features and all three dimensions.
3. View the radiographs in a quiet area with subdued lighting.
4. The viewbox should provide a uniform degree of light; variable-intensity light should be available for illuminating darker radiographs.
5. All extraneous light should be blocked out from around the edges of the film on the viewbox.
6. View the overall image from a distance before focusing on specific areas.
7. Use a good magnifying glass.
8. Restrict the size of the viewing field to the area of interest.
9. Use supplemental studies when needed.

These viewing principles are needed to create a physical environment in which the radiologist can extract the most detail from the radiographs, to assimilate them properly for the purpose of making an accurate interpretation.

SUBJECTIVITY OF RADIOLOGIC INTERPRETATION

One might expect the interpretation of caries to be straightforward. We and our colleagues (Langlais and co-workers, 1987) conducted a study whereby several sets of bitewing radiographs were displayed for interpretation by faculty who taught operative dentistry, general practice, oral diagnosis, and radiology. The radiographic findings of the faculty members were reported on a standardized form. After analyzing the data, we found little agreement among the 35 participating faculty on the size of the carious lesions, their depth into dentin, and their proximity to the pulp. The greatest area of agreement was regarding the presence or absence of disease, whereas the greatest disagreement occurred over the degree of disease present. Later in our discussion we cite further studies in which the variability among observers was greater than that of the radiologic phenomena studied.

The primary objective of radiographic interpretation is to identify the presence or absence of disease. In dentistry, this means choosing a radiographic examination that will result in the greatest diagnostic yield with the least amount of radiation to the patient, that is, an initial examination consisting of a panoramic radiograph and possibly bitewing radiographs. On consideration of recent data from the literature, some practitioners may question the value of bitewing radiographs when one also has a properly exposed panoramic radiograph taken with modern equipment. We do not mean to infer that the practitioner should immediately dispose of existing intraoral and older panoramic equipment. We intend to show how modern panoramic equipment can save billions of grays in population dose over intraoral techniques and at the same time offer diagnostic accuracy in parts of the jaws that were heretofore considered the exclusive territory of bitewing radiography or the full mouth radiographic survey.

SELECTION CRITERIA UPDATE

In our opinion, selection criteria developed before the studies of Underhill and co-workers (1988) and others such as Gibbs and co-workers (1988) on the dosimetry and risk of panoramic radiology and selection criteria for the taking of dental radiographs based on older data detailing the diagnostic yield of panoramic images must now be reexamined in light of current knowledge. For example, the United States Department of Health and Human Services (1987) developed guidelines for prescribing dental radiographs. These guidelines do not mention the use of panoramic radiography when examining a new adolescent or adult patient for dental diseases and/or growth and developmental problems. Most general dental patients fall into these categories. The guidelines recommend an individualized radiographic examination consisting of posterior bitewing and selected periapical radiographs. Furthermore, the guidelines state that a full mouth radiographic examination is appropriate when the new adolescent or adult patient has clinical evidence of generalized dental disease or a history of extensive dental treatment. Posterior bitewing examinations are recommended at intervals of 24 to 36 months for adult or adolescent patients with no clinical caries and no high risk factors for caries; bitewings at 12- to 18-month intervals are recommended for adult or adolescent patients with clinical caries or high risk factors for caries. The high risk factors listed in the guidelines are a high level of caries, a history of recurrent caries, existing restoration(s) of poor quality, poor oral hygiene, inadequate fluoride exposure, prolonged nursing by bottle or breast, diet with a high sucrose content, poor family dental health, developmental enamel defects, developmental disability, xerostomia, genetic abnormality of the teeth, many multisurface restorations, and chemotherapy. At any time the most valid selection criterion for a specific radiologic examination consists of the **ALARA** principle, which, according to Preece (1984), states: the selection of radiologic examinations shall be based on obtaining the greatest diagnostic yield while delivering radiation doses to the patient that are **A**s **L**ow **A**s **R**easonably **A**chievable.

Historically, the primary argument for taking an intraoral full mouth survey was that this imaging method was widely believed to be more sensitive for the detection of common dental disorders such as caries, periodontal disease, and periapical disease. In many studies of the diagnostic yield from panoramic radiographs, these three categories of dental disease are excluded on this assumption, or only the negative aspects of the data are emphasized when these categories of disease are compared. For example, Valachovic and colleagues (1986) concluded the following: "for dental caries, and (to a lesser extent) periodontal disease, the panoramic radiograph was inferior to the full mouth intraoral series in its ability to correctly detect evidence of the disease." Our interpretation of their data was different because a large part of their results actually favored the panoramic radiograph. In addition, when common diagnoses such as caries, periodontal disease, and periapical disease are excluded, all other pathologic conditions such as supernumerary teeth or impacted teeth or diseases within the jaw bones such as tumors and cysts purportedly show no increase in diagnostic yield when panoramic and full mouth surveys are compared. For example, Gratt (1987) has cited studies showing that when a full mouth set of radiographs is available for a patient receiving a general screening examination, little or no additional useful information is gained from a panoramic examination. Even though all the references cited were 8 to 15 years old, these beliefs still persist among some authors, educators, and practitioners. In light of current dose information, the question should read: "If a panoramic radiograph is available, how much additional information can be obtained from the full mouth survey?"

The detection of caries in anterior teeth is generally believed to be a clinical diagnosis, and radiographs of these teeth are rarely taken for this purpose. On the other hand, radiographs of posterior teeth are frequently taken for the detection of caries. Valachovic and colleagues found that panoramic radiographs demonstrated the highest positive predictive values (PPV) for the detection of caries in posterior teeth as compared to the full mouth survey including bitewing radiographs and combined panoramic and bitewing radiographs. The PPV is the probability that a patient with a positive radiographic finding actually has the disease. These values were 77% in premolars and 67% in molars as interpreted from panoramic radiographs; 75 and 65% in the premolars and molars, respectively, as viewed in full mouth survey including bitewing radiographs; and 63% each in the premolars and molars when panoramic and bitewing radiographs were viewed together. Valachovic and colleagues thus found that the panoramic radiograph alone was the most effective for detecting caries that were actually present in posterior teeth. From these data we have concluded that, not only were the periapical and bitewing radiographs less effective with respect to the PPVs of caries in posterior teeth, but also the bitewing radiographs had a negative effect on the PPVs of caries detection in posterior teeth when they were viewed in conjunction with panoramic radiographs. Valachovic and colleagues also showed that the negative predictive value (NPV) for the detection of caries in anterior teeth was equal to that of the panoramic, full mouth survey including bitewings and the panoramic and bitewing radiographic surveys. The NPV is the probability that a patient with a negative radiographic finding actually does not have the disease. The NPVs were 98% for all three imaging meth-

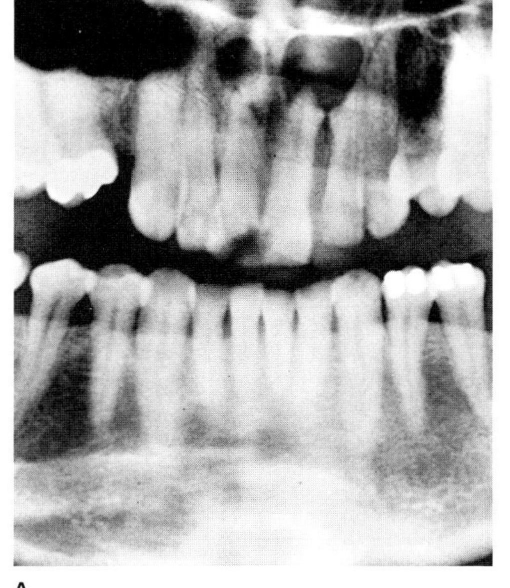

A

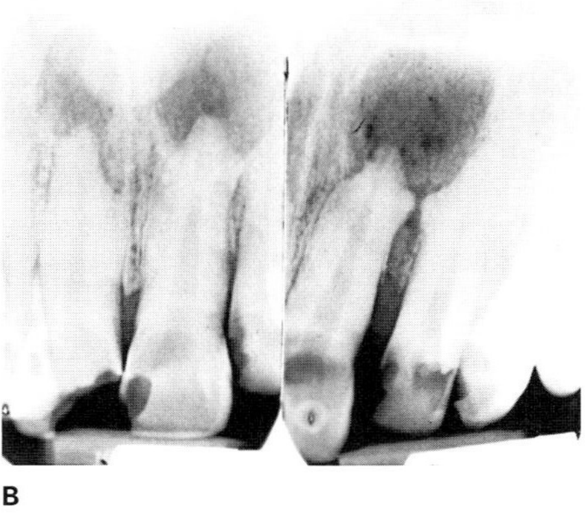

B

FIGURE 1–1.

Anterior Periapical Disease: maxillary. A and B, The lesions are well visualized in the panoramic radiograph as compared to the intraoral views.

ods of the anterior teeth. Valachovic and co-authors also showed that the PPVs for periodontal disease detection were almost exactly equal between the low-dose single panoramic radiograph and the higher-dose full mouth survey including bitewing radiographs. The PPVs for the molars, premolars, and anterior teeth were 79%, 72%, and 57%, respectively, for the panoramic radiograph and 80%, 73%, and 57% for the full mouth survey with bitewing radiographs. When panoramic and bitewing radiographs were viewed together, the PPVs for periodontal disease were slightly diminished to 77%, 69%, and 51% for the molars, premolars, and anterior teeth, respectively. Thus, the use of bitewing radiographs not only doubles the dose to the patient over that of the panoramic radiograph alone, but also has a slightly negative effect on the PPVs of panoramic radiographs when viewed without bitewing radiographs. Valachovic and colleagues also showed that the NPVs for periodontal disease of a single panoramic radiograph were superior in all three anatomic areas over the full mouth survey including bitewings and the panoramic radiograph with bitewings. The NPVs averaged 85% for the panoramic, 76% for the full mouth survey including bitewings, and 79% for the panoramic with bitewings.

One may argue that panoramic radiographs generally show poor details in the anterior region of the jaws and are thus considered undiagnostic in this area (Figs. 1–1 and 1–2). Muhammed and Manson-Hing (1982), however, compared the panoramic and full mouth survey radiographs of 300 patients. They found 21 periapical radiolucencies on periapical radiographs in the anterior mandible, and fully 16 of these radiolucencies were also seen in the panoramic radiographs. In the anterior maxilla, these clinicians found

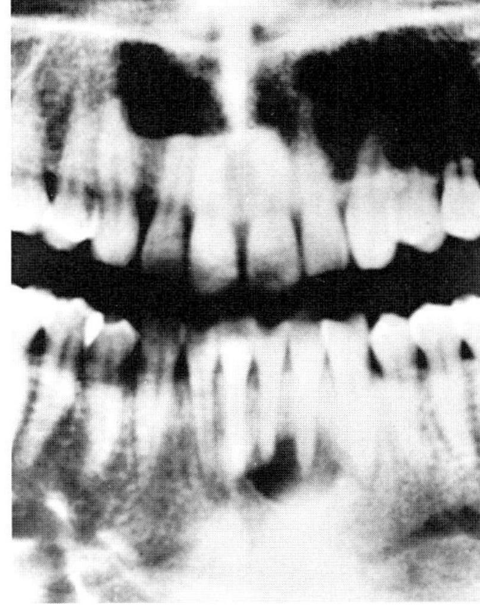

A

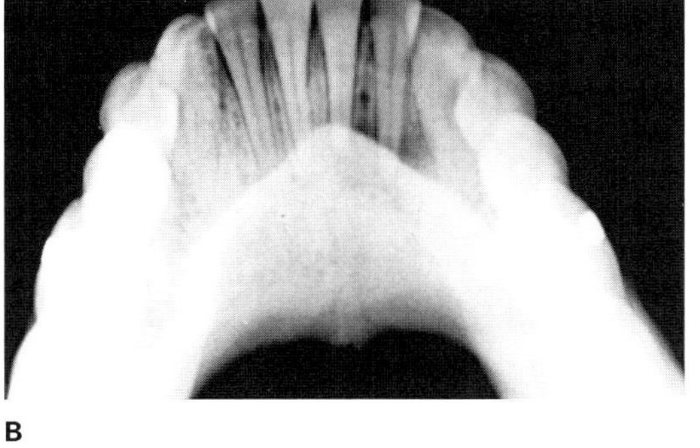

B

FIGURE 1–2.

Anterior Periapical Disease: mandibular. A, Panoramic view; B, occlusal view.

12 periapical radiolucencies, and 9 of these were also noted on the panoramic radiographs. These authors did not specify diminished panoramic image quality in the anterior region as a criterion for the rejection of cases from the study. Schiff and colleagues (1986) studied the frequency and types of panoramic errors and noted that panoramic radiographs of poor technical quality are often accepted, whereas for periapical radiographs, the policy of many institutions is that when a specific anatomic location is not diagnostic on at least one of the periapical films of the full mouth survey, the radiograph must be retaken and must continue to be retaken until the structure or region in question is diagnostic. One might also argue that the panoramic radiograph can image structures within the jaws beyond the anatomic limits of a properly exposed intraoral full mouth survey using the long-cone paralleling technique. In other parts of this text we describe cases in which tumors and other diseases were not detected because the patient was examined with intraoral radiographs only. In addition, the panoramic radiograph demonstrates structures such as the ramus, temporomandibular joint (TMJ), styloid process and styloid ligament, upper parts of the maxillary antrum, and lower orbit, which are outside the anatomic limits of the full mouth survey. The most common radiograph used in this text to illustrate the radiologic features of the various pathologic conditions of the jaw is the panoramic radiograph, including the anterior area. In fact, Ohba and Katayama (1972) examined the panoramic and full mouth surveys of 140 dental students and concluded that panoramic radiographs were preferable for the diagnosis of bone lesions in the jaws.

Indications for Panoramic Radiographs

Given that older studies emphasized the negative aspects of panoramic radiology, some authors have reasoned or assumed that because panoramic radiographs are not as sensitive as intraoral radiographs for the detection of common dental diseases such as caries, periodontal disease, and periapical disease, and because panoramic radiographs have not shown any increase in diagnostic yield over intraoral radiographs for other diseases, panoramic radiographs should be reserved only for patients who are symptomatic or who have clinical signs of jaw disease, or when signs of more extensive disease can be seen in intraoral radiographs. Gratt (1987), for example, has listed the following indications for panoramic radiographs:

1. The evaluation of trauma, third molars, extensive or unique disorders, and their associated surgical procedures.
2. The evaluation of tooth development, especially mixed dentition analysis.
3. The evaluation of developmental anomalies.

In recent studies, panoramic radiographs compared favorably with intraoral radiographs for the interpretation of caries, periodontal disease, and periapical disease. Because the savings in radiation dose is considerable, these current trends should be followed closely, and policies on the selection of radiographic studies should be reviewed and updated.

Caries

With respect to the interpretation of caries on panoramic radiographs, we have outlined the findings of Valachovic and colleagues favoring panoramic radiographs with respect to PPVs and NPVs (Fig. 1–3). Terezhalmy and colleagues (1985) used 8 raters to analyze 659 interproximal surfaces of posterior teeth for the detection of interproximal caries in bitewing and panoramic radiographs. They eliminated any panoramic or bitewing radiographs with overlapping of the interproximal surfaces of interest. Using the kappa statistic, these investigators found that the accuracy of interproximal caries detection in panoramic radiographs as compared to bitewing radiographs showed no significant variations. Currently, panoramic machines are being designed with specific projection geometry that will routinely eliminate overlapping of the interproximal areas of the posterior teeth, especially the premolars.

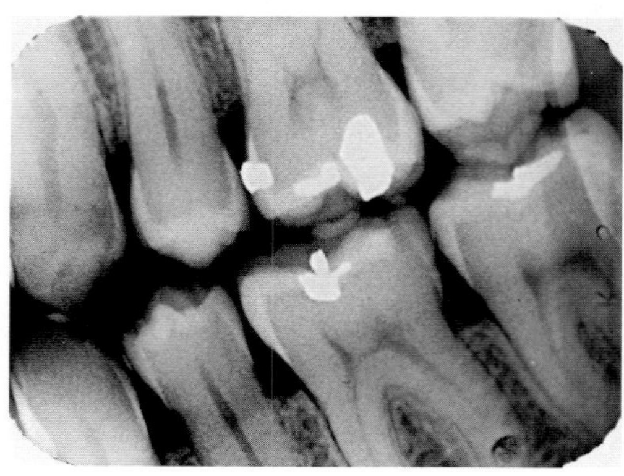

A

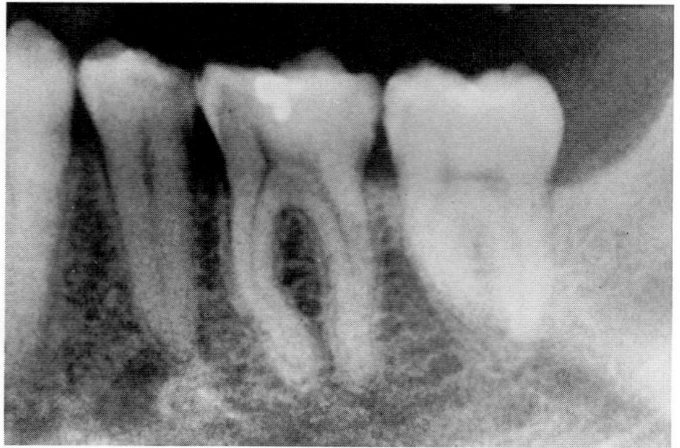

B

FIGURE 1–3.

Detection of Caries: panoramic versus bitewing radiography. A, Bitewing radiograph failed to demonstrate caries on the mesial aspect of the second mandibular molar. B, Panoramic view taken on the same day demonstrates that the lesion is through the enamel and into the dentin.

Periodontal Disease

In their classic 1967 study of periodontal disease, Ainamo and Tammisalo found that panoramic radiographs showed marginal alveolar bone loss that deviated less from the true measurements made on the teeth of skulls after they were extracted than did intraoral radiographs. Rohlin and co-workers (1989a) compared panoramic and paralleling periapical radiographs for the evaluation of marginal bone loss. They reported concordant scores in 66% of the sites in the upper arch, whereas 33% deviated by one and 3% by two score points. In the mandible, concordance was noted for 74% of the sites, whereas 25% deviated by one and 1% by two score points. One score point was approximately equivalent to a millimeter of bone loss, corrected for magnification differences between the two techniques. These investigators also noted that the panoramic radiographs more often indicated more severe bone loss than the periapical radiographs. Akesson and colleagues (1989) also compared panoramic and intraoral radiography for the assessment of marginal bone level. On the basis of their results, these investigators proposed that, in clinical practice, the panoramic radiograph should be used and then supplemented with individually selected periapical radiographs where needed. For epidemiologic studies, Akesson and co-workers recommended a panoramic radiograph in combination with a premolar bitewing radiograph. Although Rohlin and colleagues did no studies to determine truth (only agreement between imaging techniques), the full mouth survey was not designed for the accuracy of periodontal disease assessment. The technique is designed to achieve parallelism between the vertical position of the teeth and the film. The radiologic level of the alveolar bone varies with the vertical angulation of the cone and the position of the film. In addition, the alveolar bone may be considered to consist of a curved flat horizontal plane, with few variations in the vertical plane, except when disease is present. For the bisecting technique, we and our colleagues (Langland and co-authors, 1984) have recommended vertical angulation changes from +25 to +45° in the maxilla and from −15 to +5° in the mandible. These variations in the vertical angulation of the beam cause unequal differences in the projected vertical height of the alveolar bone in the radiograph. Accuracy with respect to the projection of alveolar bone height is essential when vertical bone loss associated with periodontal disease is measured. In panoramic radiography, we and our colleagues (Langland and co-authors, 1989) have reported that most manufacturers use a constant vertical angle of approximately −5 to −7° for all parts of the projection. We therefore believe that Ainamo and Tammisalo found that measurements of marginal bone loss made from panoramic radiographs were the most accurate when compared to truth. We also believe that the findings of Rohlin and colleagues (1989b) indicate that when measurements of alveolar bone height differ between panoramic and intraoral films, the intraoral films underestimate the degree of alveolar bone loss, whereas the panoramic radiograph most accurately depicts the true level of the bone. It is also probable that when machines such as the Gendex (Philips) Orthoralix SD (Gendex Corp., Des Plaines, IL) become more widely available, the supplemental periapical and premolar intraoral radiographs as recommended by Akesson and colleagues will no longer be needed.

Periapical Disease

In a study by Rohlin and colleagues (1989b), panoramic radiographs were shown to be as effective as periapical radiographs for the detection of lytic and sclerotic periapical disease. Muhammed and Manson-Hing (1982) found that the full mouth survey was deficient in identifying osteosclerosis and ectopic calcifications when compared to panoramic radiography (Fig. 1–4). In addition, when assessing early lytic periapical changes, many oral and maxillofacial radiologists and others such as endodontists have observed that such changes may be clearly seen in the panoramic radiograph when no change is visible on the corresponding periapical radiograph taken at the same time (Fig. 1–5). The authors have made this observation on a clinical basis for at least the past 12 years.

A

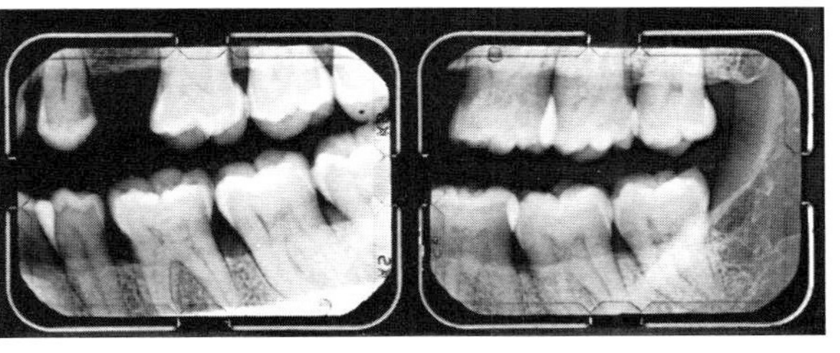

B

FIGURE 1–4.

Poorly Mineralized Tissue: A, Panoramic radiograph shows excessive calculus. B, Bitewings fail to demonstrate the calculus.

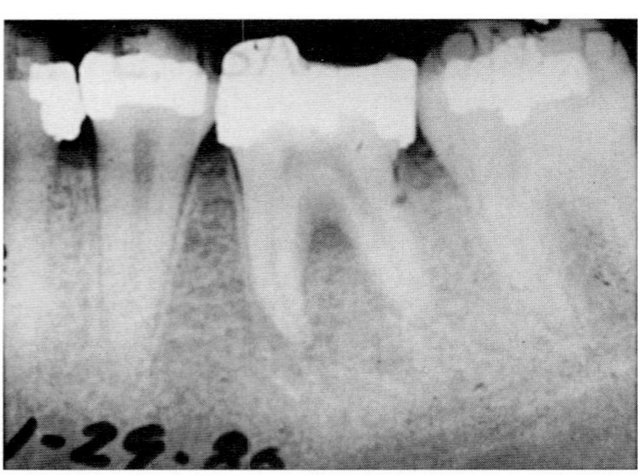

A

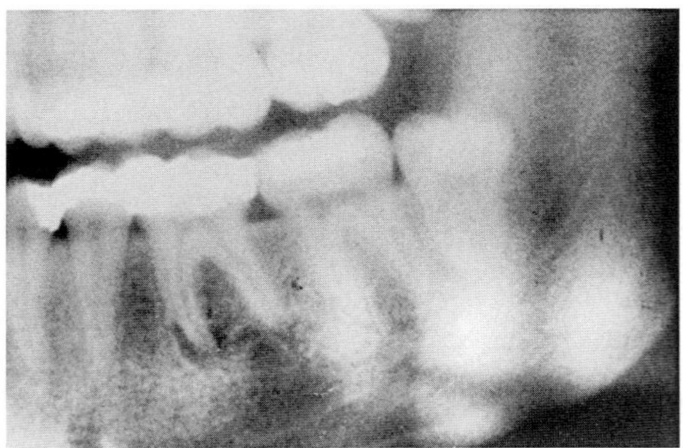

B

FIGURE 1–5.

Early Detection of Periapical Disease: A, Periapical radiograph of the first molar does not show the abscess. B, Panoramic radiograph taken the same day shows the abscess. (Courtesy of Dr. Leif Isaccson, Albuquerque, NM.)

In their classic study, Bender and Seltzer (1961) showed that periapical osteolytic lesions as viewed on intraoral films are detectable only if the inner or outer surface of the cortex is eroded or frankly perforated, and a loss of trabecular pattern is discernible only when the junction of the cortex and cancellous bone of the medullary space is eroded. Philips and Shawkat (1973) created lesions within the medullary space that did not encroach on the cortex. These investigators used dried mandibles and demonstrated that the image of the defects appeared more distinctly on panoramic than on periapical radiographs. More recently, Bianchi and colleagues (1991) reviewed the literature of the past 30 years; subsequent investigators essentially had come to the same conclusions as Bender and Seltzer in their original 1961 study. Bianchi and colleagues also showed that the detectability of a periapical lesion on a periapical film depends not only on the erosion of the cortex, but also on the density of the spongiosa and the diameter of the lesion. Information on the increased sensitivity of panoramic radiographs in the detection of periapical disease is based more on anecdotal incidences of such occurrences in practice than on studies specifically aimed at proving this theory.

Rohlin and colleagues (1989b) compared panoramic and periapical radiographs for the diagnosis of periapical bone lesions. The lesions were associated with the periapical regions of 117 teeth and were evenly divided between osteolytic and sclerotic changes. Using the receiver operating analysis (ROC), these investigators reported no overall significant difference between panoramic and periapical radiography for the detection of periapical lesions, although they reported differences in diagnostic accuracy between the two techniques, favoring periapical radiographs in the maxillary premolar region. They further explained that this difference is due to the finding of Welander and colleagues (1985), who showed that the panoramic projection deviates from the orthogonal in this area. Because the Gendex (Philips) Orthoralix SD panoramic machine has been designed with an available orthogonal projection, however, differences caused by the orthogonality of the panoramic projection should be eliminated and are currently being tested in ongoing studies.

In a study of 200 patients who were examined clinically and radiologically, Rohlin and Åkerblom (1992) concluded that the information obtained from the clinical and panoramic examinations supplemented with no more than two periapical radiographs will result in a high diagnostic yield on the periapical status; in 30% of their patients, no periapical radiographs were required. Rohlin and co-authors (1989b) also observed the following: "in radiological practice, it is not infrequent that lesions clearly depicted on the panoramic radiographs are less visible, if not totally absent in the corresponding periapical." Rohlin and colleagues theorize that such occurrences are due to the higher inherent contrast in the films used in panoramic radiology and the inherent unsharpness in the resulting image, which may increase the possibility of detecting small lesions. With respect to related studies on periapical lesions comparing other imaging methods (xeroradiography and conventional film), Gratt and co-authors (1986) found greater variation among observers than with either film system. Using subtraction radiography for the study of periapical bone lesions, Kullendorf and colleagues (1988) also noted a greater variation among observers than among the techniques studied. As enumerated by Hollender (1992), many possible variations among observers exist with respect to interpretive skill, bias toward the older, more familiar image, experience, background, and prejudice with respect to the expected outcome; the absence of such variables should be addressed by the authors of such studies.

Disease Trends

With the advent of a generation of patients who have had the benefit of fluoride, combined with other factors such as better education about oral hygiene and the value of natural dentition, better restorative procedures and materials, and more dentists than ever to deliver treatment, diagnoses such as caries, periodontal disease, and periapical disease have become less common. The dentist will become more adept at diagnosing problems in adjacent anatomic regions such as the TMJ, salivary glands, styloid process, and maxillary sinus. Ohba and colleagues (1990) noted that panoramic radiography was the method of choice for the detection of problems associated with the floor and posterior wall of the antrum. In our aging population, the reasons for taking radiographs will shift away from the detection of previously common diseases such as caries and periodontal and periapical disease to include disorders that are more occult, and more life-threatening diagnoses such as malignant diseases within the jaws will be made. Additionally, the importance of recognizing the radiologic manifestations of systemic and metabolic diseases affecting the aging or aged such as osteoporosis will have more significance to a greater number of practitioners throughout the world.

Selection Criteria Revised

The guidelines issued by the United States Department of Health and Human Services in 1987 have been widely circulated, and according to Matteson (1992), they were adopted by the American Dental Association and other professional groups. In 1992, however, Hollender found that their adoption was ''far from common, even among U.S. dental schools.'' According to Kantor (1993), who surveyed 65 dental schools in the United States and Canada, 6 of the 65 respondents explicitly mentioned use of the Food and Drug Administration guidelines. According to White (1992), dentists should use selection criteria for ordering radiographs; as ''there is no consensus on exactly what such criteria should be'' and called for continued research in this field. Therefore, we have made many literature citations concerning our recommendations for low-dose, high-yield radiologic examinations. According to Hollender, many factors may influence the decision on the time and extent of the radiographic examination and may lead to deviations from the suggested guidelines. These factors include education, peer influence, patient's preference, legal considerations, the dentist's field of interest or speciality, the training of the staff, and practice routine. As the authors of a leading textbook on panoramic radiology, now in its second edition (Langland and colleagues, 1989), we consider ourselves informed, and perhaps biased on the subject. We now believe that new early data are sufficient to allow us to state that common diseases such as caries, periodontal disease, and periapical disease can be diagnosed equally well or better on a properly exposed panoramic radiograph using modern equipment. The use of panoramic radiographs for the diagnosis of more occult pathologic processes has not been contentious. We now believe that when a dentist decides to take a radiograph in an asymptomatic patient, or when the physical findings suggest that a radiograph(s) should be taken, then the initial radiograph should be a panoramic view. All other radiographs should be considered supplemental views, including periapical, bitewing, occlusal, extraoral plain views, tomography including CT, and other more advanced imaging techniques such as MR. A much more compelling reason to select a panoramic radiograph for the initial radiologic examination exists, however. This involves an assessment of the ALARA concept and incorporating its basic tenets as it applies to the selection of dental radiographic examinations. To make an informed decision, the reader is asked to consider carefully the data presented in the following discussion.

Dosimetry and Risk Comparisons

With respect to radiation dose, no comparisons have been made between a single panoramic radiograph and the complete mouth intraoral survey. According to White (1992), panoramic radiography carries about one tenth the risk of a full mouth survey in terms of fatal malignant diseases per million persons exposed. Underhill and colleagues (1988) showed that there are several orders of magnitude less radiation with panoramic radiographs using rare earth screens and associated film as compared to the 20-film full mouth survey using the long rectangular cone and E speed film. In addition, with respect to some locations, such as the salivary glands, the diminished dose associated with panoramic radiographs is even greater still. Underhill and colleagues averaged the data obtained from 5 panoramic machines using Kodak Lanex regular screens and T-Mat G film (Eastman Kodak Co., Rochester, NY). The peak kilovoltage (kVp) ranged 73 to 80, the milliamperage (mA) ranged from 4 to 15, and the panoramic exposure cycle ranged from 12 to 20 seconds. The panoramic exposures were standardized by varying the peak kilovoltage and where possible the milliamperage such that each machine produced a calibration image of a phantom having the same density at several standardized anatomic locations. Data on the intraoral dose were obtained using the long rectangular cone and E speed film, for the 20-film full mouth survey including 4 bitewings and separate data for a set of 4 bitewings only. These investigators also obtained data using the long round cone for the full mouth survey and set of 4 bitewings. The peak kilovoltage was 65 for the bitewings, and in the full mouth survey variable peak kilovolts were used for the various anatomic regions ranging from 70 kVp in the mandibular anterior region to 90 kVp in the maxillary molar area. The milliamperage was constant for all the periapical regions and was higher for the bitewings. One millirad (1 mrad) is the same as one microgray (1 μGy). There are 100 rads in a gray.

In terms of risk from dental radiographs, the following critical organs have been implicated as the main target tissues when exposed to dental radiation and are at risk of developing disease:

1. Thyroid gland: carcinoma, adenocarcinoma.
2. Bone marrow: leukemia.
3. Salivary glands: carcinoma, adenocarcinoma.

For the thyroid gland, the data listed in Figure 1–6 indicate that the panoramic radiograph delivers a dose to the thyroid gland that is similar to that from a set of 4 bitewings using the long rectangular cone and E speed film (47 and 38 μGy, respectively). The dose to the thyroid gland from the full mouth survey is 13 times higher than that from the panoramic radiograph using the long round cone and E speed film (47 and 628 μGy, respectively). The dose for a full mouth survey using the long rectangular cone is similar to that of a set of 4 bitewings using the long round cone and E speed film (270 and 232 μGy, respectively). This same pattern was seen for all tissue doses measured.

For the bone marrow of the mandible, the data listed in Figure 1–7 indicate that the panoramic radiograph delivers a dose similar to that from a set of 4 bitewings (587 and 555 μGy, respectively) and is 12 times lower than that from the

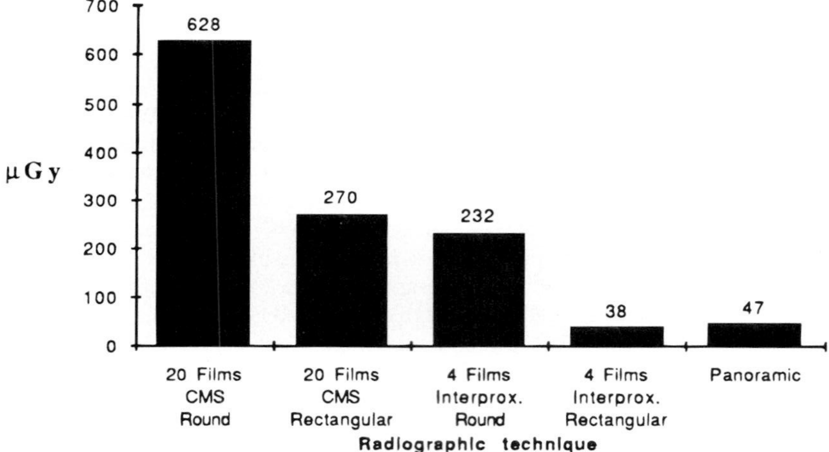

FIGURE 1–6.

Absorbed Radiation Dose to the Thyroid Gland.

full mouth survey using the long round cone and E speed film. In addition, authors such as Gratt (1987) have stated that the dose to the bone marrow in panoramic radiographs "is relatively high in the region of the centers of rotation." In their experiments, Underhill and colleagues (1988) located accurately the narrow regions within the bone marrow through which the rotation centers pass for each panoramic machine tested. Figure 1–8 demonstrates that the bone marrow doses for the panoramic machines at the narrow rotation centers is actually 2.5 to 8 times less than bone marrow dose from the full mouth survey using the long round cone (886 to 2872 and 7090 μGy, respectively). Such a small area of the bone marrow is irradiated in association with the constantly moving rotation centers of the panoramic machines, however, that such doses must be considered relatively insignificant as compared to the extensive areas of bone marrow irradiated in the full mouth survey. Only a thin slit of radiation emanates from the panoramic machine at any given time, whereas in the full mouth survey relatively large areas of bone marrow are irradiated over and over, with extensive overlapping in the process of exposing all the films. Because bone marrow is considered a circulating tissue, the risk to the bone marrow is always calculated as a percentage of the bone marrow irradiated in comparison to the total bone marrow of the whole body. To do this, Underhill and colleagues measured the bone marrow doses at 9 different sites including the mandible, cervical vertebrae, and calvarium. As a result, equivalent whole body bone marrow doses were computed. Risk to the bone marrow is estimated in this manner, not by estimating risk from doses at specific bone marrow sites. For the equivalent whole body bone marrow dose, Figure 1–9 shows that the panoramic machine delivers a dose similar to that of 4 bitewings using the long rectangular cone and E speed film (12 and 9 μGy, respectively). Moreover, the equivalent whole body bone marrow dose for the full mouth survey using the long round cone and E speed film is 12 times greater than the panoramic dose, including the doses to the rotation centers (12 and 143 μGy, respectively).

For the parotid gland, the data listed in Figure 1–10 indicate that the panoramic radiograph delivers a dose to the parotid gland that is similar to that from a set of 4 bitewings with the long rectangular cone and E speed film (670 and 611 μGy, respectively) and is 8 times lower than the full mouth survey using the long round cone and E speed film. For the submandibular glands (Fig. 1–11), the bitewing dose using the long rectangular cone is 1.7 times lower than that from the panoramic radiograph (226 and 375 μGy, respec-

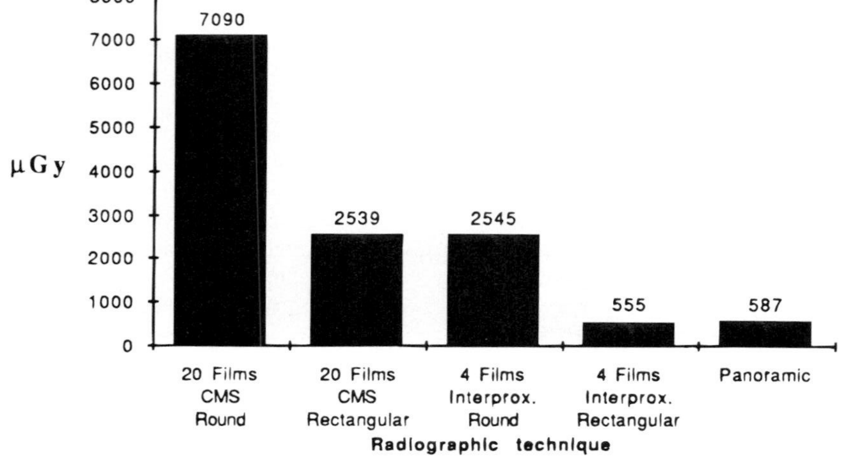

FIGURE 1–7.

Absorbed Radiation Dose to the Bone Marrow of the Mandible.

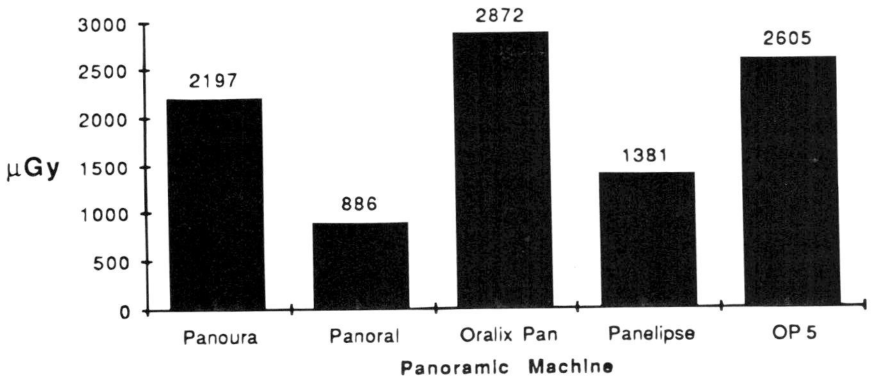

μGy
3000
2500
2000
1500
1000
500
0
2197
886
2872
1381
2605
Panoura
Panoral
Oralix Pan
Panelipse
OP 5
Panoramic Machine

Figure 1–8.

Absorbed Radiation Dose to the Bone Marrow at the Rotation Center in the Mandible.

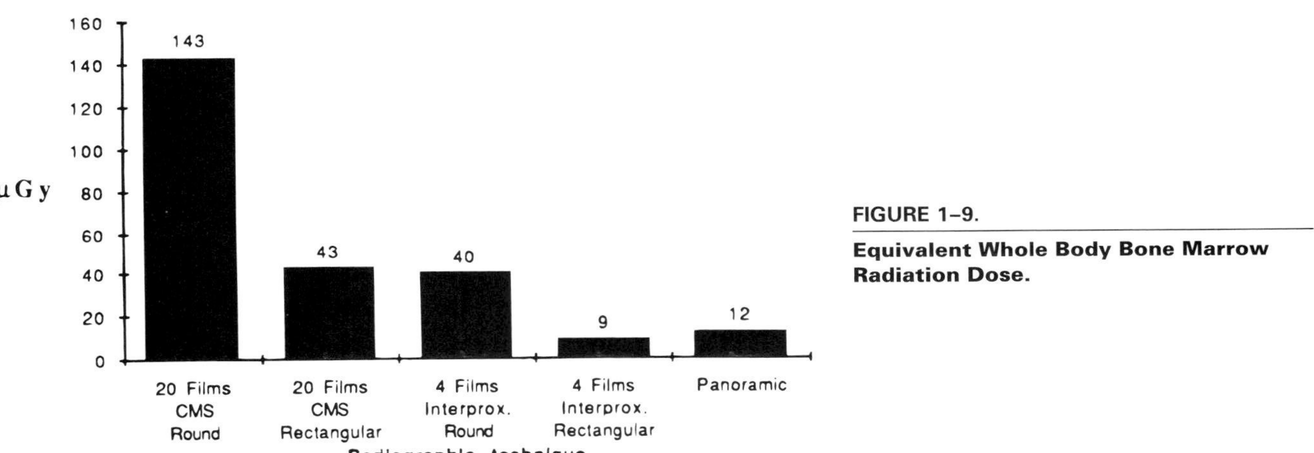

FIGURE 1–9.

Equivalent Whole Body Bone Marrow Radiation Dose.

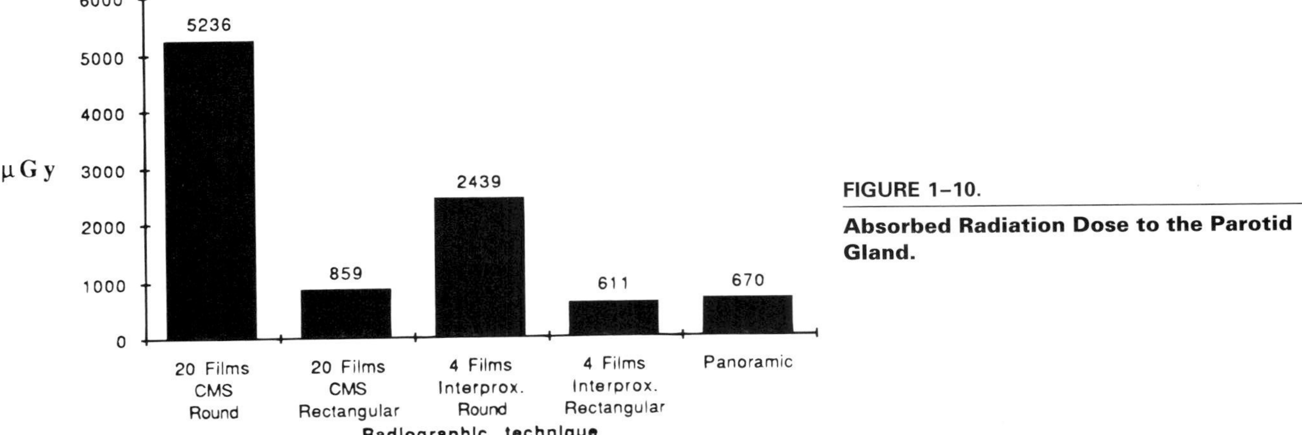

FIGURE 1–10.

Absorbed Radiation Dose to the Parotid Gland.

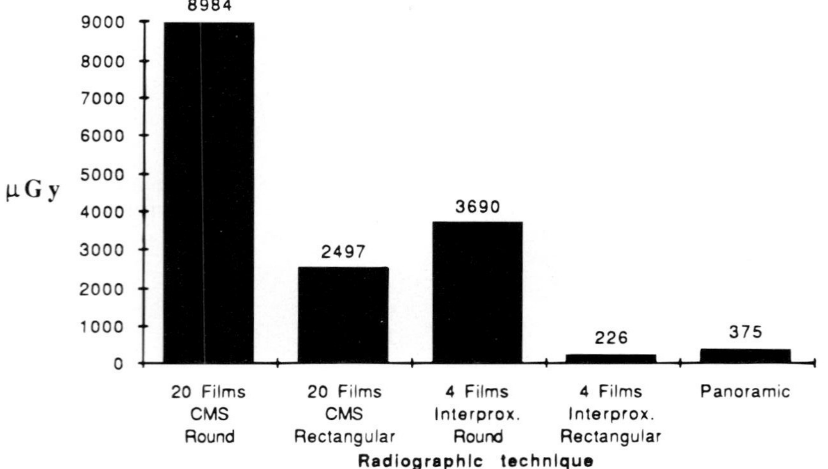

FIGURE 1–11.

Absorbed Radiation Dose to the Submandibular Gland.

tively); however, the dose from the full mouth survey using the long round cone was 24 times higher than that from the panoramic radiograph (8984 and 375 μGy, respectively). For the sublingual gland (Fig. 1–12), the dose from panoramic radiology was 3.6 times lower than that from 4 bitewings using the long rectangular cone and E speed film (134 and 484 μGy, respectively). Moreover, the dose to the sublingual gland was 58 times higher for the full mouth survey using the long round cone as compared to the panoramic film (7833 and 134 μGy, respectively).

Preston-Martin and colleagues have reported an increase in malignant parotid salivary gland tumors in patients previously exposed to radiation therapy of the head and neck, medical diagnostic radiation of the head and neck, and dental x-rays. Preston-Martin and colleagues lumped histories of panoramic and full mouth surveys together and added these to a group of patients with a history of medical diagnostic radiographs of the head and neck. Control groups were matched for age, race, sex, and neighborhood of residence. Interviews were carried out on the telephone. Some doubt existed whether other cancer risk factors in the control group were eliminated or whether other cancer risk co-factors in the tumor group were identified; one apparent exception was that a history of radiation-related work was noted in several subjects in both groups. Although the methods and data of these investigators remain to be corroborated by other investigators, and the risk to the submandibular and sublingual salivary glands remains to be determined, it seems prudent to select a radiographic examination with the least dose to the salivary glands, and that would clearly be the panoramic radiograph.

According to Eneroth (1971), 23% of all parotid gland tumors are malignant, whereas 40% of all submandibular gland tumors are malignant. Thus, one may postulate that the submandibular gland is more susceptible to developing malignant tumors than the parotid gland. Because the panoramic system delivers 8 times less radiation to the parotid and 24 times less to the submandibular glands than the full mouth survey using the long round cone and E speed film, one might conclude that the submandibular gland is at much greater risk for developing malignant tumors from the full mouth survey than from the panoramic technique. Chaudhry and colleagues (1961) reported that 39% of all intraoral minor salivary gland tumors are malignant. Thus, any method that minimizes radiation dosage to these tissues would be preferred. Recently, several panoramic machines that take partial exposures to simulate the full mouth survey have been introduced, as illustrated in Figure 1–13. These

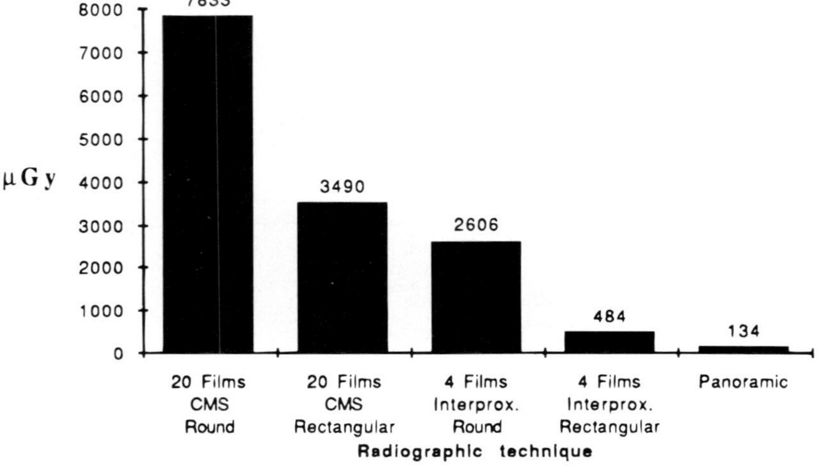

FIGURE 1–12.

Absorbed Radiation Dose to the Sublingual Gland.

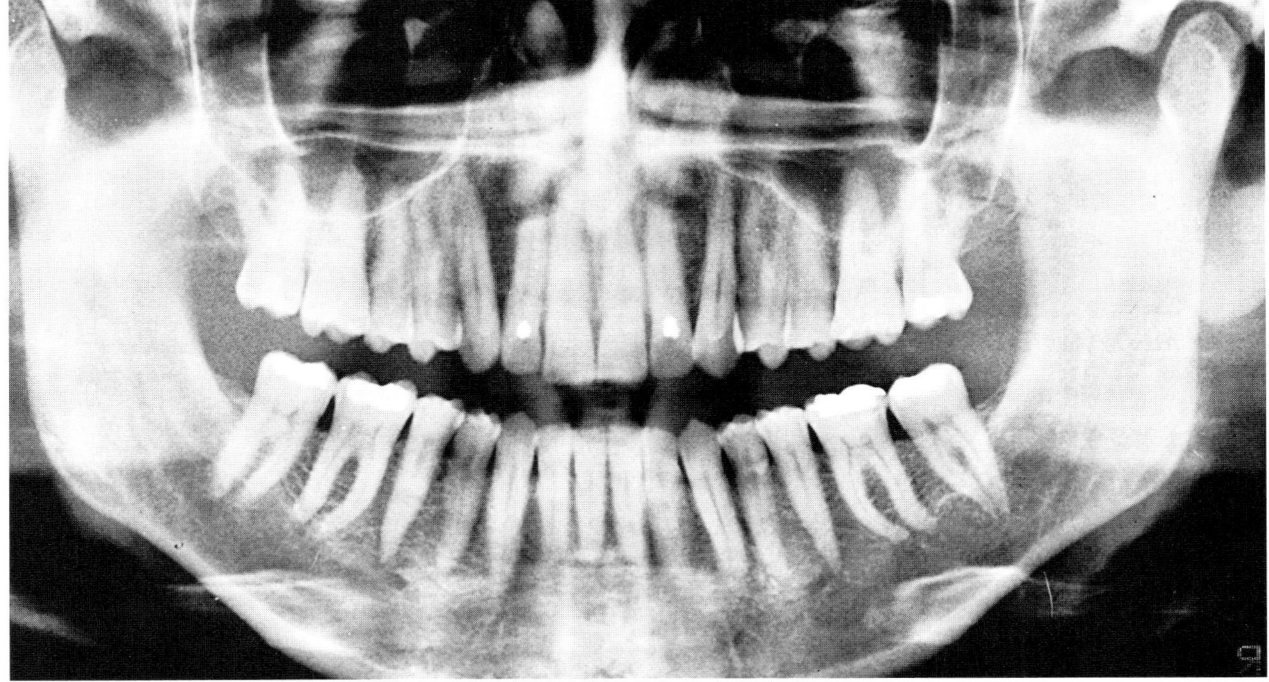

A

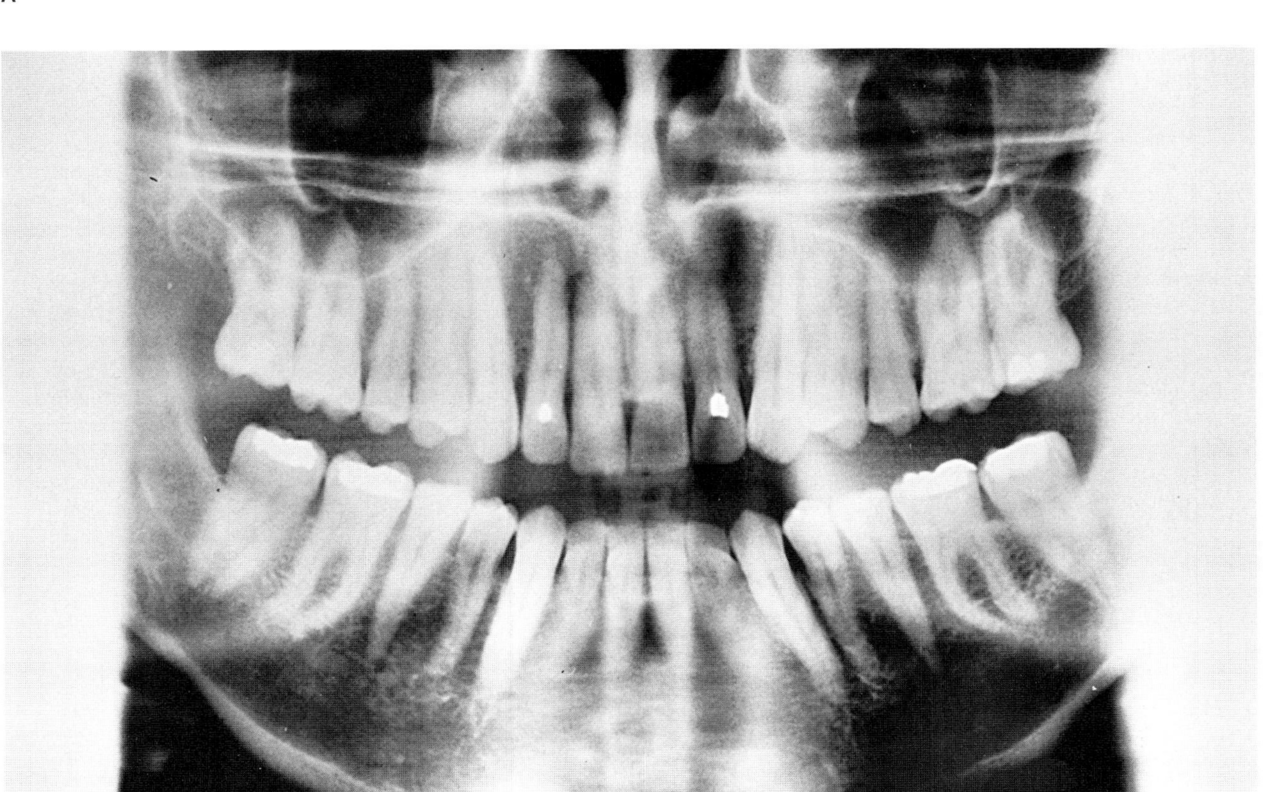

B

FIGURE 1–13.

Programmable Panoramic Exposures: Gendex Orthoralix SD. Full exposure with standard beam projection geometry; B, partial exposure using orthogonal projection geometry; absorbed doses are reduced, and interproximal overlap is minimal. (Courtesy of Gendex Corp., Des Plaines, IL.)

are the Panmecca 2002 (Panmecca OY, Helsinki) and the Gendex (Philips) Orthoralix SD (Gendex Corp., Des Plaines, IL) and Siemens Orthophos (Siemens Corp., Munich). Because the rami are not imaged in this mode, and because of the highly collimated nature of the panoramic beam of radiation, up to 80 to 90% of the exposure to the parotid glands has been postulated to be eliminated, although there are no data to support this hypothesis as yet. Lecomber and Faulkner (1993) studied the Siemens Orthophos and compared effective doses from a full panoramic exposure (program 1) to program 2, where the exposure is limited to the tooth-bearing areas. Doses to multiple tissue sites were calculated including bone marrow, 47 μSv for the program 1 full exposure and 8.9 μSv for the program 2 partial exposure; doses to the thyroid gland were 72 and 38 μSv, respectively; skin, 15 and 2.3 μSv; and bone surface, 214 and 41 μSv; all favor the program 2 partial exposure technique. Lecomber and Faulkner concluded that organ absorbed dose could be reduced by 85% and the effective dose reduced by 50%. On the other hand, no technologic development has occurred in intraoral radiography for which a similar reduction in parotid dose can be estimated.

In addition to the foregoing data, the panoramic doses obtained by Underhill and colleagues (1988) have now been reduced by 40% by adding filters made of rare earth screen material behind the narrow slit collimator of each panoramic machine used for the study. Additionally, the panoramic doses could be cut by another 50% by simply changing to Kodak OH film. On the other hand, no emerging film or beam filtration technology can produce similar decreases in dose for intraoral radiography. Digital panoramic radiology will soon become available, as it currently is on a research basis. Digital panoramic radiology will result in a fivefold decrease in radiation dose from current levels. Similar reductions in dosage might also be seen with digital intraoral systems, which are currently available from several manufacturers. These include Radiovisiography (RVG) (Trophy Radiologie, Paris), Sens-A-Ray (Regam Medical Systems, Sundsvall, Sweden), Vixa (Gendex Corp., Des Plaines, IL), and Flash Dent (Villa Sistemi Medicale, Buccimaseo, Italy). The Vixa was originally marketed as Visualix by Philips (Monza, Italy).

In this discussion we have cited dosage data that reflect the current practice in panoramic radiology. This is not so for the intraoral dose data we have cited. In current practice, E speed film is not in wide usage. D speed film, which is commonly used, delivers doses that are an average of 40% higher than E speed film. Moreover, the data presented show a significant difference in dose between the long round cone and the long rectangular cone, although the rectangular cone or rectangular collimation is rare in clinical dental practice. In addition to the cone shape, cone length also affects dose; that is, 8- and 12-inch cones give the patient a higher radiation dose than the long 16-inch cone because these shorter cones usually have less collimation. In clinical practice, shorter cones are in widespread use. In summary, our data probably overestimate the doses from panoramic radiology by 40%, whereas the data underestimate the doses from intraoral radiography by about 40%. Thus, the risks that we and other authors have calculated using these data probably overestimate the risk from panoramic radiographic examinations and underestimate the risk from intraoral radiography.

Risk Estimates

The risk in terms of new cancers per million examinations, as calculated by Underhill and colleagues (1988), is noted in Figure 1–14. A 13- to 18-fold increase in risk exists between the panoramic radiograph and the full mouth survey using the long round cone, E speed film, and variable peak kilovoltage using the UNSCEAR method (1977). In addition, the risk from a panoramic radiograph as compared to that from a set of 4 bitewings using the long rectangular cone and E speed film is similar; however, a single panoramic radiograph carries 6.5 times less probability of inducing cancer than 4 bitewings using the long round cone and E speed film. Gibbs and colleagues (1988) calculated risk using a computer simulation of a panoramic examination and the Monte Carlo method of risk estimation. This newer computer-based method is said to estimate risk more accurately than the older UNSCEAR method. In the Monte Carlo method, millions of photon histories from a simulated panoramic examination are traced throughout the body for the estimation of risk to the critical organs. Gibbs and colleagues specifi-

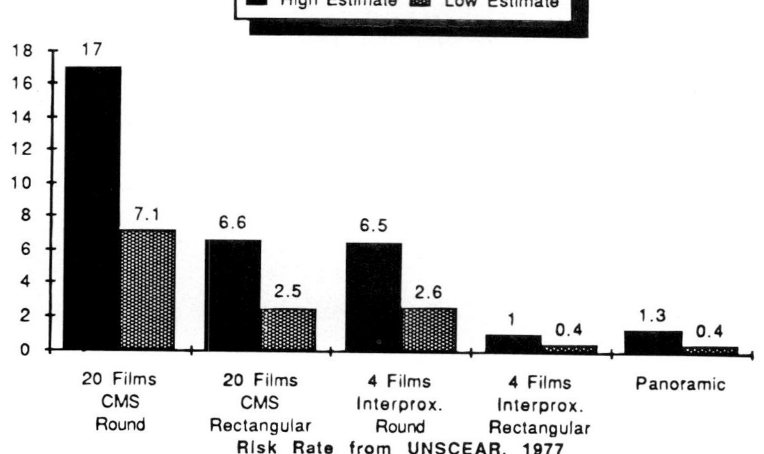

FIGURE 1–14.

Probability of Radiation-induced Cancer: cases per million examinations.

cally used the dose data as determined by Underhill and colleagues (1988) and from other reports in the literature. Gibbs and colleagues estimated the risk of developing a malignant disease from panoramic radiology at 3.2 to 5.7 times less than did Underhill and colleagues. High and low values are most often given when risk estimates are calculated. If we average these values, we can conclude that the risk of developing a fatal cancer from panoramic radiography is 4.5 times less than that reported by Underhill.

Recommendations

Dentate Patients

We recommend the panoramic radiograph as the initial radiologic examination when physical examination indicates the need for radiography. With modern equipment and good technique, this method will produce the greatest diagnostic yield with the least amount of radiation exposure to the patient (ALARA). Based on the results of this radiograph, one may determine the need for adjunctive radiographs or imaging studies, including bitewings, selected periapical radiographs, or the full mouth survey. Previously, we recommended a set of four bitewings with the panoramic radiograph. Because bitewings at the very least double the dose to the patient using the long rectangular cone and E speed film and represent a sixfold increase in risk when the long round cone and E speed film are used, and because they have a negative influence on the positive predictive values of the panoramic radiograph for both caries and periodontal disease, we recommend that the panoramic radiograph be studied first. Following this and based on the findings of this preliminary examination, other adjunctive views, including bitewings, may then be taken. Alternately, exposures recommended by the United States Department of Health and Human Services (1987) may be used, especially if panoramic radiologic examinations are not available.

Edentulous Patients

Keur (1986) recommended that a panoramic radiograph be taken on all new edentulous patients. In his study, 1135 asymptomatic edentulous patients received a panoramic radiograph. Among these, 34% (384 patients) had 465 lesions that required surgical treatment. A further 29% had abnormalities that did not require surgical intervention; and in 39% no disease was found. Keur used data from Wall and colleagues (1979), who at that time concluded that the risk of a fatal malignant tumor resulting from panoramic radiography was 1.3 per million radiographs. Keur then postulated that because substantial dosage reductions have been made since 1979 and because the age distribution of the edentulous population is much older, the risk would be reduced to 0.17 cases per million panoramic examinations. Keur's estimate is still 1.4 times higher than the average of the high and low estimates as determined by Gibbs and colleagues some 2 years later. We thus agree with Keur, who has stated that the benefits are considerable and the risk low for this group of patients. Thus, new asymptomatic edentulous patients should receive a panoramic radiograph. The United States Department of Health and Human Services (1987) recommends the full mouth survey or a panoramic examination for all new edentulous patients to assess (residual) dental diseases and growth and development abnormalities.

Trauma

Most patients with maxillofacial trauma are first taken to a local hospital emergency room. Although some facilities have panoramic radiographic machines, mandibular fractures are often studied by multiple extraoral views of the mandible. Chayra and colleagues (1986) studied 50 hospital emergency room patients with 88 mandibular fractures. These investigators found that 92% of the fractures were recognized on the panoramic radiographs, whereas only 66% were seen on the extraoral series. They concluded that the panoramic view is superior to the standard hospital series for the diagnosis of mandibular fractures. For maxillary and more complex maxillofacial fractures, we recommend CT. Various imaging methods are used; however, our emphasis is on panoramic radiography for mandibular fractures and CT for maxillary and maxillofacial trauma.

OPTIONAL VIEWS

Most intraoral films are a composite of shadows of all the tissues between the tip of the cone of the x-ray machine and the film. Because many diagnoses involving teeth do not require the third-dimensional view, the tendency is not to obtain this view when it is needed. Thus, the viewer must learn to think three dimensionally. A third-dimensional view is needed for localization procedures and for the study of pathologic changes associated with bone lesions. The two simple methods of obtaining the third-dimensional view are (1) taking a second radiograph at right angles to the existing radiograph; this usually means taking a maxillary and/or mandibular intraoral occlusal view or a submentivertex (basilar) extraoral view of the skull; and (2) taking a second radiograph at a slightly different horizontal angle for localization procedures or stereoscopic viewing.

The panoramic radiograph is a form of tomography, in that only the central layer of the jaws is imaged. Thus, structures or abnormalities falling outside the layer are not seen in the radiograph. Because the panoramic radiograph is almost invariably the initial view for the assessment of jaw abnormalities and masses, supplemental extraoral radiographs, and especially right angle views, are needed to study the abnormality accurately. The most common views include lateral, anteroposterior, posteroanterior, and basilar skull views. If the panoramic radiograph demonstrates an extensive lesion in the maxilla with involvement of the maxillary antrum (sinus), then the sinus series should be taken. These include lateral, Caldwell (posteroanterior), Waters (occipitomental), and basilar extraoral views. If the panoramic radiograph demonstrates a disorder of the TMJ, then the TMJ series should be taken. These radiographs include transcranial (open, rest, closed), transpharyngeal (open), transorbital (open), reverse Towne (open), and basilar extraoral views. If one suspects a soft tissue calcification, a low peak kilovolt (60-kVp) exposure should be taken. Depending on the circumstance, supplemental views include the lateral ramus or mandibular body radiographs, soft tissue exposures of the lip or buccal mucosa by using a number 2 intraoral or occlusal film, and soft tissue views of the tongue and floor of the mouth by occlusal radiography. We have devoted a separate chapter to soft tissue calcifications (see Chap. 19).

SPECIAL IMAGING STUDIES

Tomography

Probably the most readily available special imaging study widely used in dentistry is tomography. Tomography is often used for cases involving the TMJ and implants. Tomography consists of cutting a specific structure into thin slices that generally range from about 2 to 4 mm in thickness. Additionally, the structure can be cut along any desired axis. If two axes at right angles to each other are selected, then a three-dimensional study can be obtained. For example, coronal and sagittal cuts can be ordered. Tomographic equipment is subdivided into linear and multidirectional beam motion patterns. Thin-slice linear tomographic images are slightly blurred, whereas thicker slices are sharper; linear tomographic equipment is relatively less expensive. Multidirectional tomograms are sharper, more highly magnified, and involve longer exposure times. The result is a slightly increased radiation dose to the patient, and the equipment may be more expensive. The TMJ series consists of corrected axial lateral views in the closed, rest, and/or open positions and a corrected anteroposterior tomogram at exactly right angles to the lateral view, usually in the open position. This view shows the lateral and medial poles of the condyles. Usually, a basilar view is included in the TMJ series because this radiograph is needed to calculate the angle of the condyles with respect to the midsagittal line and the location of the central cut. For the lateral tomograms, more lateral and medial cuts can be ordered, and the same holds for the anteroposterior views (more anterior or posterior cuts can be ordered). In implant cases, tomograms must always be used to supplement information obtained from the intraoral periapical and occlusal views, the panoramic radiographs, and lateral skull extraoral views. In our opinion, the minimum standard of dental care for each posterior implant site is a panoramic radiograph, a corrected sagittal (lateral) tomographic view of each quadrant with metallic indicators showing each potential implant site, and a corrected cross-sectional (coronal) tomogram through each implant site at the location of the same metallic indicators. In the anterior region, a chin-up panoramic radiograph for the mandible and a chin-down panoramic radiograph for the maxilla and corrected cross-sectional tomograms through each implant site as shown by metallic indicators represent the minimum standard of care. The magnification factor on the tomograms must be constant and known by both the radiologist and the referring dentist. Accurate vertical measurements can only be made on the sagittal view; the width of the jaw, thickness of cortical bone, trabecular pattern type, and horizontal structural relationships can be assessed in the cross-sectional view.

Computed Tomography (CT)

In the United States, CT is widely available to medical radiologists and is slowly making its way into dental radiology. By contrast, 29 of Japan's 36 dental schools have CT. In general, the diagnosis of a lesion is usually based on plain film or panoramic radiography and is further defined by tomography; these imaging methods are widely available in dentistry. CT does not generally add to the soft tissue characterization of the lesion; however, it is useful in evaluating the extent of a lesion by detecting the presence of soft tissue extension outside of a bone or the degree of intramedullary extension within the bone.

The standard CT image is an axial cross-sectional view, oriented as if looking at the patient from the floor upward. By stacking the axial cuts within the computer's memory, reconstructions can be done in any tissue plane, the most common being coronal or sagittal. Complete three-dimensional images can also be made and adjacent structures can be disarticulated. For example, the TMJ can be viewed in the standard axial view; or coronal (anteroposterior) and sagittal (lateral) reconstructions can be done; or the joint can be viewed in three dimensions from any direction such as from below, from above, or from the side; or the three-dimensional image of the condyle can be disarticulated from the fossa and either the condyle or fossa can be viewed in any direction. Hard and soft tissue windows can be ordered, to best visualize the tissue of interest. Water is considered to have a neutral density in CT imaging. Thus, all tissues having a density greater than water have a positive (+) CT number, whereas tissues having a density less than water have a negative (−) CT number. The CT number in Hounsfield units can be used to compare the lesional tissue to that of known normal tissues such as skin, subcutaneous fat, muscle, salivary glands, or even air. Normal bone marrow contains a large amount of fat, so its density is similar to that of fat. The density of normal bone marrow ranges from −20 to −40 Hounsfield units. When tumor replaces marrow, its density is increased to that of soft tissue, well into the plus range. A cyst often has a CT number just a little above or below zero because the cystic fluid resembles water in its ability to attenuate the beam of radiation. On the other hand, a traumatic cyst may have a low density with a high negative CT number similar to that of the maxillary sinus because both contain air. Absolute CT number values cannot be assigned to each pathologic disorder because exposure factors vary from one machine to another and patients of differing size and bone density attenuate the beam of radiation differently. Within a given patient, however, comparing the CT number of the lesional tissue with that of a known tissue of similar density may give some additional information about the nature of the lesion. Lesions that are detected on scintigraphy but are inapparent on plain films are often delineated on CT.

The following is a list of indications for ordering CT in dentistry: extensive lesions in the maxilla, especially when the sinus is involved, large mandibular lesions, any suspected malignant lesion, the study of salivary gland soft tissue masses or cysts using standard techniques and CT sialography, bone lesions affecting the TMJ, and developmental disorders affecting the jaws and maxillofacial structures. Moreover, CT is the technique of choice for the assessment of trauma to the maxilla and maxillofacial complex. CT has been advocated for use in implant cases; however, we can see no advantages of CT over linear tomography. The major disadvantages of CT for implants are as follows: much higher dose of radiation because 30 to 40 cuts must be taken to give one cross-sectional view. Clark and colleagues (1990) calculated the mean absorbed doses for linear tomography and CT. The average mean absorbed bone marrow dose for a single tomographic slice was 0.5 μGy, whereas a single CT cross section of the mandible as reconstructed from 40 axial cuts was 369 μGy (738 times more radiation). The average thyroid dose for a linear tomogram was 2.7 μGy, whereas for the single CT reconstruction, the dose was 3776 μGy (1399 times more radiation). The average dose to the parotid, submandibular, and sublingual glands for a linear tomogram was 19.4 μGy, whereas on CT the dose was 30,907 μGy. Thus, for CT, a single axial cut delivers an average of 1593 times more radiation to the salivary glands than a linear tomogram. If 10 linear tomograms were taken for a single case, and 10 similar CT cuts were obtained, the CT dose would be the same as for a single CT cut, but this would still be 153 times more radiation to the salivary glands than the 10 linear tomograms. Other disadvantages of CT include the following: difficulty in orienting individual cuts with specific implant sites, poor image details because of slight movements of the patient during the procedure, difficulty in assessing bone thickness because of volume averaging of the digital image matrix, often higher cost, minimal possibility of obtaining postoperative images because of the beam scattering caused by metallic objects including implants, and in some cases the inherent communication problems that may occur when the radiologist is not a dentist. We therefore recommend tomography over CT for most implant cases.

Magnetic Resonance (MR)

This diagnostic method has recently become more widely available. MR images are obtained by measuring changes in low-frequency radio signals in a magnetic field. The resulting data can be used to create images of the structures examined or chemical profiles of the tissues. For the moment, this technology gives better soft tissue images than CT, and the patient is not exposed to radiation. MR is said to be less useful in examining cortical bone because of the lack of signal generated by this tissue. The signal strength depends on the hydrogen content of the tissue. Thus, cortex has a low hydrogen content and fat has a high hydrogen composition. Fat produces an especially strong signal on T1-weighted images. When the fatty bone marrow is replaced by tumor, infection, or hemorrhage, the strength of the signal is diminished. In current usage, adjustments can be made to obtain T1- and T2-weighted images, as well as more dynamic studies, by obtaining rapid sequences of images while an object is moving or flowing. In the future, we should be able to scan a patient for the chemical changes associated with disease, so an instant noninvasive readout of the patients' health status would be available, and the image information could be used to direct lasers and other treatment methods robotically to the exact location of the problem to treat lesions at stages so early that they would be considered undetectable with today's (1994) technology. As with CT, large amounts of metal in regions examined by MR can produce areas completely devoid of image details because metals act as an antenna to attract signal information from nearby structures. Because direct sagittal and coronal views can be easily obtained on MR, soft tissue relationships with each other and with a tumor produce images superior to those obtained by CT. The primary indication for MR imaging in dentistry is to study internal derangements of the TMJ. Other indications include soft tissue diseases in salivary glands and soft tissue lesions in the oral area such as nasoalveolar cyst, ranula, dermoid cyst, leiomyoma in the tongue, lipomas in the palate and buccal mucosa, and similar conditions.

Scintigraphy

In the field of nuclear medicine, scintigraphic images are obtained by injecting a radionuclide intravenously into a patient, waiting about 2 hours for it to be taken up in a target tissue, and assessing its uptake in that tissue by measuring the gamma radiation given off by means of a gamma camera. These radionuclides have a rapid rate of decay. Decay is a process whereby a radioactive material changes from a radioactive state to a nonradioactive condition. The process of decay is associated with a spontaneous loss of energy in the form of gamma radiation. Most radiopharmaceuticals used today have a biologic half-life of 12 to 24 hours. This means that through the process of decay combined with the biologic elimination of the material from the body, the radioactivity of these substances is reduced by 50% within 12 hours, by another 50% within the next 12 hours, and so on until the substance is completely eliminated or decays to an inert form. The radiopharmaceutical of choice for the study of both bone and salivary glands is technetium. A sample formulation is 99m (metastable) technetium MDP (methyldiphosphonate) ($^{99m/}$Tc MDP). The usual dose is 20 millicuries (mCi) given intravenously. The radionuclide may be taken up in areas where hyperemia is present because of increased metabolic activity within the bone (i.e., tumor growth) or osteogenesis (i.e., marginal reaction of bone). Decreased activity is associated with metabolically inactive bone, a lack of osteogenesis, or an absent vascular supply. Areas of increased uptake are referred to as "hot spots," whereas zones of diminished or absent activity are called "cold spots." The radionuclide is also taken up to a lesser degree by the adjacent normal bones. Thus, localization of the area of increased or decreased uptake with respect to adjacent anatomic structures is possible. The advantage of nuclear scans or scintigrams is that changes in bone can be seen early. In plain radiography, demineralization up to 60% is needed to record a change on the radiograph, whereas in the bone scan, abnormalities can be detected with 5 to 15% demineralization. Thus, scintigrams can be used to detect lesions before they become apparent in regular radiographs. The most common use of this application of nuclear medicine is the detection of metastatic lesions. An example might be a patient with deep bone pain in the left mandible and no apparent lesion on the panoramic radiograph. The patient has a 1-year history of surgery for adenocarcinoma of the colon and no further evidence of disease until this point. The patient is referred for a scintigram, and an area of increased uptake (hot spot) is seen in the left side of the jaw and in several other bones that are asymptomatic. The presumptive diagnosis is metastatic adenocarcinoma from the colon and the next step is biopsy. Invariably, the biopsy confirms the diagnosis. Other uses of scintigraphy include the localization of margins, especially in treatment planning for malignant disease where the malignant tissue has invaded beyond the apparent or visible radiologic margin. Hofer and colleagues (1985) have cited several studies where extended uptake occurred beyond the proven limits of focal bone lesions. These investigators concluded, however, that a surgical margin beyond the limits of abnormal uptake is almost always safely beyond the tumor. Scintigraphy may also be used to assess continued growth in asymmetric structures in patients with developmental disorders, especially hyperplasia of the condyle; and differential scanning is sometimes used in difficult diagnostic cases. An example might be a fragile patient who is a poor risk for biopsy but who has no contraindications against a nuclear scan. The panoramic radiographs show changes consistent with osteomyelitis or malignant disease. A technetium scan is followed several days later by a gallium scan. Technetium is taken up preferentially in association with malignant tumors and only moderately so by inflammation. Gallium is taken up rapidly at sites of infection and only weakly so in the presence of malignant disease. The scans are compared, and the nature of the bony changes can now be more accurately understood. Scintigraphy is also used to assess salivary gland disorders, and for properly trained nuclear radiologists, findings can be specific.

Hofer and colleagues (1985) compared radiographic and scintigraphic findings for a variety of lesions occurring in the jaws. A summary of their findings is presented in the hope that we may better understand what to expect from scintigrams of jaw lesions. Quiescent cysts such as large dentigerous cysts and some nonexpansile benign tumors are characterized as areas of decreased radionuclide uptake, without evidence of increased uptake at the margin. When expansion is present, the area of decreased uptake is surrounded by a zone of increased activity. Eosinophilic granuloma may show a central area of diminished uptake surrounded by a zone of increased uptake. Osteomyelitis always shows varying degrees of increased uptake, and the area of increased uptake exceeds the radiologic boundaries of bone involvement in all instances. In addition, for acute cases, when radiologic evidence of infection is absent, scans show increased uptake. In osteomyelitis, the scan may be useful as a baseline to monitor treatment. Benign tumors show slight to moderate uptake, especially at the margins of the lesion. Multilocular and expansile benign tumors such as ameloblastoma show increased uptake as compared to the surrounding tissue. Malignant neoplasms such as gingival or central squamous cell carcinoma usually demonstrate an extensively increased uptake, sometimes considerably beyond the zone of visible bone destruction on the panoramic radiograph. In a case of osteogenic sarcoma, uptake is decreased, indicating a lack of reparative response and suggesting the presence of an aggressive process. Hofer and colleagues concluded the following: (1) although the radiograph is more specific, the nuclear bone scan is more sensitive; (2) scans are especially useful in determining surgical margins; (3) scintigrams alone are especially useful in detecting early inflammatory lesions, radiographs alone are adequate for the study of cysts and benign tumors, and malignant neoplasms should be carefully followed using both imaging methods.

Digital Imaging

Digital technology, a new imaging method, has the potential of radically changing dental radiology. In digital imaging systems, the image is captured by a charge coupled device (CCD). This captor and the associated computer hardware and software replace dental film, cassettes and intensifying screens, the darkroom generally, and film processing specifically. Because the captor does not need to be removed from the patient's mouth after each exposure, as do bite blocks and film holders, the time for taking the images will be markedly reduced. Many of the infection-control problems associated with the handling and processing of x-ray film will be eliminated. The computer system consists of digital to analog and analog to digital converter boards, as well as software to process images and hardware to view it, store it, or transmit it. The advantages of this technology are as follows: (1) the system can produce images with two to five times less radiation than traditional film based methods; (2) the images can be viewed instantly on a monitor; (3) if the images are too dark, too light, or have improper contrast, they can be processed (corrected) digitally, thus saving reexposing the patient; (4) special image processing algorithms (software programs) are available to perform subtraction, whereby subtle hard tissue changes occurring over time can be detected before they are visible to the eye; (5) the images can be colorized, where thousands of colors can be substituted for the 256 shades of gray in the image; because the eye can only separate about 15 to 25 shades of gray, the multitude of available colors offers increased potential for improved visual contrast acuity; color will also be an invaluable adjunct for case presentations and patient education; (6) using teleradiology, which essentially consists of a digital fax machine connected by a modem to the computer and a high-resolution television telephone (now available as a consumer product in some areas) at the other end of the line, the image can be instantly transmitted to a colleague for consultation or referral; and (7) the images can be stored on a hard disk or a laser disk (video CD) and recalled at any time with no loss of quality. Electronic charting can become a reality because files would no longer be a necessity for storing the radiographs. Intraoral digital imaging systems are currently offered by several companies. The main disadvantages are: (1) relatively high cost, although this will invariably come down; (2) incompatibility with existing x-ray machines and computers in come cases; (3) inadequate memory for storing images; (4) insufficient image processing capability; (5) a less than ideal method for obtaining hard copies of the images; and (6) inadequate efforts to standardize so the computers can talk to each other. Although these problems may seem insurmountable, technology is currently available to solve all of them. Some predict that, by the year 2000, radiographic film in the dental office will be a thing of the past. Just think of how archaic the old 8-mm movie cameras seem now, yet home video cameras have only really come into popular use within the past decade. Currently, several prototype digital panoramic, panoramic CT, and dental tomographic machines have been built and are now in various stages of testing before their introduction on the market.

References

Ainamo J, Tammisalo EH: The orthopantomogram in quantitative assessment of marginal bone loss. Suom Hammaslaak Toim 63:132, 1967.

Akesson L, Rohlin M, Hakansson J: Marginal bone in periodontal disease: an evaluation of image quality in panoramic and intraoral radiography. Dentomaxillofac Radiol 18:105, 1989.

Bender IB, Seltzer S: Roentgenographic and direct observation of experimental lesions in bone. 1. J Am Dent Assoc 62:152, 1961.

Bianchi SD, et al: Radiological visibility of small artificial periapical bone lesions. Dentomaxillofac Radiol 20:35, 1991.

Chaudhry AP, Vickers RA, Gorlin RJ: Intraoral minor salivary gland tumors. Oral Surg 14:1194, 1961.

Chayra GA, Meador LR, Laskin DM: Comparison of panoramic and standard radiographs for the diagnosis of mandibular fractures. J Oral Maxillofac Surg 44:677, 1986.

Clark DE, Danforth RA, Barnes RW, Burtch ML: Radiation absorbed from dental radiography: a comparison of linear tomography, CT scan, and panoramic and intraoral techniques. J Implantol 16:156, 1990.

Eneroth CM: Salivary gland tumors in the parotid gland submandibular gland and the palate region. Cancer 27:415, 1971.

Gibbs SJ, et al: Patient risk from rotational panoramic radiography. Dentomaxillofac Radiol 17:25, 1988.

Gratt BM: in Goaz PW, White SC, eds. Oral Radiology: Principles and Interpretation. St. Louis: CV Mosby, 1987, p. 314.

Gratt BM, et al: A clinical comparison of xeroradiography and conventional film for the interpretation of periapical structures. J Endodont 12:346, 1986.

Hofer B, Hardt N, Voegeli E, Kinser J: A diagnostic approach to lytic lesions of the mandible. Skeletal Radiol 14:164, 1985.

Hollender L: Decision making in radiographic imaging. J Dent Educ 56: 834, 1992.

Kantor ML: Trends in the prescription of radiographs for comprehensive care patients in United States and Canadian dental schools. J Dent Educ 57:794, 1993.

Keur JJ: Radiographic screening of edentulous patients: sense or nonsense? A risk-benefit analysis. Oral Surg 62:463, 1986.

Kullendorf B, Grondahl K, Rohlin M, Henrikson CO: Subtraction radiography for the diagnosis of periapical bone lesion. Endodont Dent Traumatol 4:253, 1988.

Langlais RP, et al: Interpretation of bitewing radiographs: application of the kappa statistic to determine rater agreements. Oral Surg 64:751, 1987.

Langland OE, Sippy FH, Langlais RP: Textbook of Dental Radiology. 2nd Ed. Springfield, IL:Charles C Thomas, 1984, p. 259.

Langland OE, Langlais RP, McDavid WD, Del Balso AM: Panoramic Radiology. 2nd Ed. Philadelphia:Lea & Febiger, 1989, pp. 52 and 191.

Lecomber AR, Faulkner K: Dose reduction in panoramic radiography. Dentomaxillofac Radiol 22:69, 1993.

Matteson SR: Radiographic selection criteria: the need for continued leadership. Dentomaxillofac Radiol 21:3, 1992.

Muhammed AH, Manson-Hing LR: A comparison of panoramic and intraoral radiographic surveys in evaluating a dental clinic population. Oral Surg 54:108, 1982.

Ohba T, Katayama H: Comparison of orthopantomography with conventional periapical dental radiography. Oral Surg 34:524, 1972.

Ohba T, Ogawa Y, Hiromatsu T, Shinohara Y: Experimental comparison of radiographic techniques in the detection of maxillary sinus disease. Dentomaxillofac Radiol 19:13, 1990.

Philips JD, Shawkat AH: A study of the radiographic appearance of osseous defects on panoramic and conventional films. Oral Surg 36:745, 1973.

Preece JW: in Langland OE, Sippy FH, Langlais RP, eds. Textbook of Dental Radiology. 2nd Ed. Springfield, IL: Charles C Thomas, 1984, p. 185.

Preston-Martin S, Thomas CC, White SC, Cohen D: Prior exposure to medical and dental x-rays related to tumors of the parotid gland. J Natl Cancer Inst 80:943, 1988.

Rohlin M, Åkerblom A: Individualized periapical radiography determined by clinical and panoramic examination. Dentomaxillofac Radiol 21: 135, 1992.

Rohlin M, et al: Comparison between panoramic and periapical radiography in the diagnosis of periodontal bone loss. Dentomaxillofac Radiol 18: 72, 1989a.

Rohlin M, et al: Comparison between panoramic and periapical radiography in the diagnosis of periapical bone lesions. Dentomaxillofac Radiol 18: 151, 1989b.

Schiff T, et al: Common positioning and technical errors in panoramic radiography. J Am Dent Assoc 113:422, 1986.

Terezhalmy GT, Otis LL, Schiff TG, Langlais RP: A comparison of intraoral bitewing with panoramic radiographs for the detection of interproximal caries. Dentomaxillofac Radiol 7(suppl):Abstr 32, 1985.

Underhill TE, et al: Radiobiologic risk estimation from dental radiology. Part I. Absorbed doses to critical organs. Oral Surg 66:111, 1988.

United Nations Scientific Committee on Effects of Atomic Radiation: 1977 Report to the General Assembly with Annexes. New York, United Nations, 1977.

United States Department of Health and Human Services: The Selection of Patients for X-Ray Examinations: Dental Radiographic Examinations. Washington, DC, 1987, p. 12.

Valachovic RW, et al: The use of panoramic radiography in the evaluation of asymptomatic adult dental patients. Oral Surg 61:289, 1986.

Wall BF, et al: Doses to patients from pantomography and conventional dental radiography. Br J Radiol 52:727, 1979.

Welander U, et al: Performance with respect to an average jaw. Dentomaxillofac Radiol 8(suppl):57, 1985.

White SC: Assessment of radiation risk from dental radiography. Dentomaxillofac Radiol 21:118, 1992.

Chapter 2

Principles of Interpretation of Jaw Images

METHOD APPROACH TO RADIOLOGIC INTERPRETATION

Once the demographic information, historical data and the physical findings about the patient are known, and appropriate images have been obtained, the practitioner may begin to interpret the radiographs. The following is a series of logical steps that form the basis for our method approach to radiologic interpretation:

1. View the images under ideal conditions.
2. Interpret only from quality radiographs.
3. Order additional views and/or special images as necessary.
4. Describe the radiologic findings.
5. Explain the significance of these findings.
6. Develop a differential diagnosis.
7. State your diagnostic impression.
8. Make recommendations if appropriate.

The following sections further explain these eight logical steps.

View the Images Under Ideal Conditions

The following is a list of circumstances for ideal viewing conditions. These should be observed to create an atmosphere that allows the radiologist to extract all the information from the images.

1. The viewing area should be quiet.
2. The lighting should be subdued.
3. The viewbox should be clean.
4. The viewbox should emit an even light.
5. The viewboxes should be sufficiently large to accommodate all views of the case.
6. A variable-intensity light should be available to view dark films.
7. Extraneous light should be masked out from the edges of the radiographs.
8. Care should be taken to ensure that the radiographs are properly oriented.
9. A magnifying lens should be available.
10. The viewer should use continuous eye movements.

Continuous eye movements are the key to detecting subtle changes in lesions with a diffuse blending margin with minimal changes in density, i.e., a low contrast gradient. In these circumstances, staring at the area in question only serves to convince the viewer that an early perceived change noted at the first glance was imagined, thus leading the viewer to conclude incorrectly that no change is present. Circumstances in which this may occur include assessment of caries penetration into dentin, early periapical demineralization as a result of pulpitis, ramping of alveolar bone in periodontal disease, and the assessment of the nature of a margin of a lesion, especially malignant and inflammatory processes that may have a transitional zone between the obvious area of bone destruction and the less obvious margin of normal bone. These subtle changes may offer important information on diagnosis and treatment planning that is not readily available by other diagnostic procedures.

Interpret Only From High-Quality Radiographs

Although the foregoing statement would seem obvious, many private dental offices and even hospital and other institutional dental departments experience difficulty in achieving consistent quality. One of the ways in which this was made known to the dental profession was the data released by insurance companies on the poor quality of radiographs submitted for the approval of treatment plans. To improve this situation, the American Dental Association (ADA) established several standards for radiology instruction in dental schools. One of these was that radiology instruction shall be given under the supervision of a qualified dental radiologist. Moreover, given that many dentists delegate the taking of radiographs to the dental assistant or hygienist, many states require mandatory continuing education for the relicensure or certification of dental ancillary personnel. These and other efforts have probably improved intraoral radiographic techniques. Greater emphasis on quality assurance procedures may be needed, however, especially in automatic processor maintenance and in all aspects of panoramic radiology. These include panoramic techniques, film and cassette handling procedures, and interpretation. Especially important are the radiologic signs that identify improper operator techniques. Several textbooks by Langland and co-authors (1984, 1989) are available on these subjects. Dental radiology has become more complex in recent years, and quality is more difficult to achieve. In addition, litigation is on the rise, as demonstrated by the increasing cost of dental malpractice insurance and the advent of separate malpractice coverage for dental hygienists. The radiographs or absence thereof play a role in many court cases. As oral and maxillofacial radiologists, we have certainly acted as professional witnesses in many such instances. As a result of these and perhaps other factors, many general dentists and dental specialists are now opting to refer their patients to oral and maxillofacial radiologists or independent dental radiology laboratories for their radiographs. The strength of this trend is demonstrated by the appearance of increasing numbers of independent dental radiology practices and laboratories throughout the country and the marketing efforts of medical radiologists for dental referrals, especially in the areas of radiologic evaluation of trauma, temporomandibular (TMJ) disorders, and implants.

Order Optional Views and Special Images as Necessary

Decision making in dental radiology is usually a matter of routine. By virtue of the practitioner's professional training and judgment with the specific case at hand, correct decisions are made on a routine basis. On the other hand, new technologies, an ever more litigious society, and the trend toward continuous learning by all professionals will change the way in which decisions are made in routine practice. Accessibility to updated information by computer-linked subscriptions will help the dental profession to become more dynamic in problem solving. What must be avoided are preset solutions to problems such as fixed selection criteria in dental radiology that can become antiquated at the moment of publication, can result in excessive doses of radiation to patients, and can deprive the practitioner of the ability to consider the many variables as outlined by Hollender (1992) in making the best decision for a given individual patient or situation. In Chapter 1 we outlined the indications and contradindications and the advantages and disadvantages of the various additional views and images that are available. The ultimate goal of the decision-making process is to provide the patient with the best achievable standard of care in any given situation after consideration of all variables.

Describe the Radiologic Findings

The description of the radiologic findings should progress through an ordered series of steps with little variation from one case to the next. By establishing a pattern and sticking to it, the practitioner will have less chance of making errors of omission. Of course, allowances need to be made for differing circumstances and the possible use of multiple imaging methods, but consistency and thoroughness are still needed to describe the radiologic findings adequately. Hofer and colleagues (1985) have stated: "the vast and confusing number of pathological conditions occurring within the jaws should not deter the radiologist from a thorough diagnostic approach." Remember that the object of this step is to annotate all the findings, not to ascribe meaning or a diagnosis to them. To do this properly, the language of radiology needs to be learned. If we state that permeative changes or buttress formations are seen, these not only represent specific descriptive patterns, but they may also be of diagnostic import. Most of the necessary descriptive terms of radiology are described in this next section. Once all abnormalities have been noted, a descriptive pattern emerges. The use of proper radiologic terms is to be encouraged. This descriptive pattern is essential to developing the diagnostic impression at a later stage. The radiologic findings should contain the following information:

1. Location and extent.
2. Osteolytic versus osteoblastic.
3. Characteristics of the lesional tissue.
4. Internal margins.
5. Supporting structures of the teeth.
6. Relationship to teeth.
7. Cortical changes.
8. Periosteal reactions.

Location and Extent

The location of a lesion associated with the jaws is one of the most important specific diagnostic criteria, and one of the easiest to assess, although subtle changes can be missed. The extent of a lesion may be much more difficult to determine, and this feature may indirectly affect location. The following may be used to assess location:

1. Maxilla versus mandible.
2. Unilateral versus bilateral.
3. Incisor, premolar, molar region(s).
4. Maxilla, tuberosity; mandible, angle.
5. Maxilla: sinus, nasal fossa, orbital extension; mandible: ramus, coronoid process, condyle.
6. Location in association with teeth.
7. Central axis: central, eccentric, within cortex, parosteal.

Within this text, in the various descriptions of the jaw lesions, we usually include a specific discussion of location. Although not all the foregoing features are described for each lesion, where appropriate, any one or all of these points are discussed, if they are pertinent. Some descriptions with respect to location we have borrowed from the medical literature, because we oral and maxillofacial radiologists have been imprecise about some useful descriptive features heretofore ignored in jaw lesions. For example, the aneurysmal bone cyst that was named after its "blown out" radiologic appearance may be found in many parts of the bony skeleton, including the jaws. It tends to be centrally located in the body of the mandible, but eccentrically located in the angle and ramus areas, just as it is in the long bones. Moreover, in the body of the mandible, it may resemble certain other mandibular odontogenic and nonodontogenic lesions, whereas in the ramus, it often takes on the more typical appearance of the lesion as it occurs in other parts of the skeleton.

The ramus is a special region within the jaws. In some ways it resembles other bones. The long bones are those of the arms and legs, and each is divided into three parts: (1) the epiphysis, which includes the condyle to the epiphyseal plate and is referred to as the head of the bone; (2) the metaphysis, which is the tapered neck of the bone; and (3) the diaphysis, which is the shaft of the bone. The short tubular bones of the hands and feet have a similar configuration. There are also the flat bones such as the pelvis, ribs, and scapula. The condyles of the ramus may be affected by any of the arthridites, although such changes are often nonspecific. Thus, we recommend studying the joints of the hands in conjunction with TMJ findings. The hands are much more specific, are more easily imaged, comprise many more joints, and are often involved when the TMJ is affected. When tumors affect the condyles, however, they are much more likely to resemble those found in the epiphyseal area of the long bones rather than tumors seen in other parts of the jaws. The coronoid process is a unique part of the mandible, and although it may be compared functionally and anatomically to structures such as the greater trocanter on the upper neck of the femur, its unique motion, and the relation of the coronoid process to other maxillofacial structures, cause it to require special consideration. The coronoid process is also affected by conditions found in other parts of the skeleton, but not other parts of the jaws. The ramus itself resembles a flat bone structurally, but it may give rise to bone lesions found in both round and flat bones. Although the ramus is not thought to give rise to odontogenic lesions, odontogenic conditions may often extend into the ramus, and some conditions do so more than others. Thus, when a lesion is limited to the ramus and is not associated with a displaced tooth, such a location helps to eliminate odontogenic disorders and other conditions unique to the jaws.

The body of the mandible and most of the maxilla are radiologically different from any other bone in the skeleton. These bones contain teeth and give rise to myriad odontogenic tumors and cysts that locate uniquely in these bones. In addition, these regions give rise to most of the benign and malignant lesions of nonodontogenic origin seen in all other parts of the skeleton. Hofer and colleagues have stated that "this region of the skeleton is still neglected by (medical) radiologists, perhaps because of the overwhelming number of pathological conditions, which are very often similar in their radiological appearance."

The extent of a lesion is often ignored in the radiologic workup. In other words, as long as the diagnostic features are there, further views are not deemed necessary. From the point of view of treatment planning, however, the dentist or surgeon must know the full extent of the lesion. Thus, knowing the location also implies knowing the full extent of the lesion. This means that the lesion must be examined three dimensionally and for both hard and soft tissue changes.

Osteolytic Versus Osteoblastic

In plain film imaging, we have traditionally referred to osteolytic lesions as radiolucent and osteoblastic processes as radiopaque. With the addition of new imaging methods, other terms are used when applied to that imaging technique. On computed tomography (CT), such changes are referred to as areas of increased or diminished density. For example, osteolytic changes appear darker gray or black on CT and are referred to as areas of diminished or decreased density, whereas osteoblastic changes show as paler gray or whitish areas of increased density. These densities can be quantified and expressed as plus (+) or minus (−) Hounsfield values. Magnetic resonance (MR) imaging is different again, and changes are described in terms of signal strength. For example, bone marrow contains much fat and water, so it appears as a strong or bright signal and is whitish. Cortical bone and the articular disk, on the other hand, are fairly avascular and therefore contain little water and fat, so they appear as darker areas of low signal intensity. The strength of signal intensity for soft tissues can be altered by pathologic changes, and depending on the nature of the pathologic process, soft tissues are best visualized with T1- or T2-weighted images. Digital imaging produces images similar to plain radiographs, and the same terminology is used. In nuclear medicine, image information depends on the uptake of an injected radiopharmaceutical agent by the tissue of interest. In areas where uptake is good, the image demonstrates a black spot and is referred to as positive uptake or a "hot" spot; an area of no uptake is referred to as a "cold" spot; both cold and hot spots are significant for the presence of disease.

No matter what imaging method is used, the reader will have to determine whether the changes are osteolytic or osteoblastic, or whether they contain elements of both processes. For example, one must almost always consider these two questions: (1) What is the nature of the lesional tissue? and (2) What is the nature of the host bone's defensive reaction to the lesional tissue? In each of these two instances, the changes may be osteolytic or osteoblastic, or they may contain elements of both. In general, accurately characterizing the radiologic appearance of the lesional tissue is the first step in correctly estimating the histologic nature of the lesion; however, the appearance of the margin greatly narrows the choices because this area gives us the most information about the behavior of the lesion and thus its true histologic diagnosis. Radiopaque changes generally consist of reactive sclerosis as a host bone response to the pathologic process or mineralization of tumor matrix. The mineralized matrix may be odontogenic or nonodontogenic in origin, and the condition may be benign or malignant.

In the jaws, only 7% of the lesions are estimated to be purely radiopaque; however, this finding may be based on lesions biopsied. Because many radiopaque lesions are innocuous or do not require treatment, the incidence of radiopaque lesions is probably higher. In addition, authors have ignored the characteristic radiologic features of radiopaque jaw lesions. We have made a great effort to establish new descriptive features for some of these lesions.

Characteristics of the Lesional Tissue

The easiest way to characterize the lesional tissue is by identifying the overall pattern, such as "multilocular radiolucency" or "periapical radiopacity." These two examples specify the lesion group as lytic or blastic, and in the case of periapical, location with respect to the apices of the teeth is specified. In the other example, multilocular refers to the appearance of the lesional tissue. Further narrowing may be specified in the overall pattern, such as circumscribed radiolucencies or poorly defined radiolucencies. Most lesions in the former group are benign and often cystic, whereas most diseases in the latter group are malignant, with a few inflammatory lesions.

In this textbook, we have classified all jaw lesions into overall patterns. Our classification is based on the mature and/or most typical appearance of the condition. We have done this for the sake of simplicity, as a beginning point for the student in developing a differential diagnosis. Similar kinds of pathologic lesions tend to occur within each group. If variations in radiographic appearance exist for a given disease, we illustrate these within the same discussion. For example, a discussion of ameloblastoma is found in Chapter 13, ''Multilocular Radiolucencies.'' Similarly, the diseases in Chapter 13 form the basic list for the differential diagnosis of a multilocular lesion. The ameloblastoma, however, may also appear as a circumscribed or a pericoronal radiolucency. Thus, some conditions have secondary characteristics, and these must also be learned by the student and added to the preliminary list forming the differential diagnosis. For example, we have classified a group of lesions as pericoronal radiolucencies. This list does not include ameloblastoma, so ameloblastoma will need to be added in many instances. Hofer and colleagues (1985) stated that medical radiologists view many of the jaw lesions as similar regardless of pathologic nature. Perhaps for this reason, the differential diagnostic approach to learning the radiologic interpretation of jaw lesions has such a widely accepted initial appeal for students and their teachers alike. In addition, dental students are taught pathology by disease process, and most oral pathology instructors like to illustrate the disease process with case examples. Thus, most dental students are taught radiologic interpretation after the oral pathology course, and the differential diagnostic approach more closely simulates the perceived clinical situation. In other words, the patient's presenting condition is a multilocular radiolucency, not an ameloblastoma. The interpretation of many lesions as they appear in the jaws has not evolved sufficiently to enable the dentist to look at the radiograph, decide that a tumor is present, and state with some certainty that it is an ameloblastoma. Many practitioners are adept at differential diagnosis by pattern recognition, however.

Further to the foregoing discussion on patterns in general, purely radiolucent lesions without septations, mineralized matrix, or expansion may be divided into three patterns of medullary bone destruction: (1) geographic; (2) motheaten; and (3) permeative. Geographic areas of bone destruction tend to be single, large, mostly confined to a specific area, and clearly defined; several separate grouped or ungrouped lesions may be seen. In the jaws, these are about one or more centimeters in size. Motheaten areas consist of several or more smaller and less well defined patches of medullary destruction. Typically, these areas are about 3 to 5 mm in diameter. Permeative areas are much smaller poorly defined areas of medullary destruction and are sometimes associated with multiple areas of pinpoint destruction of the cortex. These areas are most often about 1 or 2 mm in size. Some lesions may have varying admixtures of any two or all three patterns.

A radiolucent lesion containing septa is said to be septated or multilocular. True septation occurs when trabeculae of bone or other mineralized elements are produced by the lesion. An example of true septation may be seen in some vascular lesions. In other instances, the multilocular appearance is derived from erosion, bosselation, or scalloping of the endosteal surface at the advancing margin of the lesion with the ridges of bone between the cupped out areas giving the false appearance of septa in the radiographic image. False septation occurs in ameloblastomas that appear as multilocular lesions. Another form of false septation occurs when filaments of remnant host bone appear to form locules within the lesion. This type of false septation is seen in aneurysmal bone cyst and central giant cell granuloma. Multilocular lesions in the jaws have been described as honeycomb, soap bubble, tennis racket, and scalloped (ridging, crenated). In the honeycomb type, the loculations are small and numerous; the soap bubble variant has larger, less numerous loculations; the tennis racket pattern occurs when the septa intersect at right angles, thus forming geometric forms such as squares, rectangles, triangles, and diamond shapes; and in the scalloped variant, incomplete septation gives a false impression of multilocularity. The ameloblastoma may have a honeycomb or soap bubble appearance; the tennis racket pattern is seen in the odontogenic myxoma; and the scalloped type is seen in the odontogenic keratocyst, to name three examples.

When lesional tissue is characterized by blastic changes, such changes may be entirely radiopaque, or one may see both radiolucent and radiopaque components. Although some authors classify these blastic lesions as ''mixed'', we have lumped both types into the radiopaque groups. We have done this for several reasons: First, many radiopaque lesions are associated with mineralization within the tumor matrix, especially those of odontogenic origin and some primary bone tumors. Some of these lesions may progress through an early radiolucent stage, through a mixed phase, and ultimately to a progressively more radiopaque appearance in mature lesions. This is consistent with our classification, which is based on the mature presentation of a lesion. Second, we have attempted to standardize or at least to define terms descriptive of the specific appearance or pattern of the blastic tissue. These patterns of radiopaque tissue often contain a radiolucent component and, perhaps less frequently, only radiopaque changes. For example, a cementoma progresses through radiolucent, mixed, and radiopaque stages; even in the mature radiopaque stage, however, a radiolucent outer margin may or may not be present. Thus, the mature lesion may have a mixed appearance. On the other hand, osteosclerosis is almost invariably radiopaque, with no lytic component. We have divided the basic patterns of radiopaque tissue in mixed lesions into macroscopic and microscopic subtypes. Macroscopic patterns are easily noted under nonmagnified viewing conditions. Some examples include target, coiled snake, cotton wool, mottled, washerlike, and homogeneous appearances. Microscopic features are more descriptive of the radiopaque flecks that may be seen in the lesion and are best studied under the magnifying lens. Some examples include osseous foci or flecks, spiculation, calcific foci, calcific spherules, driven snow, and nonspecific flecks of mineralization. As we shall see, accurate characterization of these macroscopic and microscopic features may be characteristic, indicating the histologic nature of the lesional tissue. In the past, these terms were used loosely and interchangeably, and varying appearances were not well characterized. We hope that these terms will be used more consistently because their diagnostic import may be considerable.

Internal Margins

The internal margin of a lesion relates to the appearance of the interface between the lesion and the host bone from which it arises. The specific changes that occur at this interface depend on the nature and behavior of the disturbance in terms of its aggressiveness and growth rate. These behavioral characteristics are related to the radiologic manifestations of the host bone's defensive reaction to the lesion. Thus, an accurate interpretation of these changes will give the reader important clues to the aggressiveness and growth rate of the disturbance. These clues are of significant diagnostic importance. The "zone of transition" refers to the margin between the lesion and the normal surrounding bone. This zone of transition consists of "narrow" and "wide" subtypes. Lesions with a narrow zone of transition may be punched out, with no rim of sclerotic bone; they may have a thin rim of sclerotic bone; or they may have a thick rim of sclerotic bone. In addition, the sclerotic rim may be described as smooth, irregular, scalloped, crenated, discontinuous, or wispy, for example. A wide zone of transition consists of an ill-defined margin of the lesion that blends more or less imperceptibly into the surrounding intramedullary bone.

Supporting Structures of the Teeth

The supporting structures of the teeth include: (1) the periodontal membrane or ligament space; (2) the lamina dura; and (3) the alveolar bone. The changes associated with these structures may cause them to become diminished or enlarged. The effects of pathologic processes on these structures are unique to the jaws. This is true whether the origin of the disturbance is odontogenic, nonodontogenic, or metabolic. These additional features with respect to jaw lesions offer important diagnostic clues not seen anywhere else in the skeleton. The periodontal membrane space (PMS) should be studied and a determination made whether it is normal, absent, or widened. Additionally, if the PMS is abnormal in dimension, is the abnormality focal or a part of a more generalized pattern? The lamina dura may be normal, absent, or widened, and these changes may also be focal or generalized. The alveolar bone may be resorbed or it may appear enlarged, and these changes may be focal or generalized. The alveolar bone, including the size of the marrow spaces and the appearance of the trabeculae, has a variety of pathologic patterns. Some conditions affect only one of the supporting structures of the teeth, whereas others may affect all three. The changes in the supporting structures may be due to the direct effects of disease, or they may be a result of fixed or removable, partial, or complete denture prostheses. The various permutations and combinations by which disease affects these structures may add considerable weight to the accuracy of the radiologic diagnosis. The meaning of these changes is discussed later in this chapter.

Relationship to Teeth

Just as the effects of pathologic processes on the supporting structures of the teeth are unique to the jaws, so too is the association of the lesion with the teeth. The relationship with the teeth may be looked at in three ways: (1) to the crown; (2) to the apex; and (3) to the tooth overall. With respect to the crown, we have divided these lesions into three groups: (1) pericoronal radiolucencies that do not tend to contain radiopaque flecks; (2) pericoronal radiolucencies containing radiopaque flecks; and (3) pericoronal radiopacities. These lesions are the subject of Chapters 11 and 12. Effects on the apex of a tooth may be characterized as resorption of the apex, deposition of material onto the root, and special relationships that root apices may have with respect to some lesions. Overall relationships with teeth include impaction, displacement, straddling, and floating. At times, these features are pathognomonic, such as hypercementosis; at other times, they suggest the nature of the lesion because pericoronal lesions are almost always odontogenic. The meaning of these various changes is discussed in a later section of this chapter.

Cortical Changes

Up to this point, the purpose of these steps has been to describe the radiologic changes. We are not yet trying to ascribe meaning to the findings. A word of caution about descriptive terms is in order, however. As the viewer scans the image, and as all the foregoing information is assimilated, one sometimes has an impression of the nature of the lesion. With experience, this impression comes more rapidly. Thus, when we are thinking of something benign, we should not be using descriptive terms inconsistent with such an impression; conversely, if we do have a description that is consistent with a malignant lesion, we should not be thinking about benign conditions, or at least it should not be at the top of our list of diagnostic possibilities.

The cortex may be affected by a lesion in the following ways:

1. Expansion with visible margins.
2. Expansion with an invisible margin.
3. Endosteal scalloping.
4. Cortical destruction.
5. Saucerization of the outer cortex.

A lesion may cause an outward expansion of the cortex, causing a distortion in the normal outline of the bone, but the cortex may remain intact. Conversely, some lesions cause expansion that produces an invisible peripheral margin of the cortical bone. In such instances, the peripheral margin is so thin that it cannot be seen on plain film, but it may be seen on tomography or CT. Other lesions cause erosion of the inner (endosteal) cortex, without appreciable expansion, whereas some produce cortical destruction seen as an irregular loss of cortical bone. Saucerization is seen in association with the outer cortex, caused by mostly benign lesions arising in the periosteum; however, some malignant lesions beneath the periosteum such as Ewing's sarcoma and juxtacortical osteosarcoma may also erode the outer cortex.

Periosteal Reactions

Periosteal reactions consist mostly of varying patterns of subperiosteal new bone formation. These patterns occur in the mandible much more frequently than in the maxilla. Periosteal reactions associated with the mandible are less common than in other bones of the skeleton, however. Periosteal reactions are more likely to be imaged with newer rare earth screens because of the lower radiation dose and consequent reduced chances of burnout. Moreover, the periosteal reaction may not be fully apparent on the panoramic radiograph, but may often be seen on a low exposure occlusal view, or the reverse Towne or posteroanterior views. When periosteal reactions are seen in the jaws, they are helpful in establishing the diagnosis. These reactions have been characterized as follows:

1. Lamellar: uninterrupted, or continuous.
2. Lamellar: interrupted, or discontinuous.
3. Onion skin or layered.
4. Solid, thick, compact, and smooth.
5. Solid, irregular mass.
6. Buttress.
7. Codman's triangles.
8. Sunburst, divergent.
9. Hair on end, parallel or spiculated.
10. Irregular.

Some of these periosteal reactions are seen much more frequently than others.

The uninterrupted lamellar type consists of a single intact layer of subperiosteal new bone appearing as a faint, radiodense (radiopaque) line about 1 to 2 mm in width. This line often parallels the outer cortical surface, or it may sometimes curve slightly outward. An important observation is that this single layer of new bone is intact, and the underlying bone may appear normal. The interrupted lamellar type is similar to the uninterrupted type and differs from it in the following ways: the single layer of new bone is interrupted; it tends to be slightly more radiodense, and there may or may not be destruction within the underlying bone. The onion skin periosteal reaction, one of the more common periosteal reactions in the jaws, consists of several parallel concentric layers of periosteal new bone laid down between the periosteum and the outer cortex. The number of layers may vary from several to a maximum of about 12. The solid, compact, and smooth type consists of multiple closely packed layers of new bone added to the cortex overlying a lesion. This type is also referred to as cortical thickening or hyperostosis. The type consisting of a solid irregular mass is often seen as an area of increased density on panoramic or periapical views. An occlusal radiograph usually demonstrates that the diffuse opacity is an irregular mass of subperiosteal new bone. This type is often associated with underlying medullary bone changes. The buttress type consists of a triangular area of periosteal new bone formation in association with cortical expansion having an invisible margin. A triangle of compact bone is seen at the edges of the expanded margin. One must distinguish this variant from Codman's triangle, which consists of several layers or a solid mass of periosteal new bone at the margins of a lesion. This new bone is triangular and does not consist of tumor bone, although it may overlie the pathologically altered bone. Thus, Codman's triangle should be avoided as a biopsy site. The sunburst reaction has been well described in association with jaw lesions. On close inspection, the radiating spicules of bone are often irregular and coarse. These spicules are thought by some to represent tumor bone growth rather than a periosteal reaction. The hair on end pattern consists of relatively short, fine, parallel striae oriented perpendicular to the underlying outer cortex. The irregular type of periosteal reaction consists of an interlacing pattern of disorganized striae associated with an underlying bone lesion.

Explain the Significance of These Findings

The information contained within this next section is vitally important to the person interpreting the radiograph. It also represents a departure from previous textbooks, where this knowledge was not fully disseminated. In the past, we looked at dental radiographs from the standpoint of recognizing broad patterns and creating a differential diagnosis. Because of our in-depth knowledge and our understanding of odontogenic pathology, we have an advantage over our medical colleagues, many of whom freely admit that the radiology of the jaws is difficult to interpret. On the other hand, our medical colleagues have a much more in-depth understanding of the basic significance of the various radiologic changes that occur in the bones of the skeleton. In other words, we of the dental profession have made some omissions, although these have not necessarily been by intent. We thus have a lot to gain if we can expand our knowledge of the significance of the radiologic changes before we consider diagnostic possibilities. Examples include radiomorphologic features suggesting a specific tissue type histologically, signs of an aggressive lesion, patterns indicating rate of growth, features predictive of recurrence for the specific case, changes indicating quiescent or active phases of a lesion, and perhaps an expanded list of alterations that separate benign from malignant conditions. The significance of this can be illustrated as follows: Using the well-tried method of overall pattern recognition, the clinician develops a differential diagnosis containing a group of five benign lesions. Generally, the radiologic diagnosis does not go much beyond this step, and the patient is sent for a biopsy. For the purposes of this discussion, let us say that the pattern of the lesion in question is multilocular, and the differential diagnosis is as follows: (1) odontogenic keratocyst; (2) ameloblastoma; (3) odontogenic myxoma; (4) central giant cell granuloma; or (5) central hemangioma. Each of these lesions has features that, when present, suggest the specific diagnosis. Although these features have been described, they have not received adequate attention, and few students have learned them well. For example, the odontogenic keratocyst is not truly multilocular; it has a scalloped margin and a few false septa; the cortication at the margin is potentially the thickest condensed type of all lesions found in the jaws, with the exception of some salivary gland depressions; expansion is often minimal or absent, although parts of the cortex may be perforated; the lumen of the cyst may be cloudy; lesions can be found in several or all quadrants; displaced teeth may be present, but root resorption is rare; and cortical perforations may be predictive of recurrence, whereas an anterior maxillary location may be predictive of nonrecurrence. The multilocular ameloblastoma usually demonstrates expansion of the cortex to an eggshell-thin or disappearing peripheral margin; there may be an admixture of the honeycomb and soap bubble patterns in parts of the lesion; the individual locules are of the false type and are well rounded with a smooth sclerotic margin, giving individual locules a cystlike appearance; the pattern of the locules may give the appearance of a central body and long legs of a huge spider; associated root tips may show a knife edge pattern of resorption, and there may be a displaced unerupted tooth; the multilocular pattern in an ameloblastoma is predictive of recurrence. The odontogenic myxoma is most easily recognized by the tendency of the septa of bone to form elongated, straight lines. These striae intersect at right angles and form geometric figures such as squares, rectangles, triangles, and diamond shapes. One clinician characterized the pattern as resembling lichen planus of the jaw bone (L. Roy Eversole), although most clinicians refer to these changes as a tennis racket pattern. The margin may be well corticated and uninterrupted in the early growth stage of the lesion; however, the margin becomes less distinct and focally absent when the lesion has reached the aggressive ''breakout'' stage; in right angle views and on axial CT, parallel radiating striae within the tumor mass can be seen to extend beyond the limits of the host bone and at right angles to it, forming a fish skeleton pattern; recognition of the breakout stage is predictive of recurrence. The central giant cell granuloma has a poorly mineralized sclerotic margin that may or may not be discontinuous. The margin may demonstrate one or several crenations, a highly characteristic feature; septation within the lesion is irregular, and the density is described as ''wispy.'' This lesion tends to occur in the mandible, anterior to the first molar, whereas the previous three lesions are often found in the posterior mandible. Resorption of adjacent tooth apices may be seen, and each individual tooth apex may be resorbed on several planes or on a different plane from an adjacent resorbed apex. Tooth resorption, size larger than 2 cm, and perforation of the expanded cortex are signs of the aggressive variant and are predictive of recurrence. Superficially, the central hemangioma may often appear initially to be a multilocular lesion. On close inspection, however, the following additional features may be visible: noncorticated afferent and/or efferent foramina, singly or in clusters; parallel radiodense lines representing corticated blood vessel channels; a pattern of radiating striae from a central hub (strongly suggestive); and phleboliths in association with an adjacent soft tissue lesion. The recognition of these and other signs of vascular lesions can be lifesaving, because several perioperative deaths have been reported. Although this example is lengthy, it demonstrates quantitatively and qualitatively the value of the specific diagnostic and behavioral characteristics of the five lesions. This additional information is invaluable to the clinician and is far more useful than a simple list of five possible histologic diagnoses. In addition, some of the information is seen uniquely in the radiographs and is not learned from the pathologist's report. In some cases, the information is needed prior to surgery because an aggressive lesion or one with more potential for recurrence might be treated differently and possibly followed up on an accelerated schedule. Postbiopsy information can be too late for a patient who exsanguinates during a surgical procedure. Some cartilaginous lesions are known to develop slowly, but metastasize relatively rapidly if the tumor is incised for biopsy. In such cases, the nature of the lesion can be suggested by the radiologic findings preoperatively, and total ablative surgery can be planned after frozen section analysis. Even under these circumstances, new, clean instruments should be used for the definitive surgical procedure, to avoid contamination or seeding of the surgical margins with tumor.

Features that indicate the rate of growth of a lesion are most important because they are indicative of the nature and aggressiveness of the lesion. Recognizing these characteristics helps one to narrow the diagnostic possibilities. According to Hofer and colleagues (1985), the predictor variables used to assess the rate of growth from a radiograph are as follows:

1. The basic pattern of bone destruction.
2. The reparative response of the host bone.
3. The behavior of neighboring anatomic structures such as the teeth, the supporting structures of the teeth, and others such as the inferior alveolar canal.

For example, conditions arising above the inferior alveolar canal may or may not be odontogenic; those arising below the canal are rarely odontogenic. We have already outlined the important descriptive features of a lesion. In the discussion that follows, we try to explain the significance of these findings.

Location

In this text, we cannot list all the lesions for which location can be significant. Some conditions, however, tend to occur in a single anatomic site. Some of these are the submandibular, sublingual, and parotid salivary gland depressions, the so-called globulomaxillary cyst and median mandibular cyst, the incisive canal cyst, and the nasoalveolar cyst. Other lesions have a strong tendency to locate in one area, although they may appear in other regions. Examples include the lateral periodontal cyst, the botryoid odontogenic cyst, the inflammatory paradental cyst, the central giant cell granuloma, and the adenomatoid odontogenic tumor. Some lesions tend to occur bilaterally, such as cherubism, some odontogenic keratocysts, and florid osseous dysplasia. Some conditions greatly resemble others, such as Paget's disease and florid osseous dysplasia; however; the maxillary location of Paget's disease strongly suggests the diagnosis.

Location may also point to the general nature of the disease. For example, location below the inferior alveolar canal usually suggests that the problem is not odontogenic, although it may still be unique to the jaws. An example is the submandibular salivary gland depression. A location above the inferior alveolar canal must certainly include odontogenic disorders, although other conditions may also be seen here. An example is the widening of the periodontal membrane space seen in scleroderma. Conditions that appear to arise within the alveolar canal may be of vascular or neurogenic origin, and the alveolar canal may be the site of the initial lesion in metastatic disease.

Osteolytic Versus Osteoblastic

Radiolucent lesions are associated with bone destruction and replacement with cystic fluid, soft tissue, unmineralized matrix of some blastic conditions, and air. The traumatic bone cyst is unique in that it is frequently filled with air, so the lesional area is often overexposed. Some radiolucent conditions that may become radiopaque include periapical cemental dysplasia, florid osseous dysplasia, Paget's disease, central ossifying fibroma (cementifying and cemento-ossifying included), many of the odontogenic tumors including the calcifying epithelial odontogenic tumor of Pindborg, the calcifying and keratinizing odontogenic cyst of Gorlin, odontomas, chondrosarcoma, mesenchymal chondrosarcoma, and osteosarcoma. All these lesions may appear as radiolucencies, mixed lesions, and radiopacities. Radiopaque lesions may then consist any of the foregoing group, although others such as osteoma, osteoblastoma, and osteoid osteoma occur rarely in the jaws. Distinguishing among osteosclerosis, condensing osteitis, and dormant cementoma is difficult. Condensing osteitis is a sequel of infection, often pulpal inflammation, and evidence of this may be seen. Osteosclerosis occurs idiopathically, but it is distinguished from a dormant cementoma by the finding of pointed spicules at the margin of the osteosclerotic area and small rounded massules of cementum at the margin of the cemental lesion.

When You See . . ., Think . . .

The "when you see . . ., think . . ." principle is a common approach to assessing the meaning of the radiologic changes. The principle assumes that all pertinent changes have been seen, but that now these changes must somehow be processed into a meaningful interpretation. At this point, we can apply our knowledge and understanding of radiologic interpretation. Sir William Osler has been credited with the following: "what the brain does not know, the eye cannot see."

Characteristics of the Lesional Tissue

Geographic, motheaten, and permeative radiolucent patterns: (Fig. 2–1). Radiolucent lesions are caused by bone destruction. Many clinicians believe that, in the jaws, medullary destruction is usually inapparent on the radiograph. As the disease begins to destroy the endosteal surface of the cortex, the lesion becomes apparent. In clinical experience, numerous authors have observed that osteolytic changes appear sooner in panoramic radiographs than on high-dose intraoral direct exposure periapical radiographs.

A **geographic pattern** of bone destruction describes a large area of lysis, implies an absence of expansion, and is not associated with a specific type of margin. It may indicate a monolocular or nonseptated benign lesion or a malignant disorder. A benign geographic pattern of bone destruction may often be consistent with an early aggressive lesion, such as a unilocular ameloblastoma. Second, it may be a slow-

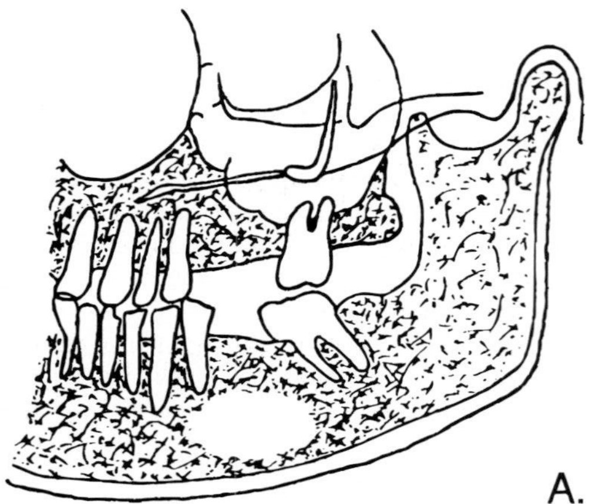

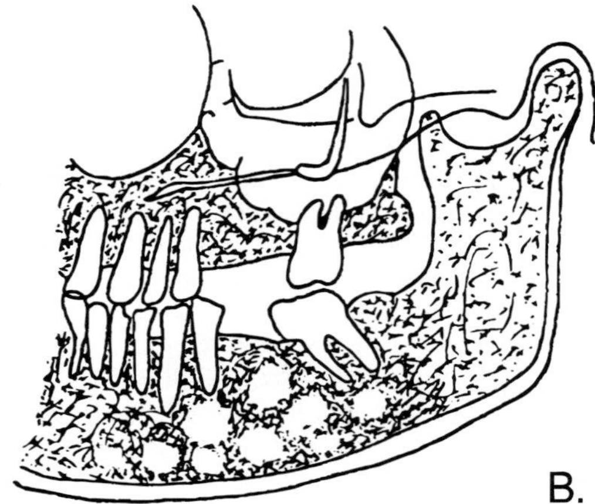

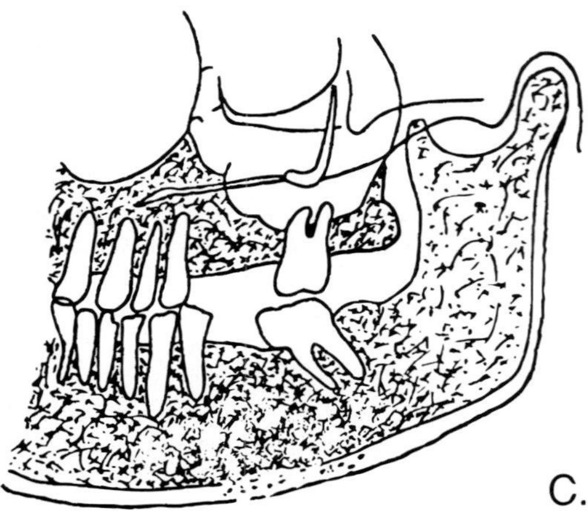

FIGURE 2–1.

Lytic Patterns: A, Geographic; B, motheaten; C, permeative.

growing, nonaggressive benign condition such as a residual cyst or a traumatic cyst. Third, it may represent an early stage of a lesion that will have a calcified tumor matrix, such as an ossifying fibroma. The term geographic is most often applied to a suspected malignant disorder and indicates slower, less aggressive growth than malignant lesions with other radiographic appearances. Some examples include solitary or multiple myeloma, central mucoepidermoid carcinoma, and metastatic disease. In their small study of 57 patients, some of whom had malignant disease, Hofer and colleagues (1985) found that the geographic pattern was the least frequent presentation of malignant jaw lesions. Distinction between benign and malignant geographic patterns depends on the appearance of the margins of the lesion.

The **motheaten pattern** of lytic bone destruction consists of several smaller areas of lysis. This pattern also implies an absence of expansion. This variant may also be seen in association with benign and malignant conditions. In this case, it is more difficult to separate these two categories of disease on the basis of the radiographs alone because the margins are similar in both instances. Motheaten patterns are seen in association with inflammatory conditions, principally chronic osteomyelitis, and also in osteoradionecrosis. Similar changes are seen in malignant disorders, especially metastatic disease. In osteomyelitis, one may see an associated single faint layer of subperiosteal new bone formation, which may only be visible on the occlusal radiograph. Sequestration is seen in more advanced cases of osteoradionecrosis. In such cases, the history and clinical findings help one to narrow the possibilities. Examples include previous radiation therapy with the jaws in the portal of irradiation, treatment for a malignant disorder almost anywhere in the body, or clinical findings of suppuration and redness in the overlying mucosa. Whether the condition is benign or malignant, a motheaten pattern of bone destruction indicates a more aggressive, rapid process than a geographic pattern.

A **permeative pattern** implies an absence of expansion and is seen almost exclusively in aggressive, rapidly destructive malignant disease. These changes may be confined to the medullary area, or one may see adjacent involvement of the cortex with similar changes. Cortical involvement in association with a permeative pattern denotes the single most aggressive, rapidly destructive change that a viewer may see on a radiograph. We have noted this pattern in association with some cases of metastatic disease and other malignant disorders. According to Hofer and colleagues (1985), lytic malignant disease in the jaws manifests mainly as motheaten and permeative patterns, although geographic changes are seen.

Honeycomb, soap bubble, tennis racket, and scalloped patterns: (Fig. 2–2). Multilocular patterns of bone destruction have been divided into honeycomb, soap bubble, tennis racket, and scalloped patterns. They are seen in association with locally aggressive benign conditions. Thus, multilocularity helps to rule out malignancy, although a few low-grade malignant conditions such as central mucoepidermoid carcinoma may appear multilocular. Multilocular patterns generally imply cortical expansion. Cortical expansion, whether it is associated with a multilocular lesion or not, implies more aggressive growth in a benign lesion. As a function of their aggressiveness, multilocular lesions have a tendency to recur. The recurrence rate of multilocular lesions is higher than that of other unilocular lesions of similar size and with an equal degree of cortical expansion. In fact, in some lesions of the exact same histologic tissue type, a multilocular pattern may someday prove to be more predictive of recurrence than a unilocular presentation. An example of this possible behavior is the ameloblastoma, in which unilocular lesions may recur less than multilocular ones. A multilocular lesion implies internal septation, although the scalloped variant has few or no septa. The presence of internal septations rules out other benign lesions without any tendency to appear in this way. Some examples of nonseptated lesions include ameloblastic fibroma and almost all cysts other than traumatic cyst. Second, septation rules out any lesions that produce a different pattern of calcification within the tumor matrix. Some examples include ossifying fibroma, cemental lesions, some osseous and cartilaginous diseases, and other lesions such as the Pindborg tumor and Gorlin cyst. On the other hand, an absence of a multilocular pattern does not rule out any of our list of diseases with a multilocular pattern. To find this list, see Chapter 13, ''multilocular radiolucencies.'' We and others have classified these diseases thus because this is their most common or classic presentation.

A **honeycomb** pattern is probably an earlier change than the soap bubble variant. Thus, a honeycomb pattern may break down and become a **soap bubble** lesion. Ameloblastomas have honeycomb and soap bubble variants, and some have a combination of these findings. In such instances, a correct diagnosis is more likely. A further variant of the soap bubble pattern is seen in some ameloblastomas in which the septa radiate from a central body, giving the appearance of a **spider**. The **tennis racket** pattern is seen in the odontogenic myxoma exclusively. A **scalloped** pattern is typically seen in the odontogenic keratocyst. The central giant cell granuloma may have multilocular or scalloped variants. We believe that the multilocular pattern occurs earlier, whereas the scalloped or crenated appearance is a later change. A scalloped margin may or may not be associated with expansion. In the case of the central giant cell granuloma, crenations may be seen with or without expansion. Some authors report significant expansion in association with the odontogenic keratocyst. In our experience, this cyst enlarges at the expense of the medullary space with generally a minimal effect on the cortex; perhaps this is the reason that these lesions can achieve a large size with a minimum of symptoms or disfigurement. In the odontogenic keratocyst one may see slight cortical bulging, although the cortex generally remains thick; however, focal areas of cortical expansion, thinning, and perforation may be present in association with the odontogenic keratocyst. These varying features all need to be recognized in a given lesion, and they contribute to the accuracy of the radiologic diagnosis.

Mineralization of tumor matrix (Fig. 2–3). Lesions with a tendency to produce mineralization within the tumor matrix generally develop a radiolucent early stage through varying degrees of mixed or radiodense appearances. We believe

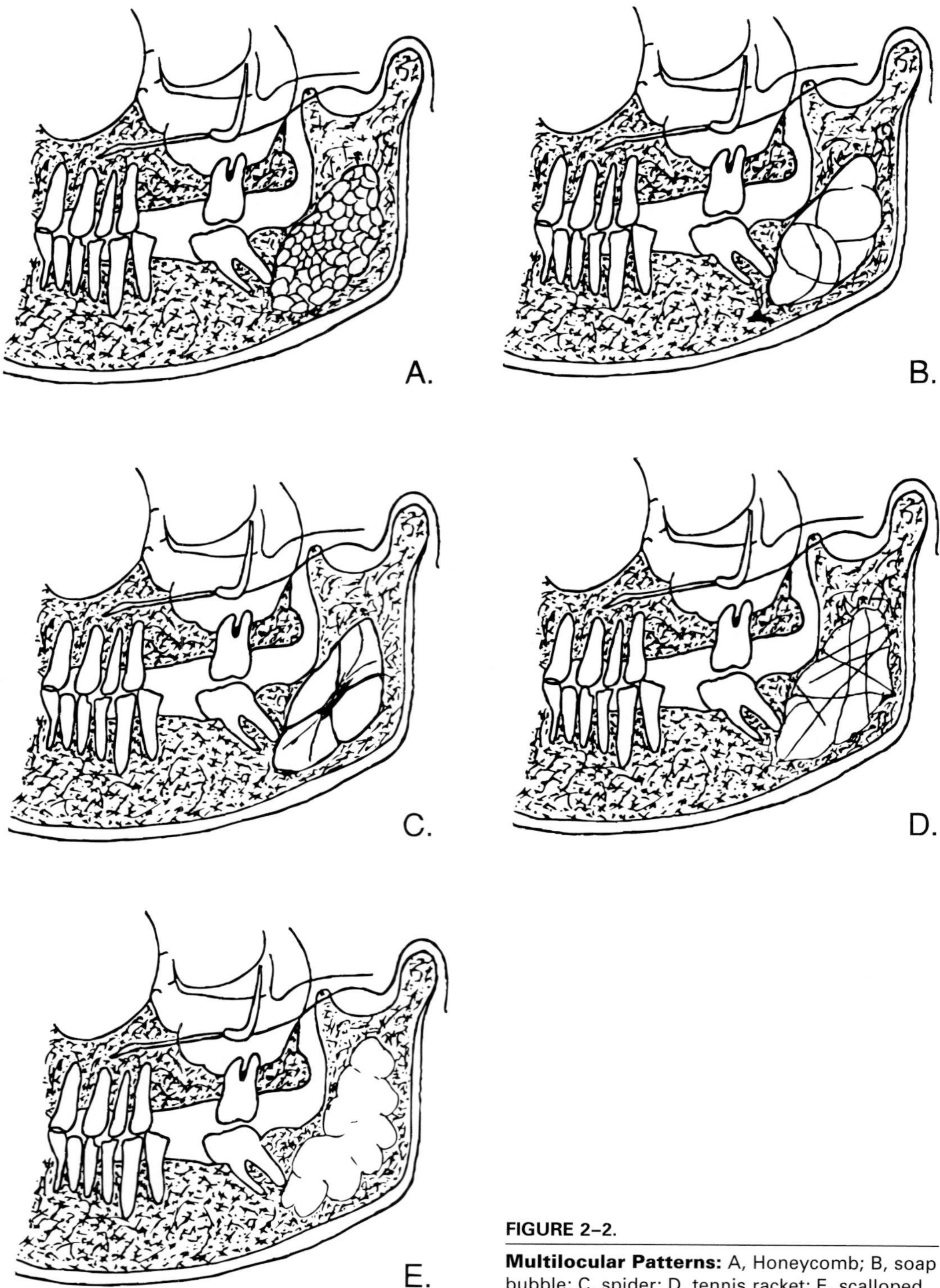

FIGURE 2–2.

Multilocular Patterns: A, Honeycomb; B, soap bubble; C, spider; D, tennis racket; E, scalloped.

that these features should be studied under the magnifying lens because the appearance of these small flecks may be indicative of histologic tissue type. We also recommend the use of standardized terminology because each term implies a specific tissue type. Although more work is needed in this area, this represents an initial effort to separate these appearances in jaw lesions.

Osseous foci or flecks suggest that the mineralized flecks within the tumor matrix represent bone or osseous trabeculae histologically. Osseous foci may aggregate into clumps; they have no tendency to locate in any specific part of the lesion or to form any pattern. They may be located more toward one quadrant, or they may spread throughout the lesion. The density of these flecks, especially when they are not clumped

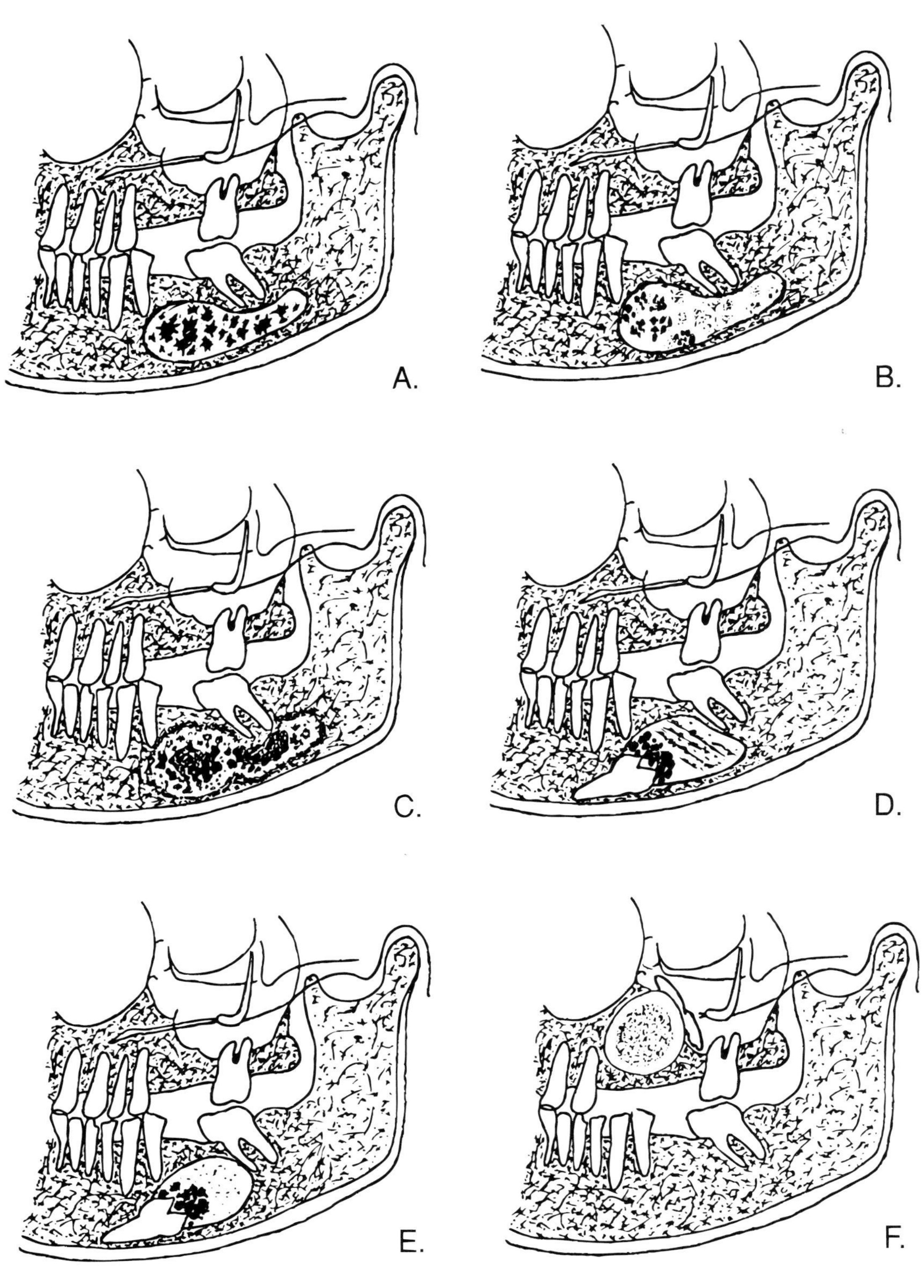

FIGURE 2–3.

Tumor Matrix Mineralization Patterns: A, Osseous foci; B, calcific foci; C, calcific spherules/massules; D, Pindborg flecks; E, Gorlin flecks; F, AOT flecks.

together, is similar to that of the surrounding bone. Osseous foci do not have smooth margins; they tend to be irregular, with small points or spicules projecting from the margins. On rare occasions, one or several small fine trabeculae of bone can be seen within osseous foci. Trabeculae may project from a spicule, or they may join several osseous foci.

Calcific foci specifically denote the mineralization of chondroid matrix. The density of these foci is often less than that of the surrounding bone, especially in benign conditions. Benign calcific foci not only have a low density, but individually, they are round, tiny, and almost invisible. What helps to make calcific foci more visible is the magnifying lens and the tendency of these foci to clump together. In small tumors or at an earlier stage of calcification, calcific foci are described as stippled or punctate, and they group together to form a faint but distinct snowflake pattern. In larger tumors, they are more easily seen because of their increased density and size. The increased density may still be less than that of the surrounding bone. In larger lesions, they form nodules, flocculent or popcornlike rings and arcs of calcific density. The presence of bizzare variations of these shapes is extremely helpful in suggesting chondrosarcoma.

Calcific spherules and **calcific massules** refer specifically to the mineralized flecks seen in cemental lesions. These flecks have not been described radiologically in the literature until now. First, calcific spherules form only during active periods of cemental lesion growth. Second, they can be seen in the central part of the early osteolytic lesion and within the outer radiolucent band of a growing or reactivated lesion. The marginal radiolucent band is divided into three activity zones: (1) the outer zone consisting of bone resorption and replacement with a fibrocemental matrix; (2) the middle zone of calcific spherule mineralization and coalescence with adjacent calcific spherules; and (3) the inner zone of coalescence of calcific spherules to form calcific massules and coalescence of the calcific massules with the central calcific mass. Calcific spherules are tiny circular structures with a radiolucent center, are only faintly radiopaque, and may only be seen under the magnifying lens. They range in size from about 0.2 to 0.5 mm. Initially, their density is much less than that of the surrounding bone. Their outer margins are smooth. They then group together to form a small circle of calcific spherules with a radiolucent center. Each calcific spherule coalesces with the adjacent one to become a small massule, perhaps 0.5 to 1.0 mm in diameter. The margins of these massules may have tiny, rounded elevations representing coalesced calcific spherules. The individual calcific spherules become radiodense in the center, as do the small massules, because of coalescence with other spherules. The small massules aggregate in a circle to coalesce with each other to form a larger massule that also loses its radiolucent center. These vary in size from 1.0 mm in diameter to about 4 mm. Therefore, from the periphery to the central mass, spherules appear, enlarge, and coalesce to form massules that progressively enlarge and ultimately coalesce with the central mass. Several small central masses, each about 0.5 cm in diameter, may form within the same lesion, and these can coalesce to form a large central mass; sometimes, several large, central masses are seen coalescing throughout a quadrant of the jaw.

If radiolucent areas are present in the zones of coalescence, calcific spherule formation can be seen. Calcific spherule formation may be observed in association with some ossifying fibromas. In this lesion, calcific spherules may be the only mineralized tissue, or they may occur in combination with osseous foci. Possibly, when the mineralized matrix consists primarily of cementum, the appearance of a mineralized mass is more toward the center, although this topic needs more study. Calcific spherule formation can be seen in association with some benign cementoblastomas, although we have much less experience in this area.

Mineralized flecks of various other tissue types may form in specific patterns that help to suggest the diagnosis. The mineralized flecks seen in the calcifying epithelial odontogenic tumor of **Pindborg** consist of calcified amyloid, which is round and like a droplet. The calcifying and keratinizing odontogenic cyst of **Gorlin** produces a **dentinoid** material that is much more irregular in its outlines. Both lesions may be associated with the crown of an impacted tooth, and in both cases, the mineralized flecks tend to be located about the occlusal area of the crown of the impacted tooth. These flecks sometimes aggregate to form smaller and larger clumps; the larger clumps usually occur toward the crown of the impacted tooth. Such findings help one to separate these two lesions from all others. In addition, the mineralized flecks in the Pindborg tumor sometimes have a streaked or "driven snow" appearance. The **adenomatoid odontogenic tumor** (AOT) contains mineralized flecks that have variously been reported as dentinoid, cementumlike, and dystrophic calcification. We have observed that, when mineralized flecks appear, they tend to be evenly distributed throughout the lesion with no tendency toward clumping. In some instances, they sometimes organize into identifiable shapes such as circles, semicircles, handprints, footprints, pawprints, and little clusters of dots. These patterns reflect the organoid arrangement of the cells producing the mineralized elements. In other lesions, we have seen clumping. A heretofore unreported feature of the AOT is a distinct radiolucent band encircling the outer margin of the lesion. The inner margin of the band is defined by the outer extent of mineralized flecks; the outer margin is delineated by the sclerotic margin of reactive host bone. This band is consistent with the thick capsule associated with the AOT. This band can only be seen when mineralized foci are present; this distinctive feature helps one to confirm the diagnosis when other similar lesions are suspected.

Odontomatous calcifications are generally considered pathognomonic. They have a density that is similar to teeth, so they tend to be denser than the surrounding bone. This is certainly true when the structures resemble little teeth. Other appearances include a washerlike radiodensity with a radiolucent center or a hodge-podge of dental structures with little to identify them as odontomatous. In such instances, identification of an array of dentinal tubules with pulplike spaces in between can be helpful. Odontomatous calcifications are associated with impacted teeth, and the complex type is especially associated with maxillary and mandibular third molars. These calcifications can be associated with dentigerous cysts, the Gorlin cyst, ameloblastic odontoma, and ameloblastic fibro-odontoma, or they may simply occur on their own as odontomas.

Dentinomatous mineralization occurs in dentinoma and ameloblastic fibrodentimoma, and these lesions are rare. Clinically, it is difficult to separate from the odontoma type.

Internal margins (Figs. 2–4 to 2–6). The internal margin relates to the appearance of the interface between the lesion and the host bone within which it occurs. The internal margin provides information on aggressiveness and growth rate, although the distinction between benign and malignant conditions is not always possible based on the appearance of the margin alone. The findings at the margin depend on the host bone's reaction to the disturbance.

A **narrow zone of transition** exists when the lesion is not aggressive or the host bone walls off the disturbance by laying down a layer of sclerotic bone (see Fig. 2–4). The four basic variations of the narrow transition zone are:

1. Thick condensed sclerotic rim.
2. Thick diffuse sclerotic rim.
3. Thin condensed sclerotic rim.
4. Punched out lesion, with no sclerosis at the margin.

Indolent or slow-growing lesions are usually marginated by sclerotic bone. When growth is more rapid, the sclerotic rim is only seen in some areas, or it is absent entirely. Moreover, when present, the sclerotic rim may be condensed, compact, or diffuse. Most benign tumors and cysts have the condensed type, whereas more reactive processes usually have a diffuse type of marginal sclerosis. For example, one sometimes sees a diffuse and thick sclerotic rim at the margin of some cementomas. These lesions are slow growing, having a maturation period in excess of 10 years. Odontogenic myxomas have an early growth stage, and these are usually marginated by the condensed type of sclerotic bone; in the aggressive breakout stage, the sclerotic margin becomes thinner, discontinuous, and absent in some cases. Punched out lesions are sharply defined, but they lack a sclerotic rim. In the jaws, this can mean a lack of a defensive response in the host bone, or it may indicate that the periosteum has been injured as a result of disease or its treatment. Myeloma

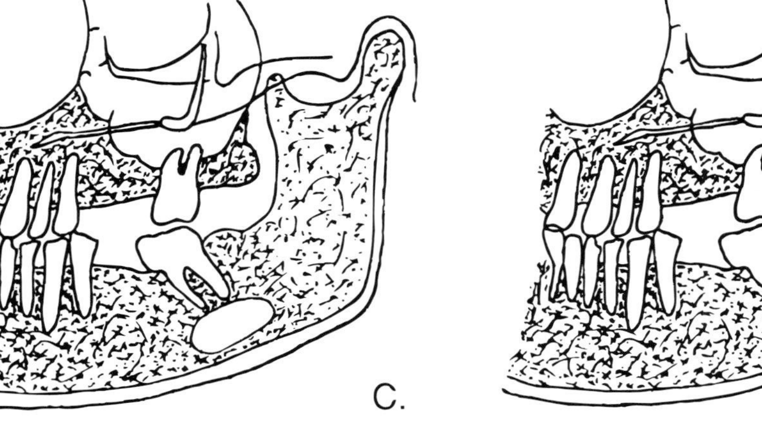

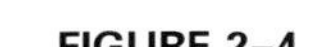

FIGURE 2–4.

Margins with a Narrow Zone of Transition: A, Thick condensed; B, thick diffuse sclerotic; C, thin condensed sclerotic; punched out.

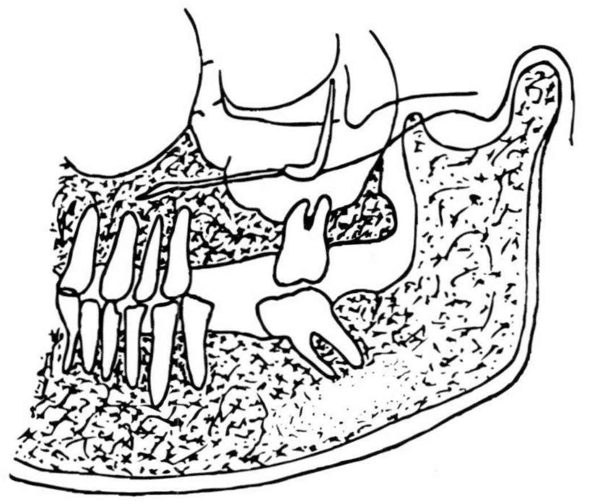

FIGURE 2–5.

Margins with a Wide Zone of Transition.

typically has a punched out appearance, as does the fibrous healing defect.

A **wide zone of transition** exists when a lesion is aggressive, and the margin between healthy and abnormal bone becomes progressively less well defined, with a wider and wider zone of transition (see Fig. 2–5). A wide zone of transition is associated with a rapid growth rate. A rapid growth rate may be seen in both benign and malignant conditions, and this is the reason that many aggressive rapidly growing benign lesions have poorly defined margins. Some examples include eosinophilic granuloma, central giant cell granuloma, and aneurysmal bone cyst. Some eosinophilic granulomas may produce a periosteal reaction, however, and others may demonstrate expansion of the cortex, thus helping to identify them as benign, because these features are absent in most malignant tumors. A wide zone of transition in the absence of expansion suggests a malignancy such as metastatic disease.

Some other jaw lesions undergo periods of **dormancy** and **reactivation** (see Fig. 2–6). Examples of such conditions include periapical cemental dysplasia, florid osseous dysplasia, and Paget's disease. Although the appearance of the margin can demonstrate growth rate, it can also indicate no growth at all. For example, in periapical cemental dysplasia and florid osseous dysplasia, the radiolucent rim at the periphery of the lesion and the sclerotic rim of reactive host bone have been described as variable features of these disorders. When the lesion is dormant, the cemental mass is in direct apposition to the adjacent normal bone; superficially, it exactly resembles idiopathic osteosclerosis. On examination with the magnifying lens, however, the peripheral margin of the cemental mass is relatively smooth, with several rounded massules on its surface; one sees a lack of spiculation at the margin, as can be seen in osteosclerosis. As the lesion reactivates, the peripheral radiolucent band containing calcific spherules reappears first, followed by an increasingly thick and diffuse outer rim of reactive bone. This is followed by a relatively short period of growth, and as activity diminishes, the outer rim of sclerotic bone followed by the peripheral radiolucent band disappears, leaving the cemental mass in direct apposition to the adjacent bone. Because lesions may be multiple, the patient may have both active and dormant lesions at any given moment. When no alveolar bone is present above the cemental mass and a peripheral radiolucent zone is seen, then the complication of osteomyelitis has probably occurred, and a further period of dormancy should not be expected. Rather, a slow sequestration of the cemental mass should now be expected. This represents the end stage of the condition, after which a normal appearance of the underlying bone can be expected.

Supporting Structures of the Teeth

The supporting structures of the teeth are the periodontal membrane space (PMS), the lamina dura, and the alveolar bone. Because these structures are unique to the jaws, changes here when affected by disease can offer additional diagnostic clues not available in any other bone.

The periodontal membrane space may disappear or it may increase in size. A loss of the PMS is associated with ankylosis. A generalized increase in width of the PMS is seen in

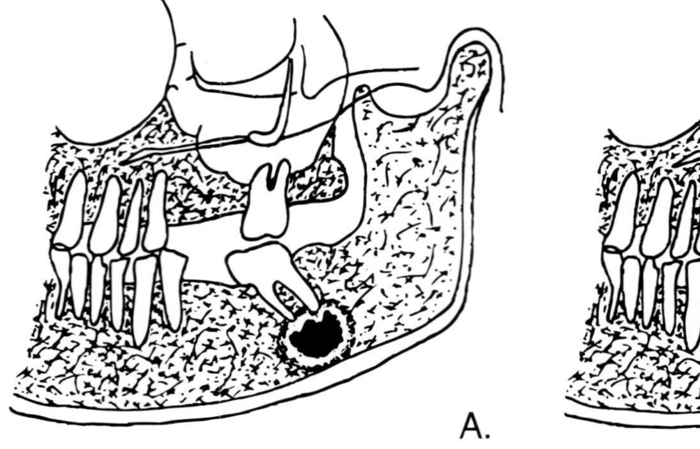

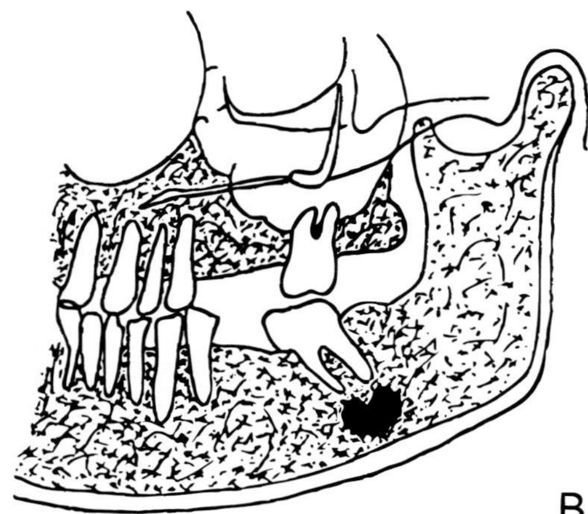

FIGURE 2–6.

Active and Dormant Phases: A, Active; B, dormant.

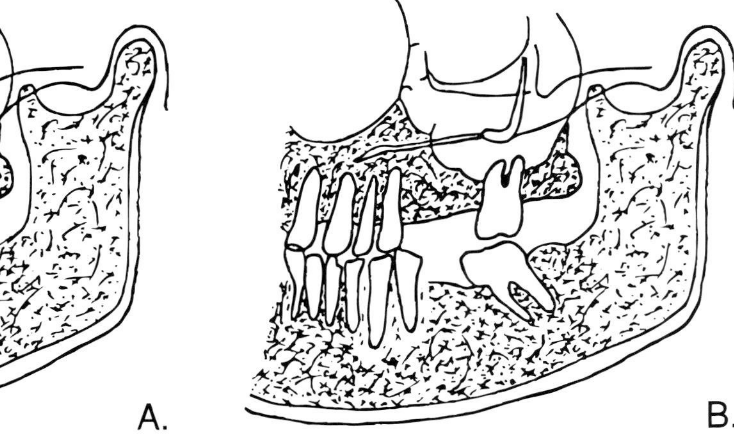

FIGURE 2–7.

Floating Tooth: A, Periodontal disease; B, gingival carcinoma.

orthodontic tooth movement and scleroderma. Severe bruxism may produce a generalized widening of the PMS along with similar widening of the lamina dura. A focal widening of the PMS may be caused by traumatic occlusion and is a helpful but seldom used adjunct to the sometimes difficult task of identifying the most significant premature occlusal contact. Localized PMS enlargement, particularly down one side of one or several roots, may be an ominous sign of aggressive malignant growth. This finding is seen in metastatic disease, gingival carcinoma, and bone sarcomas, among others. The most common cause of periodontal space widening is either local or generalized periodontal disease, principally periodontitis, invariably accompanied by an associated loss of the lamina dura.

One especially notable pattern is a uniform widening of the periodontal membrane space around the entire root, producing a **"floating tooth"** appearance (Fig. 2–7). The cause is either aggressive malignant tumor replacement of bone, as in gingival carcinoma, or bone destruction associated with a benign process, usually periodontal disease and sometimes eosinophilic granuloma. In **periodontal disease,** the following features are present: (1) reactive osteosclerosis at the remaining margin of alveolar bone; (2) a distinct margin with a narrow zone of transition; (3) the absence of trabecular remnants within the periodontal membrane space; and (4) the possible appearance of periodontal disease at other sites in the patient. In **gingival carcinoma,** the following features are present: (1) no reactive sclerotic bone at the margin; (2) an irregular margin with a wide zone of transition; (3) possible appearance of trabecular remnants within the periodontal membrane space; and (4) the possible absence of periodontal disease in other parts of the patients' dentition.

In the absence of periodontal disease, a loss of the lamina dura may be seen in association with fibrous dysplasia, hyperparathyroidism, Paget's disease, and dominant craniometaphyseal dysplasia. These findings are usually accompanied by a ground glass pattern of the alveolar bone. In fibrous dysplasia, the changes are often limited to one quadrant in a younger person. In Paget's disease, this phenomenon occurs mostly in the maxilla of older patients, and focal remnants of the lamina dura may sometimes be seen; hypercementosis and diastemas between the teeth sometimes occur. In hyperparathyroidism, the condition is generalized, and one or more geographic areas of bone destruction representing brown tumors (histologically identical to central giant cell granuloma) may sometimes be seen. A generalized enlargement of the lamina dura is seen in osteopetrosis, and focal widening occurs in traumatic occlusion.

A generalized loss of alveolar bone occurs most frequently as a result of periodontitis. Other conditions include Papillon-Lefèvre syndrome, Chédiak-Higashi disease, agranulocytosis, cyclic neutropenia, and uncontrolled diabetes. In edentulous patients, resorption of the alveolar ridge occurs slowly over time and is said to be accelerated by osteoporosis. Localized enlargement of the interdental crestal bone is an ominous sign and may be the only manifestation of early osteosarcoma or chondrosarcoma. It may also be seen in association with a peripheral fibroma with calcification. The alveolar ridge may be focally enlarged beneath a bridge pontic, but the significance of this finding is not known.

Relationship with Teeth

As with the supporting structures, the teeth offer unique diagnostic opportunities when they are affected by a disorder in the region. Conditions associated with the crown of an unerupted tooth are almost invariably odontogenic in nature. Most of these lesions are either cysts or benign tumors. The presence of characteristic radiopaque flecks within the lesion further helps to narrow the diagnostic possibilities.

Resorption of the root apex of one or several teeth in association with a lesion is usually a sign of a benign process with a more aggressive growth pattern (Fig. 2–8). On rare occasions, it is associated with a malignant lesion, and in such cases it indicates a relatively slower malignant growth pattern, similar to an aggressive benign lesion. The ameloblastoma produces a **knife edge** type of root resorption, whereas the central giant cell granuloma produces resorption along **multiple root planes,** although other lesions including ameloblastoma may also produce this pattern. Generally,

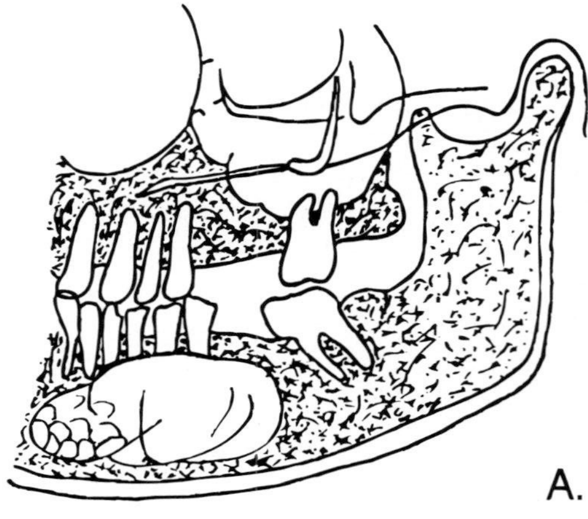

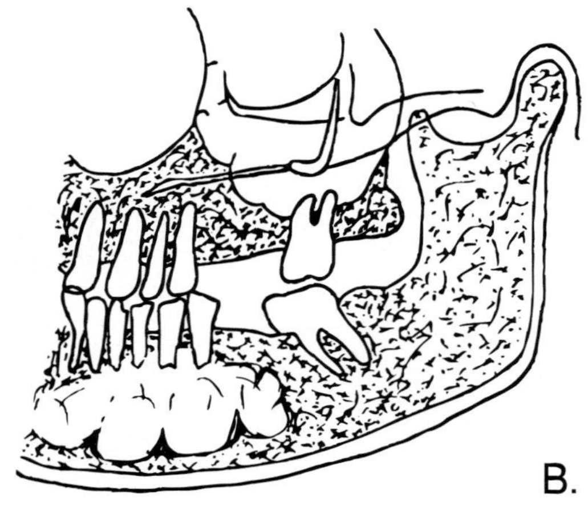

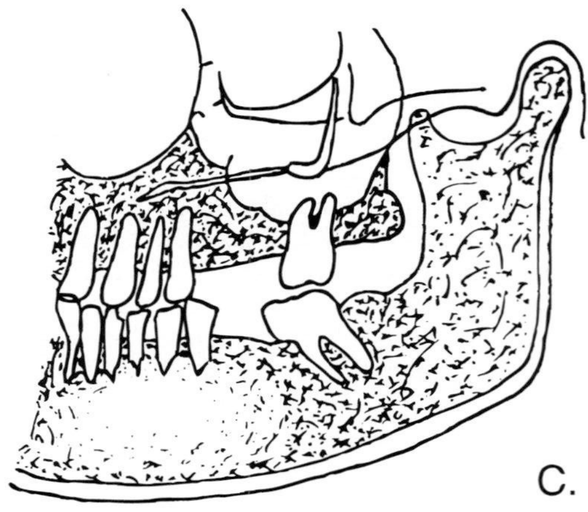

FIGURE 2–8.

Root Resorption: A, Knife edge; B, multiplanar; C, spiked.

malignant disorders are too rapidly destructive to resorb teeth. Notable exceptions are some cases of chondrosarcoma, a few instances of osteosarcoma, and myeloma. In these disorders, a nondescript pattern of root resorption may be seen, or occasionally, a characteristic finding consists of resorption at both sides of the apices to produce a pointed appearance of the roots, referred to as **"spiking."** Thus, the spiking pattern of root resorption may suggest the presence of malignant disease.

Deposition of material on the root of a tooth is usually an indication of a benign, odontogenic process. The two most common conditions are hypercementosis and benign cementoblastoma. In hypercementosis, the dentinal outline of the root can be seen, whereas in benign cementoblastoma, the dentinal outline is lost. Additionally, Paget's disease and Gardner's syndrome are said to be associated with generalized hypercementosis. Benign osteoblastoma, periapical cemental dysplasia, and ossifying fibroma do not usually alter the appearance of the apical portion of involved roots.

The relationship of the apex with a radiolucent lesion is notable (Fig. 2–9). If the apex of one or more teeth **protrudes** into a lesion, this may be a sign of neoplasia, as opposed to cyst formation. If the apices do **not protrude** into a radiolucency that closely approximates them, then the lesion may be cystic. The reason for these differences is that cysts either cut teeth off along a broad front, or the cystic margin stops at the apices of the teeth. On the other hand, tumors tend to go around teeth. This is not a hard and fast rule, but when used in combination with other features, it may be helpful. The apices may or may not be resorbed by both cysts and tumors.

Some lesions may **displace** teeth, whereas others may cause unerupted teeth to become **impacted** (Fig. 2–10). If a lesion appears to be displacing an erupted or unerupted tooth, this may be interpreted as a sign of a benign process, although exceptions do occur. The ossifying fibroma displaces adjacent erupted or unerupted teeth, whereas the benign cementoblastoma usually does not, so the presence of tooth displacement can help one to distinguish between these two lesions. Displacement of unerupted teeth is also seen with the dentigerous, Gorlin, and inflammatory paradental cysts, as well as with the odontogenic keratocyst. It is also seen in association with ameloblastoma, odontogenic myxoma, and the brown tumors of renal osteodystrophy in children. When the displaced tooth is unerupted, such an observation points to the age at which the condition arose.

Some lesions cause unerupted teeth to become impacted, without necessarily causing them to be displaced. In such circumstances, the lesion may be considered less aggressive than one that displaces unerupted teeth. Some early aggres-

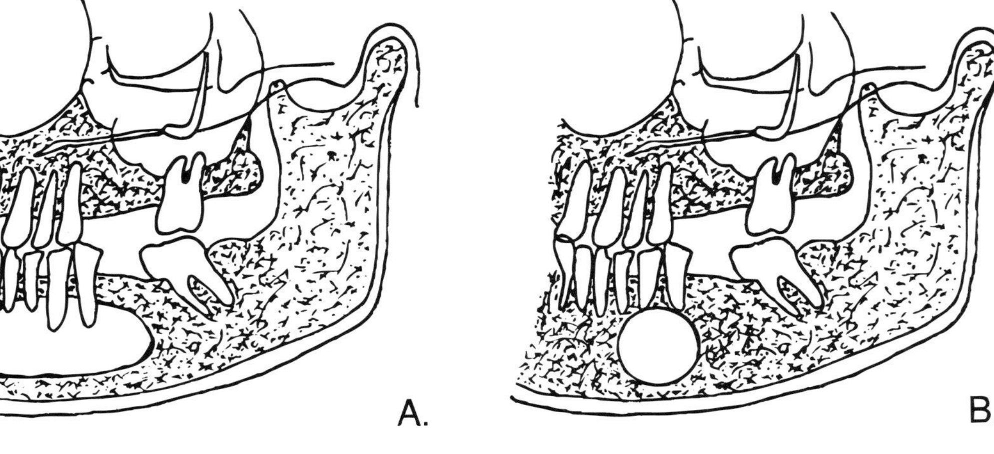

FIGURE 2–9.

Tumor versus Cyst: A, Tumor: apices protrude into lesion; B, cyst: apices do not protrude into lesion.

sive lesions, however, cause teeth to become impacted without necessarily displacing them. The odontoma is typically associated with a nondisplaced impacted tooth, although the ameloblastic fibro-odontoma and the ameloblastic odontoma are more aggressive and are often associated with a displaced tooth. Odontogenic tumors and cysts are often associated with an unerupted tooth; however, any jaw lesion that arises during odontogenesis may be associated with an unerupted tooth.

The one lesion that characteristically 'straddles' the roots of erupted teeth is the traumatic cyst. Classically, the superior portion projects up between the teeth with or without destruction of the lamina dura or displacement of adjacent teeth. The traumatic cyst is the only lesion with this presentation.

Cortical Changes (Figs. 2–11 to 2–13)

When the cortex is expanded, this is a sign of a locally aggressive benign lesion. Expansion without septation internally is considered less aggressive than expansion with septation. In fact, expansion without septation is the hallmark of a slow-growing benign lesion. The integrity of the expanded cortex may be **intact and visible, intact and invisible** on plain films, or **perforated** (see Fig. 2–11). The expanded cortex is an important indicator that the lesion is benign; however, whether it *appears* intact or not is not a particularly good predictor of recurrence. For example, the ameloblastoma may demonstrate an intact, eggshell-thin cortex and may still have a good chance of recurrence even with adequate treatment, whereas the ameloblastic fibroma is often associated with burnt out or disappearing cortical margin and has little propensity for recurrence. When the expanded cortex is visibly perforated, this is a sign of the most aggressive benign lesions, with a propensity to recur, and a few low-grade malignant conditions. Perforations are easily noted on CT. Once the lesion has destroyed the cortex, one must determine how much abnormal tissue has herniated into the extraosseous soft tissues. A soft tissue window on

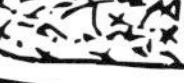

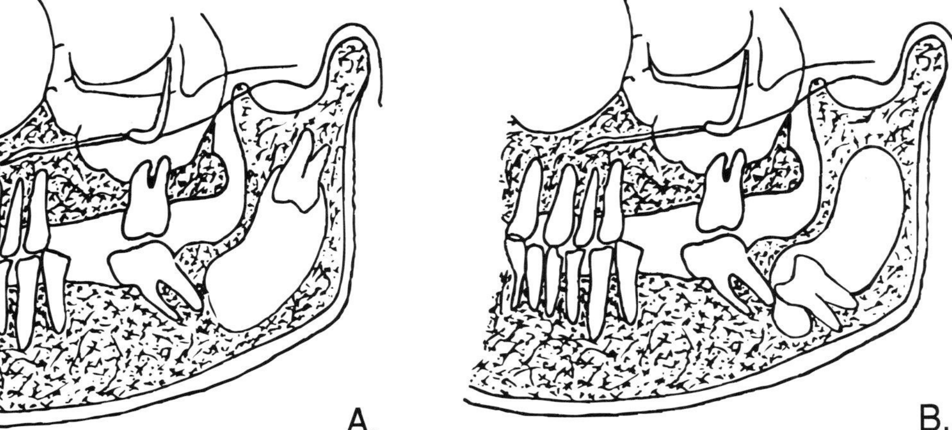

FIGURE 2–10.

Tooth Displacement versus Impaction: A, Displacement; B, impaction.

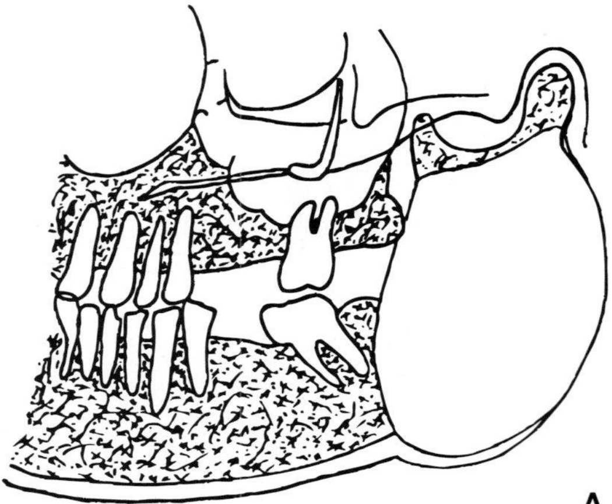

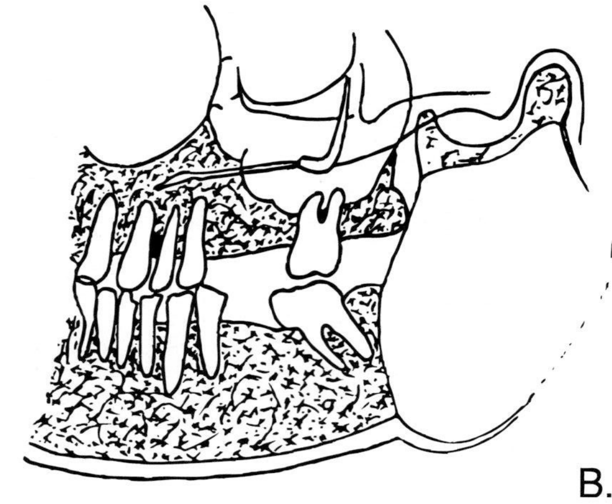

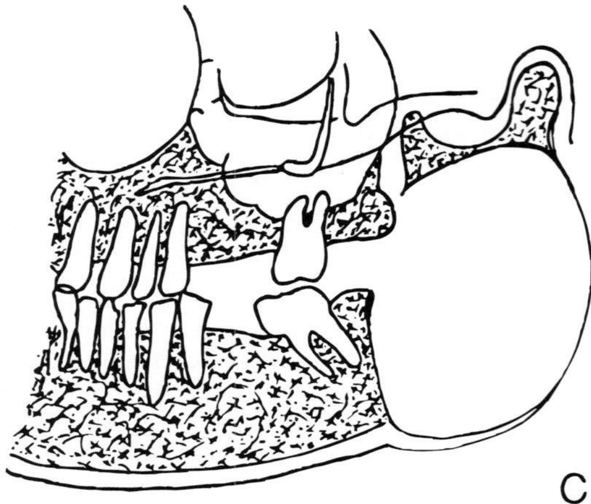

FIGURE 2–11.

Cortex Expansion: A, Intact and visible; B, intact and invisible; C, perforated.

CT or MR images is useful for this purpose. Lesions that behave in this manner are the odontogenic myxoma and the aneurysmal bone cyst.

The jaws give rise to more cystic lesions than any other bones in the skeleton. **Cystic expansion** of the cortex differs from **neoplastic expansion** (see Fig. 2–12). Cystic lesions exhibit a hydraulic effect on the cortex; that is, the cystic fluid applies pressure equally on all margins, so the cortex is expanded evenly and smoothly, with the expanded margin meeting the normal cortex at an equal obtuse angle at both sides of the cyst. Moreover, the cortex is thinned in a uniform manner such that its thickness is equal throughout the expanded margin. The cortex does not tend to disappear from excessive thinning at its greatest bulge. On the other hand, tumors produce an expanded margin that meets the normal cortex at an acute angle on one side and at a different acute or obtuse angle on the other side. The angles are rarely equal. The vector of growth of a tumor is most often not exactly perpendicular to the cortex, nor is the pressure applied equally in all dimensions. For tumors, the expanded cortex may not be of uniform thickness, it may become paper thin and seem to disappear, and it may even have a slightly wavy or irregular endosteal surface.

The cortex may also be eroded without being expanded or perforated (see Fig. 2–13). This may occur at the endosteal surface inside the bone or at the periosteal surface outside the bone. Specific terms are used to describe these two circumstances. **Scalloping** occurs at the endosteal surface of the cortex. The most typical lesions that behave in this way are the odontogenic keratocyst and the central giant cell granuloma. **Saucerization** may be seen in the outer cortex and is caused mostly by lesions arising in the periosteum or gingiva. The most common jaw lesions causing saucerization are submandibular, sublingual, and parotid salivary gland depressions. Others include scleroderma, gingival cyst of the adult, neural sheath tumors, and the sometimes minute traumatic neuroma. Another lesion that causes saucerization is the peripheral giant cell granuloma; saucerization of crestal alveolar bone in edentulous areas is typical.

Periosteal Reactions (Fig. 2–14)

Periosteal reactions are classified as follows:

1. Lamellar, uninterrupted, or continuous.
2. Onion skin or layered.
3. Solid, thick, compact, and smooth.

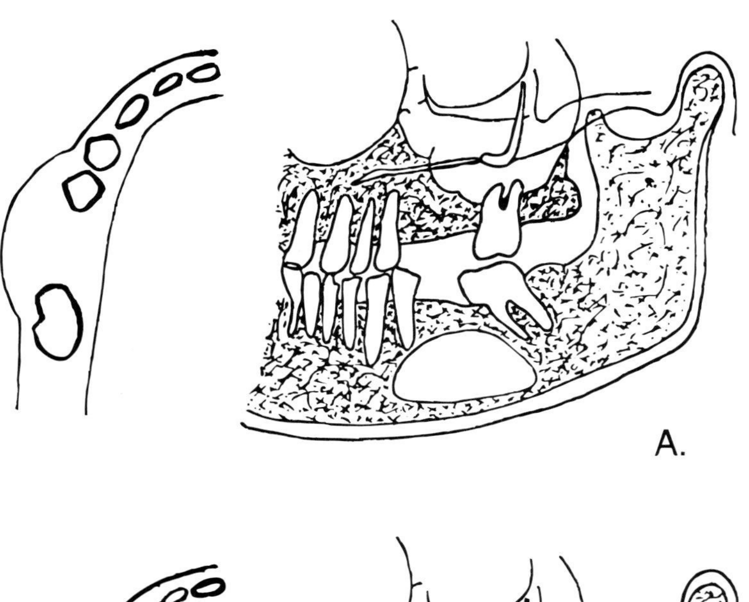

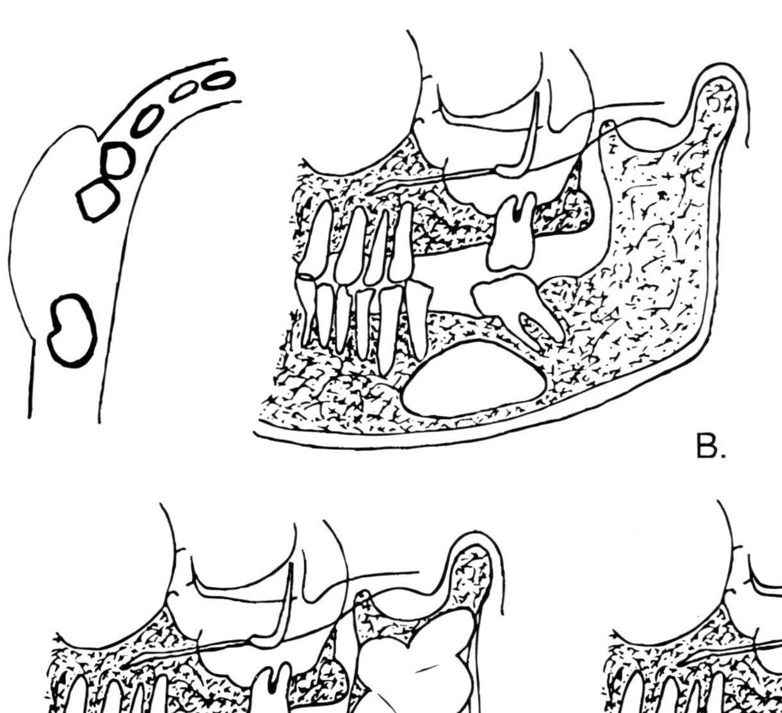

FIGURE 2–12.

Cystic versus Neoplastic Expansion: A, Cyst; B, neoplasm.

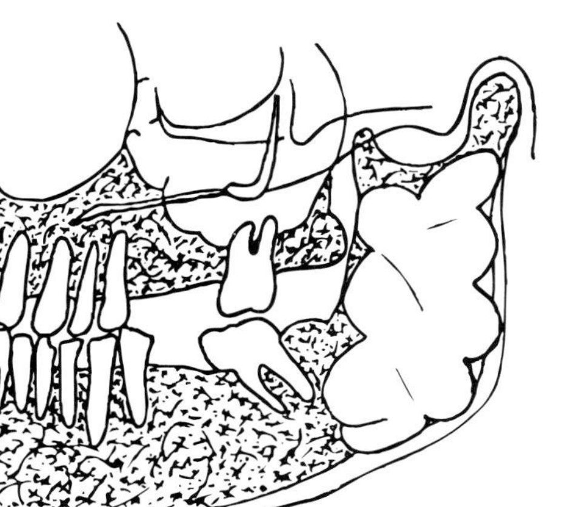

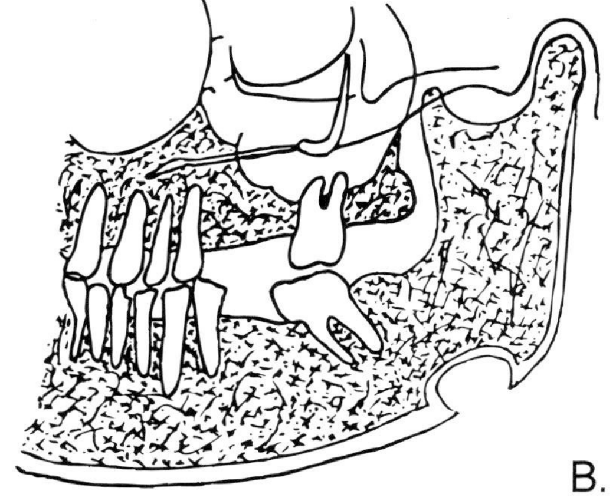
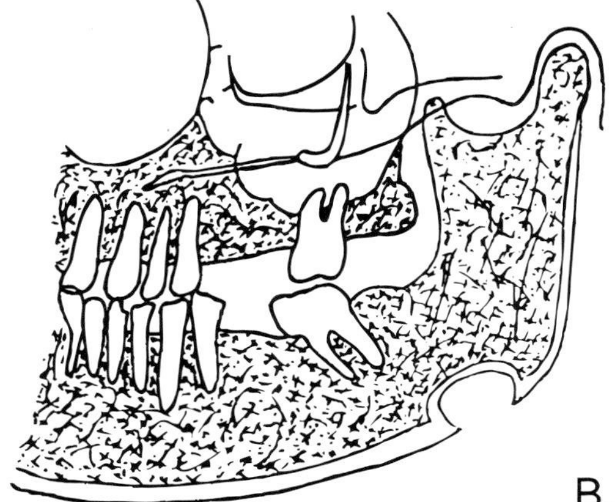

FIGURE 2–13.

Cortex Erosion: A, Scalloping; B, saucerization.

4. Buttress.
5. Lamellar, interrupted, or discontinuous.
6. Solid irregular mass.
7. Codman's triangles.
8. Sunburst, divergent.
9. Irregular spicules.
10. Hair on end.

These reactions are seen in the jaws specifically. Although such reactions in the jaws have been considered rare, we theorize that they probably occur more frequently than previ-

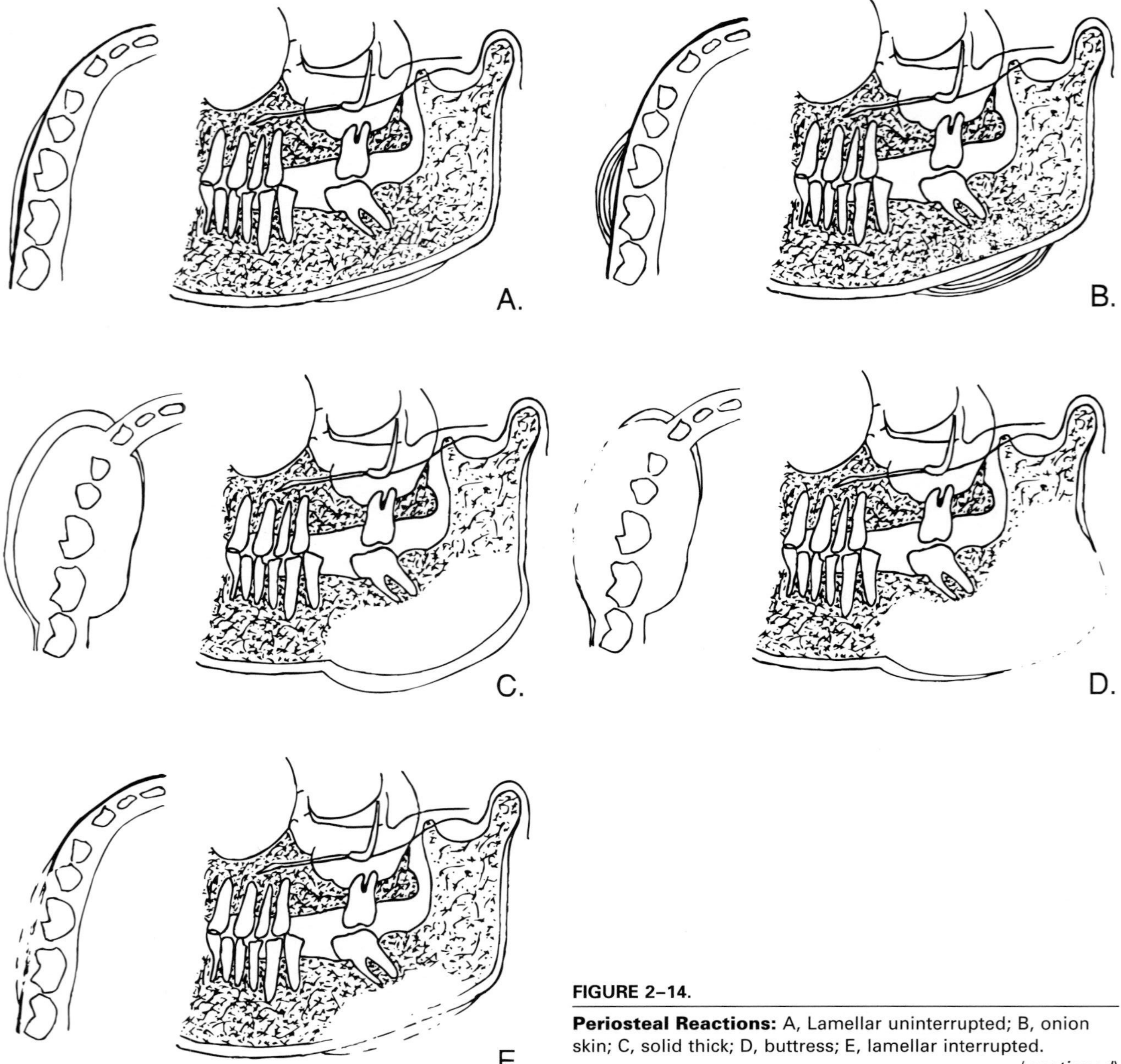

FIGURE 2–14.

Periosteal Reactions: A, Lamellar uninterrupted; B, onion skin; C, solid thick; D, buttress; E, lamellar interrupted.
(continued)

ously believed. In the past, these changes may have gone unnoticed, or most likely, imaging to detect such changes was inadequate. Each of the foregoing reactions is illustrated in some part of this text.

The **uninterrupted lamellar** type is the hallmark of a benign process. In the jaws, it is seen in association with osteomyelitis and may be the only radiologic manifestation of acute osteomyelitis. The osteomyelitis may be the primary problem, or it may occur as a complication in a preexisting lesion.

The **onion skin** pattern implies a more aggressive process, and it is seen in association with both benign and malignant diseases. In the jaws, it is perhaps the most common periosteal reaction when it occurs in association with Garrè's osteomyelitis. As many as 12 laminations have been observed. Only about half these reactions can be seen on the panoramic radiograph; the remainder are seen in the occlusal and reverse Towne or posteroanterior views. This pattern is also seen in Ewing's sarcoma, osteosarcoma, and chondrosarcoma.

The **thick compact** type of cortical thickening is occasionally associated with jaw lesions. It is most commonly noted in cases of resolving Garrè's osteomyelitis, in which the individual laminations become indistinct. This appearance may persist for several months during the healing process. It is also seen in association with osteoid osteoma, and we have seen this reaction in a patient with odontogenic fibroma.

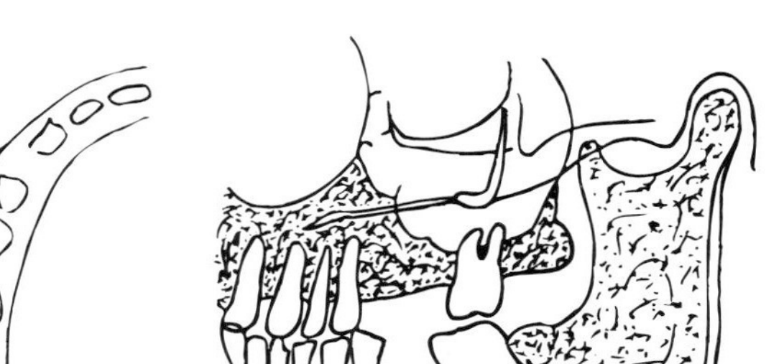
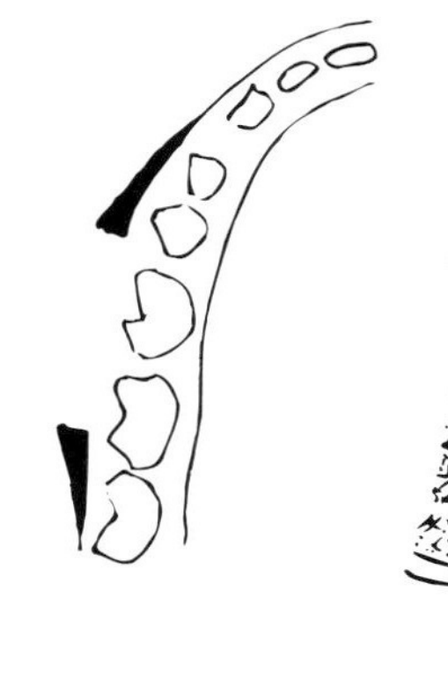

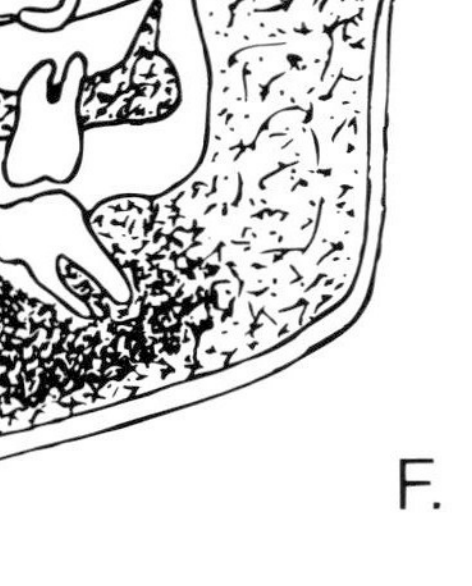
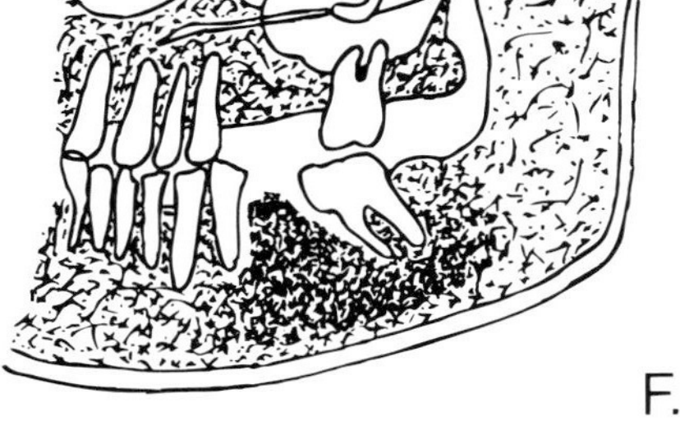
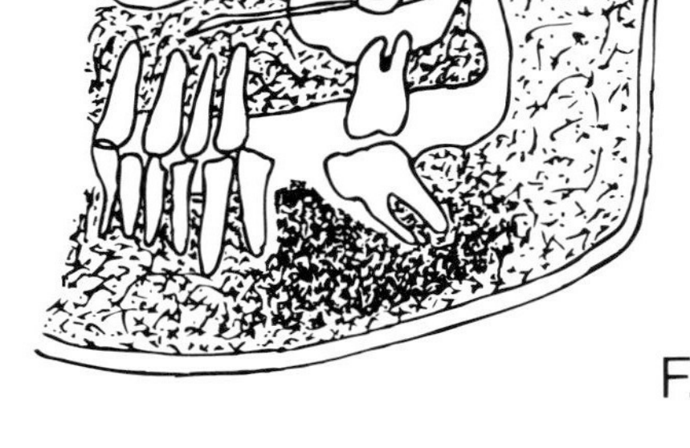
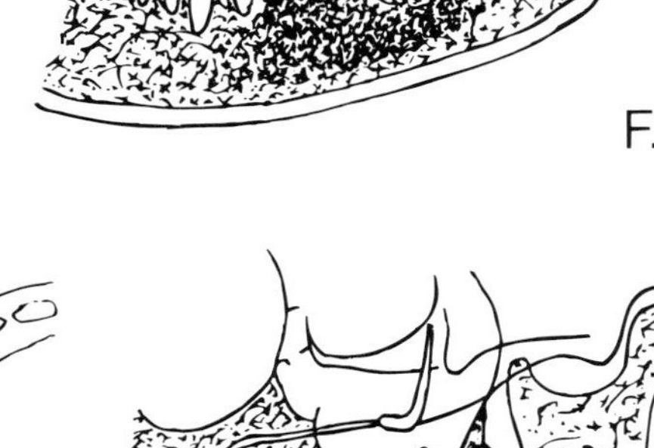
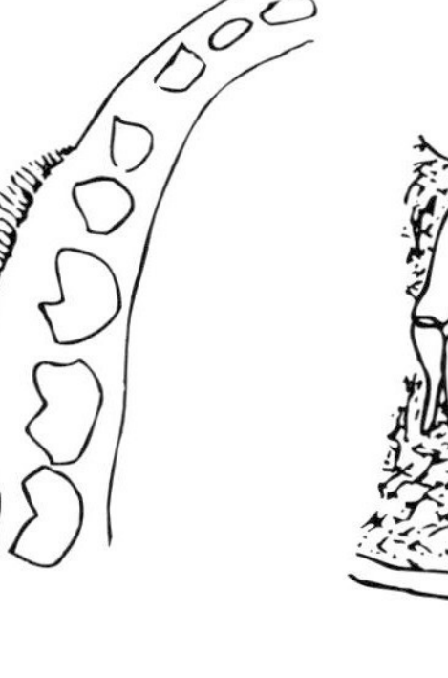
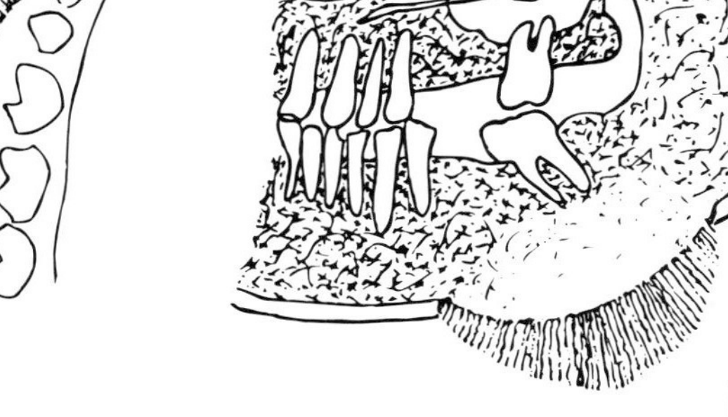
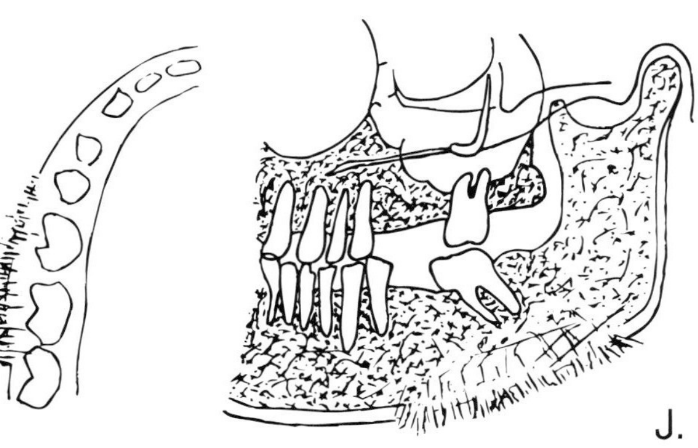

FIGURE 2–14. *(continued)*

Periosteal Reactions: F, irregular mass; G, Codman's triangle; H, sunburst; I, irregular spicules; J, hair on end.

Buttress formation is associated with slow-growing benign lesions, especially tumors. It produces a triangular area of cortical bone at the margins of a lesion with the invisible expanded cortical margin. Buttress formation is especially prone to occur in some ameloblastomas and the ameloblastic fibroma. With correct windowing for bone, the margin that appears invisible on plain radiographs can be seen on CT.

The **interrupted lamellar** type is seen in association with osteogenic sarcoma, so its distinction from the uninterrupted type is important. Underlying bone changes consistent with osteosarcoma are usually apparent. Because reactive sclerosis sometimes occurs in osteomyelitis and blastic neoplastic bone can be produced in osteosarcoma, whether the single layer of subperiosteal new bone is intact helps one to make the diagnosis.

The **solid irregular mass** is seen in osteosarcoma. It is not as closely associated with the inferior cortex as it is with the lingual or buccal cortical plates, however. In lateral views, it appears as a diffuse, mottled area of increased density (radiopaque) and takes on its characteristic appearance in the occlusal view.

Codman's triangles are highly suggestive of bone sarcomas and consist entirely of periosteal bone. Thus, they should be avoided as biopsy sites.

The **sunburst** pattern is a classic finding in bone sarcomas such as osteosarcoma and chondrosarcoma. On close examination, these spicules are not truly straight, but instead form irregular, slightly wavy lines. Some authors claim that this is not actually a true periosteal reaction, but an outgrowth of tumor matrix. We have also seen a report of a case of multiple myeloma involving the mandible with this finding. Some odontomas, odontogenic myxomas, and benign cementoblastomas may also mimic this pattern in some views. In these instances, individual spicules are difficult to separate from the associated radiopaque mass, and the spicules are not usually wavy or irregular.

Irregular spicules form a pattern of interlacing and relatively coarse spicules, a pattern seen in bone sarcomas, especially osteosarcoma. These spicules are similar to those seen in the sunburst pattern, except they are arranged in a much more disorganized, bizzare pattern.

The **hair on end** appearance, rarely seen in the jaws, may occur in Ewing's sarcoma, where the bone spicules are fine and short. In some cases of odontogenic myxoma, the appearance is similar; the spicules are also fine, but they may be coarser and probably represent soft tissue extension of the tumor mass rather than a periosteal reaction. The hair on end appearance is well known as a skull finding in cases of sickle cell anemia and thalassemia; however, this reaction has not been reported in the jaws.

Develop a Differential Diagnosis

The differential diagnosis simply consists of a listing of lesions that may generally resemble a given pattern. For example, multilocular radiolucencies all superficially resemble each other, as do pericoronal radiolucencies. The diseases in this book are discussed in groups by differential diagnosis. Thus, the student must learn to list all the diseases in each group. In addition, some conditions have several radiographic appearances, and these must also be added to the list. At this point, one could state: "when you see a multilocular radiolucent lesion, think odontogenic keratocyst, botryoid odontogenic cyst, ameloblastoma, odontogenic myxoma, central giant cell granuloma, and central hemangioma." If an accurate description of the lesion has been made, it should be easy to categorize it into one of the differential diagnostic groups.

State Your Diagnostic Impression

A diagnostic impression gives the radiologist's opinion of the identity of the lesion. The diagnostic impression can be made based on one of three levels of confidence:

1. The appearance is pathognomonic of a specific condition.
2. The findings are sufficiently characteristic for a probable accurate diagnosis.
3. A tissue diagnosis cannot be established with assurance.

The first group has been referred to by Murray and Jacobson (1977) as "leave me alone lesions." Many of the conditions in this group of pathognomonic lesions rarely require treatment. Examples of leave me alone lesions include salivary gland depressions, fibrous healing defect, cherubism, idiopathic osteosclerosis, osteoma, Gardner's syndrome, and osteopetrosis. Others that are also pathognomonic but that may require treatment include incisive canal cyst, benign cementoblastoma, periapical cemental dysplasia, florid osseous dysplasia, and compound odontomas.

The second group presents such characteristic findings that one has a high level of confidence in the diagnosis. Some of these lesions include the traumatic cyst, lateral periodontal cyst, most other odontogenic cysts such as the dentigerous cyst, multilocular lesions such as ameloblastoma, fibro-osseous conditions such as fibrous dysplasia and ossifying fibroma (which are histologically indistinguishable), and many benign odontogenic tumors such as adenomatoid odontogenic tumor and complex odontoma. One's level of confidence in the diagnosis varies among these lesions; some presentations are almost pathognomonic, whereas others are not as definitive.

In the third group, it is difficult to establish a tissue type with confidence. In such cases, the features should be studied carefully for signs of a benign or malignant process. Additionally, an attempt should be made to differentiate tumors and cysts from inflammatory, metabolic, and dysplastic processes.

Making Recommendations

Depending on the certainty of the radiologic diagnosis, and/or its nature, any recommendations made should be given from the perspective of the person reading the film. In dentistry, all dentists read radiographs. Some are more adept at interpreting them than others. The radiologist may recommend more in terms of diagnostic considerations, whereas the surgeon contemplates the surgical implications. Because recommendations are not binding, one must have them in writing; the radiograph often becomes an important piece of evidence in cases of litigation. This is equally important for recommendations made to other colleagues as well as those made to the patient.

USING THIS TEXTBOOK

The reader can become frustrated if the terminology discussed in this chapter is not clearly understood and learned. It is not practical to explain over and over again the meaning of descriptive terms such as zone of transition or periosteal reaction. On the other hand, many lesions have unique features that we have not described here, and it is appropriate to do so when the lesion is discussed in later chapters.

The student may question the need to read descriptions of radiologic changes outside the jaws, some of which are included in this text. For lesions that may affect other parts of the skeleton, the radiologist first learns the basic kinds of changes produced by the condition in a general way. Then there are the most common location and presentation, and these findings are learned next. Then one learns the differences and variations occurring in specific bones. The medical radiologist learns about the jaws last, if at all. In dentistry, we have been trying to learn the appearances of jaw lesions as though they were the only bones in the body. Where applicable, it is more efficient to learn the basic radiology of a condition first and then to determine whether the changes in the jaws are typical, similar to changes seen in other conditions, or unique to that condition. In our experience, diseases of bone occurring in the jaws are similar to those seen elsewhere in the skeleton, whereas odontogenic tumors and cysts are often unique.

The reader may also wonder about the inclusion of the descriptions of skull, facial, and sometimes vertebral changes described in this text. The dentist often takes radiographs of these structures, however, and so is responsible for recognizing any pathologic changes in them, or, having recognized a jaw lesion, such as Paget's disease or myeloma, the dentist will often order appropriate extraoral views.

Another feature of this text is the inclusion of descriptions of the findings on tomography, CT, MR, or scintigraphy. Although we have shown mainly plain radiographs available in most dental offices, we have also gone to great lengths to obtain the additional features of advanced imaging where appropriate. We have searched the world for the cases described in these pages and are extremely thankful to our colleagues who so willingly provided them.

We recognize that this book will be used on many different levels, from the beginning dental student to the board-certified oral and maxillofacial radiologist. When multiple descriptions of different bones are included, the section dealing with jaw changes is always clearly marked; our emphasis here is clearly on this section. If the condition is odontogenic or unique to the jaws, we always begin with the discussion of the jaws. If the condition can occur in other bones as well as the jaws, we may begin with the jaw changes and progress to other bones; conversely, we may start with the descriptions of other bones then move on to the jaws. Whatever we have done is based on what we believe will make learning easiest. As a result of our research, much of it unpublished, the reader will discover new features of jaw lesions that have not been described before.

With all the foregoing, the reader has various options. For example, this text has enough illustrations so one can learn much from simply studying the cases and reading the legends. Some believe (and rightly so) that the pathologic process determines the effects on a bone, and thus they will learn the radiology in conjunction with the pathologic descriptions. Others are more clinical in their orientation because they must examine patients, make diagnoses, and plan treatment; for these readers, the clinical and demographic features in conjunction with the radiologic findings are best. Surgeons especially appreciate the value of studying the third dimension, as we have illustrated in many of our cases. Others still are course directors and must decide on curricular content. Recognizing that the needs of the sophomore dental student are different from those of an oral surgeon or radiologist, we have taken great pains to indicate how common a condition is. For some readers, it may be appropriate to delete certain diseases from a course outline or from a specific discussion. Although it is easy to delete, it is impossible to add.

Finally, whatever the interest or objective of the reader, the quality and quantity of the illustrations reproduced here should help to make dental radiology more easily learned and understood. The illustrations have been selected on the basis of their representative nature or to demonstrate a specific radiologic manifestation. The illustrations should be studied with attention to detail. Radiology is a pictorial science, so looking at the pictures is what this book is all about.

References

Hofer B, Hardt N, Voegeli E, Kinser J: A diagnostic approach to lytic lesions of the mandible. Skeletal Radiol 14:164, 1985.

Hollender, L: Decision making in radiographic imaging. J Dent Educ 56: 834, 1992.

Langland OE, Langlais RP, McDavid WD, Del Balso AM: Panoramic Radiology. 2nd Ed. Philadelphia:Lea & Febiger, 1989, pp. 38 and 183.

Langland OE, Sippy FH, Langlais RP: Textbook of Dental Radiology. 2nd Ed Springfield, IL:Charles C Thomas, 1984, p. 206.

Murray RO, Jacobson HG: The Radiology of Skeletal Disorders. Vols. 1 to 3. New York:Churchill Livingstone, 1977.

Chapter 3

Normal Anatomy of the Jaws

The tooth substance is the densest structure of the human body, and consequently it absorbs more x-rays than does any other tissue in the body of comparable size and thickness.

ENAMEL (Fig. 3–1)

Enamel is the hardest calcified tissue in the human body. The enamel consists mainly of inorganic material (96%) and only a small amount of organic substance and water (4%).

DENTIN (Figs. 3–1 to 3–3)

The greater portion of the tooth is made up of dentin. Dentin and cementum present a uniform, gray radiographic image on the radiograph (Fig. 3–1). In its physical and chemical qualities, dentin closely resembles bone. Both are considered vital tissue because they contain living protoplasm. Dentin is harder than bone, but considerably softer than enamel. The smaller content of mineral salts (65% inorganic and 35% organic matter and water) renders dentin more radiolucent than enamel.

Under normal conditions, the odontoblasts of the dentin are active, and the formation of dentin may continue throughout one's life. Dentin formed in later life is called "secondary dentin" and forms pulpward on the entire pulpal surface of the dentin, thereby narrowing the pulp cavity. Secondary dentin formation is observed best in the premolars and molars, where more secondary dentin is produced on the floor and the roof of the pulpal chamber than on the side walls. In time, the entire pulpal chamber may be closed completely by secondary dentin (Fig. 3–2).

Reparative dentin is "hard tissue" dentin formed as a result of extensive wear, erosion, caries, or operative procedures. Damaged or newly differentiated odontoblasts are stimulated in a defensive reaction whereby the hard reparative dentin seals off the area of injury. Secondary and reparative dentin cannot be differentiated from primary dentin on the radiograph.

Sometimes, severe stimuli to the dentin such as caries or operative procedures induce changes in the dentin itself. Calcium salts may be deposited in or around degenerating odontoblastic processes and may obliterate the tubules. This condition is called dentinal sclerosis and may start at the dentinoenamel junction and proceed toward the pulp. In advanced cases, selerotic dentin can be detected in a regular radiograph as a radiopaque structure (Fig. 3–3).

CEMENTUM (Fig. 3–4)

Cementum is the mineralized dental tissue covering the anatomic roots of human teeth. Cementum forms the attachment of collagen fibers that bind the tooth to surrounding structures. It is a specialized connective tissue that is similar to compact bone; unlike bone, however, human cementum is avascular. Although fully mineralized cementum is not as hard as dentin, their physical properties are similar; that is why the two tissues cannot be differentiated on the radiograph. Cementum is formed on permanent teeth throughout one's life. Under certain circumstances, the formation of cementum may exceed physiologic limits and may cause an increased deposition of cementum called "hypercementosis." The increased formation of cementum occurs mainly on the apical two thirds of the roots and can be recognized on the radiograph (Fig. 3–4).

PULP CHAMBER AND ROOT CANALS (Figs. 3–5 and 3–6)

Each pulp organ is composed of a coronal pulp, located centrally in the crowns of teeth, and the root or radicular pulp. The pulp chamber and root canal(s) are continuous cavities within the teeth that are filled with soft tissue and absorb fewer x-rays than surrounding dentin. Therefore, the pulp is more radiolucent than dentin, and it appears as a dark image within the tooth on the radiograph. The young pulp has pulp horns, which are protrusions that extend into the cusp of each tooth. Because of the continuous deposition of dentin, the pulp becomes smaller with age.

In the developing tooth, the pulp chamber and pulp canals are wider. The lumen at the apex of a younger tooth root diverges at the apical end. This feature gives this portion of the tooth a "funnel shape." The wide apex of a maturing tooth contains the dental papilla (Fig. 3–5). The tooth pulp is initially called the dental papilla. This tissue is designated as "pulp" only after dentin forms around it.

The lumen of the root canal of a mature tooth usually converges toward the apex, but appearances vary. In some teeth, the root canal can be traced to the extreme apex, and the foramen is visible. In others, the foramen is not visible. In still others, the root canal is clearly visible to within a few millimeters of the apex, but beyond this point there is no evidence of a foramen. Although the foramen is present, it cannot be seen on the radiograph. If the tooth is vital, it must have a foramen. This narrowing at the apex of the root is caused by deposition of cementum within the canal. Occasionally, the apex is situated at the side of the tooth rather than at the extreme tip of the tooth.

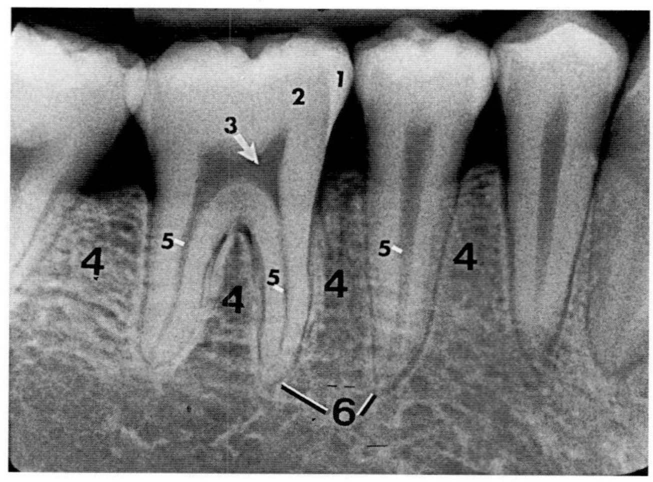

FIGURE 3–1.

Radiographic Normal Anatomy of Tooth and Supporting structures: The enamel and dentin line of demarcation is very sharp. The enamel is whiter than dentin because enamel is much denser. Enamel (1), dentin (2), pulp chamber (3), alveolar bone (4), pulp canal (5), root apex (6).

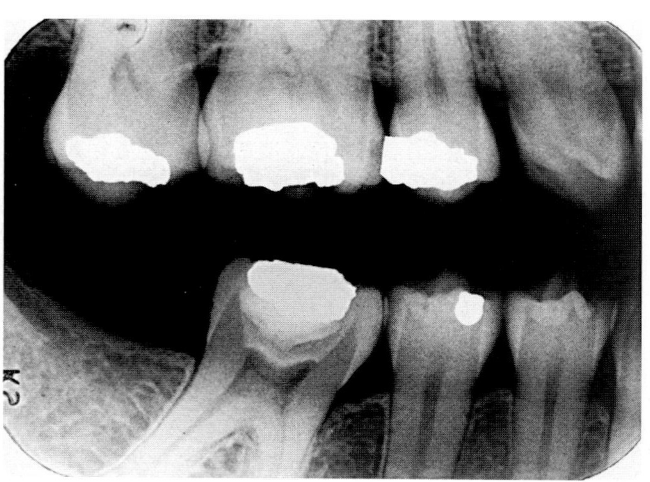

FIGURE 3–3.

Sclerotic Dentin: Sclerotic dentin as result of caries beneath restoration in lower first molar.

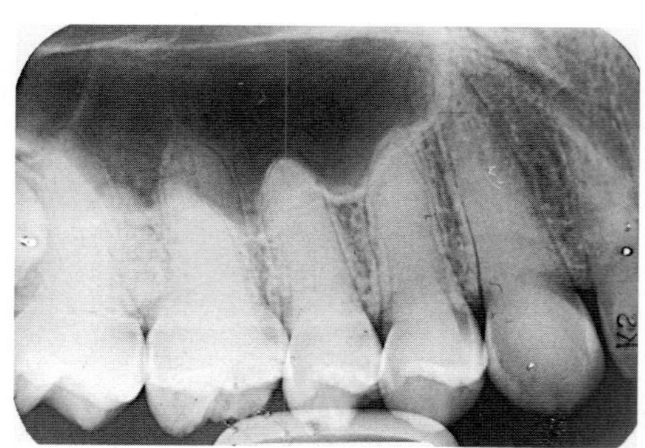

A

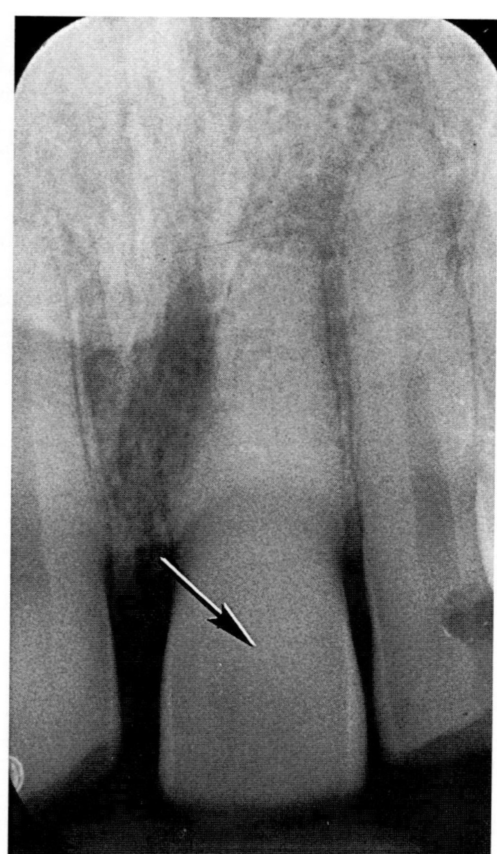

B

FIGURE 3–2.

Secondary or Reparative Dentin: A, Radiograph of reduced pulpal chambers by deposition of secondary dentin in maxillary teeth as a result of the normal aging process. B, Radiograph of a maxillary central incisor with severely reduced pulpal chamber and canal from previous trauma to the tooth.

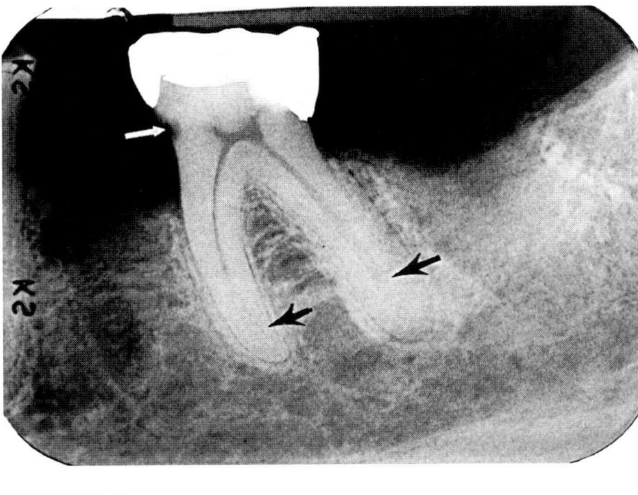

FIGURE 3–4.

Hypercementosis: Hypercementosis present in excessive amounts in this case cannot be distinguished from dentin in mandibular first molar in a 70-year-old man (black arrows). The distal root is larger than the mesial root. Note root caries (white arrow.)

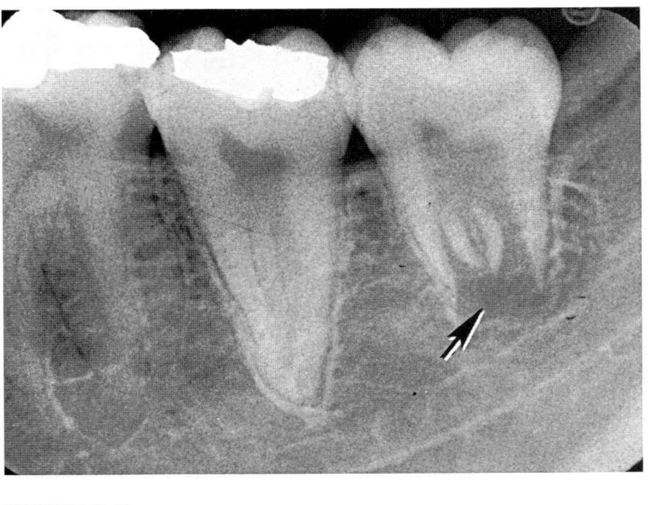

FIGURE 3–5.

Pulp and Dental Papilla of a Young Person: Developing roots in an erupting third molar tooth. The pulp chamber and root canals are large (arrow), and the dark spaces at the apices of the tooth are occupied by dental papilla.

Accessory root canals are not ordinarily apparent in radiographs. Rarely, one sees a larger aberrant canal on the radiograph that has come to surface below the cementoenamel junction. When accessory canals are located near the coronal part of the root or in the bifurcation area, a deep periodontal pocket may cause inflammation of the dental pulp. Conversely, a necrotic pulp can cause disease of the periodontal tissue through an accessory canal.

Pulp stones or denticles are nodular, calcified masses appearing in either or both the coronal or root portions of the pulp. They appear as radiopaque masses within the pulp (Fig. 3–6A). The incidence and the size of pulp stones increase with age. Hill (1934) reported that pulp stones occur in 66% of all teeth between the ages of 10 and 20 years, and the incidence rises to 90% when the age group is between 50 and 70 years.

Diffuse calcifications appear as irregular calcific deposits in the pulp tissue, usually following collagenous fiber bundles or blood vessels. Sometimes, they develop into larger masses, but usually they persist as fine spicules (Fig. 3–6B). Diffuse calcifications usually are found in the root canal and less often in the coronal area, whereas the pulp stones (denticles) are seen most often in the coronal pulp.

Barabas (1969) reported a high incidence of large pulp

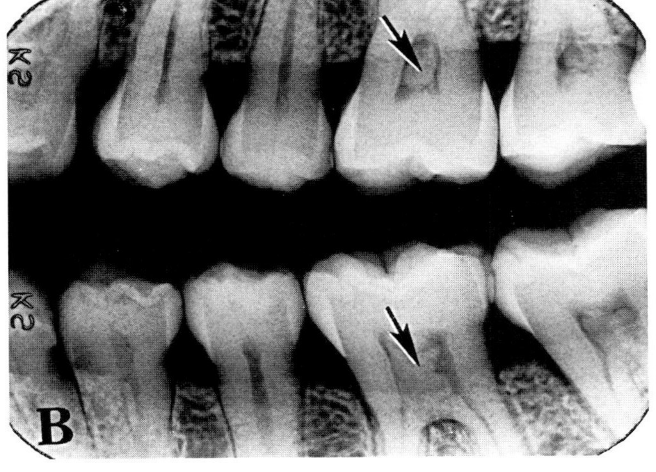

FIGURE 3–6.

Pulp Stones (denticles) and Diffuse Calcifications: A, Radiograph of tooth with a pulp stone or denticle in a mandibular canine tooth (arrow). (From Langland OE, Langlais RP, Morris CR: Principles and Practice of Panoramic Radiology. Philadelphia:WB Saunders, 1982, p. 223.) B, Periapical radiograph of diffuse calcification of the pulp in upper and lower first molars (arrows).

stones in Ehhers-Danlos syndrome. Shields et al. (1973) reported that multiple pulp stones occur in patients with type 2 dentinal dysplasia.

ALVEOLAR PROCESS AND PERIODONTAL LIGAMENT SPACE (Figs. 3–7 to 3–10)

The alveolar process may be defined as the part of the maxilla or mandible that forms and supports the sockets of the teeth (Fig. 3–7). As a result of adaptation and function, two parts of the alveolar process can be distinguished. The first part consists of a thin layer of dense bone, called the alveolar bone proper or the lamina dura, which lines the tooth socket and gives attachment to the principal fibers of the periodontal ligament (Fig. 3–9). The second part is the bone that surrounds the lamina dura and gives support to the socket. This is called the supporting alveolar bone. It consists of the cortical plates and the spongy bone between the cortical plates. The cortical plates consist of compact bone and form the outer and inner plates of the alveolar process. The spongy bone fills the area between the cortical plates and the lamina dura (alveolar bone proper). In the region of the anterior teeth in both jaws the supporting bone is usually very thin; the cortical plates are fused with the lamina dura, and the spongy bone is absent (see Fig. 3–7).

Immediately adjacent to the tooth surface lies the periodontal ligament, a composite of tissues surrounding the root of the tooth and serving as the attachment of the tooth to the alveolar bone proper (see Fig. 3–8). The periodontal ligament consists primarily of bundles of continuously intermingling collagen fibers arranged into a network running from the tooth to the lamina dura. These fibers are called principal fibers of the periodontal ligament. The average width of the periodontal ligament of an adult tooth in function is 0.18 mm. It has an hourglass shape, however, it is widest in the coronal aspect, slightly narrower near the apex, and narrowest in the middle of the alveolus in the area of rotation. The periodontal ligament tissue is of a density insufficient to absorb any appreciable amount of x-rays. On the other side of the periodontal ligament lies the lamina dura, which is radiopaque (Fig. 3–9). With a dense structure on either side of the periodontal ligament, the space the ligament occupies appears as a thin, hourglass-shaped dark line. The periodontal ligament has also been known as the periodontal membrane, but because its principal structures and functions resemble those of a ligament more than those of a membrane, the preferred term is periodontal ligament.

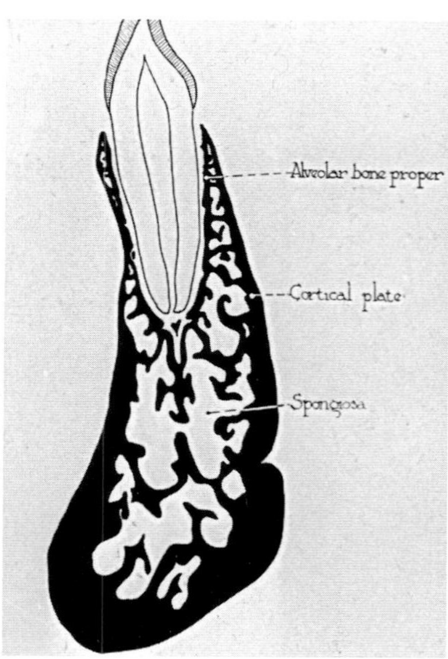

FIGURE 3–7.

Alveolar Bone and Tooth: Cortical bone (inner and outer plates), spongiosa (cancellous bone), and alveolar bone proper (lamina dura).

In younger persons, the periodontal ligament spaces are usually thicker; they become thinner in the elderly (see Fig. 3–8B and C). When the teeth are mobile or loose, the periodontal ligament space usually appears wider (see Fig. 3–8D). If the teeth receive undue mechanical stress during orthodontic treatment, the periodontal ligament space will appear thickened. In the presence of some diseases, the periodontal ligament space thickens. These diseases are scleroderma and early malignant disorders such as osteogenic sarcoma, chondrosarcoma, fibrosarcoma, and metastatic disease (see Fig. 3–8E). In ankylosis, the periodontal ligament space is invisible.

The spaces in the alveolar bone proper (lamina dura) that accommodate the roots of the teeth are known as alveoli. The tooth sockets are lined with a layer of bone known as the alveolar bone proper or the lamina dura. It is perforated by many small openings (cribriform plate) that carry branches of the intra-alveolar nerves and vessels and Sharpey's fibers to the periodontal ligament and cementum. This layer of dense bone appears as a white line on radiographs and is called the lamina dura (Fig. 3–9).

The alveolar processes are subdivided into various parts depending on their anatomic relationships with the teeth they surround. The bone located between the adjacent teeth is known as the interproximal bone or interdental septum (see Fig. 3–1). The bone located between the roots of multirooted teeth is known as the interradicular bone. The alveolar process located on the facial or lingual surfaces of the roots of teeth is known as radicular bone. In healthy teeth, the alveolar processes surround the roots to within 1 to 2 mm of the cementoenamel junction. The crest of the interproximal bone is normally more coronally positioned than the adjacent radicular bone. The coronal margin of the alveolar bone processes are called the alveolar crests. The width of the crests depends on the distance between the teeth; the crests are narrower as the roots of adjacent teeth which approximate each other more closely.

Between the molars and premolars, the alveolar crests are flat and horizontal (Fig. 3–10B and D). In the incisor regions, the teeth are closely set, with room for the alveolar crests to rise only as points, to which some observers have applied the term "alveolar interdental septal spines" (Fig. 3–10A and C).

The surfaces of the alveolar crests are smooth and formed by the continuation of the lamina dura from the sockets of

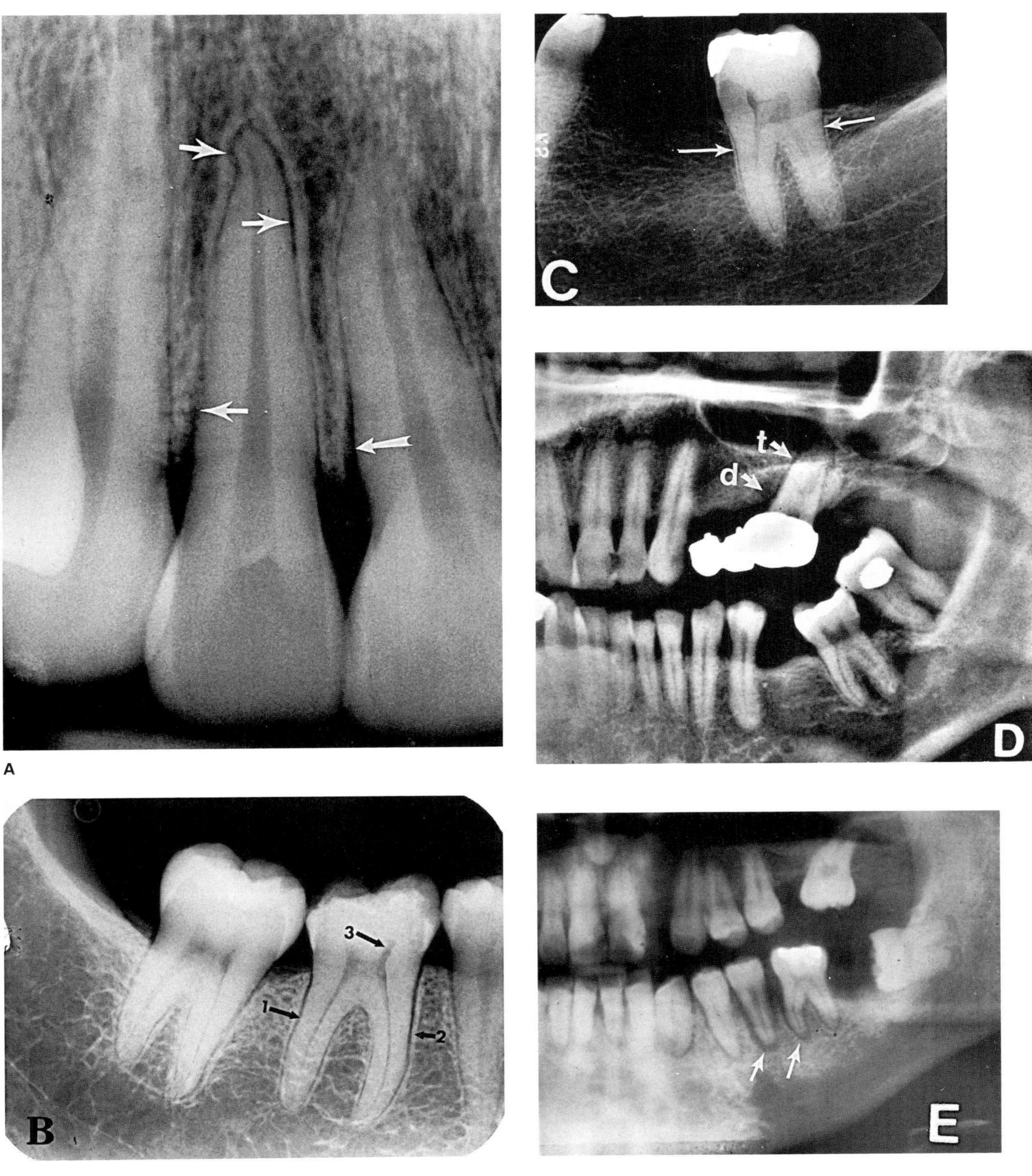

FIGURE 3–8.

Periodontal Ligament Space: A, Adult normal periodontal ligament space (arrows: dark thin line). B, Adult normal periodontal ligament space: periodontal ligament space (1), lamina dura (2), and pulp horn (3). C, Periodontal ligament space narrowing seen in patient with advancing age (arrows). D, Thickened periodontal ligament space (t) with periodontal destruction (d) in a maxillary molar with a cantilever bridge. The maxillary molar is extremely mobile. (From Langland OE, Langlais RP, Morris CR: Principles and Practice of Panoramic Radiology. Philadelphia: WB Saunders, 1982, p. 252.) E, Chondrosarcoma: note the localized widened periodontal ligament spaces in the lower left quadrant (first and second premolars and first molar) in a patient who was diagnosed as having chondrosarcoma in this region of the mandible.

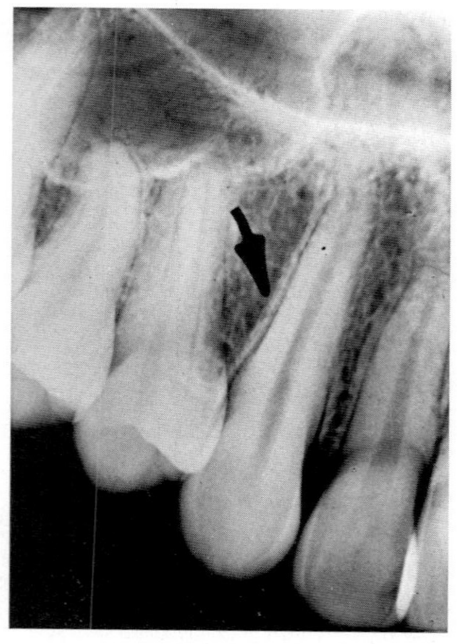

FIGURE 3–9.

Lamina Dura: It is a thin layer of dense bone (cribriform bone) that lines the tooth socket (arrow).

the teeth and the facial and lingual cortical bone. They are sometimes covered with a thin layer of dense bone that may be seen as a thin, white line on the radiograph. In radiographs of premolars and molars, however, normal alveolar crests most commonly show flat, smooth surfaces with no evidence of condensation of bone on the surface. In the incisor region, the sharp, pointed crests are normally covered by dense bone that is actually a continuation of the lamina dura.

CORTICAL BONE

The facial and lingual cortical plates produce no images on the radiograph and hence are not identifiable. The cortical plates are identifiable, however, on the inferior border of the mandible and at the alveolar bone crests between the teeth of both jaws. In patients with an anatomic depression or destruction of some portion of the cortical plates, radiographic appearances sometimes mimic the radiolucency produced by pathologic changes in the deeper parts of the bone.

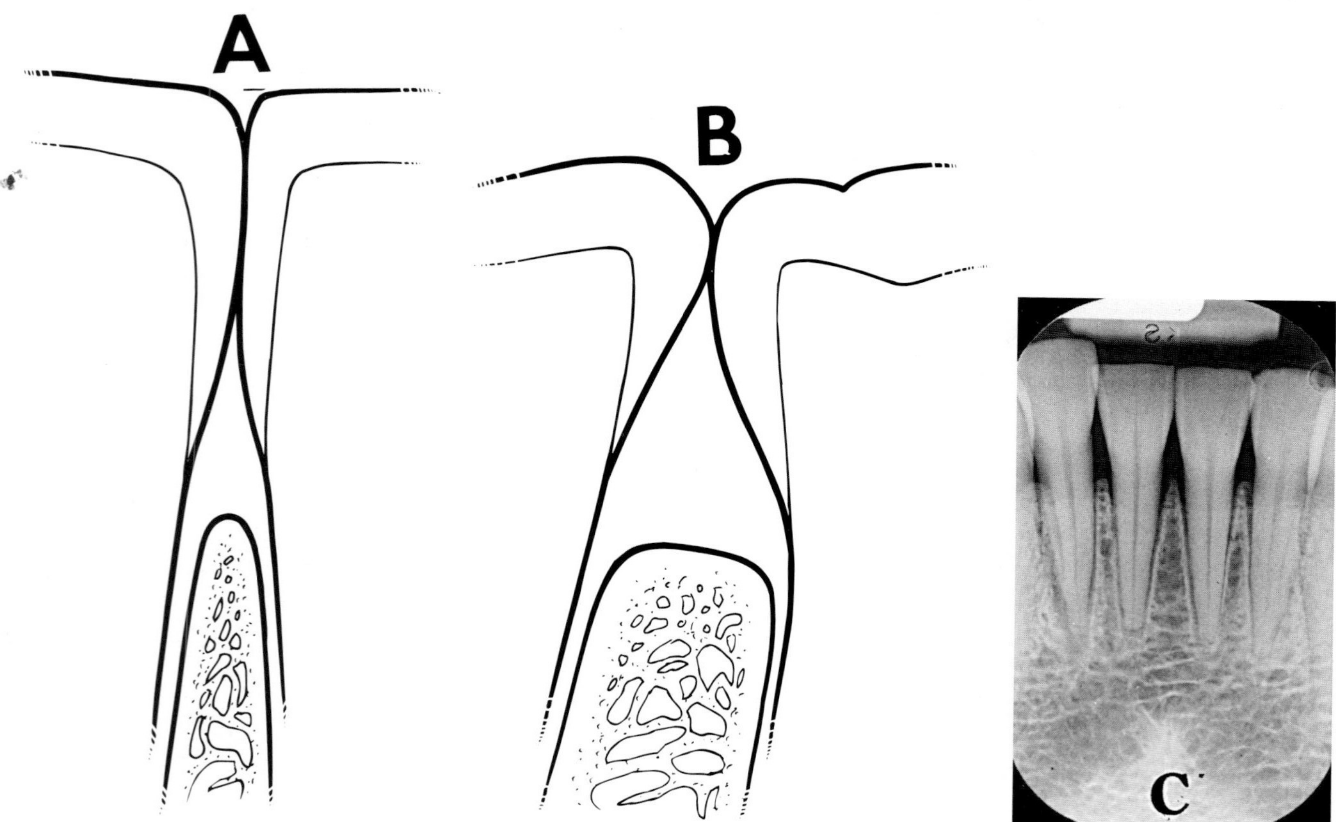

FIGURE 3–10.

Effect of Tooth Form on Alveolar Bone Crest: A, A relatively flat proximal tooth surface as seen in the incisor region goes together with narrow pointed septa. B, A wide, flat alveolar crest is usually present with an extremely convex tooth surface as seen in molar regions. C, Narrow pointed alveolar bone crests in the incisor region go together with flat interproximal tooth surfaces or contact areas.

(continued)

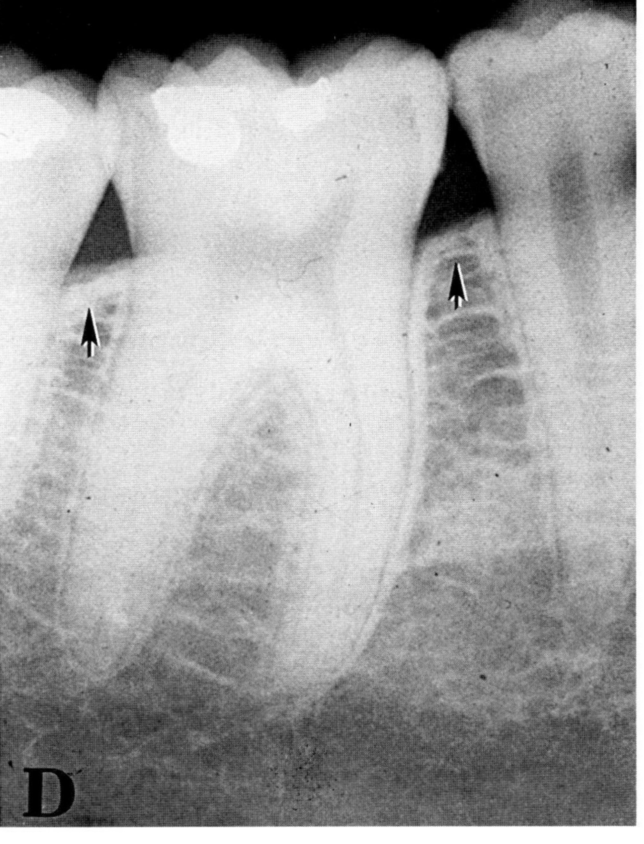

FIGURE 3–10.

(continued) D, Flat interproximal alveolar bone crest in the molar and premolar regions (arrows).

Depressions in the cortical plates that can produce radiolucencies are anatomic conditions such as the submandibular fossa, incisive fossae, and salivary gland depressions. The cortical plates on the inferior border of the mandible are evaluated on the radiograph for fractures and a variety of destructive processes. Moreover, some diseases may reveal subperiosteal reactions, such as Garrè's osteomyelitis, osteogenic sarcoma, and Ewing's sarcoma.

Depressions in Cortical Plates That Can Mimic Pathologic Processes (Figs. 3–11 and 3–12)

Anatomic depressions in the maxilla are thin, and this thinness causes darker or radiolucent images that could be misinterpreted as a pathologic process. One of these depressions in the bone is the maxillary incisive fossa just mesial to the canine eminence, the anatomic prominence labial to the maxillary canines (Fig. 3–11). Sometimes, the radiolucency or darkness of this depression in the bone (incisive fossa) is arranged such that it may give the impression of disease of the bone (Fig. 3–12).

Mandibular Radiolucencies Due to Thinness of Bone (Fig. 3–13)

When anatomic structures are thicker, more x-rays are absorbed, and this increased absorption, in turn, produces more radiopaque (white) areas in the radiograph. Thinner anatomic areas produce radiolucent or darker shadows. In the mandible, the very thin labiolingual bone of the mandibular incisive fossa region is sometimes extremely radiolucent (dark) and mimics disease (Fig. 3–13A). The submandibular gland fossa beneath the mylohyoid ridge is much thinner than the bone above it. Therefore, the submandibular fossa

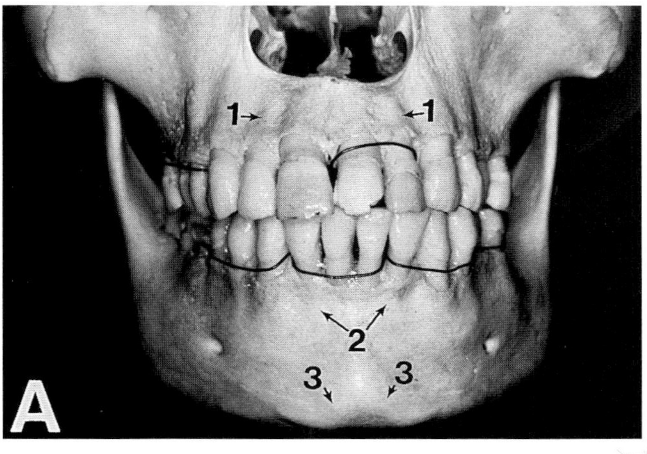

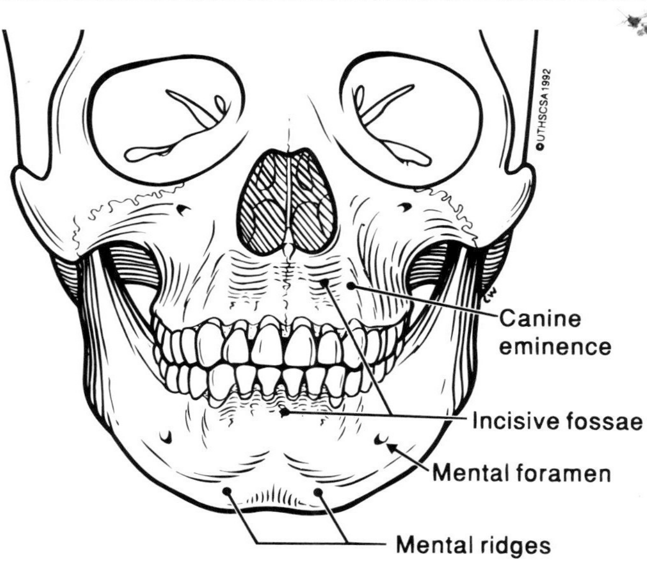

FIGURE 3–11.

Maxillary and mandibular incisive fossae: A, Skull, frontal view, showing the anatomic locations of the maxillary incisive and mandibular incisive fossae: maxillary incisive fossae (1), mandibular incisive fossa (2), and mental ridges (3). B, Diagram of a front view of the skull showing the maxillary and mandibular incisive fossae, mental ridges, canine eminences, and mental foramen.

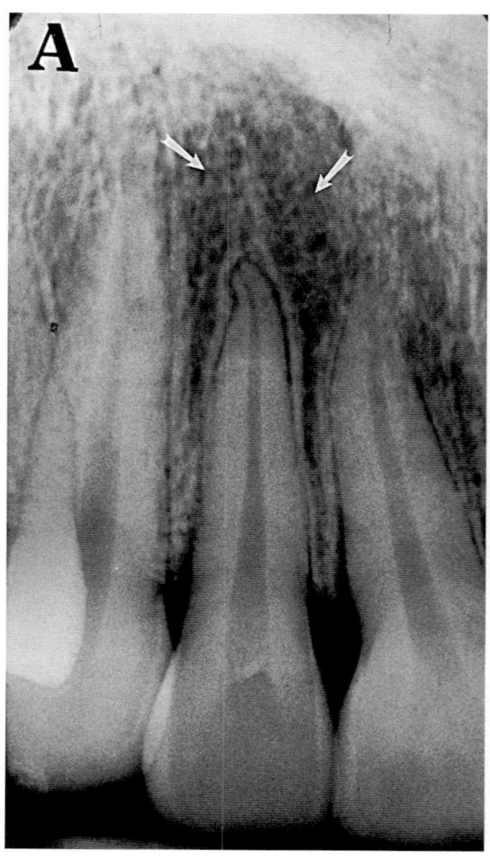

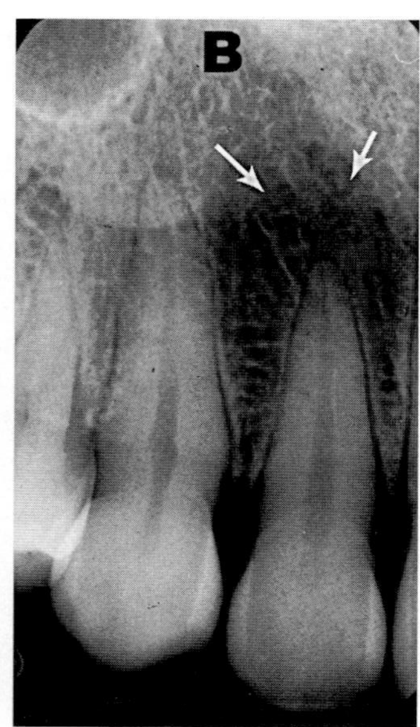

FIGURE 3–12.

Maxillary Incisive Fossa Radiolucency: A, Radiolucency (darkness) in the globulomaxillary region (arrows) that in reality is the depression of the incisive fossa. B, The incisive fossa (depression) is revealed as a radiolucent halo above the maxillary lateral incisor (arrows) and gives the impression of disease arising from the tooth.

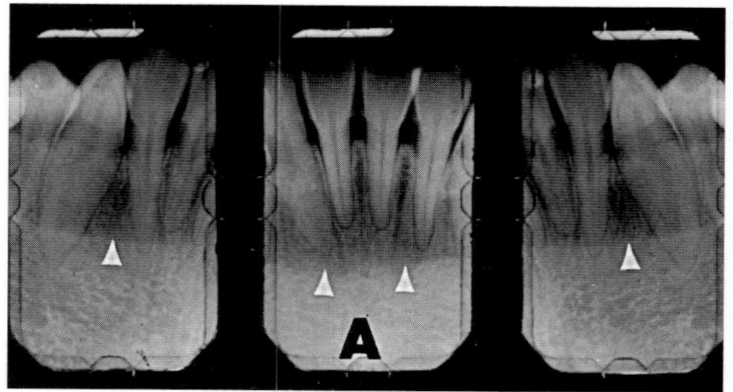

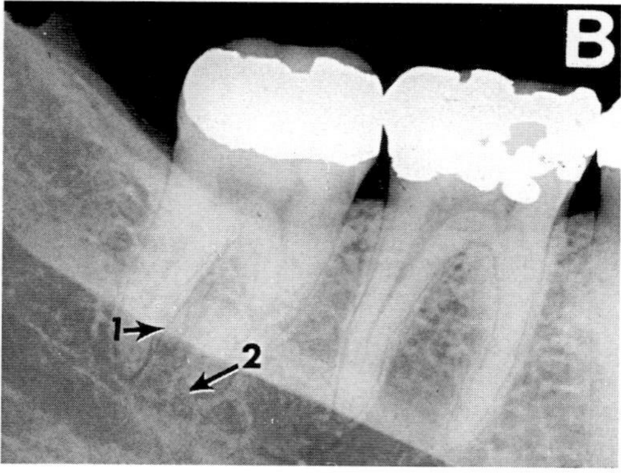

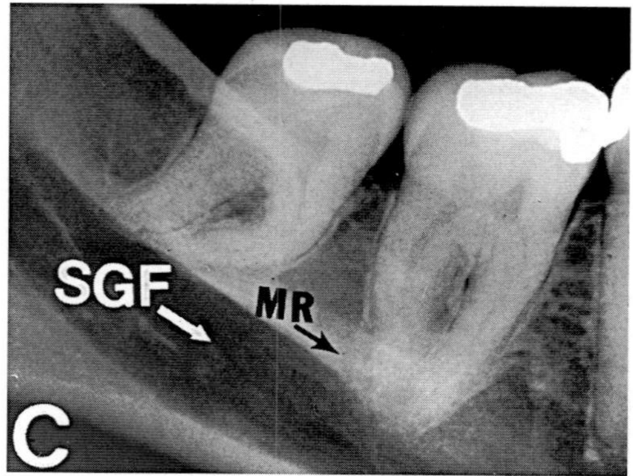

FIGURE 3–13.

Mandibular Radiolucencies from Thinness of Bone: A, Very thin labiolingual bone of the mandibular incisive fossa region producing a very dark radiolucency (arrowheads). B, Radiolucency indicating submandibular gland fossa area could be mistaken for a pathologic process: mylohyoid ridge (1) and submandibular gland fossa (2). C, Radiolucency below the mylohyoid ridge (MR) could mimic a pathologic process. It is actually the submandibular gland fossa (SGF).

area is sometimes extremely radiolucent (dark) and may be mistaken for a pathologic process (Fig. 3–13B).

CANCELLOUS OR SPONGY BONE

The cancellous or spongy bone surrounding the lamina dura and tooth socket is made up of thin strands of bone called trabeculae that cross one another in an irregular manner. Separating the trabeculae, as revealed in the radiographs, are dark spaces that contain the bone marrow. The white strands (trabeculae) and these dark spaces (medullary spaces) produce a network pattern with wide normal variations in size and shape in different persons. The marrow spaces in the alveolar process may contain hematopoietic marrow, but usually they contain fatty marrow. In the condylar process, the angle of the mandible, and the maxillary tuberosity, hematopoietic cellular marrow is found. Various pathologic trabecular patterns of the alveolar process have been described as ground glass, salt and pepper, orange peel (peau d'orange), granular, permeative, geographic, honeycomb, and motheaten.

Maxillary Trabecular Pattern (Fig. 3–14)

In the maxilla, the supporting bone commonly presents an overall uniform appearance. The trabecular arrangement produces smaller marrow spaces than in the mandible of the same person. The network pattern of the maxilla is almost always finer than that in the mandible. One sees numerous, delicate interdental and interradicular trabeculae. The size of the maxillary bone spaces, or the mesh of the network, may vary from less than 1 to 4 mm. Although the network pattern of the maxilla lacks the distinct trajectory pattern seen in the mandible, it seems to be compensated for by a greater number of trabeculae in any given area.

Mandibular Trabecular Pattern (Fig. 3–15 to 3–17)

In the mandible, the cancellous bone varies considerably in different parts of the same bone, as well as in different persons. Rarely is the pattern uniform throughout the greater part of the bone. The network pattern in the cancellous bone around the teeth may present a linear trabeculation with strands running in a relatively horizontal direction, with little or no crossing. This fits the general idea of trajectory pattern of spongy bone well. A variation of this mandiblar network trabecular pattern consists of a stepladder pattern and occurs most frequently between the roots of the mandibular first molars (Fig. 3–15) and between the mandibular central incisors. The interdental and interradicular trabeculae are regular and horizontally arranged in a ladderlike arrangement. Patients with sickle cell anemia and thalassemia sometimes have a ladderlike arrangement of the trabeculae in the jaws. This pattern is also described as a ''honeycomb'' configuration.

In many mandibles, one sees a marked trabeculation around the teeth themselves, but the bone below the roots is much less patterned and may be devoid of any trabeculation (Fig. 3–16). In large persons with large jaws, the mandibular bone has thicker trabeculae and smaller medullary spaces (Fig. 3–17), and in smaller adults and children, the bone is more radiolucent throughout.

Senile Bone (Fig. 3–18)

As a person grows older, bone loses some of its calcific content for various reasons, such as nutritional causes, disease atrophy, hormonal changes, and osteoporosis. The bone of the elderly (75 years and older) is often more radiolucent with thinner trabeculae and wider medullary spaces (see Figs. 3–8C and 3–18).

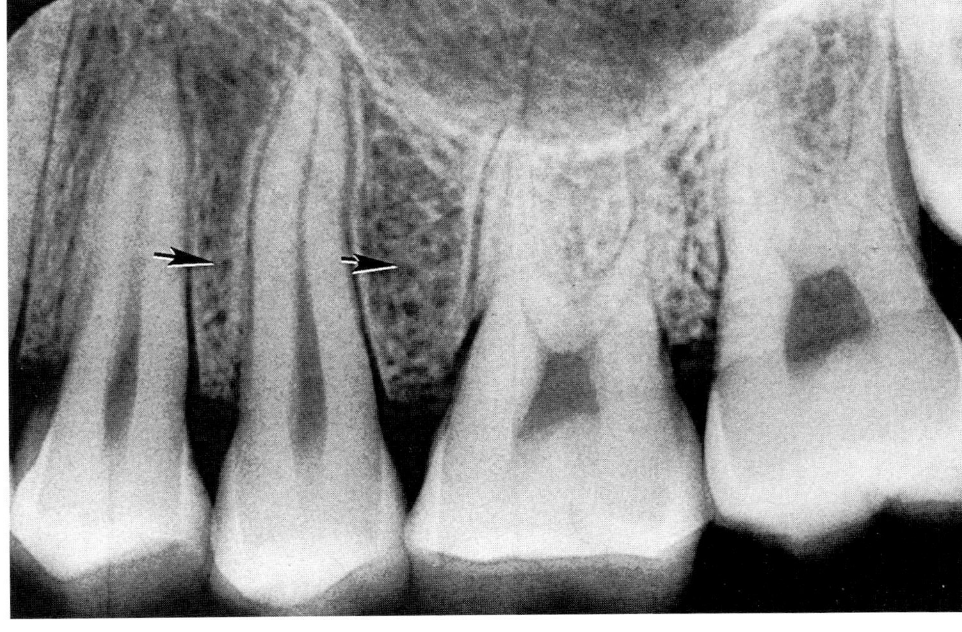

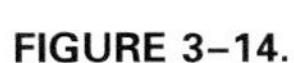

FIGURE 3–14.

Maxillary Alveolar Bone: The overall picture is one of uniformity of the trabecular pattern (arrows). The size of the maxillary bone spaces, or the mesh of the network, may vary from less than 1 to 4 mm. The trabecular network in the maxilla produces smaller medullary spaces than the mandible of the same person.

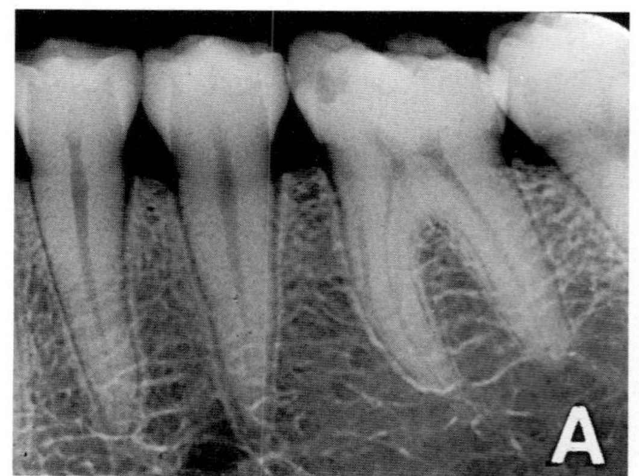

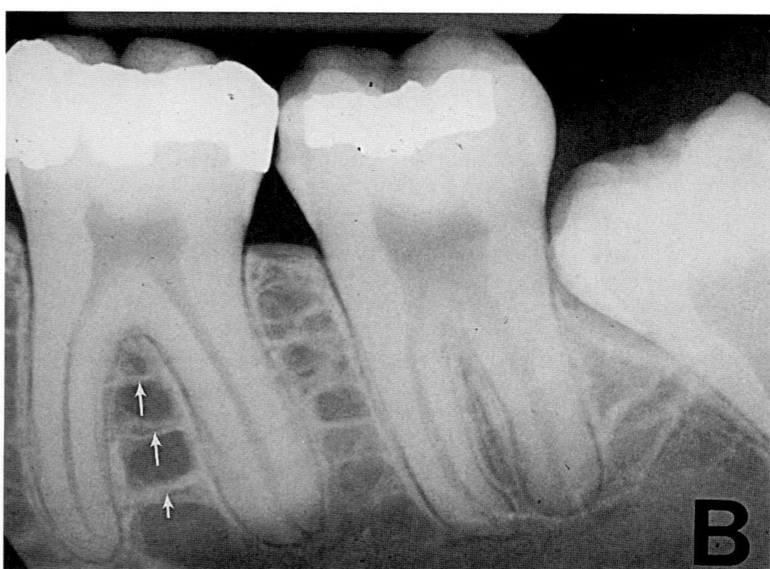

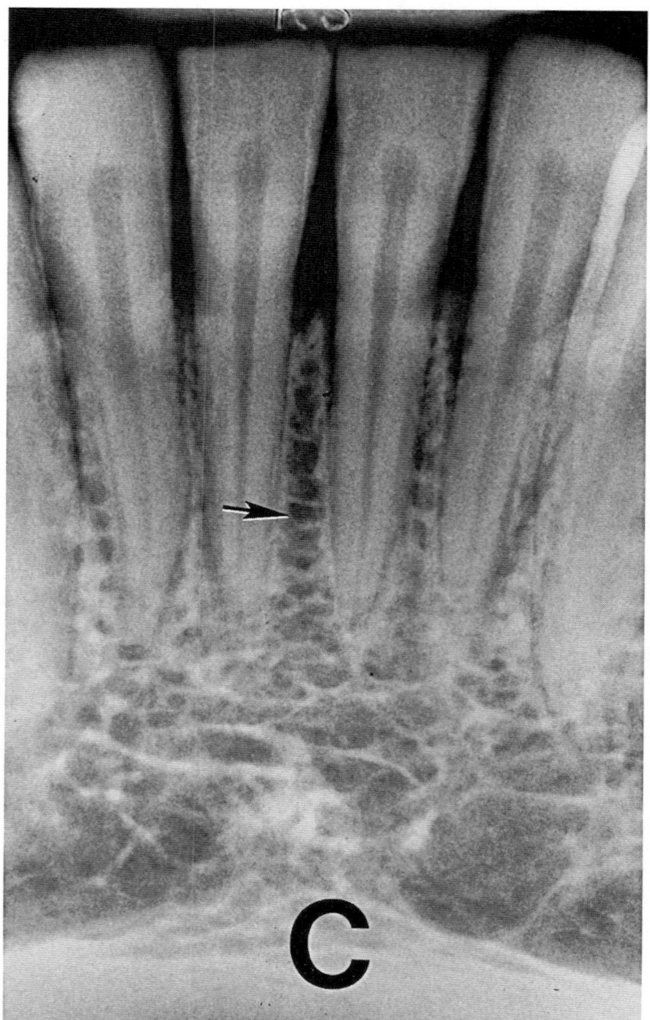

FIGURE 3–15.

Mandibular Linear Network Pattern: A, Linear trabeculation with strands running in relatively horizontal directions, with little or no crossing. B, Stepladder trabeculation pattern (arrows) in the first molar. C, Lower incisor region. Note stepladder trabeculation between central incisors (arrows).

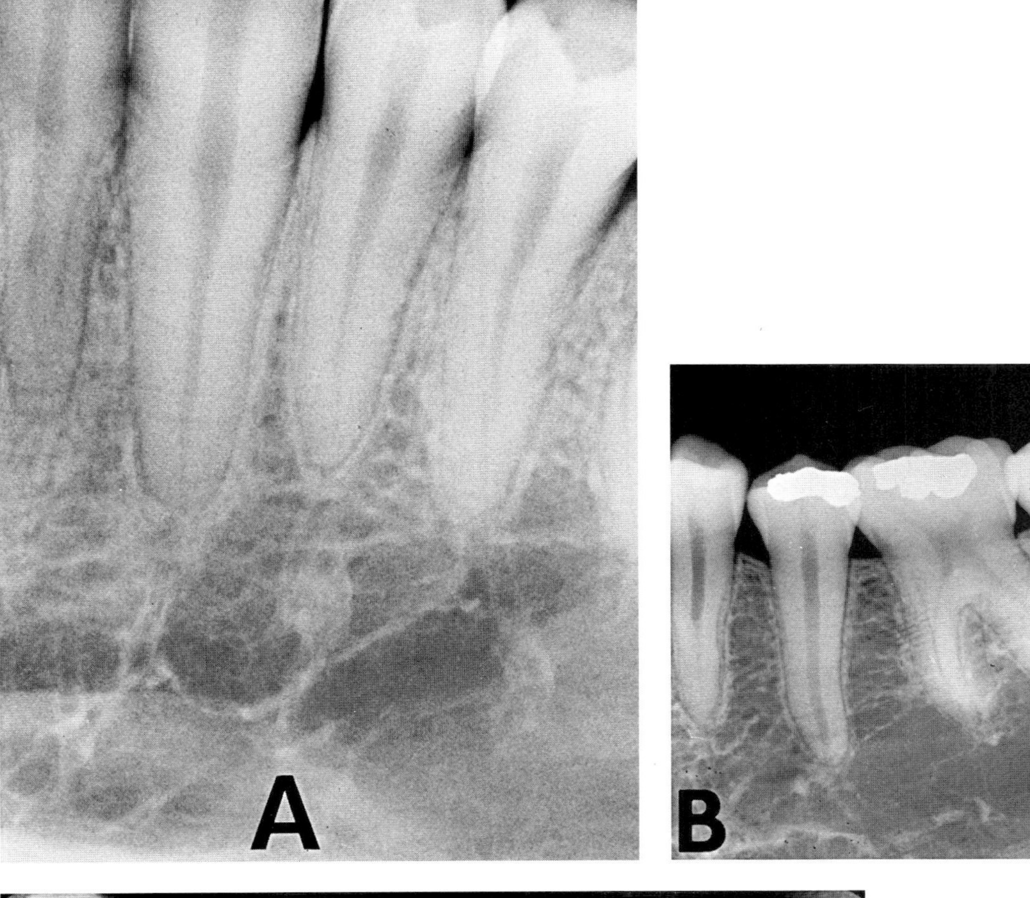

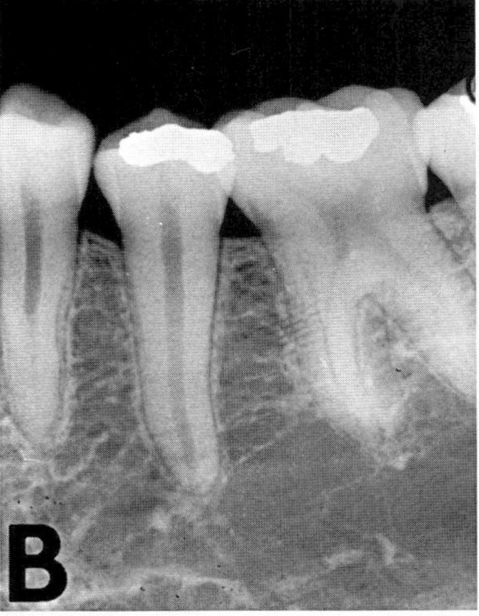

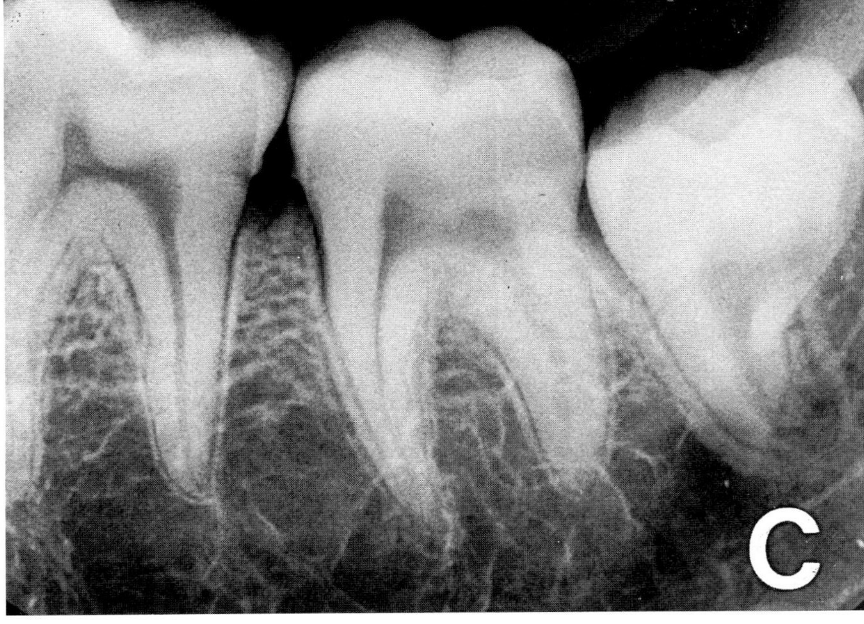

FIGURE 3–16.

Mandibular Trabeculation: A, Lower premolar region (note the larger bone spaces below the roots of the teeth). This is a normal variation. B, Some variations in bone trabeculae in the lower molar region. Normal amounts of trabeculation are between the molars, but there are areas of sparse amounts of trabeculation at or below the roots. C, In this case there is a gradual transition from trabeculated bone into a structureless area. In others, the line of demarcation may be relatively abrupt or extremely sharp; however, these are all normal variations in trabecular patterns.

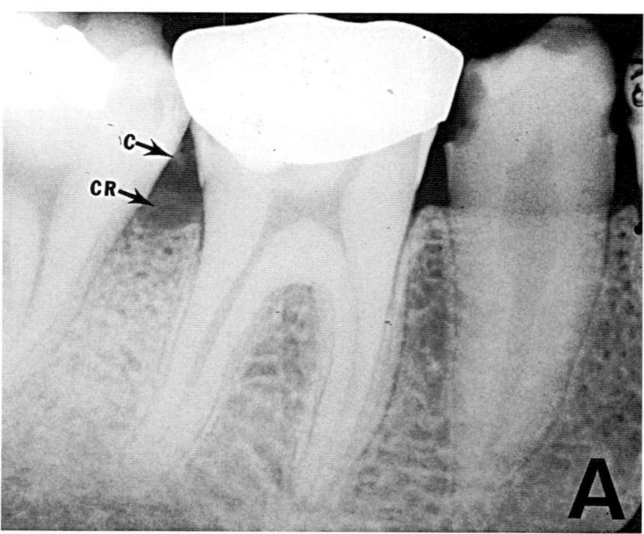

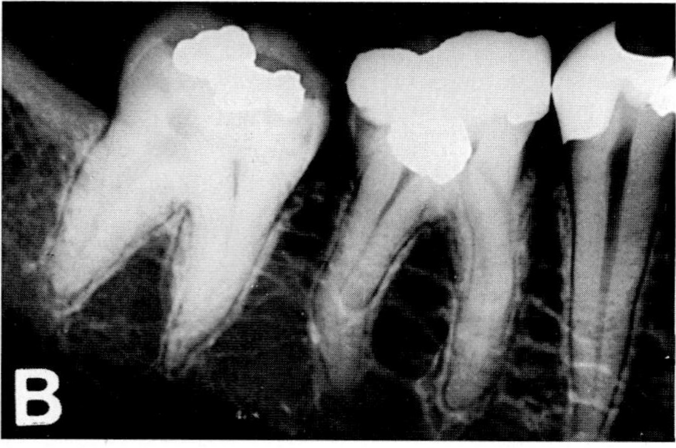

FIGURE 3–17.

Mandibular Bone in a Large Jaw: A, Mandibular bone with thick trabeculae and small medullary spaces in a former professional football player (6′5″ tall and 260 lb). Calculus (C); crater bone deformity (CR). B, Alveolar bone of a small adult reveals larger medullary spaces and smaller trabeculae.

Wolff's Law (Fig. 3–19)

Localized anatomic variations in the bone structures are common. Most of the variations are developmental, but some result from acquired influences such as the removal of teeth.

In regard to acquired anatomic changes in bone pattern, it is pertinent to mention Wolff's law, which states in effect "that the number and the distribution of the bony trabeculae are dependent on the strains and stresses to which the bone is subjected." Alteration in direction or degree of stresses or strains on bone results in changes in trabecular pattern. When a tooth is removed, the bone from which the tooth

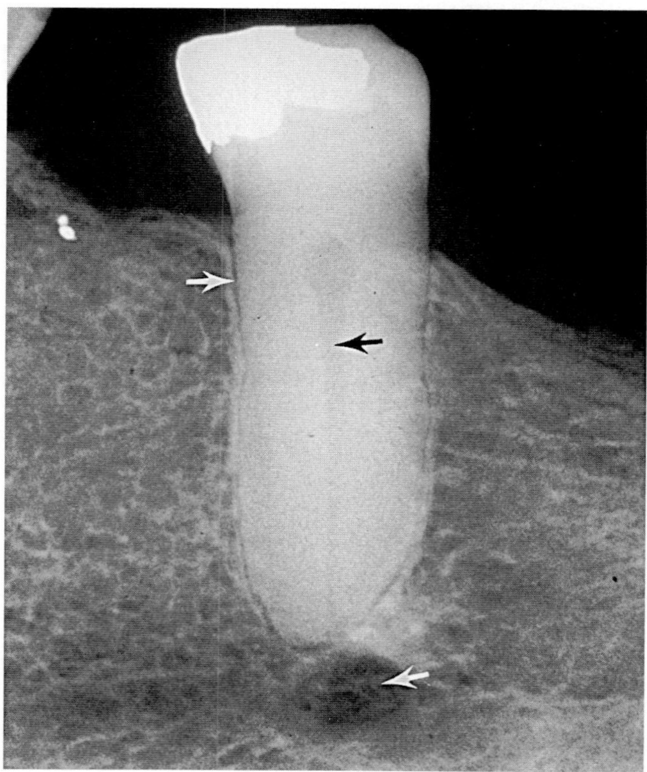

FIGURE 3–18.

Senile Mandibular Bone: The alveolar bone of this older person (75 years or older) is osteoporotic (radiolucent), as seen in the radiograph. The periodontal ligament space has narrowed (upper white arrow) as well as the pulp canal (black arrow). Note the mental foramen (lower white arrow) just inferior to the root apex of the premolar.

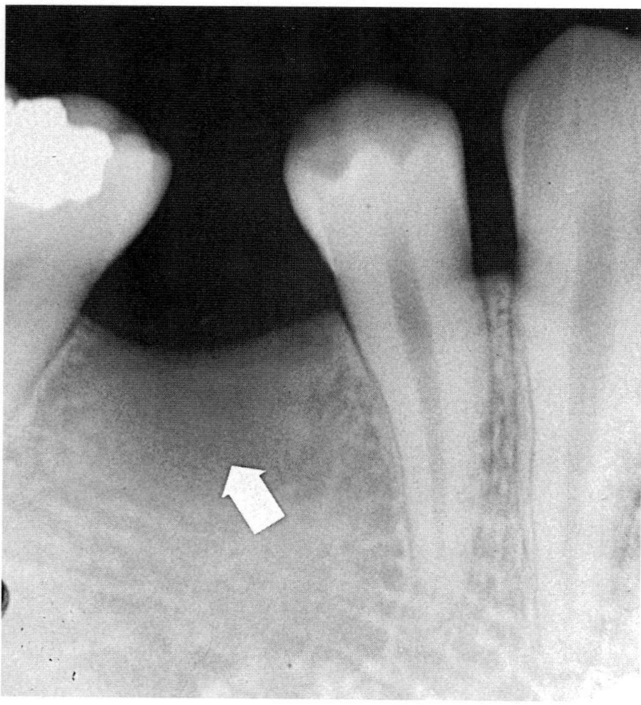

FIGURE 3–19.

Bone Atrophy and Osteoporosis after Tooth Extraction: Radiolucent bone (osteoporosis) after extraction of a second premolar. This is more radiolucent because of altered function (arrow).

was removed will usually experience less strain as when the tooth was in full function. Therefore, bone is expected to be more radiolucent and trabeculae less organized to withstand stress (Fig. 3–19).

Bone Remodeling (Fig. 3–20)

When a tooth is removed, healing normally takes place and the bone is restored, but not always with the same arrangement of the trabeculae as before the extraction. This process is called remodeling. The time that any socket takes to heal varies from a few weeks to as long as a year. In the remodeling process, there is a gradual loss of density of the lamina dura, and at the same time, bone develops at the base and sides of the socket. By the time the socket is filled with bone, all trace of the lamina dura is gone (Fig. 3–20).

Osteosclerosis (Fig. 3–21)

In certain circumstances, increased pressure and stress on the bone may produce increased bone formation. The trabeculae increase in number, size, and density. When pressure on the bone is less severe, it may be borne a long time. Later, it may be associated with sclerosis or condensation of bone around the whole tooth socket and extending into the adjacent bone for a short distance (Fig. 3–21).

Fibrous Healing (Fig. 3–22)

Healing of any alveolar bone will proceed normally if the cortical plates are intact and if they are covered by healthy periosteum. When the cortical plate and periosteum are destroyed by a pathologic condition or surgical procedure, the probability of developing a fibrous healing defect is increased. Fibrous healing defects occur at sites of previous injury. They may be well corticated and are usually well demarcated from surrounding bone. These defects have a distinct radiolucent punched-out or see-through appearance, which is usually characteristic (Fig. 3–22).

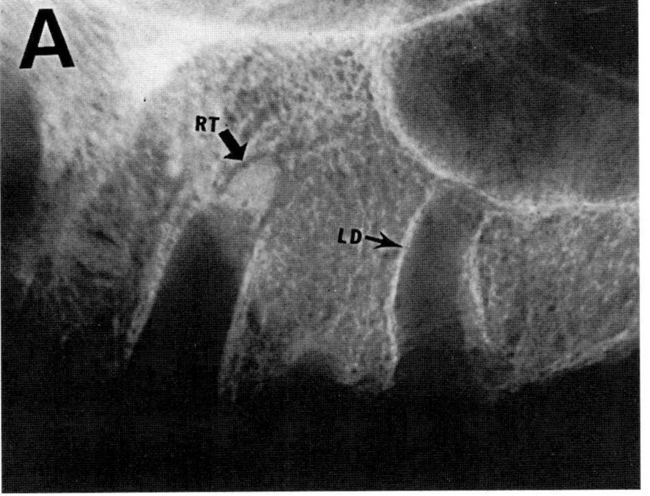

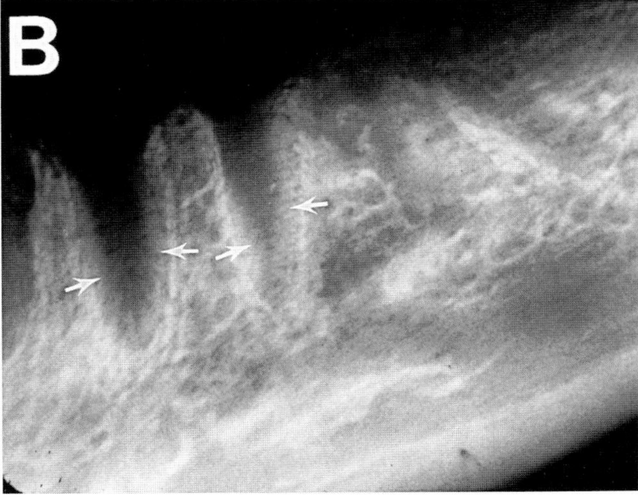

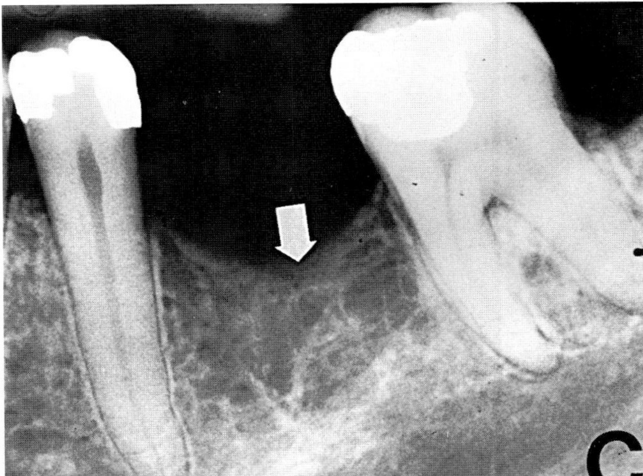

FIGURE 3–20.

Bone Remodeling after Tooth Extraction: A, Recent maxillary canine and second premolar socket extraction sites with the root tip (RT) still retained in the canine socket. Note that the lamina dura (LD) is still present. B, Healing of extraction sockets (arrows) by granulation tissue with subsequent conversion into new bone with a gradual loss of the lamina dura. C, Socket site completely healed with complete restoration of bone without a trace of lamina dura. Note the reduction in height of bone (arrow).

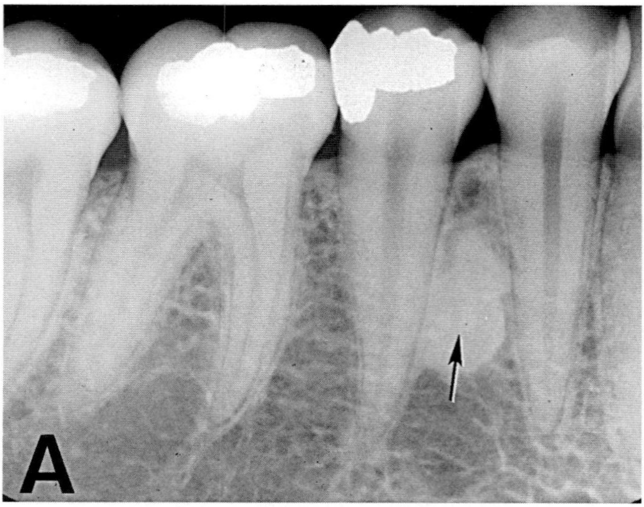

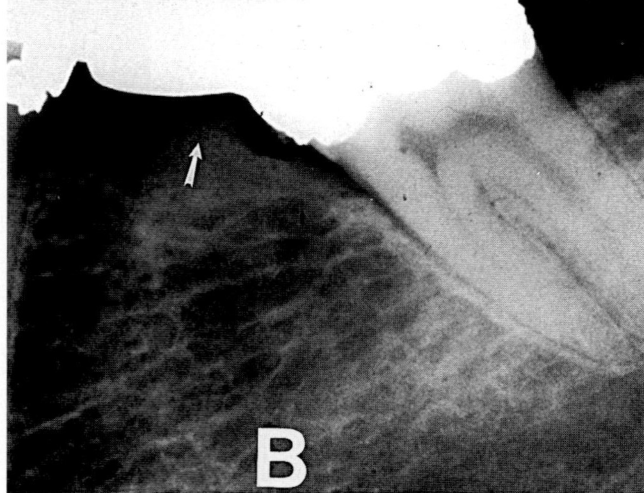

FIGURE 3–21.

Bone Condensation or Osteosclerosis: A, Osteosclerosis between premolars (arrow). B, Alveolar crestal cortical bone growth underneath a bridge with a posterior abutment that is severely inclined (arrow).

LAMINA DURA (Fig. 3–23)

The lamina dura is a thin layer of dense bone that lines the normal tooth socket. On the radiograph, it is revealed as a thin white or radiopaque line (see Fig. 3–9). The appearance of the normal lamina dura varies widely: some are thin and of poor density, whereas others are thick and relatively dense. Because the lamina dura always conforms to the shape of the teeth, the width of the lamina dura as seen on the radiograph differs, depending on the variations of the shape of the teeth. Differences in thickness, density, shape, and number of lamina dura images can be estimated from a study of cross-sections of sockets seen in dry skulls. All these differences in the radiographic appearances of the lamina dura have no clinical significance so long as the lamina dura is continuous around the root because, with few exceptions, discontinuity

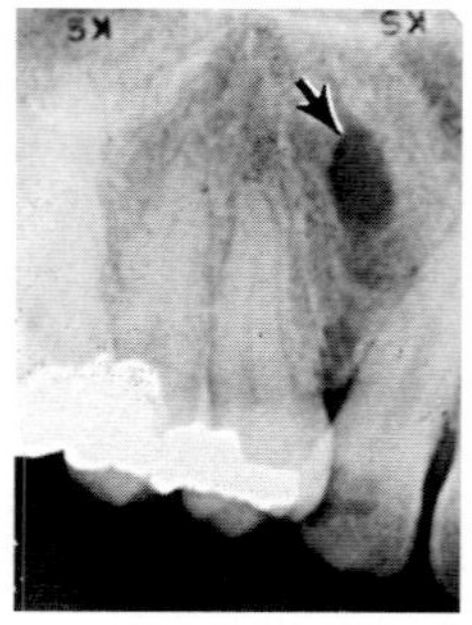

FIGURE 3–22.

Fibrous Healing Defect: In the removal of an impacted canine tooth, a portion of the cortical bone periosteum was destroyed, creating a fibrous healing defect (arrow).

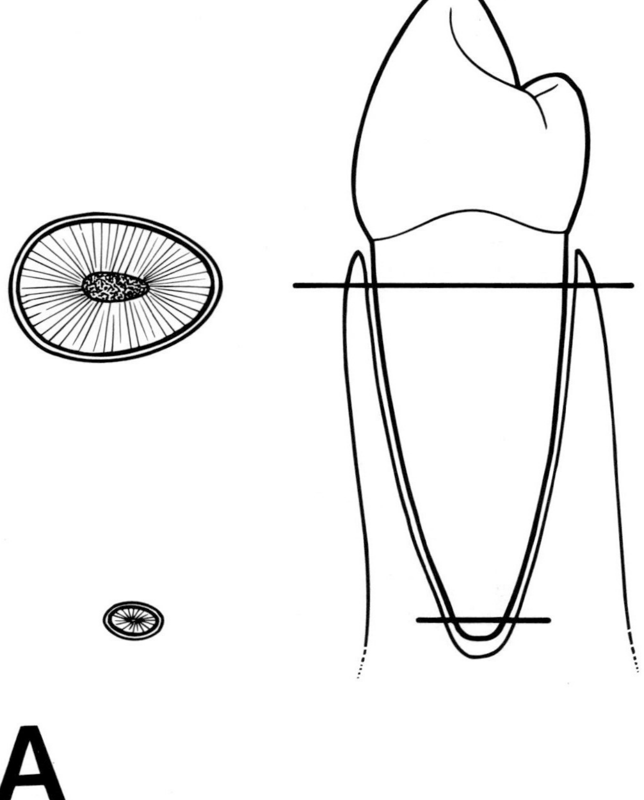

FIGURE 3–23.

Variation in Apical Appearance of Normal Lamina Dura: A, Apical portion of lower second premolar root is dense and thick, allowing the structure to absorb x-rays. *(continued)*

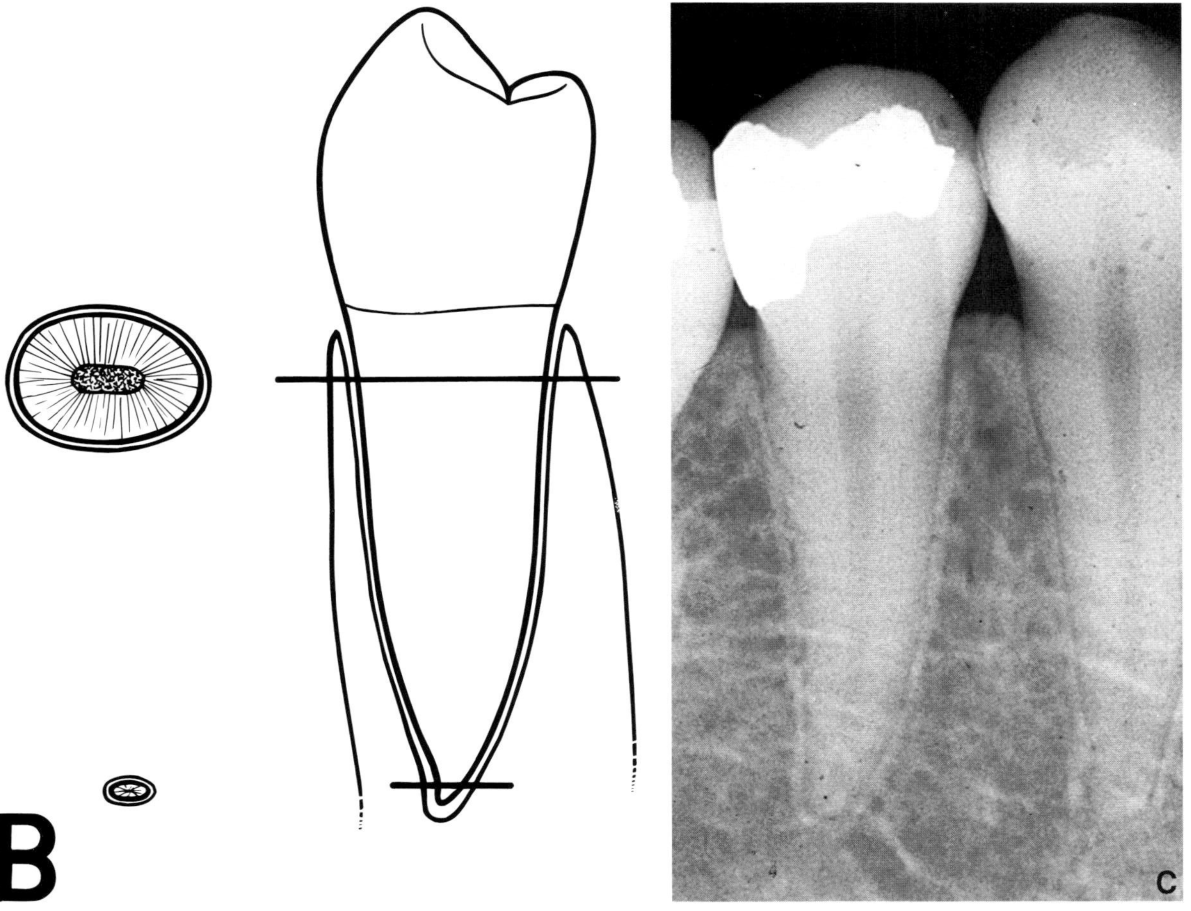

FIGURE 3–23.

(continued) B, Apical portion of the first premolar is slender and pointed, with a small circle of lamina dura around the apices. When this condition is present, one is unable to trace the lamina dura at the apex of the tooth. C, Radiograph of the lower first and second premolars. The lamina dura can be traced around the apex of the second premolar, but it cannot be seen at the apex of the first premolar.

is evidence of an abnormality, usually disease (see Fig. 3–9). Teeth that end in slender apical points, however, may have only a small circle of lamina dura surrounding the apices. The circle of lamina dura may be so small that its thickness at any given point may be insufficient to produce a radiographic image. In such a case, there may be an apparent absence of lamina dura without disease. The teeth that are most likely to present difficulty in tracing the lamina dura around the apex are the canines and first premolars (Fig. 3–23).

The integrity of the lamina dura is important in the evaluation of early periapical pathologic processes, periodontal disease and other disorders in which the lamina dura is lost, such as hyperparathyroidism, renal osteodystrophy, Paget's disease, fibrous dysplasia, osteomalacia, osteoporosis, and Pyle's disease. In osteopetrosis, there is a generalized increased density of bone, leading to absence of any distinction between lamina dura and adjacent bone.

ALVEOLAR BONE CREST (Fig. 3–24)

Effect of Variation in Buccolingual Width and Contour on Radiographic Appearance

The alveolar bone crests are the gingival margins of the interseptal bone. Normally, these crests are situated near the cementoenamel junction. They are covered with a thin layer of dense cortical bone, which may be seen as a thin white line (Fig. 3–24A). The bony cortices may not be seen even in normal cases, depending on the configuration of the interproximal cementoenamel junction of the teeth. The alveolar bone crest appears radiopaque when the cementoenamel junction line is straight and wide buccolingually (Fig. 3–24B). The alveolar bone crest appears less radiopaque when the cementoenamel junction line is peaked and is thin buccolingually (Fig. 3–24B and C). If the alveolar crestal

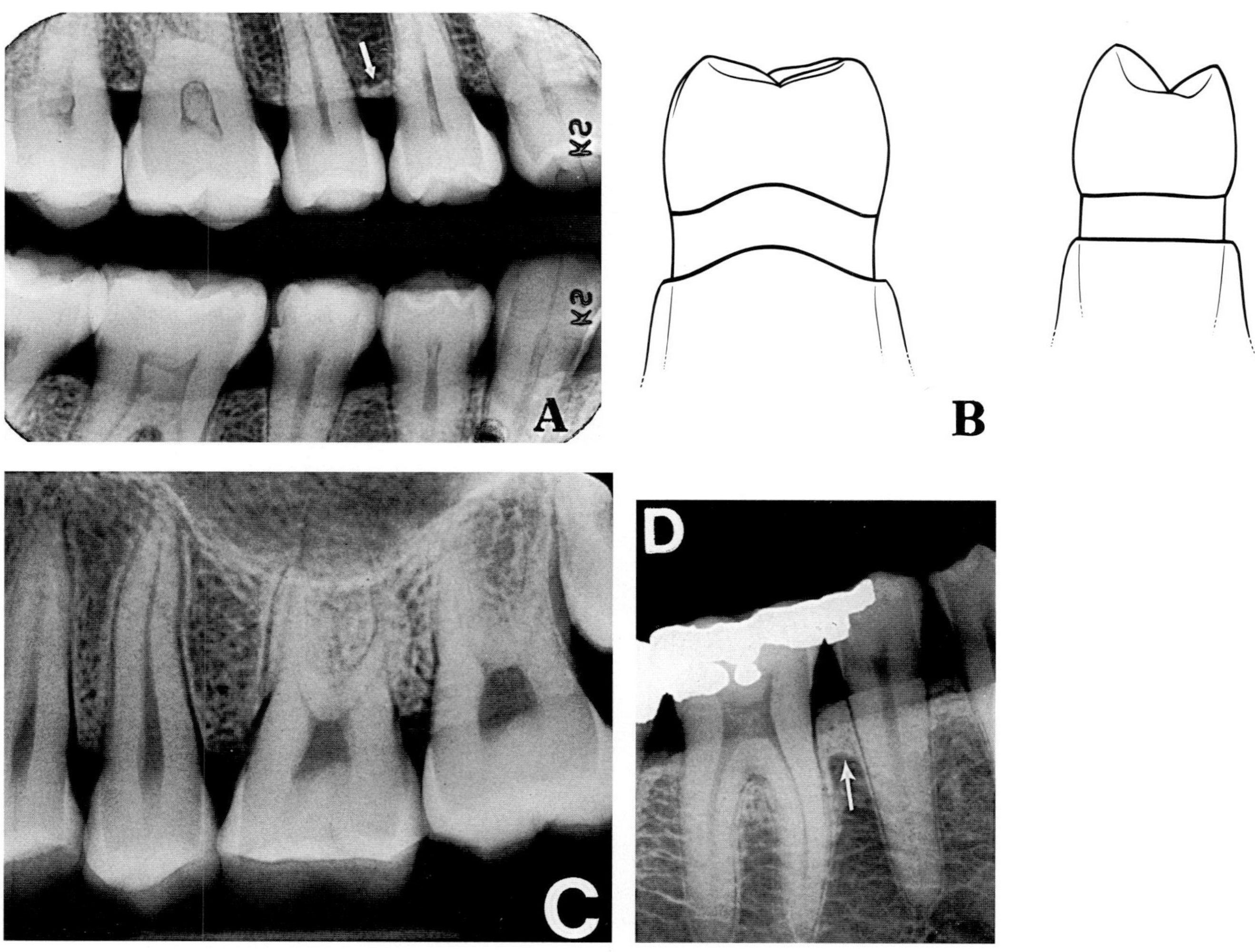

FIGURE 3–24.

Alveolar Bone Crest: A, Normal alveolar crest covered with a fine layer of dense cortical bone (arrow). B, Diagram illustrating variations in the interproximal cementoenamel junction configuration. On the left is a contoured interproximal bone crest, and on the right is a flat interproximal bone crest. C, The alveolar crests are less radiopaque because the interproximal cementoenamel line is probably peaked and thin, as in B left. D, The alveolar crests are radiopaque as in A because interproximal cementoenamel junction lines are probably flat, as in B right.

bone is radiopaque, the cementoenamel junction line will usually be straight and flat and wide buccolingually (Fig. 3–24B and D).

Influence of Tooth Inclination on Shape of Alveolar Crest (Fig. 3–25)

Horizontal alveolar bone crests are present when teeth are positioned vertically. As a person becomes older, there is a normal mesial shift of the posterior teeth because of the wearing away of the contact points and normal occlusal function. This normal mesial oblique drift of the teeth causes the alveolar crests to deviate from their usual vertical position to an oblique position simulating vertical bone loss (Fig. 3–25).

Alveolar Bone Crest Configuration Influenced by State of Eruption of Teeth (Fig. 3–26)

Alveolar bone follows the eruption pattern of the teeth. The configuration of the alveolar bone crest differs depending on whether the tooth is undererupted, normally erupted, or supraerupted. Sometimes, supraerupted teeth cause the alveolar bone crest to take on an oblique shape simulating vertical bone loss from periodontal disease (Fig. 3–26).

Variations in Individual Bone Spaces (Fig. 3–27)

Large localized areas in cancellous bone without bone trabeculation, sometimes with sharp, corticated margins, may

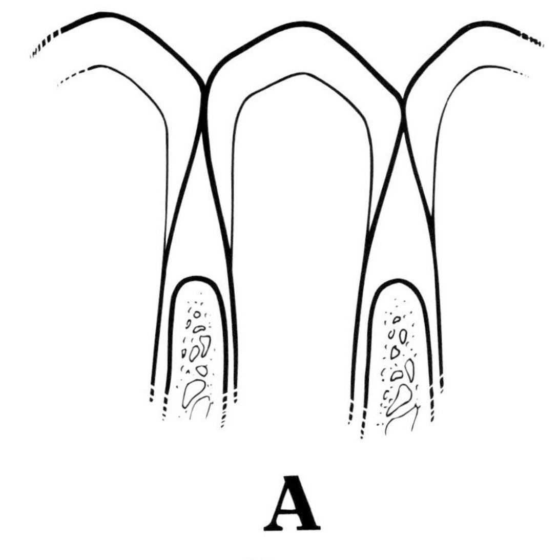

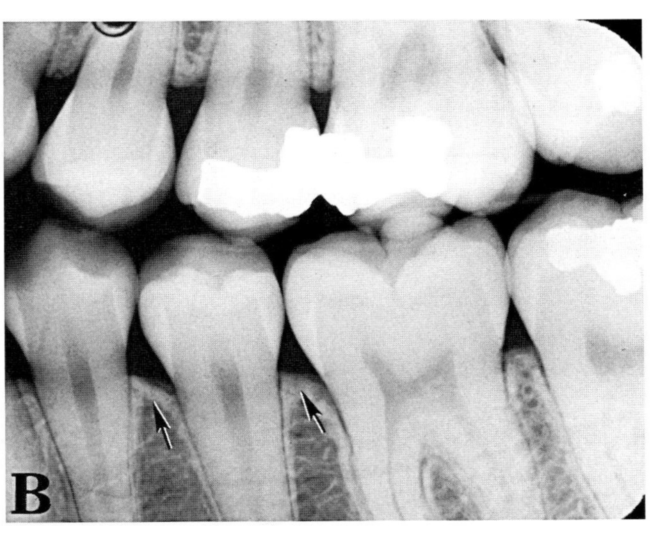

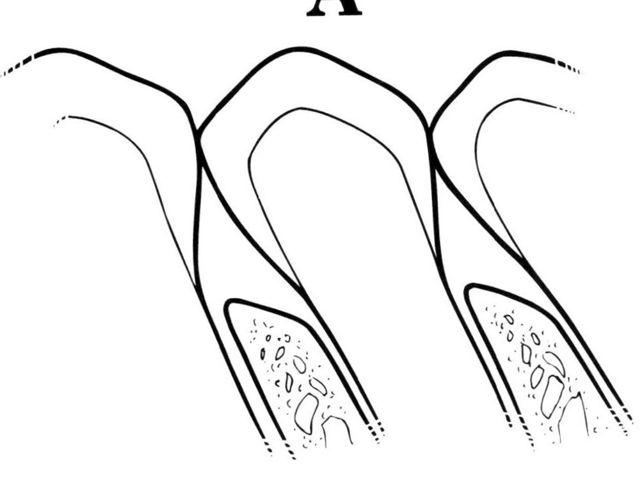

FIGURE 3–25.

Influence of Tooth Inclination on the Shape of the Alveolar Crest: A, Horizontal alveolar bone crests are present when teeth are positioned vertically (upper illustration). The normal mesial drift of the posterior teeth with aging produces oblique alveolar bone crests, as shown (lower illustration). B, Bitewing radiograph showing oblique alveolar bone crests resulting from normal mesial drift that may simulate vertical bone loss from periodontal disease.

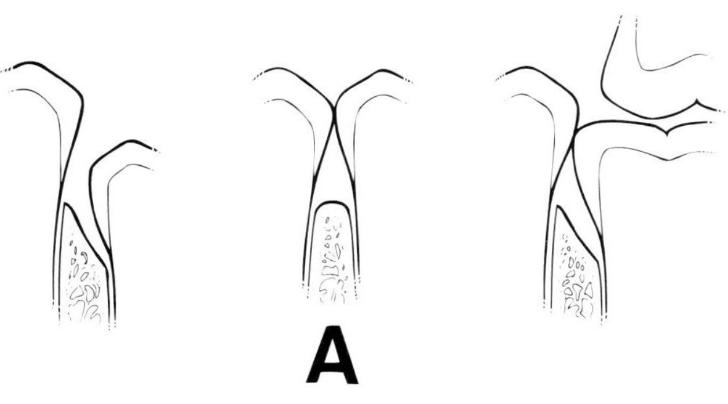

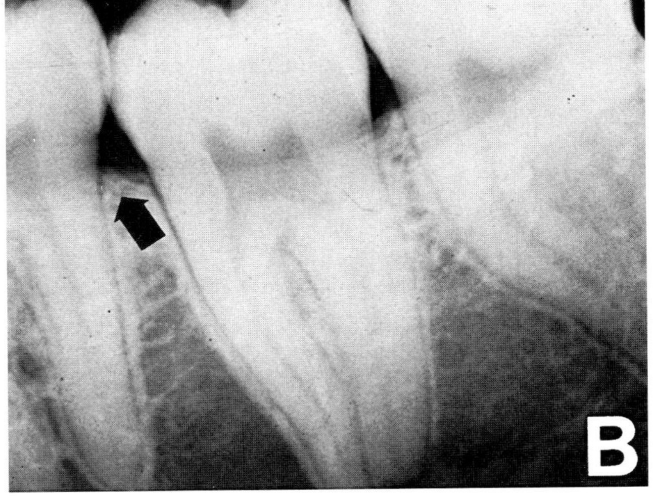

FIGURE 3–26.

Alveolar Bone Crest Configuration: A, Alveolar bone crest configuration as influenced by the state of tooth eruption, as shown on the diagram. B, Supraerupted first and third molars cause a change in the usual vertical shape of the alveolar crests (arrow).

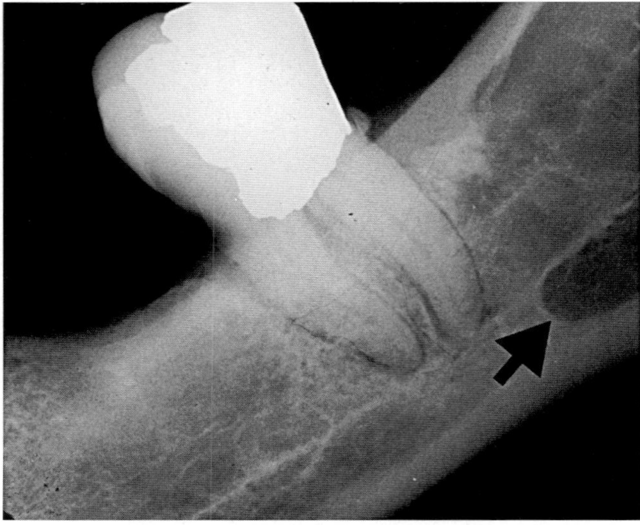

FIGURE 3–27.

Large Medullary Spaces Simulating Disease: Large radiolucent medullary space seen below this single molar with a large metal restoration (arrow).

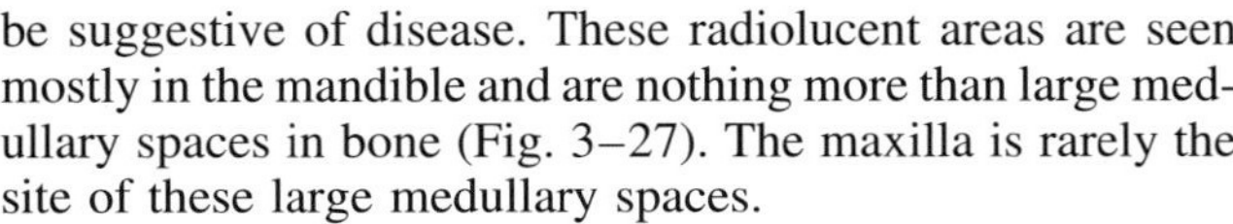

be suggestive of disease. These radiolucent areas are seen mostly in the mandible and are nothing more than large medullary spaces in bone (Fig. 3–27). The maxilla is rarely the site of these large medullary spaces.

NUTRIENT CANALS (VASCULAR CHANNELS) (Figs. 3–28 to 3–31)

Blood vessels, lying in channels or grooves, traverse the alveolar bone of the jaws to supply nutrients to the teeth and gingival spaces. In width, the canals vary from the thickness of a hair to a little over 1 mm. In the mandible, they arise from the mandibular canal vessels, extend upward through the interdental bone, and exit through foramina at the superior surface of the interdental alveolar bone to supply the gingiva with nutrients (Fig. 3–28). The nutrient canals are seen in the mandible most frequently in the incisor region, followed by the premolar region. These vascular channels are spaces in bone and appear as dark linear shadows situated between the roots of adjacent teeth, more or less parallel to them. In edentulous areas and in the maxillary sinus, nutrient canals persist as vertical dark lines (Fig. 3–29). The nutrient

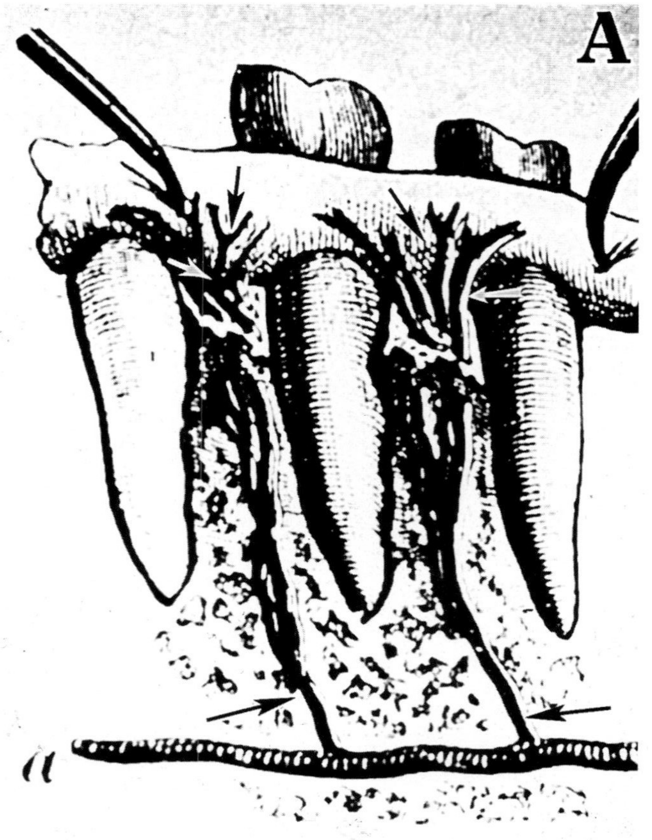

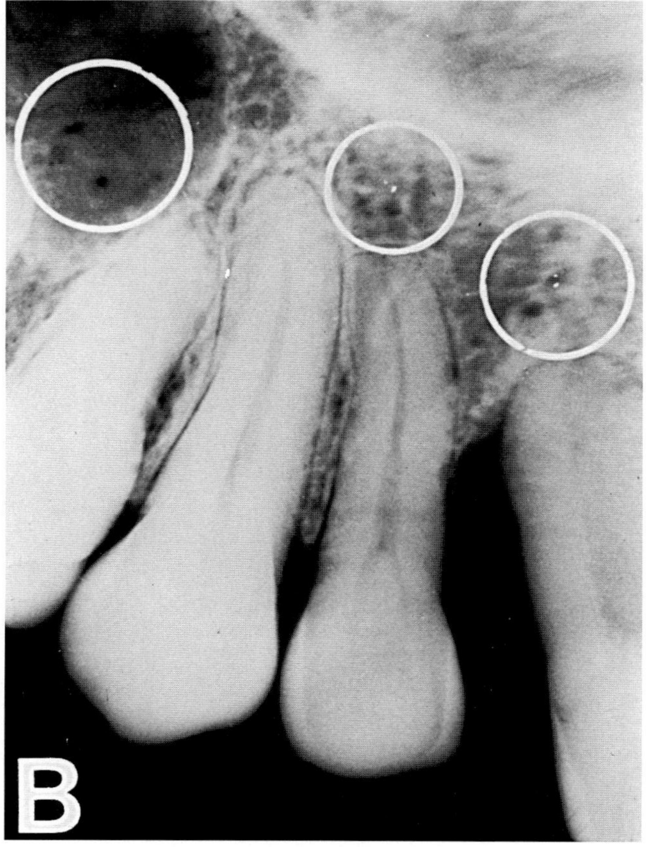

FIGURE 3–28.

Nutrient Canals and Foramina: A, These vascular channels (arrows) arise from the mandibular canal vessels, traverse the interdental alveolar bone, and exit foramina at the superior portion of alveolar bone to supply nutrients to gingiva. B, Multiple nutrient foramina in anterior maxillary alveolar bone (circles).

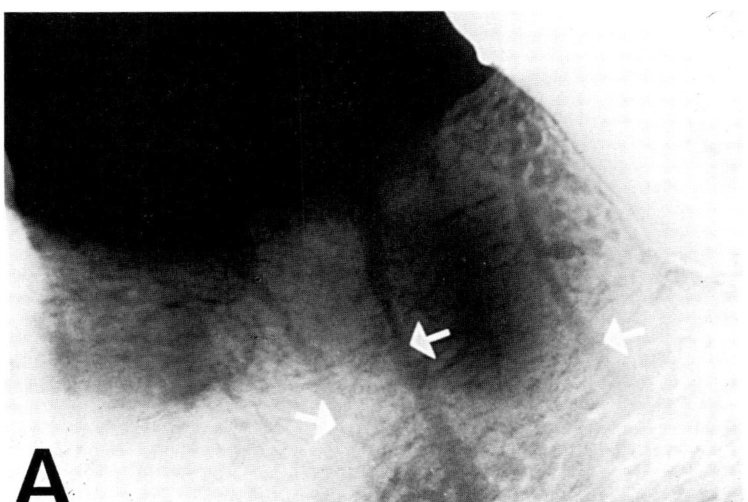

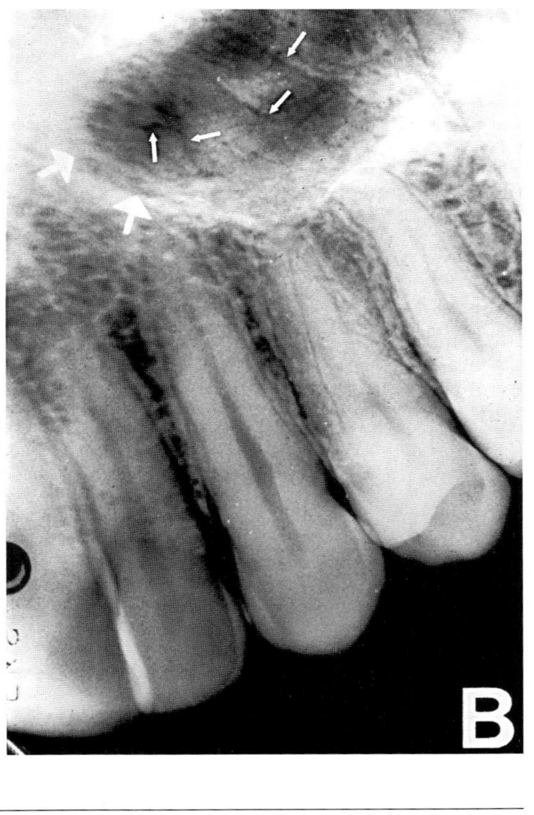

FIGURE 3–29.

Nutrient Canals: A, Nutrient canals in an edentulous area revealed as vertical dark lines (arrows). B, Nutrient canals in the anterior wall of the maxillary sinus (small arrows). The large arrows identify the palatal extension of the maxillary sinus.

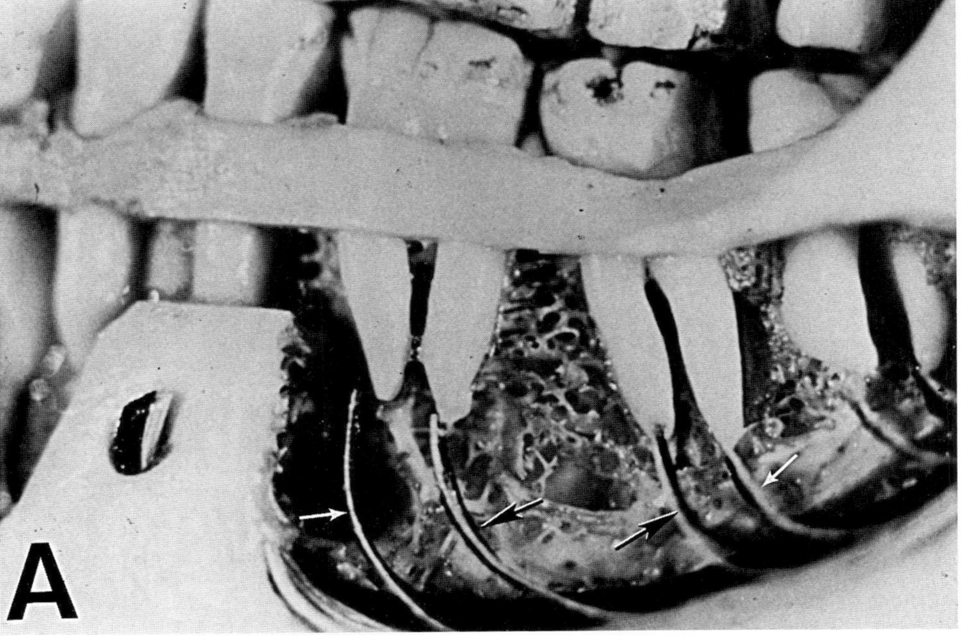

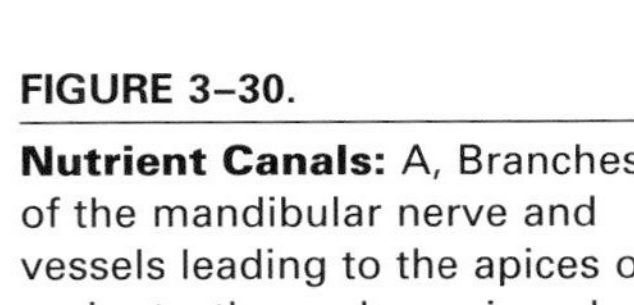

FIGURE 3–30.

Nutrient Canals: A, Branches of the mandibular nerve and vessels leading to the apices of molar teeth, as shown in a dry mandible (arrows). (*continued*)

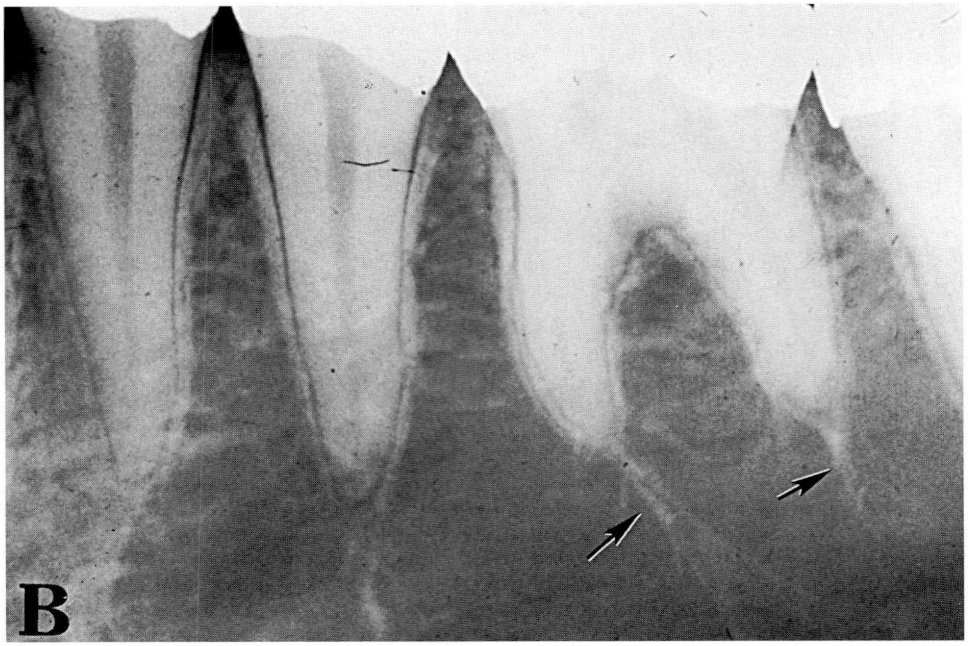

B

FIGURE 3–30.

(continued) B, Nutrient canal (arrows) revealed as radiopaque lines leading to the apices of the roots of the mandibular first molar.

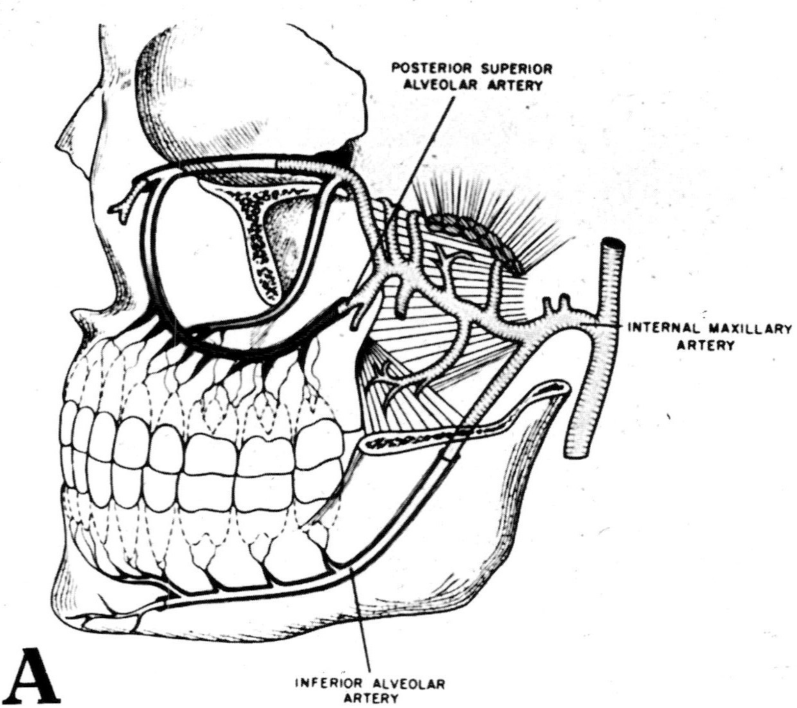

FIGURE 3–31.

Posterior superior alveolar canal: A, The posterior superior alveolar artery originates from the internal maxillary artery and passes through the alveolar foramina on the infratemporal surface of the maxilla. The artery is accompanied by the posterior superior alveolar vein, which empties into the pterygoid plexus and the posterior superior alveolar nerve, which is a branch of the maxillary nerve of the fifth cranial nerve. (Courtesy of Eastman Kodak Co., Rochester, NY.) *(continued)*

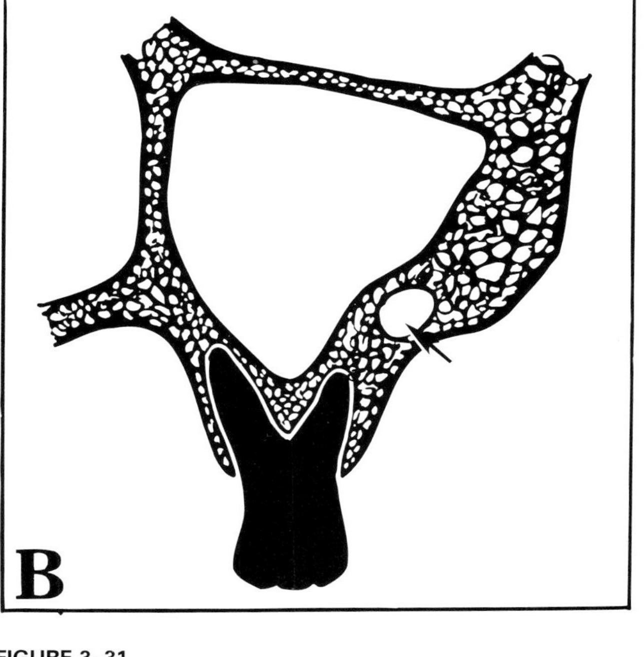

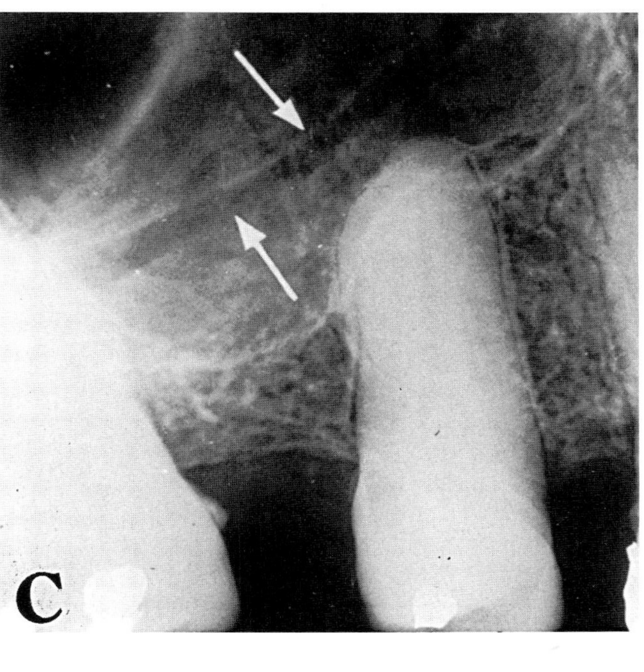

FIGURE 3–31.

(continued) B, Diagram showing the posterior superior alveolar canal (arrow) in the bone on the outer surface of the maxillary sinus. (From Poyton HG: Maxillary sinus and oral radiologist. Dent Radiol Photogr 45:46 1972.) C, Periapical radiograph showing the posterior superior alveolar canal in the maxillary sinus wall (arrows).

canals leading to the periapical foramina of posterior teeth of the mandible are sometimes revealed as radiopaque vertical lines extending down from the apices of teeth.

In the maxilla, nutrient canals are less frequently seen outside the radiographic image of the maxillary sinus. They are mostly seen in the premolar-molar region. The blood supply to the maxillary molars comes from the posterior superior alveolar artery, from which branches pass along grooves of the outer wall of the maxillary sinus and extend to the teeth (Fig. 3–30). Sometimes, the posterior superior alveolar canal can be seen above the maxillary premolar and molar teeth (Fig. 3–31). Determining whether the radiolucent cavity of the maxillary sinus is pathologic is sometimes difficult. The appearance of radiolucent lines or grooves of nutrient canals in the cavity serves to confirm that the cavity is the maxillary sinus.

ANATOMIC STRUCTURES OF THE MAXILLA

Aside from the teeth and their supporting structures, any anatomic structure that produces an image in radiographs should be identified.

Intermaxillary Suture (Median Maxillary Suture) (Fig. 3–32)

The suture between the two maxillary processes of the maxilla in the midline of the palate is usually visible in radiographs. It appears in intraoral radiographs as a dark line in the midline from the alveolar crest between the central incisors and extending back to the posterior portion of the palate (Fig. 3–32). The width of the suture is almost uniform individually, but it differs slightly from person to person. Radiographic studies show extreme variation in the age at which the suture undergoes fusion. There is no clinical significance in the observation that the suture is closed.

Nasal Fossae (Fig. 3–33)

The nasal fossae, being cavities in bone, appear in radiographs as dark images, and because they contain air, they are radiolucent or dark, at least in some part. The nasal fossae are roughly pear shaped when seen in large posteroanterior extraoral radiographs. In intraoral periapical radiographs, only portions of the fossae are seen. These images resemble the letter W, but with rounded inferior margins; the nasal septum forms the central portion of the letter W. The margins of the fossae are lined with compact bone. Therefore, the dark radiolucencies of the cavities are lined with a narrow white line radiologically.

The nasal septum commonly presents a wide image because the septum usually deviates from the midline. Hazy gray images may be seen arising from the lateral wall of both fossae, and these images may extend almost to the septum. They represent the anterior portions of the inferior turbinate (concha) bones. In the midline at the inferior aspect of the nasal fossae, one can usually see a small, white, inverted V, which represents the anterior nasal spine (Fig. 3–33).

The floor of the nasal cavity, which is also the superior

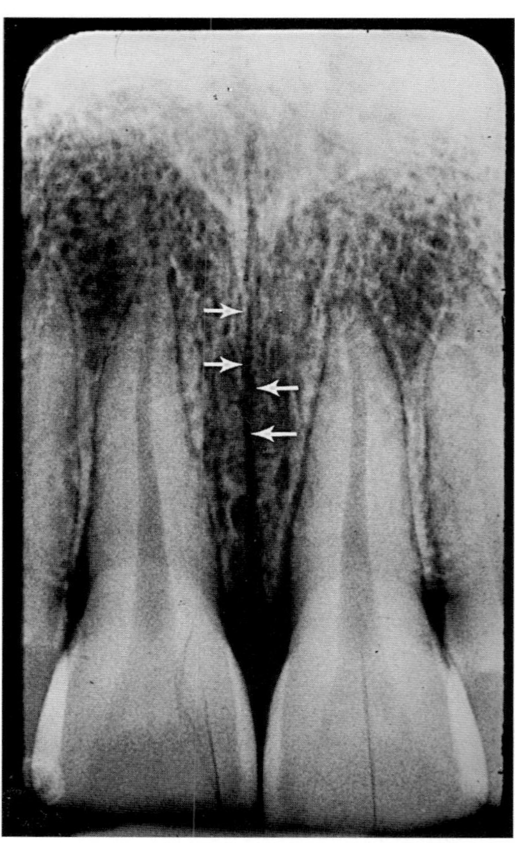

FIGURE 3–32.

Intermaxillary Suture (Median Maxillary Suture): The thin dark line in the center of the periapical radiograph is the intermaxillary (midpalatal) suture (arrows). The two curved white lines coming together in the midline above roots of teeth represent the cortical lining of the floor of the nasal fossae. The V-shaped image where these lines meet is the inferior nasal spine.

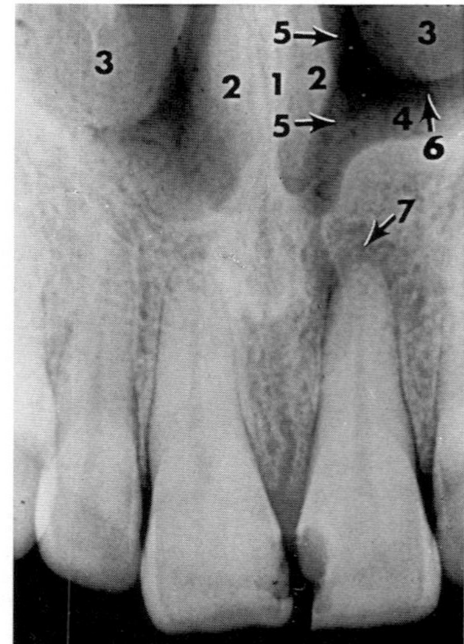

FIGURE 3–33.

Maxillary Midline Region: Nasal septum (1), soft tissue lining of nasal septum (2), inferior turbinate (3), soft tissue of the floor of the nose (4), common meatus (5), inferior meatus (6).

aspect of the hard palate, is covered by mucosa. The inferior meatus is situated between the floor of the nasal cavity and the inferior turbinate bone (Fig. 3–33). Anteriorly, just behind the nostrils, small depressions in the mucosa lining the nasal floor are foramina that lead into the nasopalatine canals. The nasolacrimal duct also opens into the inferior meatus.

Nasopalatine Foramen (Incisive Foramen) (Figs. 3–34 and 3–35)

The foramen is located behind the maxillary central incisors, formed by the union of the palatal processes of the maxillae. The nasopalatine or incisive foramen varies widely in size and shape. It may be a mere slit in the sagittal plane, or it may be round, oval, heart shaped, or diamond shaped. It may also appear as four small holes situated between the apices of the maxillary central incisors.

Most of the time, the nasopalatine foramen does not have a cortical outline (Fig. 3–34). This normal structure should be distinguished from an incisive or nasopalatine cyst, which it may resemble if the foramen is large. The size of the incisive foramen varies greatly; the diameter ranges from 2 mm to 1 cm or more. Roper-Hall (1938) studied over 2000 skulls and concluded that the average dimension was 3 × 3 mm, and an image less than 6 mm wide may be considered within normal limits.

The nasopalatine nerve, a branch of the sphenopalatine

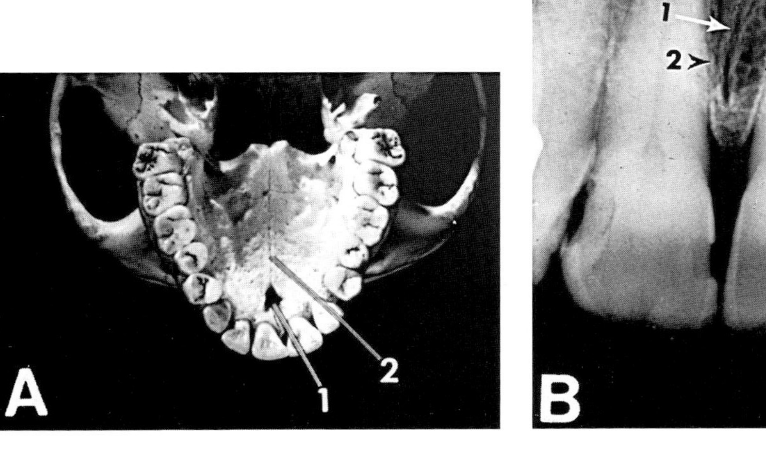

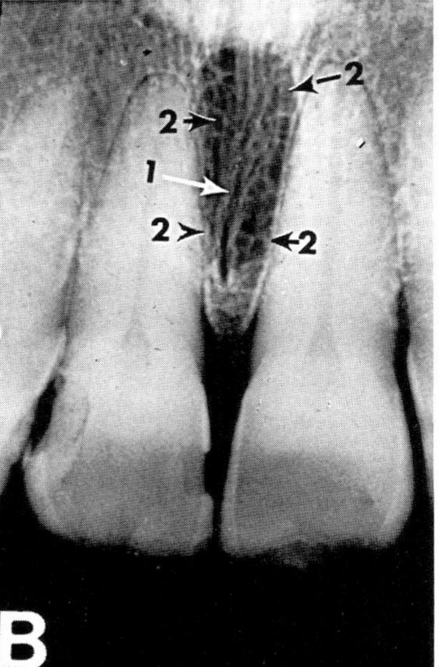

FIGURE 3–34.

Nasopalatine foramen: A, Dry skull showing the nasopalatine foramen (1) and the median palatine suture (2). B, Nasopalatine or incisive foramen, the large, dark, elliptical area between the central incisors (arrows): incisive suture (1) and nasopalatine foramen (2).

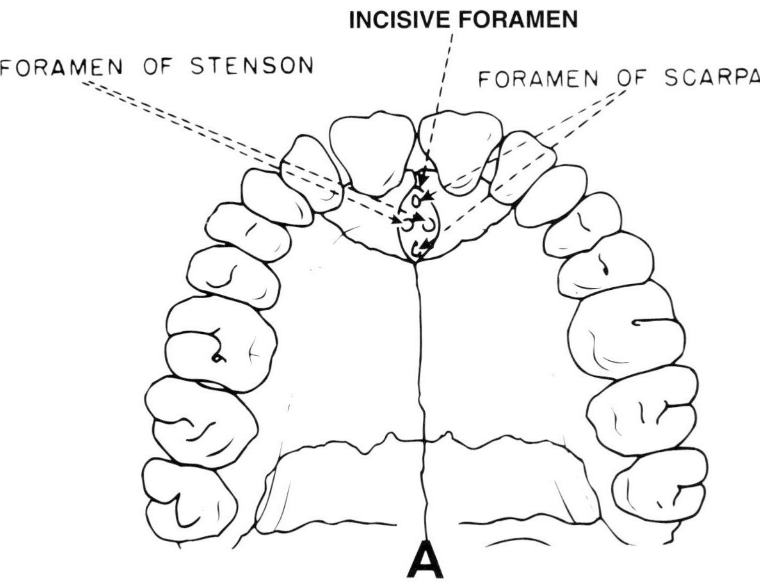

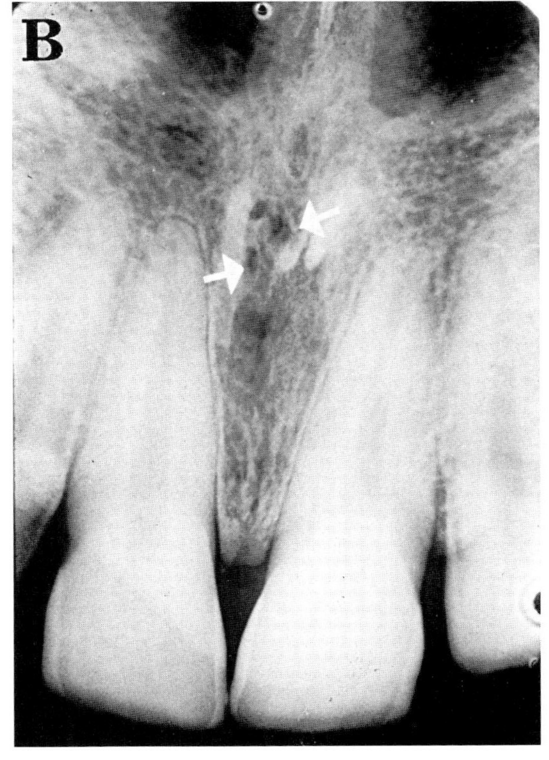

FIGURE 3–35.

Foramina of Scarpa and Stensen: A, The incisive foramen, just behind the upper central incisors, is formed by the union of halves of the maxilla. Lateral canals within this fossa, on each side of the midline (foramina of Stensen), transmit the nasopalatine nerves and the terminal branch of the descending palatine artery. In some individuals, additional canals within the fossa (canals of Scarpa) are found in the midline. When present, these also serve as passages for the nasopalatine nerves. B, Radiograph revealing four small radiolucent holes (arrows) representing the foramina of Stensen and Scarpa. (A and B, Courtesy of Eastman Kodak Co., Rochester, NY.)

ganglion, supplies the nasal roof and septum and extends down and forward in a groove in the vomer bone and the cartilaginous septum. On reaching the anterior portion of the floor of the nose, the nasopalatine nerve enters and traverses the canal of Stensen, finally emerging on the hard palate through the nasopalatine or incisive foramen. There is one Stensen canal on each side of the nasal septum, and both lateral canals terminate in the foramina of Stensen. The two foramina of Stensen transmit the nasopalatine nerves and the terminal branches of the descending palatine artery. Sometimes, the two foramina of Stensen further subdivide into the four canals of Stensen and Scarpa. When the additional two smaller canals of Scarpa are found, they are seen more toward the midline and serve as passageways for the nasopalatine nerves (Fig. 3–35).

Maxillary Lateral-Canine Area (Fig. 3–36)

The inverted Y is an important anatomic landmark in this region and is especially useful in locating the canine area in edentulous surveys. It is formed by the cortical lining of the anterior wall of the maxillary sinus and the floor of the nasal fossa (Fig. 3–36). The Y-shaped landmark is of value in differentiating some dental cysts in this region because it tends to be obliterated in such conditions.

Maxillary Sinus Area (Figs. 3–37 to 3–44)

The maxillary sinus, or antrum, is a cavity in bone that contains air and therefore is revealed in radiographs as a dark radiolucent image. As in all normal cavities in bone, at the margins of the cavity is a thin layer of dense cortical bone, which appears as a thin white line in radiographs (Fig. 3–37).

A lack of continuity of the floor of the maxillary sinus is seen in the antro-oral fistula. The most common antro-oral fistula arises during tooth extraction, but the removal of cysts or benign tumors may be associated with an artificial opening between the maxillary sinus and the oral cavity (Fig. 3–38).

In posterior periapical radiographs, the maxillary sinus cavity is usually seen extending from the premolar area to the maxillary tuberosity (see Fig. 3–37). The size of the

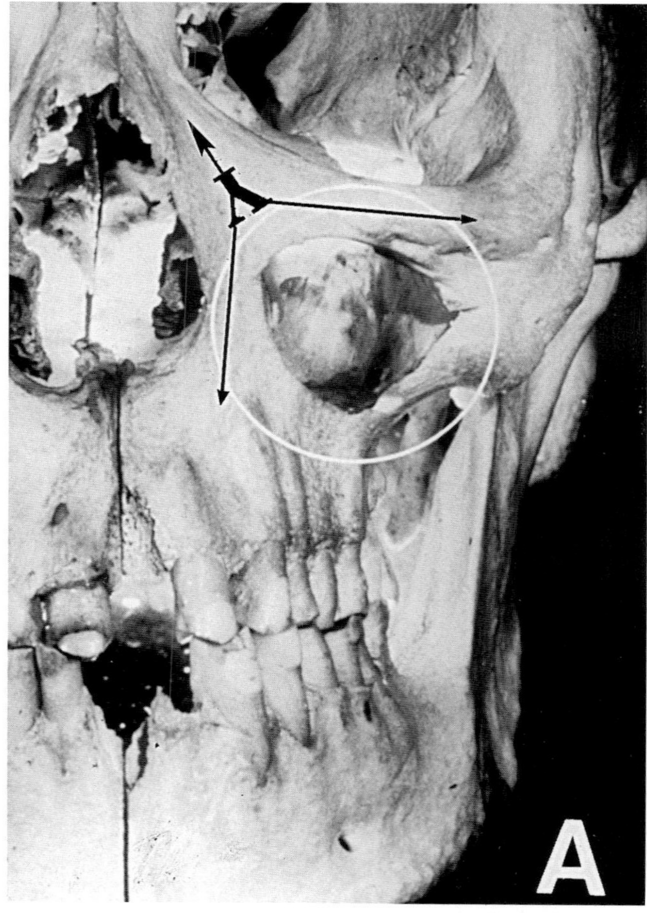

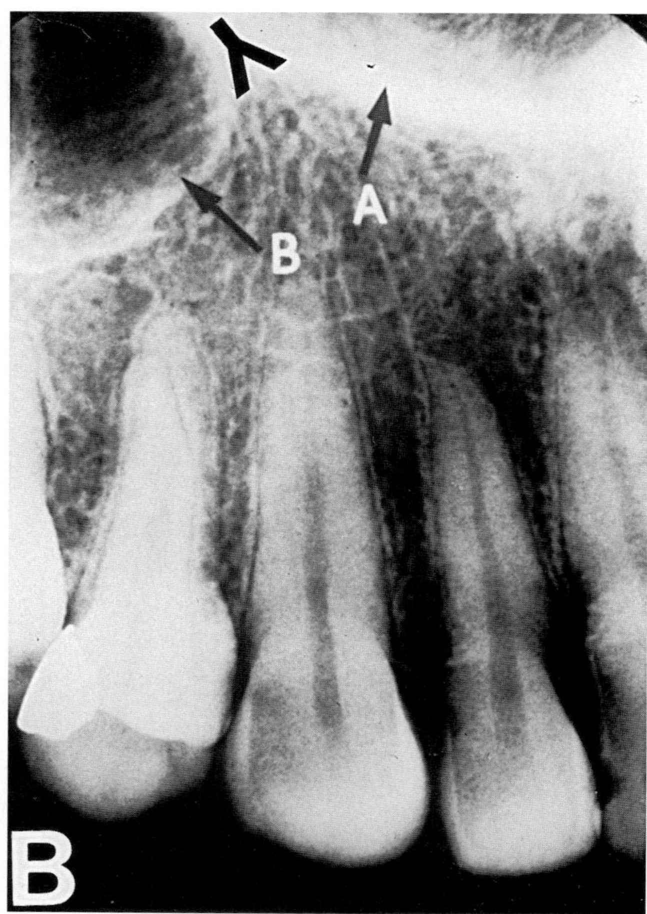

FIGURE 3–36.

Maxillary Lateral-Canine Region: A, Human skull: the anterior or facial bony wall of the maxillary sinus has been removed (circle). An inverted Y formation is created by bony structures between the maxillary sinus and the nasal cavity. B, An inverted Y is formed by the floor of the nasal fossa (A) and the floor of the maxillary sinus (B).

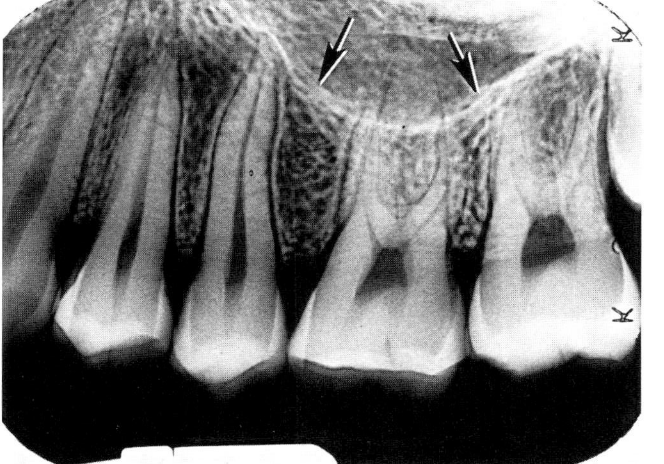

FIGURE 3–37.

Maxillary Sinus: The floor of the maxillary sinus is revealed as a white line (arrows) on the radiograph.

maxillary sinus is variable. Some are so small that evidence of them does not appear in the dental radiograph. A small maxillary sinus is situated well superiorly and posteriorly and may be obscured from view by the superimposition of the zygomatic bone, for instance (Fig. 3–39A). Other maxillary sinuses are so large that they extend well downward into the interseptal alveolar bone spaces between the posterior maxillary teeth (Fig. 3–39B).

The tuberosity of the maxilla may be completely occupied by the maxillary sinus, so one sees only thin cortices, which attach the tuberosity to the maxilla (Fig. 3–40A). Under such circumstances, as sometimes happens in extracting the third molar, the whole body of the tuberosity is removed with the tooth. To prevent such an occurrence, a preoperative radiograph should be made.

During development, the sinus may extend into the alveolar process and from there into the palate. In such a case, the palatal extension occupies a position well below the nasal floor and approaches the midline, past the maxillary canine tooth (Fig. 3–40B). From a small, elongated cavity on the lateral wall of the middle meatus at birth, the maxillary sinus enlarges by pneumatization, which is proportional to the growth of the maxilla and alveolar process. Pneumatization is the formation of pneumatic air cells or cavities in tissue.

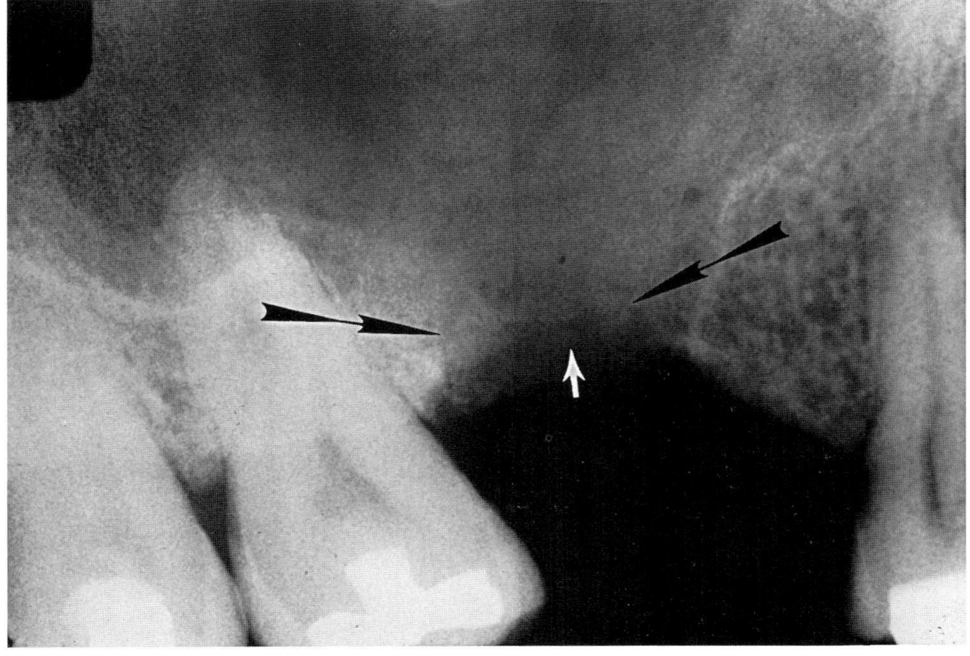

FIGURE 3–38.

Antro-oral Fistula: This abnormal communication (arrows) between the maxillary sinus and the oral cavity is a result of surgical procedures. Notice the gap in the continuity of the white line (cortical bone), which represents the floor of the maxillary sinus.

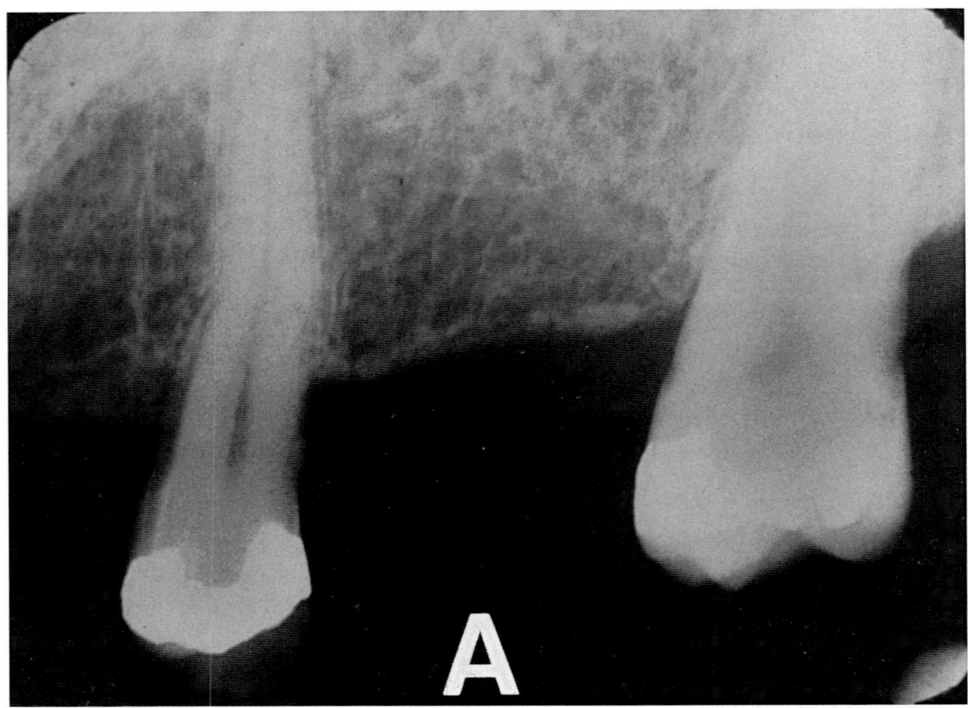

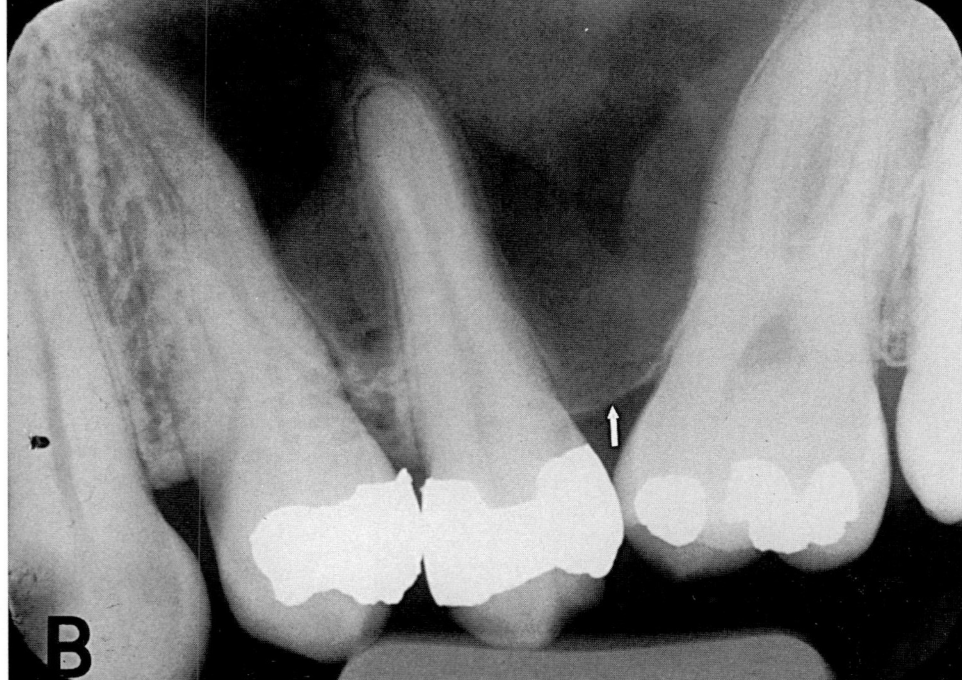

FIGURE 3–39.

Maxillary Sinus: A, Dental radiograph of the posterior maxillary region in which a small maxillary sinus image does not appear on the periapical radiograph. B, Enlarged maxillary sinus extending into the alveolar bone (arrow).

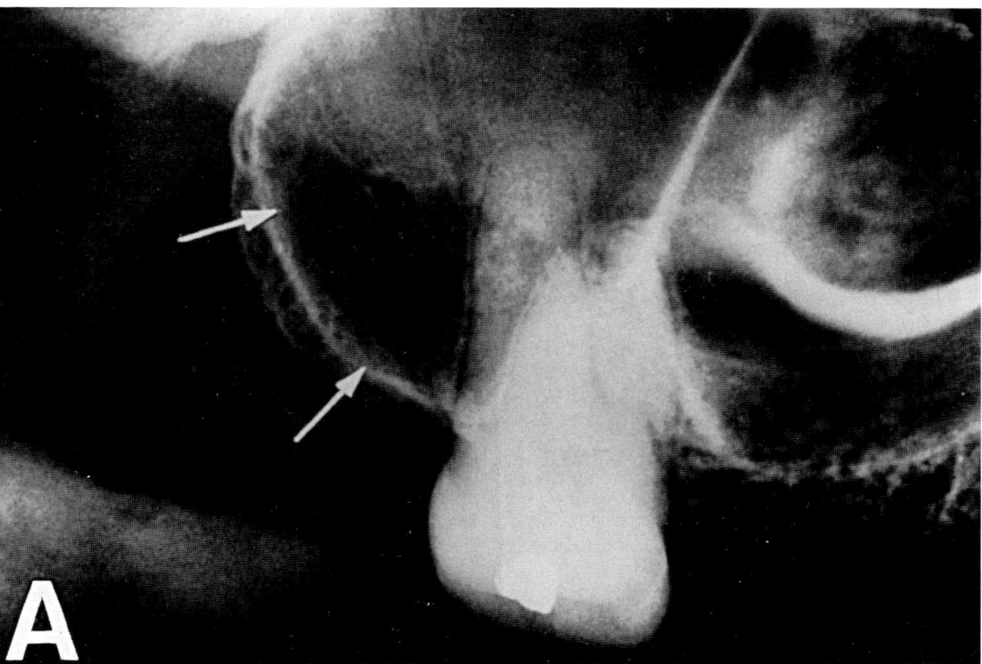

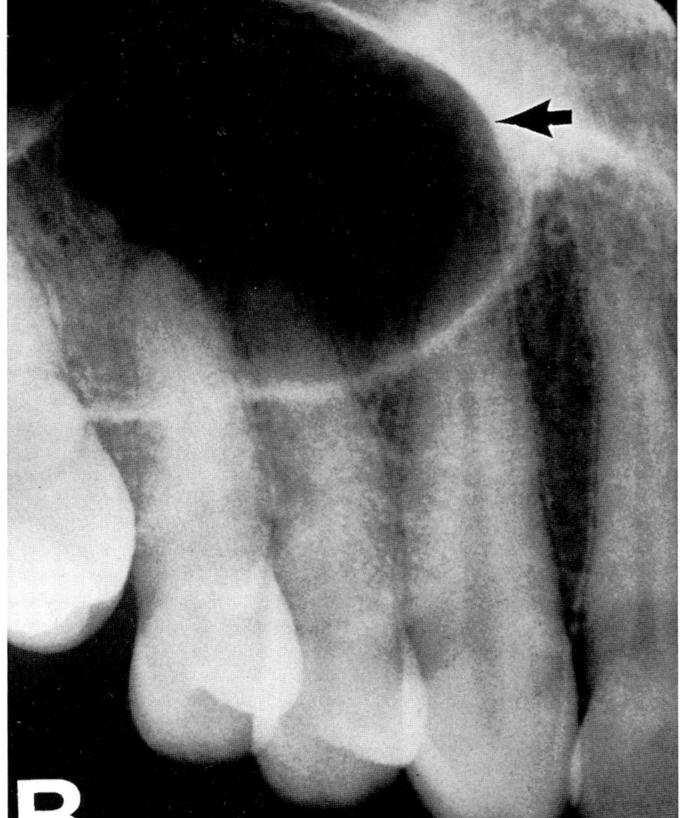

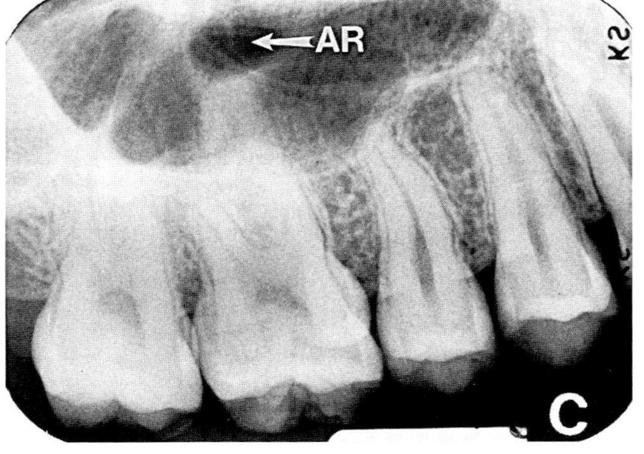

FIGURE 3–40.

Large Maxillary Sinuses: A, Large maxillary sinus in which the sinus has extended into the region of the maxillary tuberosity (arrows, alveolar recess). B, Palatal extension (recess) of the maxillary sinus (arrow) past the maxillary canine tooth into an area well below the floor of the nasal cavity. C, Antral recess (AR) or outpouching of the antrum appears dark when associated with a ridge or septum. These structures resemble cysts.

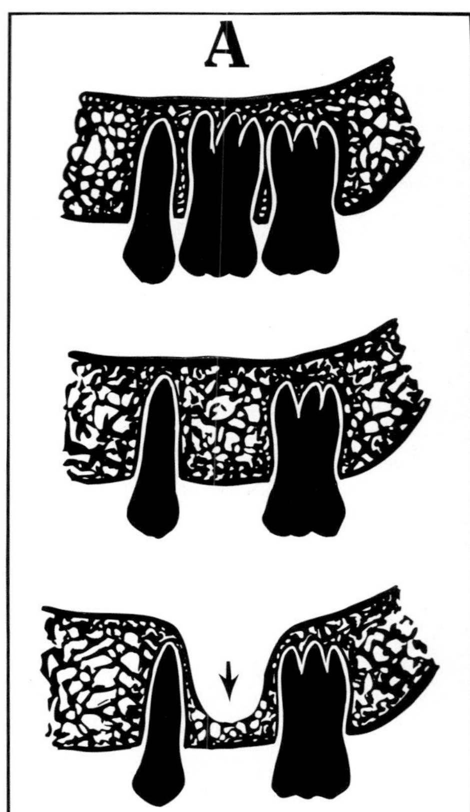

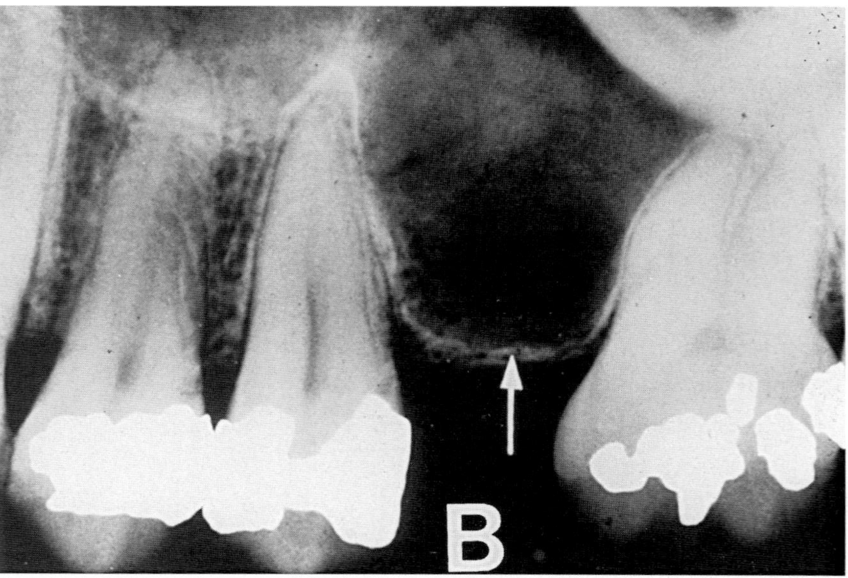

FIGURE 3–41.

Pneumatization of Maxillary Sinus: A, Following the removal of teeth, especially during the earlier decades of life, it is not uncommon for the antrum to extend down to the alveolar crest in the premolar and molar areas (arrow). (From Poyton HG: Maxillary sinuses and the oral radiologist. Dent Radiol Photogr 45:46, 1972.) B, Radiograph showing pneumatization of the maxillary first molar area by the antrum into alveolar bone (arrow) after removal of the tooth in this area. The white arrow identifies the floor of the maxillary sinus.

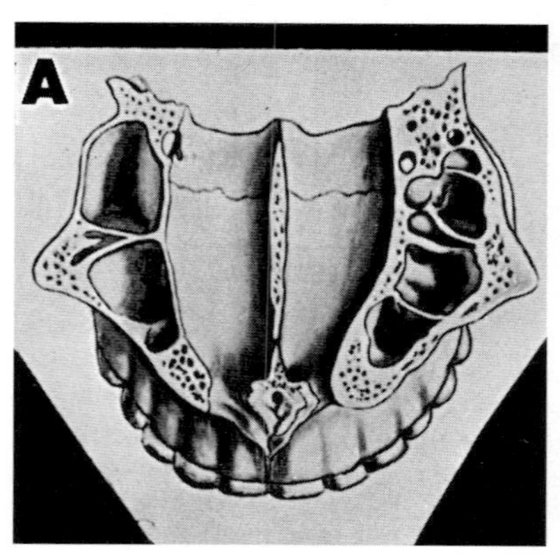

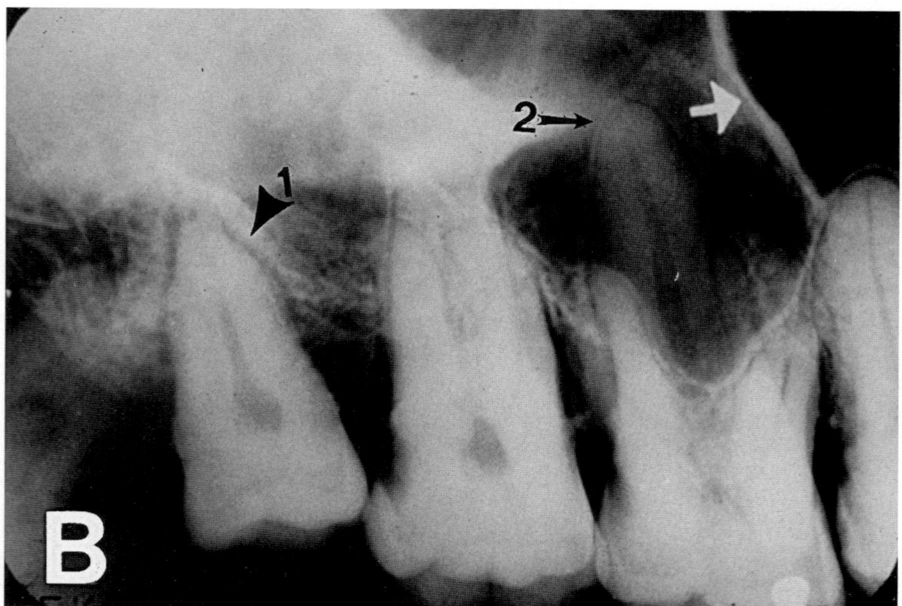

FIGURE 3–42.

Maxillary Sinus Septa: A, Cross-sectional diagram of maxillary sinuses illustrating various compartments made by bony partitions or septa that vary in size and thickness. B, Thick septum (white arrow) dividing the maxillary sinus into two loculi that resemble cystic formation: periodontal ligament thickening of the third molar (1) and normal continuous periodontal ligament and lamina dura around the palatal root of the first molar (2).

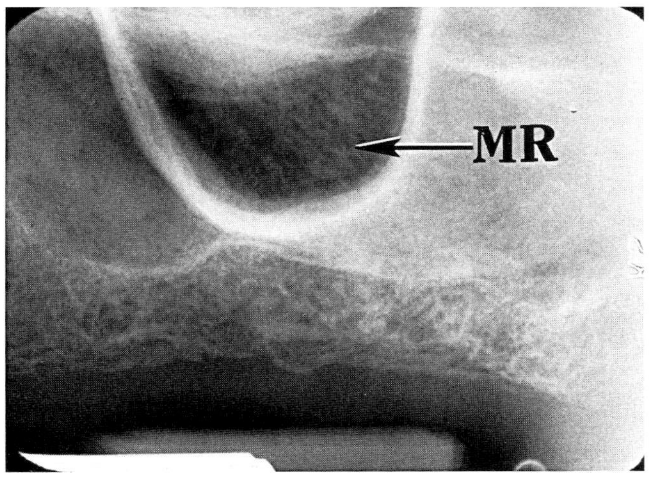

FIGURE 3–43.

Maxillary Sinus Recess: Maxillary sinus recess (MR, arrow) into the zygomatic bone.

The growth of the maxillary sinus continues in all directions until the fifteenth to eighteenth year, when the approximate adult size is reached. The maxillary sinus may extend by pneumatization into an alveolar space previously occupied by teeth, and the floor of the sinus will be represented by the alveolar crest. A thin cortex remains over the alveolar ridge to maintain normal contour. It is due in part to the resorption of bone after the removal of teeth. In some cases, it is due to the actual extension of the air sinus into the bone previously occupied by the teeth, particularly when teeth are removed during the earlier decades of life, when the supporting bone is healthy and normal (Fig. 3–41).

Many sinuses are partially divided into compartments by bony partitions or septa that vary greatly in length and thickness. Some septa are little more than ridges, whereas others are well-developed partitions that fall just short of completely partitioning off the sinus. Rarely, one sees a complete division of the maxillary cavity into separate compartments, in which case an extra ostium (opening) leads into the nasal cavity. Most commonly, only one septum is present in an antrum, but there may be two or more. Septa appear as straight or curved white lines extending up from the antral floor more or less vertically. Septal images are important only because they sometimes simulate the images of dental cysts (Fig. 3–42).

Outpouching or partially compartmentalized areas of the antrum are called recesses. These appear dark or gray and, when associated with a ridge or septum, they may suggest the presence of disease. When these ridges accentuate the radiolucency of the recess, and especially when recesses are projected over the apex of a tooth, they may mimic a periapical pathologic process (Fig. 3–43).

The antral wall often passes well below the apices of the posterior teeth. This gives an impression that the tooth roots actually protrude or project into the antrum with no bone between the tooth and the sinus. This is not the case, because a normal tooth rarely protrudes into the antrum without a bony covering. The covering is frequently very thin, but it is always there, unless disease has caused it to disappear.

The antrum sometimes dips down between the buccal and lingual (palatal) roots of the first molar. This gives the appearance that the lingual root protrudes into the sinus with-

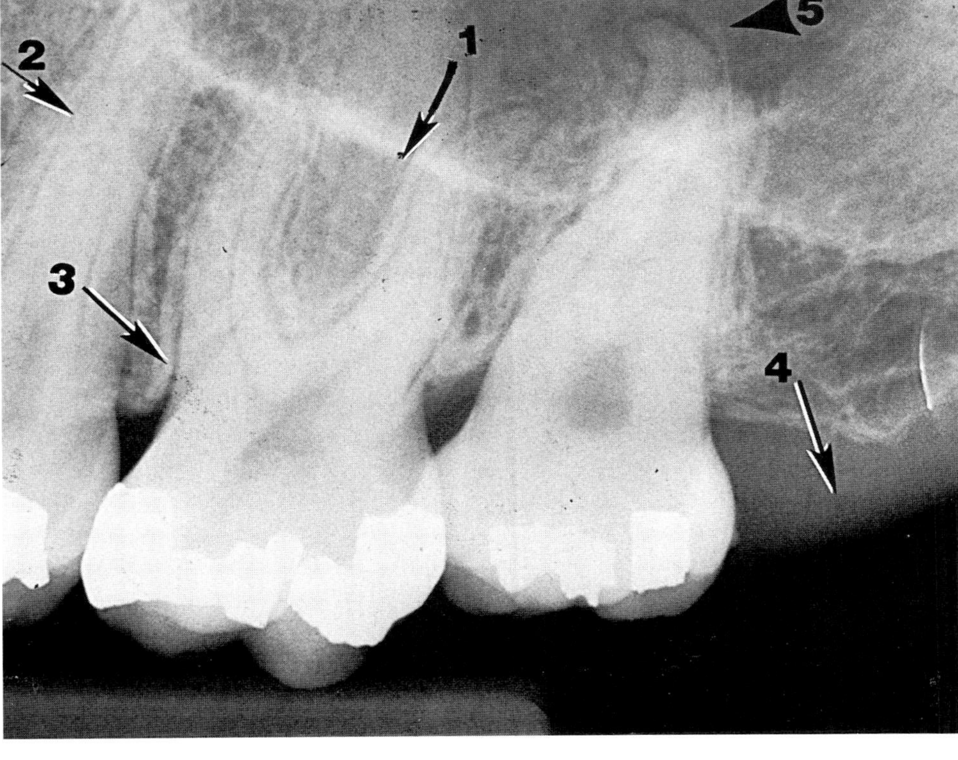

FIGURE 3–44.

Relationship of the Maxillary Sinus with the Roots of the Maxillary Molar Teeth: Floor of the maxillary sinus (1), periodontal ligament of the maxillary second premolar (2), lamina dura and periodontal ligament space of the maxillary first molar (3), soft tissue of the maxillary tuberosity (4), and palatal root showing the periodontal ligament space at the apex of the maxillary first molar (5).

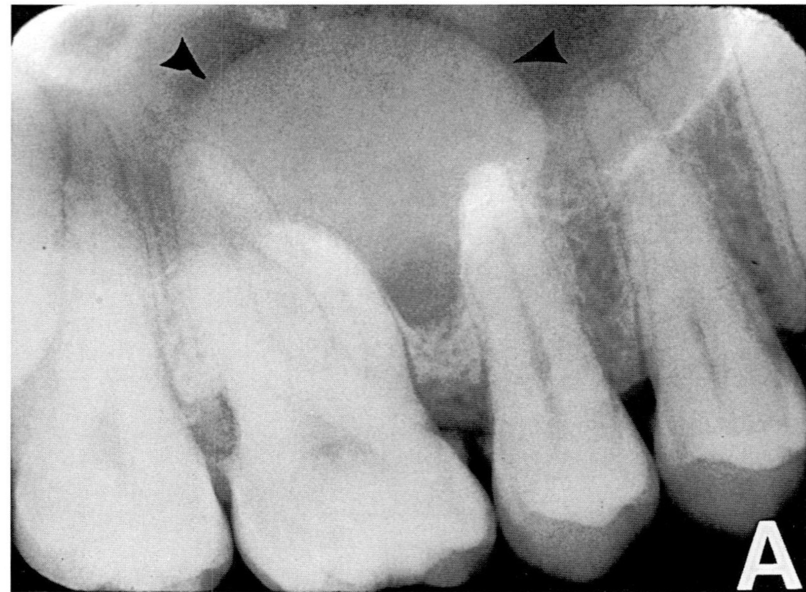

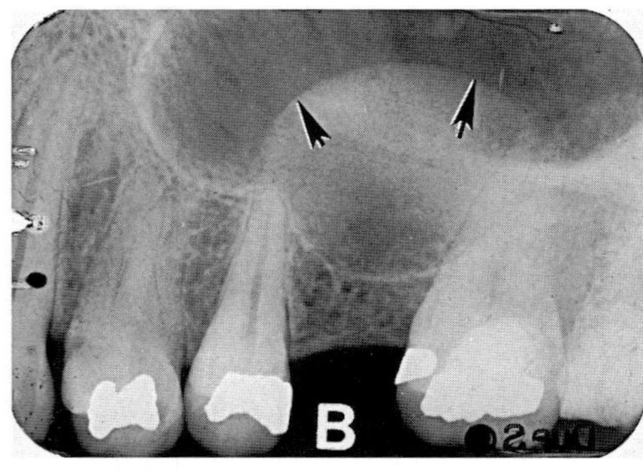

FIGURE 3–45.

Mucous Retention Cyst: A, The domelike image arising from the floor of antrum (arrows) is a mucous retention cyst. B, Mucous retention cyst of the maxillary sinus (arrows). (From Poyton HG: Maxillary sinus and oral radiologist. Dent Radiol Photogr 45:46, 1972.)

out a bony covering, when actually the root is located on the lingual side of the sinus. Most often, the lamina dura and periodontal ligament space can be seen on the radiograph completely surrounding the lingual root (Fig. 3–44).

Mucous Retention Cysts of Maxillary Sinus (Fig. 3–45)

Mucous retention cysts that have their origin in the mucosal lining of the maxillary sinus appear frequently in dental intraoral and panoramic radiographs. They are a result of distention (enlargement) of a mucous gland from blockage of a mucous gland duct in the floor of the maxillary sinus. In the radiograph, mucous retention cysts are radiopaque and dome shaped or hemispherical, with the antral floor as a base (Fig. 3–45). Most of these cysts are asymptomatic. They have no bony cortex and do not destroy bone, and they may remain stationary for years before they rupture and disappear completely. If symptomatic, they are usually removed by cannulation (tube inserted into cavity usually by means of trocar) and drainage.

Stalagmites of Maxillary Sinus (Fig. 3–46)

Small osseous excrescences resembling stalagmites (inverted stalactite formed on floor of cave) are sometimes revealed in dental radiographs of the antral floor. They are formed on the floor of antrum and are revealed as small white masses that seldom reach 3 mm in height. They have no pathologic significance except they may mimic a root fragment. Differentiation between a root tip and one of these "stalagmites" may be difficult and may depend on the knowledge that, in a root fragment, a small canal is visible or there is a free margin on all sides of the image (Fig. 3–46).

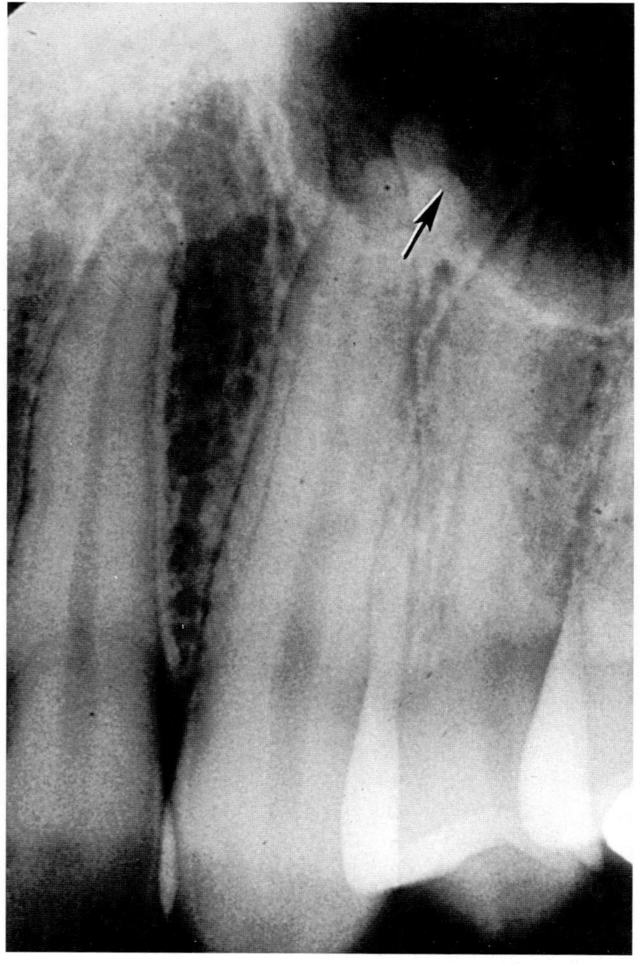

FIGURE 3–46.

Antral Stalagmites: These small, bony masses (arrow) attached to the antral floor resemble root fragments.

Nasolacrimal Canal (Fig. 3–47)

The nasolacrimal (tear duct) canal is not revealed in periapical radiographs, but it may be visible in a maxillary occlusal view. This structure is an osseous canal formed by the

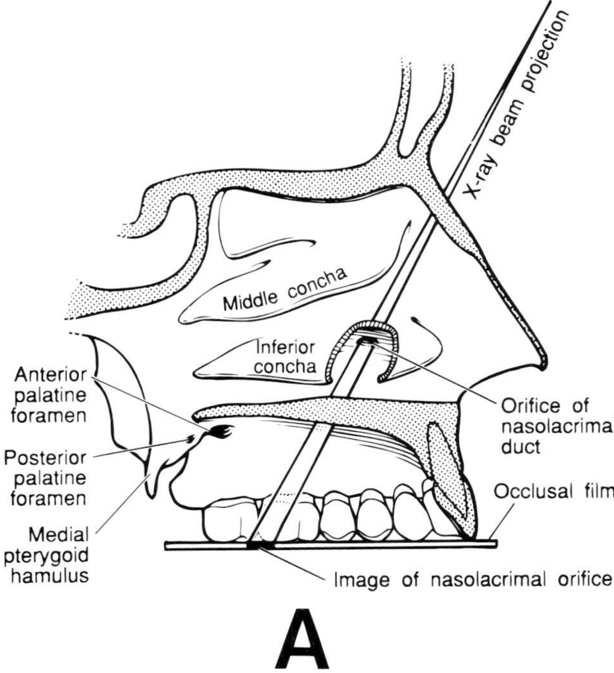

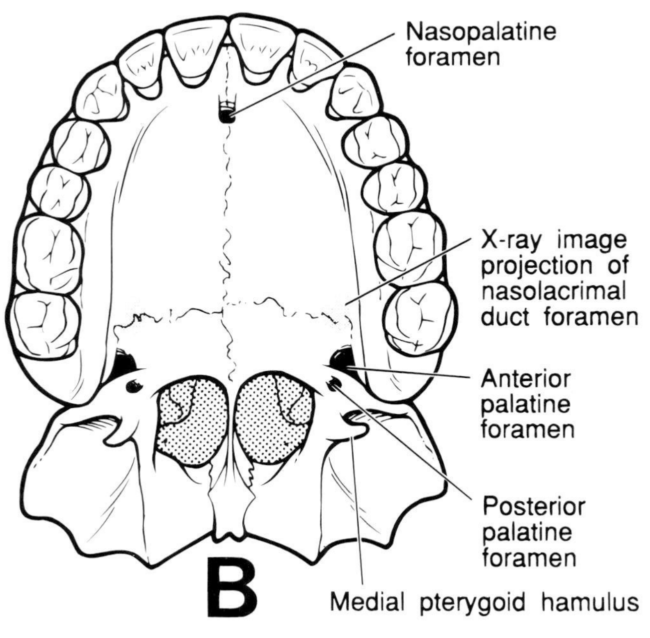

FIGURE 3–47.

Nasolacrimal Canal: A, Diagram showing a projection of an image of a nasolacrimal duct onto a maxillary occlusal radiograph. B, Palatal view of the maxilla showing the position of the x-ray image of a nasolacrimal duct. C, Occlusal radiograph showing nasolacrimal canals (NL) in an adult.

maxilla, the lacrimal bone, and the inferior nasal turbinate. It extends (18 mm in length) from the lower part of the lacrimal (tear) sac to the inferior meatus of the nose, where it terminates at an expanded orifice. The radiolucent images of the nasolacrimal canal in the occlusal film are considerably enlarged and may be mistaken for a cyst. This canal is seen on an occlusal film, particularly when excessive vertical angulation is used (Fig. 3–47).

Posterior Maxillary Area

Maxillary Tuberosity (Fig. 3–48)

The terminal enlargements or protuberances on each side of the maxillae are called maxillary tuberosities. The size of the tuberosities appears relatively larger when the third molars are absent. Destruction or absence of the tuberosities interferes with the retention of maxillary complete dentures, however. If the tuberosity is larger than usual, there may be impingement of the maxillary complete denture on the coronoid process of the mandible when opening and closing or on insertion of the complete maxillary denture. When a periapical survey is taken of the posterior maxillary region, the maxillary tuberosity region should always be included in the molar periapical radiograph because of the possible presence of third molars or pathologic processes such as odontomas or primordial cysts in these areas (Fig. 3–48).

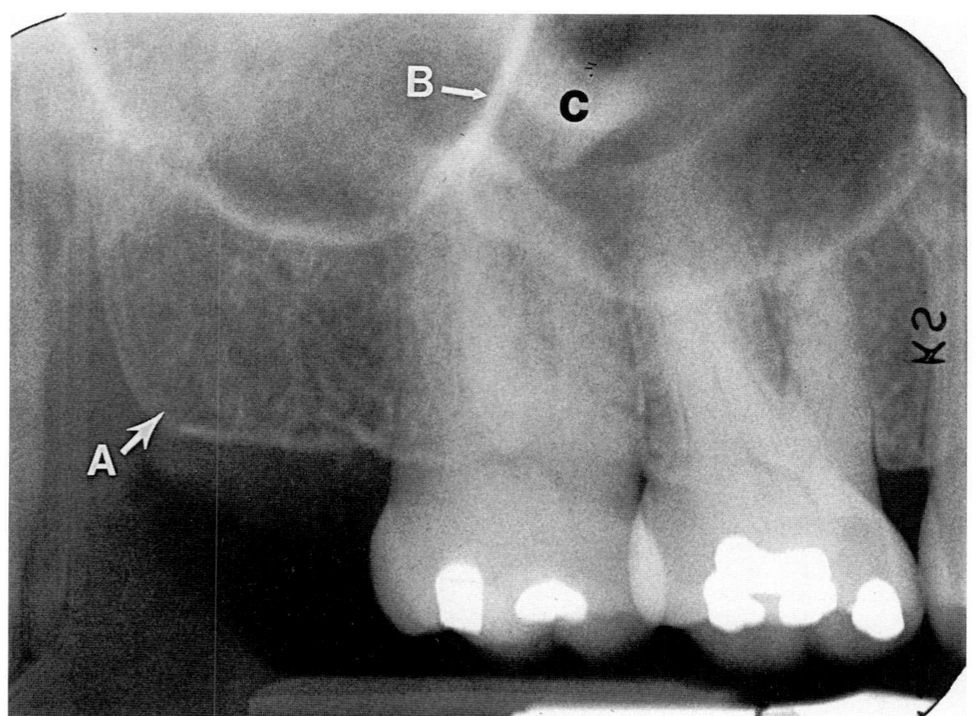

FIGURE 3–48.

Maxillary Tuberosity Region: Maxillary tuberosity (A), maxillary sinus septum (B), and inferior border of the zygomatic (malar) bone (C).

Greater Palatine Foramen (Figs. 3–47B and 3–49)

The anterior palatine nerve, a branch of the sphenopalatine ganglion, and the descending palatine artery descend the pterygopalatine canal, exit through the greater palatine foramen, and pass forward in the groove of the hard palate, as far as the nasopalatine foramen, where the anterior palatine nerve anastomoses with filaments of the nasopalatine nerve. The descending palatine artery sends a terminal branch through the incisive canal and anastomoses with posterior septal branches of the sphenopalatine artery (Fig. 3–47B). Sometimes, the greater palatine foramen can be seen as a small radiolucent area above the maxillary molar teeth (depending on x-ray tube angulation) that may mimic apical

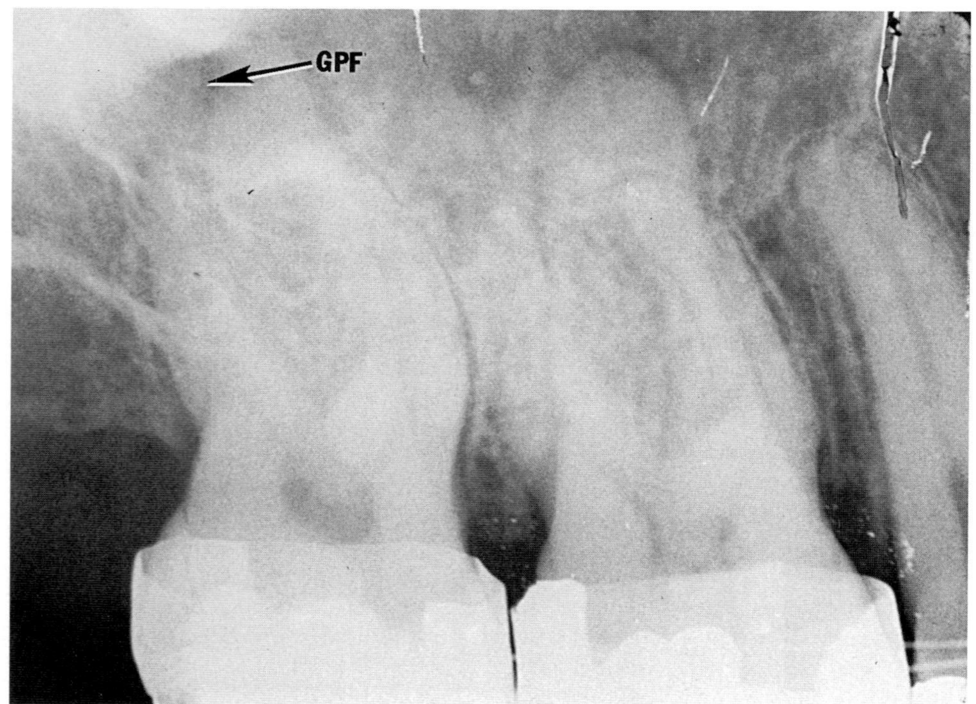

FIGURE 3–49.

Greater Palatine Foramen: Periapical radiograph revealing a radiolucent greater palatine foramen (GPF) superimposed above the palatal root of maxillary second molar. The tooth is vital.

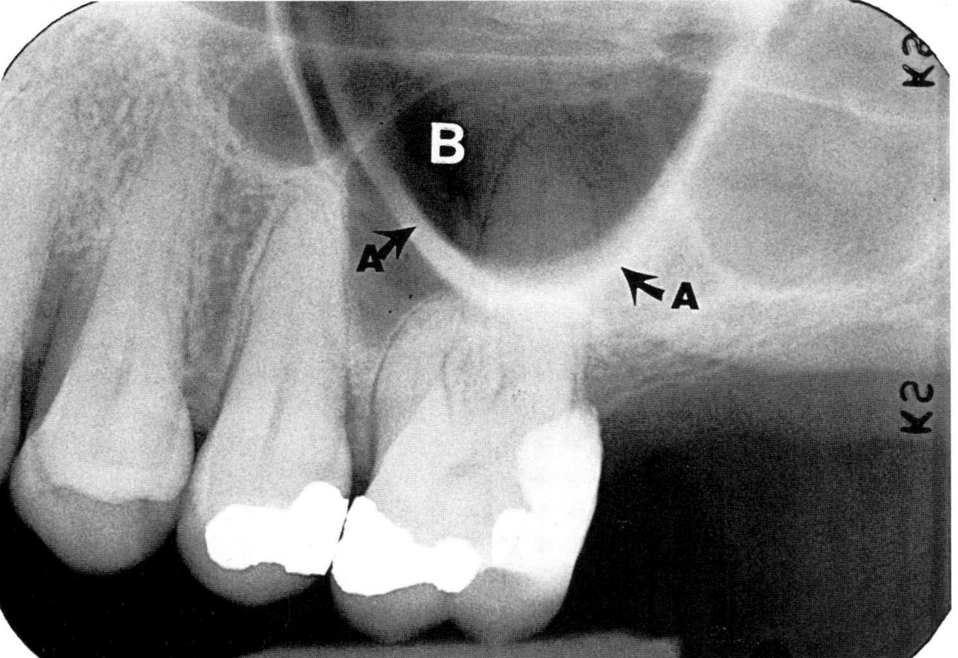

FIGURE 3–50.

Maxillary Region: The radiopaque U represents the inferior border of the zygomatic (cheek) bone (A). The dark area (B) represents the zygomatic recess of the maxillary sinus.

disease (Fig. 3–49). One rarely sees the greater palatine foramen in a periapical radiograph.

Zygomatic (Malar) Bone (Figs. 3–43, 3–48, 3–50, and 3–51)

The prominence of the cheek is produced by the zygomatic (malar) bone and the zygomatic process of the maxilla. The zygomatic arch is formed by the zygomatic process of the temporal bone (zygoma) and the temporal process of the zygomatic bone (Fig. 3–51A).

An anatomic factor of great importance is the extent of the antral recess that protrudes into the zygomatic (malar) bone. Some antra do not develop malar recesses, whereas others extend into and involve the greater part of the body of the bone (see Fig. 3–43). All these differences are reflected in radiographs. Only the inferior portion of the malar bone appears in intraoral radiographs, and it appears as a gray or white image, depending on the thickness of the bone and the proportion of dense bone. The extent of the inferior border varies, commencing over the second premolar or first

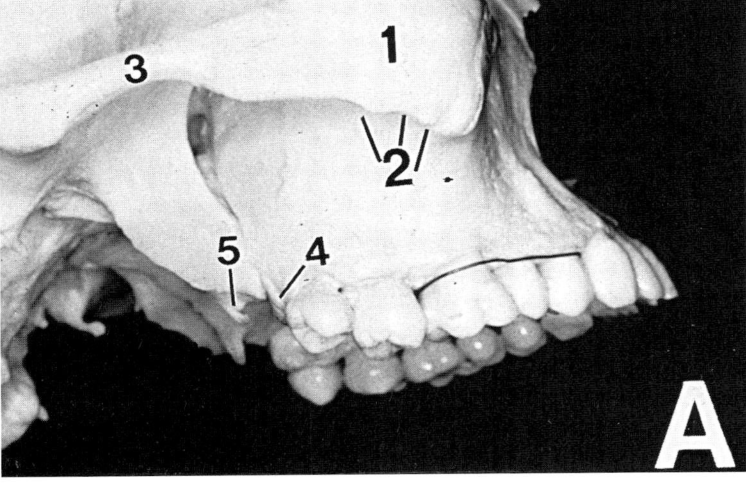

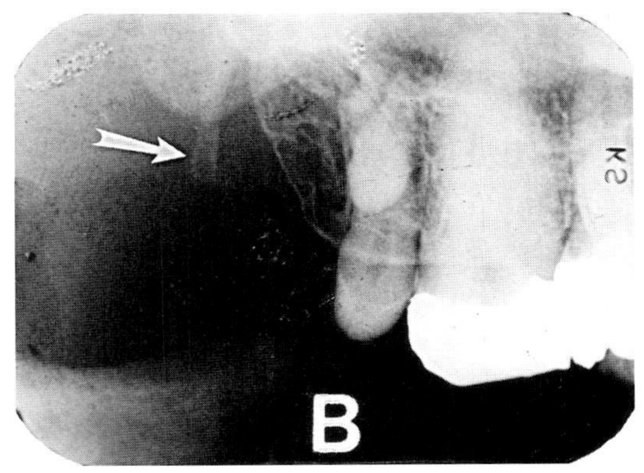

FIGURE 3–51.

Zygomatic bone and Related Structures: A, Lateral facial view of a skull: zygomatic (malar) bone (1), inferior border of the zygomatic bone (2), zygoma (3), maxillary tuberosity (4), and hamular process of the medial pterygoid plate of the sphenoid bone (5). B, Hamular process of the medial pterygoid plate (arrow). Note the microdontic third and fourth molars.

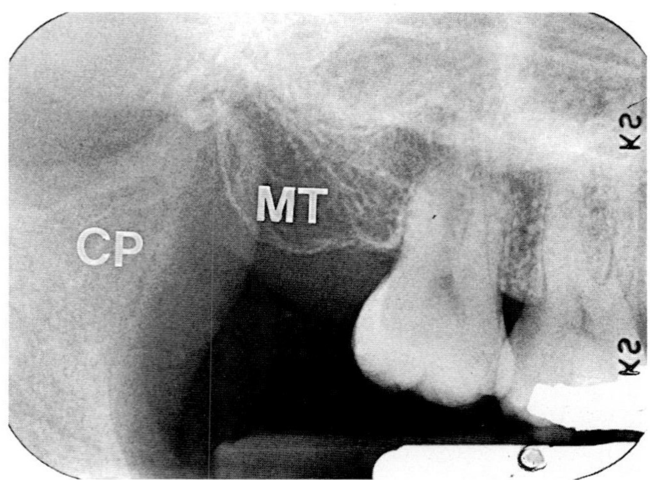

FIGURE 3–52.

Maxillary Molar Posterior Region: Coronoid process (CP) of the mandible and maxillary tuberosity (MT).

molar area and extending posteriorly, usually beyond the limits of the film. The general shape of the inferior border of the malar bone on the radiograph roughly resembles the letter U. The limbs of the letter U represent the walls of the maxillary sinus and the dark area between these limbs represents the antral recess of the malar bone. When the recess air space is deep, the image is dark; when there is little or no aeration, it is gray or white (see Figs. 3–48 and 3–50).

Hamulus (Fig. 3–51)

The hamulus is a hooked process extending from the medial pterygoid plate of the sphenoid bone. The tensor veli palatini muscle arises from the medial pterygoid plate and ends in a tendon that winds around the pterygoid hamulus and finally inserts into palatine aponeurosis and the horizontal plate of the palatine bone. In between the hamulus and maxillary tuberosity is the pterygomaxillary notch or fissure, an important prosthodontic landmark forming the periphery of the edentulous maxillary impression (Fig. 3–51). Sometimes, the hamulus can be seen in the intraoral radiograph.

Coronoid Process (Fig. 3–52)

The coronoid process is a thin, triangular eminence of the mandible that is flattened from side to side and varies in size and shape. Its medial surface gives insertion to the temporalis muscle. Sometimes, the coronoid process is seen on the maxillary molar intraoral projection (Fig. 3–52).

ANATOMIC STRUCTURES IN THE MANDIBLE

Mental Ridges or Tubercles (Figs. 3–53 and 3–54)

The mandible develops originally from lateral bones that unite in the midline. On the outer surface of the body, the mark of this union (the symphysis) is usually indicated by a groove or ridge. At the side of the symphysis, just above the base of bone, is an elevation (the mental protuberance) that terminates laterally on each side by tubercles or ridges (the mental tubercles) (Fig. 3–53). In conventional intraoral radiographs, the apex of the triangle (the mental protuberance) may or may not be apparent, depending on the vertical angulation of the x-ray beam (Fig. 3–54).

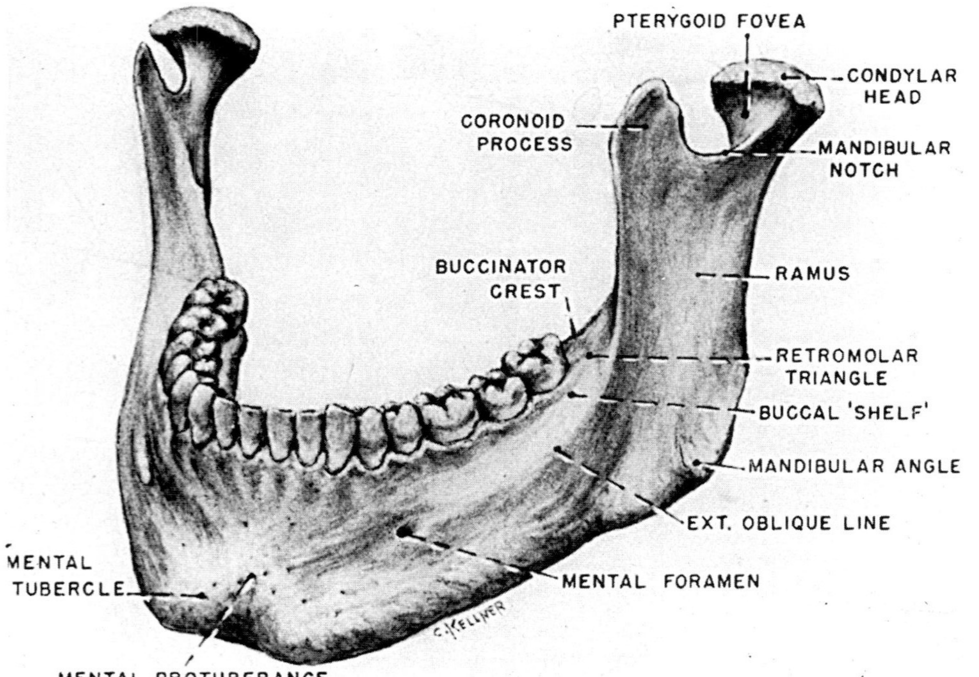

FIGURE 3–53.

Mental Ridges or Tubercles: Mental tubercle, mental protuberance, mental foramen, external oblique line. (From Shapiro H: Applied Anatomy of the Head and Neck. 2nd Ed. Philadelphia:JB Lippincott, 1947, p. 89.)

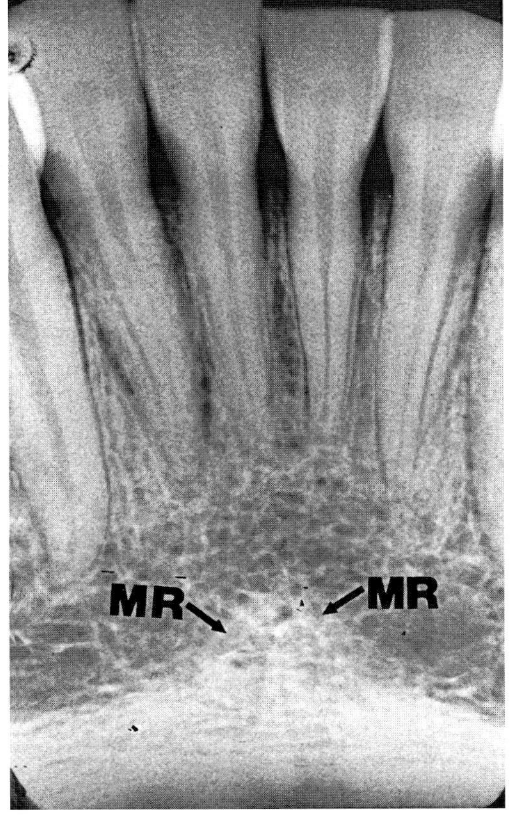

FIGURE 3–54.

Mental Ridges or Tubercles: Mental ridges (MR).

Genial Tubercles (Mental Spine) (Figs. 3–55 and 3–56)

Located on the inner surface of the body of the mandible, in the midline behind the symphysis, is the mental spine, sometimes paired and referred to as the genial tubercles (Figs. 3–55 and 3–56A and C). The genioglossus and geniohyoid muscles are attached to the upper and lower portions, respectively, of the genial tubercles. Below the mental spine or genial tubercles, and lateral to the midline, is the digastric fossa, the area of attachment for the anterior belly of the digastric muscle (Fig. 3–55).

Radiographically, the genial tubercles produce a doughnut-shaped radiopacity, usually well below the apices of the mandibular central incisors. The lingual foramen lies between the upper and lower pairs of genial tubercles and is the radiolucent center of the doughnut-shaped genial tubercles. This foramen transmits a small lingual nutrient artery that is a branch of the incisive artery and is not the larger lingual artery, which is a branch of the external carotid and supplies the tongue and sublingual glands (Figs. 3–55 and 3–56B).

External Oblique Line or Ridge (Figs. 3–57 and 3–58)

This ridge may be followed in an obliquely upward direction from the mental tubercle to the anterior border of the ramus. It is visualized as a radiopaque line of varied width and density that passes anteriorly and across the molar region. The triangularis and inferior labial quadratus muscles are attached along the anterior portion of this landmark. The oblique ridge also serves as a line of division between the reticular (netlike) portion of the bone above and the denser bone below. In addition, the inner aspect of the ridge serves to limit the lateral attachment of the buccinator muscle, which rises from the outer alveolar process just below the molar teeth (Figs. 3–57 and 3–58).

Mylohyoid Ridge (Internal Oblique Ridge) (Fig. 3–59)

This structure, which extends obliquely upward from just above the digastric fossa to the anterior border of the ramus, serves as the point of attachment of the mylohyoid muscle (Fig. 3–59). Radiographically, it is a radiopaque line, often seen below the apices of the molar teeth (Fig. 3–59). The mylohyoid ridge varies greatly in size, and its posterior portion is much more prominent. A dense mylohyoid ridge and a deep submandibular fossa may produce an abnormally radiolucent area beneath the mylohyoid ridge. This radiolucent area could be mistaken for a cystic lesion (Figs. 3–58 and 3–59).

Mental Foramen (Fig. 3–60)

The mental foramen is on the buccal surface of the body of the mandible below the second premolar tooth on either side, midway between the upper and lower borders of the mandible (Fig. 3–60A). The mental foramen affords passage of the mental nerve and blood vessels to the outside of the mandible. Its image may be superimposed on the apex of the root of a tooth, especially the second premolar, and may be mistaken for a periapical lesion (Fig. 3–60B). If the alveolar bone has marked resorption, the foramen may be situated near the crest of the ridge.

Mandibular Canal (Figs. 3–61 to 3–68)

The mandibular canal is an important structure because it transmits the inferior alveolar vessels and nerve. The internal maxillary artery, arising from the external carotid artery within the parotid gland, gives rise to the inferior alveolar artery, which enters the mandible through the mandibular foramen. It runs along the mandibular canal in the substance of the bone, accompanied by the vein and nerve and, opposite the first premolar tooth, divides into the incisive and mental branches (Fig. 3–61). The incisive branch is continued forward beneath the incisor teeth as far as the midline, where it anastomoses with the artery on the opposite side. The mental branch emerges with the nerve and vein from the mental foramen and anastomoses with branches of the facial or external maxillary artery.

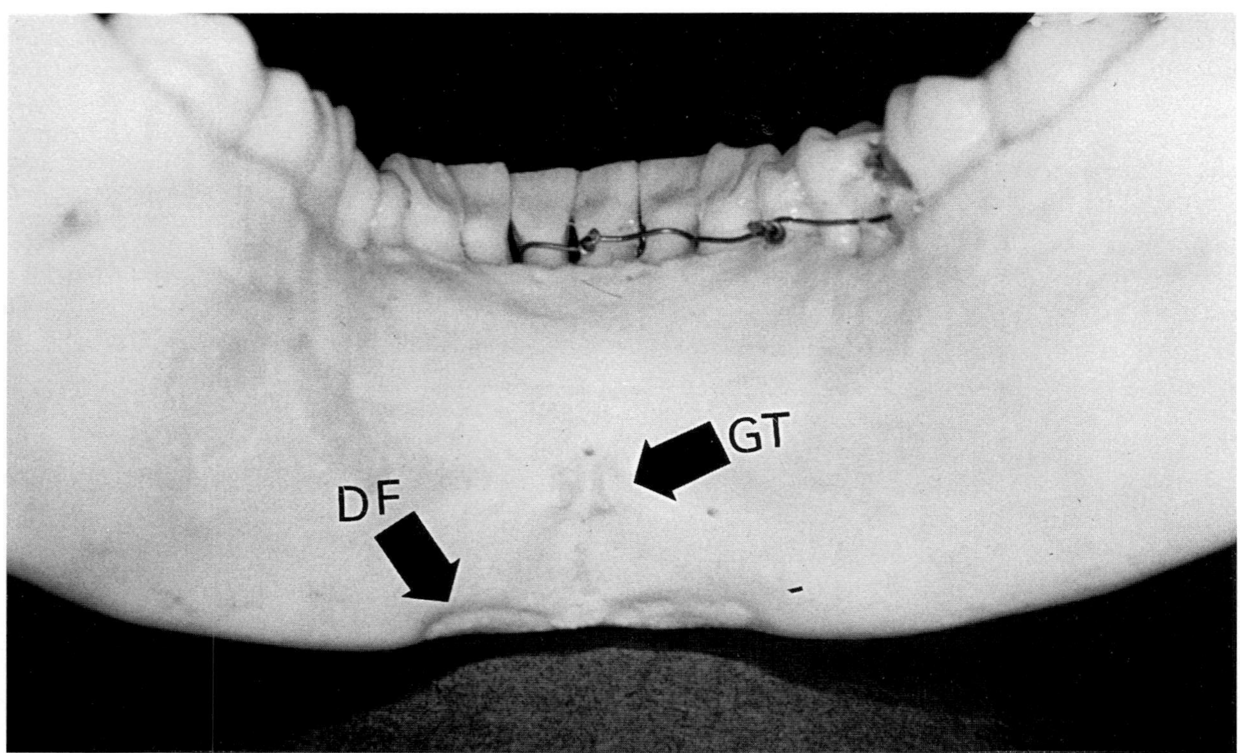

FIGURE 3–55.

Lingual View of the Mandible: Genial tubercles (GT) and (DF) digastric fossa.

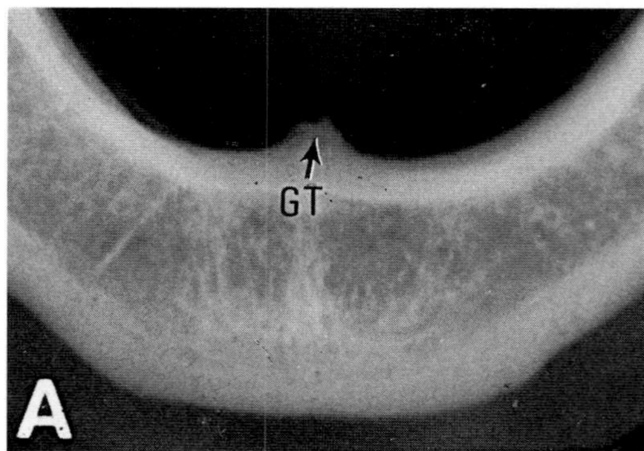

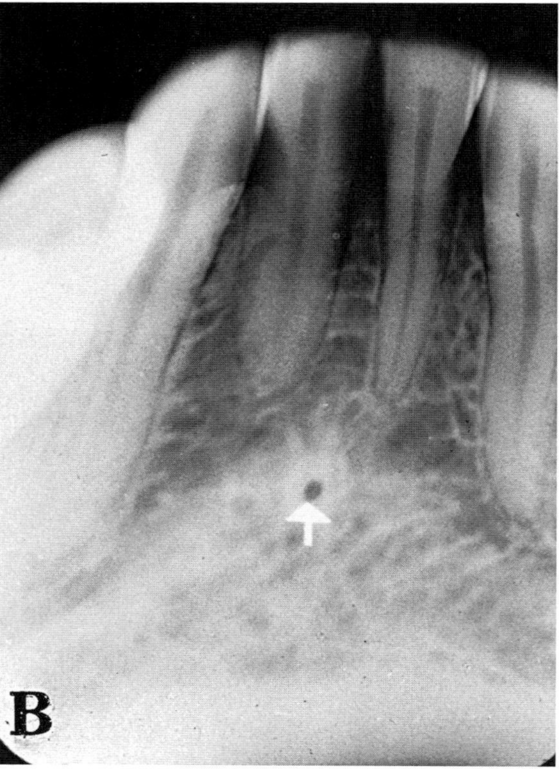

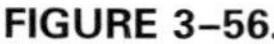

FIGURE 3–56.

Genial Tubercles: A, Occlusal radiograph showing genial tubercles (GT). B, Mental spine or genial tubercles. The doughnut-shaped radiopacity (arrow) is the mental spine (genial tubercles), and the radiolucent center is the lingual foramen, which transmits a small lingual nutrient artery. *(continued)*

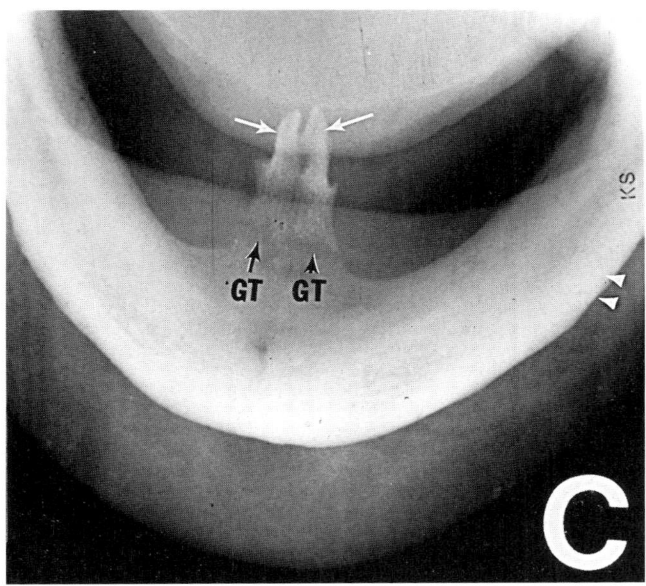

FIGURE 3–56.

(continued) C, Enlarged genial tubercles (GT, arrows) or spines fractured from accident. (Courtesy of Dr. Luis Alfaro, Pathology Referral Center, University of Chile Dental School, Santiago, Chile.)

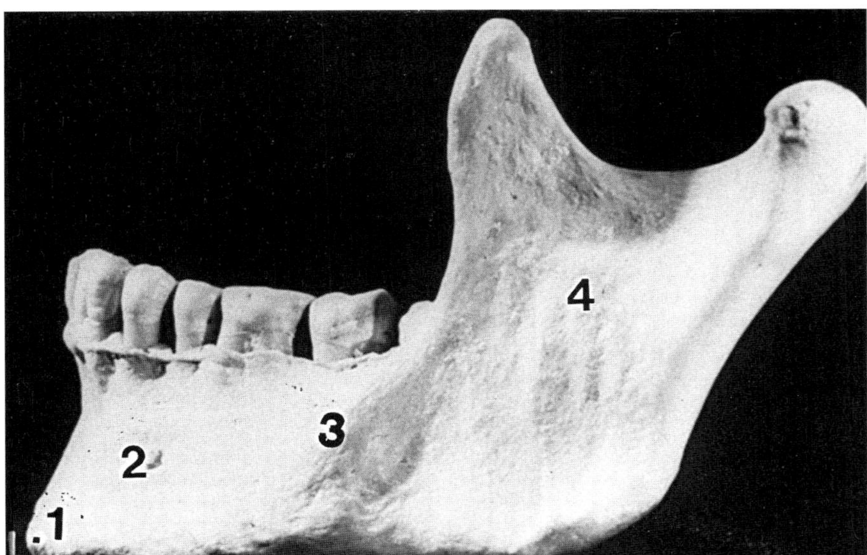

FIGURE 3–57.

Lateral View of the Mandible: Mental protuberance (1), mental foramen (2), external oblique ridge (3), and ramus (4).

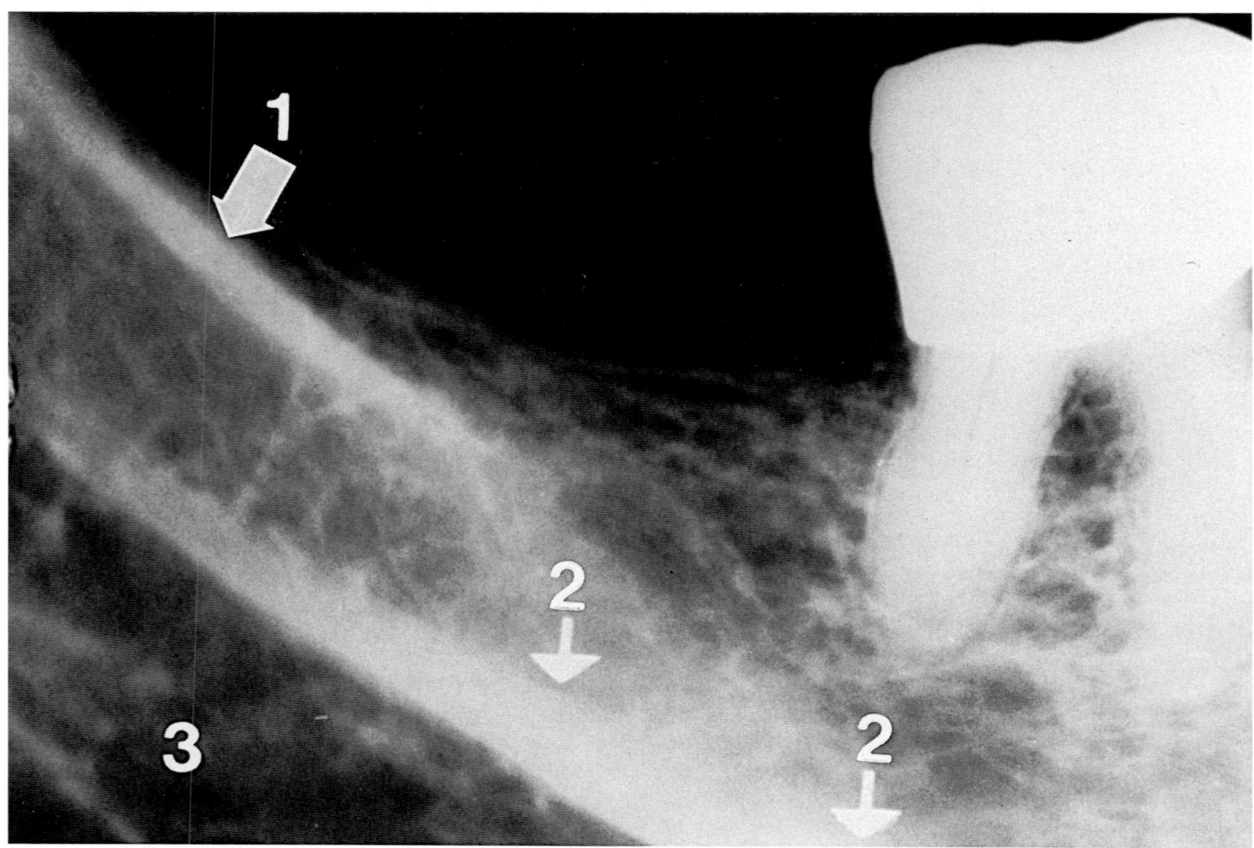

FIGURE 3–58.

Mandibular Posterior Region: External oblique ridge (1) and mylohyoid ridge (2) below. Note the abnormally dark submandibular gland fossa (3) below the mylohyoid ridge (2).

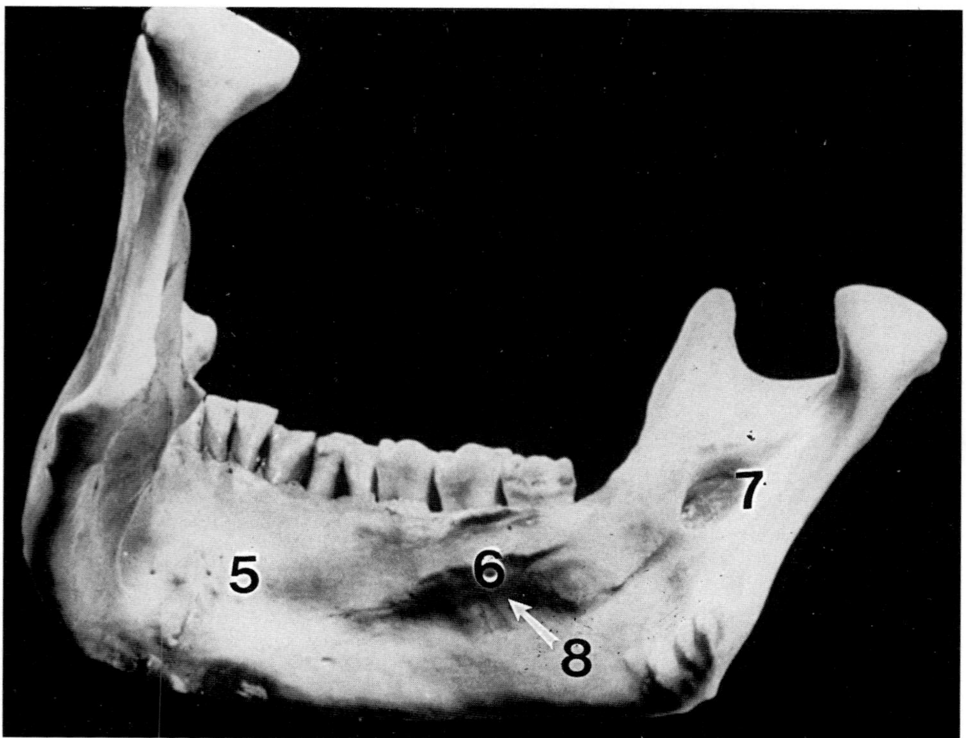

FIGURE 3–59.

Medial Surface of the Mandible: Mental spine or genial tubercles (5), mylohyoid ridge (6), mandibular foramen with small, tonguelike structure of bone, the lingula, which guards the foramen on its anterior aspect (7), and submandibular fossa (8).

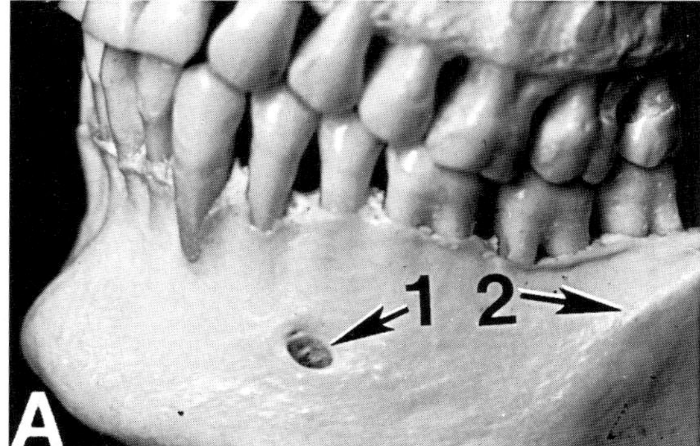

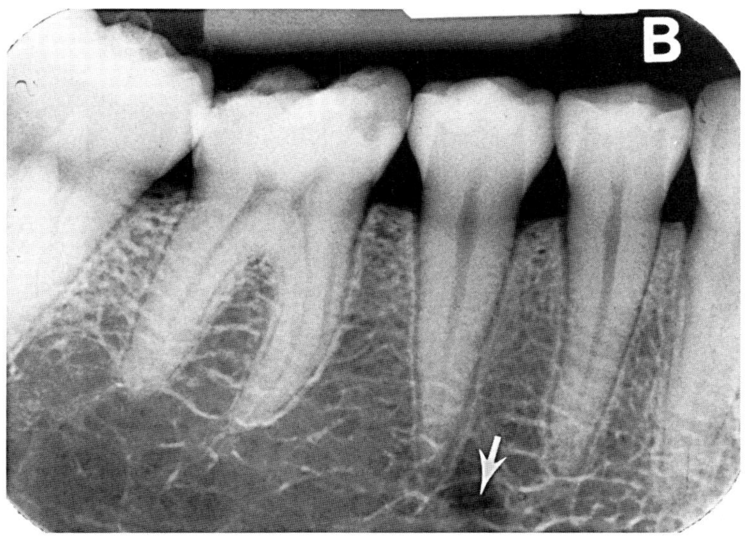

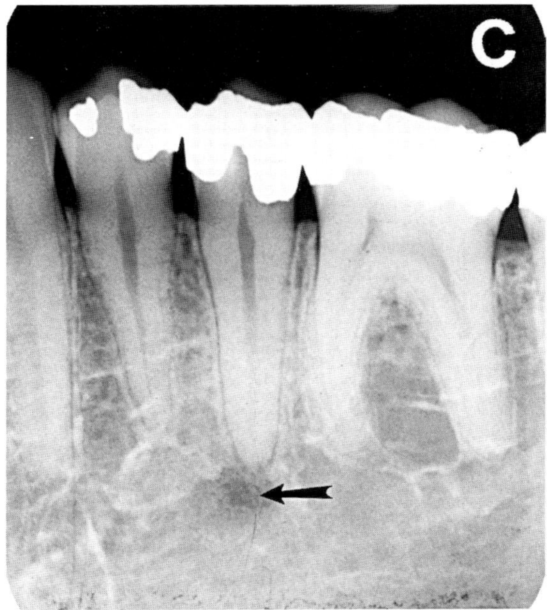

FIGURE 3–60.

Mental foramen: A, Mental foramen on a dry mandible specimen (1); external oblique ridge (2). B, Radiograph of the mandibular premolar region showing the mental foramen mimicking periapical disease (arrow). The second premolar is vital, and the lamina dura can be seen completely surrounding the tooth. C, Mental foramen (arrow) at the apex of a vital second premolar. Note that the periodontal ligament is separate from the radiolucency.

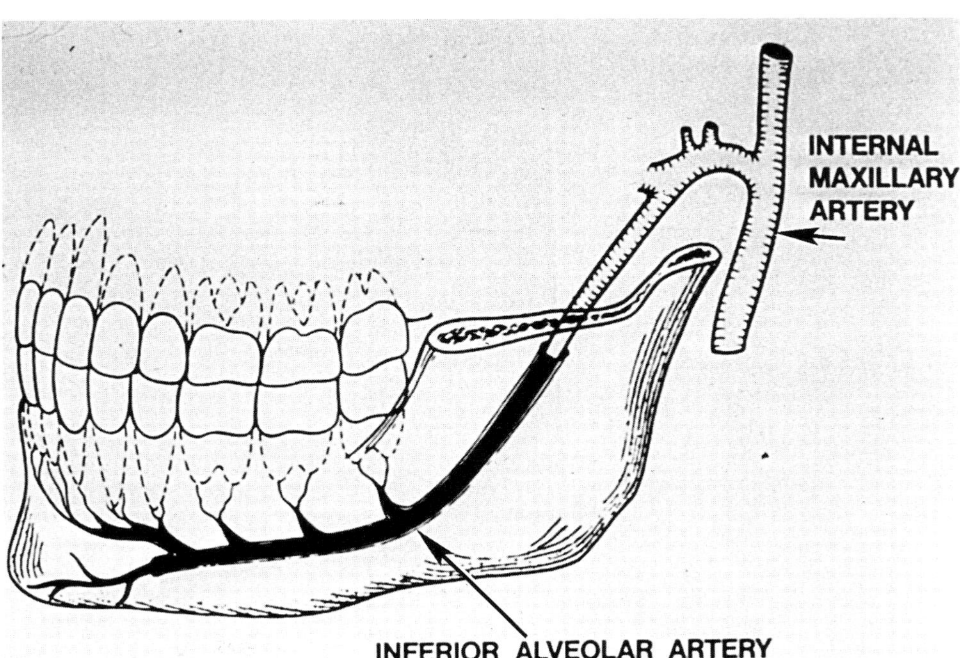

FIGURE 3–61.

Mandibular Canal (Inferior Alveolar Canal): The inferior alveolar (mandibular) artery descends with the inferior alveolar nerve to the mandibular foramen on the medial surface of the ramus of the mandible. It runs along the mandibular canal and is accompanied by nerve and vein. It gives off a few branches that are lost in the cancellous tissue and a series of branches that correspond in number to the roots of the teeth. Opposite the first premolar tooth, the nerve and vessels divide into the incisive and mental branches. (Courtesy of Eastman Kodak Co., Rochester, NY.)

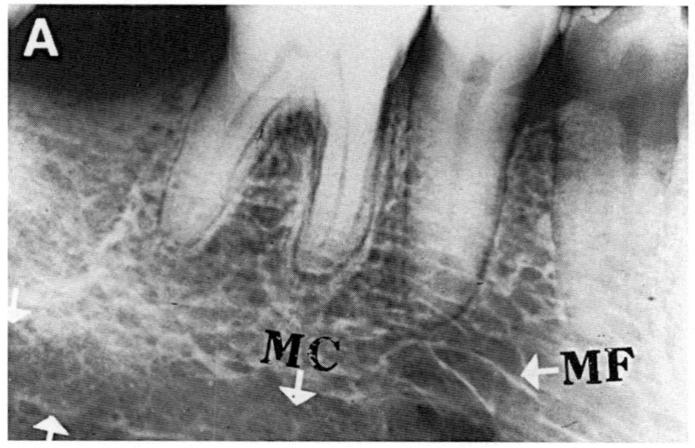

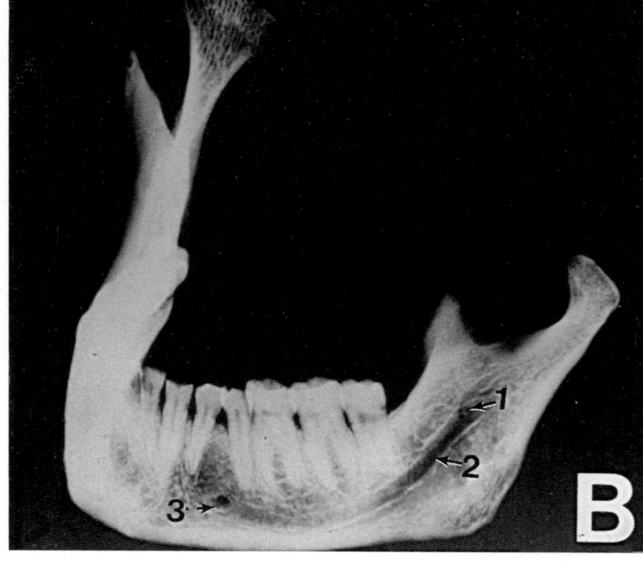

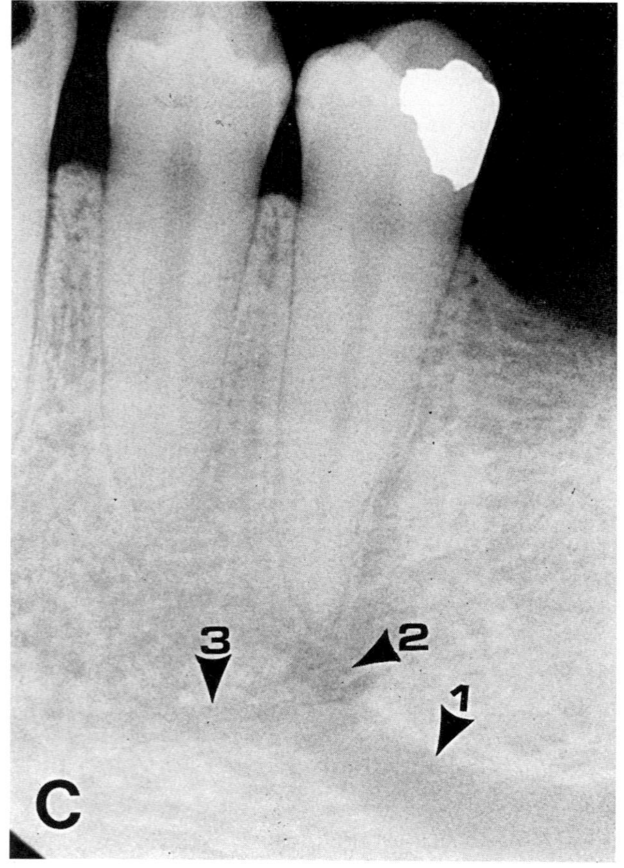

FIGURE 3–62.

Mandibular Canal, Mental Foramen and Incisive Canal: A, Radiograph of the mandibular canal (MC, arrows). The mandibular canal transmits the inferior alveolar nerve, artery, and vein. The mental foramen (MF) is a distorted radiolucent area. B, Radiograph of a dry mandible revealing the mandibular foramen (1), mandibular canal (2), and mental foramen (3). C, Mandibular canal (1), mental foramen (2), and incisive canal (3).

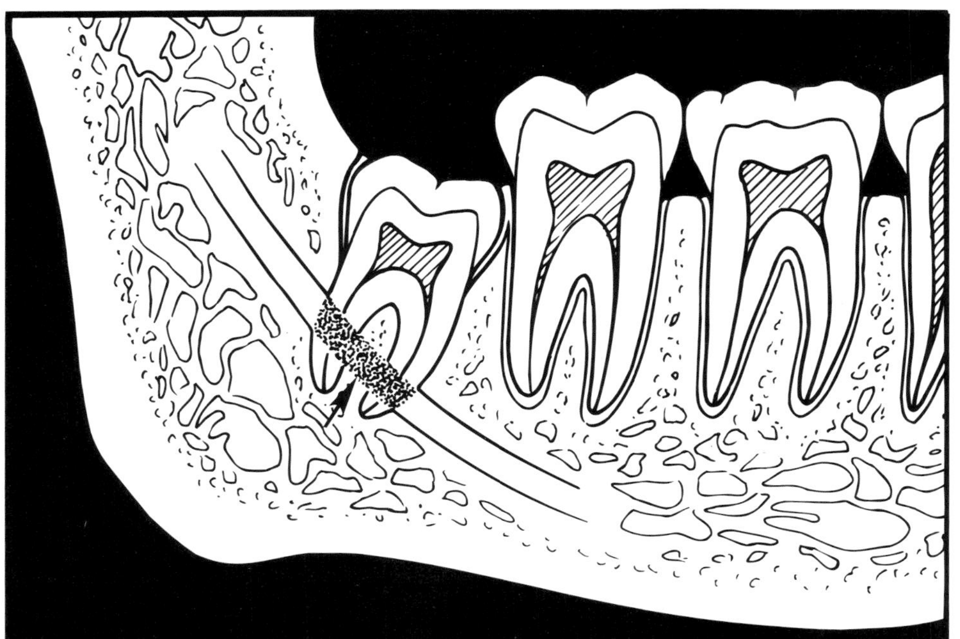

FIGURE 3–63.

Close Proximity of the Mandibular Canal to the Roots of an Impacted Third Molar: Illustration of "dark band phenomenon" indicating a close proximity of the mandibular canal to an impacted third molar (arrow).

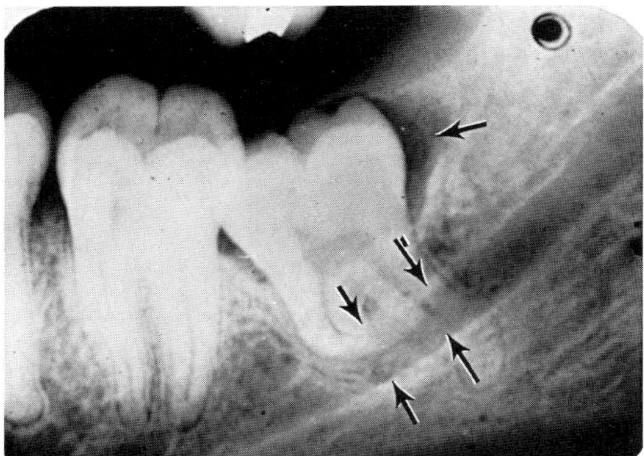

FIGURE 3–64.

Dark Band Phenomenon: Radiograph of an impacted third molar. The mandibular canal appears as a dark band crossing the roots of the third molar (arrows); this feature indicates that the canal is probably in close proximity to the roots. Enlarged follicle of the third molar area (arrow on upper right).

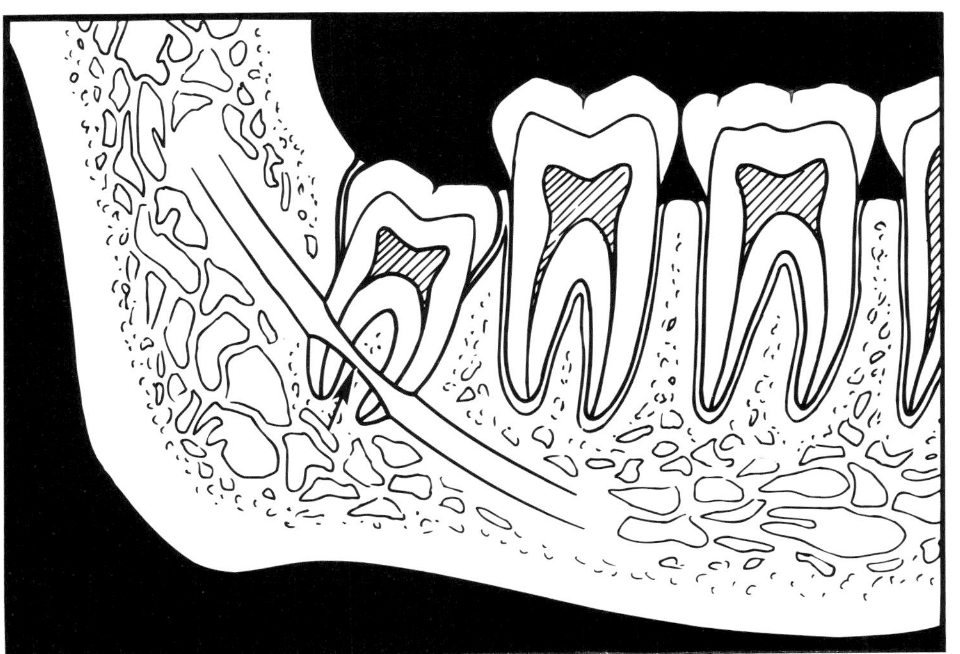

FIGURE 3–65.

Close Proximity of Mandibular Canal to Roots of Impacted Third Molar: Illustration of constriction of the canal diameter as the mandibular canal crosses the roots of impacted third molar, indicating a close proximity of the mandibular canal to an impacted third molar (arrow).

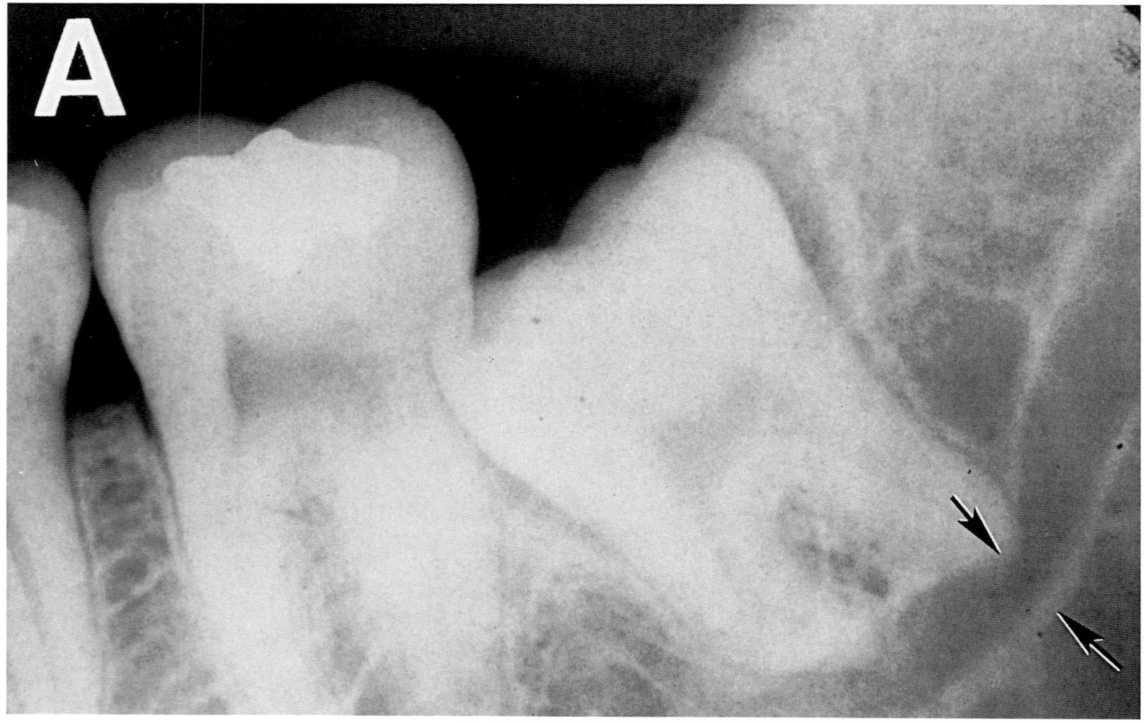

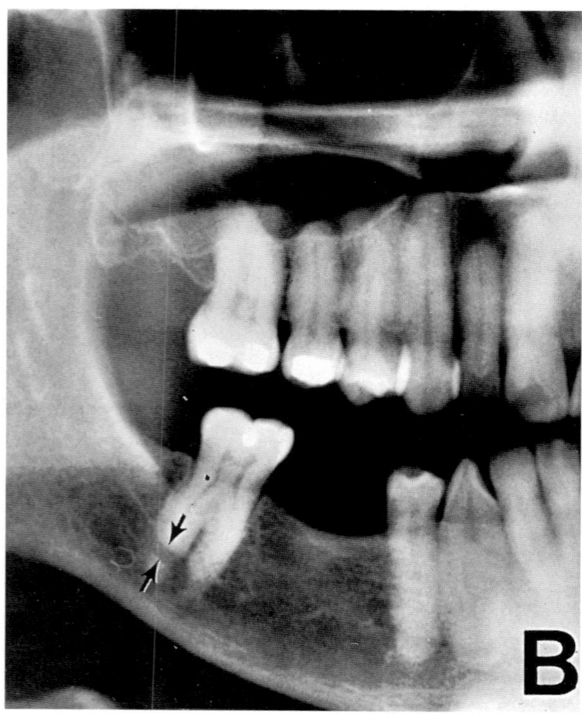

FIGURE 3–66.

Mandibular Canal Constriction: A, Radiograph of a mesioangular impacted third molar. The mandibular canal appears to become constricted (arrows) as it crosses the lower portion of the roots of the impacted third molar, indicating that the canal is most likely in close approximation to the third molar roots. B, Narrowing of the canal across the distal root of the molar. The darkened canal (arrows) means that the roots are deeply notched by the canal.

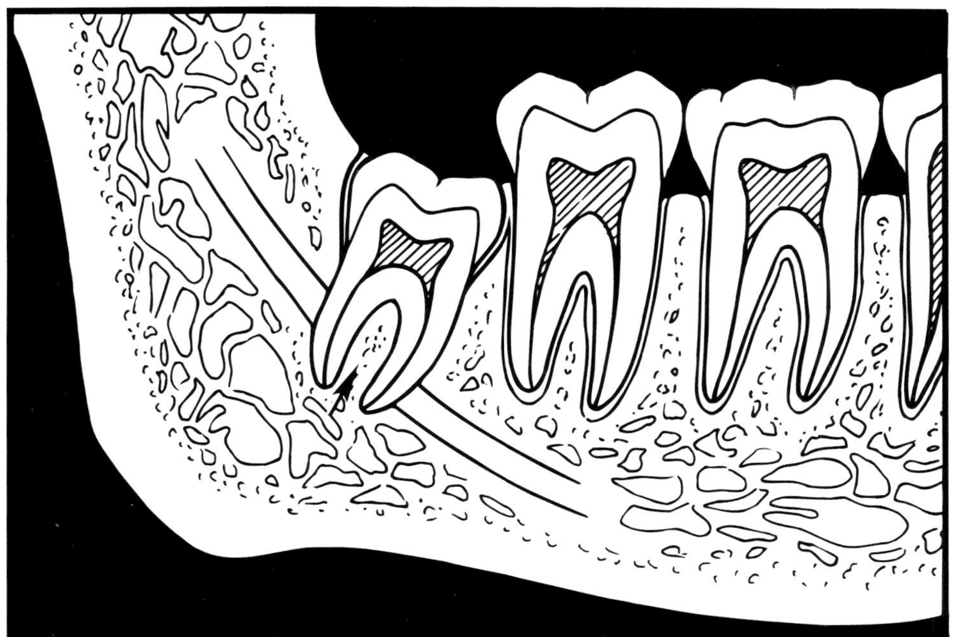

FIGURE 3–67.

Canal Discontinuous Phenomenon: Illustration of a discontinuous image of the mandibular canal as it crosses the roots of the impacted third molar, indicating a close proximity of the mandibular canal to an impacted third molar (arrow).

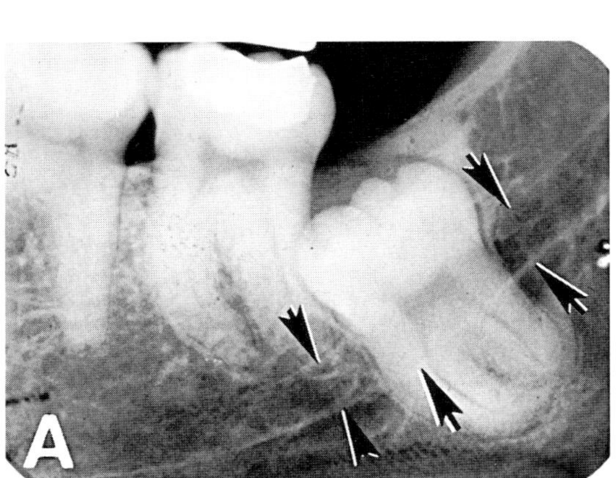

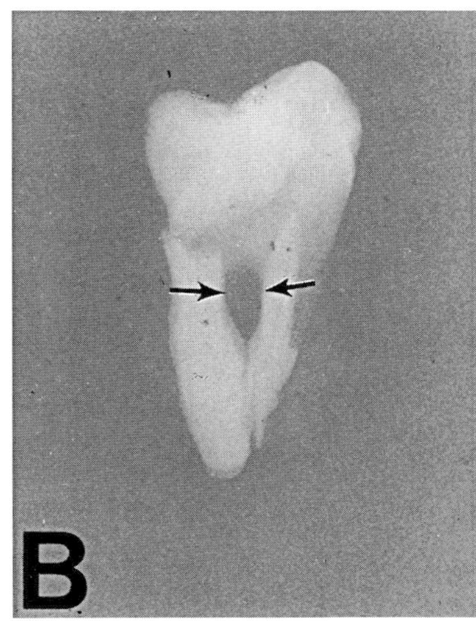

FIGURE 3–68.

Mandibular Canal in Relation to Third Molar: A, Radiograph of a deeply mesioangular impacted third molar. The mandibular canal is discontinuous on the superior wall of the canal (arrows). B, Extracted third molar oriented in a buccal-lingual view in which the mandibular canal went through the root of the tooth (arrows).

The inferior alveolar nerve, the largest branch of the mandibular nerve, enters the mandibular foramen midway up the medial aspect of the ramus, a landmark sometimes seen on panoramic films. It continues its passage through the bony mandibular canal beneath the roots of the teeth and gives off filaments that supply the molar and the premolar teeth and the adjacent gingival tissue.

In the radiograph, the mandibular canal appears as a dark or radiolucent ribbon between two white lines. It passes in a downward and forward direction (Fig. 3–62). In the region of the mental foramen, the inferior alveolar nerve bifurcates into its terminal branches, the incisive and mental nerves. The incisive canal is sometimes seen on a radiograph (Fig. 3–63).

The relationship of the mandibular canal with teeth that are to be removed or with pathologic lesions that are to be excised is important. The mandibular canal is in close proximity to the third molar roots if a dark band is seen crossing the roots (Figs. 3–64 and 3–65), and if a constriction of the canal can be seen (Figs. 3–66 and 3–67). Sometimes, the canal appears as an interrupted outline as it crosses the root of the tooth; this feature indicates a close proximity of the mandibular canal to the root of the tooth (Fig. 3–68).

REFERENCES

Barabas GM: The Ehlers-Danlos syndrome. Br Dent J 126:509, 1969.

Hill TJ: Pathology of the dental pulp. J Am Dent Assoc 21:820, 1934.

Roper-Hall HT: Br Dent J Oct. 24–25, 1938.

Shields ED, Bixler P, El-Kafawy AM: A proposed classification for heritable human dentin effects with a description of a new entity. Arch Oral Biol 18:543, 1973.

Chapter 4

Normal Panoramic Anatomy

A CONCEPTUAL APPROACH TO UNDERSTANDING THE PANORAMIC IMAGE

Certain peculiarities of the panoramic system result in a unique projection of many anatomic structures in the image. This produces numerous anatomic relationships in the image that are not found in any other kind of radiographic projection. These peculiarities must be understood as part of the process of learning normal structural relationships; otherwise, it would be impossible to accurately interpret pathologic conditions as they differ from normal structures.

Over the past decade or so, we have developed a conceptual approach to understanding the panoramic image. We have found that most peculiarities of normal structural relationships can be explained by one or more of the following seven concepts. For example, consider the following questions: Why is the cervical spine sometimes seen or not seen in the image? Because the spine is in the midline, halfway between the two rami of the jaws, why does it show up posterior to the right and left rami bilaterally? Why does the spine sometimes produce a ghost that ends up in the midline of the image? These and other similar questions can be answered by the application of one or more of these several concepts.

Concept 1: Structures are Flattened and Spread Out (Fig. 4–1)

This concept states that the jaws and structures of the maxillofacial complex, as well as the spine, are portrayed as if they were split vertically in half down the midsagittal plane, with each half folded outward such that the nose remains in the middle, the right and left sides of the jaws are on each side of the film, and the spine, having been split in half, appears beyond the rami at the extreme right and left hand edges of the film. This simple explanation should suffice for the novice, but it is strictly limited to the understanding of this first concept. As we describe other concepts, it will be seen that specifics of the projection geometry are responsible for this effect. In some instances, this feature of the panoramic projection produces desirable results; however, sometimes undesirable effects are also seen.

The first desirable effect is our understanding that the midline of the film corresponds to the anterior midline of the patient and that the right and left hand edges of the film correspond to the posterior midline of the patient. The second desirable effect is that we can see the right and left halves of the jaws and maxillofacial complex side by side on the film without one half being superimposed on the other and without the distortions that normally occur in plain films when one side is projected out of the image, as in the lateral jaw view. Thus, we can easily study the teeth, mandible, nasal fossa, maxillary sinus, zygomatic bone/arch, and maxilla without one side being superimposed on the other (Fig. 4–1A).

In this concept, we refer to the formation of "real" images, as opposed to "ghost" images. Further, we have subdivided real images into "single" and "double" images. To understand the differences between real and ghost images and single and double real images, an understanding of the following two concepts is needed.

Undesirable effects of this concept occur when the patient is improperly positioned in the machine. For example, when the patient's chin is tipped too low and the patient is positioned a little back in the machine, the hyoid bone is spread out and projected up, right on top of the mandible. In the same way, the turbinate and meatus of the nose are spread out and projected across the maxillary sinus (Fig. 4–1B). To explain why these undesirable effects occur, one needs to understand the second concept.

Concept 2: Midline Structures May Project as Single Images and Double Images (Figs. 4–2 to 4–6)

A real image is formed when the object is located between the rotation center of the beam and the film (Fig. 4–2). An object is portrayed with minimal unsharpness and distortion when it is close to the plane at the center of the layer. On the other hand, it is portrayed with considerable unsharpness and distortion when it is far away from this focal plane or trough. In either case, the image is "real" as long as it depicts an object located between the rotation center and the film. The regions where real images are formed relative to typical continuous movement patterns are shown in Figure 4–3.

In the central portion of the oral and maxillofacial region is a zone where points are intercepted twice by the beam. In the diagram (Fig. 4–3), this area is dotted and diamond shaped and corresponds to the patient's midline from about the middle of the image to the most posterior extent of the radiograph. A double image is a pair of real images formed by an object lying within these zones. An example of a double image is shown in Figure 4–4. Here, a single radiopaque tube inserted in the nasal passage appears in two locations (double real images) on the panoramic radiograph.

The structural configuration of such double images may

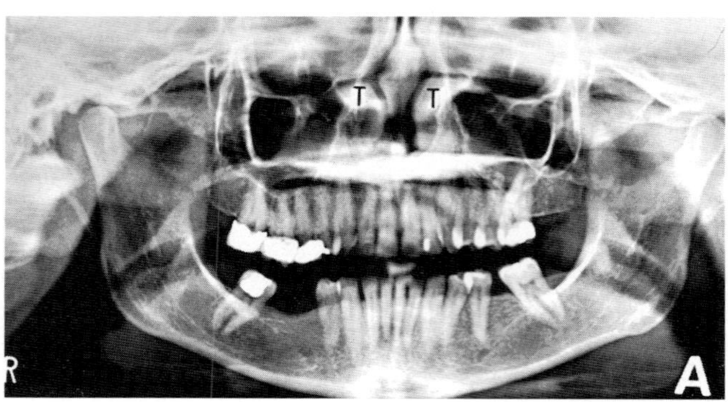

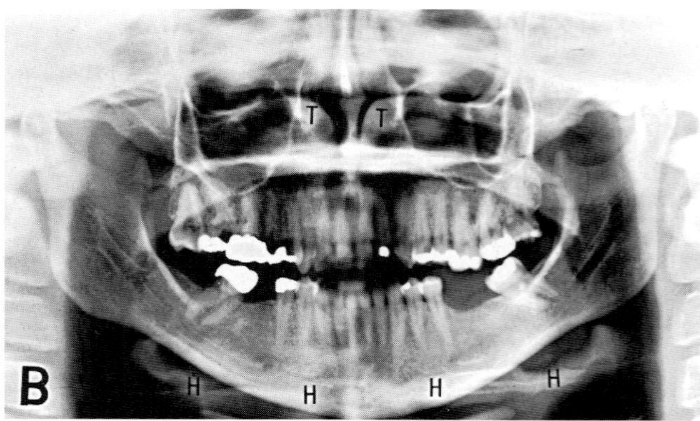

FIGURE 4–1.

Concept 1. Structures are flattened and spread out: A, Notice that the soft tissue of the inferior turbinate (T) and the air space (meatus) around it is entirely within the nasal fossa. B, The soft tissue shadow of the inferior turbinate (T) is spread out across the maxillary sinus. In addition, the hyoid bone (H) is spread out across the inferior portion of the mandible. These undesirable effects can be avoided by proper patient positioning. Note the narrow mandibular anterior teeth.

be understood by examining the sequence in which the beam intersects an object during its projection onto the film. Figure 4–5 shows the formation of the double image of two adjacent points A and B. In the formation of the first image, the beam first intercepts A and then B. On the opposite side of the scan, B is intercepted before A. The result is that double images are reversed with respect to one another. Some examples of structures that produce double images are the hard palate, the palatal tori, the body of the hyoid bone, and the epiglottis (Fig. 4–6). When the patient is positioned too far back in the machine, the turbinates and meatus enter the diamond area, and double images are produced. These spread across the maxillary sinus. The same may be said for the greater horns of the hyoid bone, which are spread across the mandible. When the patient is positioned too far forward, the spine enters the diamond area and is projected as a double image on the film (see Fig. 4–5C); it is sometimes superimposed on the styloid process, ramus, and temporomandibular joint areas. Thus, the undesirable effects of concepts 1 and 2 result from patient positioning errors by the operator.

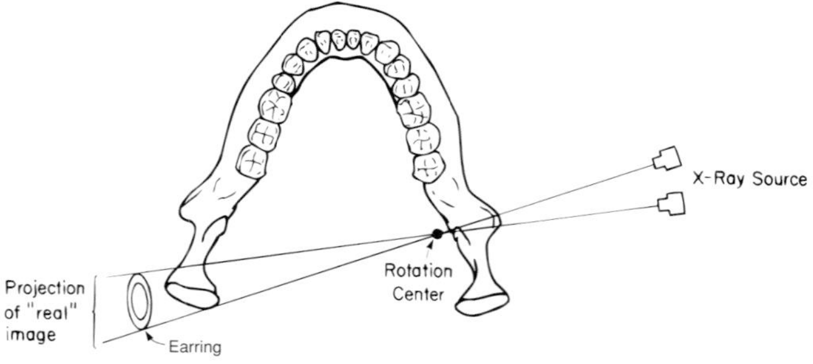

FIGURE 4–2.

Real Images: Formation of the real image of an earring. The earring is located between the rotation center of the beam and the film. (From Langland OE, et al: Panoramic Radiology. 2nd Ed. Philadelphia:Lea & Febiger, 1989, p.185.)

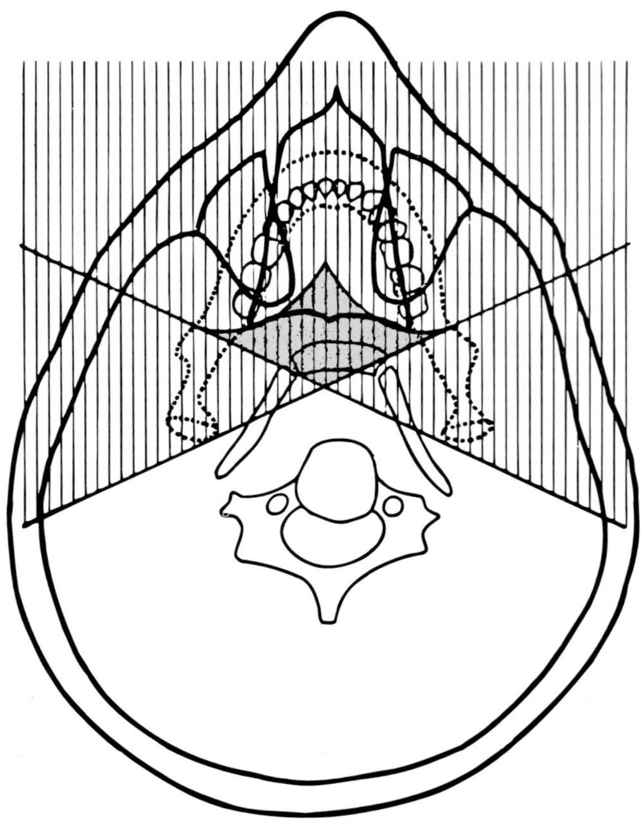

FIGURE 4–3.

Region Where Real Images Are Formed: The zone where real images are formed when a continuous movement pattern is used (vertical hatch marks). Double images are formed in the central diamond-shaped region (shaded pattern). (From Langland OE, et al: Panoramic Radiology. 2nd Ed. Philadelphia:Lea & Febiger, 1989, p. 186.)

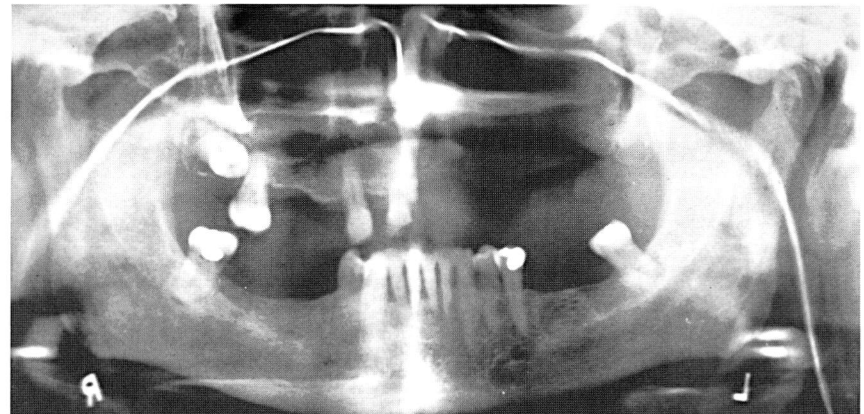

FIGURE 4–4.

Double Image: Double image of a single radiopaque tube inserted into the right nasal passage. (From Langland OE, et al: Panoramic Radiology. 2nd Ed. Philadelphia:Lea & Febiger, 1989, p. 186.)

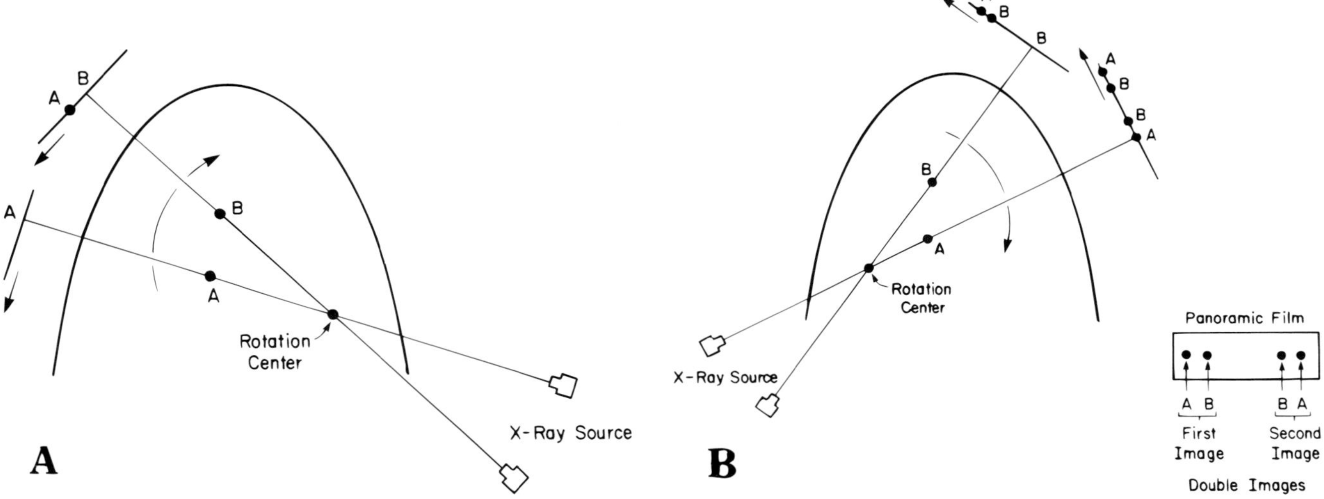

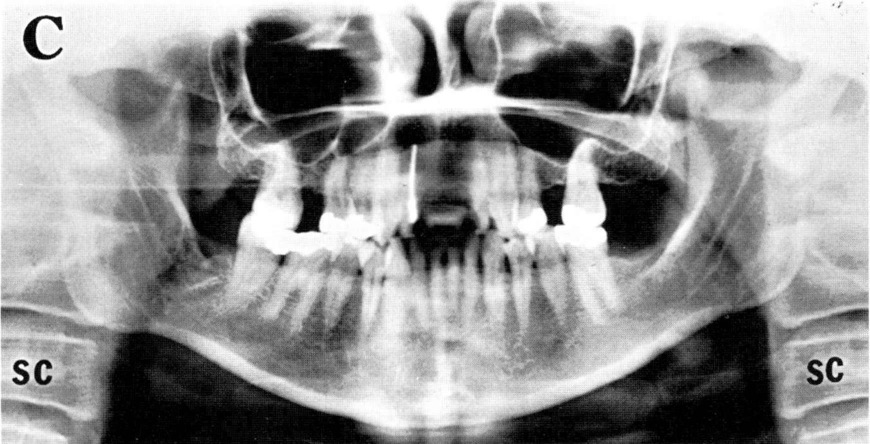

FIGURE 4–5.

Double Images: Formation of double images of points A and B. A, Formation of double images of points A and B; formation of the first image. B, Formation of double real images of points A and B; formation of the second image. C, Double real images of the spinal column (SC) caused by positioning the patient too far forward. (A and B, From Langland OE, et al: Panoramic Radiology. 2nd Ed. Philadelphia:Lea & Febiger, 1989, p. 187.)

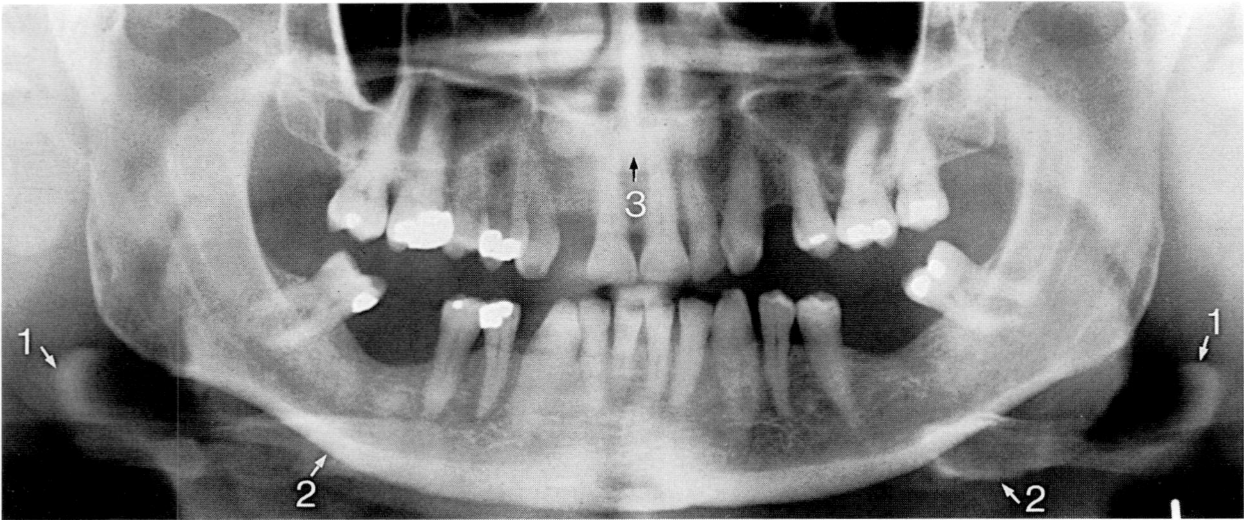

FIGURE 4–6.

Double real images: Epiglottis (1), hyoid bone (2). Both are in the midline and fall in the diamond area. Note the single real image of the nose, which is in the midline of the patient, but does not fall in the diamond area (3). (From Langland OE, et al: Panoramic Radiology. 2nd Ed. Philadelphia:Lea & Febiger, 1989, p. 188.)

Concept 3: Ghost Images are Formed (Figs. 4–7 to 4–18)

A ghost image is formed when the object is located between the x-ray source and the center of rotation (Fig. 4–7). The radiograph in Figure 4–8A shows two ghosted earrings. Each ''ghost'' corresponds to the earring on the opposite side. The regions satisfying the preceding requirement for the formation of ghost images are shown in Figure 4–9. Structures situated within this region can appear as ghosts,

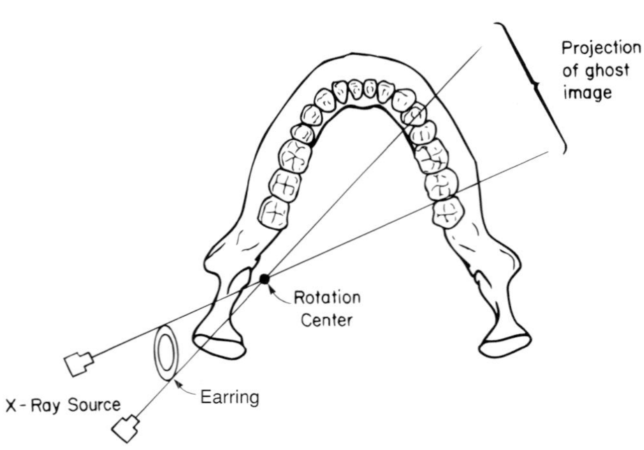

FIGURE 4–7.

Ghost Images: Formation of the ghost image of an earring. The earring is now located between the x-ray source and the center of rotation. (From Langland OE, et al: Panoramic Radiology. 2nd Ed. Philadelphia:Lea & Febiger, 1989, p. 188.)

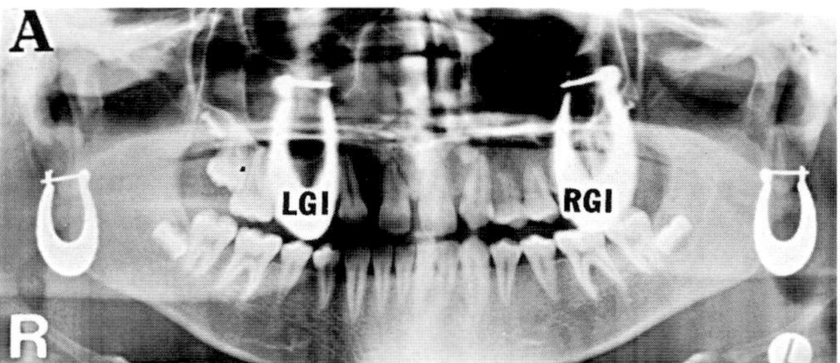

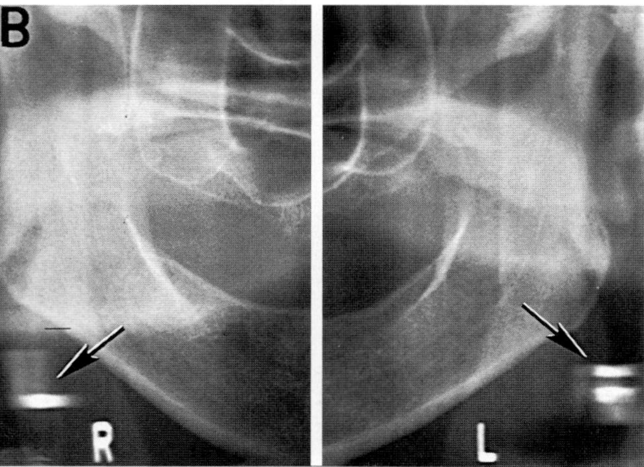

FIGURE 4–8.

Ghost Images: A, Radiograph containing ghost images of two earrings LGI, Left ghost image of the left real image; RGI, right ghost image of the right real image. B, The vertical component of the right and left ghost images (arrows) is more blurred (effaced) than the horizontal component. In addition, the ghost images of the right and left markers are magnified and appear higher than their real counterparts.

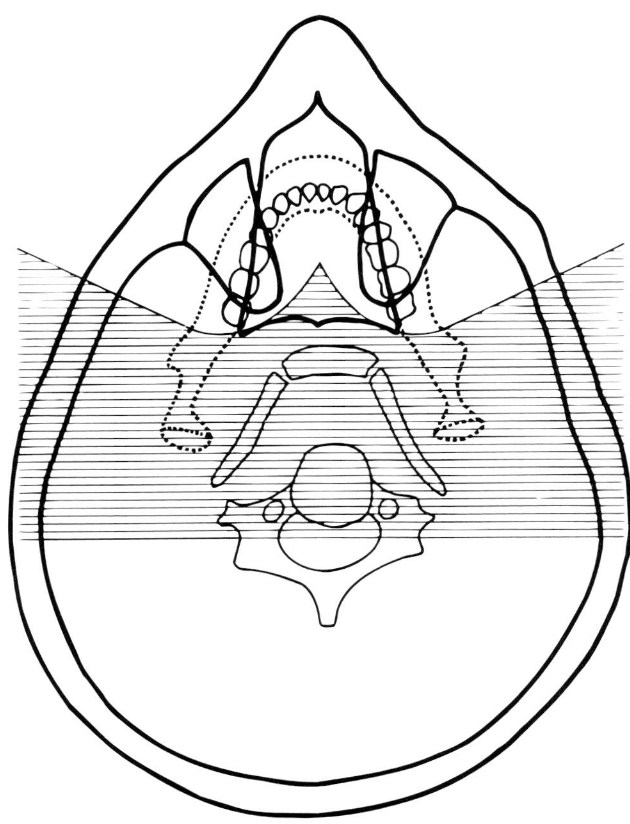

FIGURE 4–9.

Ghost Images: The region where ghost images are formed when a continuous movement pattern is used (horizontal hatch marks). (From Langland OE, et al: Panoramic Radiology. 2nd Ed. Philadelphia:Lea & Febiger, 1989, p. 189.)

whereas structures situated elsewhere cannot. Ghost images have the following characteristics:

1. The ghost image has the same morphology as its real counterpart.
2. The ghost image appears on the opposite side of the radiograph from its real counterpart.
3. The ghost image appears higher up on the radiograph than its real counterpart.
4. The ghost image is more blurred than its real counterpart.
5. The vertical component of a ghost image is more blurred than the horizontal component.
6. The vertical component of a ghost image is always larger than its real counterpart, whereas the horizontal component of a ghost image may or may not be severely magnified.

Each of these characteristics of ghost images is discussed in the paragraphs that follow.

Figure 4–10 shows the formation of a single real image and a ghost image of two adjacent points located in the lateral portion of the ghosting zone. In this example, the real image is formed first, the beam initially intercepting A and then B. The result is that structures appearing as ghosts retain the same morphology as their real counterparts. Although they are displaced, blurred, and magnified, their internal configuration remains the same. Thus, the ghost images of the right and left markers are still recognizable as an R and an L, respectively, but the vertical component of the R and L ghost images is more blurred than the horizontal component (see Fig. 4–8B). Moreover, the ghost image appears on the reverse side of the radiograph from its real counterpart.

In the vertical dimension, the ghost image invariably appears higher than the real image, because structural details lying between the radiation source and the rotation center are projected at higher levels than structural details at the same height, which lie between the rotation center and the film (Fig. 4–11).

For objects between the x-ray source and the rotation center (objects producing ghost images), blurring is especially severe, because the images and the film are actually moving in opposite directions relative to the beam (Fig. 4–12). This results in the extreme blurring seen in ghost images. Double real images are always blurred because they

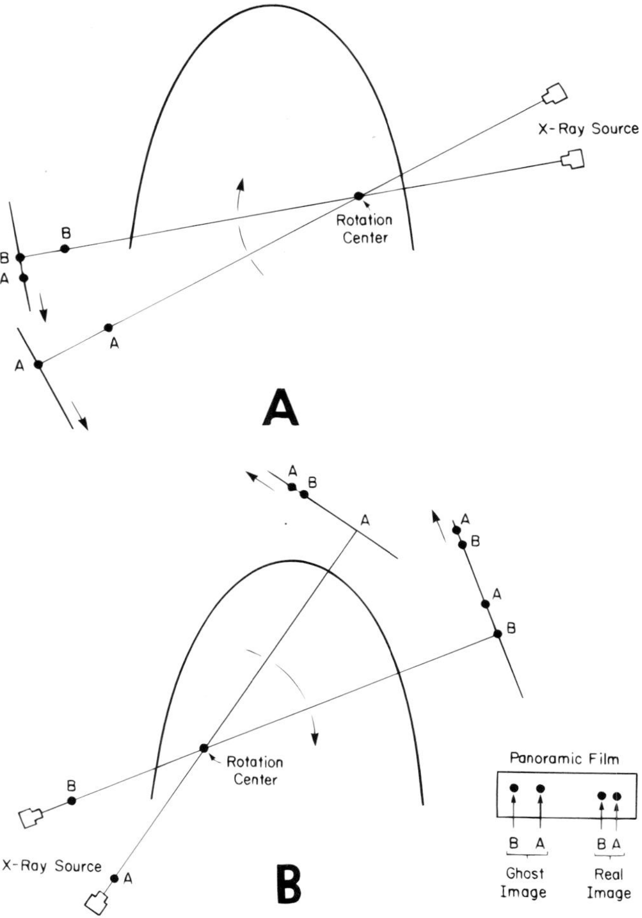

FIGURE 4–10.

Real Images and Ghost Images: A, Formation of real images of points A and B. B, Formation of ghost images of points A and B. (A and B, From Langland OE, et al: Panoramic Radiology. 2nd Ed. Philadelphia:Lea & Febiger, 1989, p. 190.)

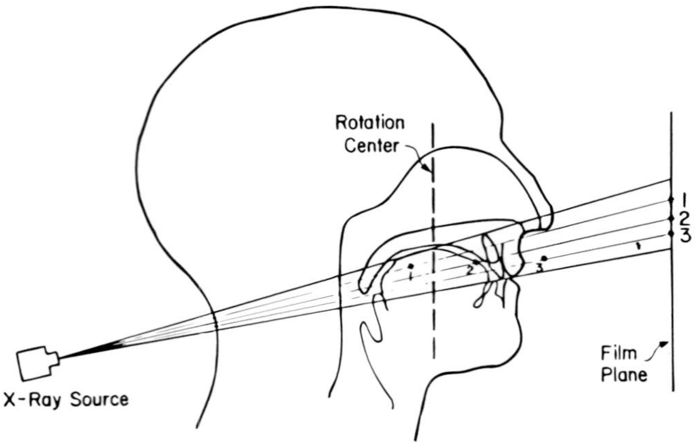

FIGURE 4–11.

Ghost Images: Because the x-ray beam is directed from below, posterior features are projected higher than anterior features at the same height. (From Langland OE, et al: Panoramic Radiology. 2nd Ed. Philadelphia:Lea & Febiger, 1989, p. 191.)

correspond to a region between the rotation center and the central plane of the image layer.

Narrow structures are more severely affected by motion blurring than wide structures because the shadow of a narrow structure, moving a distance with respect to the film that is large relative to its width, has its density "spread out." A wide object, on the other hand, moving a distance with respect to the film that is less than its own width, overlaps itself as it is radiographed, with the result that only the extremes are blurred. This is seen in the ghost images of the right and left markers in Figure 4–8B. The vertical, narrow details almost are effaced from sight, whereas the horizontal, wide details are clearly portrayed, but are elongated.

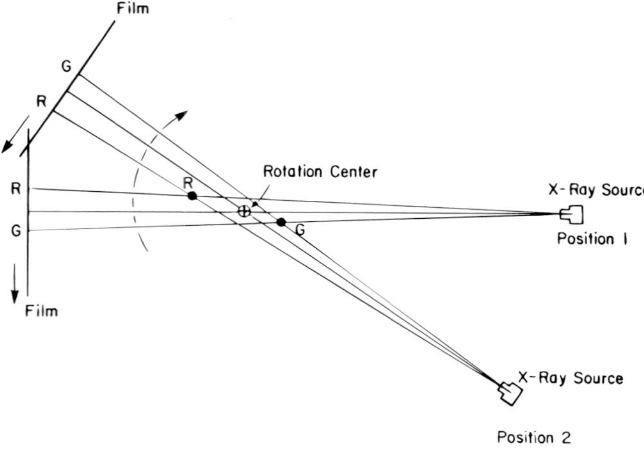

FIGURE 4–12.

Real and Ghost Images: The projected shadow at point R in the real image zone moves in the same direction as the film, relative to the beam. The projected shadow of point G in the ghost image zone moves in the opposite direction as the film, relative to the beam. (From Langland OE, et al: Panoramic Radiology. 2nd Ed. Philadelphia:Lea & Febiger, 1989, p. 192.)

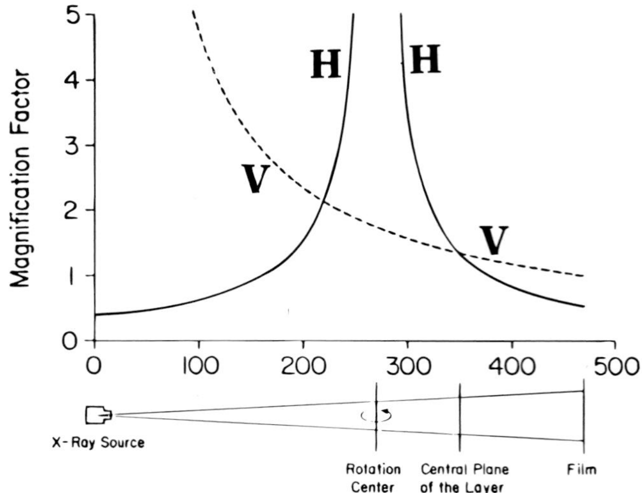

FIGURE 4–13.

Magnification Factors: Typical horizontal (H) and vertical (V) magnification factors in rotational panoramic radiography as a function of distance from the rotation source. Where the lines meet at the central plane of the layer, the horizontal and vertical dimensions of the image on the film are proportional. (From Langland OE, et al: Panoramic Radiology. 2nd Ed. Philadelphia:Lea & Febiger, 1989, p. 192.)

Panoramic radiographs are characterized by different magnification factors for horizontal and vertical dimensions. The magnification factors in the two dimensions are equal for those structures lying in the sharply depicted plane at the center of the layer (Fig. 4–13). The vertical magnification factor increases continually as an object is moved closer and closer to the x-ray source. The horizontal factor also increases and does so faster than the vertical magnification. As a result, objects appear too wide when they are displaced towards the source. Because double images in continuous systems are formed in the region between the rotation center and the plane at the center of the layer, they always appear widened. Further on in the same direction, the horizontal magnification factor increases greatly close to the rotation center of the beam. This results in images that are markedly widened whenever the object is intercepted by the rotation center. On the other side of the rotation center, in the region where ghost images are formed, the horizontal magnification factor decreases again. At one position on this side, once again the horizontal and vertical magnification factors are equal. These complex relationships explain why it is not easy to predict what kind of distortion will be seen in a ghost image. In the vertical dimension, a ghost image always appears larger than its real counterpart. The horizontal dimension may be more or less magnified than the vertical dimension, depending on the location of the object between the center of rotation and the x-ray source. This is further complicated by the fact that, in the horizontal dimension, the image is affected by both magnification and the blurring effects.

Anatomic structures that are often ghosted include the

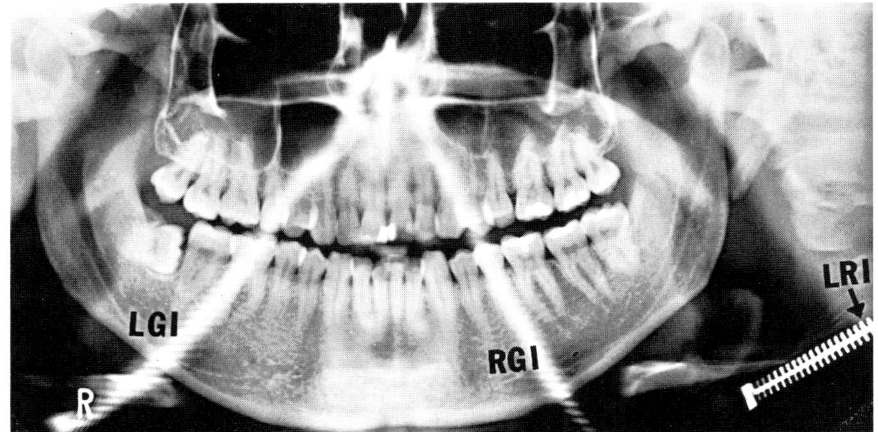

FIGURE 4–14.

Real and Ghost Images: Note the real image of a coat zipper on the patient's left side (LRI). The ghost image of the zipper (LGI) on the left is seen on the patient's right and is projected toward the image of the patient's nasal fossae. The real coat zipper image on the patient's right is not seen, but the right ghost image (RGI) of the zipper is seen on the patient's left.

hyoid bone, the cervical spine, the inferior border of the mandible, the posterior border of the ramus, the condyles, and the turbinates. Other objects that create ghost images are the chin rest and right and left markers of some machines, as well as earrings, napkin chains, neck chains, and the shoulder straps of protective aprons. If such an object is intercepted by the portion of the beam between the rotation center and the film, the ghost will have a real counterpart. This may or may not be visible depending on the distance to the central plane of the layer and on the contrast of the object. An example is seen in Figure 4–14, where the patient's right coat zipper is visible as a ghost but not as a real image. The left zipper, on the other hand, gave rise to both real and ghost images. The difference was simply the region of the horizontal plane within which the two zippers were positioned. Note that napkin chains, coat zippers, neck chains, earrings, and improper apron placement can all produce ghost images, which can be eliminated by proper preparation of the patient before taking the radiograph. When the patient is slumped in the machine, the patient's spine enters the diamond area, and a ghost image is produced in the midline of the film (Fig. 4–15). This error can be avoided by proper patient positioning.

To understand the differences among these last three concepts, study Figure 4–16A, which is a composite diagram showing the areas giving rise to single and double real images and ghost images. Note that two areas in the horizontal plane contain structural details that project only real or ghost images, as the case may be. This diagram depicts the properly positioned patient. Where only vertical hatch marks are seen, structures such as the body of the mandible, the teeth, and the antrum may only produce real images. In the area of the horizontal hatch marks, the spine, neck chains, and the greater horns of the hyoid bone may produce only ghost images. The projection geometry of most machines is such that these latter ghosts are not usually projected onto the

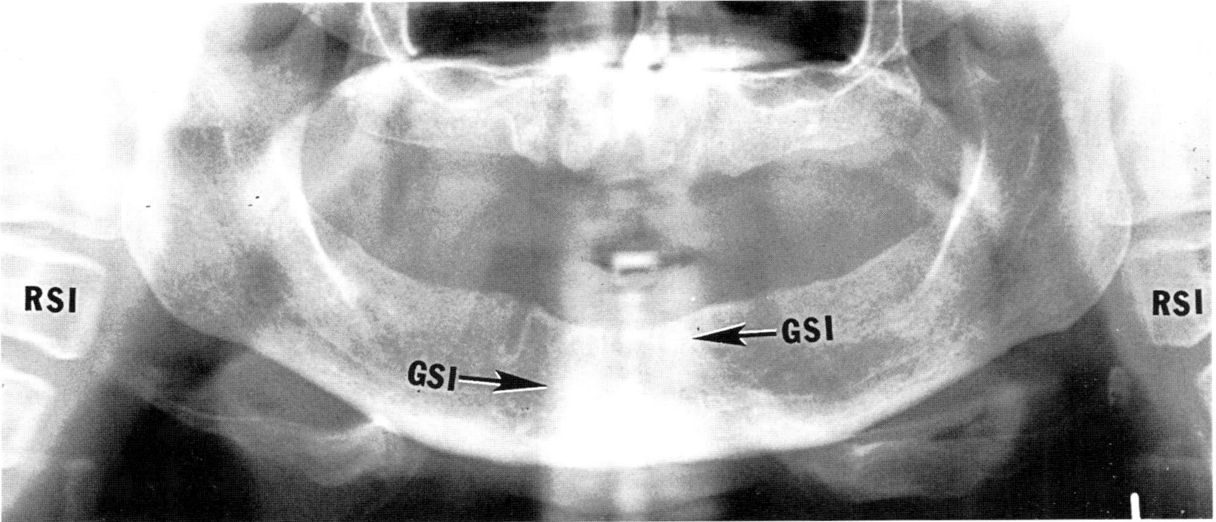

FIGURE 4–15.

Ghost Image of the Spine: The shadow of the ghost image of the spine (GSI) is in the middle of the image, especially the lower two thirds of the radiograph. A double real image (RSI) of the spine in the slumped position (not straight) can be seen at the right and left edges of the image. (From Langland OE, et al: Panoramic Radiology. 2nd Ed. Philadelphia:Lea & Febiger, 1989, p. 193.)

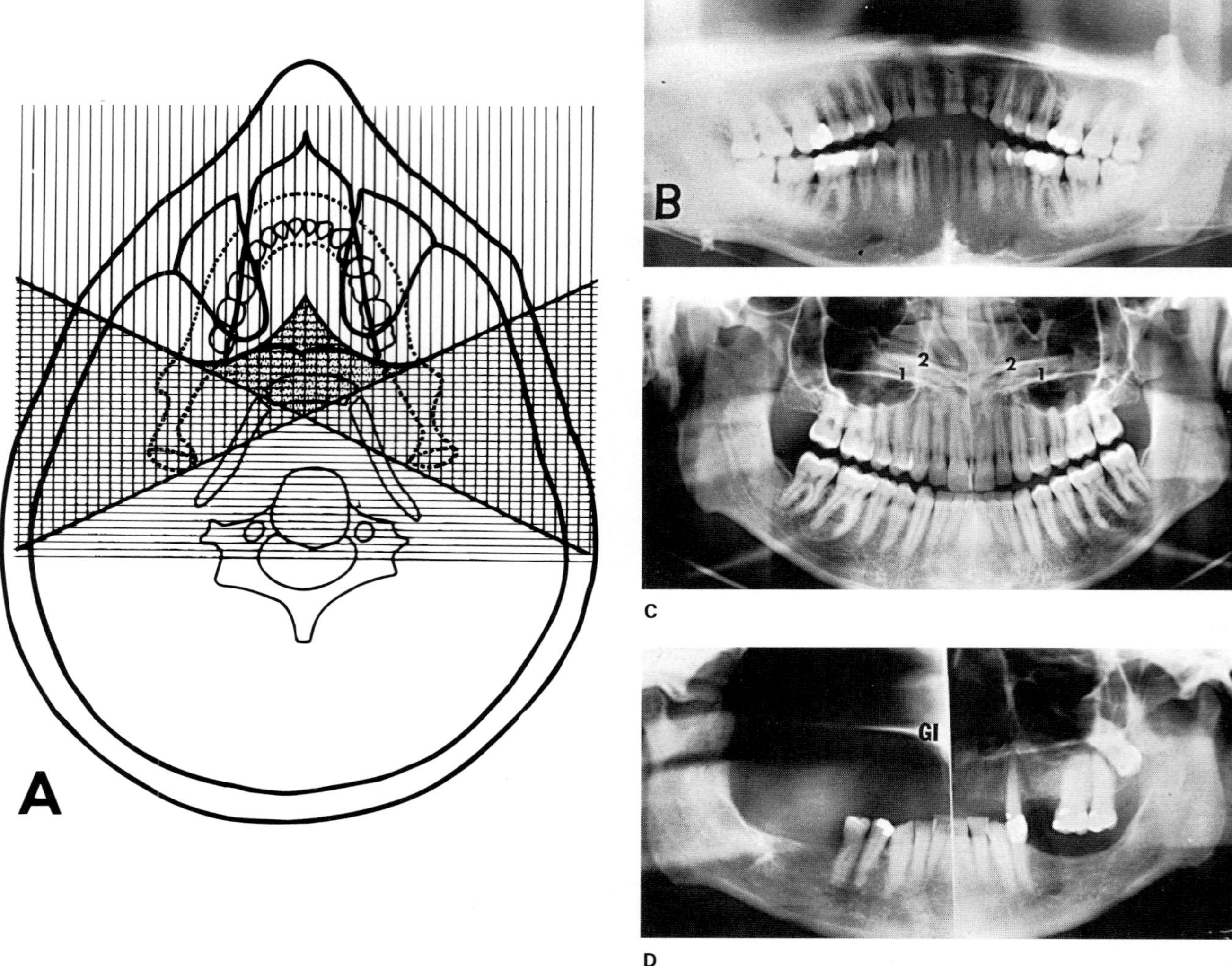

FIGURE 4–16.

Real and Ghosted Images: A, Composite diagram showing the zones giving rise to real (single and double) and ghost images in continuous image machines. The zones are marked as in the previous figures. (From Langland OE, et al: Panoramic Radiology. 2nd Ed. Philadelphia:Lea & Febiger, 1989, p. 194.) B, Note the ghosted condyles on this panoramic radiograph of a dry specimen of the mandible and maxilla. C, Real hard palate image (1) and ghost images of contralateral portions of the hard palate (2). D, Ghost image of the hard palate. This panoramic radiograph is of patient with a previous right maxillectomy (no hard palate); however, notice the ghosted image (GI) of the real hard palate on the left.

image. In the "X" area where vertical and horizontal hatch marks are seen, both single real and ghost images of the structures included therein may be produced in the same image. These include the greater horns of the hyoid bone, the ramus/condyle (Fig. 4–16B) of the mandible, and earrings. In the diamond area, real double and ghost images may be produced. Examples include the body of the hyoid bone (see Fig. 4–27), the epiglottis, and the posterior aspect of the hard palate (Fig. 4–16C and D). To further illustrate this phenomenon, we placed a napkin chain in a panoramic machine, as seen in Figure 4–17. The resulting radiograph may be seen in Figure 4–18. Using Figures 4–17 and 4–18, begin at the bottom of the radiograph in the midline. We see that the most anterior parts of the chain are projected as a single image, which is within the layer. The first two or three spheres appear round, however, because the chain is in the central plane of the layer. The next five or six spheres become more and more widened. As the chain enters the

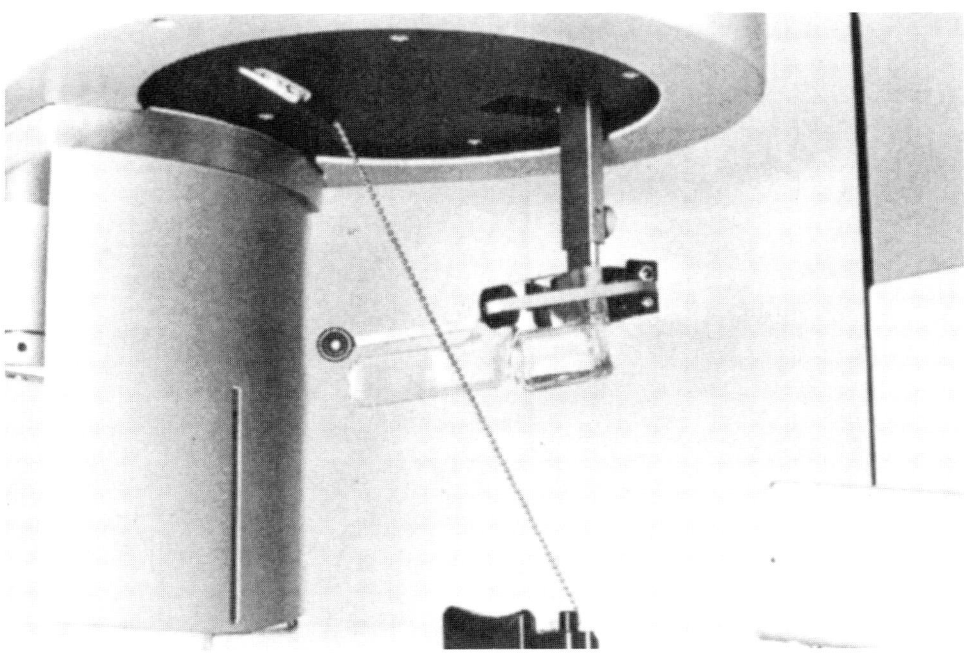

FIGURE 4–17.

Ghost Image: A napkin chain positioned in the Siemens OP5 so it passes along the midline, through the various zones in the center of the patient depicted in the diagram in Figure 4–16. (From Langland OE, et al: Panoramic Radiology. 2nd Ed. Philadelphia:Lea & Febiger, 1989, p. 195.)

area corresponding to the anterior part of the diamond, a double real image is seen on either side of the midline, and at the same time a ghost image is seen in the middle. Because the chain was positioned superiorly toward the posterior, its image moves up on the film toward the posterior portions of the image of the right and left sides. The chain was positioned in the midline, so it did not enter the "X" area shown in Figure 4–16A where it may have produced single real and ghost images, such as in the case of earrings. Because the "ghosting only" zone does not normally fall within the beam of radiation, there was no corresponding "ghost-only" image of the chain.

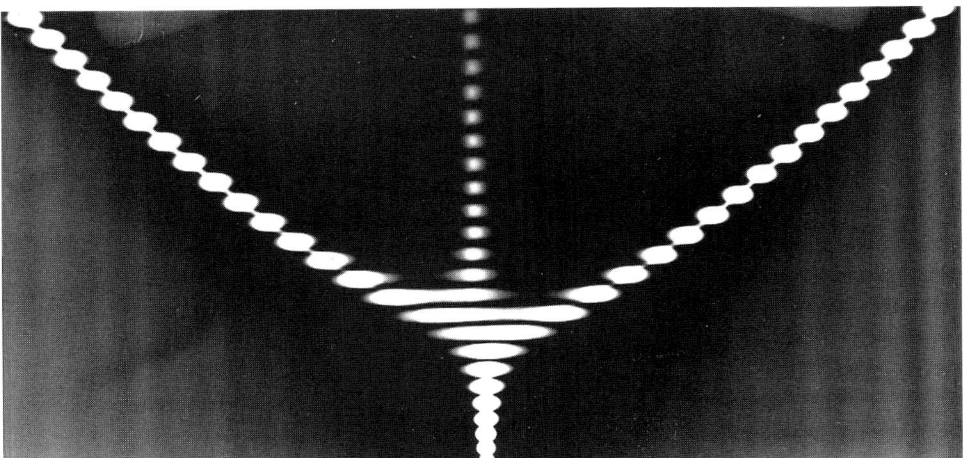

FIGURE 4–18.

Ghost Image: A single chain positioned in the midline appears different, depending on the zones through which it passes. (From Langland OE, et al: Panoramic Radiology. 2nd Ed. Philadelphia: Lea & Febiger, 1989, p. 195.)

Concept 4: Soft Tissue Outlines are Seen (Fig. 4–19)

One of the unique advantages of panoramic radiology is that some soft tissue structures attenuate the beam of radiation to a sufficient degree to become visible in the radiograph. This is especially true in the posterior and superior regions, where there are no teeth, and in all regions of edentulous patients. We also include fluids and cartilaginous tissues such as the ear, nose, and epiglottis in this concept. Others include the soft palate and uvula, dorsum of the tongue, posterior pharyngeal wall, lips, nasolabial fold and soft tissue of the nasal turbinates, and septum. Additionally the gingiva, retromolar pad, and operculum of erupting teeth may be seen. In some instances, visualization of the tongue, soft palate, lips, and nasal turbinates represents an error in technique (Fig. 4–19).

Concept 5: Air Spaces are Seen (Fig. 4–20)

Some of the air spaces that may be seen include those of the hypopharynx, oropharynx, and nasopharynx, the maxillary sinus, and the nasal fossa. One may also see the mastoid air cells, the external auditory canal, and occasionally, the ethmoid sinuses. If an air space is noted above the dorsum of the tongue, the periapical region of the maxilla will be difficult to interpret. This represents an error in technique and can be avoided by asking the patient to place his or her tongue against the palate while the radiograph is being taken. If an air space is noted in the region of the anterior teeth, the crowns of these teeth will be difficult to interpret. This represents an error in technique and can be avoided by asking the patient to close his or her lips around the bite block during the exposure. Asking the patient to swallow just be-

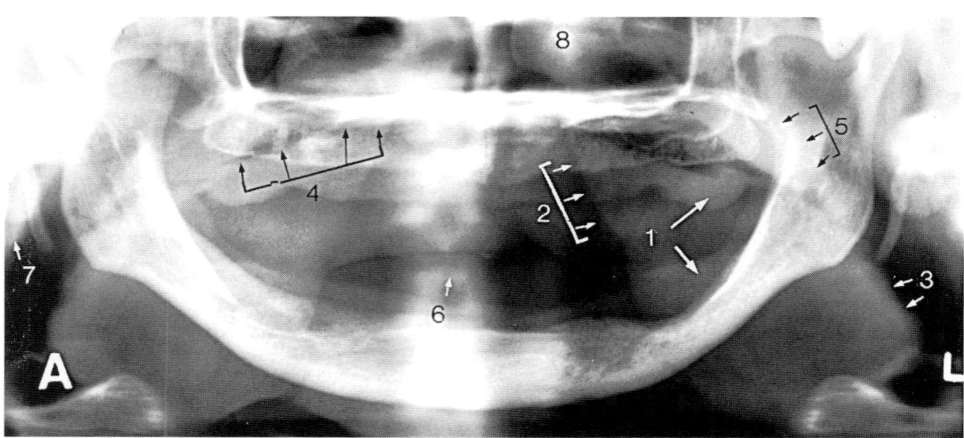

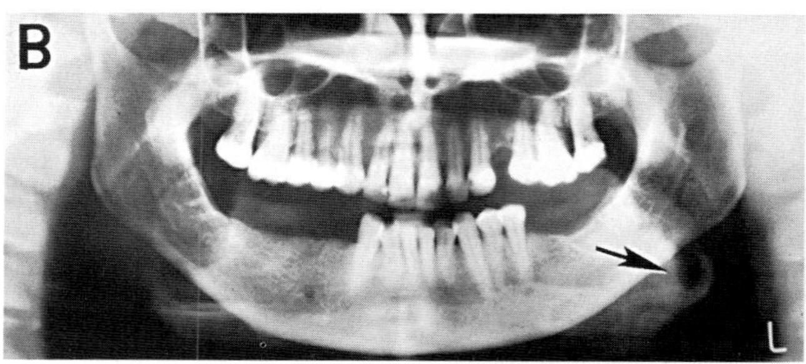

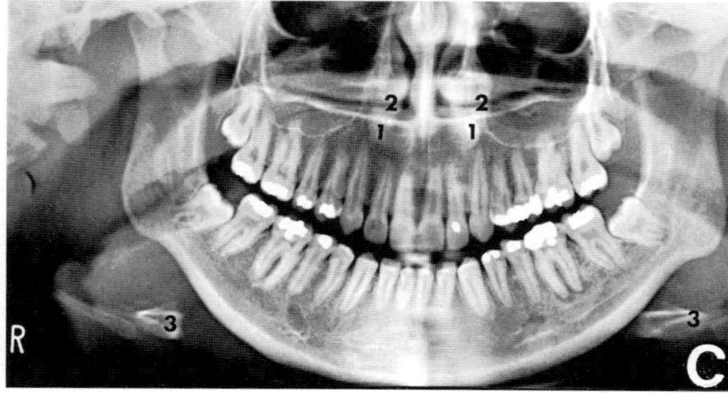

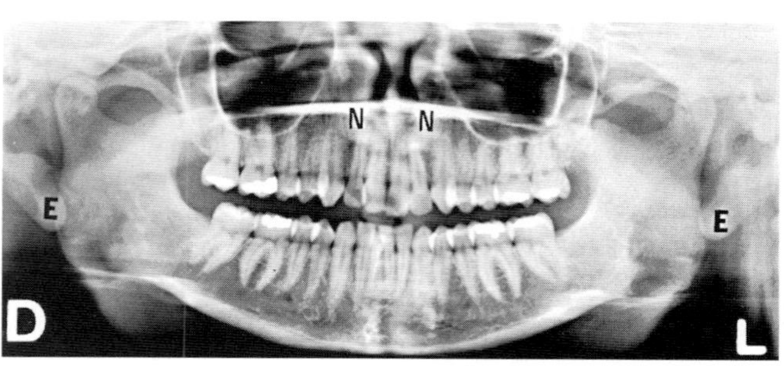

FIGURE 4–19.

Soft Tissue Shadows and Outlines: A, Soft tissue shadows. Soft tissue of the ridge (1); nasolabial fold (2); base of the tongue (3); dorsum of the tongue (4); soft palate (5); lips (6); posterior pharyngeal wall (7); turbinates (8). All these structures may be seen bilaterally. (From Langland OE, et al: Panoramic Radiology. 2nd Ed. Philadelphia:Lea & Febiger, 1989, p. 195.) B, Soft tissue shadows; epiglottis (arrow). C, Soft tissue outlines of nose (1), spreading of the middle meatus across the maxillary sinuses (2), and the double real images of the hyoid bone (3). D, Soft tissue outlines of ear lobes (E) and nose (N).

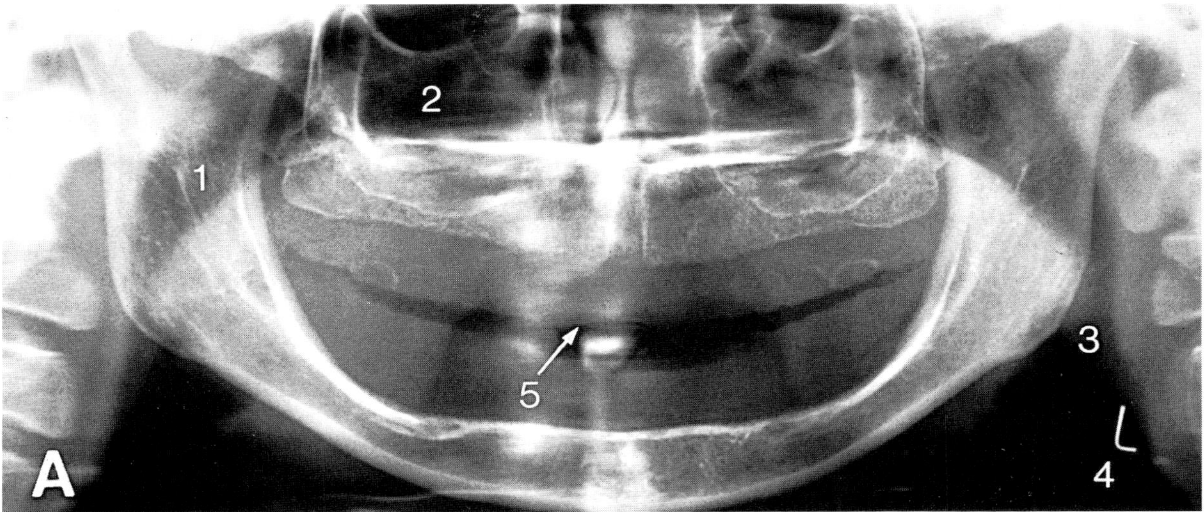

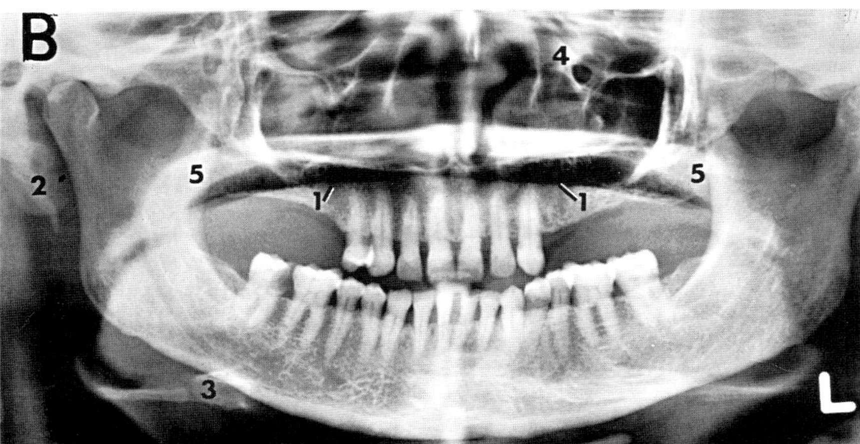

FIGURE 4–20.

Air Spaces: A, Air spaces: nasopharynx (1), maxillary sinus (2), oropharynx (3), hypopharynx (4), air space between the lips (5). Note that the upper and lower dentures are in place and resemble soft tissue in density. (From Langland OE, et al: Panoramic Radiology. 2nd Ed. Philadelphia:Lea & Febiger, 1989, p. 196.) B, Air space above the tongue (1), styloid process (2), hyoid bone (3), infraorbital foramen (4), and soft palate (5).

fore taking the film will usually cause the person to place the tongue against the palate and to close his or her lips. When the soft tissue outlines of the turbinates are projected across the maxillary sinus, the patient probably has been placed too far back in the machine, a position that causes the turbinates to enter the diamond region and produce double images (Fig. 4–20).

Concept 6: Relative Radiolucencies and Radiopacities are Seen (Figs. 4–21 to 4–23)

In any image, it is important to separate shadows originating from parts of the machine from those coming from the patient. Machine components seen in the image are made of plastic, have a density similar to that of soft tissue, and are usually easy to identify because of their geometric or linear configuration. One may think of the patient as being made of three basic components: hard tissue (teeth and bone), soft tissue (including cartilage and fluid), and air. All these machine and patient components may produce single and/or double real images and/or ghost images. If our basic objective is to obtain a single real image of the three patient tissue components, then all other possible shadows must be recognized and mentally subtracted before any added changes due to a pathologic process can be recognized. Thus, multiple areas consisting of relative density changes are produced. If an area of hard tissue is intersected by an air space, it will appear relatively more radiolucent than an adjacent area that is interrupted by a soft tissue shadow. For example, in the ramus area, the outline of the air space of the nasopharynx and oropharynx can be seen because of the soft tissue outline of the dorsum of the tongue and soft palate superimposed on the ramus and the posterior wall of the pharynx on the spine shadow when present. Ghost images and machine components produce further relative density changes.

This concept ties the previous five together and can allow the clinician to use the panoramic radiograph in a meaningful way to detect disease. To obtain the ideal single real image of the patient's three basic tissue components, one must identify all other shadows that can be caused by machine components, double images, and ghosts. If a pathologic process is present, it will consist either of hard tissue or soft tissue and it will affect one or more of the three tissue components in

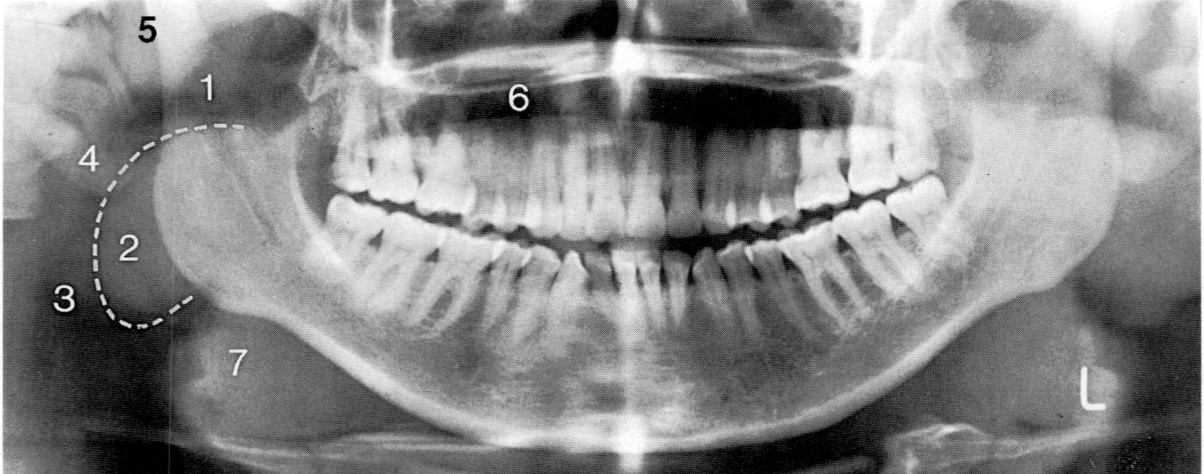

FIGURE 4–21.

Relative Radiolucencies and Radiopacities: The ramus is relatively more radiolucent because of superimposition of the nasopharyngeal air space (1); the oral and nasopharyngeal air spaces are interrupted by a soft tissue mass consisting of a hyperplastic palatine tonsil (2); the air space of the oropharynx (3); the soft tissue of the ear lobe superimposed on the air space of the nasopharynx (4); the hyperplastic adenoid tonsil causes the condylar neck and head to appear relatively radiopaque (5); the artifactual palatoglossal air space obliterates bony details in the apical region of all the upper teeth and represents an error in technique (6); soft tissue of the base of the tongue (7). Note that each numbered item can be seen bilaterally in the image because of either double image formation or paired structures. (From Langland OE, et al: Panoramic Radiology. 2nd Ed. Philadelphia:Lea & Febiger, 1989, p. 197.)

the patient, as follows: Conditions producing hard tissue cause all three patient components to become relatively more radiopaque in the region of the disorder. A soft tissue pathologic condition within the mineralized component causes it to become more radiolucent, whereas the soft tissue and air components become more radiopaque when a soft tissue disorder is present. Thus, when a soft tissue lesion encroaches on an air space such as the nasopharynx or maxillary sinus, it becomes visible as an opacity superimposed on the air space (Fig. 4–21). Note that when errors are present, further relative radiolucencies and opacities may also appear. The recognition of these is essential, to identify and correct operator errors.

Some years ago, a president of the United States was retiring from office. As a part of the administrative process of retiring, the president was scheduled for an extensive physical examination including a dental check-up. Eventually, a panoramic radiograph was taken, and a radiolucency similar to the one in Figure 4–22 was noted at the apices of the lower anterior teeth. There was a sudden flurry of interest and concern for the president, and a bevy of consultants was surreptitiously called in while the examination was completed. Everybody seemed to have differing opinions about the nature of the "lesion," but all agreed that it most certainly appeared to be pathologic. Finally, it was decided that intraoral periapical radiographs should be taken. These radiographs appeared completely normal (Fig. 4–22B). This panoramic pseudoradiolucency occurs in individuals with a prominent depression in the midline of the labial mental area (Fig. 4–23).

Concept 7: Panoramic Radiographs are Unique (Fig. 4–24)

From the discussion of our previous concept, it is obvious that the scope of interpretive potential from panoramic radiographs far exceeds that of the full mouth intraoral survey alone. Even in the study of teeth, angular interrelationships of structures are anatomically accurate in panoramic radiographs. Therefore, the relationships of teeth with each other and with other structures may be studied in treatment planning for crown and bridge abutment tooth parallelism, the path of insertion of partial dentures, the orthodontic tipping of teeth, and the surgical removal of impacted teeth. Because each intraoral film is taken individually, these interrelationships cannot be studied using full mouth intraoral surveys. Our studies have shown that panoramic radiographs are not significantly different from bitewings for the detection of caries. Impacted teeth can be localized as lateral or medial to the central plane in a single panoramic film by observing a widening (lingual) or narrowing (buccal) of their horizontal dimension.

In addition, areas such as the ramus, the styloid process (Fig. 4–24C), the temporomandibular joint, upper portions of the sinus, and the tissues below the jaws all give rise to the many pathologic conditions discussed in the remaining chapters of this book. We describe the radiographic features that distinguish such pathologic disorders as calcified lymph nodes, phleboliths, and sialoliths. We discuss the mucocele and mucous retention cyst as they affect the maxillary sinus. The panoramic radiograph is an excellent resource in patients with trismus or trauma because patients are not

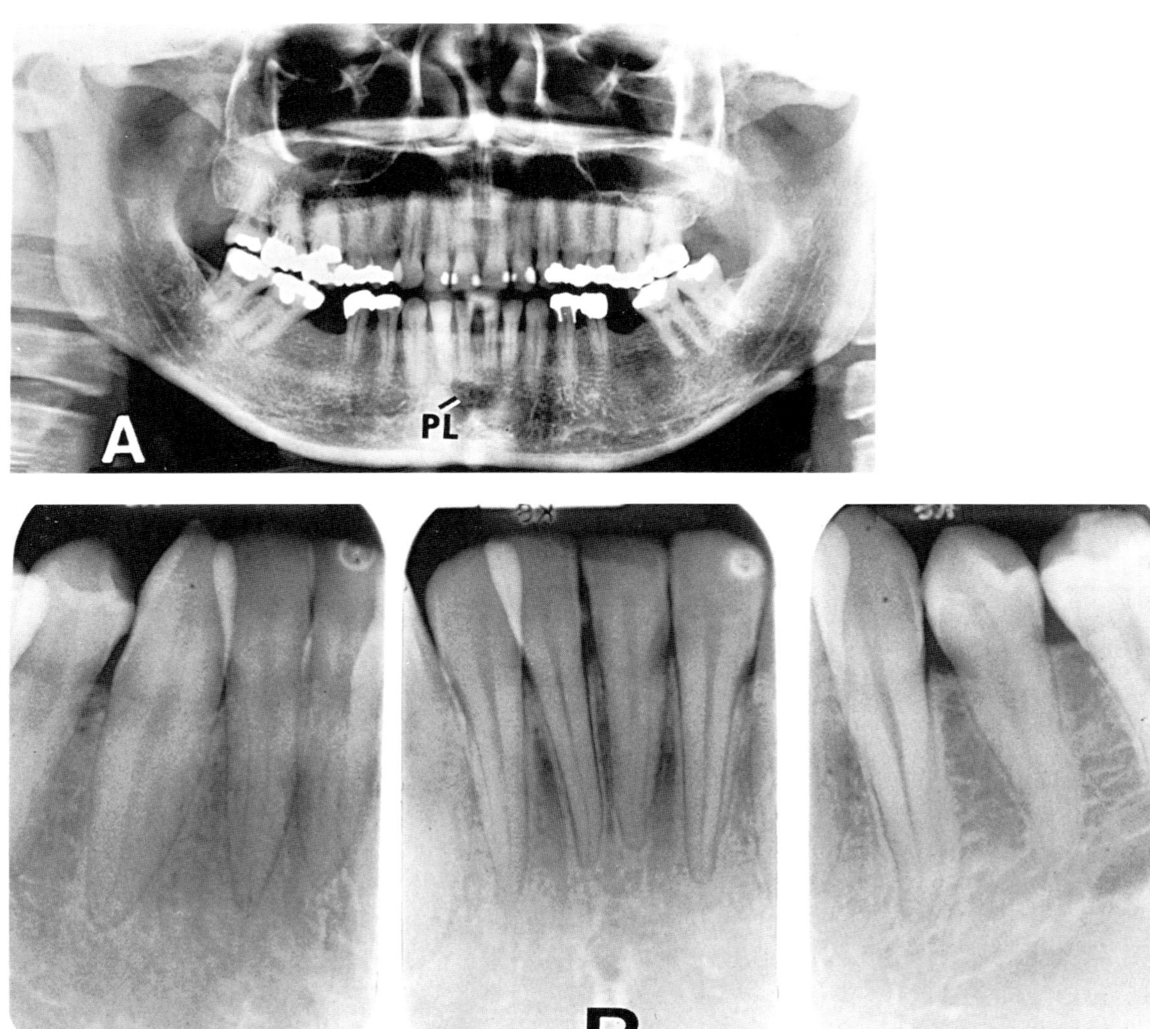

FIGURE 4–22.

"Pseudolesion:" A, Panoramic radiograph of radiolucent "pseudolesion" (PL) at the periapical region of the lower anterior teeth. B, Periapical radiographs of a patient with a radiolucent "pseudolesion" usually reveal a normal condition of the bone in the area where the radiolucency was noted in the panoramic film shown in A. (B, From Langland OE, et al: Panoramic Radiology. 2nd Ed. Philadelphia:Lea & Febiger, 1989, p. 209.)

required to open their mouth for a panoramic film. The uniqueness of the panoramic technique is that it results in an excellent projection of a variety of structures on a single film, which no other imaging system can achieve. Individual structures may be imaged in other ways once pathologic conditions have been detected using the panoramic radiograph (Fig. 4–24).

ATLAS OF ANATOMIC STRUCTURES (Figs. 4–25 to 4–27)

Most clinicians prefer the continuous image. All machines other than the older Panorex machines (SS White) produce continuous images. To obtain a continuous image, the distance between the center of rotation and the teeth is greatly diminished on many machines, thus producing a narrower image layer. Some manufacturers have overcome this compromise to a greater degree than others. In all continuous image machines, care must be taken to position the patient properly and to place the anterior teeth within the central plane of the layer. For this reason, many newer machines have convenient position-indicating light beams that are helpful in diminishing positioning errors. For an atlas of anatomic panoramic structures see Figures 4–25, 4–26 and 4–27.

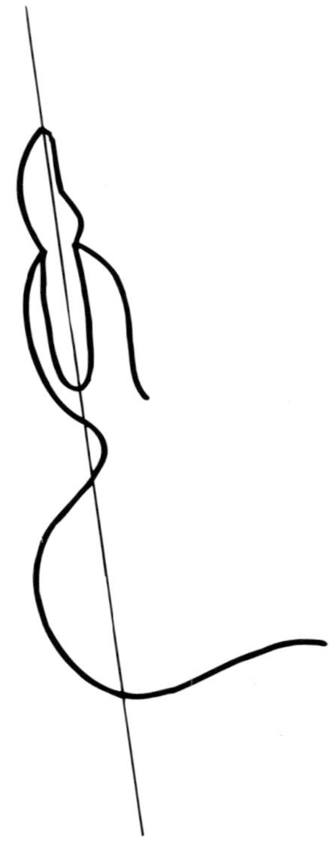

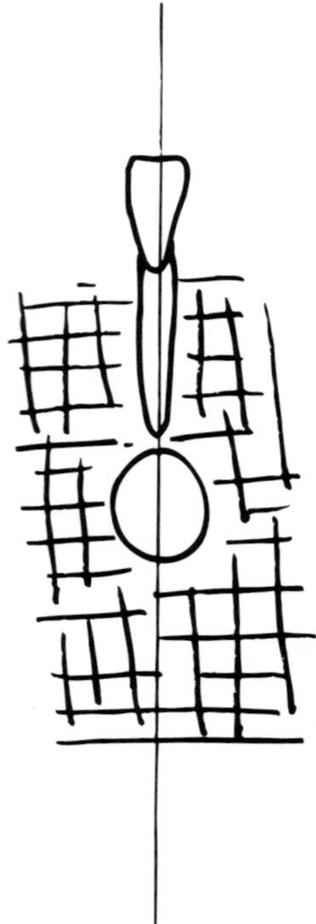

FIGURE 4–23.

Anterior Depression: Schematic drawing illustrating the anterior depression within the central plane of the layer. (From Langland OE, et al: Panoramic Radiology. 2nd Ed. Philadelphia:Lea & Febiger, 1989, p. 210.)

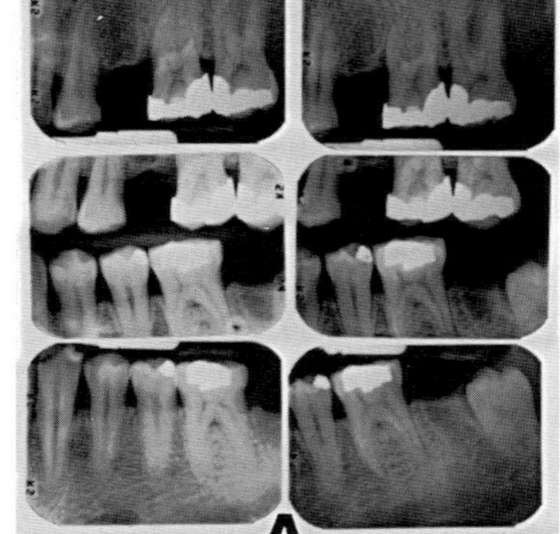

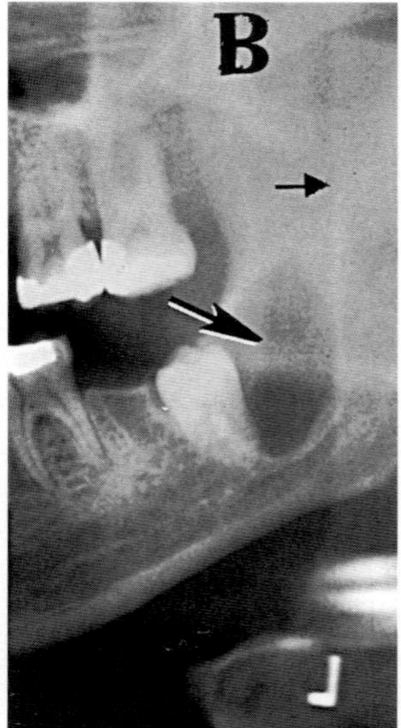

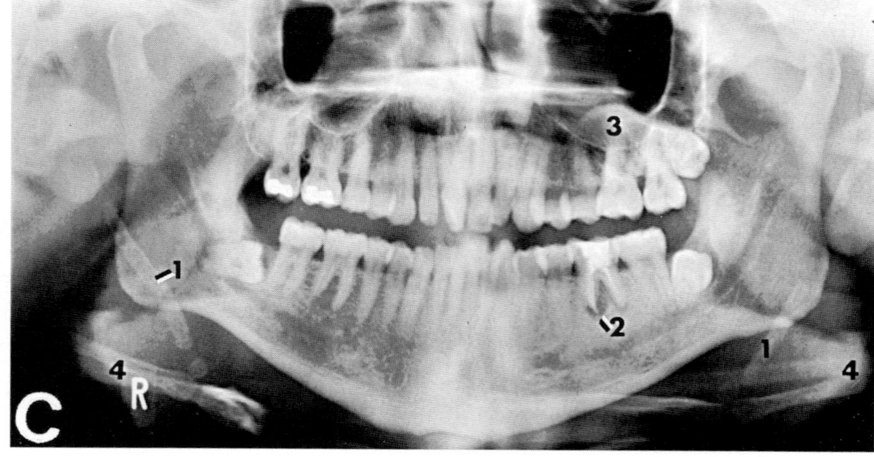

FIGURE 4–24.

The panoramic image is unique: A, The full mouth survey fails to detect the dentigerous cyst. B, Panoramic radiograph of the same patient. Note the relative radiopacity produced by the vertical head positioning bar (upper arrow). C, Bilateral elongated and mineralized stylohyoid ligament complex (1), periapical lesion of lower left first molar previously treated endodontically (2), mucous retention cyst in left maxillary sinus (3), and hyoid bone (4).

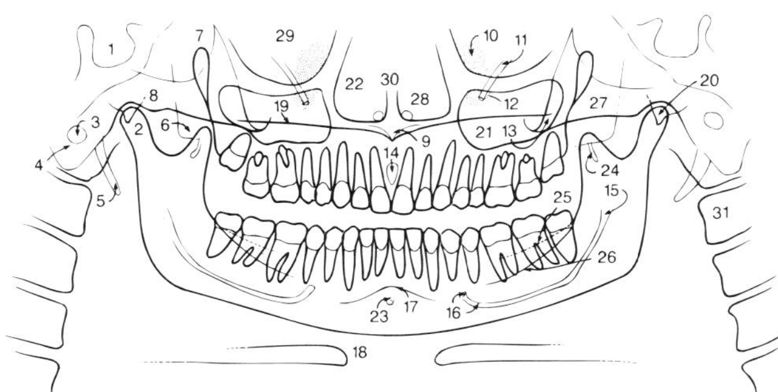

FIGURE 4–25.

Continuous Image: Common anatomic structures: sella turcica (1), mandibular condyle (2), external auditory meatus (3), mastoid process (4), stylohyoid ligament (5), lateral pterygoid plate (6), pterygomaxillary fissure (7), articular eminence (8), anterior nasal spine (9), ethmoid sinuses (10), infraorbital canal (11), infraorbital foramen (12), zygomatic process of the maxilla (13), incisive foramen (14), mandibular foramen (15), mandibular canal and mental foramen (16), mental ridge (17), hyoid bone (18), hard palate (19), spine of the sphenoid bone (20), maxillary sinus (21), nasal fossa (22), genial tubercles (23), hamular process (24), external oblique ridge (25), internal oblique ridge (26), zygomatic arch (27), superior foramen of the incisive canal (28), orbit (29), nasal septum (30), second cervical vertebra (31). (From Langland OE, et al: Panoramic Radiology. 2nd Ed. Philadelphia:Lea & Febiger, 1989, p. 222.)

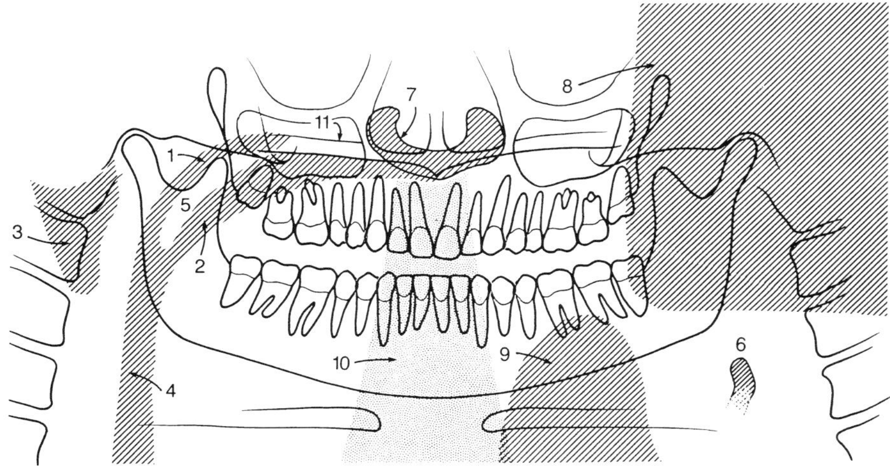

FIGURE 4–26.

Continuous Image: Common soft tissue shadows and areas of radiographic artifact. All artifact areas and shadows are bilateral. Nasopharyngeal air space (1), palatoglossal air space (2), shadow of the ear (3), glossopharyngeal air space (4), soft palate (5), epiglottis (6), soft tissue of the ear (7), ghost image of the contralateral mandible (8), ghost image of an apron too high on the shoulder (9), ghost image of the spine because of the slumped position of the patient (10), ghost image of the contralateral hard palate (11). (From Langland OE, et al: Panoramic Radiology. 2nd Ed. Philadelphia:Lea & Febiger, 1989, p. 222.)

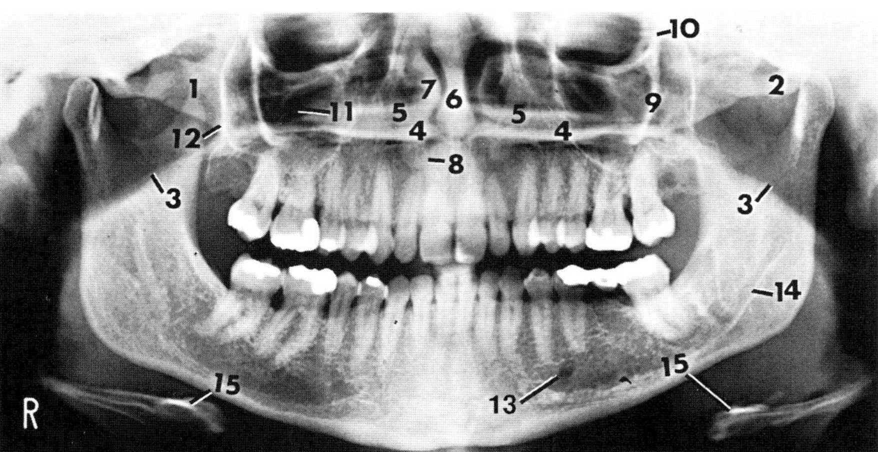

FIGURE 4–27.

Panoramic Radiograph: Common anatomic structures are identified: zygomatic bone (1), zygomatic arch (2), nasopharyngeal air space (3), hard palate (4), ghosts of the hard palate (5), nasal septum (6), turbinate (7), nose (8), zygomatic process of the maxilla forming an innominate line (9) with the frontal process of the zygomatic bone (10), maxillary sinus (11), posterior border of the maxillary sinus (12), mental foramen (13), mandibular canal (14), hyoid bone (15).

SUGGESTED READINGS

Akinosi JO: A new approach to the mandibular nerve block. Br J Oral Surg 15:83, 1977–78.

Britt GN: A study of human mandibular nutrient canals. Oral Surg 44:635, 1977.

Chiles JL, Gores RJ: Anatomic interpretation of the orthopantomogram. Oral Surg 35:564, 1973.

Christen AG, Segretto VA: Distortion artifacts encountered in Panorex radiography. J Am Dent Assoc 77:1096, 1968.

Farhood VW, Steed DS: Pseudocysts: two cases. Oral Surg 48:491, 1979.

Gow-Gates GA: Mandibular conduction anesthesia: a new technique using extraoral landmarks. Oral Surg 36:321, 1973.

Greer DF, Wege WR, Wuehrmann AH: The significance of nutrient canals appearing in intra-oral radiographs. *In* International Association of Dental Research Programs and Abstracts of Papers. March, 1968, p. 62.

Higashi T, Iguchi M: "Ghost images" in panoramic radiograph. Oral Surg 55:221, 1983.

Katayama H, Ohba T, Ogawa Y: Panoramic innominate line and related roentgen anatomy of the facial bones. Oral Surg 37:131, 1974.

Kaugars GE, Mercuri LG, Laskin DM: Pneumatization of the articular eminence of the temporal bone: prevalence, development and surgical treatment. J Am Dent Assoc 113:55, 1986.

Knight N: Anatomic structures as visualized on the Panorex radiograph. Oral Surg 26:326, 1968.

Knight N: Reverse images and ghost of Panorex radiography. J Am Soc Prev Dent 3:53, 1973.

Kulikowski BM, Schow SR, Kraut RA: Surgical management of a pneumatized articular eminence of the temporal bone. J Oral Maxillofac Surg 40:311, 1982.

Langlais RP, Kasle M: Exercise in Dental Radiology. Vol. 1. Intra-oral Radiographic Interpretation. Philadelphia:WB Saunders, 1978, pp. 82, 138.

Langlais RP, Broadus R, Glass BJ: Bifid mandibular canals in panoramic radiographs. J am Dent Assoc 110:923, 1985.

Langlais RP, Miles DA, Van Dis ML: Elongated and mineralized stylohyoid ligament complex: a proposed classification and report of a case of Eagle's syndrome. Oral Surg 61:527, 1986.

Langlais RP, Glass BJ, Bricker SL, Miles DA: Medial sigmoid depression: a panoramic pseudoforamen in the upper ramus. Oral Surg 55:635, 1983.

Langland OE, Sippy FH: Anatomic structures as visualized on the orthopantomogram. Oral Surg 26:475, 1968.

Langland OE, Sippy FH, Langlais RP: Textbook of Dental Radiology. 2nd Ed. Springfield, IL:Charles C Thomas, 1985, p. 402.

Lundeen RC: Spine of the sphenoid: varying presentation in panoramic radiology. Presentation at the 36th Annual Meeting of the American Academy of Dental Radiology, November 1, 1985.

McDavid WD, Langlais RP, Welander U, Morris CR: Real, double and ghost images in rotational panoramic radiography. Dentomaxillofac Radiol 12:122, 1983.

McVaney TP, Kalkwarf KL: Misdiagnosis of an impacted supernumerary tooth from a panoramic radiograph. Oral Surg 41:678, 1976.

Nortje CJ, Farman AG, Grotepass FW: Variations in the normal anatomy of the inferior dental (mandibular) canal: a retrospective study of panoramic radiographs from 3,612 routine dental patients. Br J Oral Surg 15:55, 1977.

O'Carroll MK: Interpretation of Panorex radiographs. J Oral Med 6:86, 1971.

Patel JR, Wuehrmann AH: A radiographic study of nutrient canals. Oral Surg 42:693, 1976.

Pernkopf E: Atlas of Topographical and Applied Human Anatomy. Vol. 1. Head and Neck. Philadelphia:WB Saunders, 1963, p. 123.

Perrelet LA, Garcia LF: The identification of anatomical structures on orthopantomographs. Dentomaxillofac Radiol 1:11, 1972.

Roser SM, Rudin DE, Brady FA: Unusual bony lesion of the zygomatic arch. J Oral Med 31:72, 1976.

Shapiro SD, et al.: Neurofibromatosis: oral and radiographic manifestations. Oral Surg 58:493, 1984.

Smith CJ, Fleming RD: A comprehensive review of normal anatomic landmarks and artifacts as visualized on Panorex radiographs. Oral Surg 37:291, 1974.

Tebo HG: The pterygospinous bar in panoramic roentgenography. Oral Surg 26:654, 1968.

Turk MH, Katzemell J: Panoramic localization. Oral Surg 29:212, 1970.

Turvey TA, Fonseca RJ: The anatomy of the internal maxillary artery in the pterygopalatine fossa: its relationship to maxillary surgery. J Oral Surg 38:92, 1980.

Tyndall DA, Matteson SR: Radiographic appearance and population distribution of the pneumatized articular eminence of the temporal bone. J Oral Maxillofac Surg 43:493, 1985.

Tyndall DA, Matteson SR: Zygomatic air cell defect (ZACD) on panoramic radiographs. Oral Surg 64:373, 1987.

Walton RE, Abbott BJ: Periodontal ligament injection: a clinical evaluation. J Am Dent Assoc 103:571, 1981.

Chapter 5

Developmental and Acquired Abnormalities of the Teeth and Jaws

A developmental abnormality is a departure or divergence from what is considered the normal process of growth and differentiation. A developmental disturbance or abnormality may be classified according to severity. A variation is a minor deviation from the normal; examples are a large oral orifice or enlarged medullary spaces. Anomalies are more severe deviations, but they do not interfere with function; examples are enamel hypoplasia and peg laterals. Malformations are even more severe deviations and do interfere with function; examples are cleft lip and cleft palate. Monstrosities are extreme deviations that severely interfere with function; examples are agnathia and dicephalus.

Anomalies may be caused by local conditions, they may arise as inherited dental tendencies, or they may be manifestations of systemic disturbances. Most dental defects discussed in this chapter are familial or follow definite mendelian patterns of inheritance. Some are associated with life-threatening diseases.

The most common oral anomalies are those that affect the teeth; rarer are those that result from faulty development of the supporting structures of the teeth. The anomalies of the teeth have been classified conventionally to include defects or alterations in numbers, morphology, hard tissue structure, and eruption. In addition, acquired defects of the teeth such as abrasion, attrition, erosion, and resorption are discussed.

VARIATIONS IN NUMBER OF TEETH (Figs. 5–1 to 5–4)

Hypodontia (Agenesis of teeth, anodontia, oligodontia, partial anodontia)

Hypodontia is best defined as agenesis of one or more teeth. An acceptable, but less clear, definition is congenital absence of one or more teeth. Jorgenson (1980) stated that this latter definition is less clear because teeth are rarely evident clinically at birth, and many teeth do not begin to develop until after birth. Congenital refers to a condition that exists at, and usually before, birth, and therefore the best criterion for agenesis of a tooth is its clinical and radiographic absence at an age when it is ordinarily expected to be present. Adequate latitude must be given for individual, familial, racial, and sexual variations, however.

Hypodontia may be total or partial. It may involve both primary and permanent teeth, but it is far more often encountered in the permanent teeth. Total hypodontia of the permanent teeth is extremely rare (Fig. 5–1), although acquired hypodontia is not uncommon. Anhidrotic ectodermal dysplasia is one of the most probable causes of serious or complete suppression (failure to develop) of teeth (Fig. 5–4).

Idiopathic hypodontia is much more common and refers to one or several missing teeth (Figs. 5–2 and 5–3). Any tooth in the dental arch may fail to develop; however, the order of frequency in which teeth are absent is as follows: third molars, premolars, and maxillary lateral incisors. Absence of 1 or more of the third molars occurs in approximately 1 in 10 persons, whereas absence of the canine tooth is rare. The results from 6 large studies of children under the age of 18 years by Dolder (1936; Switzerland), Werther and Rothenberg (1939; United States), Rose (1967; England), Grahnen (1956; Sweden), Niswander and Sujaku (1963; Japan), and Volk (1963; Austria) indicated that the prevalence of hypodontia ranged from 2.3 to 9.6%. These studies did not include the third molars and primary teeth.

Volk (1963) reported that the frequency and pattern of hypodontia differ among sexes. In some populations, females have a higher frequency of hypodontia. In the population from nine studies reviewed by Jorgenson (1980), hypodontia was almost twice as common in females, and agenesis

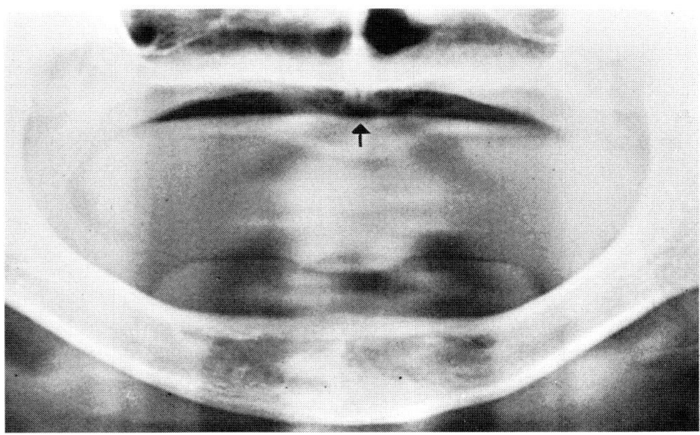

FIGURE 5–1.

Hypodontia. Congenital anodontia in a 5-year-old boy. The arrow shows the dorsum of the tongue. (Courtesy of Drs. M. Araki and K. Hashimoto, Nihon University, Tokyo, Japan.)

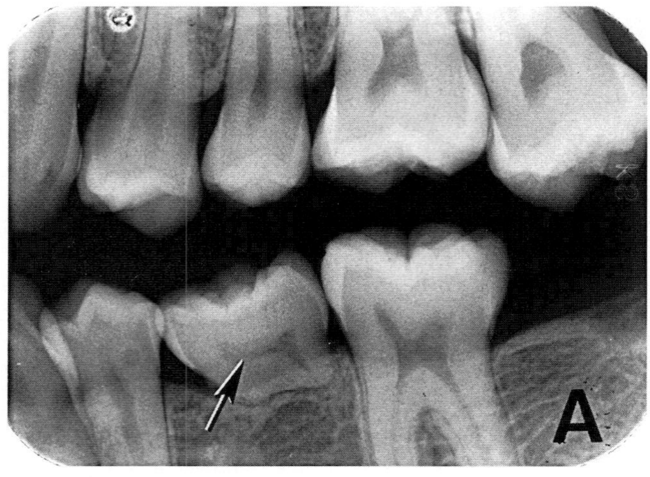
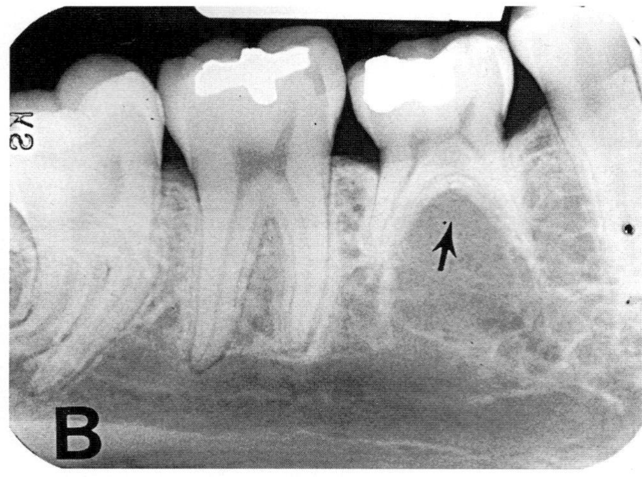
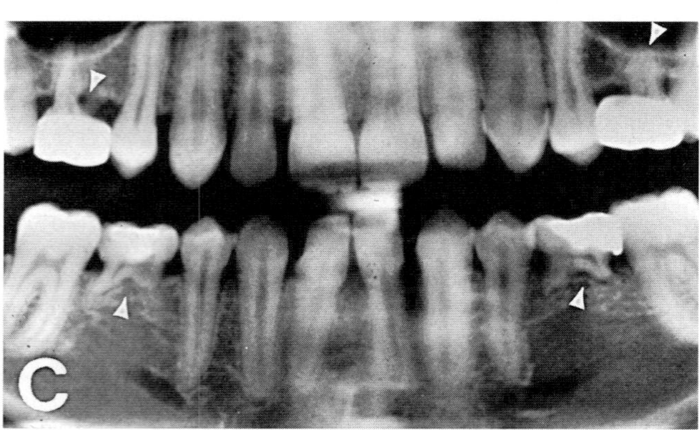
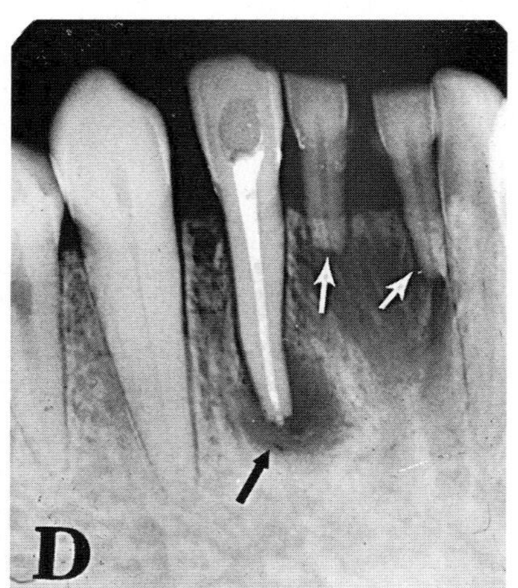

FIGURE 5–2.

Hypodontia. A, Congenitally missing second mandibular premolar and a retained primary second molar with resorbed roots (arrow). B, Congenitally missing second premolar with a retained primary second molar (arrow). C, Congenital absence of all four second premolars (arrowheads). D, Congentially missing mandibular central incisors and retained primary central incisors (white arrows); a permanent lateral incisor has the radiographic appreance of chronic apical periodontitis (black arrow).

of the maxillary lateral incisors was more frequent in males than agenesis of the mandibular second premolar.

Cases of hypodontia may be divided into two major groups. The first, symmetric hypodontia, comprises cases of hypodontia involving particular teeth or groups of teeth, usually symmetrically, whereas the second group is characterized by haphazard involvement, although the hypodontia may still occur symmetrically. In the symmetric type of hypodontia, the following teeth are most often missing: third molars, maxillary lateral incisors, and second premolars.

A sequela of missing second premolars is the ankylosed, submerged, second primary molar. If this condition is present, the submerged tooth will render the involved arch more susceptible to periodontal disease, owing to its altered interproximal contact (Fig. 5–3B). Additionally, its antagonist, especially in the case of the maxillary second premolar, may extrude and is also more susceptible to periodontal disease because of its altered interproximal contact.

Grahnen and Granath (1961) reported that hypodontia is rare among primary teeth. In the few epidemiologic studies done so far, the prevalence has ranged between 0.1 and 0.7%. In primary teeth, hypodontia especially affects the maxillary lateral and mandibular central and lateral incisors; the maxilla is more often affected than the mandible. Hypodontia may be an isolated tract or one manifestation of a syndrome of multiple systems.

There are few documented pedigrees of agenesis of the mandibular second premolars, but a high frequency of concordance among monozygous twins suggests a genetic cause. Agenesis of the premolars is constant in PHC syndrome (P-premolar hypodontia, H-hyperhidrosis, C-canities, i.e., white hair; also known as Book's syndrome) and is occasionally present in syndromes such as otodental dysplasia and Rieger's syndrome.

Woolf (1971) reported that agenesis of the maxillary lateral incisors is one of the most common single gene traits

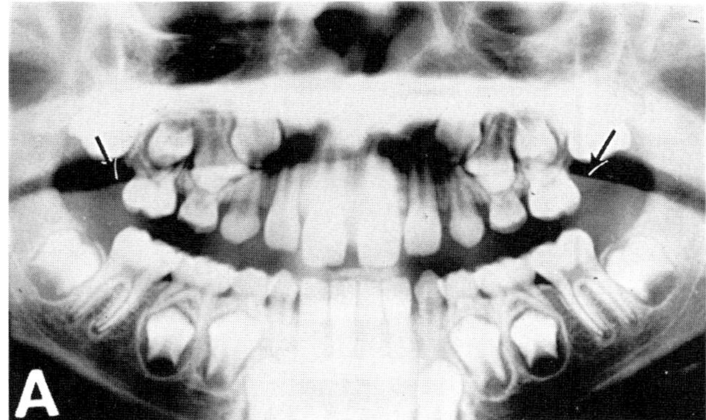
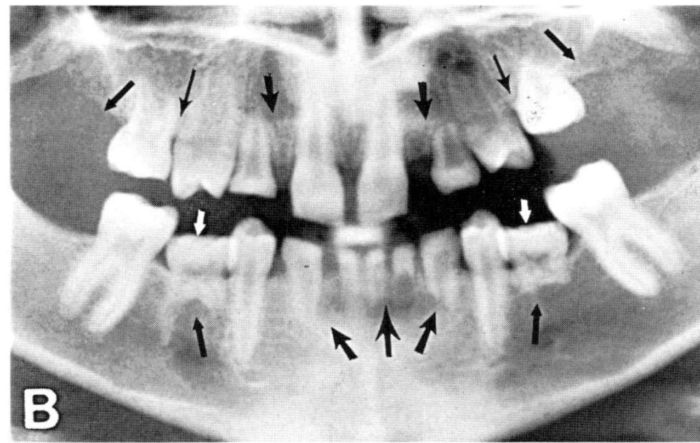
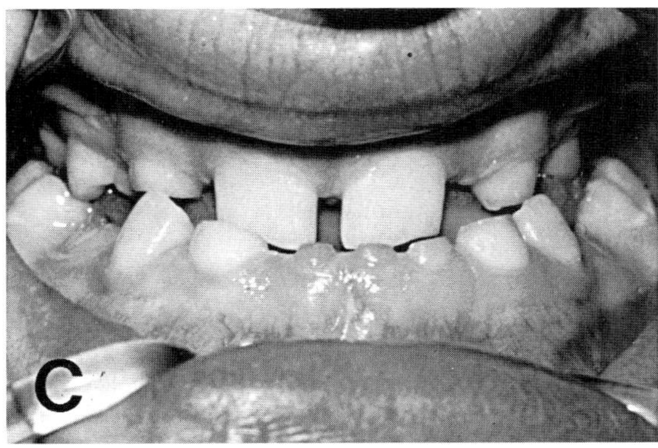

FIGURE 5–3.

Hypodontia. A, Rare congenitally missing maxillary first permanent molars (arrows); the second molars had not yet erupted. B, Panoramic radiograph of a teenage female patient with congenitally missing second premolars, maxillary first molars, maxillary canines and lateral incisors, and all mandibular anterior teeth (arrows). C, Clinical photograph of the patient in B with multiple congenital missing teeth.

in humans; it is an autosomal dominant trait with high penetrance (frequency with which heritable trait is manifested) and wide variability. Jorgenson (1980) reported that this disorder occurs with a higher than expected frequency in persons with Down's syndrome (15%), in the mentally retarded (11%), and in patients with cleft palate. Agenesis and pegging of the maxillary lateral incisors are phenomena caused by the same gene. Agenesis of the mandibular central incisors and agenesis of the maxillary canine teeth are well-known autosomal dominant traits, according to Gruneberg (1936) and Kurtz and Brownstein (1974) (Fig. 5–2D)

Gorlin and co-workers (1976) reported that hypodontia is often seen in certain syndromes. Jorgenson and co-workers (1978, 1980), McKusick (1978), and Witkop and associates

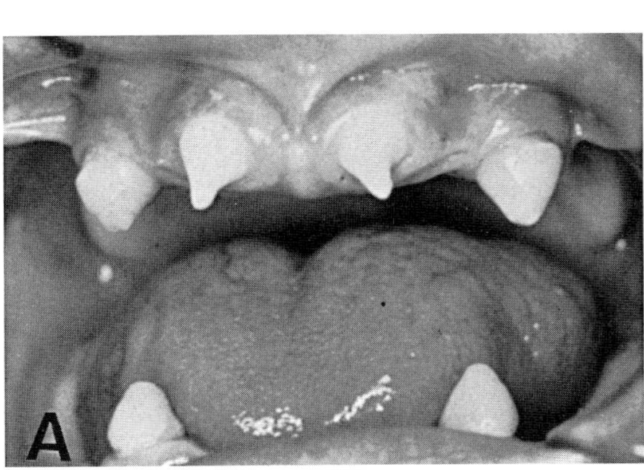
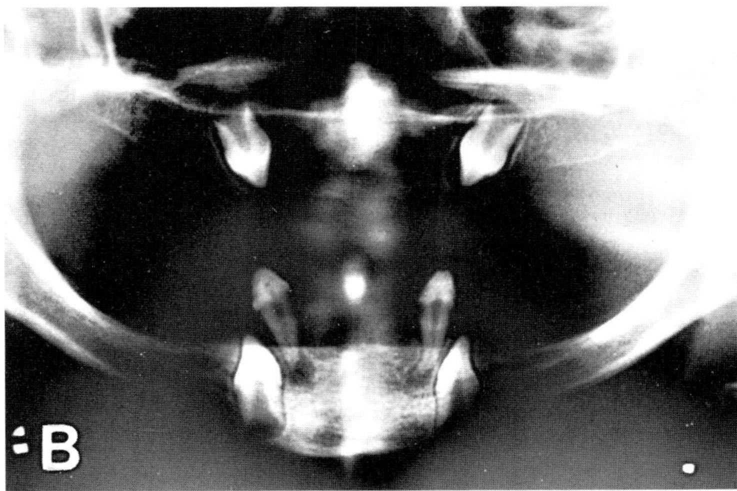

FIGURE 5–4.

Hypodontia: ectodermal dysplasia. A, Clinical photograph of a patient with ectodermal dysplasia. B, Panoramic radiograph of another patient with all permanent teeth congenitally missing except the canines.

(1975) reported at least 35 syndromes with hypodontia as a component.

The hypodontia observed in patients with anhidrotic ectodermal dysplasia is an outstanding feature of the syndrome. Occasionally, one sees a total absence of teeth. Witkop and associates (1975), after reviewing the literature extensively, found 40 distinct syndromes under the category of ectodermal dysplasia and added a new one. An abnormal dentition has been associated with 33 of these conditions, including oligodontia and/or conical teeth in 19. Some of the syndromes are inherited as an autosomal dominant or recessive trait, whereas others have a sex-linked mode of transmission. As stated by Freire-Maia (1971), to fulfill the criteria for ectodermal dysplasia, the syndrome must demonstrate at least 2 of the following features: (1) abnormal hair (trichodysplasia); (2) abnormal or missing teeth (anodontia or oligodontia); (3) abnormal nails (onchodysplasia); and (4) abnormal or missing sweat glands (dyshidrosis) (Fig. 5–4).

In chondroectodermal dysplasia (Ellis-Van Creveld's syndrome; Ellis and Van Creveld, 1940), in which ectodermal dysplasia is associated with polydactyly, chondrodysplasia, and heart malformations, there is often a deficiency in the number of teeth, especially in the lower anterior ridge. The alveolar ridge is often serrated because of pronounced vestibular frenula.

Book of Sweden (1950) noted, in 25 individuals of 4 generations with the PHC or Book syndrome, that 9 of them showed a total lack of premolars, whereas the rest had hypoplasia of a lesser number of premolars. In half these patients, the third molars failed to develop.

Hypodontia may also be seen as part of other syndromes such as incontinentia pigmenti (Bloch-Sulzberger's syndrome; Bloch, 1926; Sulzberger, 1928), orodigitofacial dysostosis, Down's syndrome (trisomy 21, mongolism), cheilognathopalatoschisis, hyalinosis cutis et mucosae, and progeria. Rieger's syndrome should be suspected in any patient with hypodontia, particularly when the permanent maxillary central and lateral incisors are missing. This syndrome is associated with congenital glaucoma, which may produce blindness by age 6 or 8 years.

◆ *RADIOLOGY (Figs. 5–1 to 5–4)*

Panoramic radiographs are particularly useful in evaluating the number of missing teeth and the collapse of the arches, which may occur as a consequence. No difficulty exists in the radiographic recognition of absent teeth, but when single teeth are concerned, it is wise to allow a wide margin of variation before stating that such teeth will not develop. A year or more may separate the appearance of some teeth compared with their development on the opposite side of the mouth. If many teeth fail to develop, it is common for those that do to be defective, the most frequent deformity being small, cone-shaped teeth, which are usually markedly spaced. Gross deficiency in dentition is often accompanied by abnormalities in other parts of the body.

The dental findings of hereditary anhidrotic ectodermal dysplasia, incontinentia pigmenti (Bloch-Sulzberger Syndrome; Bloch, 1926), and chondroectodermal dysplasia (Ellis-Van Creveld Syndrome) are radiographically identical and consist of hypodontia and a mixture of normal and conical tooth shapes. The teeth also show delayed eruption in incontinentia pigmenti and chondroectodermal dysplasia. Incontinentia pigmenti is seen only in females because it is lethal in males.

Hyperdontia (Supernumerary, Supplemental, and Accessory Teeth) (Figs. 5–5 to 5–9)

The presence of teeth in excess of the normal complement is referred to as hyperdontia, accessory or supernumerary. Bhaskar (1961) suggested the term "accessory" for teeth that do not resemble the normal form, whereas a supernumerary tooth is one that mimics the normal shape. Worth (1963) suggested that the word "supplemental" be used for teeth that are extra but have the shape and size of normal teeth. Pindborg (1970) also used Worth's terminology of supplemental for supernumerary teeth that resemble a normal set of teeth. Most supernumerary teeth, however, have a morphology that deviates from the normal appearance of the teeth.

A supernumerary tooth between the maxillary central incisors is called a mesiodens (Fig. 5–5). A supernumerary tooth distal to the third molars is a distodens (fourth molar) (Fig. 5–8), whereas one that is buccal or lingual to the molars is called a paramolar (peridens) (Fig. 5–7). Because many supernumerary teeth are completely buried, a full mouth radiographic survey or panoramic radiograph is mandatory to determine the exact prevalence of hyperdontia (supernumerary teeth) in a given study population.

Pindborg (1970), in a review of seven hyperdontia incidence studies of Rosenzweig and Garbaski (1965), Stafne (1932), Parry and Lyer (1961), LaCoste and associates (1962), Niswander and Sujaku (1963), and Lind (1959), gave the prevalence as ranging between 0.1 and 3.6%. Dixon and Stewart reported a prevalence of supernumerary teeth in the Caucasian population of 1 to 3%, and a frequency higher than 3% in Mongoloid races.

In Stafne's study (1932) of 48,550 patients, 446 patients had supernumerary teeth. Of these patients 382 (87%) had a single supernumerary tooth, 54 (12%) had 2 extra teeth, and 5 (1%) had 3 supernumerary teeth. Primosch (1981) reported that 90 to 98% of supernumerary teeth occur in the maxilla, with a particular predilection for the premaxilla.

Supernumerary teeth in the primary teeth are less common than in the permanent dentition, according to studies of Grahnen and Granath (1961). According to epidemiologic studies by Clayton (1956) and Magnusson (1959), the prevalence of primary supernumerary teeth ranges from 0.1 to 1.9%. Ravin (1971), Brook (1974), Parry and Lyer (1961), Egermark-Eriksson and Lind (1971), and Sarto (1959) reported that although there is no sex distribution in primary supernumerary teeth, and males are affected approximately two to five times as frequently as females in the permanent dentition.

Although the etiology of supernumerary teeth is still obscure, several theories have been proposed. Gardiner (1961)

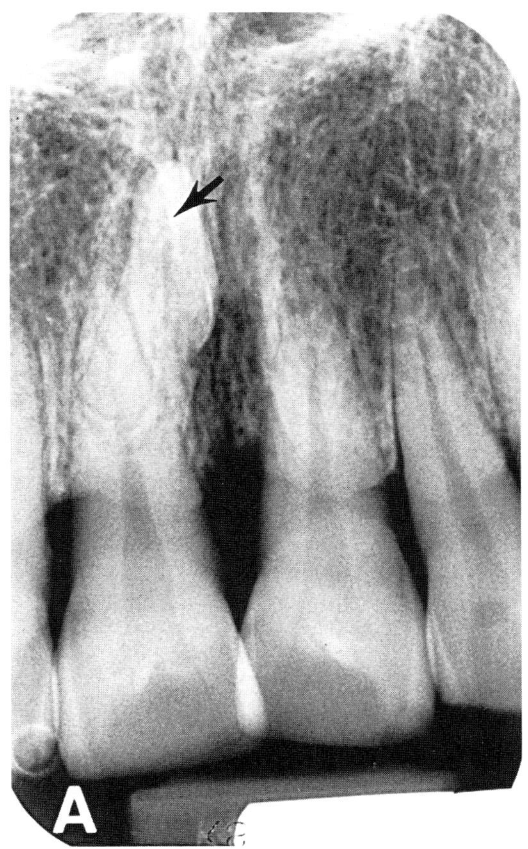

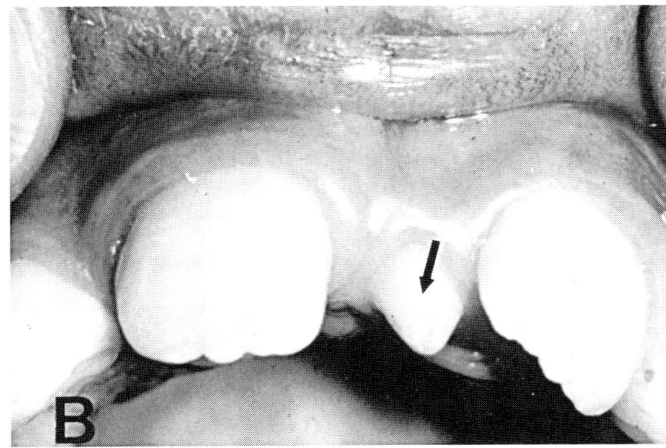

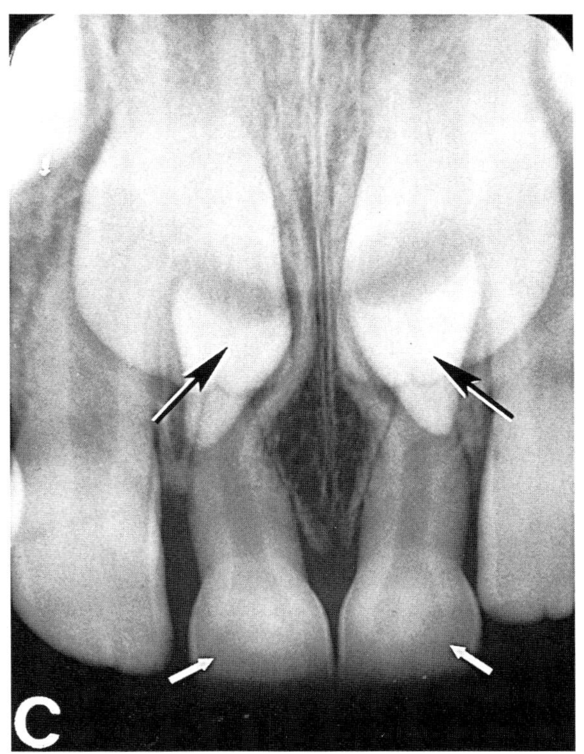

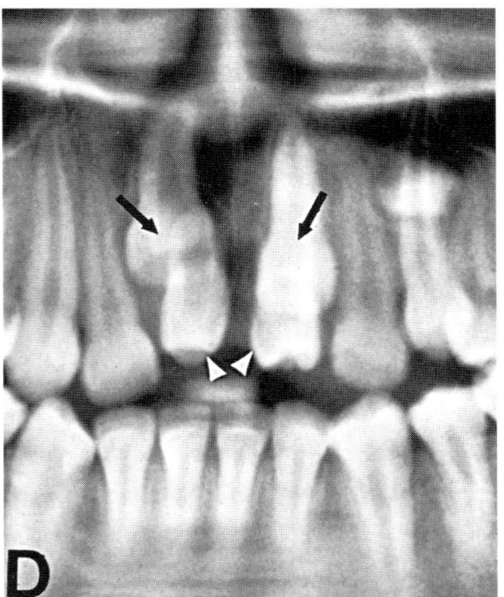

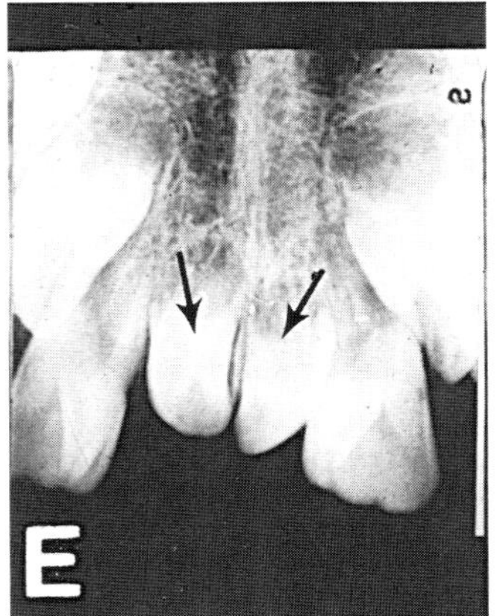

FIGURE 5–5.

Mesiodens. A, At the apex of the right central incisor (arrow). B, Clinical photograph of an erupted mesiodens (arrow). C, Double mesiodens (black arrows) blocking erupting permanent central incisors with retained primary central incisors (white arrows). D, Double mesiodens (white arrowheads) erupting to block erupting maxillary central incisors (black arrows). E, Double mesiodens (arrows) erupting between erupted maxillary central incisors.

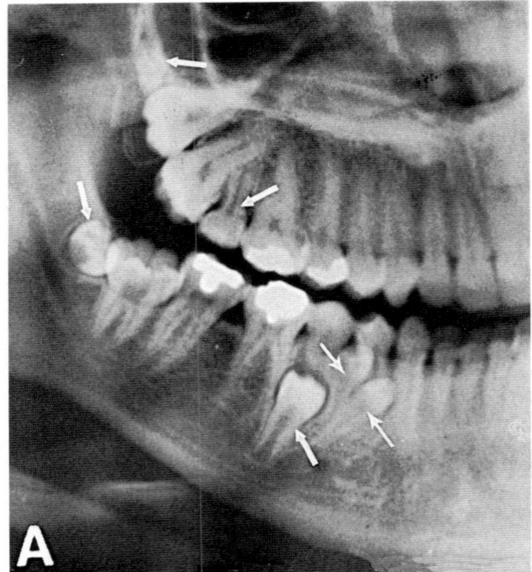

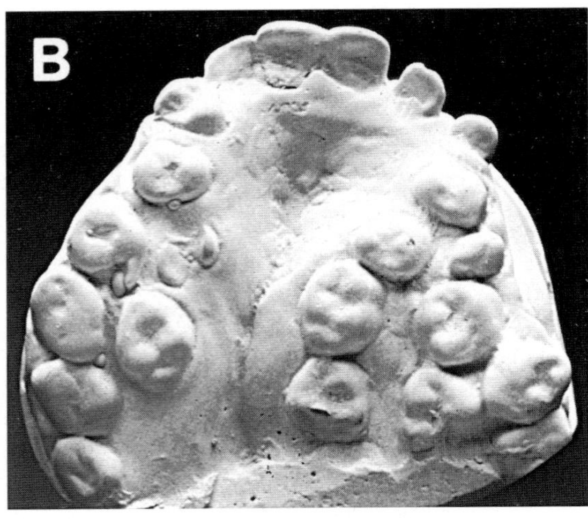

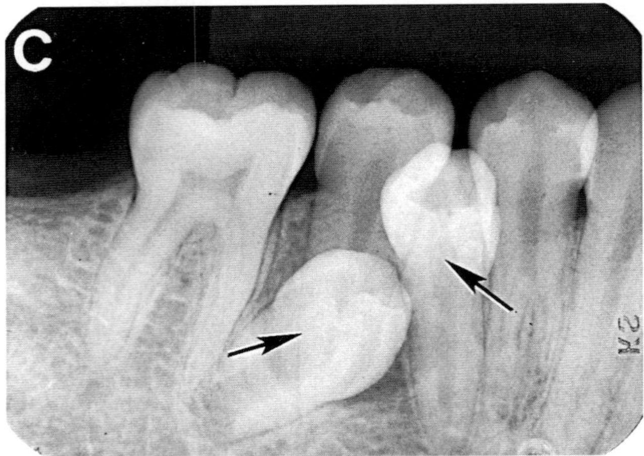

FIGURE 5–6.

Supernumerary Teeth. A, Multiple supernumerary teeth (arrows): one extra mandibular molar, two extra maxillary molars, and three extra mandibular premolars. B, Multiple erupted supernumerary maxillary teeth (plaster cast). C, Two supernumerary unerupted premolars (arrows).

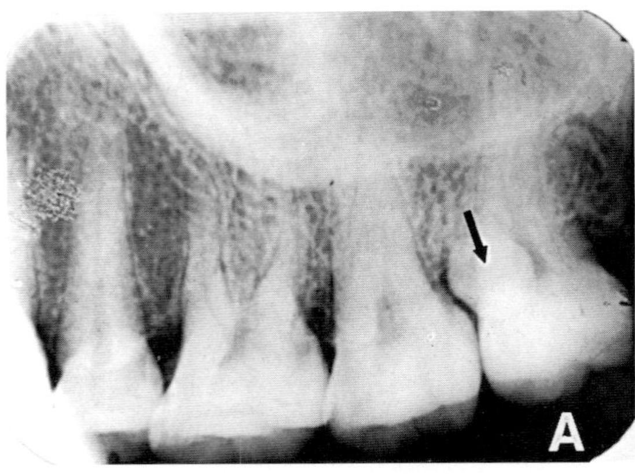

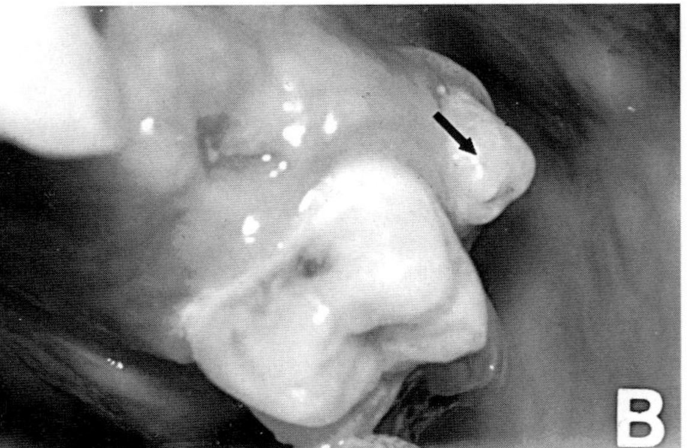

FIGURE 5–7.

Paramolars. A, Paramolar (arrow), buccal to a maxillary third molar. B, Clinical photograph of a paramolar (arrow). (Courtesy of Dr. P. Dhiravarangkura, Chulalonghorn University, Bangkok, Thailand.)

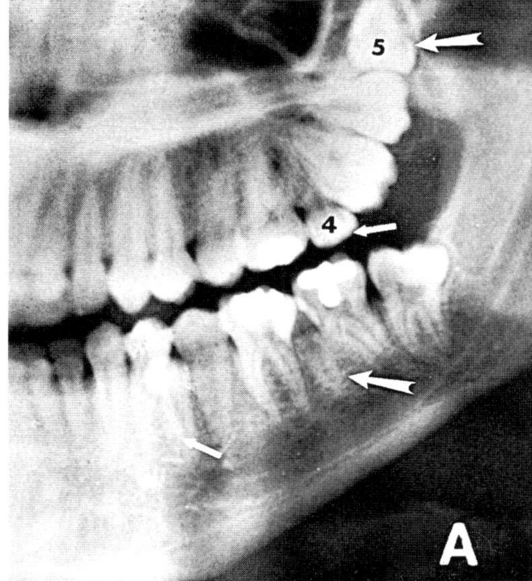

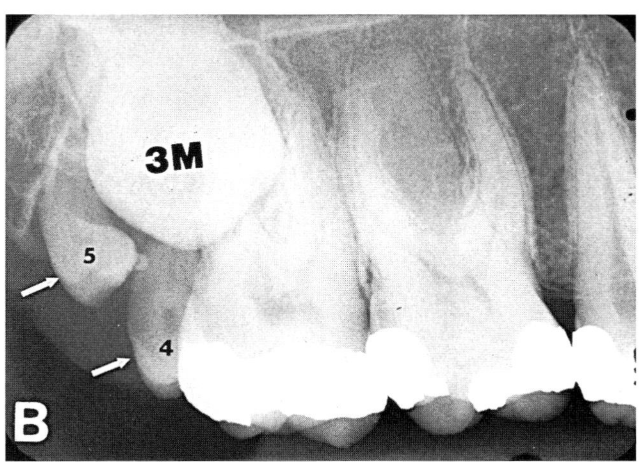

FIGURE 5–8.

Distomolar. A, Fourth and fifth maxillary molars (arrows) and two supernumerary mandibular premolars (arrows). B, Fourth and fifth maxillary molars (arrows).

reported that hyperdontia can be explained by dichotomy (schizodontia) of the tooth germs, a hypothesis supported by experiments in which split germs have been cultivated in vitro. This dichotomy theory, according to Brook and Ekanayake (1980), constitutes the basis for the hypothesis that hyperdontia is a polygenically determined, quasicontinuous variable based on the underlying distribution of tooth size.

According to Primosch (1981), hyperdontia may be caused as a result of local, independently conditioned hyperactivity of the dental lamina. In contrast to hypodontia, hyperdontia only rarely shows a dominant inheritance. Sedano and Gorlin (1969) and Hammond-Williams (1934) reported a familial tendency in hyperdontia.

Although hyperdontia can be found in any location, it has an apparent predilection for certain sites. The most common supernumerary tooth is the "mesiodens." One or two round, small, peg-shaped supernumerary teeth are located either in the bone above the roots of the central incisors or behind or between the central incisor teeth. Kronfeld (1939) stated that this form of supernumerary tooth called "mesiodens" was named by Bok.

In a Swedish study by Billberg and Lind (1965) comprising 11,400 children, 7 to 15 years of age, mesiodens were found in 1.4% of the children. Among those children with mesiodens, 80% had 1 and 20% had 2 or 3 mesiodens. The anomaly was more common in boys, who also had the largest mesiodens. In approximately 75% of cases, a mesiodens is buried and may cause retarded eruption, dislocation, or resorption of the roots of the permanent incisors. A mesiodens is most often located palatally to the permanent incisors and may be totally inverted. It usually has a conical crown and a short root.

Hyperdontia in the premolar region is more frequent in the mandible than in the maxilla. Usually, the supernumerary teeth in the premolar region are similar to normal teeth. There is rarely sufficient space for them to undergo complete eruption, although premature loss of the first molar may afford space for them to do so (Fig. 5–6).

Hyperdontia is more frequent in the maxillary molar region than in the mandibular molar region, and the supernumerary teeth are most often reduced in size and have an abnormal appearance when compared with the normal molars. The maxillary fourth molar, called a distomolar, is the second most common supernumerary tooth and is situated distal to the third molar. It is usually a small, rudimentary tooth, but it may be of normal size. A mandibular fourth molar or distomolar is also seen occasionally, but this is much less common than the maxillary distomolar. Nordenram (1968) reported on a case with a fifth molar in the ramus of the mandible.

Other supernumerary teeth seen with some frequency are maxillary paramolars. The paramolar is a supernumerary molar, usually small and rudimentary, which is situated buccally or lingually to one of the maxillary molars or interproximally between the first and second or second and third maxillary molars.

Supernumerary maxillary lateral incisors are not always conical; they often resemble the normal tooth in form, although rarely in size. There is a relatively high incidence of supernumerary lateral incisors associated with cleft palate. These teeth were present in 22 of 60 cases of cleft palate reported by Millhon and Stafne in 1941. The overproduction of teeth in these patients may be due to (1) cleavage of the tooth germ caused by the cleft or (2) an extension or folding of the oral mucosa whereby the supernumerary teeth are a product of the correspondingly extended dental lamina.

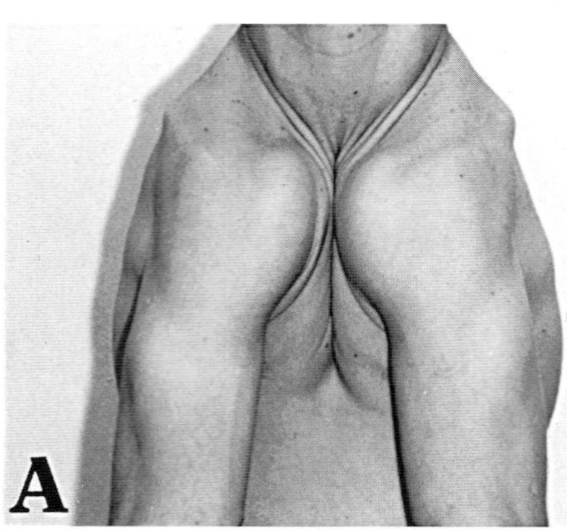

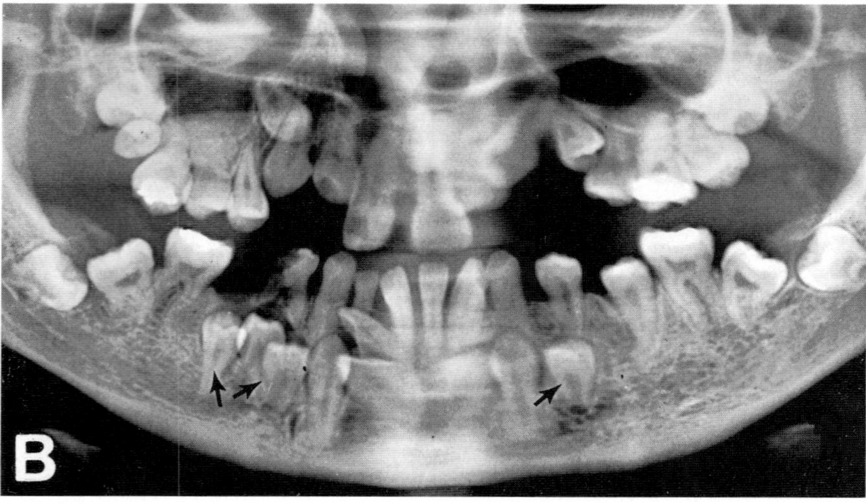

FIGURE 5–9.

Cleidocranial Dysplasia. A, Clinical photograph of a patient with cleidocranial dysplasia who has no clavicles. B, Radiograph of a 20-year-old woman with cleidocranial dysplasia revealing multiple supernumerary teeth and multiple unerupted teeth (arrows). (Courtesy of Drs. K. Hashimoto and M. Araki, Nihon University, Tokyo, Japan.)

◆ RADIOLOGY (Figs. 5–5 to 5–9)

Supernumerary teeth are easily detected in the absence of superimposition of other structures (Figs. 5–5 and 5–6). The paramolar (Fig. 5–7) is often difficult to detect because it may be superimposed on the molars and may resemble an odontoma, gemination or concrescence.

Hyperdontia is associated with other defects of the oral and maxillofacial complex. In cleidocranial dysplasia (aplasia or hypoplasia of clavicles, brachycephalic skull, delayed ossification of the fontanels, and hereditary transmission), one of the most striking features is the number of supernumerary teeth (Fig. 5–9). These teeth may be so numerous that the jaws appear to have a third dentition. There are multiple crown and root abnormalities, crypt formation around impacted teeth, ectopic location of teeth, and lack of tooth eruption. Winter (1943) reported that extraction of primary teeth does not promote eruption of permanent teeth. Rushton (1937) and Hitchin and Fairley (1974) attributed noneruption of teeth to the failure of bone to resorb. The bizarre supernumerary crown and root morphology appears to be related to spacial crowding. The abnormalities of root morphology in the permanent dentition are thought to be secondary to arrested eruption.

The following features may be seen in Gardner's syndrome: (1) retention of several primary teeth, with delayed eruption of their permanent successors; (2) multiple unerupted supernumerary teeth and odontomas; and (3) osteomas of the jaws, sinuses, and facial bones. The osteomas in the jaws may be distinct, well-delineated radiopaque lesions, or they may be diffuse, sclerotic masses that appear to affect the entire jaw. Other features of Gardner's syndrome include multiple skin lesions consisting of epidermoid and sebaceous cysts and fibrous (desmoid) tumors. The most significant feature is a tendency to develop polyps in the colon and rectum that usually undergo malignant transformation. Because this disorder is hereditary, siblings and other family members should be investigated and should receive genetic counseling. The disorder is due to a single pleiotropic gene and has an autosomal dominant pattern of inheritance, with complete penetrance and variable expression. This disease is of interest to the dental profession because the impacted teeth and osteomas of the jaws may lead to early diagnosis of the entire syndrome. In addition, patients with the orodigitofacial dystosis (OFD) syndrome and the Hallermann-Streiff syndrome (dicephalia, parrot or beaked nose, mandibular hypoplasia, nanism, i.e., dwarfism, hypertrichosis, and blue sclerae) may have hyperdontia.

VARIATIONS IN SIZE OF TEETH: MICRODONTIA AND MACRODONTIA (Figs. 5–10 to 5–15)

The size of teeth is predominantly genetically determined. A sex difference in tooth size exists in that males have larger teeth than females. Garn and co-workers (1966) reported that when the buccolingual and mesiodistal tooth diameters are measured, a major sex difference in tooth shape is found, with males tending toward more nearly square dimensions and females from the same families showing greater size reduction buccolingually than mesiodistally.

The size of teeth also depends on race. Pedersen (1944) reported that the crowns of the molars in Eskimos are larger than in Caucasians, but at the same time the third molars in Eskimos show a tendency to reduction in size.

Microdontia is a term used to describe teeth that are smaller than normal, such as outside the usual limits of variation. Microdontia is much more common than macrodontia. Three types of microdontia are recognized: (1) true generalized microdontia; (2) relative generalized microdontia; and (3) microdontia involving a single tooth (Fig. 5–10).

In true generalized microdontia, all the teeth are smaller than usual. This disorder is exceedingly rare and is seen in dwarfism (hypopituitarism and gonad hypofunction), with the teeth conforming in size to the skeleton. Microdontia of an entire dentition may also be associated with other defects such as congenital heart disease or Down's syndrome. Microdontia is not an uncommon finding in osteogenesis imperfecta and in hemiatrophy of the face, in which there is an associated underdevelopment of the jaws. Dwarfing of teeth also may be produced by irradiation used in treatment of tumors of the jaws (Fig. 5–13).

In relative generalized microdontia, normal or slightly normal teeth present in jaws are somewhat larger than normal. This gives an illusion of true microdontia. In reality, the person has inherited the jaw size from one parent and the tooth size from the other.

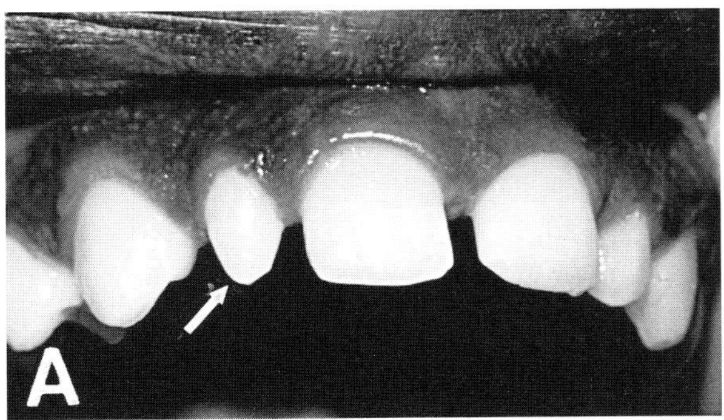

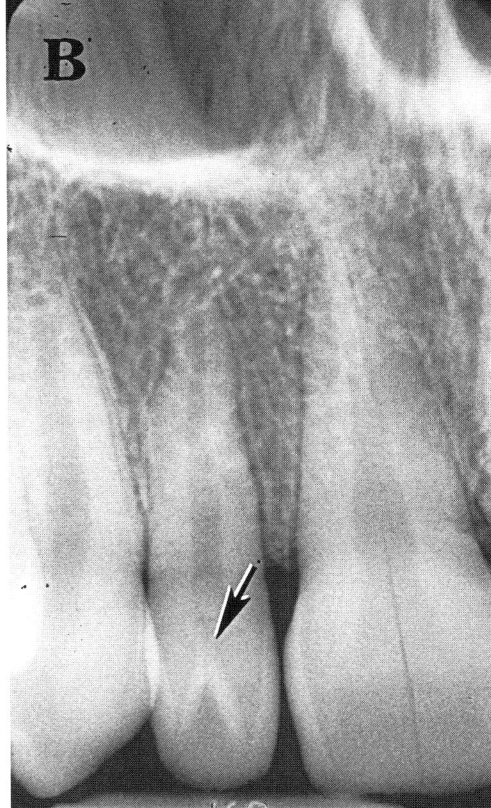

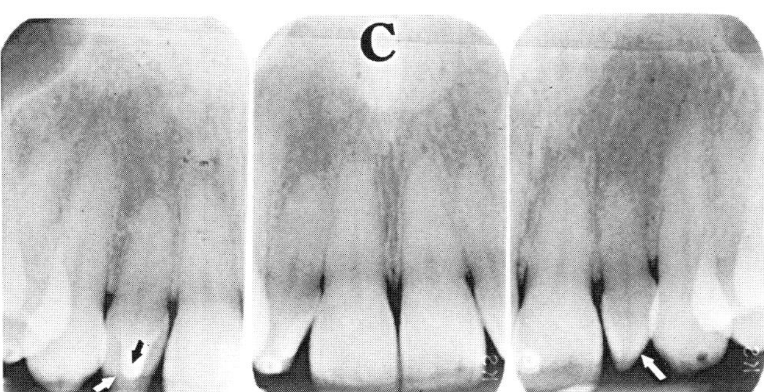

FIGURE 5–10.

Microdontia. A, Clinical photograph of a "peg" lateral (arrow; maxillary right lateral incisor). B, Radiograph of a maxillary right peg lateral with a shovel-shaped lingual surface (arrow). C, Double peg laterals (white arrows) with a talon cusp on the right maxillary peg lateral (black arrow).

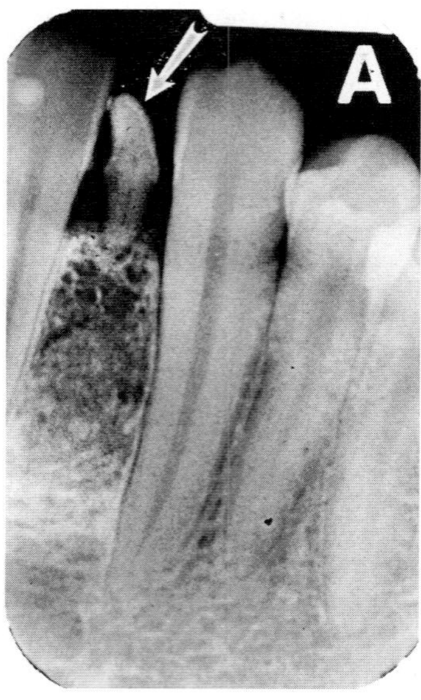

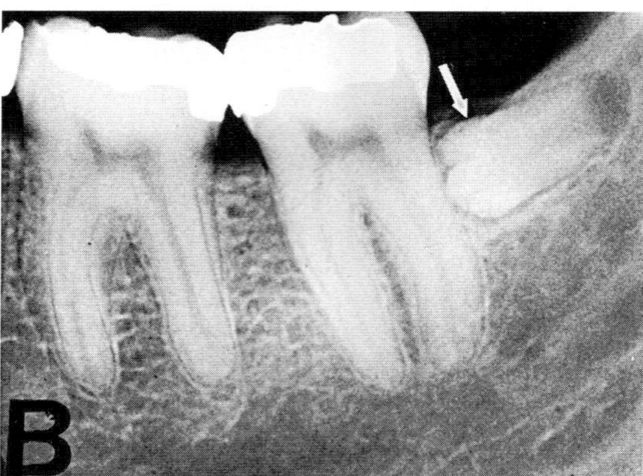

FIGURE 5–11.

Microdontia. A, Microdontic extra tooth (arrow) between a mandibular canine and a lateral incisor. B, Microdontic horizontally impacted third molar (arrow).

More often, microdontia involving a single tooth is a common condition. Microdontia, like other dental defects, is often found in the so-called variable teeth, those teeth that are more prone to congenital failures to develop. Hence, there is a greater frequency of discovery of microdontia of maxillary incisors and maxillary third molars. Other teeth that are often congenitally absent, however, the maxillary and mandibular second premolars, for some reason seldom exhibit microdontia. Supernumerary teeth, in contrast, are frequently small (Fig. 5–11). One of the most common forms of localized microdontia is that which affects the maxillary lateral incisor, called a "peg lateral" (Fig. 5–10).

A peg-shaped lateral incisor has a marked reduction in diameter, extending from the cervical region to the incisal

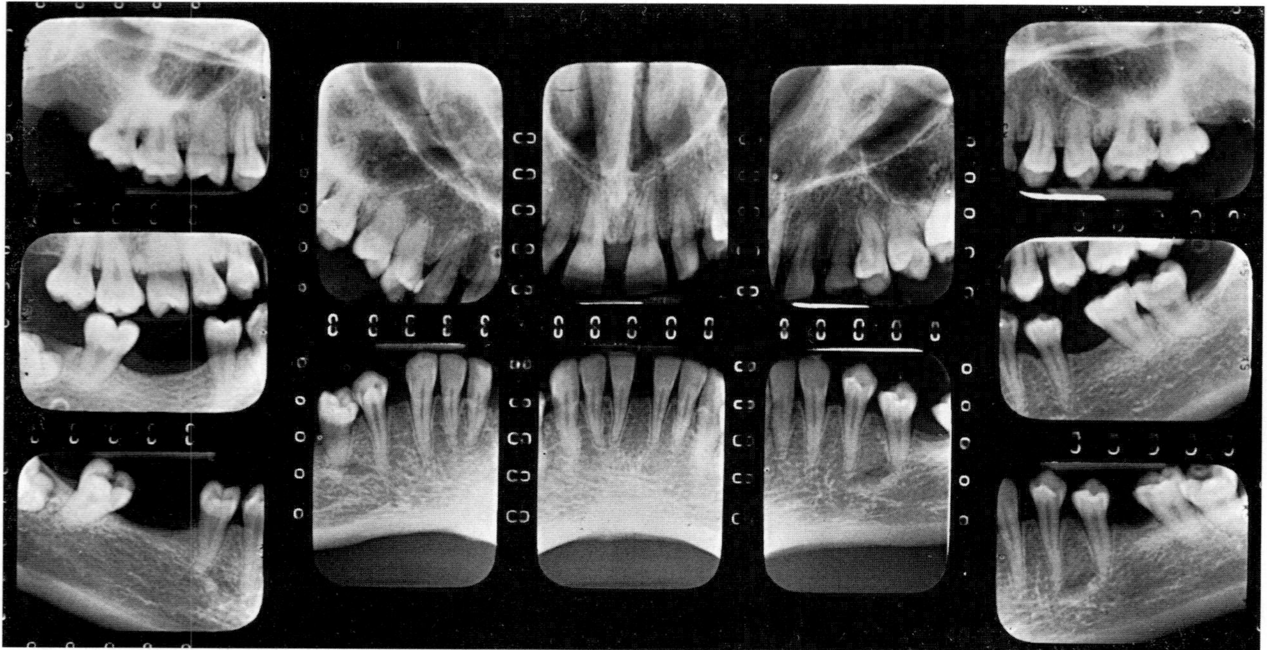

FIGURE 5–12.

Microdontia. Generalized microdontia.

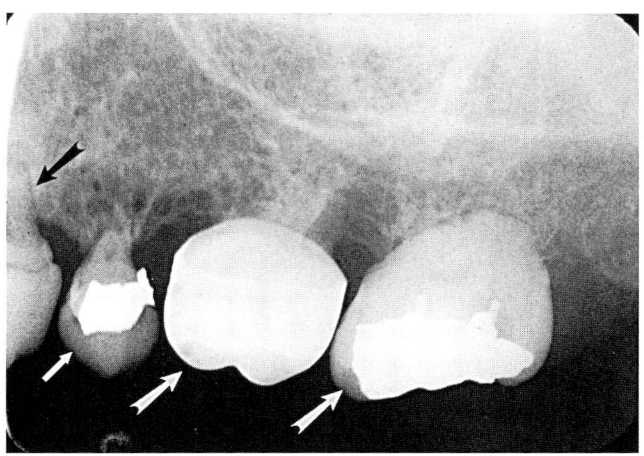

FIGURE 5–13.

Microdontia. Dwarfing of teeth (arrows) can be produced by irradiation used in treatment of malignant tumors of the jaws, as had occurred in this 18-year-old male patient when he was a child.

edge. Buenviaje and Rapp (1984) reported, from a sample of 1500 males and 879 females ranging in age from 2 to 12 years of age, 8 individuals (0.34%) having a total of 13 peg-shaped lateral incisors in the permanent dentition. LeBot and Salmon (1979) observed the prevalence of (peg-shaped) upper lateral incisors to be 1.59% in 5738 French men aged 18 to 25 years.

"Dwarfed roots" is a term used for teeth with normal crowns and unusually small roots. Unfortunately, this condition often goes undetected until discovered during routine dental radiographic examination, or until loose teeth begin to appear in what might have been considered a healthy dentition. When dwarfed roots are seen in association with normal clinical crowns, it is evident that odontogenesis has been disturbed only during the period of root formation. Smaller roots than normal (rhizomicry) are usually found in the premolars and third molars. Dwarfed roots are seen in dentinal dysplasia and dentinogenesis imperfecta.

In our clinical experience, an idiopathic generalized shortening and/or tapering of the roots of any or all of the teeth has been noted among Mexican Americans, the lower premolars being the most commonly affected. The crowns are normal, except for prominent marginal ridges in the maxillary central and lateral incisors, often referred to as shovel-shaped incisors. This combination of findings has been loosely named the shovel-shaped incisor syndrome.

In addition, roots of the maxillary central incisors may be short, a feature frequently reported among the Japanese. A study of 300 Japanese children by Ando and co-workers (1967) revealed that 10% had bilateral short-rooted upper central incisors. The reason for these short-rooted teeth is ascribed to a heavy occlusal load sustained by the teeth during root formation. In addition, undo pressure put on teeth during root formation by orthodontic appliances can cause dwarfing of the roots of teeth, especially the maxillary anterior teeth.

Macrodontia is the opposite of microdontia and refers to teeth that are larger than normal. Macrodontia may be classified in the same manner as microdontia. True generalized macrodontia, the condition in which all teeth are larger than normal, has been associated with pituitary gigantism, but is extremely rare. Relative generalized macrodontia is more common and is a result of a normal or slightly larger than normal teeth in small jaws, giving the appearance of generalized macrodontia. Of course, this condition does not represent true macrodontia.

Macrodontia of single teeth is relatively uncommon. The tooth may appear normal in every respect except for its size. In the primary dentition, the maxillary canine tooth and mandibular second molar are sometimes observed to be larger than normal; the latter may resemble the permanent first molar. In the permanent dentition, macrodontia is most frequently noted in the maxillary central incisors, the canine teeth, and the molars, and in the mandible, the second premolar and third molar.

True macrodontia of a single tooth should not be confused with fusion of the teeth (the union of two or more teeth), which results in a single large tooth. In some instances, the root alone shows variation in size. Larger roots than normal (rhizomegaly) are frequently seen in maxillary canine teeth, in which the root may reach the length of 43 mm.

◆ *RADIOLOGY (Figs. 5–10 to 5–15)*

As the names of these conditions imply, an alteration is size is noted in one tooth or several teeth. When macro- or microdontia affects one tooth or a few teeth, the condition is generally considered to be of no clinical significance, and treatment would only be an esthetic or restorative consideration. When the condition is generalized, however, there may be some significant underlying systemic or developmental disorder such as pituitary dwarfism or giantism. Moreover, generalized shortening of the roots must be distinguished from dentinal dysplasia and orthodontic root resorption.

VARIATIONS IN SHAPE OF TEETH

Gemination (Schizodontia)

Gemination is an attempt by the tooth bud to divide. This partial division is halted before development is completed. Colyer (1926) was the first to show an irregular epithelial invagination on the enamel organ that seemed to be an attempt to divide it and form two teeth.

Gemination is more prevalent among primary than permanent teeth. The favorite location is the incisor and canine regions, but gemination may also be seen among premolars. It is not always possible to differentiate between gemination and fusion in a case where there has been fusion between a normal tooth and a supernumerary tooth.

According to Tannenbaum and Alling (1963), the term "twinning" means that the tooth bud cleavage is complete,

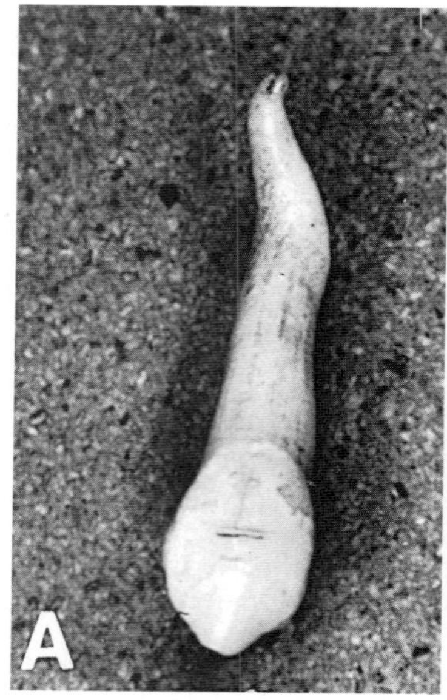

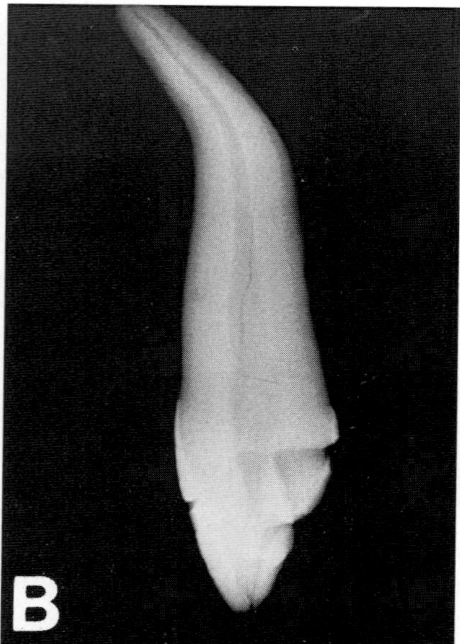

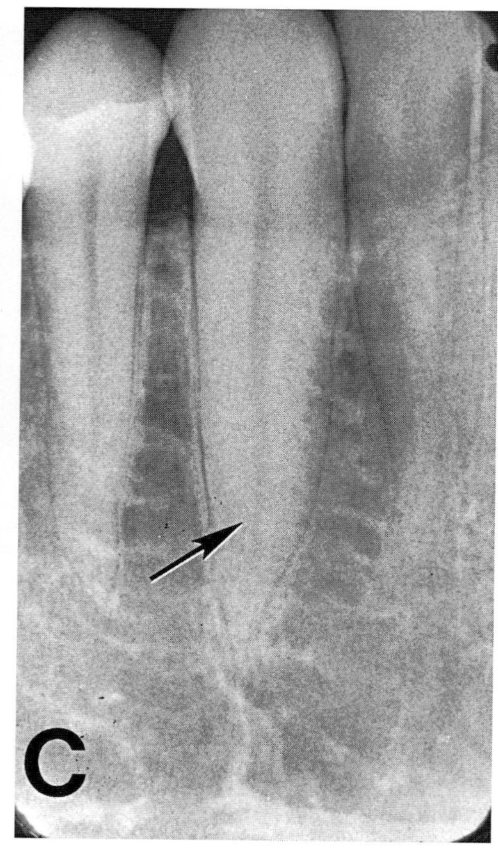

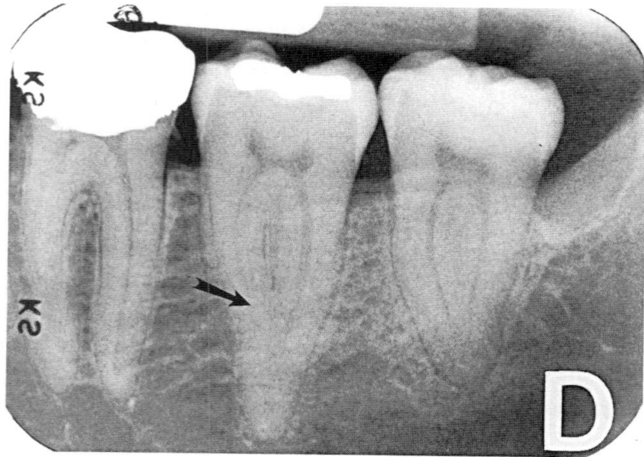

FIGURE 5–14.

Macrodontia. A, Clinical photograph of an extracted maxillary canine tooth (37 mm long; the average length is 27.3 mm). B, Radiograph of the maxillary canine in A. C, Very long canine tooth (arrow; length, 32 mm; the average length is 26.0 mm). D, Extremely long mandibular second molar; note that the roots are fused (arrow).

resulting in formation of an extra tooth in the dental arch that is usually a mirror image of its adjacent partner. De Jong in 1957 called this condition schizodontia (schizo: to split), a term applied to geminated teeth that originate by a division of the tooth anlage into a mesial and distal component. Levitas (1965) believed schizodontia or twinning does not fit the criteria suggested for geminated teeth. He believed that this condition more properly should be placed under the heading of supernumerary teeth.

As to prevalence of joined teeth, various writers agree that the condition of gemination and fusion constitutes a problem in the primary dentition and occurs rarely in permanent teeth. Tannenbaum and Alling (1963), in a study of 2000 men, disclosed but 2 instances of gemination, a prevalence of 0.1%. Menczer reported 2209 clinical examinations of preschool children (aged 2 to 6 years) in which he found 11 instances of joined teeth, or a prevalence of 0.5%. Buenviaje and Rapp (1984), in an examination of 2439 children, found 2 instances of gemination, for a prevalence of 0.08%. Clayton (1956), in an examination of 3557 children, found a prevalence of 0.47% for joined teeth (fusion, gemination, and concrescence).

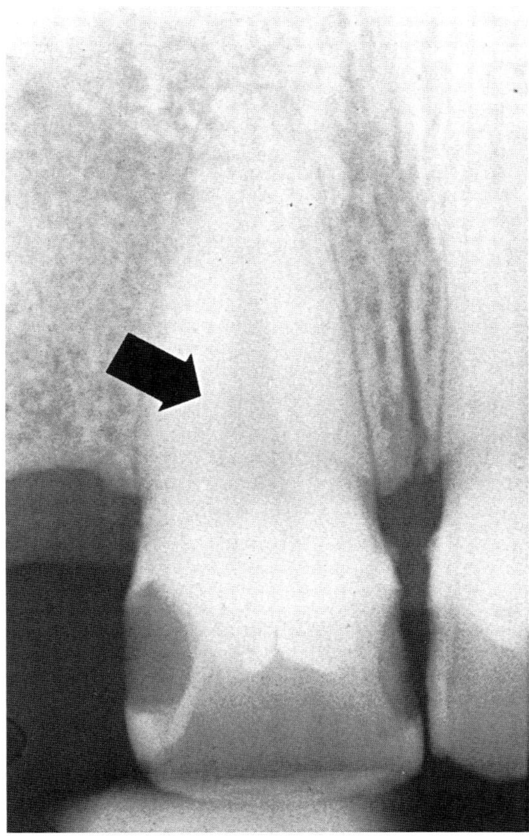

FIGURE 5–15.

Macrodontia. Radiograph of a maxillary central incisor 11 mm wide (arrow). The average normal size is 9.0 mm.

◆ *RADIOLOGY (Figs. 5–16 to 5–18)*

Radiographs are especially helpful in distinguishing gemination from fusion. A normal complement of teeth must be established, confirmed by an accurate history. An enlarged notched crown with two pulp chambers and a single root and pulp canal are often noted in gemination. As Tannenbaum and Alling (1963) suggested, a radiograph to count the number of roots is helpful. Heslop (1954) stated that the radiograph has value in the diagnosis of gemination.

Fusion (Syndontia)

Fusion may be defined as a union between the dentin or enamel of two or more separate developing teeth (tooth buds). Rarely, however, are two teeth united by enamel only. There may be complete union to form one abnormally large tooth, union of crowns, or union of roots only. A supernumerary tooth is frequently one of the affected teeth. Fusion of teeth leads to a reduced number of teeth in the dental arch. Sometimes, the term synodontia is used for fusion of teeth. As a rule, there are two distinct pulp chambers, although occasionally one large, irregular pulp cavity may extend through the fused teeth. Fusions are more frequent among primary than permanent teeth. Clayton (1963), Grahnen and Granath (1961), Toth and Csemi (1967), and

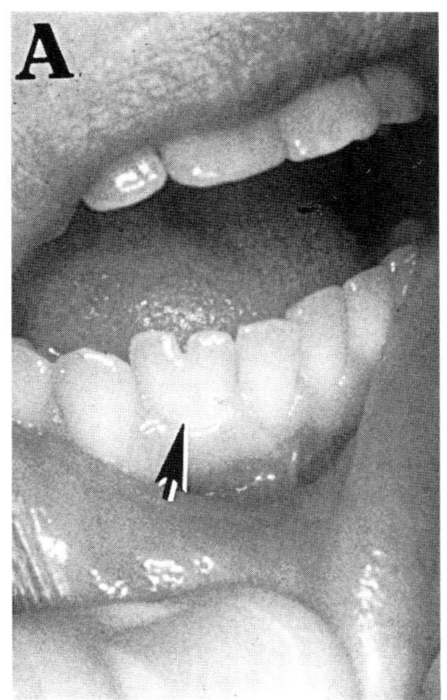

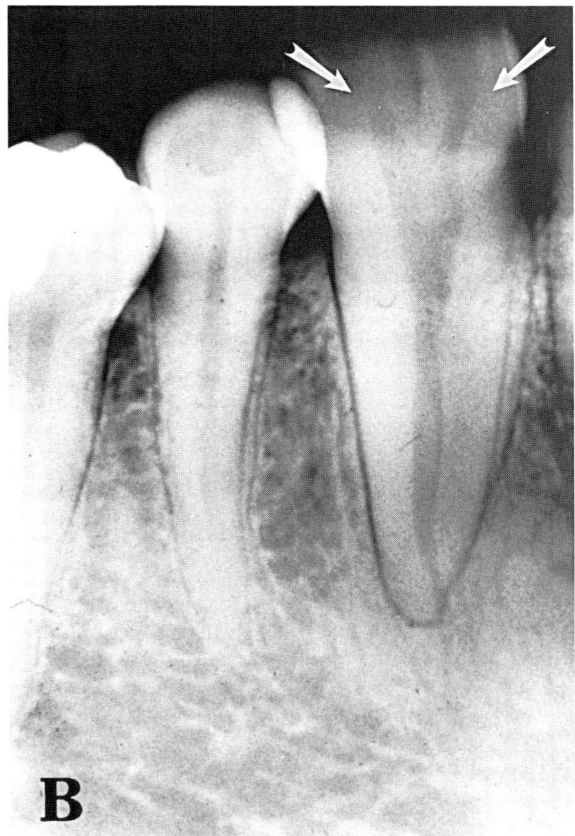

FIGURE 5–16.

Gemination. A, Clinical photograph of a patient with gemination of the lower right lateral incisor (arrow). B, Erupted geminated mandibular canine tooth (arrows).

(continued)

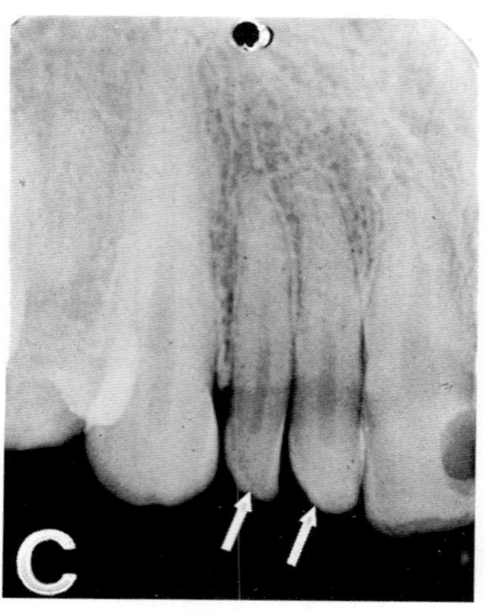

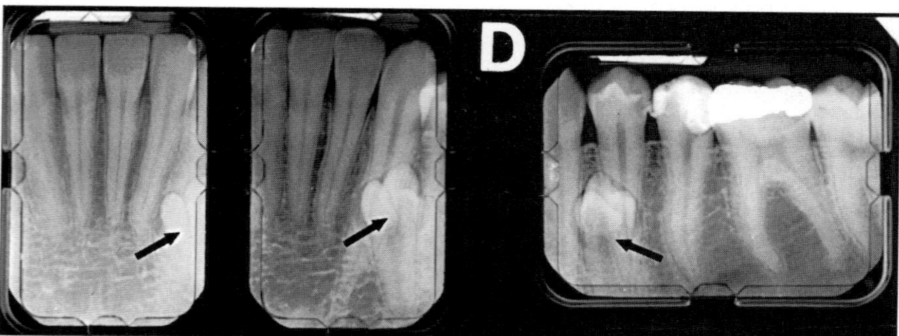

FIGURE 5–16.

(continued) C, Twinning (gemination) of two maxillary microdontic lateral incisors from one tooth bud (arrows). D, Gemination of a supernumerary premolar (arrows), which is lingual to other mandibular teeth (Clark's rule).

Niswander and Sujaku (1963) reported that the prevalence of fused and geminated primary teeth varies between 0.5 to 2.5%. Buenviaje and Rapp (1984) found that 10 children (0.42%) had fused teeth among 2439 children examined. In 9 instances, the primary central and lateral incisors were fused, and 1 child exhibited a fusion of the permanent mandibular left central and lateral incisors.

Fusion of primary teeth in children with thalidomide-induced embryopathy was reported by Gysel (1965). In the permanent dentition, fused teeth are also frequent in the incisor region. A fusion of maxillary central incisors has been reported, but it is extremely rare. A dominant trait of fused teeth has been found in some families.

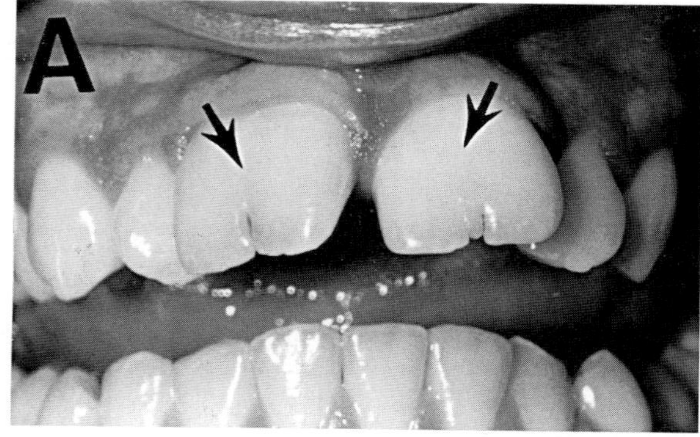

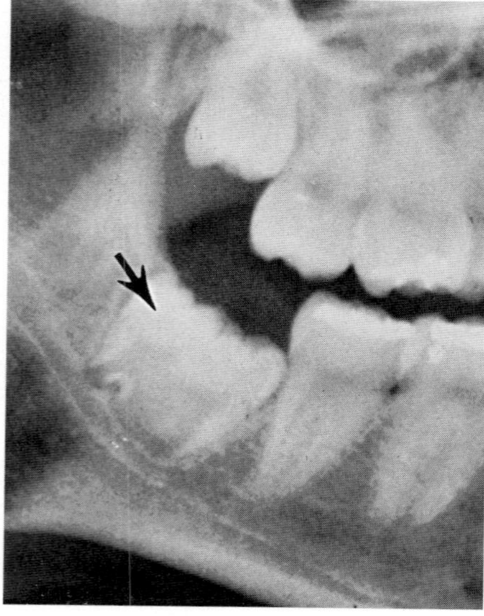

FIGURE 5–17.

Posterior Gemination. Gemination of the mandibular third molar (arrow). (Courtesy of Dr. J. Ribamar De Azevedo, Instituto Odonto-Radiologico, Brasilia, Brazil.)

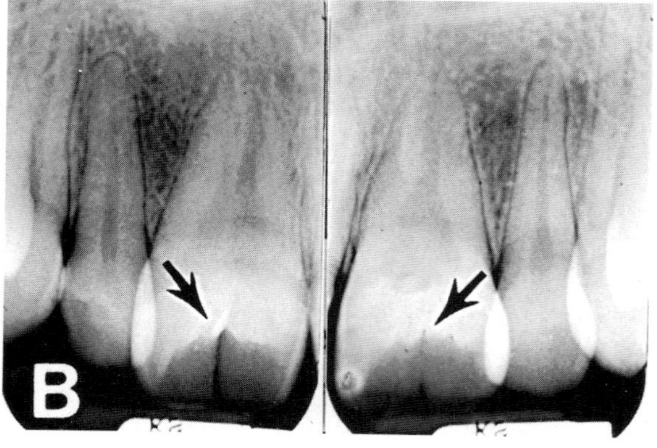

FIGURE 5–18.

Bilateral Gemination. A, Clinical photograph of bilateral gemination of the maxillary central incisors (arrows). B, Radiographs of bilateral gemination of the maxillary central incisors (arrows) in the patient in A. (Courtesy of Dr. S. Bricker, University of Indiana School of Dentistry, Indianapolis, IN.)

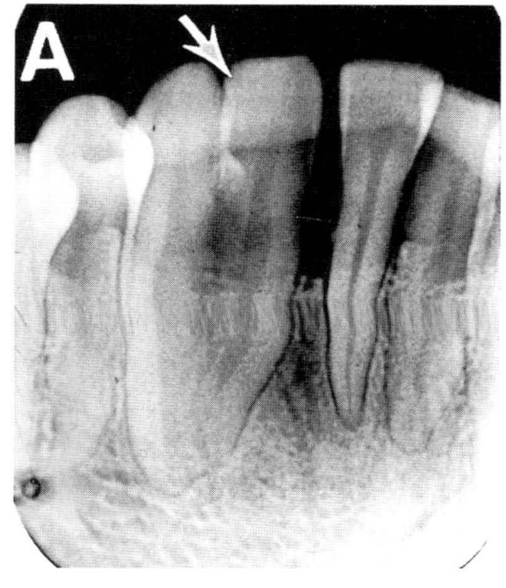

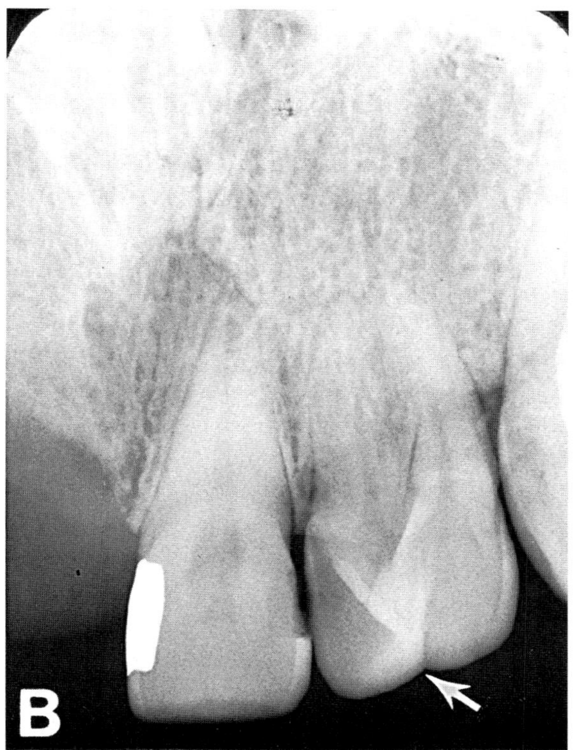

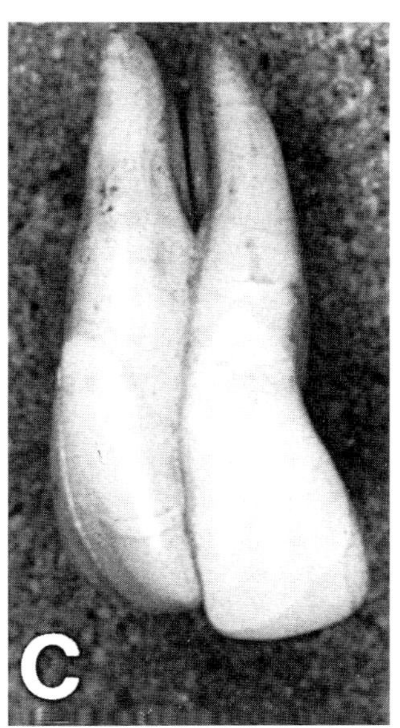

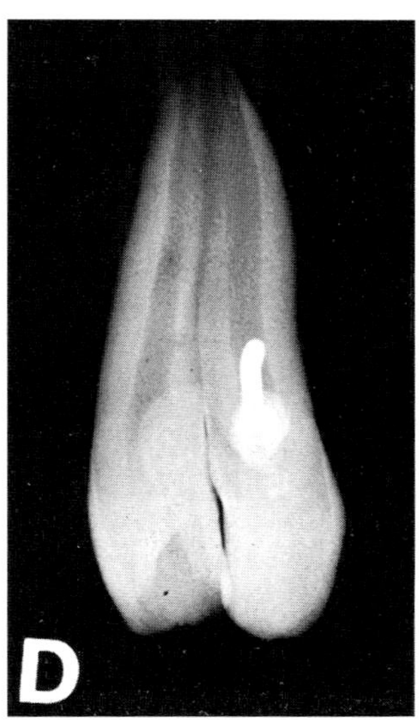

FIGURE 5–19.

Fusion. A, Fusion between a mandibular canine tooth and a lateral incisor (arrow). (Courtesy of Drs. L. Archilla, F. Erales, and R. Carlos, Guatemala City, Guatemala.) B, Fusion between a maxillary lateral incisor and a supernumerary lateral incisor (arrow). C, Clinical photograph of fusion between maxillary incisors. D, Radiograph of fusion of the maxillary incisors in C.

◆ *RADIOLOGY (Figs. 5–19 and 5–20)*

It is important to count the teeth. If one tooth appears to be missing, fusion may be suspected. Usually, fused teeth look like two teeth stuck together, and often the dentin is confluent. The diagnosis is easier when there are two separate pulp chambers and root canals (Fig. 5–19). A single, confluent pulp chamber and root canal in an oversized tooth may also be seen (Fig. 5–20).

Concrescence (Figs. 5–21 and 5–22)

Concrescence of teeth is actually a form of fusion that may be defined as a condition in which the roots of two or more teeth have been united by cementum alone after formation of the crown (Fig. 5–21). The condition is thought to arise as a result of traumatic injury or crowding of teeth with resorption of the interdental bone, so the two roots are in

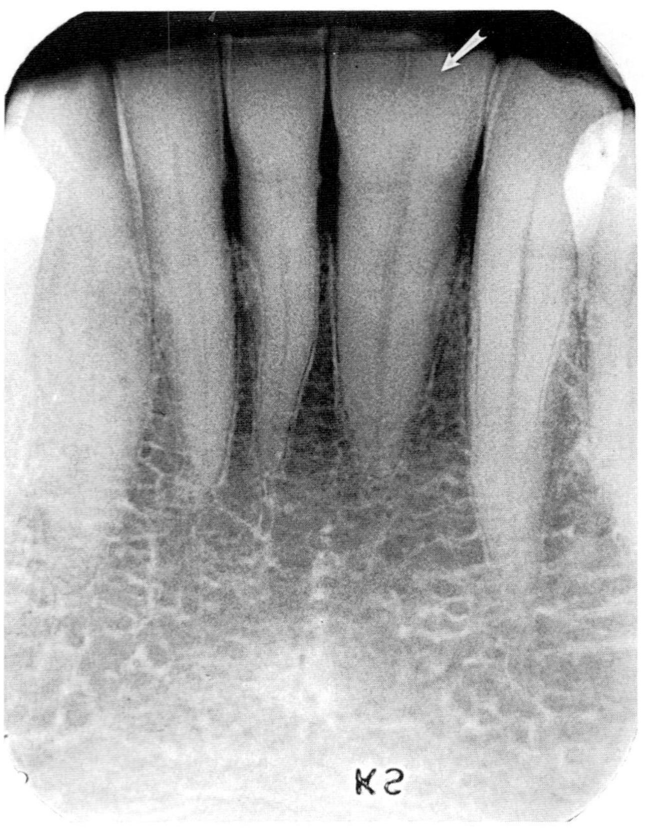

FIGURE 5–20.

Fusion. Fusion between the left mandibular lateral and central incisors forming one large tooth (arrow). (There is one less tooth in the mandibular incisor region.)

approximate contact and become fused by the deposition of cementum between them.

If the union has occurred during tooth development, the condition is called **true concrescence.** Reasons for this type of cemental union include lack of space and distortion of tooth germs. True concrescence is most often seen between second and third molars in the maxilla, where lack of space may be responsible for the anomaly (Figs. 5–21 and 5–22).

If the union has occurred after completion of root formation, the condition is called **acquired concrescence.** Such a condition may be the result of union of hypercementosis associated with chronic inflammation. Concrescence may take place between normal teeth, between normal and supernumerary teeth, or between two or more supernumerary teeth.

◆ *RADIOLOGY (Figs. 5–21 and 5–22)*

More often than not, one or both of the united teeth remain unerupted; therefore, in most instances, they are first recognized incidental to a radiographic examination. Because in concrescence the extraction of one tooth may result in the extraction of the other, it is desirable that the dentist be forewarned of the condition and advise the patient. However, it is not always possible to distinguish between actual concrescence and images of teeth that are in close contact, but are merely superimposed. Concrescence, if not recognized, presents a hazard in extraction, particularly if undue and indiscriminate force is applied. Pindborg (1970) reported a case of a 50-year-old man who had acquired concrescence of three molars and one premolar in the maxilla.

Dilaceration

The term "dilaceration" refers to an angulation, or sharp bend or curve, in the root or crown of a formed tooth. Minor root curvature is sometimes called "flexion," which is distinguished from dilaceration by being a deviation involving the root alone. However, the term dilaceration is applied to all teeth having seriously deflected or angulated roots. Any tooth may show this type of defect. It is frequently seen in mild to severe form in roots of mandibular third molars, maxillary lateral incisors, and maxillary premolars.

The condition is thought to be due to trauma during the period in which the tooth is forming, with the result that the position of the calcified portion of tooth is changed and the

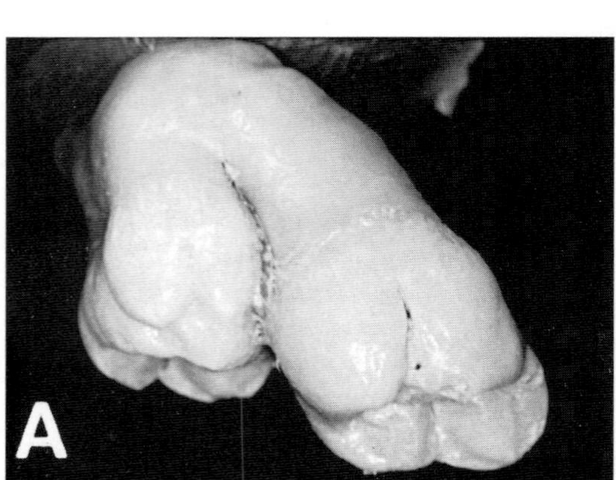

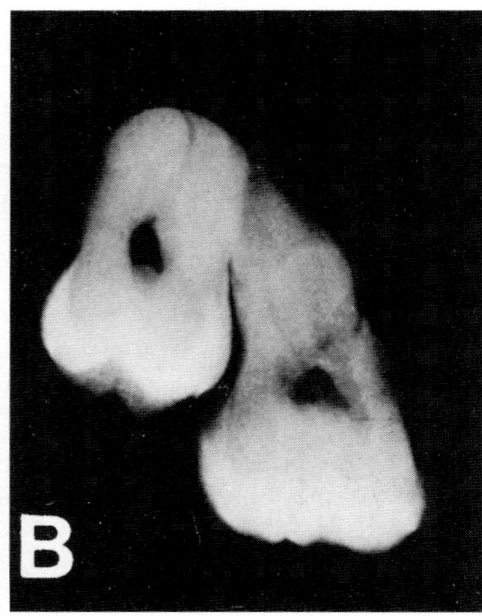

FIGURE 5–21.

Concrescence. A, Gross specimen (second and third molars). B, Radiograph of the gross specimen (second and third molar concrescence) in A. (Courtesy of Dr. J. D'Ambrosio, University of Connecticut, Farmington, CT.)

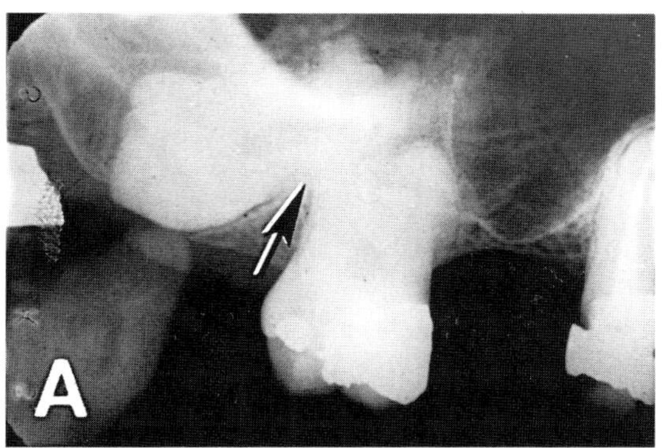

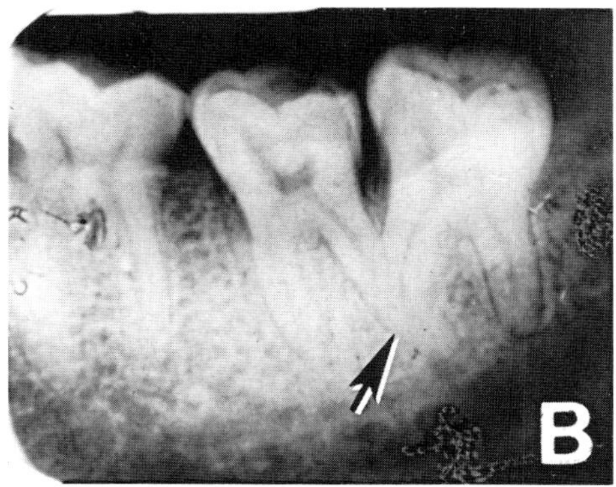

FIGURE 5–22.

Concrescence. A, Concrescence of the second and third mandibular molars (arrow). (Courtesy of Dr. P. Dhiravarangkura, Chulalonghorn University, Bangkok, Thailand.) B, Concrescence of the second and third mandibular molars (arrow). (Courtesy of Dr. J. D'Ambrosio, University of Connecticut, Farmington, CT.)

remainder of the tooth is formed at an angle. The curve or bend may occur anywhere along the length of the tooth, sometimes at the cervical portion, at other times midway along the root or even just at the apex of the root, depending on the amount of root formed when the injury occurred. Some dilacerations are undoubtedly unrelated to sudden physical trauma, but are bent and distorted by the crowding of teeth into an arch that is too small to permit full dental root development. Of course, the slight natural distal curvature of some dental roots should not be mistaken for malformation. Dilacerated roots display sharp and obvious bends.

According to Wheeler (1965), the permanent maxillary lateral incisors are second only to third molars in exhibiting shape and form variation. In addition, Sommer and co-workers (1966) reported that the roots of these teeth, when dilacerated, tend to curve in a distal direction; or, as pointed out by Weine (1989), root dilaceration can occur in distolabial and distolingual directions.

Chohayeb in 1983 examined 480 extracted permanent upper lateral incisors and found that 52.1% of the roots of these teeth were distolabially dilacerated. In this study, the root dilaceration was defined as a deviation of 20° or more of the apical end of the root from the normal long axis of the tooth. Chohayeb (1983) proposed that the oversight of the distolabial direction of root dilaceration of the upper lateral incisor could be a contributing factor in the failure of endodontic treatment of these teeth. In fact, Grahnen and Hansson (1961) reported a higher rate of failure of endodontic treatment of the single-rooted maxillary lateral incisor teeth when compared to the treatment failure of multirooted teeth.

◆ *RADIOLOGY (Fig. 5–23)*

Because dilacerated teeth frequently present problems at the time of extraction if the dentist is unaware of the condition, the obvious need for adequate preoperative radiographic visualization of the entire root structure of such teeth cannot be overemphasized. Moreover, the radiograph is the best available guide to a treatment plan if it should be necessary to compete a root canal procedure on a dilacerated tooth.

One or more curve or bend may be present in the same root (Figs. 5–23 and 5–25C). The change in direction is sometimes sharp, even as great as a right angle. The deformity is best seen in radiographs when it is situated at the mesial or distal aspect of the tooth; if the abnormality is toward the facial or lingual aspect, it may not be apparent radiographically.

The apex of the lower molar may be at right angles to the root, and this is apparent in the radiograph irrespective of the direction of the root, even when buccal or lingual. Consideration of the anatomic arrangement when the apex is directed buccally or lingually enables the radiographic appearance to be understood. The deflected portion of the root lies in the axis of the x-rays that pass directly through the length of that portion of the root; consequently, it will appear in the radiograph as a more or less rounded opacity; in the center is the dark spot for the root canal. Surrounding the apex is the lamina dura, which appears as a white ring around the root separated from it by the dark ring of the periodontal ligament space. It is not possible to determine the direction of the apex, except it is at right angles to the tooth. The apex may be buccal or lingual and may produce an identical appearance in radiographs, but when the root is deflected lingually, it is much more defined. In the maxilla, a different set of circumstances holds. The x-rays for the most part are directed more buccally, and only when the inclined x-rays happen to coincide in direction with the axis of the dilacerated portion of the root are the characteristic radiographic appearances seen. Nevertheless, on many occasions, the images described previously for mandibular molars do appear in the maxillary teeth.

Supernumerary Roots (Fig. 5–24)

This developmental condition is not uncommon and may involve any tooth. Teeth that are normally single rooted may

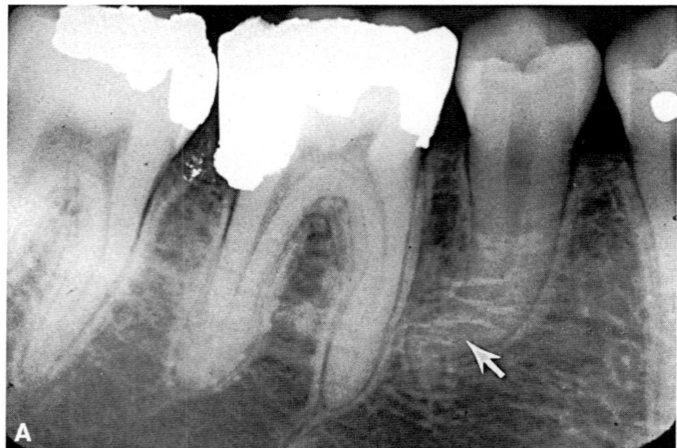

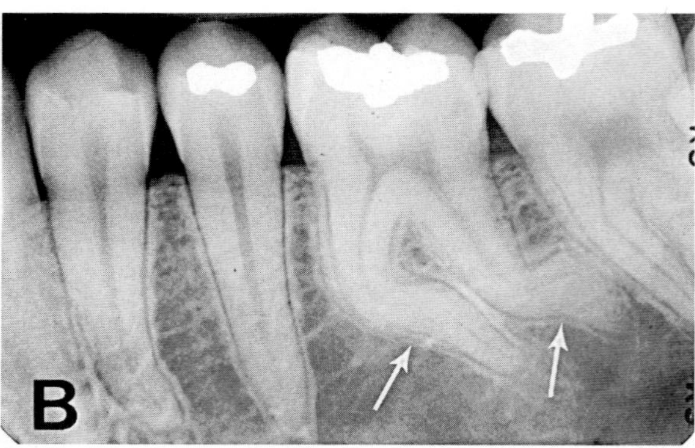

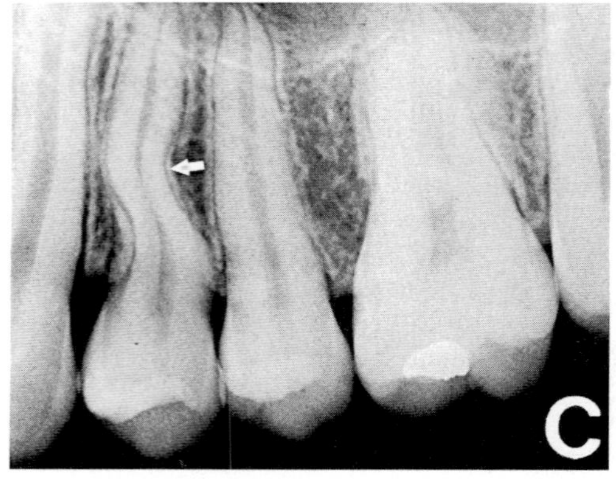

FIGURE 5–23.

Dilaceration. A, Erupted dilacerated root of a mandibular second premolar (arrow). B, Distally inclined root tips of a mandibular first molar (arrows). C, Dilaceration of a maxillary first premolar (arrow).

have two or more roots or apices. The lower canine tooth is often bifid (Fig. 5–24). Harboro (1934) has made a special study of two-rooted mandibular canine teeth and gives many interesting illustrations.

The upper first premolar, normally two rooted, may have three roots that are arranged in a manner similar to those of the upper first molar. The upper second premolar may have two roots instead of the normal one. The lower premolars may be two rooted (Fig. 5–24B). Freenezy reported that a bifurcation of the root canal is seen in 13% of mandibular first premolars, but only in 1% of the mandibular second premolars. Bifid roots of lower premolars occur when there is an abrupt termination of the pulp chamber into two fine root canals for each root. The lower molar usually has two roots, and it may have a third (Fig. 5–24C). The mesial root usually has two separate canals, but on occasion the roots are bifid and separate.

The prevalence of the three-rooted lower first molar varies from 1% in Caucasians to 20% in Mongolians, as reported by Pindborg (1970). Pedersen (1949) reported this trait of 16% in one Native North American population. Turner obtained a remarkably high figure of 43.6% for trifurcate mandibular molars in Aleuts. The frequency of this trait in Mongoloid races must be considered a genetically determined characteristic.

Because many of the people in ''Chinatowns'' throughout the world have migrated from Hong Kong, practitioners in these areas should be aware of the possibility of the lower 3-rooted first molar. Walker and Quackenbush (1985) found, in a radiographic survey of 2131 Hong Kong Chinese patients, a 14.6% prevalence of this anomaly. The need to diagnose this variation is important in both endodontics and oral surgery. In radiographs, careful examination of the radiolucent lines of the pulp spaces and the periodontal ligament spaces can lead to identification of most trifurcated lower molars. The roots of the maxillary third molar may, after an initial spreading, unite to form a taproot whereby the roots have a common layer of dentin.

◆ *RADIOLOGY (Fig. 5–24)*

Supernumerary roots can be either fully developed in size and shape or small and rudimentary. Sometimes, they are fused to the other roots, but they may be bifid and widely separated. The presence of supernumerary roots is established by radiographic examination. Two radiographs may have to be made from slightly different angles to reveal hidden supernumerary roots.

When supernumerary roots are not superimposed on other roots, they are easier to detect. An extra root canal or double periodontal membrane space may be a clue. Supernumerary roots may be suspected when there is a sudden diminution in the size of the root canal space or when it appears to divide into several smaller root canal spaces.

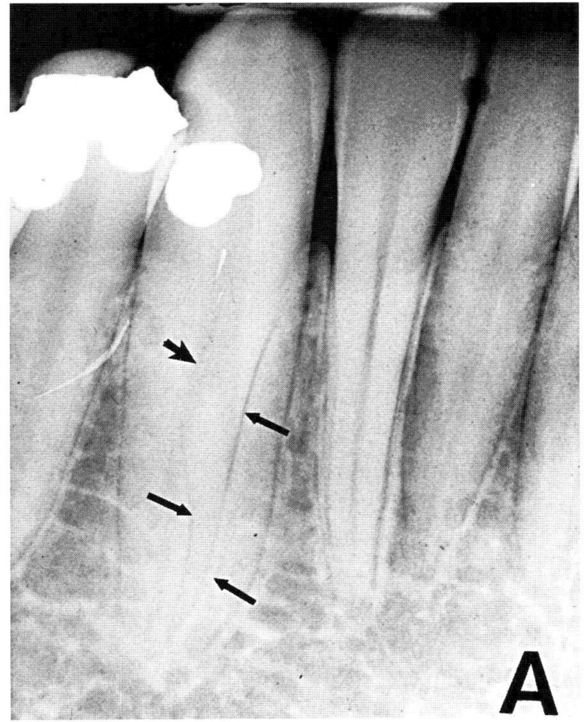

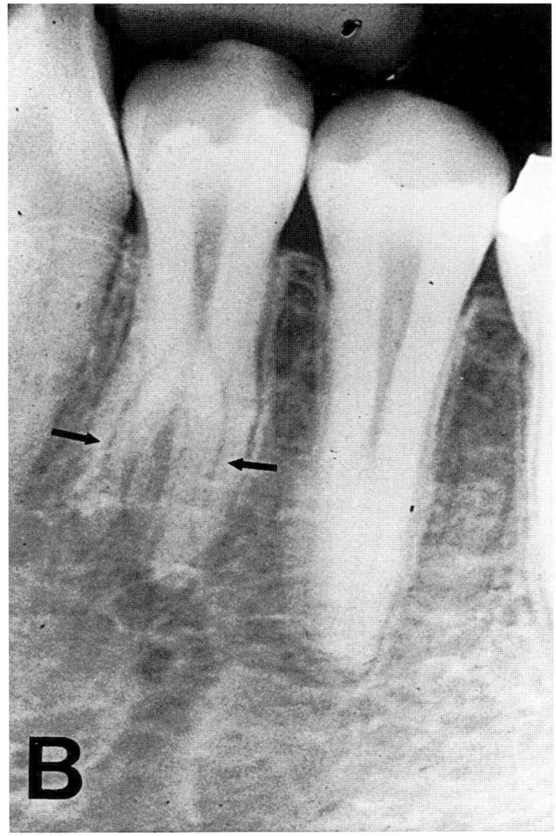

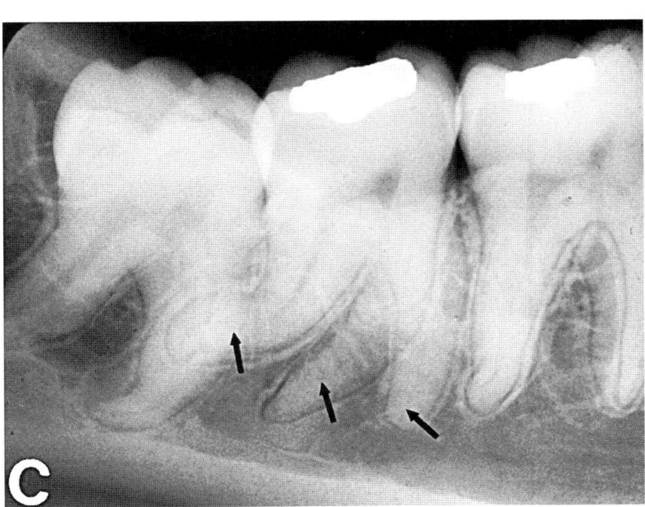

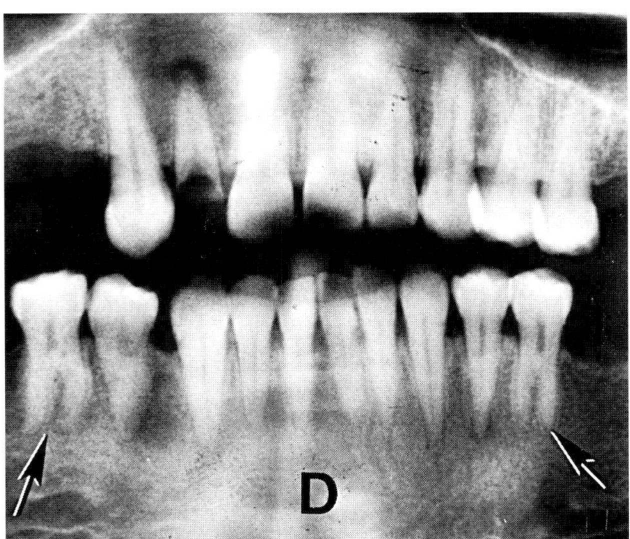

FIGURE 5–24.

Supernumerary Roots. A, Two-rooted canine tooth. Note that the canine tooth shows the periodontal ligament space crossing the roots (thin arrows) and the inverted Y shape of the root canal (thick arrow). B, Multirooted mandibular premolars. C, Three-rooted mandibular second molar (arrows). D, Bilateral mandibular two-rooted second premolars (arrows).

Supernumerary Cusps (Figs. 5–25 and 5–26)

Mellor and Ripa (1970) described the talon cusp as a markedly enlarged cingulum on a maxillary incisor tooth, a rare finding in the normal population. This anomalous structure resembles an eagle's talon and projects lingually from the incisor teeth (Fig. 5–25A). The talon cusp blends smoothly with the tooth, except for a deep developmental groove where the cusp blends with the sloping lingual tooth surface. It is composed of normal enamel and dentin and contains a horn of pulp tissue. The fissure between the enlarged cingulum and the lingual surface of the tooth is particularly susceptible to dental caries that may rapidly involve the pulp, resulting in loss of the tooth if endodontic therapy is not instituted. It is therefore wise to restore this fissure as a prophylactic measure. Talon cusps may also interfere with the occlusion of the teeth. If this becomes a problem, the cusp may have to be removed. Mellor and Ripa (1970) reported that this procedure may also expose the dental pulp and may necessitate endodontic therapy.

Fortunately, this anomaly is uncommon in the general population. Gardner and Girgis (1979) found that talon cusps appeared to be more prevalent in persons with the Rubinstein-Taybi syndrome. The main clinical features of the Rubenstein-Taybi syndrome, which was first described in 1963 by Rubinstein and Taybi, are developmental retardation, broad thumbs and great toes, characteristic facial features, delayed or incomplete descent of testes in males, and bone age below the fiftieth percentile. The talon cusp has not been reported as an integral part of any other syndrome, although Mader (1979), in his review, suggested that it may be associated with other somatic and odontogenic anomalies.

In canine teeth, the palatal (lingual) tuberculum may be so accentuated that the teeth resemble premolars. Therefore, the term "premolarization of the canines" is sometimes applied to these teeth. By analogy with the canine teeth, the premolars may "molarize" and may therefore cause difficulties in eruption. The premolars may show a significant reduction in size, especially the maxillary second premolar. An extra cusp may occur, usually on the buccal aspect of the premolars.

The maxillary first molar may have an extra tuberculum located on the mesial part of the palatal surface. These extra cusps are called "cusps of Carabelli." Pindborg (1970) reported that when the cusps of Carabelli is present it is seen on both right and left sides, and the prevalence varies from 10 to 36%, depending on the population studied.

Dens evaginatus represents an accessory cusp emanating occlusally from the central groove of premolars and molars. This anomaly is rare and is most often encountered among Eskimos. A pulp horn may extend into this central occlusal cusp.

Dahlberg (1951) reported a shovel-shaped incisor that is

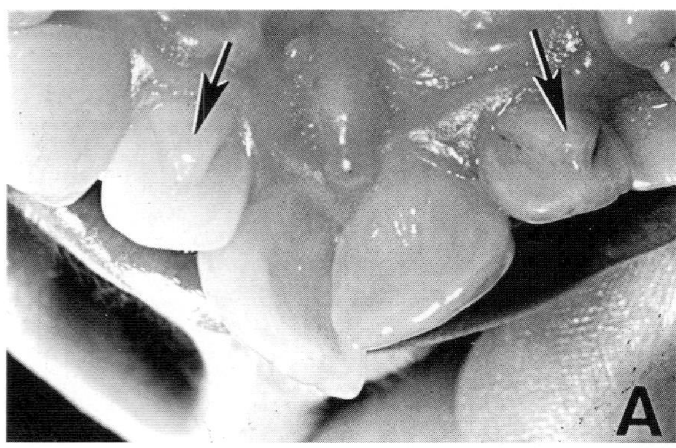

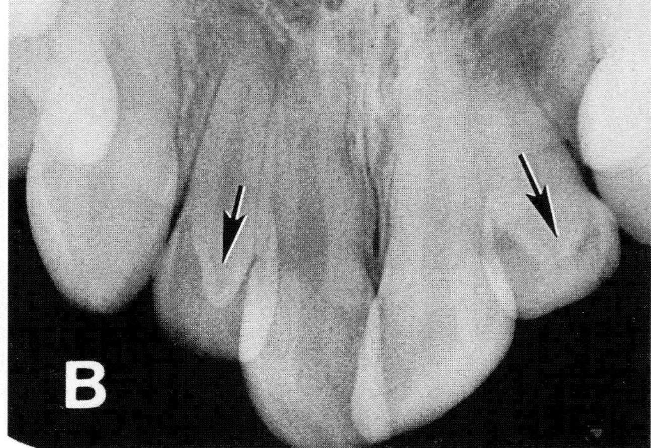

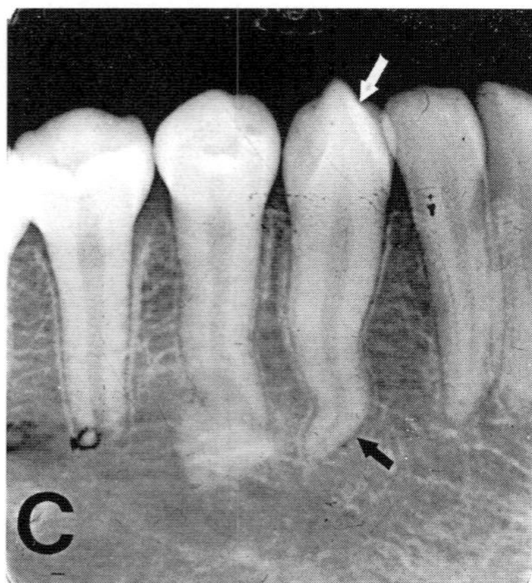

FIGURE 5–25.

Supernumerary Talon Cusps. A, Clinical photograph of bilateral talon cusps (arrows) on the lingual surface of the maxillary incisors. B, Radiograph of bilateral talon cusps (arrows) of the maxillary lateral incisors in A. (Also see Fig. 5–10C.) C, Radiograph of a talon cusp of a mandibular canine tooth (white arrow). Also note the dilaceration (black arrow) of the first premolar. (Courtesy of Dr. P. Dhiravarangkura, Chulalonghorn University Bangkok, Thailand.)

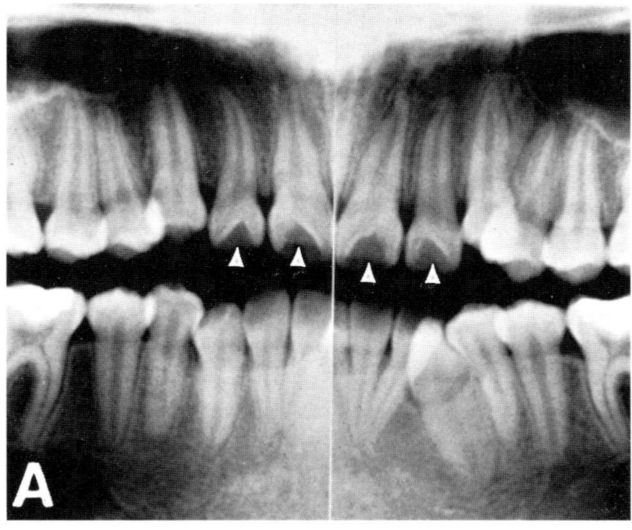

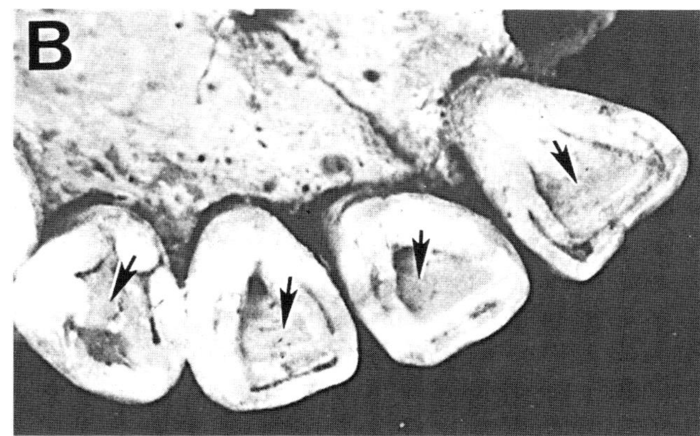

FIGURE 5–26.

Shovel-Tooth Incisors. A, Shovel-tooth maxillary incisors (arrowheads) in a Mexican-American patient. B, Clinical photograph of shovel-tooth maxillary incisors (arrows) in a dry skull of a Native North American.

racially determined and may be seen in Mongoloid races such as Eskimos and Mongolians, Native North and South Americans, Chinese, Japanese, Polynesians, and Melanesians. The crowns are normal except for prominent lingual marginal ridges in the maxillary central and lateral incisors, often referred to as shovel-shaped incisors. Occasionally, the shovel shape is associated with accentuated marginal ridges, providing what might be termed a "double shovel."

◆ *RADIOLOGY (Figs. 5–25 and 5–26)*

The talon cusp enlargement sometimes is so great that the cingulum reaches the incisive edge. When the talon cusp is seen before eruption, this is likely to be mistaken for a supernumerary tooth superimposed by the crown of the incisor. The cingulum is sometimes represented by two or more elevations varying in size by small clefts of variable depth between them. Radiographs made from different angles help in the identification of such unusual teeth before eruption. The enamel covering of these pronounced tubercles may appear as thin white lines seen through the crown of the incisor and converging toward the incisal margin. The cingulum that extends to the incisal edge has curved mesial and distal margins, covered by enamel, with the concavities backing each other. The images of the enamel suggest the presence of a small extra tooth. Accessory cusps are rarely in occlusion, so no treatment is required except in the case of buccal accessory cusps, in which periodontal pocket formation is encountered.

Dens evaginatus may pose a problem because the cusps are in occlusion and the pulp horns extend into these areas. The radiograph is most helpful in revealing the extent of the pulpal horn into these central supplemental cusps (dens evaginatus) of the premolars. Sometimes, premolars with extra cusps have difficulties in eruption. The radiograph aids in the diagnosis of this problem.

When shovel-shaped incisors are seen on radiographs (Fig. 5–26A), the clinician should look for the following abnormalities in the maxillary incisors: interproximal caries, lingual pit caries, and periapical lesions of pulpal origin. Additionally, the presence of shortened or tapered roots is of significance in planning treatment, especially in prosthodontics and periodontics. This combination of findings has been loosely named the **shovel-shaped incisor syndrome.**

Taurodontism

Taurodontism is an apical extension of the pulp chamber of molar teeth that results in a proportionately shortened root and enlarged pulp in the affected dentition. Teeth with pulp chambers extending below the cementoenamel junction and lacking constriction at this level are said to have the condition of taurodontism. The teeth also have apical displacement of the bifurcation or trifurcation of roots. The diagnosis of taurodontism depends on the degree to which the pulp chamber occupies the overall length from the cementoenamel junction to the root apex. This feature is common to nearly all definitions of taurodontism. Reports have indicated that taurodontism may not be limited to molar involvement because it occurs in the premolar teeth. This condition was recognized in Neanderthal teeth from Krapina in Croatia after a radiographic study by Kallay (1949, 1963) and also in studies of modern man by Garcia-Godoy and Armach (1977), Bruszt (1953), Brabant and Kovacs (1960), Ferenczy (1962), and Bernick (1970).

The term "taurodontism" (tauros: bull; and odous: tooth), was coined in 1913 by Sir Arthur Keith to describe a peculiar dental anomaly in which the body of the tooth is enlarged at the expense of the roots. The term means "bull-like" teeth, and its usage is derived from the similarity of these teeth to those of ungulate or cud-chewing animals. In contrast, Keith used the term cynodont (doglike tooth) to describe the normal condition in which the body of the tooth is above the border of the alveolus.

The prevalence of taurodontism reported in modern populations has varied from 0.54% in primary dentitions of Japanese children, as reported by Daito and Hieda (1971), to 5.6% in the permanent dentitions of Israeli adults, as reported by Shifman and Chanannel (1978). Jaspers and Witkop (1980) reported that taurodontism is not a rare trait in modern man, as indicated by a majority of the recent reports (1980), but it occurs in approximately 2.5% of adult Caucasians.

Madeira and associates (1986) examined 4459 premolar and molar teeth and revealed that 0.25% of them (all mandibular premolars) showed distinctive characteristics of taurodontism. None of the maxillary premolars exhibited this condition. This was probably the first report on the prevalence in premolar teeth in a contemporary population.

Theories concerning the pathogenesis of root formation in taurodontism are varied. Hamner and associates (1964) believed that taurodontism is caused by failure of Hertwig's epithelial sheath to invaginate at the proper horizontal level.

Taurodontism may be an isolated, singular trait, according to Winter and co-workers (1969), Crawford (1970), and Parker and associates (1975), or it may occur in association with syndromes and anomalies. Some of the syndromes and anomalies associated with taurodontism have been reported by the following: amelogenesis imperfecta by Winter and associates (1969), Crawford (1970), Parker and co-workers (1975), and Congleton and Burkes (1979); Down's syndrome by Witkop (1976) and Jaspers (1981); ectodermal disturbances by Levin and associates and Stenvik and co-workers (1972); Mohr syndrome by Goldstein and Medina (1974); osteoporosis by Fuks and others (1982); and tricho-dento-osseous syndrome by Jorgenson and Warson and Lichtenstein and associates (1972). Jorgenson and co-workers (1982) believe that these malformations suggest than an ectodermal abnormality may be the cause of taurodontism.

In addition, Keeler (1973), Mednick (1973), and Stewart (1974) reported that many patients with Klinefelter's syndrome (males whose sex chromosome constitution includes one or more extra X chromosomes) exhibit taurodontism. For this reason, Gardner and Girgis (1978) recommended that male patients exhibiting taurodontism should undergo chromosomal studies, especially if there is any nonspecific diagnosis of mental retardation, and if the patient is tall and thin, with long arms and legs and a prognathic jaw.

Jaspers and Witkop (1980), in a review of the literature of taurodontism to date, indicated that the condition occurs as an isolated trait with greater frequency in certain populations with common racial, geographic, and ethnic backgrounds.

Taurodontism may affect either the deciduous or permanent dentition, although permanent involvement is more common. The molars are almost invariably involved, sometimes a single tooth, and at other times several molars in the same quadrant.

◆ *RADIOLOGY (Fig. 5–27)*

The defect is observable only in dental radiographs because no obvious clinical malformation exists. There is a markedly elongated pulp chamber with rudimentary root formation mimicking to some extent the normal morphology of the ungulate (hoofed mammal) dentition. Involved teeth frequently tend to be rectangular rather than tapering toward the roots. The pulp chamber is extremely large, with a much greater apico-occlusal height than normal. In addition, the pulp lacks the usual constriction at the cervical region of the tooth, and the roots are exceedingly short. The bifurcation or trifurcation may be only a few millimeters above the apices of the roots. The radiographic picture is characteristic.

The diagnosis of taurodontism depends on the degree to which the pulp chamber occupies the overall root length from the cementoenamel junction to the root apex. Sometimes, the mandibular second molar varies morphologically, forming a conical root form with the pulp chamber extending to the apex. This should not be confused with taurodontism.

Enamel Pearls (Enamel drop, enameloma)

Enamel pearls are called enamelomas by some authors; however, they are not true neoplasms. They are droplets of white, dome-shaped calcific concretions of enamel, usually located at the furcation areas of molar teeth. Enamel pearls are most often attached to the surface of the root of the tooth at or close to the cementoenamel junction. In some instances, they are attached to the dentin, and in others, to cementum. Those attached to the cementum most likely arise in the periodontium and become fused to the root of the tooth following complete development of the root. Clinically, it may be impossible to distinguish an enamel pearl from a small supernumerary tooth fused to the root. They vary in size, occasionally reaching the size of a pea. Cavanha (1965) found pearls that contain enamel only, others that contain a small core of dentin, and rarely, a small strand of pulp tissue extending from the pulp chamber or root canal of the tooth. Worth (1963) stated that there is no pulp cavity in an enamel pearl, and if it contains a pulp cavity, it is a geminated tooth.

The figures for prevalence of enamel pearls vary considerably; according to Pedersen (1949), the higher prevalence is found in Eskimos. Turner (1945) reported observing 23 enamel pearls in 1000 maxillary molars, but only 3 in 1000 mandibular molars. In addition, he found no enamel pearls on teeth anterior to the molars. Thus, the enamel pearl is not a common finding, and its clinical significance depends entirely on the site. If it happens to occupy such a position at the cementoenamel junction that it leads to pocket formation, then it is important in predisposing the patient to periodontal disease, and the mass may have to be removed with dental burs or stones. Apart from this potential problem, the enamel pearl has no importance, although it may occasionally be mistaken for calculus.

Enamel pearls are most frequently seen on maxillary teeth, usually mesially or distally on the upper second and third molars. On mandibular teeth, enamel pearls are usually found buccally or lingually.

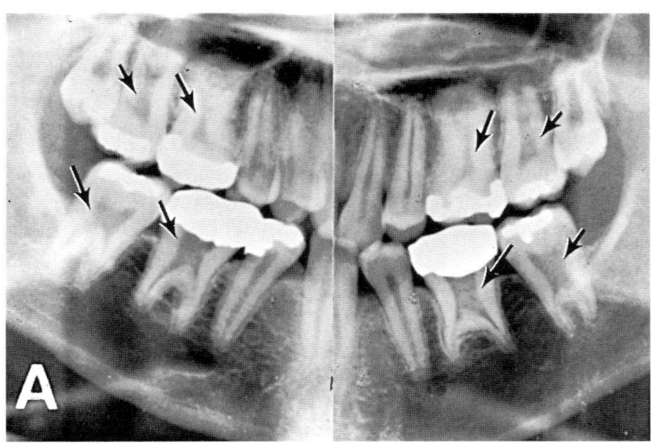

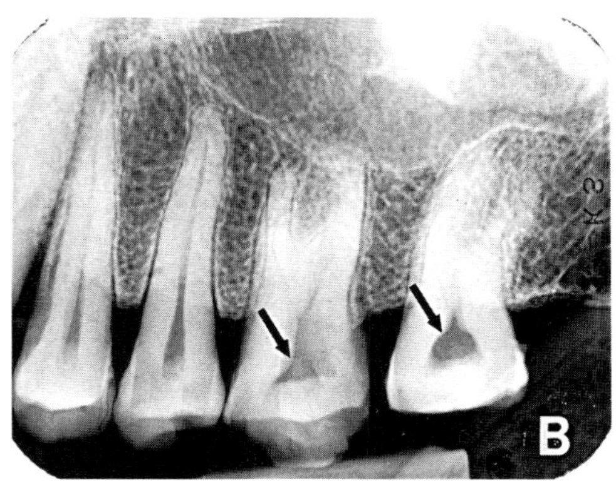

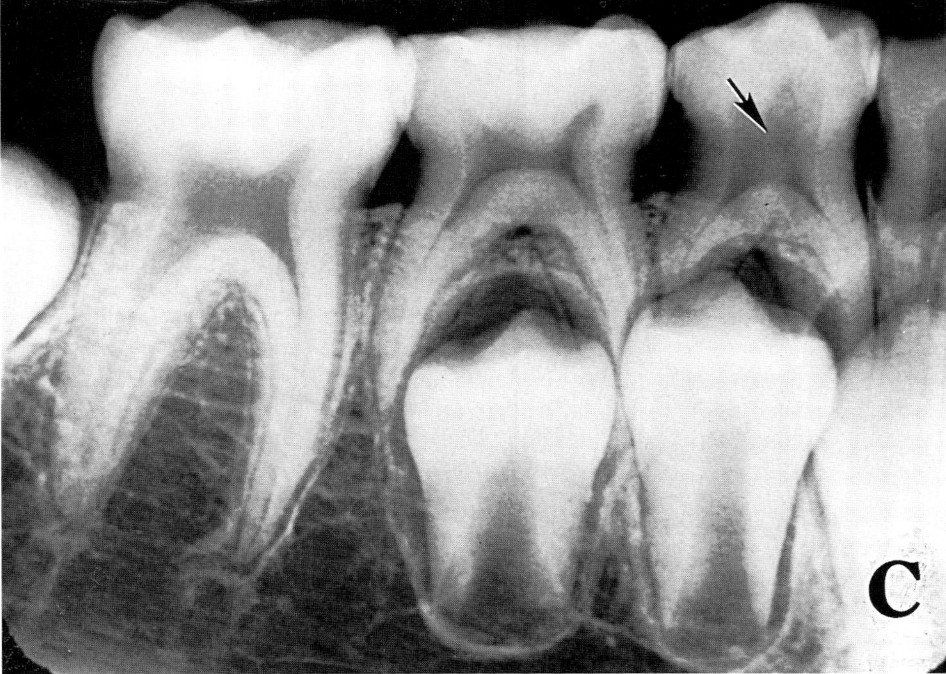

FIGURE 5–27.

Taurodontism. A, Radiograph of taurodontism of maxillary and mandibular first and second molars (arrows). B, Taurodontism of maxillary first and second molars (arrows). C, Taurodontism in a primary first molar (arrow). Note the large pulp chamber with a greater apico-occlusal height than normal.

◆ *RADIOLOGY (Figs. 5–28 to 5–30)*

The little mass is made up of enamel that absorbs more x-rays than the adjacent dentin, so it appears as a white image that is usually hemispherical and varies in size from 1 to 3 mm or more. The radiographic appearance of enamel pearls depends on the site and is best when they are situated on the mesial or distal aspect of the tooth, so they appear in profile. The typical appearance of an enamel pearl is a circular, dense, smooth projection at the cementoenamel junction (Fig. 5–28A). Enamel pearls may involve any part of the root. When attached below the gingival crest and on the mesial or distal aspect, an enamel pearl is covered by the periodontal ligament space image, beyond which is the lamina dura.

An enamel pearl situated on the lingual or the buccal surface is partially obscured by the mass of the crown or root, as the case may be, and its presence will probably escape recognition. If the pearl is large, the added density will usually be apparent on the radiograph, but this is unusual.

The only appearance that is likely to be mistaken for an enamel pearl is one that is due to projection effects, a common phenomenon. In the case of the mandibular molar and much less frequently the maxillary molar, in projecting the image of the roots in the radiographs, the angulation of the x-rays may be such that they do not pass freely between the roots where they approximate the bifurcation. The result is that a portion of the distal aspect of the mesial root is projected over the mesial portion of the distal root. The images of the superimposed portions of the adjacent roots reinforce one another and add to their radiographic density. The result is a rounded shadow of greater density where the roots converge at the bifurcation. The image is commonly seen in relation to the mandibular first molar, and less often the maxillary molar, and may be mistaken for an enamel pearl or pulp stone (Fig. 5–29). It is too low in position and outside

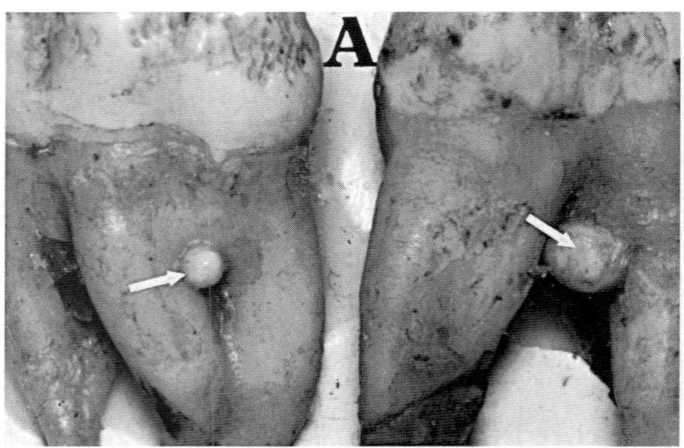

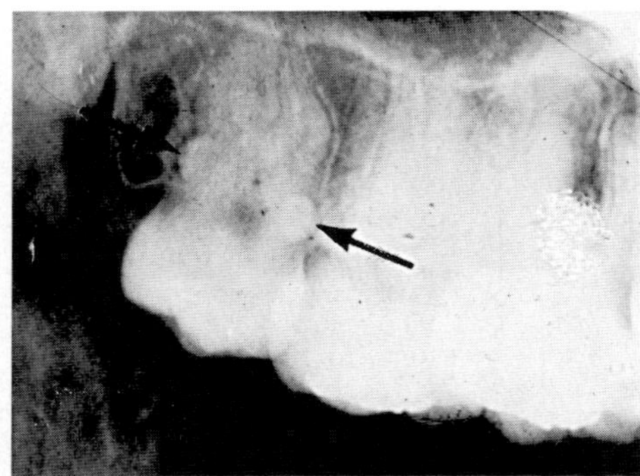

B

FIGURE 5–28.

Enamel Pearls. A, Enamel pearls (arrows) in gross specimens in furcations of maxillary and mandibular molars. B, Double enamel pearls of a maxillary second molar (arrows). (Courtesy of Dr. P. Dhiravarangkura, Chulalonghorn University, Bangkok, Thailand.)

the pulp to be a pulp stone. The proof of the nature of the image is demonstrated by making radiographs in such a way that the x-rays pass between the contentuous portions of the roots, and the radiopaque images then disappear. It is a common source of error.

Dens Invaginatus (Palatal invaginations, dens in dente, bilateral composite odontome, gestant odontome)

Tomes in 1859 was the first to describe a case of coronal dens in dente. Since that time, both coronal and radicular invagination types have been described by Swanson and McCarthy (1947). Dens invaginatus is a developmental variation thought to arise as a result of an invagination in the surface of a tooth crown before calcification has occurred.

The term ''dens in dente'' originally applied to a severe invagination that gave the appearance of a tooth within a tooth, which is actually a misnomer, but the term is still in use. In the classic form, there is a deep invagination in the lingual pit area that may not be evident clinically. Radiographically, it is recognized as a pear-shaped invagination of enamel and dentin with a narrow constriction on the surface of the tooth and closely approximating the pulp in its depth.

British authors often classify the anomaly among odontomes (defined as a tumor that contains enamel and dentin). The condition is not a tumor and is most probably caused by an invagination of the enamel. The origin is certainly not a tooth within a tooth because the enamel is located centrally and the dentin peripherally, so the term ''dens invaginatus'' introduced by Hallet in 1953 is preferred.

Previously, the anomaly was considered rare, but the present widespread use of radiography has disclosed that dens invaginatus is not a rare phenomenon. Any type of tooth may have an invagination, but the majority of cases are located in the maxillary lateral incisors, sometimes bilaterally.

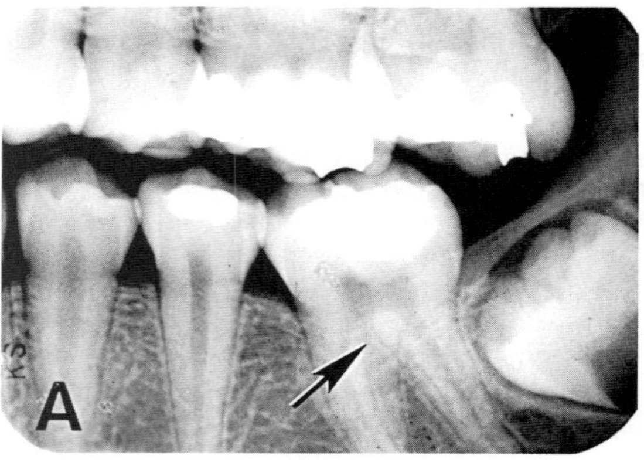

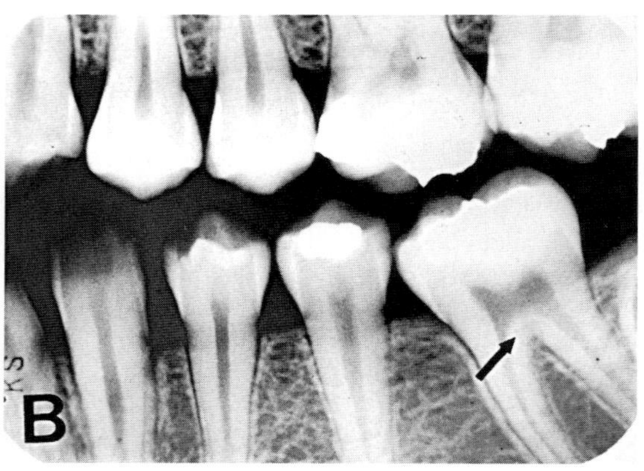

FIGURE 5–29.

Disappearing Pearl. A, Possible enamel pearl (arrow) at the bifurcation of a mandibular first molar in a radiograph with faulty horizontal angulation; note the overlapping of the crowns in both arches. B, Same patient as in A; the radiograph was taken with correct horizontal angulation, and the enamel pearl has disappeared (arrow). (Courtesy of Dr. G. Kaugers, Medical College of Virginia, Richmond, VA.)

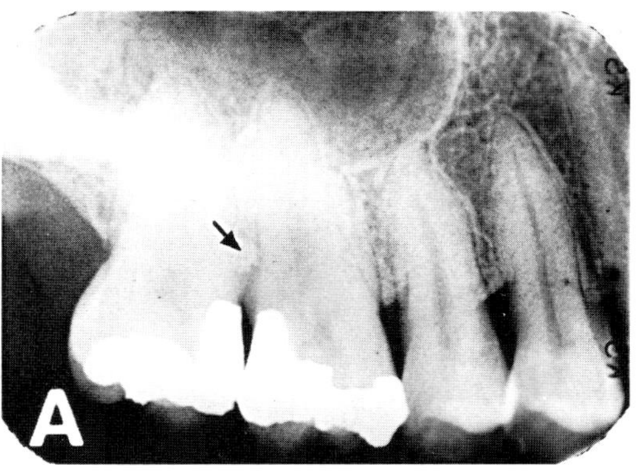

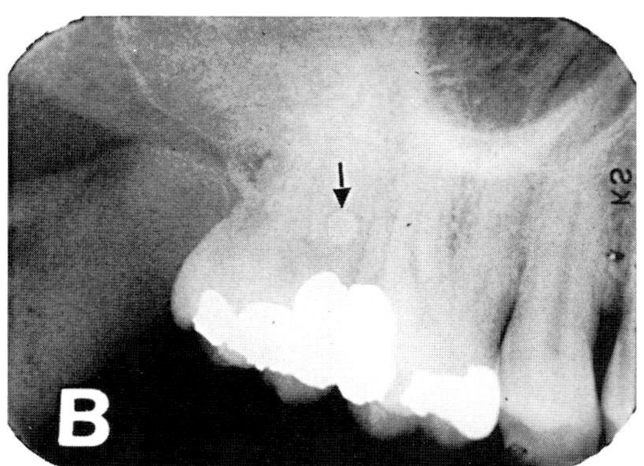

FIGURE 5–30.

Locating Enamel Pearl by "Buccal Object Rule." A, Accurate periapical radiograph revealing a possible enamel pearl on the surface of a second maxillary molar (arrow). B, Periapical radiograph of the same patient as in A taken with the x-ray beam directed more toward the mesial. (Note that the zygomatic bone and buccal cusps in B move toward the mesial.) Because the enamel pearl (arrow) moved in the opposite direction of the x-ray beam (distal instead of mesial), the enamel pearl is on the lingual surface of the second molar (buccal object rule).

In a review of the literature by Pindborg (1970), the prevalence of the condition affecting the maxillary lateral incisors among several population groups ranged from 0.25 to 5.1%. The large variation in prevalence can be in part explained by differences in criteria for dens invaginatus, applied by the various investigators.

Following the maxillary lateral incisors in order of decreasing frequency are: central incisors, premolars, canine teeth, and molars. The anomaly is rare in the mandible, and few cases have been reported among primary teeth. Supernumerary teeth, especially mesiodens, often have invaginations. Morgan and Poyton (1960) reported that bilateral occurrence is not uncommon.

Clinically, the suspicion of an invagination may arise if the foramen caecum is extremely marked. The foramen caecum is a small pit often present on the palatal surface of the upper incisors in the midline of the base of the crown. It appears on the radiographs as a dark spot that is variable in size and darkness. The depth of the foramen varies from a barely perceptible indentation to a definite cleft that is lined with and demarcated by two white lines representing the enamel margins. If the cleft is more than 1 mm deep, Hallet has suggested that it be termed an invagination of the enamel. Invagination is really an extension of the foramen caecum into an abnormal cleft or cavity. A deep foramen caecum is associated with caries and early loss of the pulp. Therefore, a deep invagination predisposes patients to early death of the pulp, even in the absence of caries. The mere presence of a well-formed invagination may lead to death of the pulp before the root of the tooth is complete.

A histologic examination will show that, whereas the enamel and dentin of the "outer" tooth are not affected, the enamel covering the invagination is more defective (poorer mineralization) at the bottom of the invagination, and the invagination has one or more thin routes to the dental pulp. In some areas, enamel as well as dentin will be completely missing, causing a direct communication between the bottom of the invagination and the dental pulp of the tooth. Lucas (1972) stated that the communication may consist of a single wide opening or several small canals. To prevent caries, pulp infection, and premature loss of the tooth, the condition must be recognized early and the tooth prophylactically restored. Fortunately, the defect may be recognized radiographically before the teeth erupt.

Oehlers and associates (1960) presented an excellent discussion on the three variant crown forms related to the permanent maxillary lateral incisor, the tooth in which invagination occurs most frequently. However, these variant crown forms may apply to other incisor teeth.

Besides the coronal type of dens invaginatus, there is a radicular variety. The radicular variety of dens invaginatus has been discussed by Bhatt and Dholakia (1975), who pointed out that the radicular dens invaginatus usually results from an infolding of Hertwig's sheath and originates at the root after the development of the crown is complete. Radicular dens invaginatus appears to be extremely rare and is represented as an enamel-lined invagination within the root, originating at an opening on the root itself. From a clinical point of view, as long as there remains no communication between the invagination through its opening on the root surface and the oral cavity, no complications such as those commonly associated with coronal dens invaginatus are likely to arise. If the opening is situated close to the anatomic neck of the tooth, then infection from the gingival sulcus may pass into tissues within the core of the invagination causing pulpal necrosis and other complications in the same way as with coronal invaginations.

◆ *RADIOLOGY (Figs. 5–31 to 5–33)*

The most common radiographic form is a pear-shaped invagination of enamel and dentin with a narrow constriction at the opening on the surface of the tooth and closely approximating the pulp in its depth (Fig. 5–31A).

More severe forms of dens invaginatus may exhibit an invagination that extends nearly to the apex of the root and

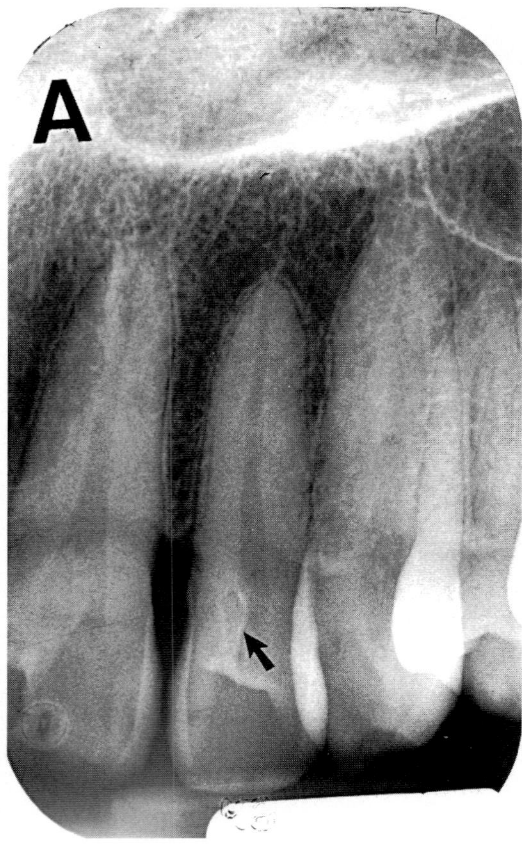

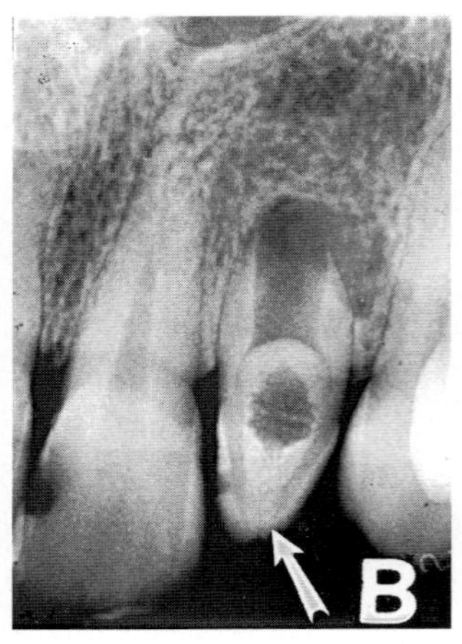

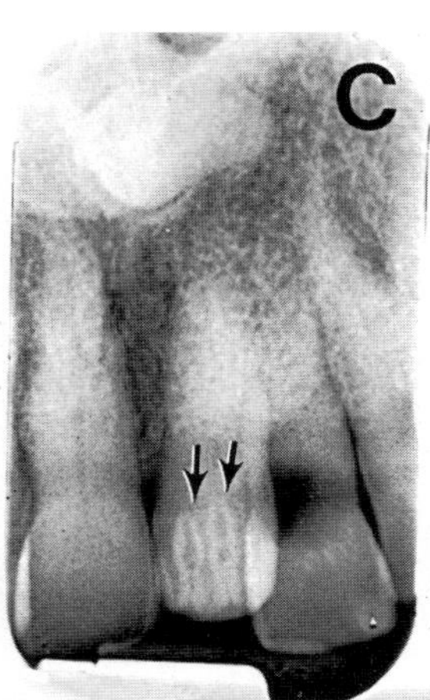

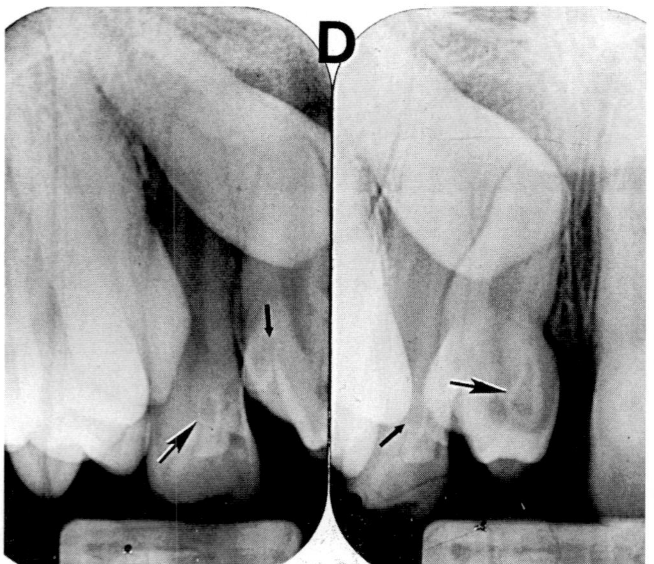

FIGURE 5–31.

Dens Invaginatus. A, Dens in dente (dens invaginatus) of a maxillary lateral incisor (arrow). B, Marked invagination of a peg-shaped lateral incisor (arrow). C, Double dens invaginatus of an erupted mesiodens between central incisors (arrows). D, Erupted maxillary lateral incisor with dens invaginatus and a partially erupted mesiodens with dens invaginatus (arrows); the maxillary central incisor has been blocked from erupting by the mesiodens. (Note there are two radiographs of same region.)

presents a bizarre radiographic picture reflecting a severe disturbance in the normal anatomic and morphologic structure of the teeth (Fig. 5–31B).

Prior to classifying the crown form variants of the permanent maxillary incisor with invaginations in 1960, Oehlers (1957) grouped the invaginations into three types: (1) those invaginations that are enamel lined and confined within the crown of the tooth; (2) those that invade the root but remain within it as a blind sac; and (3) those that penetrate the surface of the root and ''burst'' apically or laterally to produce a second foramen in the root. This third invagination may appear to be completely lined by enamel, but more often a portion of it is lined by cementum instead. It may or may not be dilated.

Radiographically, it is impossible accurately to determine the precise relationship of the invaginated portion with the pulp chamber or pulp canal, nor is it possible to define the invagination in the faciolingual dimension, that is, how much

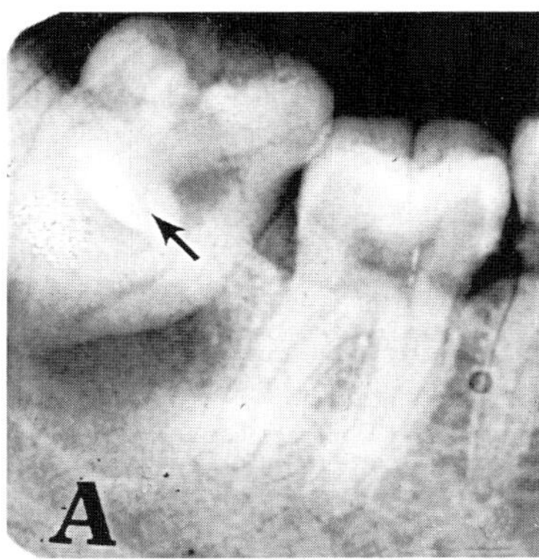

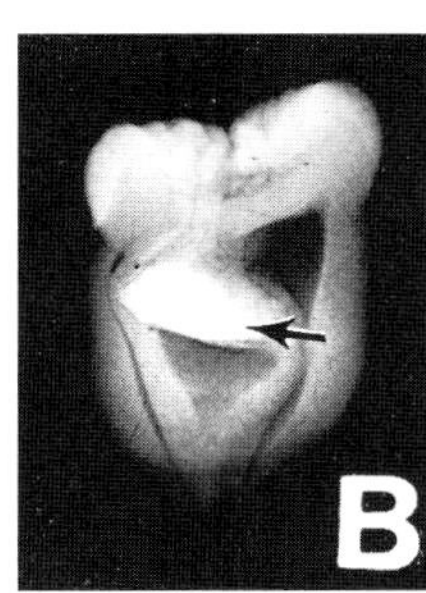

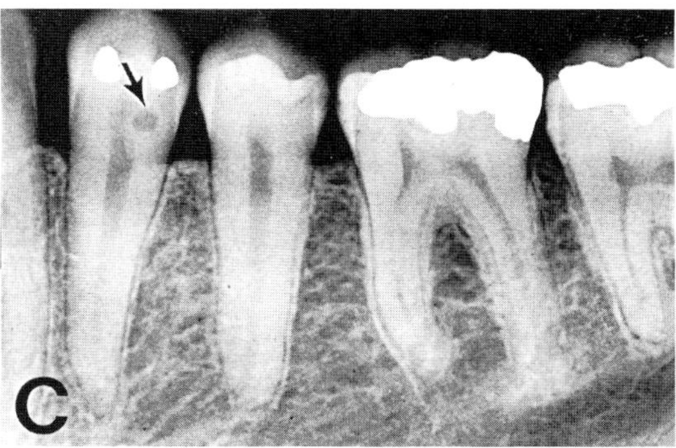

FIGURE 5–32.

Dens Invaginatus (Posterior Teeth). A, Dens invaginatus (arrow) of a mandibular third molar. B, Radiograph of the extracted mandibular third molar in A (arrow). (Courtesy of Dr. P. Dhiravarangkura, Chulalonghorn University, Bangkok, Thailand.) C, Dens invaginatus of a mandibular first premolar (arrow).

pulp space has been encroached on by the invagination. It may not be important that these points be answered because a deep foramen caecum is often associated with caries, and if the tooth is not restored, there will be an early loss of vitality of the pulp. Even in the absence of caries, the invagination predisposes the tooth to an early death of the pulp.

A palatogingival groove in the maxillary incisors was described among Chinese and East Indian populations by Lee and colleagues (1968). The defect commences at the junction of the cingulum and one of the lateral marginal ridges and extends on to the root. The groove probably represents an infolding of the enamel organ and the epithelial sheath of Hertwig and is similar to the pathogenesis of the dens invaginatus.

Dens Evaginatus

(Occlusal tuberculateral premolar, Leong's premolar, evaginated odontome, odontome of axial core type, occlusal enamel pearl, oriental premolar)

While the term "dens invaginatus" signifies the result of an infolding of the enamel organ, the term "dens evaginatus" means an outfolding of the enamel organ leading to the so-called tuberculated premolar. Oehlers and co-workers (1967) and Pedersen (1949) reported the anomaly to occur in people of Mongoloid racial stock, with a prevalence ranging from 1 to 4%.

Oehlers and associates (1967) reported that the essential feature of the anomaly is an enamel-covered, slender supernumerary tubercle that projects from the occlusal surface between the buccal and lingual cusps of an otherwise normal premolar. In rare instances, canine teeth and molars may be affected. The condition may occur unilaterally or bilaterally.

As reported by Oehlers (1967), Merrill (1964), Senia and Regezi (1974), and Curzon and associates (1970), the occlusal tubercle is large enough to cause interferences in occlusion. In addition, Trautman (1949), Yip (1974), Yong (1974), and Sykaris (1974) reported that fracture or attrition of the dens evaginatus, with either dentinal tubules or pulpal extension into the tubercle, may be exposed. The result may be pulp necrosis and periapical infection. The fate of the involved premolars depends on the degree of development of the anomaly and, to a certain degree, the extent of the

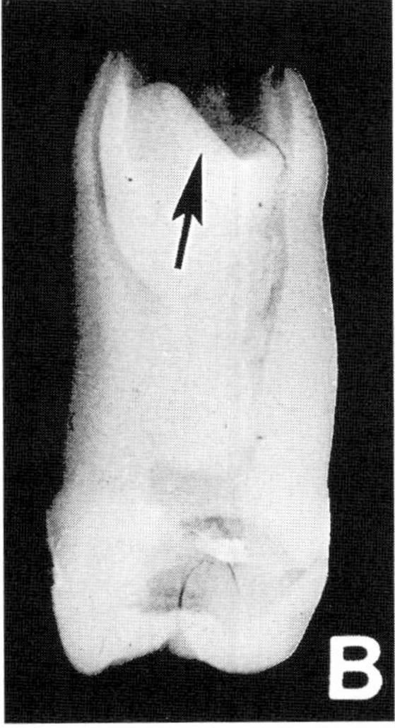

FIGURE 5–33.

Dens in Dente. A, Extracted premolar with dens in dente (arrow). B, Radiograph of A with dens in dente (arrow). This really looks like a "tooth within a tooth," rather than invagination. What do you think?

pulp horn. Teeth with thin, well-developed tubercles are more prone to fracture. Those with pulp tissue extending into the tubercle allow bacteria to involve the pulp more easily than those in which the roof of the pulp chamber is located far away from the tubercle. Secondary dentin usually occurs in teeth with a wide pulp horn.

When the dentin is exposed after fracture or attrition of the tubercle, bacteria may enter the pulp via the dental tubules. The lack of secondary dentin is significant because it usually indicates sudden death of the pulp. Pulpal death may occur before or after complete root formation.

Death of the pulp can be associated with the cessation of root development. This usually occurs at the level of about two thirds of its normal length, corresponding to the time when the tooth reaches normal occlusion. These root canals remain wide open.

Reports on dens evaginatus were made as early as 1929 in Japan by Joyojima, in 1936 by Yumikura and Yoshioa, and in 1937 by Kato. Trautman of England described evaginatus in a paper in 1949. He referred to the structure as the simplest type of dilated composite odontome. (British authors often classified these anomalies among odontomes.) The anomaly had first drawn Trautman's attention by a paper presented by Leong at the meeting of the Malayan Dental Association in August, 1946. According to Leong, the condition occurred only among the Chinese and involved only the mandibular premolars. In every case Leong examined, the premolars were free of caries and appeared clinically normal except for this occlusal anomaly. All these teeth were pulpless, with either an acute or a chronic alveolar abscess. The occlusal defect in each case was a small pit in the central ridge of the crown joining the buccal and lingual cusps. Leong stated that these defects were not exceedingly rare and probably arose from a narrow extension of the pulp occlusally through the enamel.

According to Merrill (1964), the various clinical types of dens evaginatus fall into two basic groups: one in which the protuberance arises from the lingual ridge of the buccal cusp and another in which the protuberance arises from the center of the occlusal surface and usually obliterates the central grove.

The anomaly seems to be the reverse of dens invaginatus and is caused by the folding of the inner enamel epithelium into the stellate reticulum in the early stages of the development of the tooth. Lau (1955) and Merrill (1964) reported that the evaginated enamel epithelium and the underlying cells of the dental papilla form an enamel tubercle with a dentin core that usually has a central canal connected with the pulp.

Once thought to be limited to persons of Asian ancestry (Chinese, Japanese, Eskimos, American Indians, Malayans, Aleuts, and Filipinos), dens evaginatus has been reported in Caucasians by Palmer (1973), Ekman-Westborg and Julin (1974), and Sykaris (1974). The occurrence of dens evaginatus seems to differ with racial background. In Japan, Kato reported an incidence of 1.09%, and Yoshioka and Urano (1963) noted an incidence of 1.66%. In China, Lau (1955) discovered an incidence of 1.29%, and Wu (1955) reported an incidence of 1.5%. Merrill (1964) reported an incidence of 4.3% in a group of Alaskan Eskimos and American Indians, whereas Curzon and associates (1970) found a 3.0% incidence in Keewatin Eskimos.

Merrill (1964) reported that the prevalence of dens evaginatus among American Eskimos and American Indians was greater in females (2.6%) than in males (1.87%). Curzon and associates (1970) stated that the prevalence of dens evaginatus in Eskimos was in the ratio of one male to three females. By contrast, Yip (1974) found no sex-related prevalence in his observation of Chinese and Malayan children. Yoshioka and Urano (1963) in Japan also reported no significant difference in distribution between sexes. Kato (1937) and Yoshioka and Urano (1963) reported that the incidence is more frequent in the mandibular second premolars, followed by the first premolar, and finally the maxillary second premolar and the maxillary first premolar. Yip (1974) stated that the anomaly more often involved the mandibular first premolar than the mandibular second premolar.

The most common complications of the anomaly are pulpal inflammation and necrosis, followed by periapical inflammatory lesions resulting from irritation of the pulp within the damaged tubercle. In his report of 110 cases, Oehlers (1956) noted that 40% of the evaginated teeth had periapical radiolucencies. Apparently, the pulp need not be exposed for pulpal necrosis to take place. Merrill's (1964) histologic examination of 2 nonvital teeth revealed a layer of dentin overlying the evaginated pulp thin enough to allow bacterial entry. Once the evaginated tubercle is damaged and pulp becomes inflamed, root canal therapy or extraction becomes necessary.

Yong (1974) treated 39 vital and asymptomatic teeth with dens evaginatus in children by removing the tubercles at the tooth bases under sterile conditions and treating the teeth with direct and indirect pulp capping techniques. All 39 teeth remained vital and pain free throughout the evaluation period of up to 30 months. Normal root development with closure of the apices occurred in 37 teeth; the root canals in 2 teeth were obliterated. Yong concluded that direct and indirect pulp capping was the prophylactic treatment of choice in evaginated teeth with incomplete root formation. Senia and Regezi (1974) recommended removal of opposing occlusal interferences to avoid wear of the protuberance, and pulpectomy if the vitality of the pulp could not be maintained.

◆ RADIOLOGY (Figs. 5–34 and 5–35)

In dens evaginatus, a tubercle on the surface of the premolar may be evident, and extensions of the pulp into the tubercle may be clearly visible on the radiograph (Fig. 5–34). Many of these teeth have a radiolucency or a thickened periodontal ligament at the apex of the tooth that can only be confirmed by a radiograph (Fig. 5–35). Radiographic examination must be performed to confirm the presence and extension of the pulpal horn into the tubercle. Moreover, the radiograph is useful in determining whether the roots and root canals of teeth with the anomaly are fully formed.

Many of these teeth have dilacerated roots and are tilted or rotated because of traumatogenic occlusion. Oehlers (1956) reported that abnormal occlusal forces on the crown can produce subluxation (partial dislocation), leading to dilaceration of the root at the apical one third level. This corre-

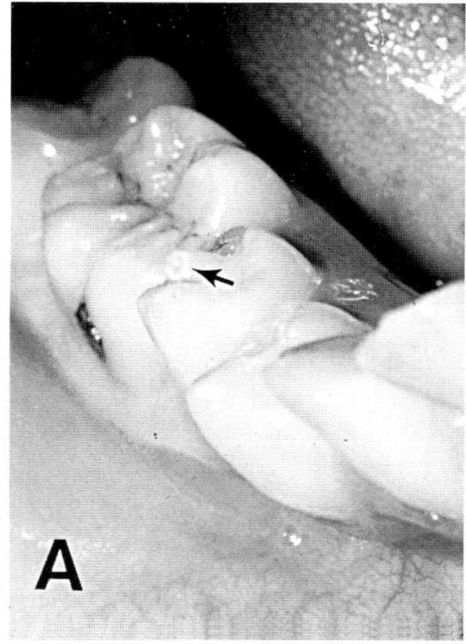

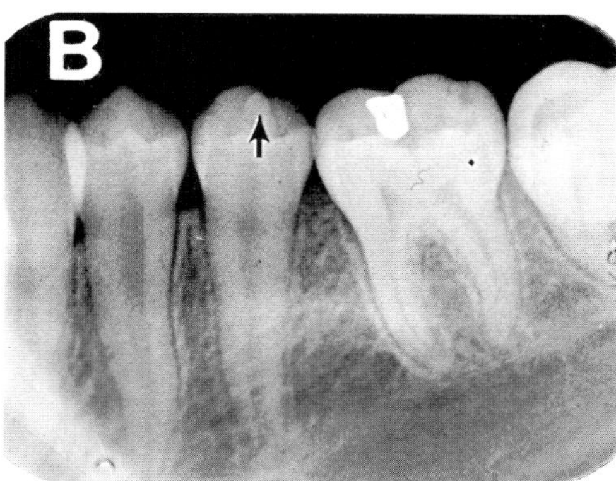

FIGURE 5–34.

Dens Evaginatus. A, Clinical photograph of dens evaginatus (arrow) of the occlusal surface of a mandibular second premolar. B, Radiograph of dens evaginatus (arrow).

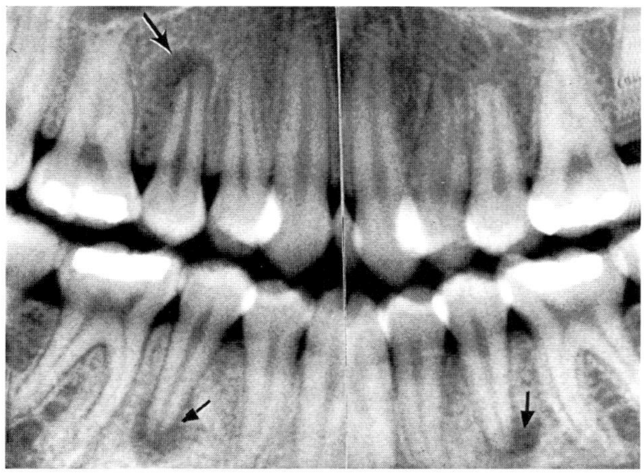

FIGURE 5–35.

Sequelae of Dens Evaginatus. Three second premolars with dens evaginatus of their occlusal surfaces have periapical radiolucencies (arrows).

sponds to the stage of root formation when the crown reaches occlusion. Geist (1989) reported that one of the evaginated teeth in his case report demonstrated dilaceration and displacement, correlating with the patient's complaint of improper occlusion. The radiograph is most helpful in determining whether endodontic therapy can be successful in these particular cases mentioned previously.

VARIATIONS IN STRUCTURE

Enamel Hypoplasia (Figs. 5–36 to 5–40)

Enamel hypoplasia may be defined as an incomplete or defective formation of the organic enamel matrix of the primary and permanent teeth. Two basic types of enamel hypoplasia exist: (1) a type caused by environmental factors; and (2) a hereditary type (amelogenesis imperfecta). When the hypoplastic defect is caused by environmental factors, either dentition may be involved, and sometimes only a single tooth. Both enamel and dentin are usually affected at least to some degree. When the defect is caused by hereditary factors, both deciduous and permanent dentitions usually are involved and generally only the enamel is affected. Sarnat and Schour (1942) reported that one of the earliest references to enamel defects of the teeth is from 1743, when Bunon described "erosion" of teeth due to rickets, measles, and scurvy. "Enamel hypoplasia," first used by Zsigmondy in 1894, has been the most generally accepted term.

Hypoplasia is preferable to the old term "enamel atrophy" because the condition is characterized by an underdevelopment of the enamel, whereas the word "atrophy" indicates a wasting or reduction in size of a fully developed tissue or organ.

Many studies, both experimental and clinical, have been carried out in an attempt to determine the cause and nature of environmental enamel hypoplasia. Certain factors, each capable of causing injury to the ameloblasts, may give rise to enamel hypoplasia. They include: (1) nutritional deficiency (vitamins A, C, and D); (2) exanthematous diseases (such as measles, chickenpox, and scarlet fever); (3) congenital syphilis; (4) hypocalcemia; (5) birth injury; (6) Rh hemolytic disease; (7) local infection or trauma; (8) ingestion of chemicals (chiefly fluoride); and (9) idiopathic causes.

In mild environmental hypoplasia, only a few small grooves, pits or fissures may be present on the enamel surface. If the condition is more severe, the enamel may exhibit rows of deep pits arranged or a linear smooth surface fissure horizontally across the surface of the tooth. There may be only a single row of such pits or fissures or several rows indicating a series of injuries. In severe cases, a considerable portion of enamel may be absent, suggesting a prolonged disturbance in function of the ameloblasts. Usually, a narrow zone of hypoplastic defects is indicative of enamel formation affected for a shorter time (acute); a wide zone indicates

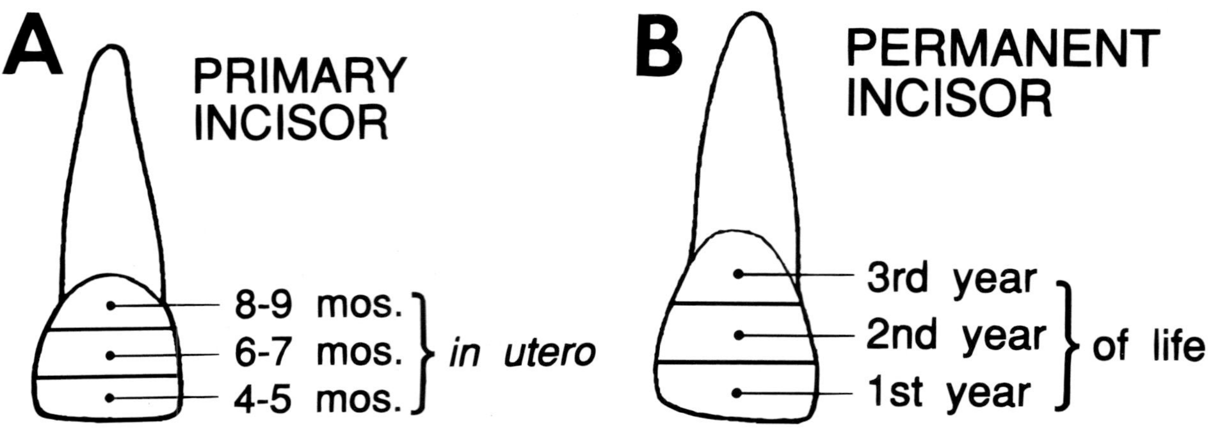

FIGURE 5–36.

Enamel Hypoplasia. Diagram indicating the time frame and area on the tooth in which enamel hypoplasias occur from serious nutritional deficiency or systemic disease states. A, Primary incisor. B, Permanent incisor.

that enamel formation has been affected for a longer time (chronic). Multiple zones indicate that enamel formation was probably affected on more than one occasion. Occasionally, the enamel defects may be the site of secondary discoloration.

Enamel hypoplasia is a result of disturbance of enamel formation. The enamel prisms in the involved areas remain permanently in the state of development they had reached when the disturbance occurred. After the disturbance subsides, normal enamel may again be formed. If the disturbance is repeated, a zone of missing or undeveloped enamel will again result; hence, an alternating distribution of the hypoplastic areas on the surface of the crown is observed. From the chronology of the enamel formation of the human primary and permanent teeth, it is possible to estimate the age of the child when the disturbance or injury occurred (Fig. 5–36).

If the interference takes place in the first year (called the infancy period), the permanent teeth affected are the first molars, the incisors (except the maxillary lateral incisors), and the canine teeth. It is striking that the maxillary lateral incisors mineralize after the central incisors and canines, approximately after the age of 10 months. It is characteristic that the mesial cusps of the first molars, formed prior to birth, are not affected by enamel hypoplasia. Sarnat and Schour (1942) reported that two thirds of the enamel hypoplasias of permanent teeth have their origin during the first 10 months after birth.

Nearly one third of the enamel hypoplasia found by Sarnat and Schour (1942) occurred in portions of the teeth formed in early childhood (approximately 13 to 34 months). Thus, the upper lateral incisors and the premolars that begin to calcify during this period are also affected. Only 2% of the time does enamel hypoplasia originate between 35 and 80 months (late childhood), and then it involves the second molars. Sarnat and Schour found no instance where the third molars had enamel hypoplasia.

With regard to enamel hypoplasia in the primary dentition, Pedersen (1949) reported that the incisors have severe structural defects more rarely than the molars and canine teeth.

Stein (1936) pointed out that the primary teeth of prematurely born children are frequently hypoplastic; they develop more slowly and are more subject to illness of all kinds. Worth (1963) reported that infants who have survived hemolytic disease of the newborn are likely to have hypoplasia of the primary dentition. The discoloration of the teeth that results from the hemolytic disease is not revealed in radiographs, but the hypoplasia is apparent.

Because of scarcity of clinical data, our knowledge of enamel hypoplasia is meager, and several hypotheses have been proposed for its etiology and pathogenesis. The most likely theory holds that (1) the primary changes occurs in the ameloblasts, and (2) enamel hypoplasia can occur only during matrix formation.

In a review of the literature, Sarnat and Schour (1942) reported that rickets (deficiency of vitamin D) was the most common cause of enamel hypoplasia. For example, in a series of rachitic children reported by Shelling and Anderson (1936), 43% of the teeth showed hypoplasia. At present, however, rickets is not a prevalent disease. In addition, deficiencies of vitamin A and C have been reported as causes of enamel hypoplasia.

Some studies have indicated that exanthematous (high fever) diseases, including measles, chickenpox, and scarlet fever, are etiologic factors; however, Sarnat and Schour (1942) were unable to confirm this finding. In general, Shafer and associates (1983) stated that any serious nutritional deficiency or systemic disease is potentially capable of producing enamel hypoplasia because the ameloblasts are one of the most sensitive groups of cells in the body in terms of metabolic function.

The type of hypoplasia occurring from these deficiencies or disease states is usually of the pitting variety. Because the pits tend to stain, the clinical appearance is unsightly. Although the introduction of antibiotics has drastically reduced the number of new cases of congenital syphilis in most countries, the disease is not yet completely controlled.

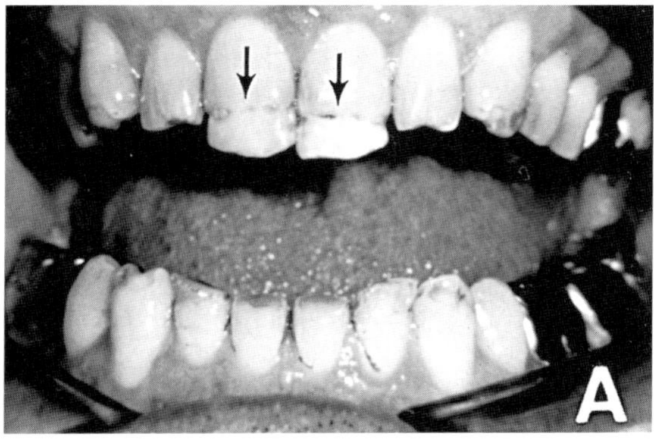

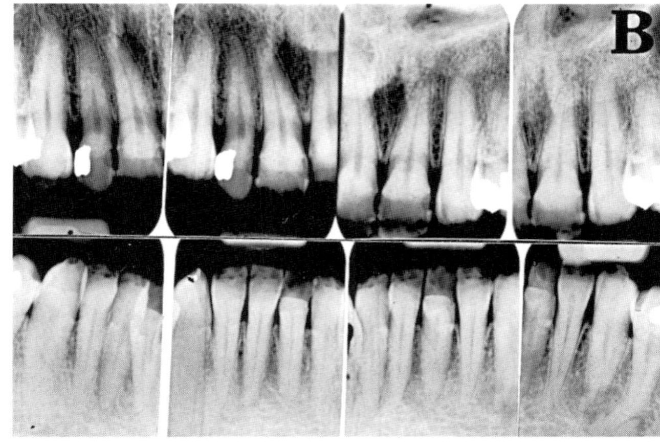

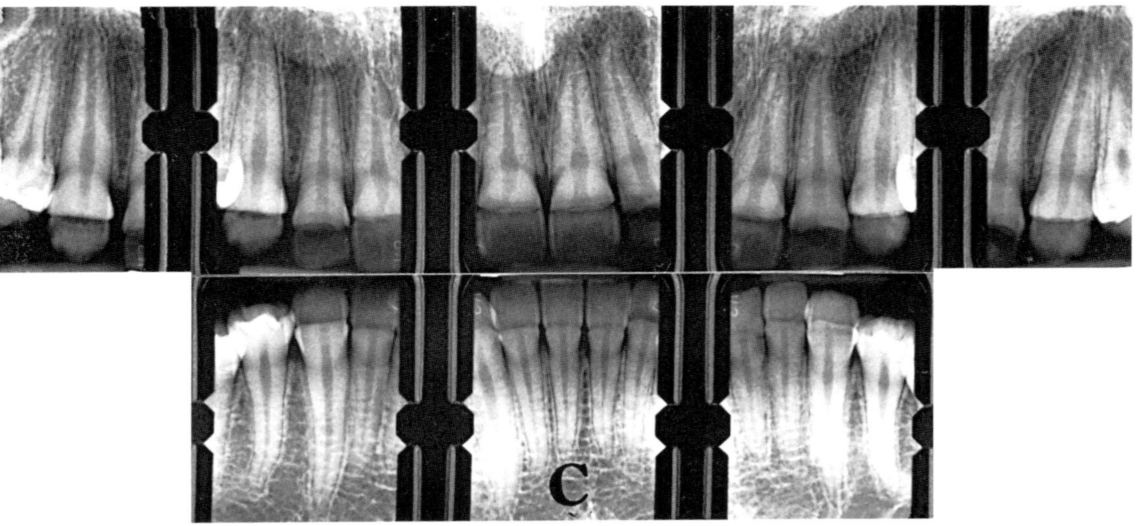

FIGURE 5–37.

Enamel Hypoplasia (Pit and Groove Type). A, Note the severe enamel hypoplasia, with rows of deep pits arranged horizontally across the surfaces of the anterior teeth (arrows), except the maxillary lateral incisors. If the disturbance takes place in the first year, all incisors except the maxillary lateral incisors will be affected. B, Radiographs of pit-type enamel hypoplasia of all maxillary and mandibular teeth, except the right maxillary lateral incisor (the left maxillary incisor is missing). C, Anterior radiographs of the grooved type of enamel hypoplasia of all mandibular and maxillary teeth, including the maxillary lateral incisors. The disturbance must have taken place during the second year of the patient's life (see Fig. 5–36B).

Hutchinson's triad was first described by Jonathan Hutchinson, an English surgeon, in 1858 as being pathognomonic for congenital syphilis. The triad consisted of (1) diffuse interstitial keratitis (deep deposits in substance of the cornea, which becomes hazy throughout), (2) disease of the labyrinth (canals of inner ear) and (3) hutchinsonian teeth (permanent maxillary incisors).

After Hutchinson's description, it was later recognized that changes might also occur in other permanent incisors, canines, and first molars. The "mulberry" molar was first described by Fournier in 1884. Sometimes, these molars are called Fournier molars.

The typical "hutchinsonian incisor" is smaller than a normal incisor, and the sides of the crown usually converge from the cervix to the incisal edge. As a result, the tooth is narrower at the cutting edge than at the normal-sized gingival margin. This gives the tooth a barrel or screwdriver form that prevents proximal contact between the teeth. In addition, the incisal edge is usually notched. The cause of the tapering and notching has been explained on the basis of the absence of the central tubercle or lobe or calcification center. One third of these patients have an anterior open bite.

According to Putkonen (1962), the first molar typical of congenital syphilis, the so-called mulberry molar, is considerably smaller than the normal first molar and also is smaller than the second molar. The mulberry molar is covered on the sides with normal, smooth enamel, but the occlusal surface is pinched together, dwarfed, rough, and hypoplastic, often pigmented. From it extend the elongated nodules or domes representing poorly developed cusps, huddled together.

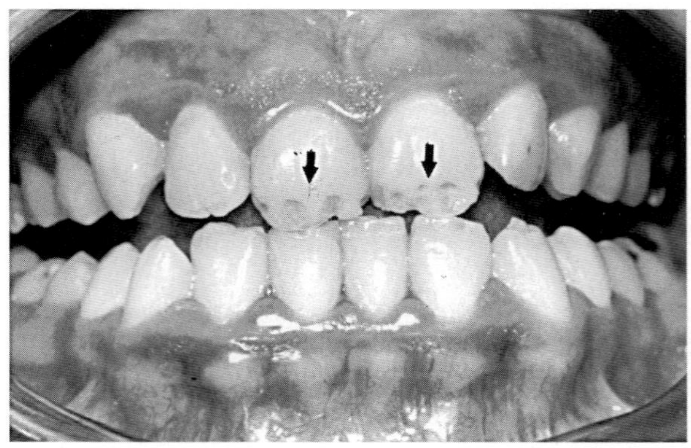

FIGURE 5–38.

Localized Enamel Hypoplasia. Localized group of pit-type enamel hypoplasia at the incisal (arrows) portion of the central incisors indicating that the hypoplastic defect was acquired in the first year of the patient's life (see Fig. 5–36B).

Often, a supernumerary nodule or pseudocusp appears that clinicians emphasize as an important feature of the mulberry molar.

The prevalence of syphilitic dental changes in patients with congenital syphilis varies greatly. Sarnat and Shaw (1942), in a sample of 36 American children with congenital syphilis, found that 67% had dental changes, whereas Putkonen (1962), in a Finnish sample of 254 patients, found that 45% had incisor changes and 22% had molar changes.

Fiumara and Lessell (1970) reported that, between 1958 and 1969, there was over a 200% increase in reported cases of primary and secondary syphilis in the United States and that, consequently, syphilis in children under 1 year of age increased 117% during the 10-year period from 1960 to 1969. Investigating 271 patients with congenital syphilis, these workers found that over 63% had hutchinsonian incisors, but because some of the teeth had already been extracted, this may not be a true incidence. In addition, approximately 65% of this group of patients with congenital syphilis had the characteristic mulberry molars.

Enamel hypoplasia affecting only a single tooth is occasionally seen, most commonly in one of the permanent maxillary incisors or a maxillary or a mandibular premolar. There may be any degree of hypoplasia, ranging from a mild, brownish discoloration to irregularity of the tooth crown. These single teeth are often called "Turner's teeth" and the condition is called "Turner's hypoplasia." In 1912, Turner described two patients with local hypoplasia in the premolars and associated the defects with the occurrence of periapical infections in the primary molars. Since that time, Turner's name has been widely used to designate such defects (see Fig. 5–39).

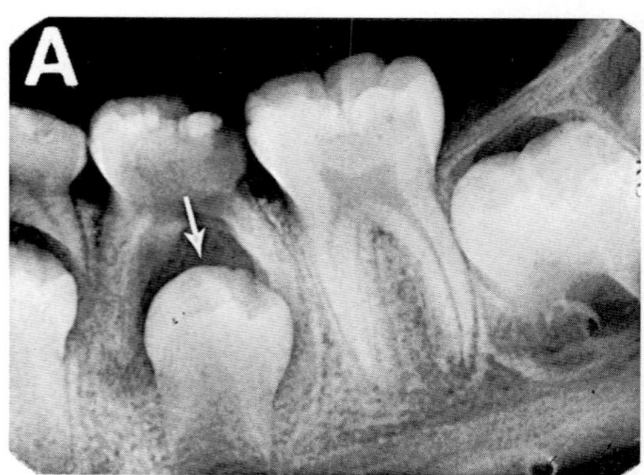

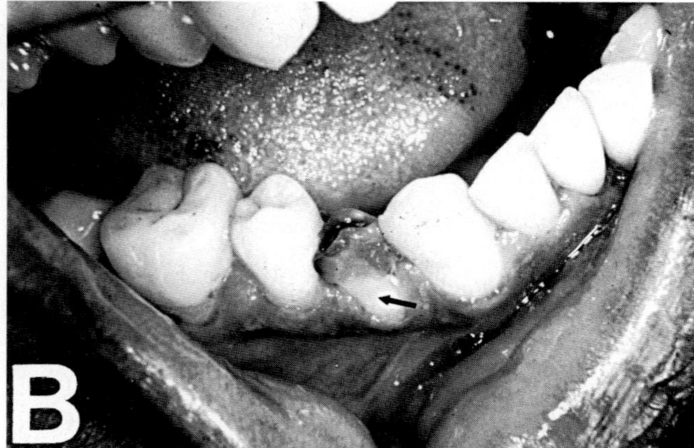

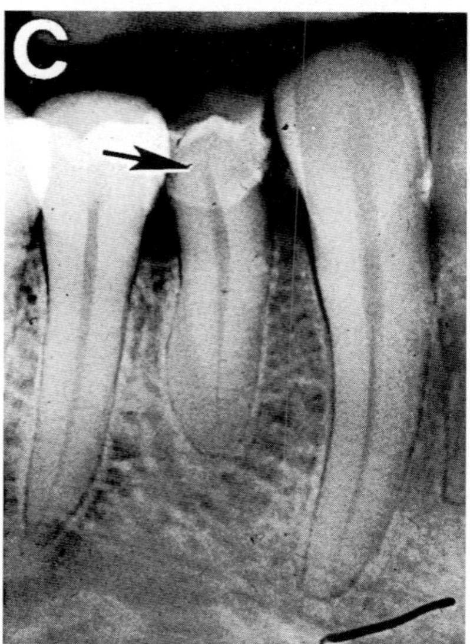

FIGURE 5–39.

Turner's Tooth. A, Turner's localized hypoplasia can be caused by trauma or periapical infection of a primary molar, as shown here (arrow). B, Clinical photograph of Turner's tooth, a mandibular right first premolar (arrow). C, Radiograph of the Turner's tooth in B (arrow). Hypercementosis is present.

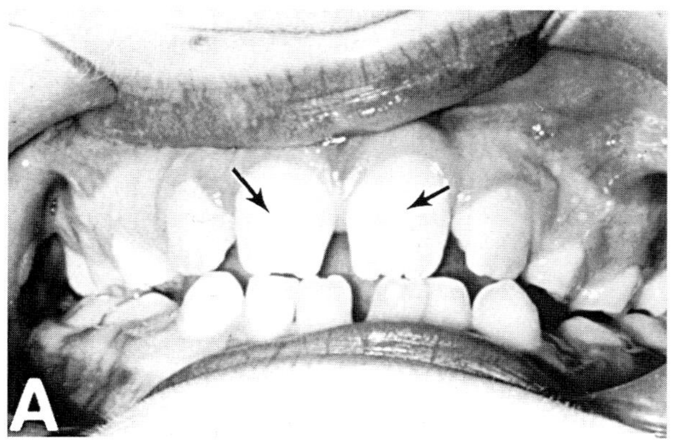

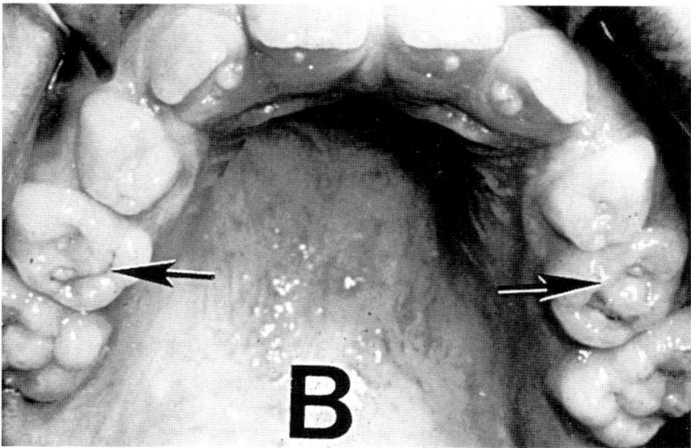

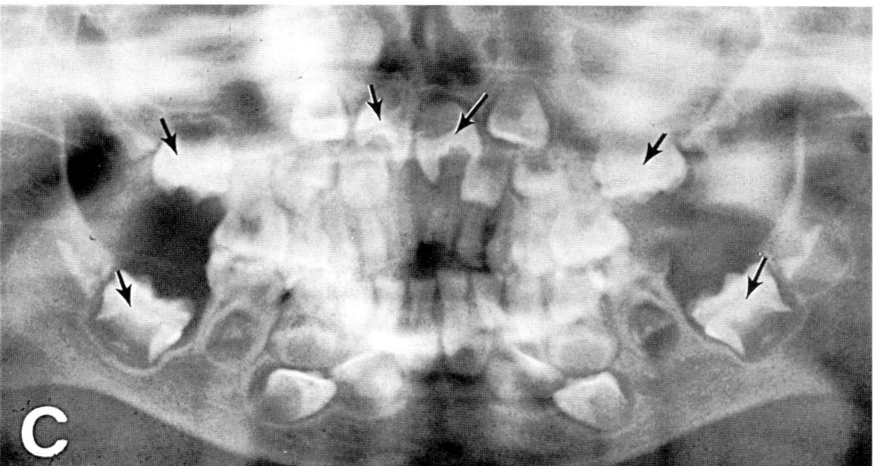

FIGURE 5–40.

Congenital Syphilis (Enamel Hypoplasia). A, Notched screwdriver-shaped central incisors (arrows) in a patient with congenital syphilis (Hutchinson's incisors). B, Mulberry molars of congenital syphilis (arrows). C, Panoramic radiograph of a 4-year-old girl with congenital syphilis. Note the unerupted notched central incisors (Hutchinson's incisors) and unerupted mulberry-shaped first molars (arrows). (Courtesy of Drs. L. Archilla, F. Erales, and R. Carlos, Guatemala City, Guatemala.)

The pathogenesis of this disturbance was described by Bauer (1946) and Morningstar (1937). The defect is seen as partial or complete localized absence of enamel at the affected part because of destruction of the enamel organ and the ameloblasts by the inflammatory reaction. On return to normal, the tissue in contact with the bare dentin attempts to repair the damage by a deposition of cementum or osteocementum to the surface (Fig. 5–39c).

Clinically, Hals and Orlow (1958) reported that the crowns of Turner's teeth are smaller than normal, and the entire tooth may be undersized. The crown exhibits defects that partly comprise loss of enamel and are partly due to deposition of cementum on the crown. The normal morphology of the crown and root may be lost. If the periapical inflammation associated with the primary tooth has acted before the root of the succedaneous permanent tooth is fully formed, the root shape may be altered.

Dental fluorosis or mottled enamel is a type of enamel hypoplasia caused by excessive fluoride intake; it usually occurs in well-defined geographic areas. Mottled enamel was first described in the United States by Black and McKay in 1916 in individuals born and raised from 1910 in Colorado Springs, Colorado and northwest Texas. Actually, dental fluorosis was first described in 1888, in a family from Mexico, and in 1891 it was found in and around Naples, according to Pindborg (1970). It was not until some years later that Smith, Lanz, and Smith (1931) established that the presence of excessive amounts of fluorine in the water was the primary etiologic factor in mottling of enamel.

The severity of the mottling increases with the increasing amount of fluoride in the water. Investigations by Dean and others (1941, 1942) have furnished evidence that a significant reduction of dental caries could be obtained with water fluoride levels in the range of 1.0 to 1.5 parts per million (ppm). This has become the accepted optimum range.

Spouge (1973) reported that the ingestion of more than 1.8 ppm of fluoride in the water is associated with mottled enamel that varies from localized white, opaque spots to generalized white or brown discolorations. At concentrations of 1.8 ppm, approximately 10% of the population has some degree of mottling, whereas 90% of those exposed to higher levels, up to 6 ppm, have mottling. There is no clear association between the fluoride content and the degree of mottling, a phenomenon based on individual predilection for drinking water and other aspects of health and diet. Primary teeth are usually less mottled than permanent teeth. Even when all teeth are affected, there may be horizontal lines across the tooth surface that demarcate the times of high and low ingestion. Very high levels of fluoride may produce enamel hypoplasia or hypocalcification, showing pitting, brownish staining, and a corroded appearance of the teeth.

Clinically, the brown stain of dental fluorosis is not present when the teeth erupt into the mouth. Later, the white cloudiness of the enamel gives way to a brownish mottled appearance because the poorly calcified areas are relatively porous and quickly acquire stains of absorbed extrinsic materials. Dental fluorosis occurs symmetrically in the dental arches. Moller (1965) reported that the premolars are the teeth most severely affected by dental fluorosis, followed by the second molars, maxillary incisors, canines, first molars, and mandibular incisors.

In 1956 came the first report that tetracyclines may cause discoloration of teeth if given during the dental formation period. Shortly after, it was reported that tetracyclines may also give rise to enamel hypoplasia. Tetracyclines react with calcium to form a tetracyline-calcium orthophosphate complex that is incorporated into the teeth if the drug is given when the teeth are undergoing mineralization.

In a Finnish study by Hakala and Makela (1963), enamel hypoplasia was observed among 79% of tetracycline-treated premature children, whereas only 8% of the control group showed enamel hypoplasia. The enamel hypoplasia was located in the areas exhibiting staining by tetracycline.

Enamel hypoplasia has been associated with cerebral palsy, congenital heart disease, gastrointestinal disturbances, erythroblastosis fetalis, and therapeutic irradiation to the head and neck at an early age.

◆ *RADIOLOGY (Figs. 5–36 to 5–40)*

The radiographic appearance of hypoplasia of enamel depends on the anatomic abnormality present and varies from a barely perceptible change to a gross deformity. The more extensive lesions appear as deformities of the mesial and distal margins of the crown or as a series of rounded dark images crossing the tooth in a straight line.

Grosser deformities produce absence of tooth substance leading to a marked radiolucency that may be strikingly localized, so the dental tissue immediately adjacent to the deformity is normal. An extremely gross deformity produces a crown that is markedly shriveled at its incisal and occlusal surfaces. Such teeth may appear as a small spike of dental tissue arising from a short, stunted base, with a series of pits at the cervical portion of the crown. A shallow groove or line of small pits may cross the crown of the tooth well away from the occlusal or incisal surface, and the dental tissue above and below may be normal. The bottom of the groove or pits may be devoid of enamel, or there may be a thin covering of enamel. Like the clinical manifestations of enamel hypoplasia, the radiographic appearances are equally varied. One striking feature may be the sharp definition of the abnormality within normal dental tissue, above and below. The diagnosis of enamel hypoplasia is clinical, but students frequently fail to identify hypoplasic changes in radiographs.

In localized hypoplasia (Turner's teeth), the bone surrounding the follicle of the developing permanent tooth may show evidence of bone disease. The follicle wall is either present normally or shows evidence of having been destroyed or partially destroyed. The infection may lead to death of the dental papilla, or the tooth may continue its growth and at eruption reveal the deformity. Hals and Orlow (1958) stated that, clinically, the crowns of Turner's teeth are smaller than normal, and the entire tooth may be undersized (Fig. 5–39B).

The radiographic appearances of localized hypoplasia depend on the severity of the changes. In the grosser lesions, all the formed portion of the crown is poorly calcified. There may be only a ghostlike representation of a part of a crown or several small opacities in a dark space of the follicles.

Hereditary Enamel Hypoplasia: Amelogenesis Imperfecta (Hereditary enamel dysplasia, hereditary brown enamel, hereditary enamel aplasia, hereditary brown opalescent teeth)

Amelogenesis imperfecta represents a group of hereditary defects of enamel unassociated with any other generalized defects. Apart from the hereditary background, they occur in the primary as well as the permanent dentition and show a tendency to impaction, normal dentin structure, and resistance to caries. The tendency to multiple impactions has been explained by the fact that the reduced enamel epithelium appears to be defective (occasionally completely lacking) and therefore unable to contribute to eruption in a normal way. Witkop, in a survey of amelogenesis imperfecta in the United States in 1958, found the prevalence to be 1:14,000 to 1:16,000.

Amelogenesis imperfecta is a term introduced by Weinmann and associates in 1945. It is entirely an ectodermal disturbance, since the mesodermal components of the teeth are basically normal.

Weinmann and associates (1945) divided the condition into two types: enamel hypoplasia and enamel hypocalcification. The difference was thought to be due to the stage of enamel development at which the defect occurs. The development of normal enamel occurs in three stages: 1) the formative stage, during which there is deposition of the organic matrix, 2) the calcification stage, during which this matrix is mineralized and the 3) maturation stage, during which crystallites enlarge and mature.

In the enamel hypoplasia type of amelogenesis imperfecta, the enamel matrix appears to be imperfectly formed and, although calcification (mineralization) subsequently occurs in the matrix so the enamel is hard, it is because of its thinness that it can be recognized on radiographs. In some cases, the hypoplastic type of amelogenesis imperfecta may resemble enamel hypoplasia. Usually, the affected teeth are yellowish brown.

In the hypocalcification (hypomineralization) type, the matrix formation appears to be normal, so the enamel is normal in thickness, but calcification (mineralization) is deficient and the enamel is soft. This soft enamel wears or chips away from the tooth because of its chalky consistency. The surface of the enamel is uneven and soft, and the teeth are usually dark brown. It is difficult to recognize the enamel on the radiograph because of the low mineral content.

In 1958, a new heritable form of amelogenesis imperfecta was suggested by Witkop, who considered the defect to be a result of defective maturation of enamel in which the enamel crystallites remain immature. An updated classification of amelogenesis imperfecta based on clinical, histologic, and genetic criteria was established by Witkop and Sauk in 1976 and Jorgenson and Yost in 1982.

As an aid in the diagnosis for the clinician, the general clinical features of the three major types of amelogenesis imperfecta were established in 1976 by Witkop and Sauk:

1. Hypoplastic type. The enamel has not formed to full normal thickness on newly developing teeth. They are pitted, rough, and smooth (anaplastic) types.
2. Hypocalcified (hypomineralized) type. The enamel is so soft that it can be removed by a prophylaxis scaler.
3. Hypomaturation type. The enamel can be pierced by an explorer under firm pressure and can be lost by chipping away from the underlying normal-appearing dentin. There are pigmented and snow-capped teeth types.

All teeth of both dentitions are affected to some degree by amelogenesis imperfecta. In some cases, the teeth may appear essentially normal, whereas in others, they may be extremely unsightly. The crowns of the teeth may or may not show discoloration. If present, it varies depending on the type of the disorder and ranges from yellow to dark brown. In some cases, the enamel may be totally absent; in others, it may have a chalky texture or even a cheesy consistency or it may be relatively hard. Sometimes, the enamel is smooth, or it may have numerous parallel vertical wrinkles or grooves. No treatment exists, except to improve function and cosmetic appearance.

◆ *RADIOLOGY (Figs. 5–41 to 5–44)*

The overall shape of the tooth may or may not be normal, depending on the amount of enamel present on the tooth and the amount of occlusal wear. In the **hypoplastic type** of amelogenesis imperfecta, the enamel is very thin, giving the crowns a tapered appearance with a lack of contact between teeth. The developing and erupting teeth appear as though they have been prepared for full crown restorations. Although the enamel is thin, it does contrast with the dentin, but the enamel sometimes can be hardly recognized. In some cases, the enamel may be congenitally absent. The crowns of the teeth tend to be square, devoid of the normal mesial and distal contours. The cusps are sometimes absent, or they may be represented by a series of serrations of varying sharpness, although often the occlusal surfaces are worn down by the time the patient comes under examination. The teeth are often worn down early, even to the gingival margins. There is a tendency for multiple impacted resorbing teeth. In the hypoplastic type of amelogenesis imperfecta, all the teeth are affected irrespective of the chronologic differences in development.

The **hypocalcified type** of amelogenesis imperfecta, which is more common than the hypoplastic type, is primarily due to a disturbance in mineralization of the enamel. When the teeth erupt, the crown may have a normal shape and size; before long, however, the enamel fractures away from the teeth because of its chalky consistency. It is difficult to recognize the enamel on radiographs because of its low mineral content. On radiographs, there is no contrast between the enamel and dentin. In some cases, the dentin may even be denser than usual. The enamel looks motheaten because of areas of pitting and lost enamel. Marked attrition of the crowns is found in some cases, probably because of softness of the enamel.

In the **hypomaturation type** of amelogenesis imperfecta, the enamel crystallites remain immature, causing the enamel to be soft and not to contrast well with the dentin on the radiograph. The enamel chips and abrades, but not as fast as in the hypocalcified type of the disorder. The enamel is of normal thickness, but it chips, especially around restorations. Resorption of the enamel may occur on the incisal and occlusal surfaces prior to eruption. There is a "snow-capped" type (Fig. 5–43).

Dentinogenesis Imperfecta (Transparent enamel, dysplasie de Capdepont, hereditary opalescent dentin, hereditary dentin hypoplasia)

This abnormality differs from amelogenesis imperfecta, as the name would indicate, in that the dentin rather than the

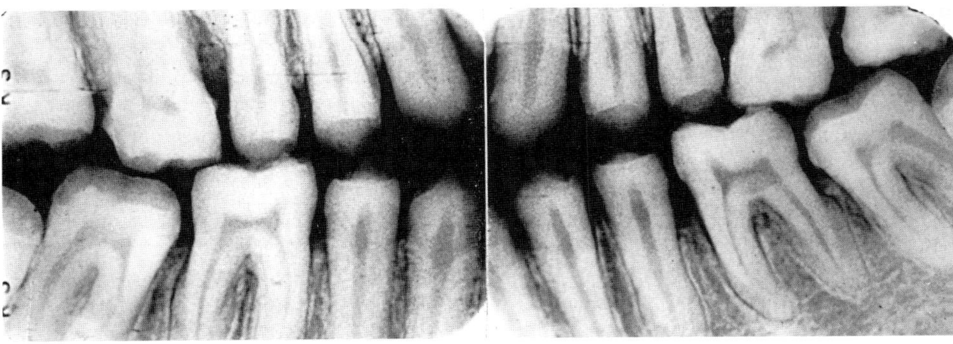

FIGURE 5–41.

Amelogenesis Imperfecta (Hypoplastic, Smooth Type). Left and right bitewing radiographs are shown here.

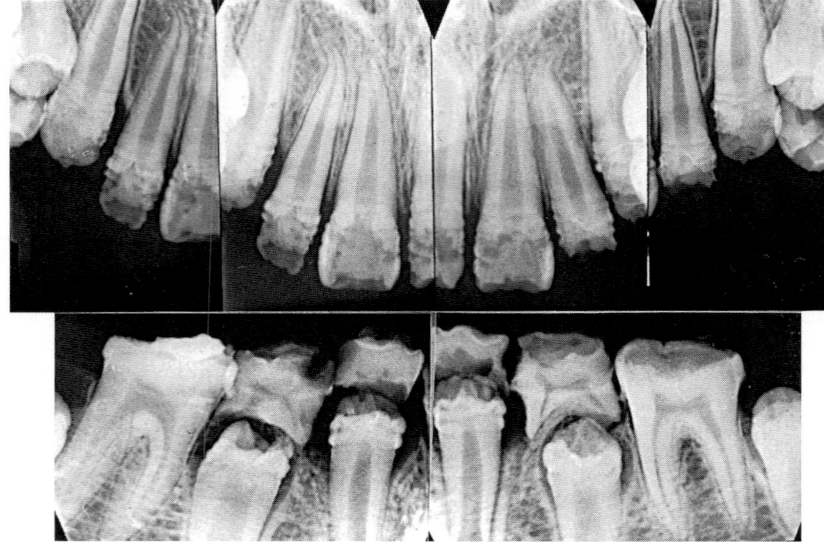

FIGURE 5–42.

Amelogenesis Imperfecta (Hypoplastic, Pitted Type). Maxillary anterior teeth, as well as right and left mandibular posterior teeth are affected. These are permanent and primary teeth.

enamel is defective. Originally, the condition was considered to be an enamel defect because the teeth may have extreme attrition. The condition is hereditary and is found in the primary as well as the permanent dentition. Witkop (1956) reported that the prevalence of dentinogenesis imperfecta is higher than that of amelogenesis imperfecta (1:14,000); 1 case is observed per 8000 individuals. Hursey and others have found dentinogenesis imperfecta to occur more frequently in inbred groups of Caucasian, Negro, and Native American ancestry.

As its name suggests, dentinogenesis imperfecta results in the production of imperfect dentin. Like bone, dentin is of mesodermal origin, and disorders of dentinogenesis may occur as part of the syndrome osteogenesis imperfecta. The color of the teeth in dentinogenesis imperfecta may range from gray to brownish violet to yellowish brown, but the teeth have a characteristic unusual translucent or opalescent (milky iridescence, rainbow colors) hue that is perhaps the most striking clinical finding in hereditary dentinogenesis imperfecta. Of course, this is soon matched by the almost inevitable and striking chipping and shearing away of enamel from its underlying dentin. The usual scalloping of the dentinoenamel junction that tends to form an interlocking union between the enamel and dentin is reportedly absent, although this finding is refuted by others. Enamel loss in this disorder has nothing to do with defects of the enamel. The enamel is of good quality and is normal in both composition and contour.

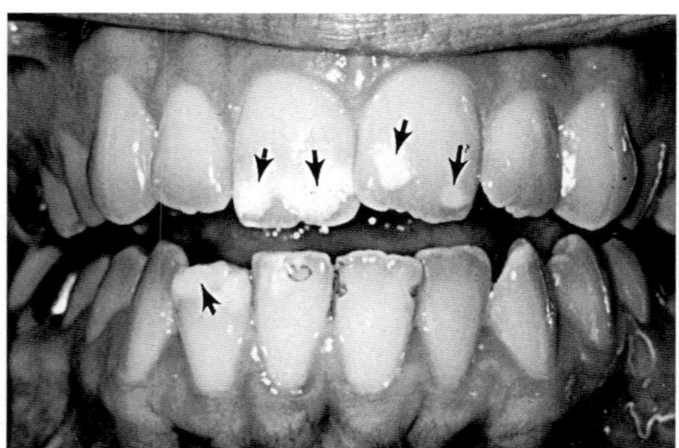

FIGURE 5–43.

Amelogenesis Imperfecta, Hypomaturation Type. Snow-capped crowns (arrows) on the maxillary central incisors and on the mandibular right lateral incisor and mandibular left canine tooth.

Among the earliest reported cases were those of Wilson and Steinbrecher (1929), who traced this condition through four generations of one family. Excellent studies of the chemical, physical, radiographic, and clinical aspects of dentinogenesis imperfecta were made by Finn in 1938 and by Hodge and his co-workers in 1939 and 1940. A racially isolated inbred group of persons with an unusually high incidence of dentinogenesis imperfecta was investigated by Hursey and co-workers in 1956 and reported a wide variation in the manifestations of the dentinal disturbance among the cases studied.

The variability in expression of various cases of dentinogenesis imperfecta has made it clear that several forms of the disease apparently exist. To separate these forms for clarity, Shields and his co-workers (1973) have suggested the following classification:

Type I dentinogenesis imperfecta includes dentinogenesis imperfecta that always occurs in families with osteogenesis imperfecta, although the latter may occur without dentinogenesis imperfecta. Type I dentinogenesis imperfecta segregates as an autosomal dominant trait (expected to be passed on to half the children of a dentinogenesis imperfecta-dominant gene parent) with variable expressivity, but it can be recessive if accompanying osteogenesis imperfecta is recessive. Osteogenesis imperfecta is a rare genetically heterogenous group of heritable bone diseases affecting the mesenchyme and its derivatives. It results in the clinical entities of fragility of bones, blue sclera and laxity of the joints. Progressive deafness and crippling deformities are present throughout life.

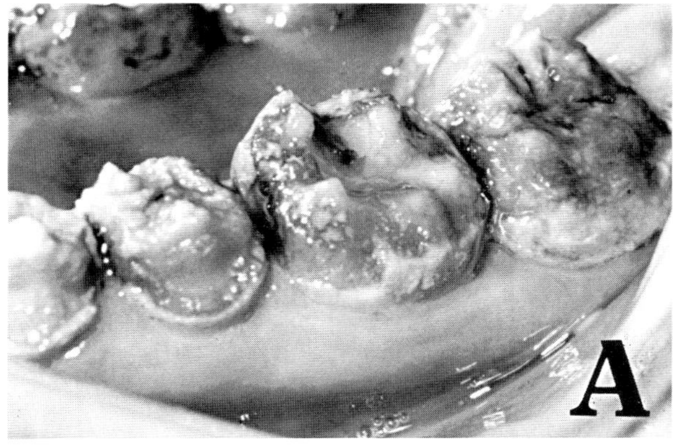

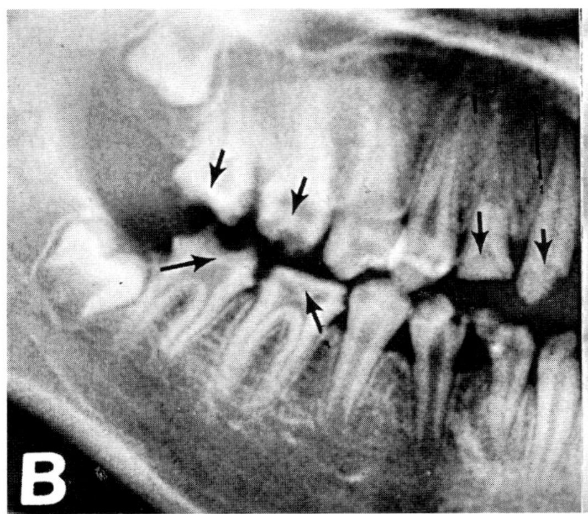

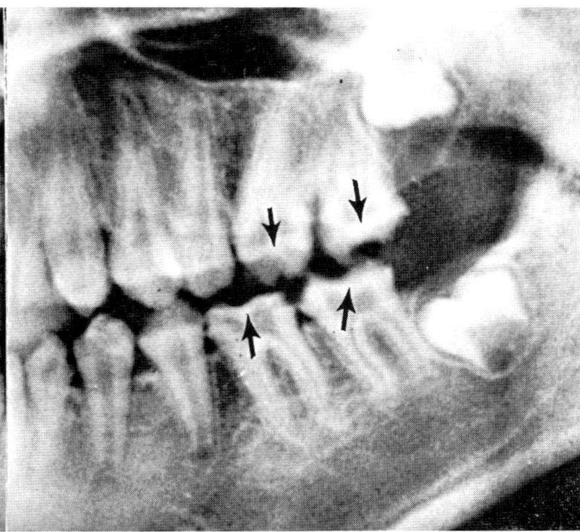

FIGURE 5–44.

Amelogenesis Imperfecta (Hypomineralized Type). A, Clinical photograph of the hypomineralized type of amelogenesis imperfecta. B, Radiograph of the hypomineralized type of amelogenesis imperfecta (arrows).

The dental changes are similar to those seen in dentinogenesis imperfecta, where the teeth are the chief target of the degeneration of their mesodermal origin. Gorlin and Pindborg (1964) reported that the primary teeth are involved in about 80% of patients, whereas the permanent teeth are involved in only 35% of patients with osteogenesis imperfecta. The documented dental findings associated with the expression of dentinogenesis imperfecta in patients with osteogenesis imperfecta as reported by Pindborg (1947), Stafne (1952), Epstein (1973) and Listgarten (1960) are as follows: blue to brown opalescent teeth, early obliteration of pulpal tissues, severe microscopic disturbances of the dentin as early as the germ stage, increased constriction of the cementoenamel junction, short and narrow roots, and excessive wear (attrition) of teeth. Crowns have been described as short, normal, abraded, and bell shaped or as having several of these characteristics.

Type II dentinogenesis imperfecta is dentinogenesis imperfecta that never occurs in association with osteogenesis imperfecta unless by chance. This type is the most frequently referred to as hereditary opalescent dentin. It is inherited as autosomal dominant defect and in fact is one of the most common dominantly inherited disorders in humans, affecting approximately 1 in every 8000 persons. Sporadic cases are virtually unreported. The dental defects of type II dentinogenesis imperfecta are similar to those found associated with osteogenesis imperfecta. However, both dentitions are affected equally. The color changes of the teeth may vary in the same dentition and also individually. Rushton (1954) reported that, soon after eruption, the color is almost normal. Later, translucency appears and is followed by a brownish color; this is not caused by the obliteration of the pulp chamber, but is due to deposits of minerals in the few dentinal tubules.

Bixler and associates (1969) reported that dentinogenesis of the type seen in patients with osteogenesis imperfecta and isolated dentinogenesis imperfects (hereditary) opalescent dentin may someday be proven to be the same genetic entity; however, until specific biochemical evidence supports one theory or another, the available clinical and family data dictate the recognition of two entities.

Type III dentinogenesis imperfecta is dentinogenesis imperfecta of the "Brandywine type." Brandywine is a racial isolate in Maryland in which this unusual form of dentinogenesis imperfecta is found. The shape and color of the teeth are much more variable than in dentinogenesis imperfecta types I and II. Unlike in types I and II, multiple pulp exposures are observed in the primary teeth of dentinogenesis imperfecta type III. The Brandywine type of dentinogenesis imperfecta was first described by Witkop and others (1956), Hursey and associates (1956), and Witkop and colleagues (1966) as an autosomal dominant condition in an inbred population of white, black, and Native American ancestry from southern Maryland. It is characterized by amber opalescent primary and permanent teeth that wear easily on their occlusal and incisal surfaces. Some of the primary teeth have pulps that are larger than normal, whereas others have obliterated pulp chambers and root canals. Crowns of newly erupted permanent teeth are bulbous, and enamel is of normal thickness, although enamel hypoplasia has been noted. Pulp chambers of permanent teeth are obliterated, and areas of rarefaction may occur at the apices of the worn permanent teeth. The findings in dentinogenesis imperfecta type III are enamel pitting, enlarged pulps early in tooth development, and radiolucencies at the apices of teeth with and without pulp exposures. The primary teeth, even within a single individual, show considerable variation in appearance, ranging from normal to dentinogenesis imperfecta type II, and even to "shell teeth."

Witkop and associates (1966) reported on eight subjects in the Brandywine isolate with teeth characterized as those in which dentin formation ceased after the mantle layer was formed. Hence, the term "shell teeth" was coined to describe their hollow appearance. There are two other reports of shell teeth, a single adult case reported by Rushton (1954) and one family reported by Schimmelpfennig and McDonald (1953). This second case was found to be related to the Brandywine isolate by Witkop in 1971. None of the patients with dentinogenesis imperfecta type II had a reported instance of shell teeth.

The treatment of patients with dentinogenesis imperfecta is directed primarily toward preventing the loss of enamel through attrition. The preparation of the teeth for crowns must be done with care. Partial dentures may exert too much stress on the abutment teeth because the roots are short and easily fractured. Restorations usually do not stay permanently because of the softness of the dentin.

◆ RADIOLOGY (Figs. 5–45 to 5–47)

The teeth in type I and II dentinogenesis imperfecta present an unusual and pathognomonic appearance on the radiograph. The most striking feature is the partial or total obliteration of the pulp chamber and root canals by early formation of dentin without any indication of the change in density of the dentin in any part of the teeth. This is seen in both the primary and permanent teeth.

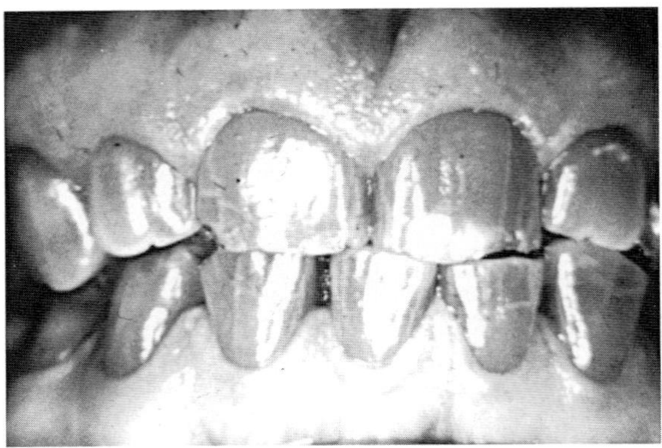

FIGURE 5–45.

Dentinogenesis Imperfecta. The color of the teeth ranges from gray to brownish violet to yellowish brown, but the teeth have a characteristic translucent or opalescent (milky iridescence) hue, which is perhaps the most striking clinical finding in dentinogenesis imperfecta.

The crowns of the teeth are excessively bulbous, with a marked cervical constriction, and the roots are unusually short, slender, and blunted. The cementum, periodontal ligament space, and supporting bones appear normal. In a proportion of the affected patients, the teeth undergo rapid attrition, with considerable loss of coronal tooth structure by the time adolescence is reached, often affecting the anterior teeth to a greater extent than the posterior. Occasionally, spontaneous root fracture occurs, and multiple areas of rarefaction may be seen on the radiograph.

Levin and associates examined the teeth of seven patients from the Brandywine isolate who had dentinogenesis imperfecta type II. They reported that the primary and permanent teeth were opalescent, and there was marked attrition. Enamel pitting was present on some permanent teeth. Anterior open bites were found in all persons with complete permanent dentitions. Pulps of the developing teeth were larger than normal during early development but rapidly became almost completely obliterated. There was increased constriction at the cementoenamel junctions. Although radiolucen-

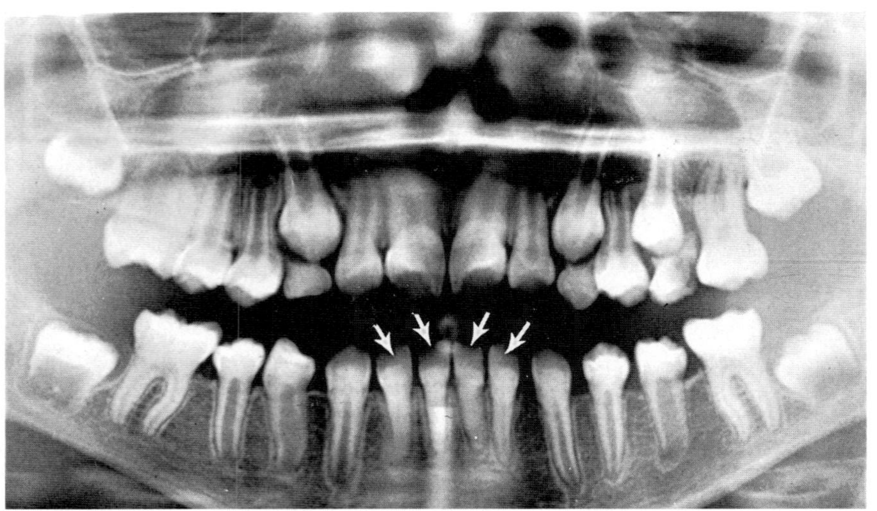

FIGURE 5–46.

Dentinogenesis Imperfecta (Type I). Panoramic radiograph of dentinogenesis imperfecta type 1 in a 9-year-old girl with osteogenesis imperfecta, blue sclera, multiple fractures, and scars. The pulps of the mandibular anterior teeth (arrows) are obliterated at an early age in this disorder.

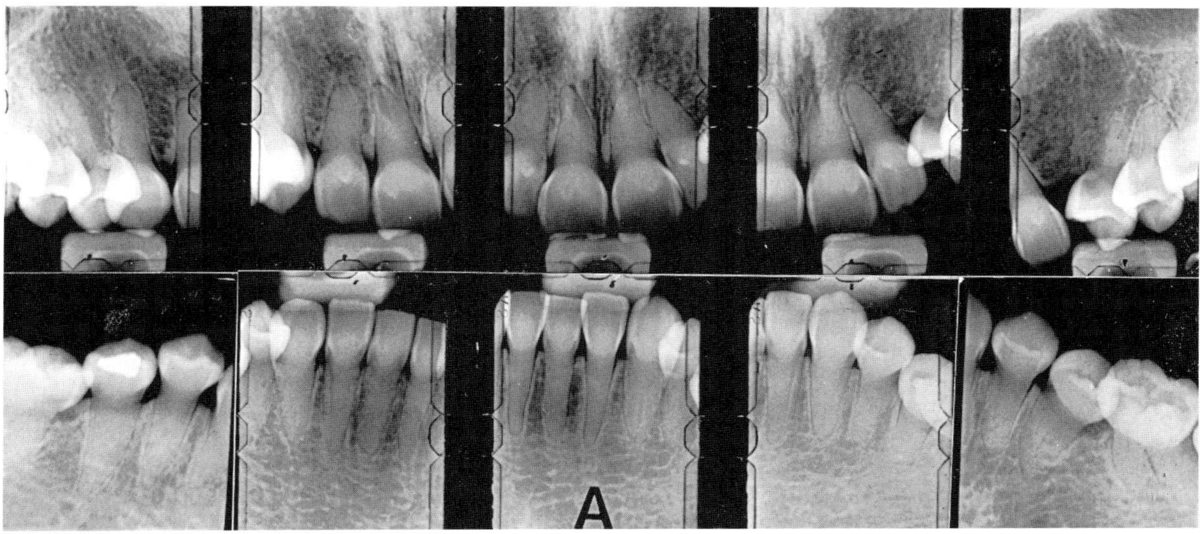

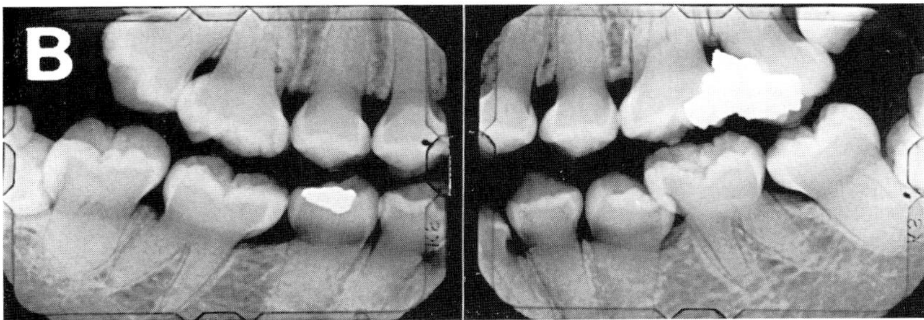

FIGURE 5–47.

Dentinogenesis Imperfecta (Type 2). This type of dentinogenesis imperfecta does not occur in association with osteogenesis imperfecta. This type is most frequently referred to as hereditary opalescent dentin. A, Maxillary and mandibular anterior teeth of a 21-year-old woman with dentinogenesis imperfecta type 2. Note the total obliteration of the pulps, the bulbous crowns, the short and slender roots, and evidence of early attrition. B, Bitewing radiographs of the patient in A.

cies were noted at the apices of teeth that had pulp exposures due to attrition, several patients had similar radiolucencies that could not be attributed to caries or attrition.

Witkop and associates (1966) and Kamen and co-workers (1980) reported the patients with dentinogenesis imperfecta type III (Brandywine isolate) had features characterized as shell teeth. These teeth consist of normal enamel lying over a thin layer of dentin surrounding an enormous pulp chamber. The large size of the pulp chambers was not due to internal resorption, but rather to insufficient and defective dentin formation. On the radiograph, the teeth appeared as "shells" of enamel and dentin surrounding extremely large pulp chambers and root canals.

Dentinal Dysplasia (Rootless teeth, familial genuine malformation of roots, radicular dentinal dysplasia type 1, and coronal dentinal dysplasia type 2)

Dentinal dysplasia is a rare disturbance of dentin formation characterized by apparently normal enamel formation with an underlying bizarre whorl-like spherical dentinal pattern, partial or complete pulpal obliteration, defectively formed roots, and a predisposition for abscess and cyst formation without an obvious inciting factor.

Ballschmiede's description in 1922, of a case of "rootless teeth," was the first published report of such an entity; short roots, pulpal occlusion, and early exfoliation were observed in six of seven children of one family. The first concise description of the disease was published in 1939 by Rushton, who was first to designate it as "dentinal dysplasia." In Rushton's case of dentinal dysplasia, the radiographs revealed a peculiar radiolucent horizontal line in obliterated pulp cavities, defective root formation, and the presence of cysts.

At one time, dentinal dysplasia was thought to be single disease entity, but it was separated by Shields and his associates (1973) into type 1 (radicular dentin dysplasia) and type 2 (coronal dentin dysplasia). Type 1 (radicular) is by far the more common disorder. Dentinal dysplasia, both type 1 and type 2, appears to be a hereditary disease, transmitted as an autosomal dominant characteristic.

Shields and associates (1973) reported that in **type 1 (radicular) dentinal dysplasia,** both the primary and permanent dentitions are affected, although clinically the teeth appear of normal size, shape, and consistency. Witkop and Sauk (1971) reported that in some cases the teeth may vary from normal and may display a slight, amber translucency. The teeth generally exhibit a normal eruption pattern; however, a delayed eruption pattern has been reported in some cases. The teeth are frequently malaligned, characteristically exhibit extreme mobility, and are commonly exfoliated prematurely or after only minor trauma as a result of their abnormally short roots.

In **type 2 dentinal dysplasia,** the primary teeth have an amber, translucent appearance, similar to the appearance of dentinogenesis imperfecta. The permanent teeth are usually normal in coloration. Both dentitions are affected in type 2 dentinal dysplasia, although the involvement in each dentition is different clinically, radiographically, and histologically. The primary teeth exhibit amorphous and atubular dentin in the radicular portion, whereas the coronal dentin is relatively normal. The permanent teeth also show relatively normal coronal dentin, but the pulp has multiple pulp stones or denticles.

No treatment exists for dentinal dysplasia, and its prognosis depends on the occurrence of periapical lesions necessitating tooth extraction as well as the premature exfoliation of teeth due to increased mobility because of short roots.

◆ *RADIOLOGY (Figs. 5–48 to 5–55)*

Radicular Dentinal Dysplasia (Type 1)

The radiographic examination is important in the identification of this anomaly. Wegner and Mannkopf (1958), Bernard (1960), and Stafne and Gibilisco (1975) reported that the teeth of both dentitions have short roots, typically with sharp, conical apical constrictions.

With the possible exception of the canine teeth, the roots are abnormally short; those of the single-rooted teeth are tapered, and those of the molars usually are blunt and stubby. No pulp chambers or root canals are in evidence because of pre-eruptive pulpal obliteration. The most characteristic radiographic feature, which is peculiar to this anomaly, is the presence of one or more horizontal radiolucent lines situated near the base of the crown. This could be called a pathognomonic sign of this disorder. These lines correspond to and represent the space between layers of the spherical bodies that are arranged in horizontal rows. Rushton (1939) reported that there are usually numerous periapical radiolucencies in noncarious teeth that are also essentially diagnostic of dentinal dysplasia.

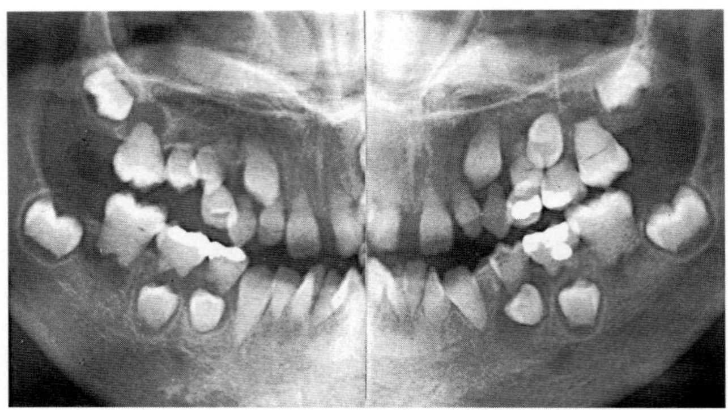

FIGURE 5–49.

Dental Dysplasia (Type 1a). A young patient with dentinal dysplasia type 1a. This is the most severe form of dentinal dysplasia and appears to develop before the sheath of Hertwig has begun the process of root development. One sees complete obliteration of the pulp, and minimal root development.

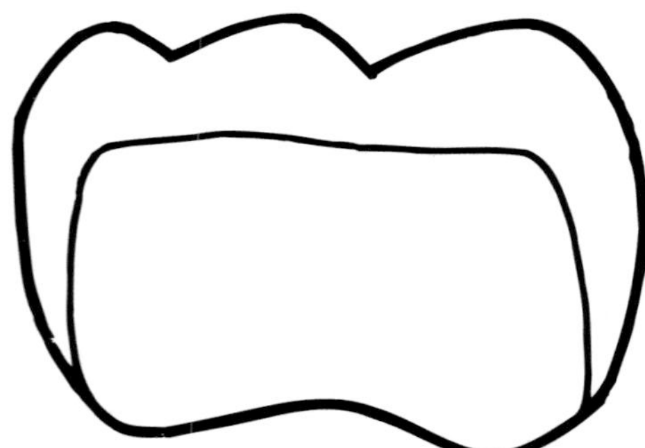

FIGURE 5–48.

Dental Dysplasia (Type 1a). Diagram illustrating O'Carroll's proposed classification of dental dysplasia type 1a, which shows a pulp completely obliterated with little or no root formation. (From O'Carroll MK, Duncan WK, Perkins TM: Dentin dysplasia: review of literature and a proposed subclassification based on radiographic findings. Oral Surg 72: 121, 1991.)

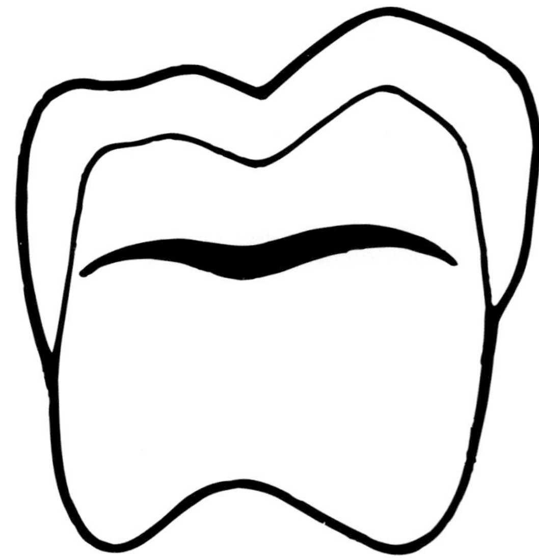

FIGURE 5–50.

Dental Dysplasia (Type 1b). Diagram illustrating O'Carroll's proposed classification of dentinal dysplasia type 1b. Pulpal remnant is minimal, showing only a curved line at the cementoenamel junction. The roots are extremely short, with no visible root canals. (From O'Carroll MK, Duncan WK, Perkins TM: Dentin dysplasia: review of literature and a proposed subclassification based on radiographic findings. Oral Surg 72:121, 1991.)

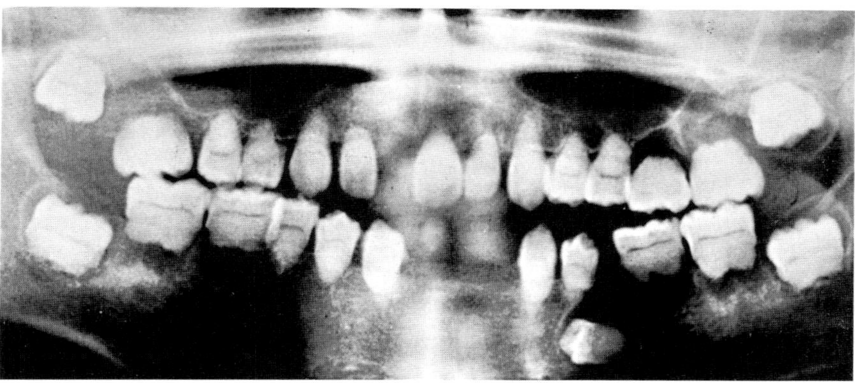

FIGURE 5–51.

Dentinal Dysplasia (Type 1b). Panoramic radiograph of a patient with dentinal dysplasia type 1b. There is a horizontal, crescent-shaped, radiolucent line along the cementoenamel junction. One usually sees a short, conical root or roots a few millimeters in length. The teeth are commonly exfoliated prematurely because of the short roots. Note the great prevalence to periapical disease and misalignment. (Courtesy of Dr. K. O'Carroll, University of Mississippi Dental School, Jackson, MS.)

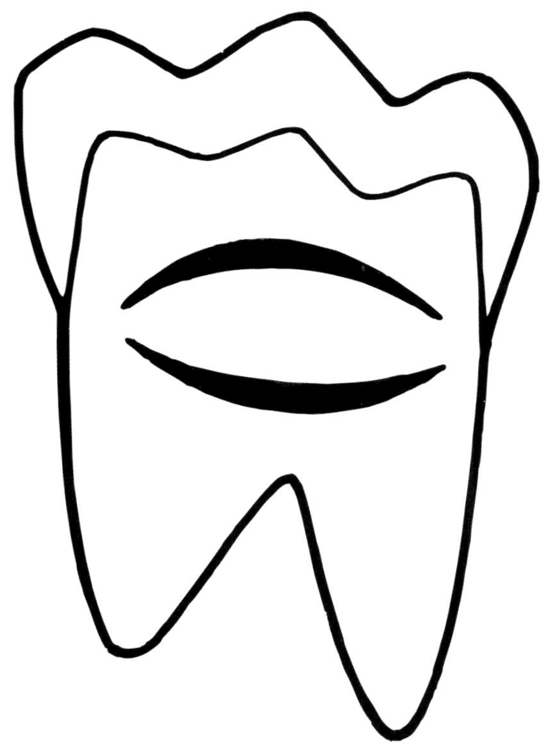

FIGURE 5–52.

Dentinal Dysplasia (Type 1c). Diagram illustrating O'Carroll's proposed classification of dentinal dysplasia type 1c. The disorder is represented by two crescent-shaped, horizontal lines, instead of only one, each concave to the other. The horizontal lines are at the cementoenamel junction, and the root is about half the normal length. Usually, there is no evidence of a pulp canal in the root. (From O'Carroll MK, Duncan WK, Perkins TM: Dentin dysplasia: review of literature and a proposed subclassification based on radiographic findings. Oral Surg 72:121, 1991.)

In their review of the literature, O'Carroll and associates (1991) identified four broad categories of variations in the radiographic appearance of radicular dentin dysplasia (type 1).

In the first type of dentinal dysplasia 1, called DD1a, there is complete obliteration of the pulp and usually little or no root development. This first category of radicular dentinal dysplasia is supported by reports of Logan and associates (1962), Perl and Farman (1977), Morris and Angsburger (1977), Bakaeen and colleagues (1985), Luffingham and Noble (1986), Witcher and co-workers (1989), and Duncan and associates (1991). This is the most severe form of DD1 and appears to develop before the sheath of Hertwig has begun the process of root development. It has the greatest prevalence for periapical pathosis, tooth exfoliation, and extraction.

In the second category (DD1b), one sees a single horizontal, crescent-shaped, radiolucent pulpal remnant and a few millimeters of root development with many periapical radiolucent areas. These roots are short and conical. This form appears to occur slightly later in development of the tooth than does DD1a and results in less than complete obliteration of the pulp and some rudimentary root structure, as if the sheath of Hertwig was severely limited in the formation of a tooth apex.

Dentin dysplasia type 1b is supported by reports of Hoggins and Marsland (1952), Logan and associates (1962), Miller (1970), McFarlane and Cina (1974), Morris and Angsburger (1977), Tidwell and Cunningham (1979), Melnick and associates (1977, 1980), Steidler and co-workers (1984), Luffingham and Noble (1986), Scola and Watts (1987), Witcher and colleagues (1989), Brenneise and associates (1989), Van Dis and Allen (1989), and Duncan and co-workers (1991).

The third category of DD1 is called DD1c and is represented by two crescent-shaped, horizontal lines (instead of only one), each concave to the other. The horizontal lines are at the cementoenamel junction, and the root is about half its

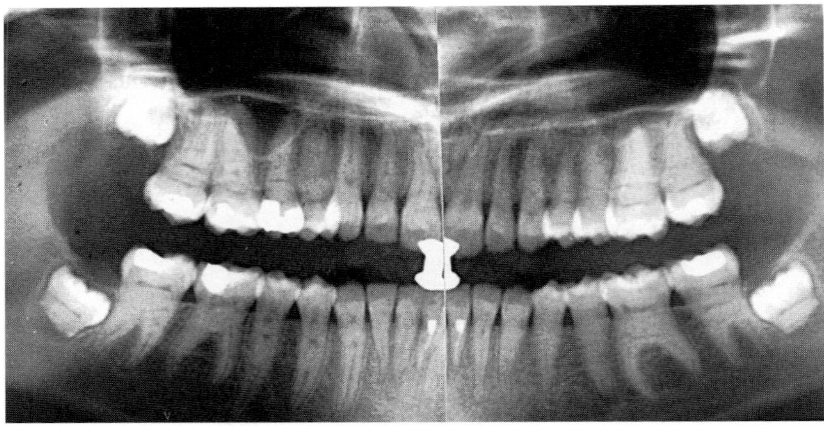

FIGURE 5–53.

Dentinal Dysplasia (Type 1c). Panoramic radiographic survey of a patient with evidence of dentinal dysplasia type 1c. The maxillary premolars and molars and the mandibular left premolars and molars are represented by two crescent-shaped, horizontal lines, each concave to the other. There is no evidence of pulp canals in the roots, which are smaller than average. (From Langland OE, Langlais RP, Morris CR: Principles and Practice of Panoramic Radiology. Philadelphia:WB Saunders, 1982, p. 178.)

normal length. This form appears to develop sufficiently late in individual tooth development, to allow for significant growth to take place without abnormality. Usually, there is no evidence of a pulp canal in the root. The DD1c category is supported by the studies of Rushton (1939, 1955), Logan and associates (1962), Graham and co-workers (1965), Brookeson and Miller, Wesley and colleagues (1976), Ciola and associates (1978), Tidwell and Cunningham (1979), and Van Dis and Allen (1989).

The fourth category of DD1 is called DD1d; there is some evidence of a pulp chamber at the level of the cementoenamel junction. The roots are of normal length but may be bulbous in the coronal third, where a large pulp stone is seen within the root canal. This type of DD1 appears to arise latest in the life of the tooth because the pulp chamber is usually not obliterated, and the least severe form in that normal completion of root formation occurs. In many instances, the pulp appears to be intact around the pulp stone. In others, the pulp is seen intact above and below the pulp stone, which seems to be continuous with the dentin mesially and distally. The fourth category of DD1 is supported by studies of Weiss (1927), Hutchin (1936), Rushton (1939, 1955), Stafne and Gibilisco (1961, 1975), Graham and associates (1965), Elzay and Robinson (1967), Petersson (1972), Hunter and colleagues (1973), Ciola and co-workers (1978), Coke and associates (1979), Rankow and Miller (1984), Nakata and colleagues (1985), Diamond (1989), and Van Dis and Allen (1989).

Dental dysplasia 1 (radicular type) seems to occur at different stages of tooth development, and the earlier it occurs, the more severe is the pulpal obliteration and the stunting of the roots.

Coronal Dentinal Dysplasia (Type 2)

The pulp chambers of primary teeth become obliterated as in type 1 (radicular) and dentinogenesis imperfecta; however, this does not appear before eruption. The permanent teeth in DD2 have normal root development with a thistle-tube-shaped pulp chamber extending into the root and containing pulp calcification in the chamber rather than in the root canal, and a sudden constriction where the chamber becomes the root canal, which is very narrow. Usually, no multiple radiolucencies are seen, unless, of course, there is an obvious reason, such as deep caries.

Dental dysplasia 2 (coronal dysplasia type) has been supported by the studies of Borkenhagen and Elfenbaum (1955), Grimer (1956), Richardson and Fantin (1970), Rao and associates (1970), Shields and colleagues (1973), Giansanti and Allen (1974), Diner and Chous (1978), Melnick and associates (1980), Burkes and co-workers (1979), Rosenberg and Phelan (1983), Steidler and associates (1984), Wetzel and Weckler (1985), Hoff and colleagues (1986), and Jasmin and Clergeau-Guerithault (1984).

The distinction between DD1 and DD2 appears to be significant enough to classify them as two distinct forms of the disease. The four types of DD1 listed here are radiographic distinctions and are not histopathologic or genetic findings.

Regional Odontodysplasia (''Ghost teeth,'' odontogenic dysplasia, odontogenesis imperfecta)

Odontodysplasia is a rare developmental anomaly characterized by defective dentin and enamel formation and by calcifications within the pulp and dental follicle.

McCall and Wald first described the condition as ''arrested tooth development'' in 1947. Neupert and Wright (1989) noted that 68 cases had been reported in the literature. Zegarelli and Kutscher introduced the term ''odontodysplasia'' in 1963 because the condition tends to affect several adjacent teeth within a particular segment or region of the

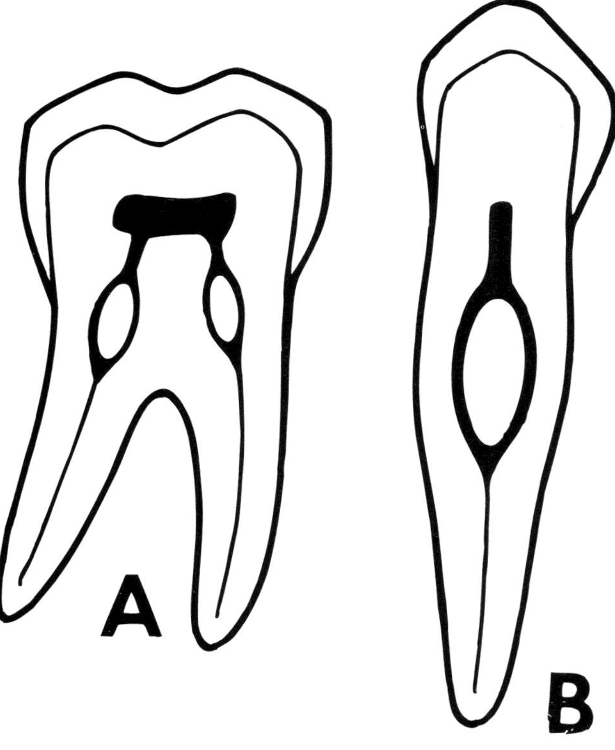

FIGURE 5–54.

Dentinal Dysplasia (Type 1d). Diagrams illustrating O'Carroll's proposed classification of dentinal dysplasia type 1d. The root canals are visible in roots of normal length. The roots may be bulbous in the coronal third, where a large pulp stone is seen within the root canal. The pulp appears to be intact around the pulp stone, and in other cases, the pulp is seen intact above and below the pulp stone, which seems to be continuous with the dentin mesially or distally. A, Molar tooth, dentinal dysplasia type 1d. B, Premolar tooth, dentinal dysplasia type 1d. C, Complete radiographic survey of a patient classified as having dentinal dysplasia type 1d. Note the multiple pulp stones (arrows). (From O'Carroll MK, Duncan WK, Perkins TM: Dentin dysplasia: review of literature and a proposed subclassification based on radiographic findings. Oral Surg 72:121, 1991.)

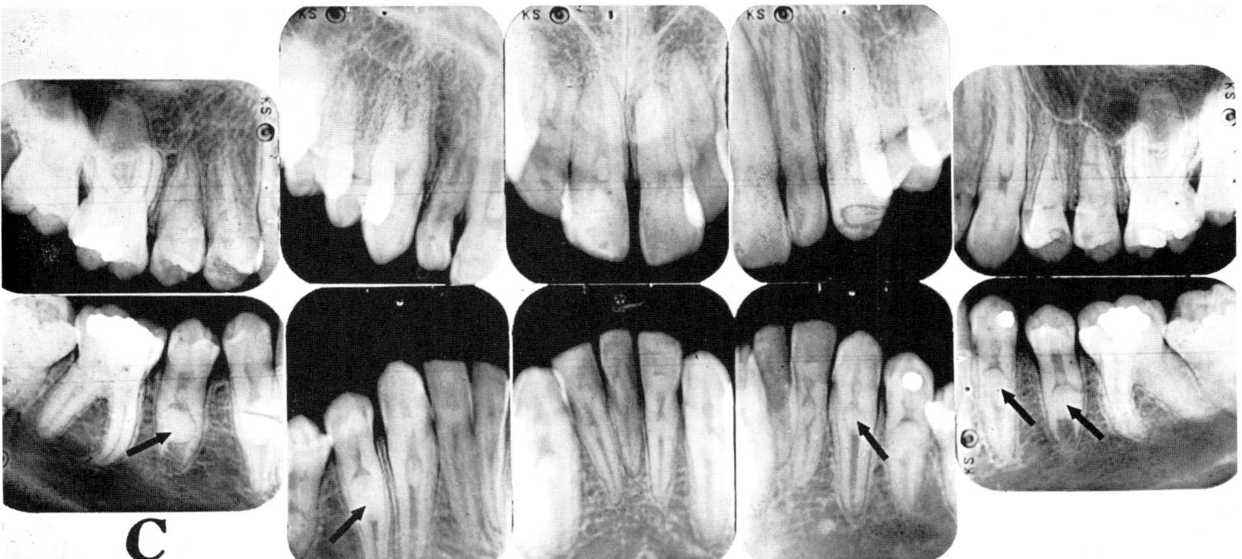

jaw. The term "regional odontodysplasia" has become the accepted terminology.

Lustman and associates (1975) reported that approximately two thirds of the affected teeth are found in the anterior segments, with the maxilla involved roughly twice as often as the mandible. Odontodysplasia is usually seen first in the primary or early mixed dentitions and is often accompanied by abscess formation adjacent to the affected teeth. Lustman and associates (1975) reported that females are more often affected than males. However, Pindborg (1970) reported no evidence of sex or site predilection, and although both primary and permanent teeth may be involved, the primary teeth are most often affected. There is no tendency toward a specific race or ethnic group.

The etiology of the anomaly has not been determined. There have been numerous theories, including local circulatory disorder, latent virus in tooth germs, genetic transmission, local infections, somatic mutation, radiation, and vascular nevi.

Microscopically, the most characteristic features of the abnormality are the marked reduction in the amount of dentin, the widening of the predentin layer, the presence of inter-

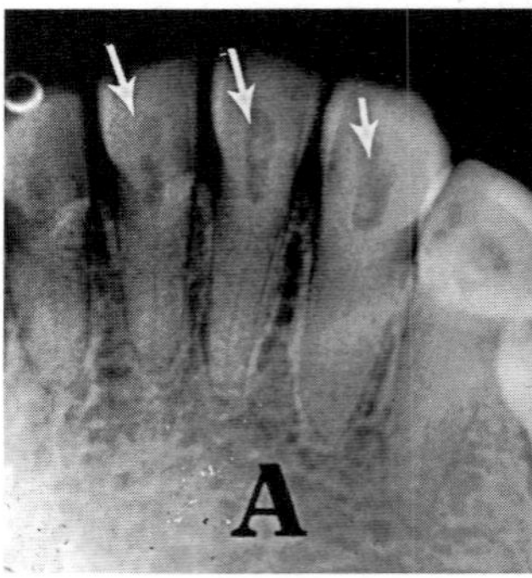

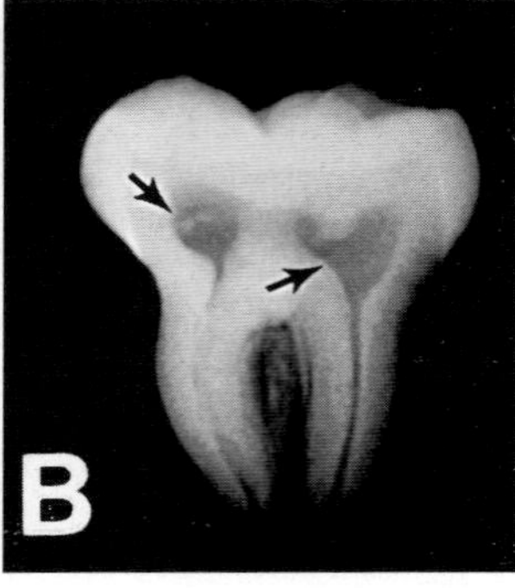

FIGURE 5–55.

Dentinal Dysplasia (Type 2 Coronal). A, Dentinal dysplasia type 2 (coronal). Radiograph of a patient with dentinal dysplasia type 2 with thistle-shaped pulp chambers of the lower anterior teeth (arrows). (From Langland OE, Langlais RP, Morris CR: Principles and Practice of Panoramic Radiology. Philadelphia:WB Saunders, 1982, p. 179.) B, Dentinal dysplasia type 2 (coronal). Extracted molar of a patient with dentinal dysplasia type 2 (coronal). Note that the pulp chamber narrows suddenly at its base into a slim canal forming a thistle-shaped pulp chamber (arrows).

globular dentin, and an irregular tubular pattern of dentin. These pulp chambers are large. The reduced enamel layer around the nonerupted teeth is attenuated and disrupted. The follicular connective tissue contains many irregular enameloid droplet calcifications.

Treatment of odontodysplasia has been extraction of the involved teeth. Many times, affected teeth are painful and abscessed. Sadeghi and Ashrafi (1981) reported that the aberrant enamel and dentin are unable to resist bacterial invasion. Lowe and Duperon (1985) suggested saving the affected teeth and including them in prosthetic reconstruction. Neupert and Wright (1989) believed that necrosis and facial cellulitis may appear as a complications if these teeth are retained.

◆ *RADIOLOGY (Figs. 5–56 and 5–57)*

Radiographic examination reveals that the radiodensity of the teeth is greatly reduced, the normal demarcation between enamel and dentin is absent, and the pulp chambers appear widened. The enamel layer often is not evident. These features contribute to the ''ghost'' appearance, hence the name ''ghost teeth.'' The affected teeth are most often localized in one of the jaws (regional), and eruption of teeth may be delayed, partially erupted, or not erupted at all.

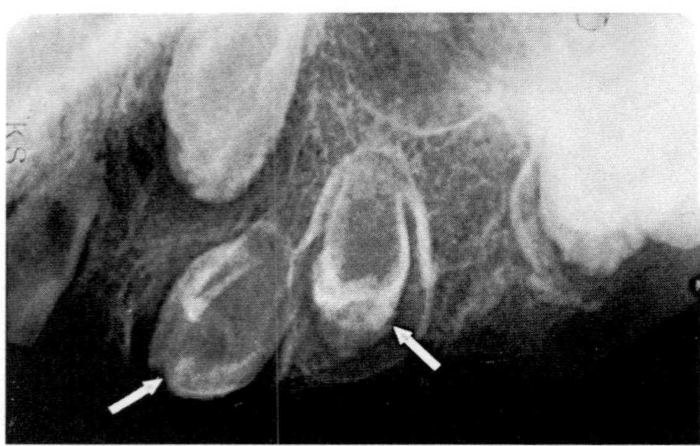

FIGURE 5–56.

Regional Odontodysplasia (Ghost Teeth). The radiodensity of teeth is greatly reduced, the normal demarcation between enamel and dentin is absent, and the pulp chambers appear widened. These features contribute to the "ghostlike" appearance of the teeth (arrows). (From Langland OE, Langlais RP, Morris CR: Principles and Practice of Panoramic Radiology. Philadelphia:WB Saunders, 1982, p. 180.)

ACQUIRED DEFECTS OF THE TEETH

Attrition

Attrition is the physiologic wearing away of tooth structure as a result of normal mastication. It affects the incisal, occlusal, and interproximal surfaces. It begins as a small, polished, wear facet and may advance to a degree whereby the occlusal and incisal edges are completely flattened with cupped-out areas of shiny, stained, exposed dentin. In patients with mandibular prognathism, an unusual form of attrition occurs on the incisal-labial surface of the maxillary anterior teeth, whereas persons having an angle class II division 2 malocclusion with a deep overbite develop a similar form of attrition on the incisal-labial surfaces of the mandibular anterior teeth. Both the primary and permanent teeth may be affected by attrition. The teeth are usually not sensitive.

◆ *RADIOLOGY (Figs. 5–58 and 5–59)*

Attrition may be seen on dental radiographs. Once noted, a careful history will be required to rule out abrasion. Prior to complete flattening of the occlusal plane, the cuspid inclines may be worn flat but may still form inclined planes. Because of these straight lines, the occlusal surfaces take on an angular, geometric appearance, with markedly thinner enamel.

Abrasion

Abrasion is the pathologic wearing away of tooth structure by a mechanical process. The occlusal surface may be severely worn, mimicking advanced attrition in a person who, for example, is a sand blaster. Probably the most common form of abrasion is toothbrush abrasion, caused by improper brushing. This produces a V-shaped notch in the faciocervical portion of the tooth and may eventually lead to pathologic pulp exposure and tooth fracture. Although dentinal sensitivity is common, caries is usually absent. The area most commonly affected is the cuspid-bicuspid region, owing to the prominence of these teeth and the curvature of the arch. Right-handed persons may show more toothbrush abrasion on the left side and, vice versa for left-handed persons, a fact often used in forensic odontology. Other forms of abrasion occur with pipe smoking, improper flossing, improper home use of scalers, improper utilization of toothpicks, opening of bobby pins with the teeth, holding nails by the

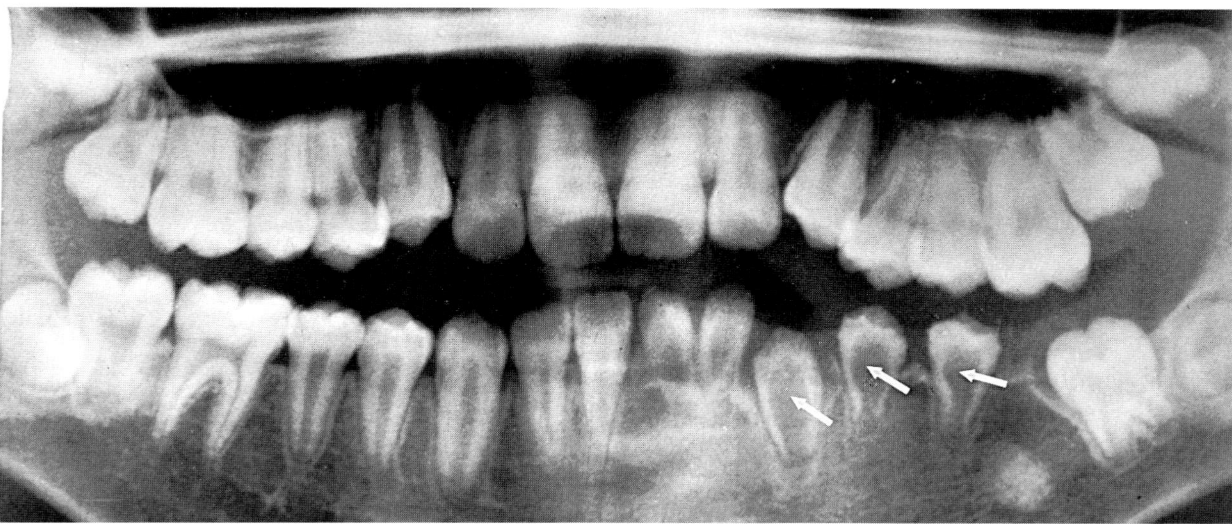

FIGURE 5–57.

Regional Odontodysplasia (Ghost Teeth). Panoramic radiograph of a patient with regional odontodysplasia in the lower left quadrant. The affected teeth are most often localized in one jaw. Eruption of the teeth may be delayed, or teeth may be partially erupted or not erupted at all (arrows). (Courtesy of Dr. P. Dhriravarangkura, Chulalonghorn University, Bangkok, Thailand.)

teeth, and so on. Abraded teeth may be sensitive, and treatment is aimed at removal of the physical source of wear. Restorative procedures may be required for esthetics, function, and comfort.

◆ *RADIOLOGY (Figs. 5–60 to 5–62)*

Localized areas of abrasion often show an unusual pattern of wear, which may alert the practitioner that further clinical investigation is necessary. Toothpick abrasion may be suspected if a circular defect in the enamel and/or dentin is seen, usually below the unaffected contact point. When more advanced, toothbrush abrasion shows a well-demarcated, horizontal radiolucent line in the cervical area of the tooth. If the tooth is slightly rotated or if the radiation is directed at the tooth from slightly off-angle, a V-shaped radiolucency may be noted, with one side of the V highly angular and well-demarcated and the other side seen as a fuzzy, indistinct outline. Other forms of wear show similar, unusual patterns, depending on the source.

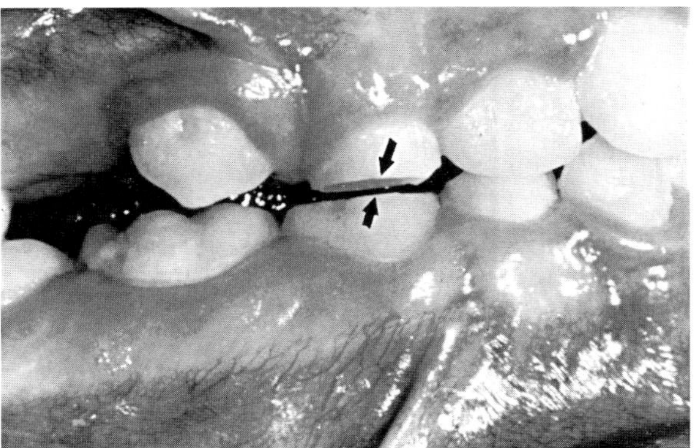

FIGURE 5–58.

Attrition in a Child. Posterior attrition in a child (arrows).

Erosion

Erosion is the loss of tooth substance by a chemical process, usually involving an acid. Clinically, the teeth appear smooth and shiny, and there may be exposed, sensitive dentin. With chronic vomiting or regurgitation and with the long-term intake of acidic carbonated soft drinks, the most involved area is usually the palatal aspect of the maxillary teeth. The erosion or gastric decalcification of teeth is a common finding in patients with anorexia nervosa with bulimia. This psychosomatic disease is characterized by induced chronic vomiting, often after bouts of uncontrolled eating that are interspersed with periods of starvation because of an inner rejection of food. In cases of chronic vomiting the lingual surfaces of teeth may show evidence of erosion. Many of these patients take excessive amounts of fruit juices in an attempt to relieve their thirst after vomiting. When the facial surfaces mainly are involved, especially the maxillary anterior teeth, lemon sucking may be suspected. Dental erosion is also well recognized in many industries involving the use of acids. Erosion may also occur idiopathically.

◆ *RADIOLOGY (Fig. 5–63)*

Only severe, advanced cases of erosion appear radiographically. The findings are vague and nonspecific. Basically, the crown looks vaguely more radiolucent than it should (Fig. 5–63). What is believed to be toothbrush abrasion on the radiograph may be due to lemon-sucking erosion. Toothbrush abrasion produces characteristic horizontal radiolucent

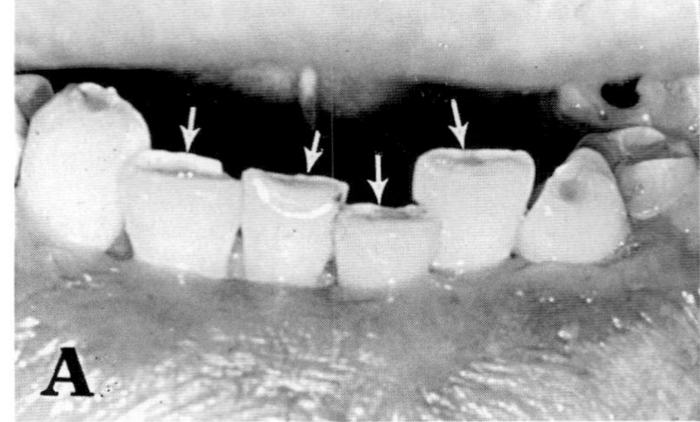

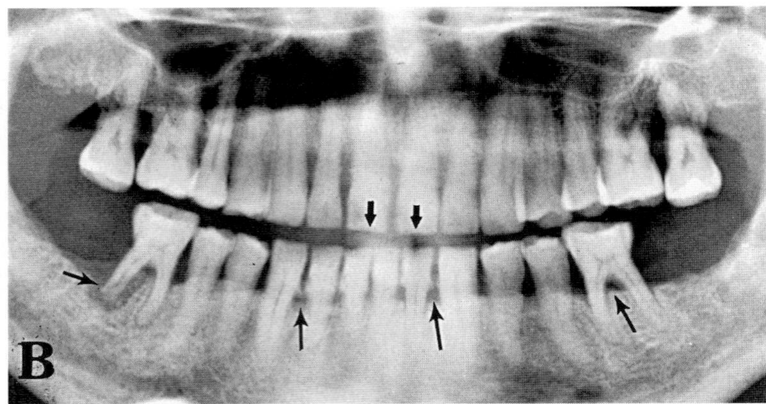

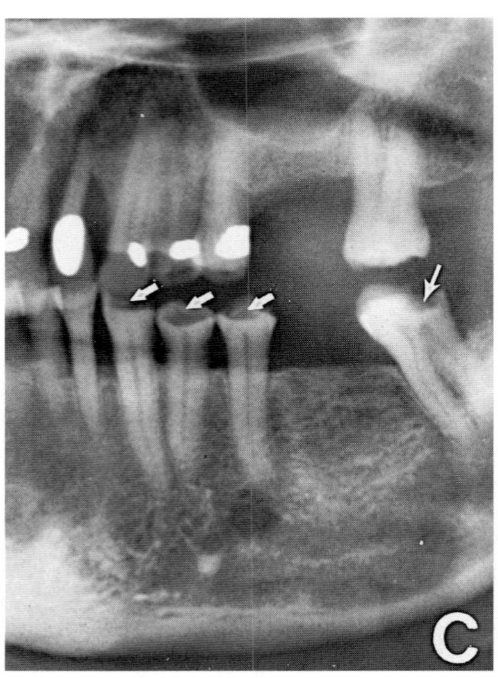

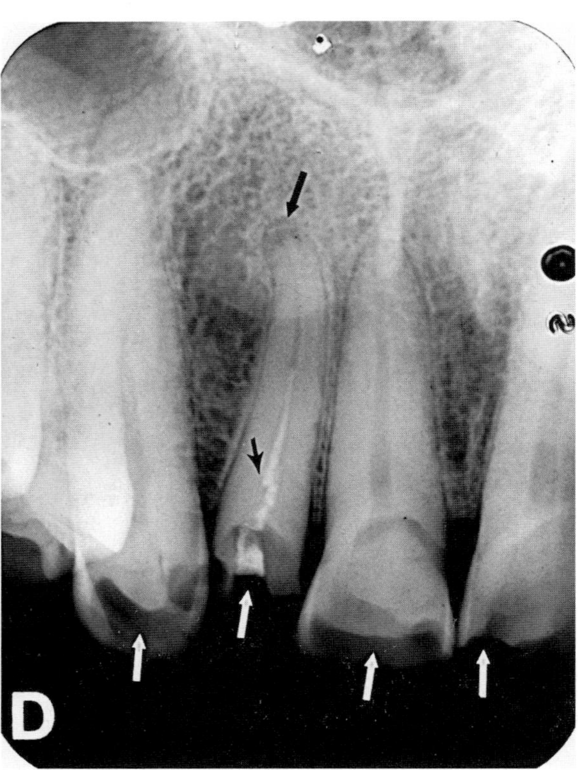

FIGURE 5–59.

Attrition in an Adult. A, Mandibular anterior attrition in an adult (arrows). B, Panoramic radiograph of an 89-year-old man with severe occlusal attrition. (Note the calculus on the lower anterior teeth, the furcation involvement of the lower left first molar, and the periodontal/periapical disease of the lower right first molar (arrows). C, Severe attrition mimicking caries (arrows). (From Langland OE, Langlais RP, Morris CR: Principles and Practice of Panoramic Radiology. Philadelphia: WB Saunders, 1982, p. 216.) D, Severe attrition (white arrows) mimicking caries. Note the incomplete root canal filling in the lateral incisor and the periodontal ligament space thickening at the apex (black arrows).

lines mesiodistally across the crowns of the maxillary anterior teeth.

Drift and Migration

Drift refers to movement of an erupted tooth when either mesial or distal contact is lost. When mesial contact is lost, mesial drift, or more commonly mesial tipping, occurs because of the mesial inclination of the occlusion forces. Permanent molars in both jaws drift mesially. In general, the maxillary permanent molars move much farther than the mandibular molars. Paradoxically, when distal contact is lost, one does not usually expect distal drift or tipping of the tooth. When distal drift does occur, it is of clinical signifi-

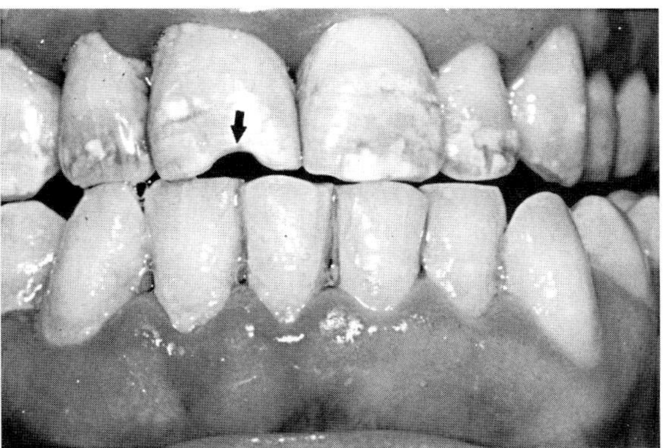

FIGURE 5-60.

Bobby-pin Abrasion Occupational abrasion of the incisive surface of the right maxillary central incisor (arrow). This is bobby-pin abrasion. The maxillary incisors show evidence of dental fluorosis.

cance, especially with respect to treatment planning. A definite difference exists in distal drifting tendencies between premolars in the maxilla and those in the mandible. The magnitude of the distal drifting is much greater in the mandible than in the maxilla, and the second premolar shows the greatest distal drift.

Kisling and Hoffding (1979) reported that tooth drifting depends mainly on the following important factors: (1) the dental age at the time of tooth extraction; (2) space conditions; (3) eruption path and time; and (4) intercuspation. Thus, the type of tooth lost is the most decisive factor in drifting. Kisling and Hoffding (1979) believed that, in general, extraction of primary molars before the first permanent molars erupt is more damaging to the dentition than extraction after eruption of the first permanent molars.

The term **migration** indicates the abnormal movement of an unerupted tooth, usually in a mesial direction. This is perhaps due to the mesial inclination of some erupting teeth, especially the canine teeth and third molars. Distal migration may also occur. Whenever migration is noted, an attempt should be made to identify an underlying cause, such as congenitally or otherwise missing teeth or displacement by a tumor mass or cyst. Migration may occur idiopathically, but when a cause is present, it may be more important to recognize and treat the cause than to remove or treat the migrated tooth. Some authors use the terms drift and migration interchangeably with respect to erupted and unerupted teeth.

◆ *RADIOLOGY (Fig. 5-64)*

In distal drift, the involved tooth occupies a position distal to where it should be. The tooth distal to the involved tooth is usually missing. We have observed this phenomenon most frequently in the mandibular second premolar. Although migrating teeth may erupt, an unerupted migrated tooth of long standing may show signs of external resorption and

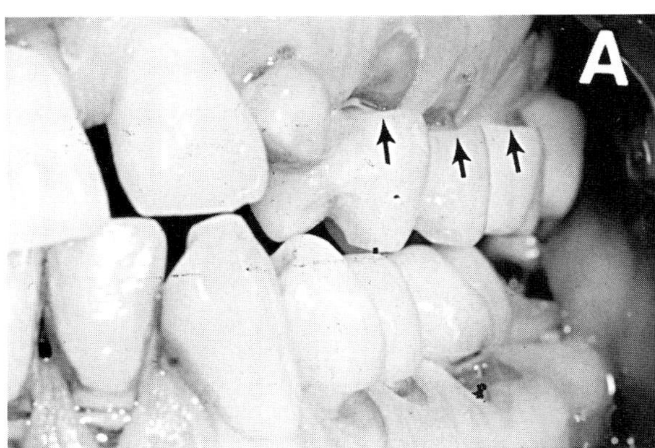

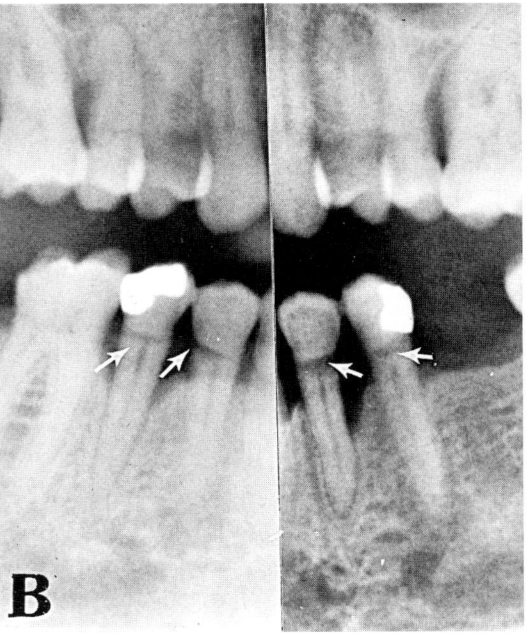

FIGURE 5-61.

Toothbrush Abrasion. This condition is caused by brushing back and forth horizontally on the cervical neck of the teeth rather than using the preferred up and down motion. A, Toothbrush abrasion at the cervical neck of the maxillary and mandibular posterior teeth (arrows). B, Radiograph of toothbrush abrasion of cervical surfaces of the right and left mandibular premolars (arrows).

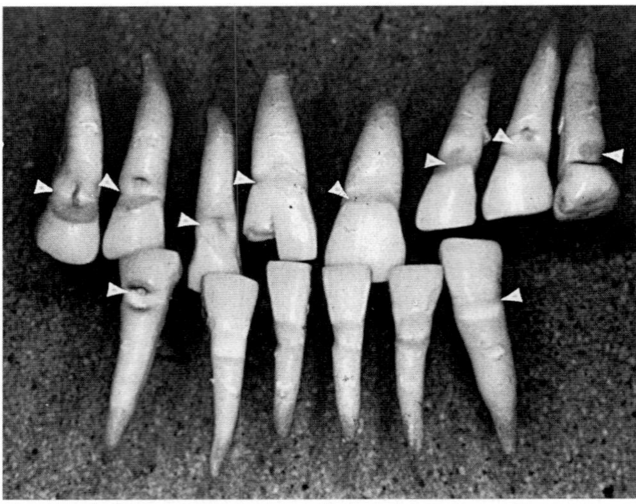

FIGURE 5–62.

Toothbrush Abrasion. Extracted teeth of a patient with severe toothbrush abrasion (arrowheads).

ankylosis. In the absence of abnormal clinical and radiographic findings, periodic radiographic observation is recommended.

Embedded and Impacted Teeth

An embedded tooth is one that has failed to erupt and remains buried in bone. An impacted tooth is one in which some physical entity has prevented its eruption.

In a study of Dachi and Howell (1961) dealing with a total of 3874 individuals, the incidence of impacted teeth was 16.7%. The third molars were most frequently impacted. The number of impacted maxillary third molars (21.9%) was significantly higher than that of impacted mandibular third molars (17.5%). The incidence of impaction among maxillary canines was 0.92%. In 1930, Mead reported on a series of radiographs of 1462 office patients. He found that 276 (18.8%) had at least 1 impacted tooth. Hellman (1936), studying a small series of university students, found the incidence of impactions to be 9.5% in men and 23.8% in women. In Mead's study, nearly 80% of the impacted teeth were third molars. The next most frequently impacted tooth was the maxillary canine.

According to Morris and Jerman (1971), 65.5% of their male patients examined from 17 to 24 years of age had at least one impacted tooth. In 22.3% of the persons studied, all four third molars were impacted.

Aitasalo and co-workers (1970) in Finland studied panoramic radiographs of 4063 individuals and found impacted teeth in 14.1% of patients. The teeth most frequently impacted were the third molars (76.1%), and of these, no difference between the maxilla and the mandible was observed. The prevalence of impacted maxillary canine teeth was higher in females than in males.

Thus, the maxillary and mandibular third molars and the maxillary canines are most frequently impacted, followed by the premolars and supernumerary teeth. Shafer, Hine, and Levy stated that the mandibular teeth are more apt to exhibit severe impaction than the maxillary teeth. Impactions of primary teeth are rare. In those cases where it does occur, impactions of the primary mandibular second molar are as numerous as impactions of all other primary teeth together.

The causes of impaction may be divided into local and systemic factors. Among the local factors, the most important is abnormal position of the tooth germ. In cases of impaction of the mandibular third molar, the space in the alveolar arch is considerably reduced. Bjork and associates (1956) reported that the lack of space for the third molar must be regarded as the essential cause of its impaction. Other local obstructing causes for impaction are abnormal size of crown, arrested tooth formation, dental ankylosis, supernumerary teeth, cysts, and tumors. Among systemic factors, especially patients with cranial defects exhibit impacted teeth. A char-

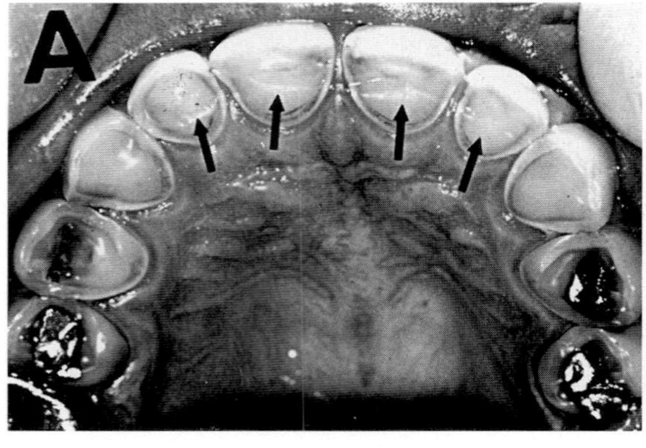

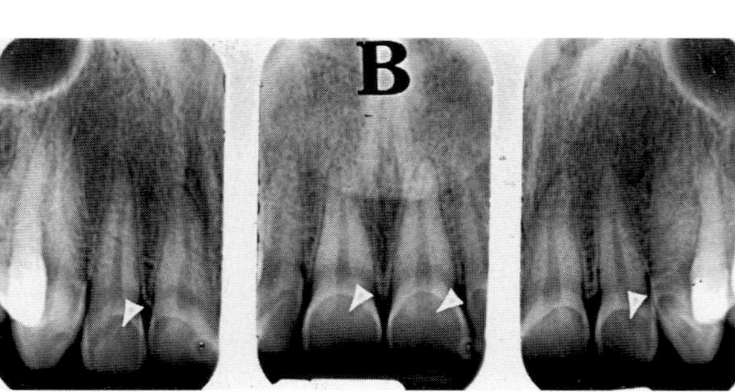

FIGURE 5–63.

Erosion. A, Photograph of a 31-year-old woman with bulimia, which causes an abnormal increase in the sensation of hunger. Note the erosion on the lingual surfaces (arrows) of the teeth of this patient. B, Radiographs of the patient in A. Note the erosion of the anterior maxillary teeth (arrowheads).

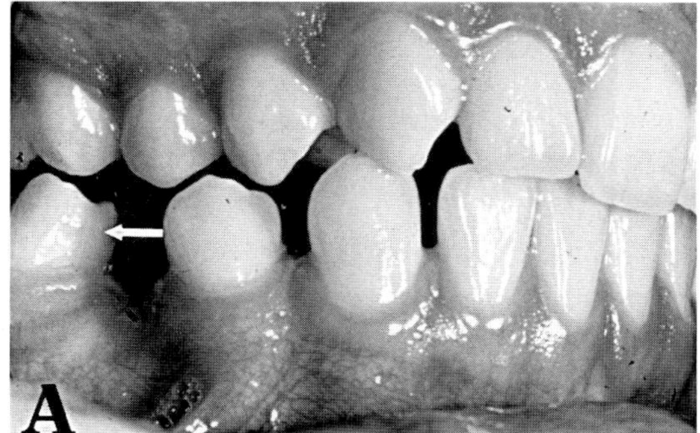

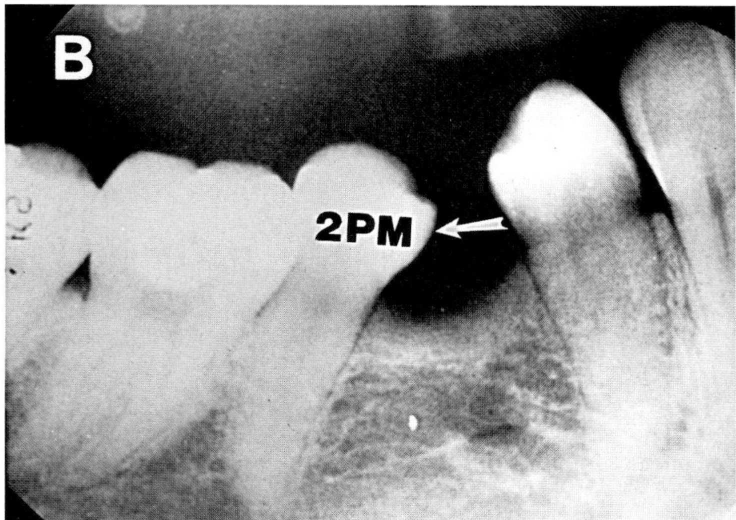

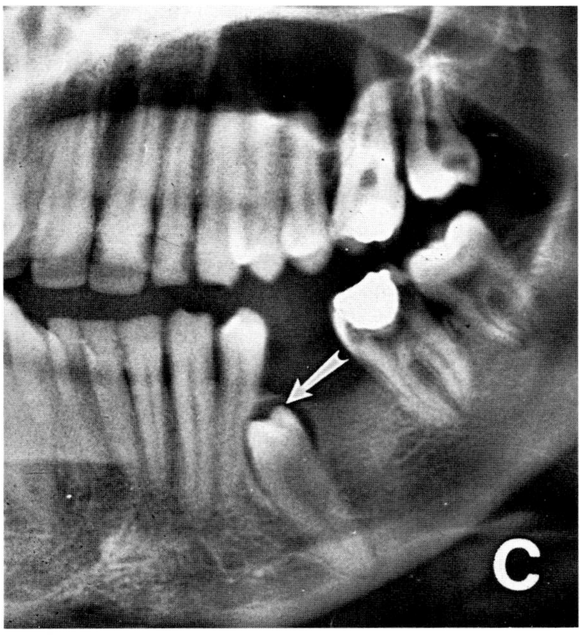

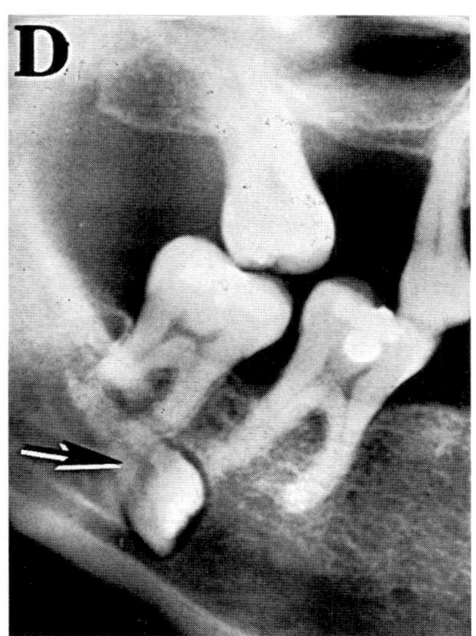

FIGURE 5–64.

Drift and Migration. A, Clinical photograph of a patient with lower second premolar distal drift (arrow). B, Radiograph showing distal drift (arrow) of a second premolar (2 PM) into a space previously occupied by a missing first molar. C, The second premolar has migrated mesially and is impacted against the first premolar (arrow). D, Migration of a premolar (arrow). (From Langland OE, Langlais RP, Morris CR: Principles and Practice of Panoramic Radiology. Philadelphia:WB Saunders, 1982, p. 192.)

acteristic example is cleidocranial dysplasia, which is almost always associated with impaction of several teeth. In cleidocranial dysplasia, the primary teeth erupt at normal rates, but they are not shed at the proper time.

Impacted teeth may cause complications. They may undergo resorption, may cause formation of dentigerous cysts or odontogenic tumors, or in cases of partial impaction, may become involved in pericoronitis. In some cases of cysts and tumors, it is difficult to determine whether these conditions have caused the impactions.

◆ *RADIOLOGY (Figs. 5–65 to 5–76)*

In evaluating impacted and embedded teeth, it is extremely helpful to determine the eruptive potential of the tooth. The earliest sign of an impending impaction may be radiographic

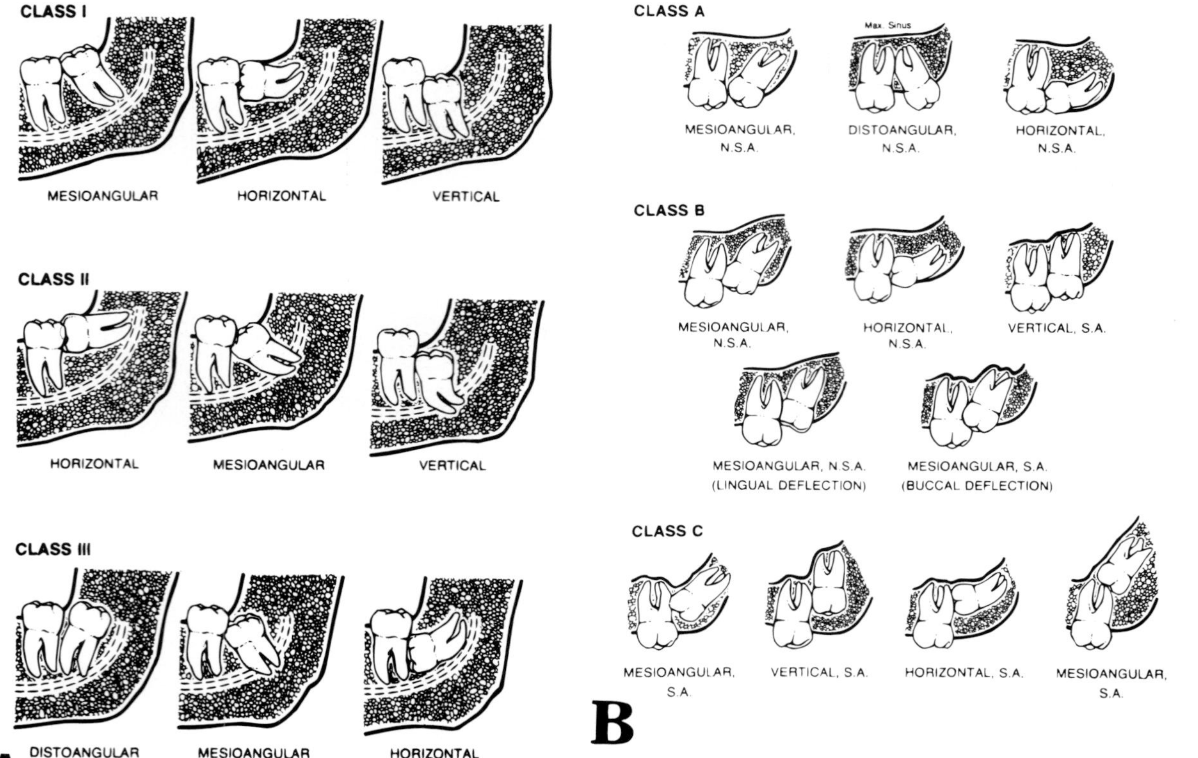

FIGURE 5–65.

Classification of Third Molar Impactions by Pell and Gregory (1942) and by Winter (1926). A, Classification of mandibular third molar impactions. The four main categories of impacted third molar teeth are (1) mesioangular, (2) horizontal, (3) vertical, and (4) distoangular. They are further classified according to the distance between the second molar and the ramus by class (I II, and III), and the depth of the third molar in bone as positions A, B, and C. B, Classification of maxillary third molar impactions. Maxillary third molar impactions occur in the same four major positions as the mandibular third molar impactions: (1) mesioangular, (2) horizontal, (3) vertical, and (4) distoangular. They are further classified according to depth of third molar in bone by classes A, B, and C, and by the relationship of the impacted third molar with sinus approximation (SA) and no sinus approximation (NSA). (From Langland OE, Langlais RP, Morris CR: Principles and Practice of Panoramic Radiology. Philadelphia:WB Saunders, 1982, p. 196.)

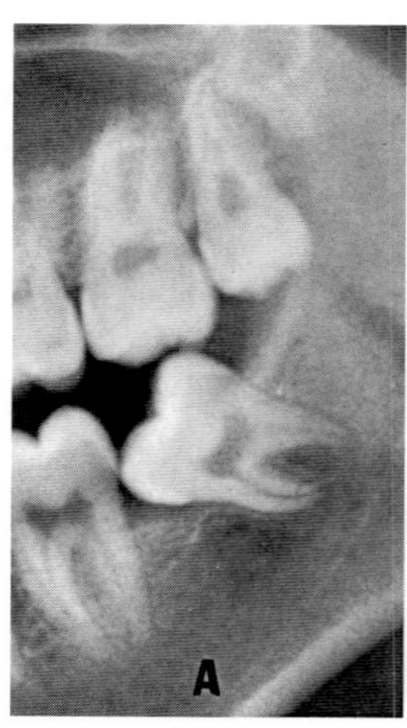

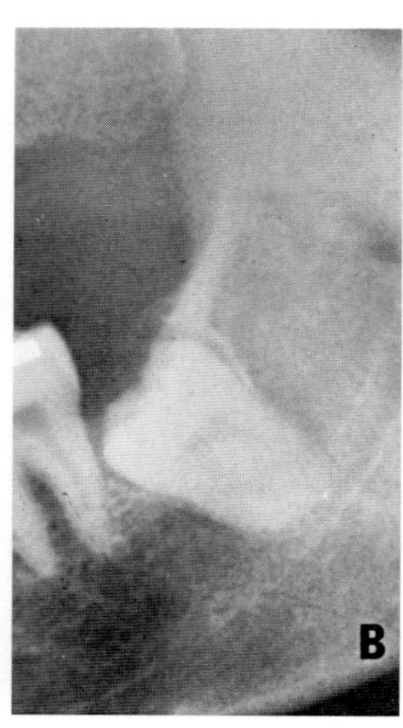

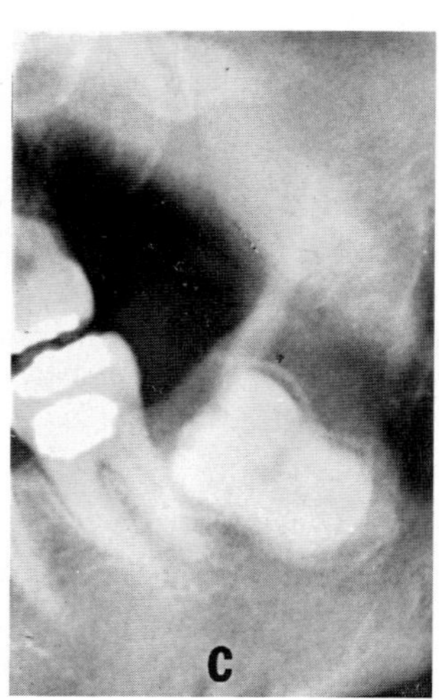

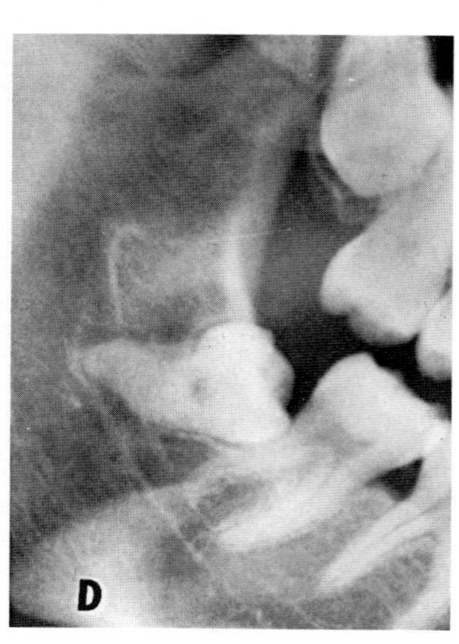

FIGURE 5–66.

Mesioangular Mandibular Third Molar Impactions. A, Class 1, position A classification of a mandibular impacted third molar. B, Class 1, position B classification. C, Class 1, position C classification. D, Class 2, position B classification with torsional deflection and possible encroachment of the root tip into the mandibular canal (note narrowing of the canal).

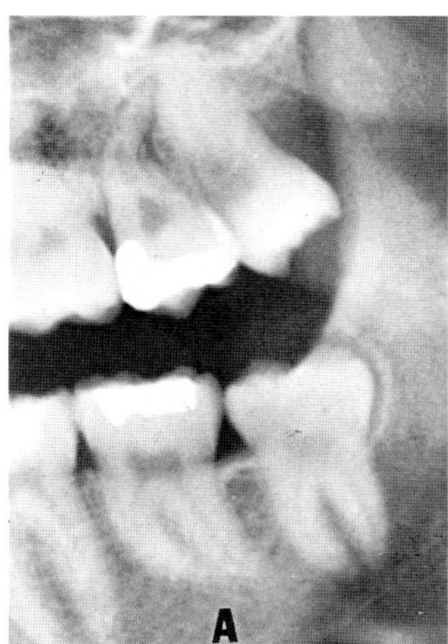

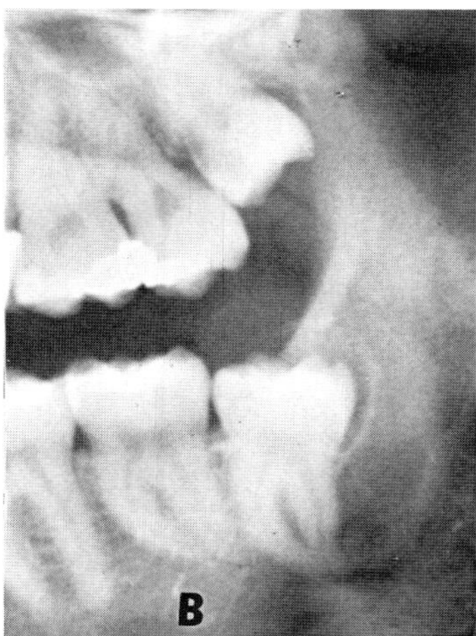

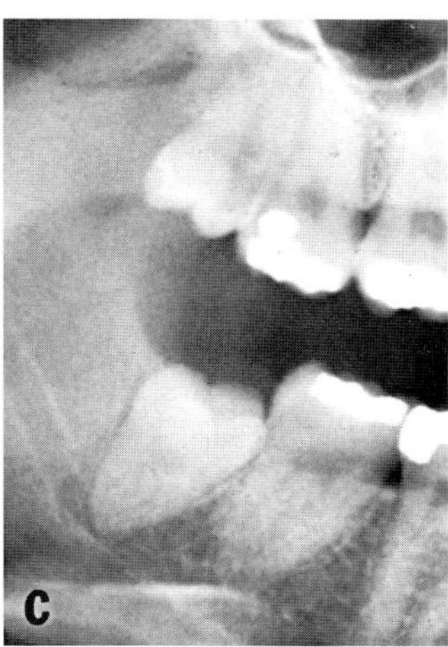

FIGURE 5–67.

Vertical Mandibular Third Molar Impactions. A, Class 2, position A. B, Class 2, position B. (The follicular sac is enlarged and could be a beginning follicular cyst.) C, Class 1, position B with torsional deflection.

evidence of delayed eruption. Barring the presence of obvious physical barriers, missing teeth, or systemic disorders such as hypopituitarism, delayed eruption may not be obvious in its early stages. Generally, if the tooth is behind its contralateral twin or if root formation has exceeded crown length, delayed eruption may exist. Delayed eruption is more obvious when the contralateral twin has erupted or when root formation and apex closure are complete. In the latter instance, the eruptive potential of the tooth is markedly reduced and may be the most important factor in distinguishing a normally erupting third molar from one that is impacted.

If the impacted tooth is a third molar, the impaction should be classified. Most classifications are based on the radiographic position of the tooth. Impacted teeth as seen on the panoramic film should sometimes be further examined with intraoral periapical views if buccal or lingual localization is necessary. In this instance, Clark's rule (1909) or the buccal-object rule of Richards (1952, 1953) may be used. Occlusal, right-angle, and maxillary crossfire views are also helpful.

Mandibular Impacted Third Molars

These impactions are classified based on the classification systems of Pell and Gregory (1942) and Winter (1926).

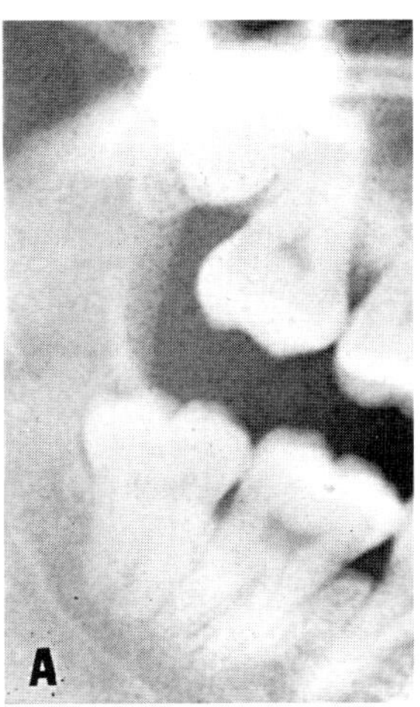

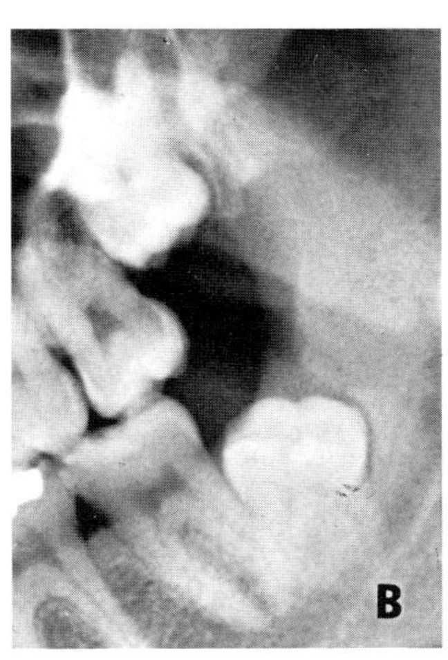

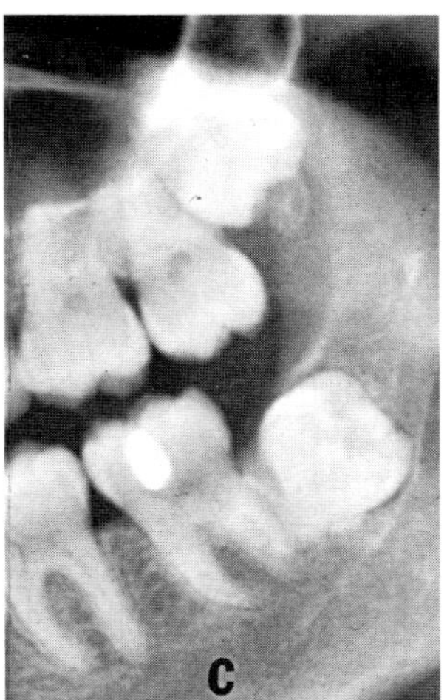

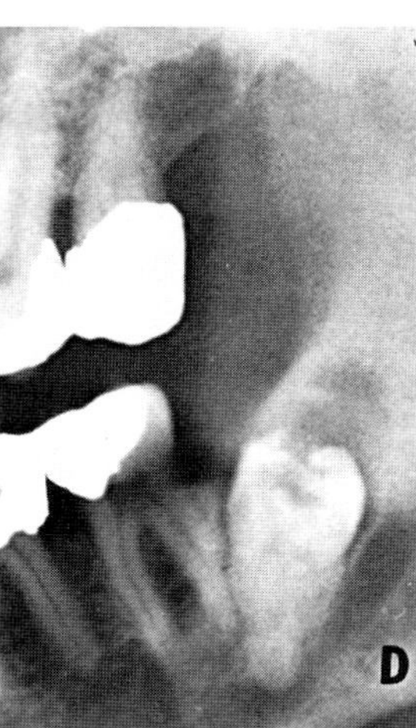

FIGURE 5–68.

Distoangular Mandibular Third Molar Impactions. A, Class 2, position A. B, Class 1, position B with torsional deflection; the patient had pericoronitis. C, Class 1, position B with buccal or lingual deflection; an occlusal radiograph is indicated to confirm deflection. D, Class 1, position C with torsional deflection; possible beginning of a dentigerous cyst.

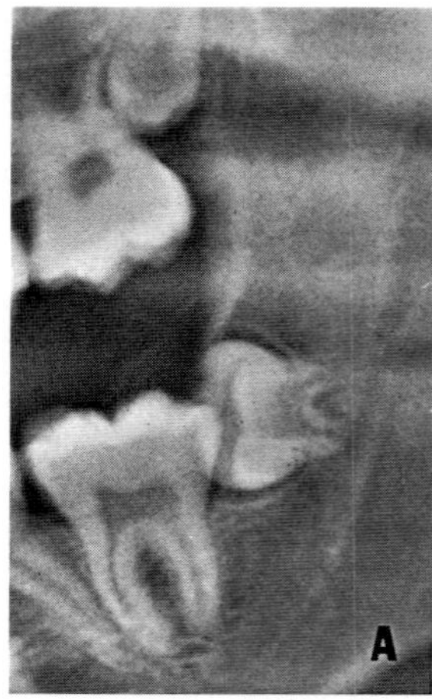

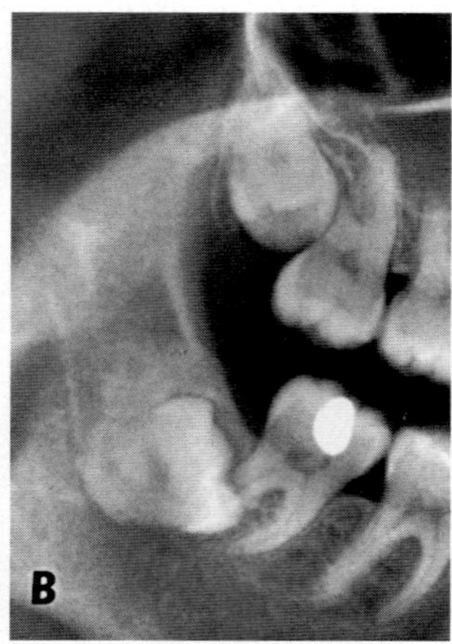

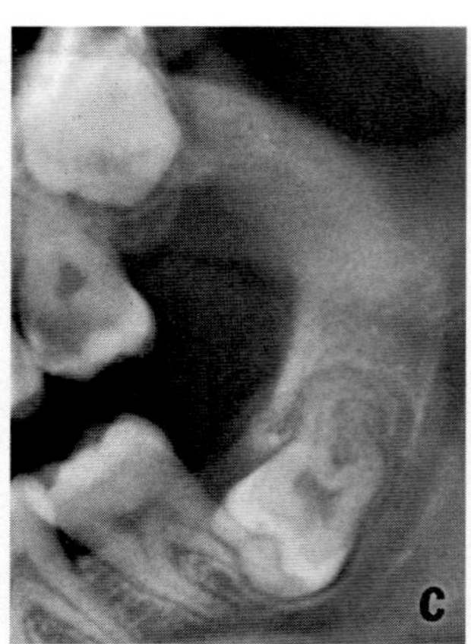

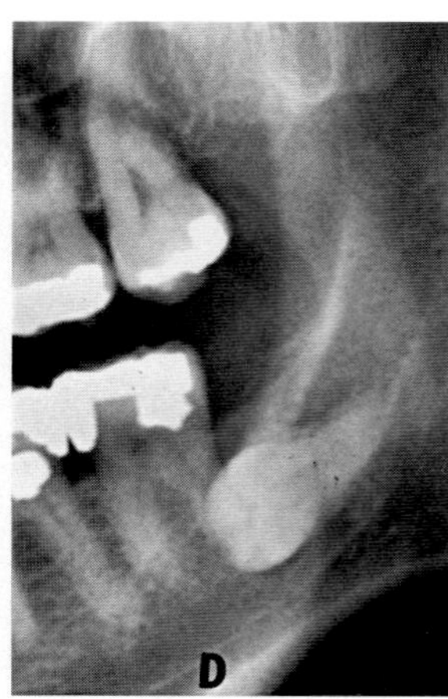

FIGURE 5–69.

Horizontal Mandibular Third Molar Impactions. A, Class 3, position A. B, Class 3, position C, buccal or lingual deflection. C, Class 1, position C, with buccal or lingual deflection and dilaceration; the patient has pericoronitis; maxillary third molar, mesioangular impaction, class C, buccal or lingual deflection, with sinus approximation. D, Class 1, position C, with buccal or lingual deflection.

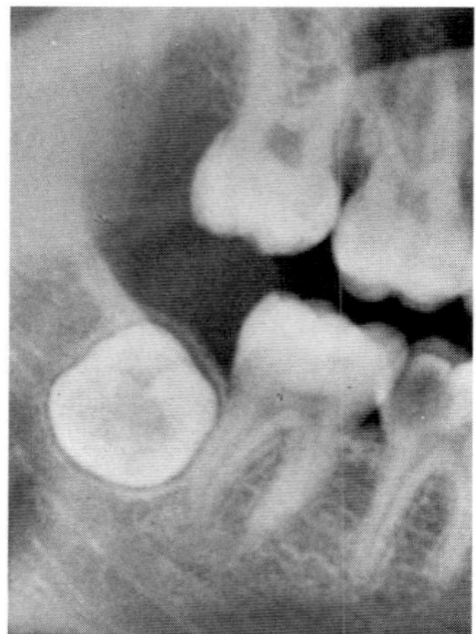

FIGURE 5–70.

Linguoangular Third Molar Impaction. Class 1, position C.

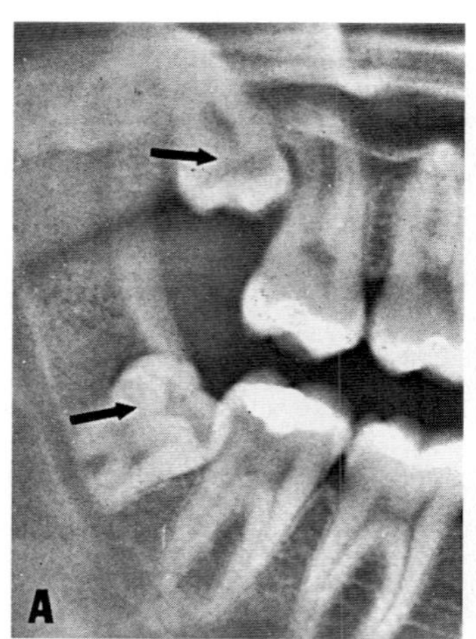

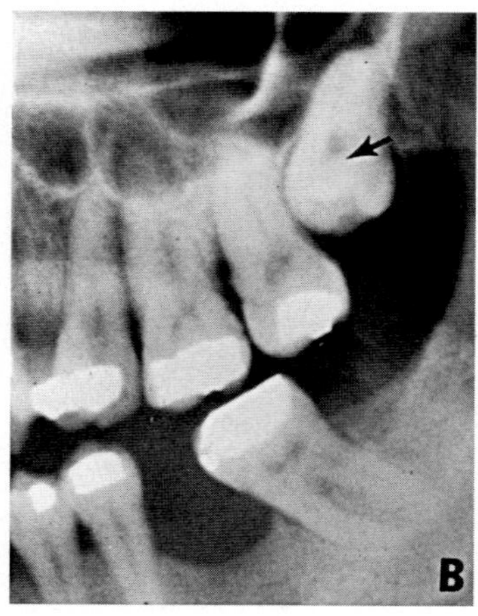

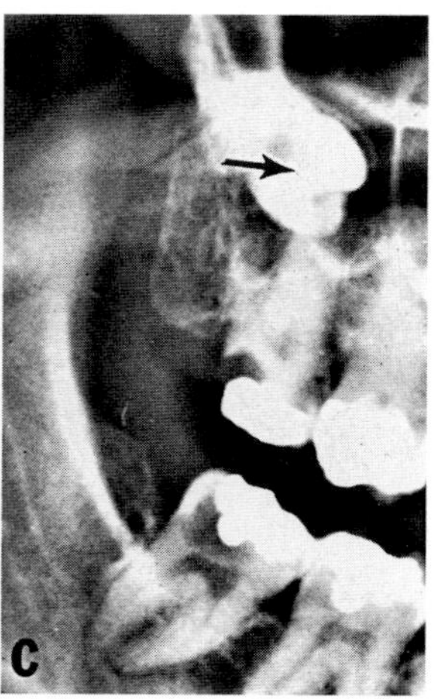

FIGURE 5–71.

Mesioangular Maxillary Third Molar Impactions. A, Mesioangular maxillary third molar impaction (arrow); class C, with sinus approximation; mesioangular impaction of a lower third molar (arrow), class 2, position B, buccal/lingual deflection. B, Class C, with sinus approximation, buccal or lingual deflection (arrow). C, Position C, with sinus approximation and buccal/lingual deflection (arrow).

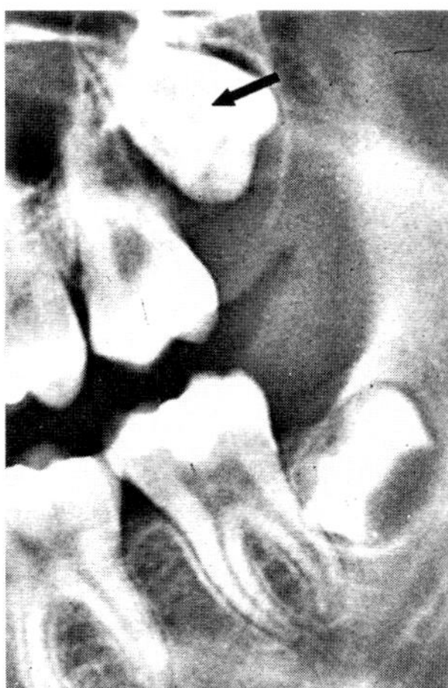

FIGURE 5–72.

Distoangular Maxillary Third Molar Impactions. Class C, with sinus approximation, buccal/lingual deflection.

Factor 1: Distance between Distal Aspect of Mandibular Second Molar and Ramus.

Class I. Space between distal aspect of second molar and ramus is equal to or larger than the mesiodistal diameter of the crown of the third molar.

Class II. Space between distal aspect of second molar and ramus is less than the mesiodistal diameter of the crown of the third molar.

Class III. All or most of the third molar is located within the ramus.

Factor 2: Depth of Mandibular Third Molar in Bone.

Position A. The most superior aspect of the third molar is level with or above the occlusal plane of the second molar.

Position B. The most superior aspect of the third molar is below the occlusal plane but above the cervical line of the second molar.

Position C. The most superior aspect of the third molar is below the cervical line of the second molar.

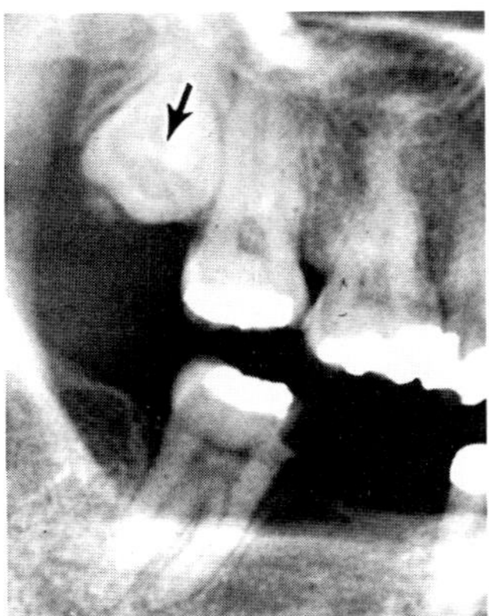

FIGURE 5–73.

Vertical Maxillary Third Molar Impactions Class C, with sinus approximation, buccal/lingual deflection.

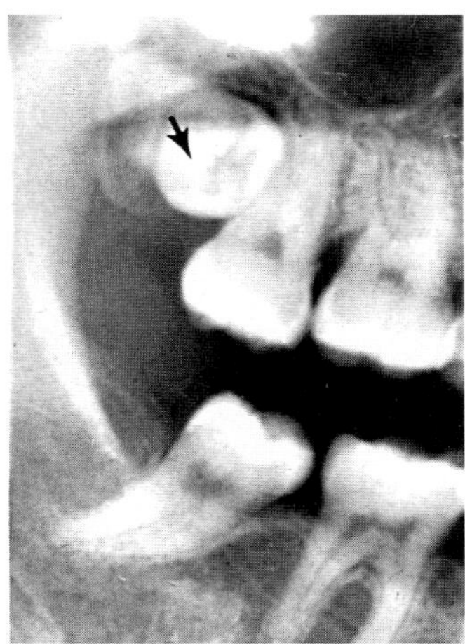

FIGURE 5–74.

Horizontal Maxillary Third Molar Impaction Class C, with no sinus approximation, torsional, and with buccal/lingual deflection (arrow).

Factor 3: Position of Long Axis of Mandibular Third Molar Relative to Long Axis of Mandibular Second Molar.

This can be vertical, horizontal, inverted, mesioangular, distoangular, buccoangular, or linguoangular. The mesioangular impaction is the most common type of impaction. The teeth may also be deflected buccally, deflected lingually, and torsioned (tooth has turned on its long axis).

Other Factors to Note Radiographically. Other considerations include dilaceration, bulbous roots, supernumerary roots, hypercementosis, ankylosis, internal and external resorption, relationship with the mandibular canal, and the presence of associated lesions or cysts.

Maxillary Impacted Third Molars

Maxillary impacted third molars are classified in the following manner, based on the classification of Archer (1956).

Factor 1: Depth of Maxillary Third Molar in Bone.

Class A. The most inferior aspect of the crown is on the level with or below the occlusal plane of the second molar.

Class B. The most inferior aspect of the crown is between the occlusal plane and the cervical line of the second molar.

Class C. The most inferior aspect of the crown is at or above the cervical line of the second molar.

Factor 2: Position of Long Axis of Maxillary Third Molar Relative to Long Axis of Maxillary Second Molar.

This position can be vertical, horizontal, mesioangular, distoangular, inverted, buccoangular, or linguoangular. The teeth may also be deflected buccally, deflected lingually, and torsioned.

Factor 3: Relationship of Maxillary Third Molar with Maxillary Sinus.

Sinus approximation (SA). Thin bone or no bone is present between the third molar and the maxillary sinus.

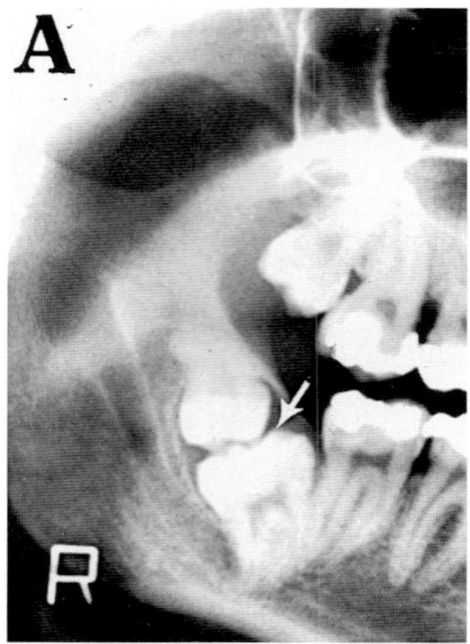

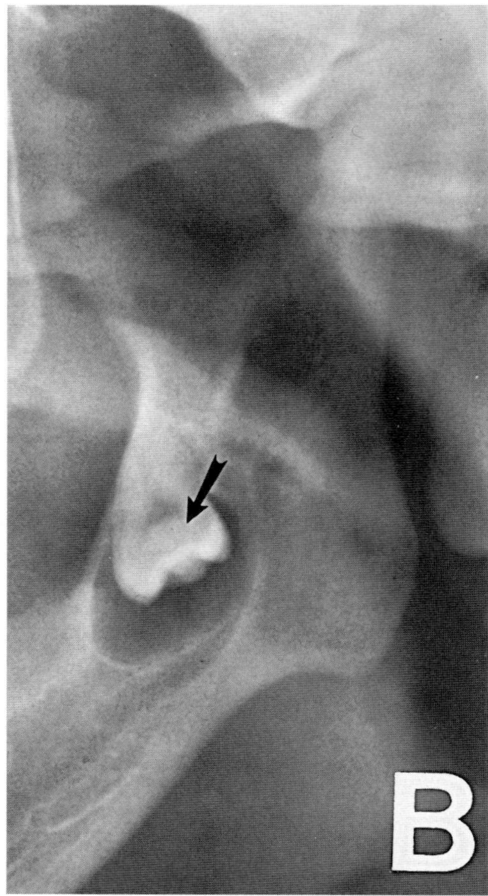

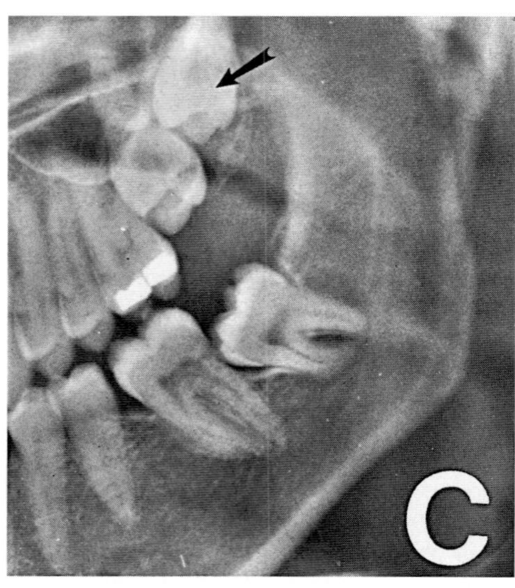

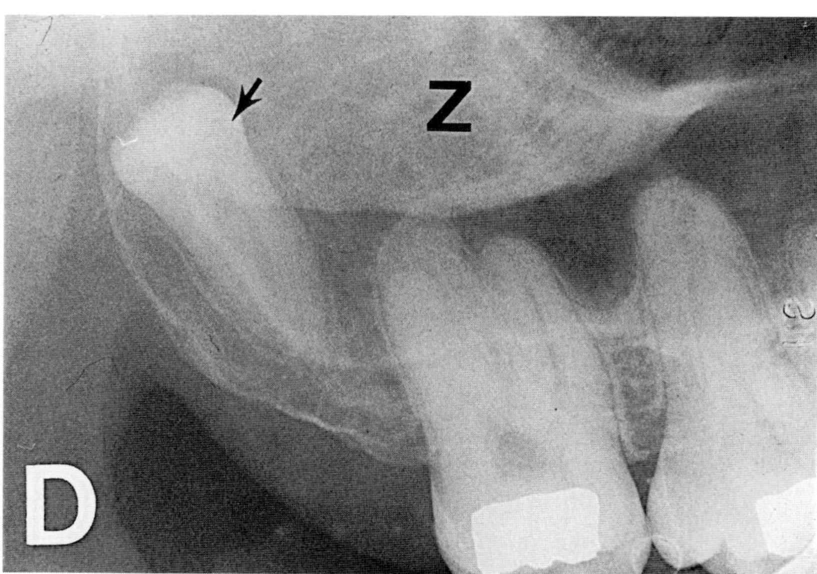

FIGURE 5–75.

Rare Impactions. A, Double impacted mandibular third molars with occlusal surfaces facing each other in so-called kissing position (arrow) and therefore called "kissing molars." B, Inverted mandibular third molar compatible with the radiographic appearance of a follicular (dentigerous) cyst (coronal type; arrow). C, Impacted maxillary second and third molars; (arrow), and mesioangular impacted mandibular third molar (class 1, position A). D, Inverted impacted maxillary third molar (arrow). Z represents the zygomatic or malar bone.

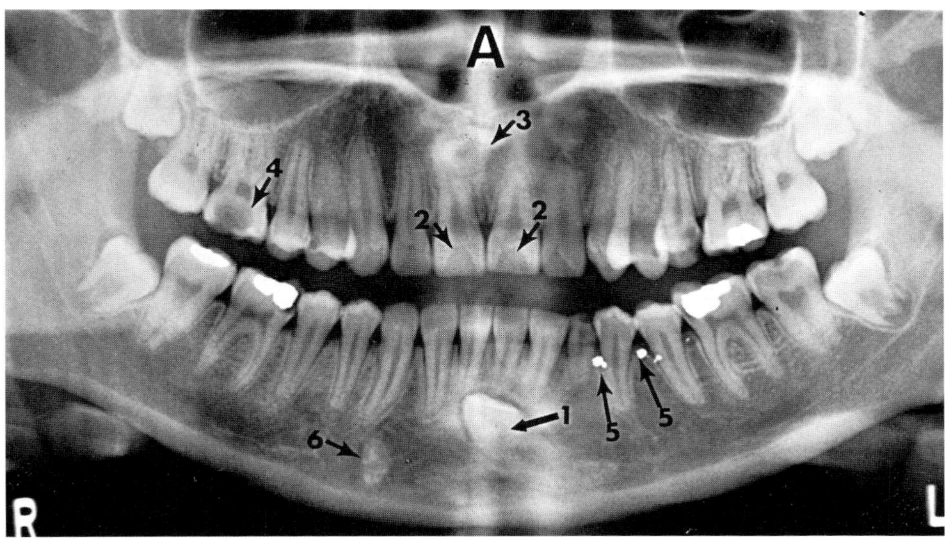

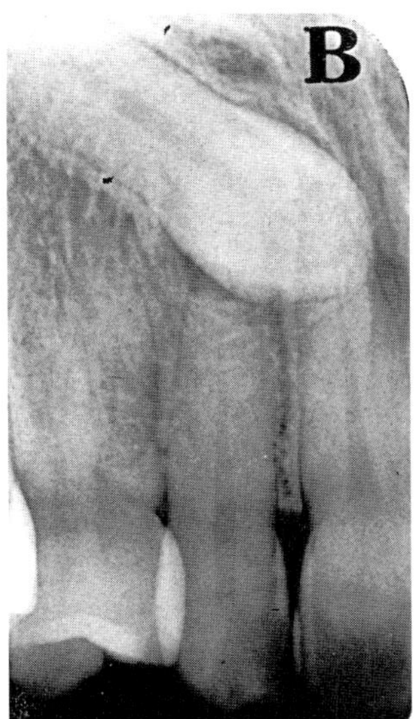

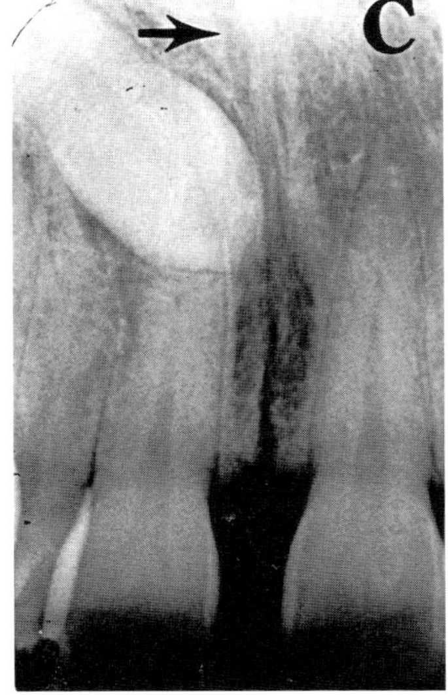

FIGURE 5–76.

Canine Impactions A, Drifting mandibular canine tooth with a retained primary canine tooth (1), shovel-toothed maxillary incisors (2), and a large carious lesion in the maxillary right first molar (4). There is possibly a mesiodens, which has a distorted image in the midline (3). One also sees amalgam debris (5) and osteosclerosis (6). B, Right maxillary canine impaction. C, By Clark's rule, the canine tooth in B is on the lingual surface because the canine tooth moved in the direction of movement of the tube (arrow) in C. (SLOB rule: Same (on) Lingual, Opposite (on) Buccal).

No sinus approximation (NSA). One sees 2 mm or more of bone between the third molars and the maxillary sinus.

Other Factors to Note Radiographically. Other considerations include dilaceration, bulbous roots, supernumerary roots, hypercementosis, ankylosis, external resorption, fusion or concrescence with the roots of the maxillary second molar, and the presence of associated lesions or cysts.

The radiographic description of any impacted or embedded tooth should include its position relative to adjacent teeth, its relationship with other anatomic structures, alterations in morphology, and the presence of other pathologic conditions. Some conditions that tend to be associated with impacted teeth include Pindborg tumor, odontomas, squamous odontogenic tumor, adenomatoid odontogenic tumor, follicular (dentigerous) cyst and its sequelae (such as ameloblastoma, squamous cell carcinoma, and mucoepidermoid carcinoma), odontogenic keratocyst, and Gorlin cyst.

References

Hypodontia

Bloch B: Eigentumliche bisher nicht beschriebene Pigmentaffekton (Incontinentia pigmenti). Schweiz Med Wochenschr 56:405, 1926.

Böök JA: Clinical and genetical studies of hypodontia: premolar agenesis, hyperhidrosis and canities premature; a new hereditary syndrome in man. Am J Hum Genet 2:240, 1950.

Dolder E: Zahn-Unterzahl. Schweiz Monatsschr Zahnheilk 46:665, 1936.

Ellis RWB, Van Creveld S: A syndrome characterized by ectodermal dysplasia, polydactyly chondrodysplasia, and congenitial morbis cordis: report of 3 cases. Arch Dis Child, 15:65, 1940.

Freire-Maia N: Ectodermal dysplasia. Hum Hered 21:309, 1971.

Gorlin RJ, Pindborg JJ, Cohen MM: Syndromes of the Head and Neck. New York:McGraw-Hill, 1976.

Grahnen H: Hypodontia in the permanent dentition. Odontol Revy 7 (Suppl 3):1, 1956.

Grahnen H, Granath LE: Numerical variations in primary dentition and their correlation with the permanent dentition. Odontol Revy 12:348, 1961.

Grahnen H, Hansson L: The prognosis of pulp and root canal therapy. Odontol Revy 12:146, 1961.
Gruneberg H: Two independent inherited tooth anomalies in one family. J Hered 27:255, 1936.
Jorgenson RJ: Clinician's view of hypodontia. J Am Dent Assoc 101:285, 1980.
Jorgenson RJ, et al: The Rieger syndrome. Am J Med Genet 2:307, 1978.
Kurtz MB, Brownstein MP: Familial absence of lower central incisors and dyslexia. Birth Defects 10:316, 1974.
McKusick VAP: Mendelian inheritance in man. Baltimore:Johns Hopkins University Press, 1978.
Niswander JD, Sujaku C: Congenital anomalies of teeth in Japanese children. J Phys Anthropol 21:569, 1963.
Rose JS: A survey of congenitally missing teeth, excluding third molars in 6,000 orthodontic patients. Dent Pract (Bristol) 17:107, 1967.
Sulzberger MB: Veber eine bisher nicht beschriebene congenitale Pigmentanomalie (Incontinentia pigmenti). Arch Dermatol Syphilol 154:19, 1928.
Volk A: Uberdie Haufegheit des Vorbomnens von fehlenden Zabnanlagen. Arch Monatsschr Zabubeilk 73:320, 1963.
Werther R, Rothenberg F: Anodontia. Am J Orthod 25:61, 1939.
Witkop CJ Jr, Brearley LJ, Gentry WC Jr: Hypoplastic enamel, onycholysis, and hypohidrosis inherited as an autosomal dominant trait: a review of ectodermal dysplasia syndromes. Oral Surg 39:71, 1975.
Woolf CM: Missing maxillary lateral incisors: a genetic study. Am J Hum Genet 23:289, 1971.

Hyperdontia

Bhaskar SN: Synopsis of Oral Pathology. St. Louis:CV Mosby, 1961, p. 117.
Billberg B, Lind V: Medfodda antalsvariationer i permanenta dentitionen: B Den overtaliga tanden i overkakens mittparti, mesiodens. Odontol Revy 16:258, 1965.
Brook AH: Dental anomalies on number, form and size: their prevalence in British school children. J Int Assoc Dent Child 5:37, 1974.
Brook AH, Ekanayake NO: The etiology of oligiodontia: a familial history. J Dent Child 48:32, 1980.
Dixon GH, Stewart RE: Genetic aspects of anomalous tooth development. In: Oral Facial Genetics (Stewart RE, Prescott GH, eds). St. Louis: CV Mosby, 1976, p. 139.
Egermack-Eriksson I, Lind V: Congenital numerical variation in the permanent dentition. D. Sex distribution of hypodontia and hyperdontia. Odontol Revy 22:309, 1971.
Gardiner JH: Supernumerary teeth. Dent Pract Dent Rec 12:65, 1961.
Grahnen H, Granath LE: Numerical variations in primary dentition and their correlation with the permanent dentition. Odontol Revy 12:348, 1961.
Hammond-Williams C: Supernumerary tooth heredity. Br Dent J 56:500, 1934.
Hitchin AD, Fairley JM: Dental management in cleidocranial dysostosis. Br J Oral Surg 12:46, 1974.
Kronfeld R: Histopathology of the Teeth. 2nd Ed. Philadelphia:Lea & Febiger, 1939, p. 24.
Lacoste L, Hirsch C, Frank R: Les inclusions dentaires surnumeraires chez l'enfant. Rev Fr Odonto-stomat 9:l967, 1962.
Lind V: Medfodda antalsvariationer i permenta dentitionen. Odontol Revy 10:176, 1959.
Magnusson B: Tandövertal: den temporära dentitionen. Svensk Tandlak T 52:357, 1959.
Millhon JA, Stafne EC: Incidence of supernumerary and congenitally missing lateral incisor teeth in 81 cases of harelip and cleft palate. Am J Orthod 27:59, 1941.
Niswander JD, Sujaku C: Congenital anomalies of teeth in Japanese children. Am J Phys Anthropol 21:569, 1963.
Nordenram A: Fourth and fifth molar in ramus mandibulae: case report. Odontol T 76:25, 1968.
Parry RR, Lyer VS: Supernumerary teeth amongst orthodontic patients in India. Br Dent J 11:257, 1961.
Pindborg JJ: Pathology of the Dental Hard Tissues. Philadelphia:WB Saunders, 1970, p. 27.
Primosch R: Anterior supernumerary teeth: assessment and surgical intervention in children. Pediatr Dent 3:205, 1981.
Ravin JJ: Aplasia, supernumerary teeth and fused teeth in the primary dentition: an epidemiologic study. Scand J Dent Res 879:1, 1971.
Rosenzweig K, Gabarski D: Numerical aberrations in the permanent teeth of grade school children in Jerusalem. Am J Phys Anthropol 23:277, 1965.
Rushton MA: The failure of eruption in cleidocranial dysostosis. Br Dent J 63:641, 1937.
Sarto T: A genetic study on the degenerative anomalies of deciduous teeth. Jpn J Hum Gen 4:27, 1959.
Sedano HO, Gorlin RJ: Familial occurrence of mesiodens. Oral Surg 27: 360, 1969.
Stafne EC: Supernumerary teeth. Dent Cosmos 72:655, 1932.
Winter GR: Dental conditions in cleidocranial dysostosis. Am J Orthod 29: 61, 1943.
Worth HM: Principles and Practice of Oral Radiologic Interpretation. Chicago:Year Book, 1963, p. 101.

Microdontia And Macrodontia

Andro S, et al: Studies of the consecutive survey of succedaneous and permanent dentition in the Japanese children. Part 4. Behavior of short-rooted teeth in the upper bilateral central incisors. J Nihon Univ Sch Dent 9:67, 1967.
Buenviaje TM, Rapp R: Dental anomalies in children: a clinical and radiographic survey. J Dent Child 51:42, 1984.
Garn SM, Lewis AB, Kerewsky RS: Sexual dimorphism in the buccolingual tooth diameter. J Dent Res 45:1819, 1966.
LeBot PL, Salmon D: Congenital defects of the upper teeth, measurements of the superior arch, head and face. Am J Phys Antropol 46:231, 1979.
Pedersen PO: Taendernes tilstand hos 2–6 arige born. Tandlagebladet 46: 485, 1944.

Gemination

Buenviaje TM, Rapp R: Dental anomalies in children: a clinical and radiographic survey. J Dent Child 51:42, 1984.
Clayton JM: Congenital dental anomalies occurring in 3,557 children. J Dent Child 23:206, 1956.
Colyer JR: Abnormally-shaped teeth from the region of the premaxilla. Proc R Soc Med (Sect Odontol) 19:39, 1926.
de Jong TE: Geminate tooth formation. Abstr Dent Alistr 2:41, 1957.
Heslop IH: True gemination in posterior teeth. Br Dent J 97:95, 1954.
Levitas TC: Gemination, fusion and concrescence. J Dent Child 33:95, 1965.
Menczer LF: Anomalies of the primary dentition. J Dent Child 22:57, 1955.
Tannenbaum KA, Alling EE: Anomalous tooth development: case reports of gemination and twinning. Oral Surg 18:885, 1963.

Fusion

Buenviaje TM, Rapp R: Dental anomalies in children: a clinical and radiographic survey. J Dent Child 51:42, 1984.
Clayton JM: Congenital dental anomalies occurring in 3,557 children. J Dent Child 23:206, 1956.
Grahnen H, Granath LE: Numerical variations in primary dentition and their correlation with the permanent dentition. Odontol Revy 12:348, 1961.
Gysel C: Diagnose en frequentie der van de eerste molar. Ned Tijschr Tandheelkd 72:597, 1965.
Niswander JO, Sujaku C: Congenital anomalies of teeth in Japanese children. Am J Phys Anthropol 21:569, 1963.
Toth A, Csemi L: Zwillingszahne im Milchgebiss. Dtsch Zahnarztl Z 22: 546, 1967.

Concrescence

Pindborg JJ: Pathology of the Dental Hard Tissues. Philadelphia:WB Saunders, 1970, p. 48.

Dilaceration

Chohayeb AA: Dilaceration of permanent upper lateral incisors: frequency, direction, and endodontic treatment implications. Oral Surg 55:519, 1983.
Grahnen H, Hansson L: The prognosis of pulp and root canal therapy. Odontol Revy 12:146, 1961.
Sommer RF, Ostrander FD, Crowley MC: Clinical Endodontics. Philadelphia:WB Saunders, 1966, p. 23.
Weine, Franklin S: Endodontic Therapy, 4th ed. St. Louis:CV Mosby, 1989, p. 314.

Wheeler RC: Textbook of Dental Anatomy and Physiology. 4th Ed. Philadelphia:WB Saunders, 1965, p 133.

Supernumerary Roots

Ferenczy K: Röntgenologische Untersuchungen über die Variationen und Anomalien der untern Pramolärenwurzeln. Dtsch Zahmartzl Z 17:623, 1962
Harboro G: The two-rooted canine. Br Dent J 56:244, 1934.
Pedersen PO: The East Greenland Eskimo Dentition. (Meddelelsen om Gronland. Vol. 42.) Copenhagen, 1949.
Pindborg JJ: Pathology of the Dental Hard Tissues. Philadelphia:WB Saunders, 1970, p. 42.
Turner CG: Three rooted mandibular first permanent molars and the question of American Indians' origins. Am J Phys Anthropol 334:229, 1971.
Walker RT, Quackenbush LE: Three-rooted lower first permanent molars in Hong Kong Chinese. Br Dent J 159:298, 1985.

Supernumerary Cusps

Dahlberg AA: The dentition of the American Indian. In: The Physical Anthropology of the American Indian. New York:Viking, 1951, p. 138.
Gardner DG, Girgis SS: Talon cusps: a dental anomaly in the Rubinstein-Taybi syndrome. Oral Surg 47:519, 1979.
Mader CL: Talon cusp. J Am Dent Assoc 98:62, 1979.
Mellor JK, Ripa LW: Talon cusp: a clinically significant anomaly. Oral Surg 29:225, 1970.
Pindborg JJ: Pathology of the Dental Hard Tissues. Philadelphia:WB Saunders, 1970, p. 42.
Rubinstein JH, Taybi H: Broad thumbs and toes and facial abnormalities: a possible mental retardation syndrome. Am J Dis Child 105:588, 1963.

Taurodontism

Bernick SM: Taurodontia. Oral Surg 29:549, 1970.
Brabant H, Kovacs I: Racine pyramidal et molaire taurodonte; leur interet pour le practicien. Acta Stomatol Belg 57:311, 1960.
Bruszt P: Oszlopos grokeru also kisorlofog. Fogorv Sz 46:55, 1953.
Congelton JE, Burkes EJ: Amelogenesis imperfecta with taurodontism. Oral Surg 48:540, 1979.
Crawford JI: Concomitant taurodontism and amelogenesis imperfecta in the American Caucasian. ASDC J Dent Child 37:85, 1970.
Daito M, Hieda T: Taurodont teeth in primary dentition. Jpn J Pedod 9: 95, 1971.
Ferenczy K: Rontgenologische Untevsuchungen uber die dtsch. Zahnarztl Z 17:65, 1962.
Fuks AB, et al: Multiple taurodontism associated with osteoporosis. J Pedod 7:68, 1982.
Garcia-Godoy F, Armach FJ: Taurodontismo en denticion temporal y permanente: reporte de casos. Rev Dent (Sant Domingo) 20:48, 1977.
Gardner DG, Girgis SS: Taurodontism, shovel-shaped incisors and the Klinefelter syndrome. J Can Dent Assoc 8:372, 1978.
Goldstein E, Medina JL: Mohr syndrome of oral facial-digital II: report of two cases. J Am Dent Assoc 89:377, 1974.
Hamner JE III, Witkop CJ Jr, Metro PS: Taurodontism: report of a case. Oral Surg 18:409, 1964.
Jaspers MT: Taurodontism in the Down's syndrome. Oral Surg 51:532, 1981.
Jaspers MT, Witkop CJ Jr: Taurodontism, an isolated trait associated with syndromes and X-chromosomal aneuploidy. Am J Hum Genet 32:396, 1980.
Jorgenson RJ, Warson RW: Dental abnormalities in the tricho-dento-osseous syndrome. Oral Surg 36:693, 1973.
Jorgenson RJ, Salinas CF, Shapiro SD: The prevalence of taurdontism in a select population. J Craniofac Genet Div Biol 2:125, 1982.
Kallay J: Some anomalies of the lower premolar roots of homoprimigenius from Krapina in Croatia. Folia Stomatol (Zagreb) 10:25, 1949.
Kallay J: A radiographic study of the Neanderthal teeth from Krapina, Croatia. In: Brothwell DR, ed. Dental Anthropology. Vol. 5. New York: Pergamon Press, 1963, p. 75.
Keeler C: Taurodont molars and shovel incisors in Klinfelter's syndrome. J Hered 64:235, 1973.
Keith A: Problems relating to the earliest forms of prehistoric man. Proc R Soc Med 6:105, 1913.
Levin LS, Jorgenson RJ, Cook RA: Otodental dysplasia: a ''new'' ectodermal dysplasia. Clin Genet 8:136, 1975.
Lichtenstein JR, et al: The tricho-dento-osseous syndrome. Am J Hum Genet 24:569, 1972.
Madeira MC, Leite HF, Filho WDN, Simors S: Prevalence of taurodontism in premolars. Oral Surg 61:158, 1986.
Mangion JJ: Two cases of taurodontism in modern human jaws. Br Dent J 115, 1962.
Mednick GA: Two case reports: taurodontism in Klinefelter's syndrome. J Mich State Dent Assoc 55:212, 1973.
Parker JL, Regattieri LR, Thomas JP: Hypoplastic hypomaturation amelogenesis imperfecta with taurodontism: report of a case. ASCD J Dent Child 42:379, 1975.
Pickerill HP: Radicular aberrations, bilateral radicular dentomata. Proc R Soc Med (Sect Odontol) 2:150, 1909.
Shifman A, Chanannel I: Prevalence of taurodontism found in radiographic dental examination of 1,200 young adult Israeli patients. Commun Dent Oral Epidemiol 6:200, 1978.
Stenvik A, Zachrisson BU, Svatun B: Taurodontism and concomitant hypodontia in siblings. Oral Surg 33:841, 1972.
Stewart RE: Taurodontism in X-chromosome aneuploid syndromes. Clin Genet 6:341, 1974.
Winter GB, Lee KW, Johnson NW: Hereditary amelogenesis imperfecta. Br Dent J 127:157, 1969.
Witkop CJ Jr: Clinical aspects of dental anomalies. Int Dent J 26:378, 1976.

Enamel Pearls

Cavanha AO: Enamel pearls. Oral Surg 19:373, 1965.
Pedersen PO: The East Greenland Eskimo Dentition. (Meddelelsen om Gronland. Vol. 42.) Copenhagen, 1949.
Turner JG: A note on enamel nodules. Br Dent J 78:39, 1945.
Worth HM: Principles and Practice of Oral Radiologic Interpretation. Chicago:Year Book, 1963, p. 425.

Dens Invaginatus

Bhatt AP, Dholakia HM: Radicular variety of double dens invaginatus. Oral Surg 39:284, 1975.
Hallet GEM: The incidence, nature, and clinical significance of palatal invaginations in the maxillary incisor teeth. Proc Soc Med 46:15, 1953.
Lee KW, Lee EC, Poon, KY: Palato-gingival grooves in maxillary incisors: a possible predisposing factor to localized periodontal disease. Br Dent J 124:15, 1968.
Lucas RB: Pathology of Tumors of Oral Tissues. Baltimore:Williams & Wilkins, 1972, p. 85.
Morgan GA, Poyton HG: Bilateral dens in dente. Oral Surg 12:65, 1960.
Oehlers FAC: Dens invaginatus (dilated composite odontome). I. Variations of the invagination process, associated anterior crown forms. Oral Surg 10:1205, 1957.
Oehlers FAC, Lee KW, Lee EC: Dens invaginatus. II. A microradiographical, histological, micro x-ray diffraction study. Acta Odontol Scand 18:305, 1960.
Pindborg JJ: Pathology of the Dental Hard Tissues. Philadelphia:WB Saunders, 1970, p. 58.
Swanson WF, McCarthy FM: Bilateral dens in dente. J Dent Res 26:162, 1947.
Tomes JA: A System of Dental Surgery. London:Lindsey and Blackston, 1859, P 266.

Dens Evaginatus

Curzon MEJ, Curzon JA, Poyton HG: Evaginated odontomes in the Keewatin Eskimo. Br Dent J 129:325, 1970.
Ekman-Westborg B, Julin P: Multiple anomalies in dental morphology: macrodontia, multituberculation, central cusps, and pulp invaginations. Oral Surg 38:217, 1974.
Geist JR: Dens evaginatus: a case report a review of literature. Oral Surg 67:628, 1989.
Joyojima T: Occlusal anomalous tubercle on premolars. Nihon Shikai 109: 257, 1929.
Kato K: Contribution to the knowledge concerning the cone shaped supernumerary cusp in the center of the occlusal surface on premolars in Japanese. Nihon Kagakudai Zassi 30:412, 1937.
Lau TC: Odontomes of the axial core type. Br Dent J 99:219, 1955.
Merrill RG: Occlusal anomalous tubercles on premolars of Alaskan Eskimos and Indians. Oral Surg 17:485, 1964.
Oehlers FAC: The tuberculated premolar. Dent Pract Dent Rec 6:145, 1956.
Oehlers FAC, Lee KW, Lee EC: Dens evaginatus (evaginated odontome):

its structure and responses to external stimuli. Dent Pract Dent Rec 17: 239, 1967.

Palmer ME: Case reports of evaginated odontomes in Caucasians. Oral Surg 35:772, 1973.

Pedersen PO: The East Greenland Eskimo Dentition. (Meddelelsen om Gronland. Vol. 42.) Copenhagen, 1949.

Senia ES, Regezi JA: Dens evaginatus in the etiology of bilateral periapical pathologic involvement in caries-free premolars. Oral Surg 38:465, 1974.

Sykaris SN: Occusal anomalous tubercle on premolars of a Greek girl. Oral Surg 38:88, 1974.

Trautman EK: An unrecorded from of the simplest type of the dilated composite odontome. Br Dent J 86:271, 1949.

Wu KL: Survey of mid-occlusal tubercle in bicuspids. China Stomat 3:294, 1955.

Yip WK: The prevalence of dens evaginatus. Oral Surg 38:80, 1974.

Yong SL: Prophylactic treatment of dens evaginatus. J Dent Child 41:289, 1974.

Yoshioka T, Urano, J: The prevalence of abnormal enamel-covered tubercle. Shikagakuho 63:476, 1963.

Yumikura S, Yoshioa K: Abnormal cusp on the occlusal surface of the human premolars. J Jpn Stomat Soc 10:73, 1936.

Enamel Hypoplasia

Bauer W: Effect of periapical processes of deciduous teeth on the buds of permanent teeth. Am J Orthod Oral Surg, 32:232, 1946.

Black GV, McKay FS: Mottled teeth: an endemic developmental imperfection of the enamel of teeth heretofore unknown in the literature of dentistry. Dent Cosmos 58:129, 1916.

Dean HT, et al: Domestic water and dental caries: a study of 2,832 white children, aged 12–14 years, of 8 suburban Chicago communities, including Lactobacillus acidophilus studies of 1,761 children. Public Health Rep 56:761, 1941.

Dean HT, et al: Domestic water and dental caries: additional studies of the relation of fluoride domestic waters to dental caries experiences in 4, 425 white children, aged 12 to 14 years of 13 cities in 4 states. Public Health Rep 57:1155, 1942.

Fiumara NJ, Lessell S: Manifestations of late congenital syphilis. Arch Dermatol 102:78, 1970.

Fournier A: Syphilitic teeth. Dental Cosmos 26:12, 81, 141, 1884.

Gorlin RJ, Meskin: Severe irradiation during odontogenesis: report of a case. Oral Surg 16:35 1963.

Hakala PE, Makela P: Tetracyclines and prematures. Suom Hammaslaak Toim 59:285, 1963.

Hals E, Orlow M: Turner teeth. Odontol T 66:199, 1958.

Hutchinson J: Report of effects of infantile syphilis in marring development of teeth. Trans Pathol Soc (Lond) 9:449, 1858.

Moller I: Dental fluorose og caries. Rhodos Kobenhavn, 1965.

Morningstar CH: Effects of infection of the deciduous molar on the permanent tooth germ. J Am Dent Assoc 24:786, 1937.

Pedersen PO: The East Greenland Eskimo Dentition. (Meddelelsen om Gronland. Vol. 42.) Copenhagen, 1949.

Pindborg JJ: Pathology of the Dental Hard Tissues. Philadelphia:WB Saunders, 1970, p. 88.

Putkonen P: Dental changes in congenital syphilis. Acta Derm Venereol (Stockh) 42:45, 1962.

Sarnat BG, Schour I: Enamel hypoplasia. J Am Dent Assoc 18:1989, 1941, and 29:67, 1942.

Sarnat BG, Shaw NG: Dental development in congenital syphilis. Am J Dis Child 64:771, 1942.

Shafer WG, Hine MK, Levy BM: A Textbook of Oral Pathology. 4th Ed. Philadelphia:WB Saunders, 1983, p. 55.

Shelling DH, Anderson GM: Relation of rickets and vitamin D to the incidence of dental caries: enamel hypoplasia and malocclusion in children. J Am Dent Assoc 23:840, 1936.

Smith MC, Lanz E.M, Smith HV: Cause of mottled enamel, a defect of human teeth. University of Arizona Agriculture Experimental Station, Technical Bulletin No. 32, 1931, p. 253.

Spouge ID: Oral Pathology. St. Louis:CV Mosby, 1973, p 162.

Stein G: Schmelzschaden and Milehgebiss and ihre klinische bedeutung. Z Stomatol 34:843, 1936.

Turner JG: Two cases of hypoplasia of enamel. Br J Dent Sci 55:227, 1912.

Worth HM: Principles and Practice of Oral Radiologic Interpretation. Chicago:Year Book, 1963, p. 425.

Zsigmondy O: Beitrage zur kenntuis der entstehungsursache der hypoplastischen emaildefecte (congenital defects of enamel). In: Transactions of the World's Columbian Dental Congress. Vol. I. Chicago, 1894, p. 48.

Amelogenesis Imperfecta

Jorgenson RL, Yost C: Etiology of enamel dysplasias. Pedodontics 4:325, 1982.

Weinmann JP, Svobuda JF, Woods RW: Hereditary disturbances of enamel formation and calcification. J Am Dent Assoc 32:397, 1945.

Witkop CJ Jr: Genetics in dentistry. Eugen Q 5:15, 1958.

Witkop CJ Jr, Sauk JJ Jr: Heritable defects of enamel. In: Stewart RE, Prescott GH (Eds): Oral Facial Genetics. St. Louis:CV Mosby Co, 1976.

Dentinogenesis Imperfecta

Bixler D, Conneally PM, Christen AG: Dentinogenesis imperfecta genetic variations in a six-generation family. J Dent Res 48:1196, 1969.

Epstein JS: Osteogenesis imperfecta and dentinogenesis imperfecta: report of a case. J Balt Coll Dent Surg 28:81, 1973.

Finn SB: Hereditary opalescent dentin. I. An analysis of literature of hereditary anomalies of tooth color. J Am Dent Assoc 25:1240, 1938.

Gorlin RJ, Pindborg JJ: Syndromes of the Head and Neck. New York: McGraw-Hill, 1964, p. 195.

Hodge H, et al: Hereditary opalescent dentin. II. General and oral clinical studies. J Am Dent Assoc 26:1663, 1939.

Hodge H, et al: Hereditary opalescent dentin. III Histological, chemical and physical studies. J Dent Res 19:3521, 1940.

Hursey RJ Jr, Witkop CJ Jr, Miklashek D, Sackett LM: Oral Surg 9:641, 1956.

Kamen S, Goodman D, Hermler A: Genetic aspects of shall teeth: report of a case. J Dent Child 48:187, 1980.

Levin LS, et al: Dentinogenesis imperfecta in the Brandywine isolate (DI type III): clinical, radiologic, and scanning election microscopic studies of the dentition. Oral Surg 56:267, 1983.

Listgarten M: Osteogenesis imperfecta with dentinogenesis imperfecta. J Can Dent Assoc 26:412, 1960.

Pindborg JJ: Dental aspects of osteogenesis imperfect. Acta Pathol Microbiol Scand 24:47, 1947.

Rushton MA: A new form of dentinal dysplasia: shell teeth. Oral Surg 7: 545, 1954.

Schimmelphennig CB, McDonald RE: Enamel and dentin aplasia. Oral Surg 6:1445, 1953.

Shields ED, Bixler D, El-Kafawy AM: A proposed classification for heritable dentine defects with a description of a new entity. Arch Oral Biol 18:543, 1973.

Stafne EC: Dental roentgenologic manifestations of systemic disease. II. Developmental disturbances. Radiology 58:507, 1952.

Wilson GW, Steinbrecher M: Hereditary hypoplasia of the dentin. J Am Dent Assoc 16:866, 1929.

Witkop CJ Jr, Sauk JJ Jr: Dental and Oral Manifestations of Hereditary Disease. (Workshop Monograph.) Washington, D.C.:American Academy of Oral Pathology, 1971, p. 28.

Witkop CJ Jr, Dyson HR, Sackett LJ: A study of hereditary defects occurring in a racial isolate residing in Southern Maryland. Clin Proc Child Hosp 12:29, 1956.

Witkop CJ, MacLean CJ, Schmidt PJ, Henry JL: Medical and dental findings in the Brandywine isolate. Ala J Med Sci 3:382, 1966.

Dentinal Dysplasia

Bakaeen G, Snyder CW, Bakaeen G: Dentinal dysplasia type I: report of a case. J Dent Child 52:128, 1985.

Ballschmiede G: Dissertation (1922). In: Steidler NE, Radden BG, Reade PC: Dentinal dysplasia: a clinicopathological study of eight cases and review of the literature. Br J Oral Maxillofac Surg 22:275, 1984.

Bernard WV: Roentgenographic and histologic differentiation of dentinogenesis imperfecta and dentinal dysplasia. J Dent Res 39:675, 1960.

Borkenhagen R, Elfenbaum A: Dentine dysplasia associated with rheumatoid arthritis and hypervitaminosis D. Oral Surg Oral Med Oral Pathol 8:76, 1955.

Brenneise CV, Dwornik RM, Brenneise EE: Clinical, radiographic and histological manifestations of dentin dysplasia, type I: report of a case. J Am Dent Assoc 119:721, 1989.

Brookerson KR, Miller SS: Dentinal dysplasia: report of a case. J Am Dent Assoc 77:608, 1968.

Burkes EJ, Aquilino SA, Bost ME: Dentin dysplasia II. J Endod 5:277, 1979.

Ciola B, Bahn SL, Goviea GL: Radiographic manifestations of an unusual combination of type I and type II dentin dysplasia. Oral Surg Oral Med Oral Pathol 45:317, 1978.

Coke JM, Del Rosso G, Remeikis N, Van Cura JE: Dentinal dysplasia, type I: report of a case with endodontic therapy. Oral Surg Oral Med Oral Pathol 48:262, 1979.

Diamond O: Dentin dysplasia type II: report of a case. J Dent Child 56: 310, 1989.

Diner H, Chous MD: Dysplasia of the dentinal pulp: follow-up of a case report. J Dent Child 45:76, 1978.

Duncan WK, Perkins TM, O'Carroll MK, Hill WJ: Type I dental dysplasia: report of 2 cases. Ann Dent 50:18, 1991.

Elzay RP, Robinson CT: Dentinal dysplasia: report of a case. Oral Surg Oral Med Oral Pathol 23:338, 1967.

Giansanti JS, Allen JD: Dentin dysplasia, type II, or dentin dysplasia, coronal type. Oral Surg Oral Med Oral Pathol 38:911, 1974.

Graham WL, Harley JB, Alberico C, Kelln EE: Absent lamina dura associated with a developmental dentin abnormality. Arch Intern Med 116: 837, 1965.

Grimer PT: An atypical form of hereditary opalescent dentin. Br Dent J 100:275, 1956.

Hitchin AD: Pulp stones in every tooth in a girl of 13 years. Br Dent J 60: 539, 1936.

Hoff M, Van Grunsven MF, van der Pel ACM, Jansen HWB: Dentinedyplasie type II. Ned Tijdschr Tandheelkd 93:45, 1986.

Hoggins GS, Marsland EA: Developmental abnormalities of the dentine and pulp associated with calcinosis. Br Dent J 92:305, 1952.

Hunter IP, MacDonald DG, Ferguson MM: Developmental abnormalities of the dentine and pulp associated with tumoral calcinosis. Br Dent J 135:446, 1973.

Jasmin JR, Clergeau-Guerithault S: A scanning electron microscopic study of dentin dysplasia type II in primary dentition. Oral Surg Oral Med Oral Pathol 58:57, 1984.

Logan J, Becks H, Silverman S, Pindborg J: Dentinal dysplasia Oral Surg 15:317, 1962.

Luffingham JK, Noble HW: Dentinal dysplasia. Br Dent J 160:281, 1986.

Melnick M, Levin LS, Brady J: Dentin dysplasia type I: a scanning electron microscopic analysis of the primary dentin. Oral Surg Oral Med Oral Pathol 50:335, 1980.

Melnick M, et al: Dentin dysplasia, type II: a rare autosomal dominant disorder. Oral Surg Oral Med Oral Pathol 44:592, 1977.

Miller AS: Case of the month for diagnosis. Pa Dent J 37:134,138 1970.

Morris ME, Angsburger RH: Dentine dysplasia with sclerotic bone and skeletal anomalies as autosomal dominant trait. Oral Surg 43:267, 1977.

McFarlane MW, Cina MT: Dentinal dysplasia: report of a family. J Oral Surg 32:867, 1974.

Nakata M, Kimura O, Bixler D: Interradicular dentin dysplasia associated with amelogenosis imperfecta. Oral Surg Oral Med Oral Pathol 60:182, 1985.

O'Carroll MK, Duncan WK, Perkins TM: Dentin dysplasia: review of literature and a proposed subclassification based on radiographic findings. Oral Surg Oral Med Oral Pathol 72:119, 1991.

Perl T, Farman AC: Radicular (type I) dentin dysplasia. Oral Surg 43:746, 1977.

Petersson A: A case of dentinal dysplasia and/or calcification of the dentinal papilla. Oral Surg Oral Med Oral Pathol 33:1015, 1972.

Rankow R, Miller AS: Dentin dysplasia: endodontic considerations and report of involvement of three siblings. J Endod 10:385, 1984.

Rao SR, Witkop CJ Jr, Yamane GM: Pulpal dysplasia. Oral Surg Oral Med Oral Pathol 30:682, 1970.

Richardson AS, Fantin TD: Anomalous dysplasia of dentin: report of a case. J Can Dent Assoc 36:189, 1970.

Rosenberg LR, Phelan JA: Dentin dysplasia type II: review of the literature and report of a family. J Dent Child 50:372, 1983.

Rushton MA: A case of dentinal dysplasia. Guys Hosp Rep 89:369, 1939.

Rushton MA: Anomalies of human dentin. Ann R Coll Surg Engl 16:95, 1955.

Scola SM, Watts PG: Dentinal dysplasia type I: a subclassification. Br J Orthod 14:175, 1987.

Shields ED, Bixler P, El-Kafrawy AM: A proposed classification for heritable human dentin defects with a description of a new entity. Arch Oral Biol 18:545, 1973.

Stafne EC, Gibilisco JA: Calcifications of the dentinal papilla that may cause anomalies of the roots of teeth. Oral Surg Oral Med Oral Pathol 14:685 1961.

Stafne EC, Gibilisco JA: Oral Roentgenographic Diagnosis. 4th Ed. Philadelphia:WB Saunders, 1975 p. 30.

Steidler, NE, Radden BG, Reade PC: Dentinal dysplasia: a clinicopathological study of eight cases and review of the literature. Br J Oral Maxillofac Surg 22:275, 1984.

Tidwell E, Cunningham CJ: Dentinal dysplasia: endodontic treatment with case report. J Endod 5:372, 1979.

Van Dis ML, Allen CM: Dentinal dysplasia type I: a report of four cases. Dentomaxillofac Radiol 18:128, 1989.

Wegner H, Mannkopf H: Zur Vererbungspatholosie der Zahn wurzeln des bleibended Gebisses. Dtsch Zahn-Mund-Kieferheilk 28:269, 1958.

Weiss LR: Unusual case of pulp stones. Dent Cosmos 69:750, 1927.

Wesley RK, Wysocki GP, Mintz SM, Jackson J: Dentin dysplasia type I: clinical, morphologic, and genetic studies of a case. Oral Surg Oral Med Oral Pathol 41:516, 1976.

Wetzel WE, Weckler C: Erbliche Dentindysplasie: type II. Dtsch Zahnarztl Z 40:1249, 1985.

Witcher SL, Dinkard DW, Shapiro RD, Schow CE: Tumoral calcinosis with unusual dental radiographic findings. Oral Surg 68:105, 1989.

Witkop CJ Jr, Sauk JJ Jr: Dental and Oral Manifestations of Hereditary Disease. (Workshop Monograph.) Washington, D.C.:American Academy of Oral Pathology, 1971, p. 28.

Regional Odontodysplasia

Lowe O, Duperon DF: Generalized odontodysplasia. J Pedod 9:235, 1985.

Lustman J, Klein, Ulmansky M: Odontodysplasia: report of two cases and review of the literature. Oral Surg 39:781, 1975.

McCall JO, Wald SS: Clinical Dental Roentgenology. Philadelphia:WB Saunders, 1947, p. 150.

Neupert EA, Wright JM: Regional odontodysplasia presenting as a soft tissue swelling. Oral Surg 67:195, 1989.

Pindborg JJ: Pathology of the Dental Hard Tissues. Philadelphia:WB Saunders, 1970, p. 120.

Sadeghi EM, Ashrafi MH: Regional odontodysplasia: clinical pathologic and therapeutic considerations. J Am Dent Assoc 102:336, 1981.

Zegarelli EV, Kutscher AH: Odontodysplasia. Oral Surg 16:187, 1963.

Drift And Migration

Kisling E, Hoffding J: Premature loss of primary teeth. Part III. Drifting patterns for different types of teeth after loss of adjoining teeth. J Dent Child 46:35, 1979.

Embedded And Impacted Teeth

Aitasalo, et al: An orthopantomographic study of prevalence of impacted teeth. Int J Oral Surg 1:117, 1970.

Archer WH: A Manual of Oral Surgery. 2nd Ed. Philadelphia:WB Saunders, 1956, p. 135.

Bjork A, Jensen E, Palling M: Mandibular growth and third molar impaction. Acta Odontol Scand 14:231, 1956.

Clark CA: A method of ascertaining the relative position of unerupted teeth by means of FIM radiography. R Soc Med Trans (Odontol Sec) 3:87, 1909.

Dachi SF, Howell FV: A survey of 3,874 routine full-mouth radiographs. II. A study of impacted teeth. Oral Surg 14:1165, 1961.

Hellman M: Our third molar teeth: their eruption, presence and absence. Dent Cosmos 78:750, 1936.

Mead SV: Incidence of impacted teeth. Int J Orthod 16:885, 1930.

Morris CR, Jerman AC: Panoramic radiographic survey: a study of embedded third molars. Oral Surg 29:122, 1971.

Pell GJ, Gregory G: Report on a ten year study of a tooth division technique for removal of impacted teeth. Am J Orthod Oral Surg 28:660, 1942.

Richards AG: Technique for roentgenographic examination of impacted mandibular third molars. J Oral Surg 10:138, 1952.

Richards AG: The buccal object rule. J Tenn State Dent Assoc 33:263, 1953.

Shafer WG, Hine MK, Levy BM: A Textbook of Oral Pathology, 4th ed. Philadelphia:WB Saunders, 1983, p. 66.

Winter GB: Principles of Exodontia as Applied to the Impacted Mandibular Third Molar. St. Louis:American Medical Book Company, 1926.

Suggested Readings

Hypodontia

Beierle LE, Jorgenson RJ: Anodontia in a child: report of a case. J Dent Child 46: 485, 1978.

Gulmen S, Pullon PA, O'Brien W: Tricho-dento-osseous syndrome. J Endod 1:117, 1976.

Hesse G: Dysostosis cleidocranialic unter besonderer Berucksicktigung des Gebisses. Vjschr Zahah 41:162, 1925.

Levin LS, Jorgenson RJ, Cook RA: Otodental dysplasia: a "new" ectodermal dysplasia. Clin Genet 8:136, 1975.

Rosenzweig K, Garbarski D: Numerical aberration in the permanent teeth of grade school children in Jerusaleum. Am J Phys Anthropol 23:277, 1965.

Hyperdontia

Andborg JJ: Pathology of the Dental Hard Tissues. Philadelphia:WB Saunders, 1970, p. 26.

Gemination

Boyne PJ: Gemination: report of two cases. J Am Dent Assoc 50:194, 1955.

Brook AH, Winter GB: Double teeth: retrospective study of geminated and fused teeth in children. Br Dent J 129:125, 1970.

Dilaceration

Miles AEW: Malformation of teeth. Proc R Soc Med (Sect Odontol) 47: 817, 1954.

Taurodontism

Garn SM, Lewis AB, Kerewehy RS: Sexual dimorphism in the buccolingual tooth diameter. J Dent Res 45:1819, 1966.

Goldstein E, Gottlieb MA: Taurodontism: familial tendencies demonstrated in eleven of fourteen case reports. Oral Surg 36:131, 1973.

Hutchinson J: Report of effects of infantile syphilis in marring development of teeth. Trans Pathol Soc (Lond) 9:449, 1858.

Karcher EW: New syphilitic dental dystrophy (similar to bud molar of Pfluger). Arch Dermatol Syphilol 31:861, 1935.

Karnosh LJ: Histopathology of syphilitic hypoplasia of the teeth. Arch Dermatol Syphilol 13:25, 1926.

Dens Invaginatus

Oehlers FAC: The tuberculated premolar. Dent Pract Dent Rec 6:145, 1956.

Dens Evaginatus

Villa VG, Bunag CA, Ramos AB: A developmental anomaly in the form of an occlusal tubercle with central canal which serves as the pathway of infection to the pulp and periapical region. Oral Surg 12:345, 1959.

Enamel Hypoplasia

Bradlow RV: The dental stigmata of prenatal syphilis. Oral Surg 6:147, 1953.

Brauer JC: Dentistry for Children. Philadelphia:Blakiston, 1939, p. 110.

Cavallaro J: Reference to syphilis in relation to dentition. Dent Cosmos 50:1325, 1908.

Dean HT: Epidemiological studies in the United States. In: Moulton FD, ed. Dental Caries and Fluorine. Washington, D.C.:Lancaster Science Press, 1946, p. 5.

Via WF Jr: Enamel defects induced by trauma during tooth formation. Oral Surg 25:49, 1968.

Amelogenesis Imperfecta

Parker JL, Regattieri LR, Thomas JP: Hypoplastic hypomaturation amelogenesis imperfecta with taurodontism: report of a case. ASCD J Dent Child 42:379, 1975.

Dentinogenesis Imperfecta

Rushton MA: Anomalies of human dentin. Ann R Coll Surg Engl 16:95, 1955.

Winter GR, Maiocco PO: Osteogenesis imperfecta and dentinogenesis imperfecta. Oral Surg 2:782, 1949.

Dentinal Dysplasia

Bruszt P: Sur deux cas dysplasie dentinare. Bull Group Int Rech Sci Stomatol Odontol 12:107, 1969.

Regional Odontodysplasia

Gardner DG, Sapp JP: Regional odonto-dysplasia. Oral Surg 34:351, 1973.

Hintz CS, Peters RA: Odontodysplasia: report of an unusual case and review of literature. Oral Surg 34:745, 1972.

Walton JL, Witkop CJ Jr, Walker PO: Odontodysplasia. Oral Surg 46:676, 1978.

Attrition, Abrasion, Erosion

Brasch SV, Lazarov JV, Abbe NJ, Forrest JO: The assessment of dentifrice abrasivity in vivo. Br Dent J 127:119, 1969.

Carlsson GE, Hugoson A, Persson G: Dental abrasion and alveolar bone loss in the white rat. IV. The importance of the consistency of the diet and its abrasive components. Odontol Revy 18:165, 1967.

Ervin JC, Bucher EM: Prevalence of toothroot exposure and abrasion among dental patients. Dent Items Interest 66:760, 1944.

Frykholm KO: Undersokning av tandforhallanden hos jarnversarbetare inom ett sinterverk med sarskild hansyn till abrasionsskador. Odontol T 71:199, 1963.

Gortner RA, Kenigsberg RK: Factors concerned with the different erosive effects on grapefruit and grapefruit juice on rat's molar teeth. J Nutr 46:133, 1952.

Hansen J: Disappearance of dental substance due to action of acid in oral cavity. JAMA 111:451, 1949.

Kitchin PC: The prevalence of tooth root exposure to the degree of abrasion in different age classes. J Dent Res 20:565, 1941.

Kitchin PC, Robinson HBG: The abrasiveness of dentifrices as measured on the cervical areas of extracted teeth. J Dent Res 27:195, 1948.

Larsson BT: Tandsubstansforluster och tandborstning i ett folktandvardsklientel. Sverig Tandlak-Forb Tidn 61:58, 1969.

Manly RS: Factors influencing tests on the abrasion of dentin by brushing with dentifrices. J Dent Res 23:59, 1944.

Manly RS, Brudevold F: Relative abrasiveness of natural and synthetic toothbrush bristles on cementum and dentin. J Am Dent Assoc 55:799, 1957.

Murphy TR: Reduction of the dental arch by approximal attrition: a quantitative assessment. Br Dent J 116:485, 1964.

Newman AT: Cervical abrasion of the teeth and their causes. Dent Items Interest 69:501, 1947.

Olesen KT, Kardel KM: Tandstikker-usur. Tandlagebladet 71:228, 1967.

Pedersen PO: Eine besondere From der Abnutzung von Eskimozahnen aus Alaska. Dtsch Zahnarztl Z 10:41, 1955.

Peter Prince of Greece and Denmark: Attrition of the teeth among Tibetans. Man 57:177, 1957.

Philips RW, Leonard LJ: A study of enamel abrasion as related to partial denture clasps. J Prosthet Dent 6:657, 1956.

Pindborg JJ: Dental mutilation and associated abnormalities in Uganda. Am J Phys Anthropol 31:385, 1957.

Rapp GW et al: Pyrophoyihate: a factor in tooth erosion. J Dent Res 39: 372, 1960.

Stafne EC, Lovestedt SA: Dissolution of tooth substance by acids. J Am Dent Assoc 34:586, 1947.

Zipkin I, McClure FJ: Salivary citrate and dental erosion. J Dent Res 28: 613, 1949.

Embedded and Impacted Teeth

Chapman H: First upper permanent molars partially impacted against second deciduous molars. Orthod Oral Surg 9:339, 1923.

Shah RM, Boyd MA, Vahel TF: Studies of permanent tooth anomalies in 7,886 Canadian individuals. I. Impacted teeth. J Can Dent Assoc 6:262, 1978.

Chapter 6

Radiologic Diagnosis of Dental Caries

Dental caries, or tooth decay, is a pathologic process of localized destruction of tooth hard tissues by organic acids in the microbial deposits adhering to the teeth. The carious lesions, or the localized destructions of tooth hard tissues, are the symptoms of the disease. The symptoms can be arranged on a scale ranging from initial loss of mineral at the ultrastructural level to total destruction of the tooth. Because of the complexity of the oral environment, a multitude of factors determines the rapidity with which the symptoms develop or the severity of the symptoms in any one person.

Dental caries is a multifactorial disease with an interplay of three principal factors: (1) the host (primarily the teeth and saliva); (2) the microflora; and (3) the substrate or diet. In addition is a fourth factor: time. When the three essential parameters of dental caries—a susceptible host, cariogenic oral flora, and a suitable local substrate—are present in a individual for a considerable time, dental caries may develop.

A susceptible host is one of the factors required for caries to occur. Tooth morphology has been recognized as an important determinant. On the basis of clinical observations, Bossert (1937) reported that accentuated pits or fissures are susceptible to dental caries. Food debris and microorganisms readily lodge in the fissures.

Individual teeth and surfaces have vastly different susceptibilities to dental caries. The most frequent site of caries attack is the occlusal surfaces of the first and second permanent molars, probably because the occlusal surfaces of these teeth have many pits and fissures. In general, the susceptibility of teeth to caries increases posteriorly in the oral cavity. This phenomenon is probably due to the anatomy of the molar teeth. The pits and fissures and the wider interproximal contact areas are not easily accessible to cleansing action.

Saliva plays an extremely important role in reducing caries activity. In part, this beneficial effect is due to the mechanical washing away of some of the food debris, bacteria, and their soluble products. Certainly, the buffering action of saliva should not be overlooked. Although certain antibacterial factors such as lysozyme are found in the saliva, organisms in the mouth manage to survive. Antibacterial factors in saliva may possibly prevent the establishment of more pathogenic transient invaders.

Caries cannot occur without microorganisms. The classic germ-free animal studies of Orland and colleagues (1954, 1955) firmly established a principle that had been debated for more than a century, namely, that dental caries is a bacterial infection. The Orland studies demonstrated that germ-free rats that rececived a highly cariogenic diet containing sucrose did not develop caries. When gnotobiotic (with known microbiota) laboratory animals receiving the same diet were infected with a combination of an enterococcus (any streptococcus of the human intestine) and a pleomorphic (various distinct forms of a single organism) bacterium, caries developed.

Newbrun (1989a) reported that a careful evaluation of studies on caries indicates that different organisms display some selectivity as to which tooth surfaces they attach, and at least four types of processes are involved.

The microflora associated with pit and fissure caries, smooth surface caries, root caries, and deep dentinal caries is not the same. Different organisms are capable of inducing caries in animals, depending on experimental conditions.

Pit and fissure caries is the most common carious lesion in modern humans. Many organisms can colonize in fissures, which provide mechanical retention for bacteria. Thylstrup and Fejershov (1986) reported that, in fissures, Streptococcus mutans is normally found in higher numbers, and S. sangius occurs in lower numbers in samples collected from the carious sites, whereas the opposite is true in caries-free fissures. Ikeda and colleagues (1973) and Loesche and Straffon (1979) reported that studies in which the microbial composition of plaque from selected occlusal tooth surfaces was observed over 12 to 18 months indicate that the initiation of caries tends to be preceded by an elevated number of both S. mutans and lactobacilli.

Fitzgerald and others (1960, 1963, 1981) stated that lactobacilli are not involved in caries initiation, but become secondary invaders that contribute to progression of already existing lesions. Lactobacillus strains may initiate caries in sites that favor their retention, however, such as deep fissures and enamel defects. Therefore, it is thought that both S. mutans and lactobacilli initiate caries in deep pits and fissures.

In smooth surface enamel caries, a limited number of organisms have proved able to colonize smooth surfaces in large enough numbers to cause dental caries in test animals. S. mutans is specific for smooth enamel surface caries. Because humans swallow every few minutes, it is obvious that unattached bacteria cannot maintain themselves on smooth enamel surfaces solely by their rates of multiplication. Bacteria are able to attach themselves to smooth enamel surfaces by means of dental plaque, however. Plaque consists of densely packed bacteria embedded in an amorphous material called the plaque matrix. A characteristic of plaque is that it resists removal by physiologic oral cleaning forces such as saliva and tongue movement, but plaque is removable by toothbrushing if the bristles can reach it. Bacterial cells have been estimated to comprise 60 to 70% of the volume of plaque, whereas the matrix makes up the remainder. The matrix consists of extracellular carbohydrate polymers synthesized by the bacteria and of macromolecules and other elements derived from saliva and crevicular fluid.

Carious lesions do not develop without plaque, and when plaque contains appreciable proportions of highly acidogenic bacteria, such as S. mutans, and is exposed to readily fermentable dietary sugars, it produces sufficient concentrations of acids to demineralize the enamel. Therefore, the pathogenicity of plaque depends on its microbial composition and on the availability of dietary sugars.

Streptococcus mutans organisms are nonmobile, catalase-negative, gram-positive cocci in short or medium chains. Several important properties account for the high cariogenic potential of S. mutans. They are acidogenic and aciduric; they rapidly synthesize insoluble polysaccharides from sucrose; they colonize on tooth surfaces; and they are homofermentative lactic acid formers.

Sumney and associates described root caries as a soft, progressive lesion of the root surface involving plaque and microbial invasion. It starts in cementum or dentin near the cementoenamel junction after the cementum is exposed as one grows older. Some of the organisms in root caries are different from those in other smooth surface lesions because the initial lesion is in dentin or cementum, not enamel. Newbrun and associates (1984) reported that the role of the various bacteria in root caries still needs clarification, and no specific microorganism has been shown convincingly to be responsible for root surface caries.

The environment in deep dentinal caries is different from that of other locations, and as expected, the bacterial flora is also different. Fairbourn and colleagues stated that the predominant organism in deep dentinal caries is lactobacillus, and it accounts for approximately one third of all bacteria. Frequently isolated gram-positive anaerobic rods and filaments are found. Actinomyces, rothia, and bacillus also occur in deep dentinal lesions.

It is generally considered that S. mutans is present in large numbers in established enamel and dentin carious lesions. However, S. mutans seems only a minor part of the flora in deep areas of carious dentin. Gram-positive anaerobic rods and filaments, specifically lactobacilli, predominate in the microbiota of deep dentinal caries. Therefore, dental caries in humans is caused by several types of microorganisms, depending on the many factors that may influence the formation, composition, and metabolism of the dental plaque.

Diet plays a central role in the development of dental caries. Observations in humans, in animals, and in the laboratory (in vitro) have clearly shown the relationship between frequent consumption (exposure) of fermentable carbohydrates (specifically sucrose) and high caries activity. The local effects of diet on plaque metabolism and specifically on acid production are considered important in the development of caries.

Different properties of the diet are important for their cariogenic effects. The most important are the type of carbohydrate, concentration of carbohydrate, stickiness, retention time, and protective compounds. Animal experiments, as well as plaque pH experiments, have clearly demonstrated that the cariogenicity or acidogenicity increases with greater amounts of fermentable carbohydrates in the food. Foods that are sticky and are retained for a long time in the mouth have a higher cariogenic potential than foods that are eliminated more quickly from the mouth.

Caries is a biosocial disease rooted in the technology and economy of our society. As living standards improve, the severity of the disease usually increases. Isolated populations that have not acquired the dietary habits of modern industrialized society retain a relative freedom from caries. In industrialized countries, dental caries is one of the most widespread and costly illnesses. Dental caries, together with periodontal disease and malocclusion, constitutes a real problem to virtually every man, woman, and child in industralized countries in the more developed countries. Billions of dollars are spent annually in repairing damage to teeth from caries. Except for mental illness, dental caries is the most costly single disease entity.

Carious lesions that result in cavitation are irreversible and therefore cumulative with age. A strong positive correlation exists between age and DMF (decayed, missing, or filled teeth) indices. Massler reported that, over a lifetime, caries incidence (new lesion per year) shows three peaks—at ages 6 to 8 years, at 11 to 19 years, and between 56 and 65 years.

The most significant recent epidemiologic event has been the dramatic decline in caries prevalence in the nations of the Western world. Barmer (1981) and the 1982 *Conference on the Declining Prevalence of Dental Caries* reported that, from 1956 to 1982, surveys among school children in many Western countries unanimously showed a fall in caries prevalence of up to 50%. These cumulative studies on children indicate that the pattern of caries is reversing, resulting in fewer carious surfaces (particularly smooth surfaces), fewer carious teeth, and more caries-free individuals. Whereas the present data pertain to children and young adults, there is every reason to expect that future studies will demonstrate similar reductions extending into adult life. A virtual elimination of smooth surface lesions, in which environmental factors are dominant, is predicted. The inherently susceptible occlusal pits and fissures will be reduced to a lesser extent.

In regions where water supply is fluoridated, it is reasonable to conclude that this measure is the major factor in the reduction of caries. The use of fluoride dentifrice, dietary fluoride supplements, and topical fluoride regimens has become widespread, and each is known to exert a significant cariostatic action. In addition, the current decline in caries prevalence could be a result of improved level of oral health care, sugar substitutes, changing patterns of sugar consumption, and improved nutrition, but data to substantiate these reasons are not available. Moreover, dental treatment of carious lesions by filling cavities eliminates stagnation areas and reduces the microbial contamination of the saliva. Therefore, dental restorative treatment of caries can terminate caries as well as prevent caries in the future.

Unlike the sharp decline in caries experienced in Western Europe and North America, caries is increasing rapidly in children in developing countries. When one considers that 1.2 billion children under 15 years of age reside in the underdeveloped countries of the world, it becomes obvious that prevention is the only hope for improved oral health in these countries in the future. Prevention of caries, not just its treatment by restorative procedures, should have a high priority in every dental office. Caries can be prevented by a combination of procedures used in the office, the home, and the community.

◆ *RADIOLOGIC FEATURES*

Several studies, such as those of Dunning and Ferguson (1946), Haugejorden and Slack (1974, 1975, 1977), and Hansen (1980), have shown that bitewing radiographs are an important aid in the interpretation of interproximal caries. In 1946, Dunning and Ferguson found that the detection of posterior interproximal dental caries increased by 215% when posterior bitewing radiographs were used in addition to the clinical examination. In a recent investigation by Hansen, four times as many posterior interproximal carious lesions were found when posterior bitewings were used as compared with the number of lesions found by clinical methods alone.

Because dental caries is essentially a process of decalcification, a certain percentage of calcium and phosphorus must be destroyed before the decreased density can be visualized on the radiograph. Early and associates (1979) estimated that bone has to be decalcified by approximately 50% before a radiolucency will be revealed on the radiograph.

The classification of the radiographic appearance of caries is discussed according to the location of caries on the tooth, such as proximal, occlusal, facial/lingual, pulpal, root or cemental, recurrent or secondary (immediate vicinity of preexisting restoration), and arrested caries (occlusal and proximal surfaces.).

Proximal Carious Lesions (Figs. 6–1 to 6–8)

More proximal lesions are usually found when the dental radiograph is used as an adjunct to the clinical examination, probably because of the lower volume of normal tooth structure through which the x-rays must penetrate to reach the carious lesion on the proximal surface than on the other tooth surfaces. The early incipient carious lesion on visible smooth enamel surface is clinically manifested as a white (loss of translucency), opaque region, which is best demonstrated when the area is air dried (Fig. 6–1).

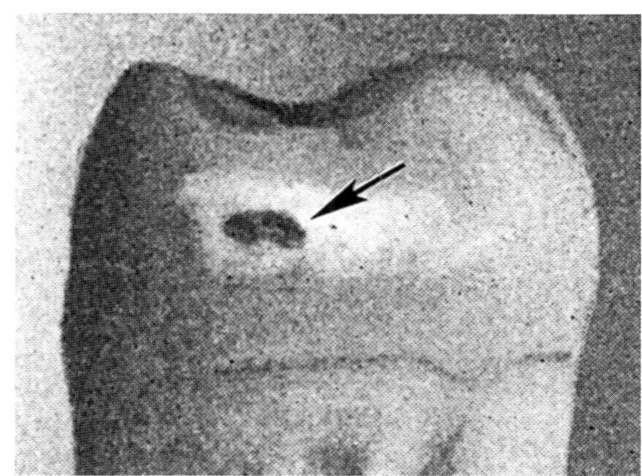

FIGURE 6–1.

White Spot Proximal Caries. Active white spot lesion on the proximal surface of a molar tooth located just below the contact point and above the cementoenamel junction. Note the stained portion in the white spot that could represent an area of arrested caries. (From Black AD: Pathology of hard tissues of the teeth. In: Oral Diagnosis. 7th Ed. Chicago: Medico-Dental, 1936, p. 346.)

Incipient Carious Lesions

Incipient interproximal lesions can be detected on a bitewing radiograph as a small, cone-shaped radiolucent area in the outer enamel (Fig. 6–2). At this stage, the incipient lesion

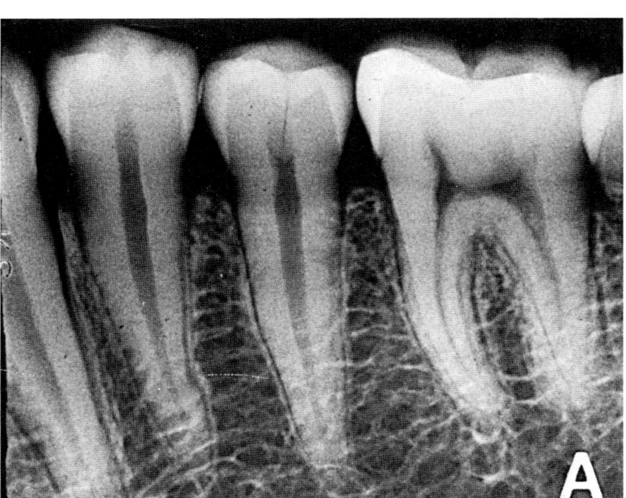

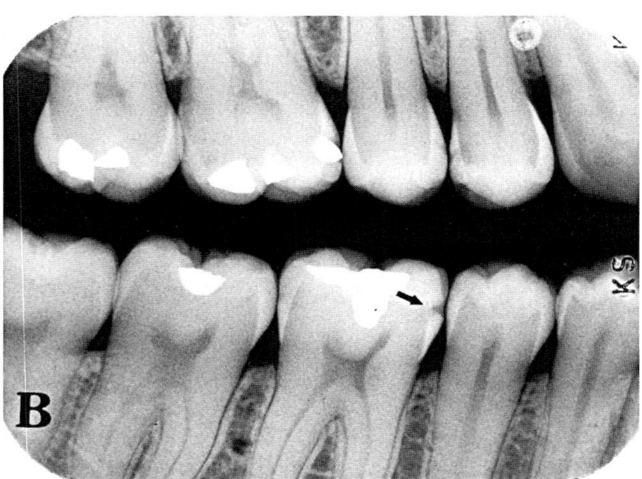

FIGURE 6–2.

Incipient Enamel Caries. A, Normal interproximal enamel surface without caries. B, Note the classic carious V-shaped lesion on the mesial surface of the lower first molar (arrow); a smaller lesion is present on the distal surface of this tooth and on the mesial surface of the maxillary second premolar.

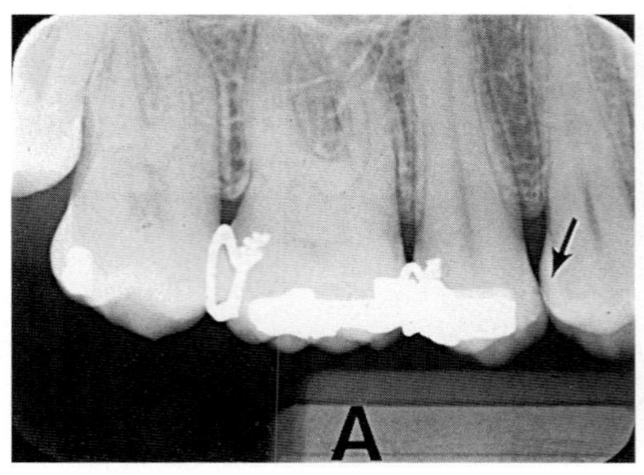

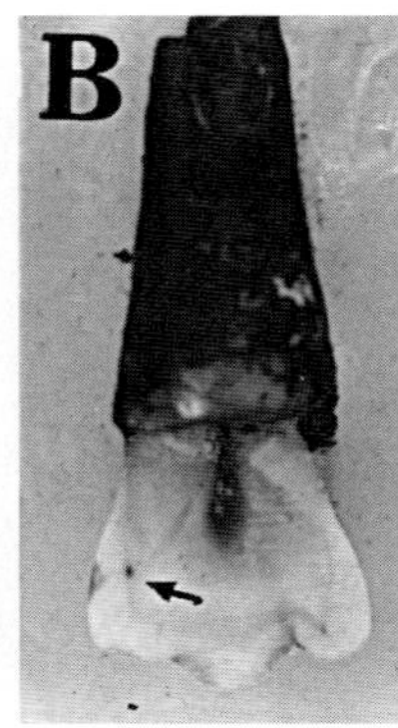

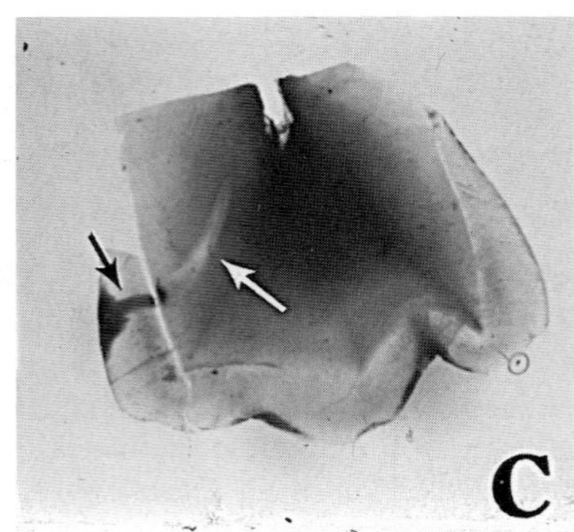

FIGURE 6–3.

Histopathology of Incipient Carious Lesion. A, Note the distal incipient carious enamel lesion of a maxillary first premolar prior to extraction (arrows). B, Longitudinal gross section of the tooth in A after extraction; it was soaked in organic dye. C, Ground thin section of the tooth in A showing an active proximal carious lesion reaching the dentinoenamel junction, followed by a sclerotic reaction or transparent zone in the dentin. The transparent zone or sclerotic dentin (white arrow) is an apparent attempt to wall off the lesion in the dentin; it extends almost to the pulp. (From Langland OE: Radiologic examination. In: Clark JW, ed., Clinical Dentistry. Hagerstown, MD: Harper & Row, 1976, p. 26.)

may be arrested or even reversed by remineralization if an effective preventive program is enacted. Restoration of an incipient lesion is an elective procedure that is generally not recommended, except in cases of high caries susceptibility.

Silverstone (1982) reported that histologic examination of a radiographically detectable incipient carious lesion shows that the carious process has penetrated the dentin, although the dentinal tissue is not invaded by bacteria (Fig. 6–3). This finding implies that carious lesions that may appear on radiographs to involve part of the enamel only may, at the histologic level, have reached the dentinoenamel junction, with a marked response from the pulpodentinal organ. A slowly progressing enamel carious lesion may be attenuated by an effective defensive response in the dentin and pulp.

The spread of the enamel carious lesion is basically determined by the distribution of plaque and the direction of the enamel rods or prisms. The enamel rods tend to converge from the convex proximal surface to the dentinoenamel junction, so they produce the classic triangular V-shaped or cone-shaped radiolucent appearance because the caries process tends to follow the course of the enamel rods (Fig. 6–4). However, many shapes and sizes of proximal enamel carious lesions may be seen radiographically (thick line-shaped, W-shaped, flame-shaped, half-moon shaped, etc). Newbrun (1989b) states that what determines the shape of the lesion is still unknown.

Lamellar Caries

At one time, the onset of caries was thought to be related to the presence of lamellae (proteolytic theory), which were considered pathways of primary invasion. Because lamellae are in all teeth, inevitably some of them may be involved in carious lesions, called lamellar caries. Scott and Wyckoff (1949), however, believed that the association between lamellae and lesions is random and is not a cause-and-effect relationship. Lamellar caries appears radiographically as a dark thin line running completely through the interproximal enamel into the dentin, where the caries spreads along the dentinoenamel junction.

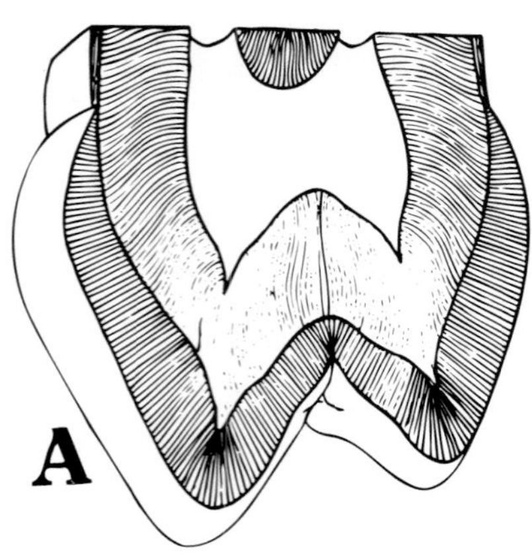

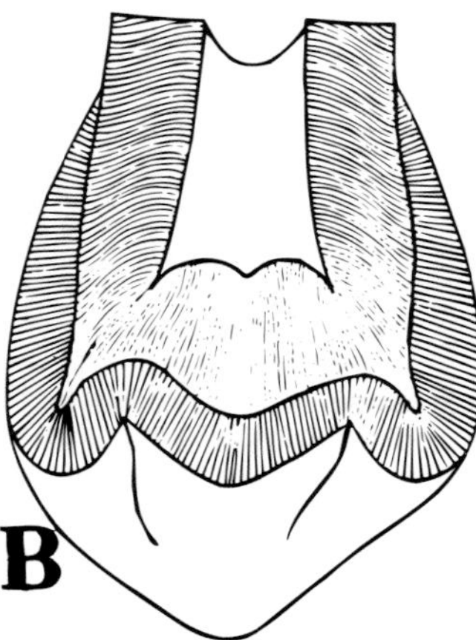

FIGURE 6–4.

Enamel Rods or Prisms. Arrangement of the enamel rods and dentinal tubules on a premolar sectioned buccolingually (A) and mesiodistally (B). (From Noyes F: Dental Histology and Embryology. Philadelphia: Lea & Febiger, 1943.)

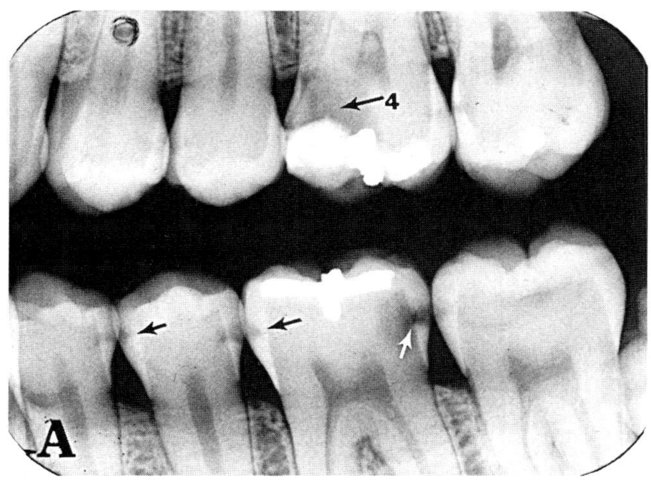

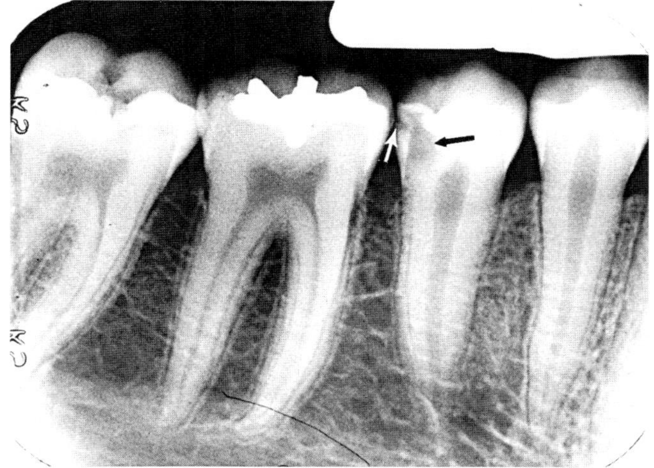

B

FIGURE 6–5.

Dentinal Caries. A, Note the spread of caries at the dentinoenamel junction of the distal surface of the lower first molar (white arrow), the classic V-shaped lesion on the mesial surface of the same tooth, and the mesial surface of the lower second premolar (black arrow). Note the class 4 caries lesion in the upper first molar (arrow). B, Enamel caries leading to the dentinoenamel junction, where it spreads and follows the dentinal tubules to the pulp (arrows).

Classification of Radiographic Caries

C-1. Enamel Caries *less* than 1/2 way through enamel (sometimes called incipient caries) Do not record these lesions if doubtful of their existence.

C-2. Enamel caries penetrating at least 1/2 way through enamel, but *NOT* involving dentino-enamel junction.

C-3. Caries of enamel and dentine definitely at or through the dentino-enamel junction extending less than 1/2 way to pulp cavity.

C-4. Caries of enamel and dentine penetrating more than 1/2 way dentine toward pulp cavity.

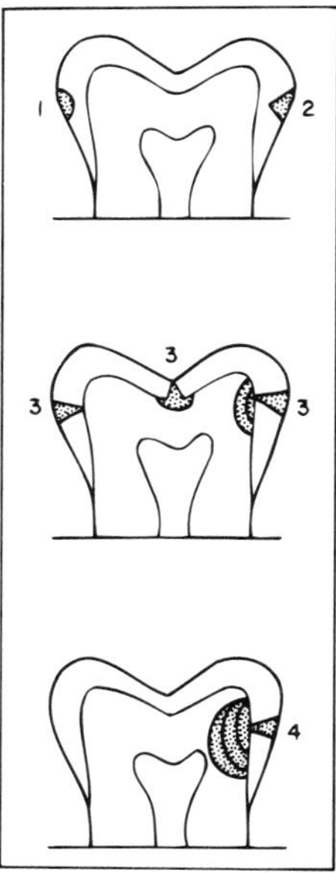

Record the lesser score if there is doubt concerning depth of lesion.

Since occlusal caries is first seen radiographically when the caries penetrates the dentine, a score of C-3 or C-4 is given for occlusal caries.

Enamel caries of C-1 and C-2 cannot be scored if overlapping of interproximal surfaces occurs.

FIGURE 6–6.

Classification of Dental Caries. A radiographic caries scoring code as recommended by Haugejorden and Slack in 1975. (From Haugejorden O, Slack GL: Progression of approximal caries in relation to radiographic scoring codes. Acta Odontol Scand 33:183, 1975.)

Dentinal Caries

As the carious lesion reaches the dentinoenamel junction, it usually first spreads laterally, undermining normal enamel. It then spreads much more rapidly toward the pulp, in a form like a mushroom, with its base on the dentinoenamel junction (Fig. 6–5).

Proximal Caries Progression

To follow the development of caries over time, one must distinguish between the initiation of lesions and the progression of lesions. Initiation is the development of new lesions and can be quantified by the number of new carious lesions developed in a certain period of time and expressed in caries increment or incidence. Registration of progression of the lesion requires a measure of size to recognize the change. Estimation of depth is the method most commonly used. Wagg (1974), Zamir and associates (1975), and Haugejorden and Slack (1975, 1977) developed methods of registration of caries progression.

Only by the use of a written description of each stage of caries penetration of the proximal surface can the clinician properly record a baseline from which to determine whether the lesion has progressed or stabilized from one office visit to the next. The prognosis of caries and hence the prognosis of the tooth depend on a large variety of clinical factors. Most recently, more conservative criteria have been used for operative treatment of caries. Many times, it may be more appropriate to institute preventive and remineralization procedures for a carious lesion than to attempt restorative treatment. At any rate, a radiographic caries classification system is shown in Figure 6–6 (as suggested by Haugejorden and Slack, 1977), and examples of each of the penetration stages of proximal caries are illustrated.

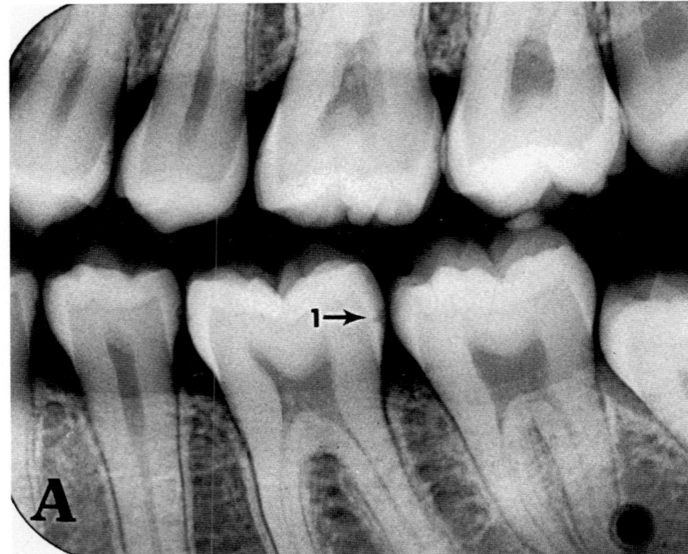

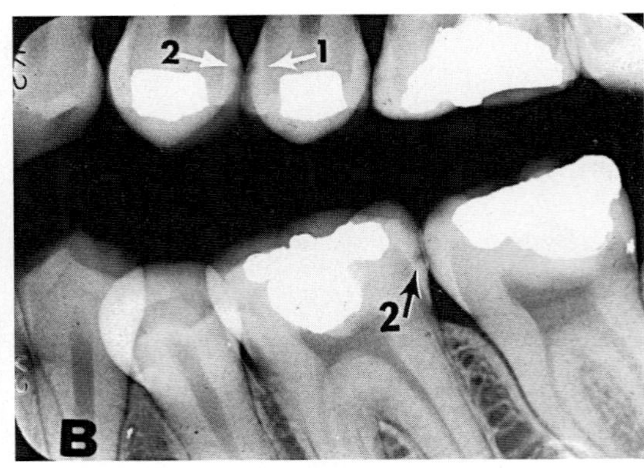

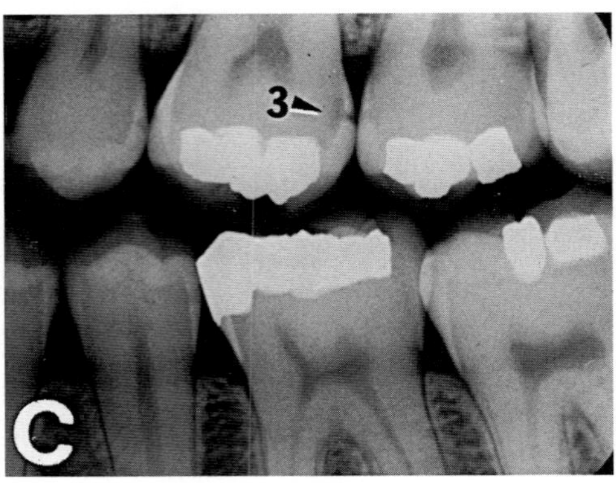

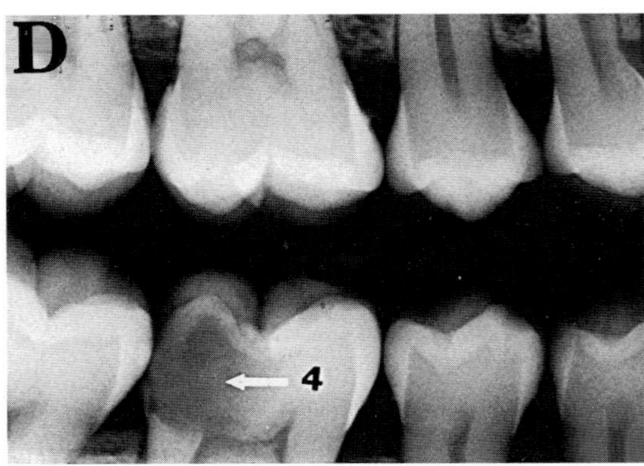

FIGURE 6–7.

Classification of Dental Caries. A, Class 2 distal caries (arrow) and class 1 on the mesial surface of the upper first molar. B, Class 3 caries of the distal surface of a mandibular first molar, and class 2 caries of the distal surface of a maxillary first premolar and class 1 on the mesial surface of a maxillary second premolar. C, Class 3 caries of the distal surface of an upper first molar and the mesial surface of a second molar. D, Class 4 caries (arrow).

For many years, proximal enamel carious lesions, when seen radiographically, regardless of their extent, have been treated by restorative measures. This philosophy of treatment of proximal caries has been based mainly on two premises: (1) the carious lesion is further advanced histologically than what is seen on the radiograph; and (2) the rate of progress of proximal lesions was commonly believed to be faster than that of more accessible lesions. For these reasons, the early identification of proximal lesions and prompt restorative treatment have been rigid principles of treatment of individual patients.

The rapid decline in the rate of caries progression recognized since 1963 underlines the importance of reviewing the newer studies on caries progression. Pitts (1983) and Schwartz and associates (1984) reported that progression of proximal carious lesions is usually a slow process, and many lesions remain unchanged for long periods of time. Using data from Sweden and the United States, Schwartz and colleagues (1984) concluded that a lesion takes an average of 4 years to progress through the enamel of permanent teeth. These investigators also concluded that progression is slower for older individuals, particularly those with long-term exposure to fluoride. In a study by Grondahl (1979), over a third of the lesions diagnosed as enamel caries did not progress beyond the dentinoenamel junction over a 6-year period. The data thus provided evidence that caries progression in many industrialized countries has slowed down, leaving adequate time for nonsurgical treatment of proximal lesions. However, the progression site of lesions varies between individuals as well as between lesions within an individual. On the basis of these observations, it is essential that decisions to treat or not to treat incipient lesions surgically and restoratively should be based on combined radiographic and clinical assessments.

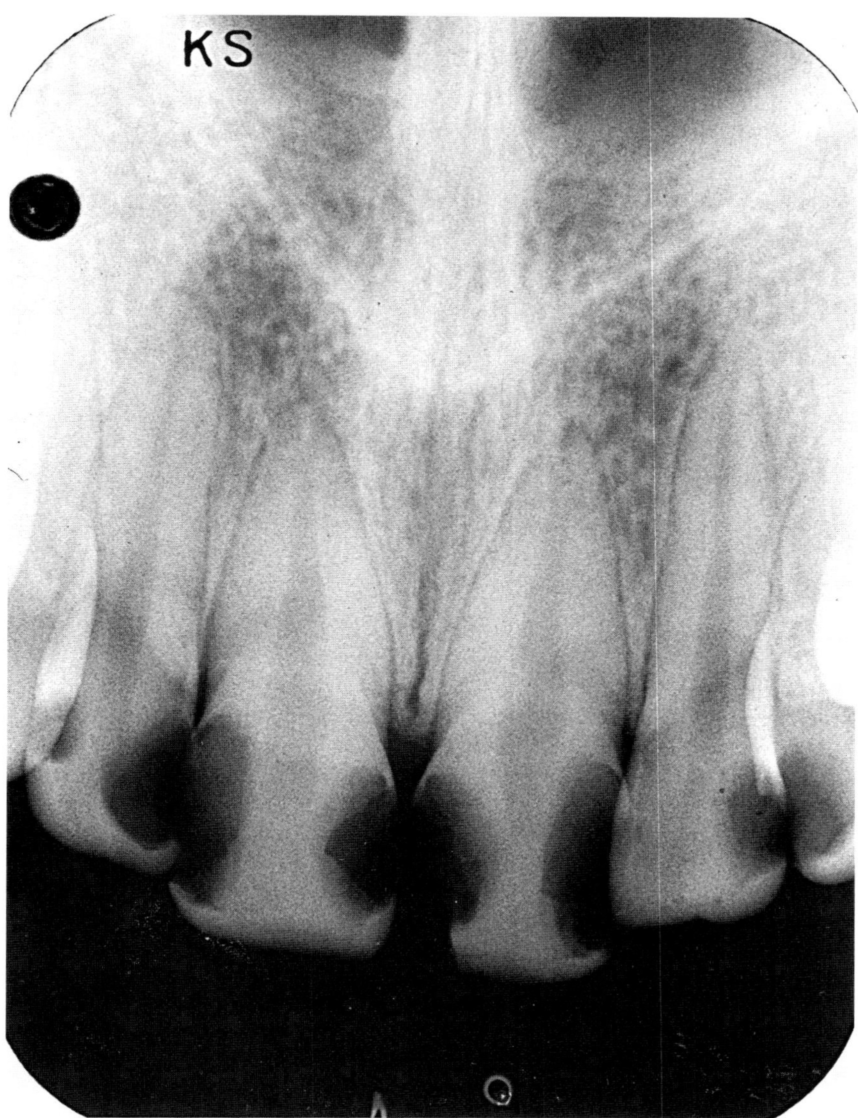

FIGURE 6–8.

Rampant Caries. This is a sudden, rapid, and uncontrollable destruction of teeth. Note the large interproximal carious lesions in the maxillary incisor teeth that, if not arrested, will amputate the crowns of these teeth.

Rampant Caries

Rampant caries is a sudden, rapid, and almost uncontrollable destruction of teeth. Rampant caries involves surfaces of teeth that are ordinarily relatively free of caries. Proximal and cervical surfaces of anterior teeth, including mandibular incisors, which are relatively caries free, may be attacked. Rampant caries is most often observed in the primary teeth of young children, in the permanent teeth of teenagers (11 to 19 years), and in patients with xerostomia (Fig. 6–8).

Acute and Chronic Caries (Figs. 6–9 and 6–10)

In most cases of acute caries, a condition commonly seen in young adults between the ages of 15 and 25 years, there is rapid penetration through the enamel, and the initial entrance of the carious process remains small (Fig. 6–9). In chronic caries, commonly seen in adults over 25, there is a slower progression of the lesion, and it has a larger entrance at the surface of the enamel (Fig. 6–10).

Occlusal Caries (Fig. 6–11)

Occlusal caries is the most prevalent caries of the oral cavity. Occlusal caries usually occurs early in life, before smooth surface lesions appear. The irregular pit and fissure surfaces of the premolar and molar teeth are inherently more prone to caries because of their mechanical characteristics, which result in poor self-cleaning features. Enamel caries that begins in the pits and fissures of occlusal surfaces of teeth takes on an appearance opposite that of proximal enamel caries in that the apex of the triangle is toward the outer surface of the tooth and the base of the triangle is at the dentinoenamel junction (Fig. 6–11). The occlusal carious lesion is usually not seen radiographically until it has reached the dentinoenamel junction and has spread in all directions. This is because of the great mass of enamel tissue superimposed over the occlusal enamel lesion. Usually, caries of the occlusal surface is initially seen as a radiolucent dark line or area just under the occlusal enamel surface (Fig. 6–11). The radiograph is not a reliable diagnostic aid for the detec-

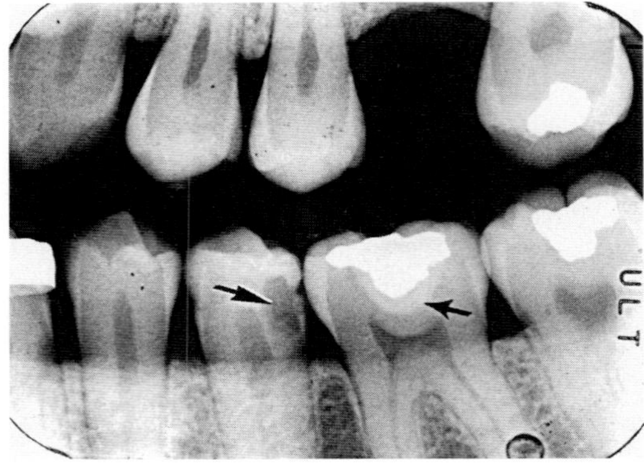

FIGURE 6–9.

Acute Caries. Small enamel entrance and a large dentinal carious lesion in the distal surface of a lower second premolar (arrow). Note the sclerotic dentin under occlusal restoration in the lower second molar.

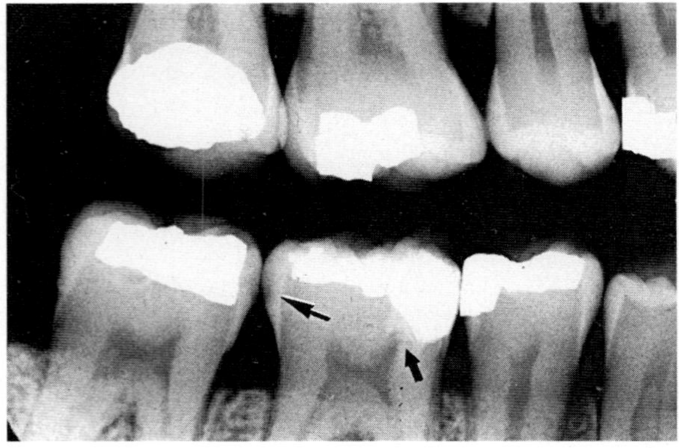

FIGURE 6–10.

Chronic Caries. Note the large enamel opening of chronic caries of the distal surface of a mandibular first molar (arrow). Also notice the flamelike sclerotic dentin under the mesio-occlusal restoration of this tooth (arrow).

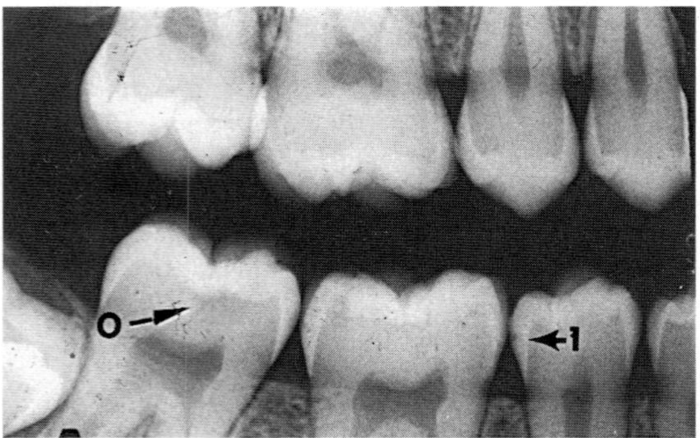

FIGURE 6–11.

Occlusal Caries. Occlusal caries (O) in the mandibular second molar and class 1 caries of the distal surface of a mandibular second premolar. (From Langland OE, Langlais RP, Morris CR: Principles and Practice of Panoramic Radiology. Philadelphia:WB Saunders, 1982, p. 214.)

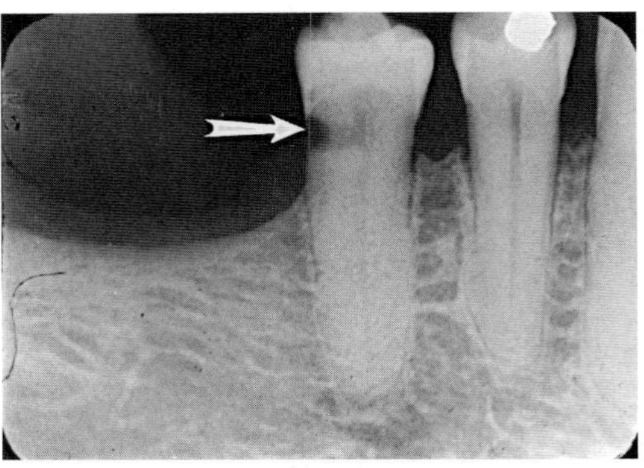

FIGURE 6–12.

Cervical Caries (Facial/lingual). Note the cervical facial/lingual caries of a mandibular second premolar (arrow). (Actually there is facial caries on both premolars.)

tion of occlusal caries. It can only alert the clinician to occlusal surfaces that should be examined more thoroughly. A mirror and now controversial sharp explorer are the traditional diagnostic aids in the detection of this type of caries.

Facial/Lingual Caries (Fig. 6–12)

Caries on the facial and lingual surfaces of the teeth begins in the pits, fissures, or cervical region of the tooth. Caries developing in pits on the facial and lingual surfaces appears on the radiograph as round dots on the tooth surface. Many times, it is like looking into a ''black hole.'' The periphery of the black hole is especially well demonstrated if the pit or fissure is on the lingual surface. Cervical caries extends laterally toward the proximal surfaces, forming a typical crescent-shaped, semilunar cavity, although the cavity may also be round or oval. It almost always seems to be a wide-open cavity unlike that found in proximal and occlusal caries, which has a narrow area of penetration. Figure 6–12 illustrates examples of facial and lingual caries. The radiographic film serves only to alert the clinician to caries of the facial or lingual surface. It does not routinely show carious lesions of these surfaces as well as a good clinical examination.

Pulpal Caries (Fig. 6–13)

The extent and/or proximity of the caries to the pulp chamber can be evaluated with only a limited degree of reliability from radiographs. This limitation stems in large part from the two-dimensional image on the radiograph trying to depict a three-dimensional tooth. The radiograph does provide some information, however, and so long as it is applied with reservation, it has a place in the evaluation of pulpal caries. If a carious lesion appears on the radiograph to have progressed right to the edge of the pulp chamber, the dentist should be forewarned of a pulp exposure during caries excavation (Fig. 6–13). Overangulation of the x-ray beam can create an appearance of pulpal exposure or abnormal apical periodontal ligament space widening. In addition, overexposure of the

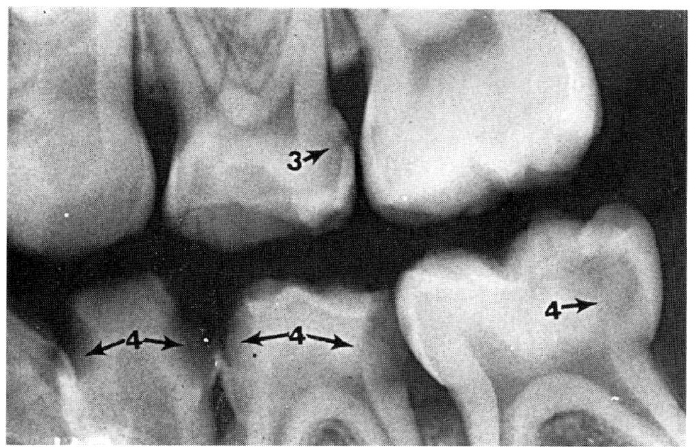

FIGURE 6–13.

Pulpal Caries. Note the large carious class 4 lesions with possible pulpal involvement in the lower primary molars and a primary canine (arrows). There is a class 3 dentinal caries lesion on the distal surface of an upper first primary molar (arrow).

film causes "burnout" of dentin between the pulp and carious lesion by enlarging the carious lesion. Moreover, the radiograph does not have depth, so a large carious lesion can be superimposed over the pulp, and in reality the caries has not penetrated the pulp.

Root or Cemental Caries (Fig. 6–14)

Root caries is known by a variety of terms including cemental caries, radicular caries, and even senile caries. Sumney and associates reported that root caries is usually seen as a shallow (less than 2 mm deep), ill-defined, softened area, often discolored, and characterized by destruction of cementum with penetration of underlying dentin. As it progresses, the lesion extends more circumferentially than in depth. Root caries starts at or near the cementoenamel junction and appears only after the cementum is exposed. It usually occurs in the elderly for three reasons: (1) cementum is exposed in most instances in the elderly because of gingival recession; (2) the elderly have many more loose contacts between adjacent teeth because of attrition, and this causes food packing areas; and (3) older people often have xerostoma (dry mouth) for various reasons (salivary gland atrophy, drugs, etc.).

When root surfaces are exposed to the oral environment as a result of recession of the gingiva, plaque retention areas increase, particularly along the cementoenamel junction. The cemental or root carious lesions start as small lesions along the cementoenamel junction and eventually coalesce and spread over the entire surface by microbial deposits. The surface becomes soft on probing, with a leathery consistency. Cementum has a laminated appearance microscopically, and when the microbial deposits reach the cemental layers, they produce caries, which tends to progress laterally

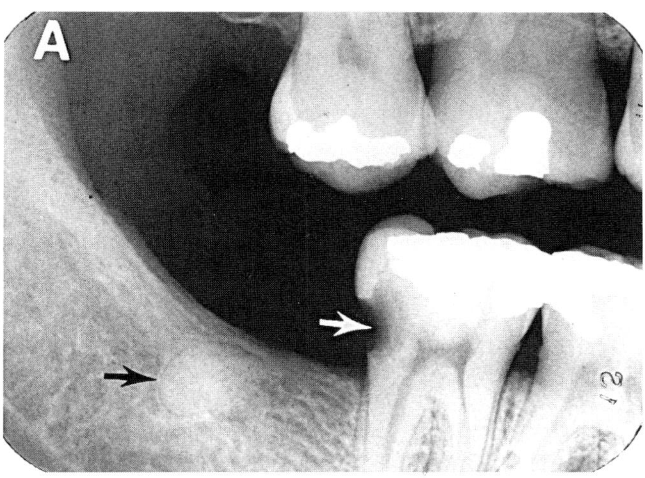

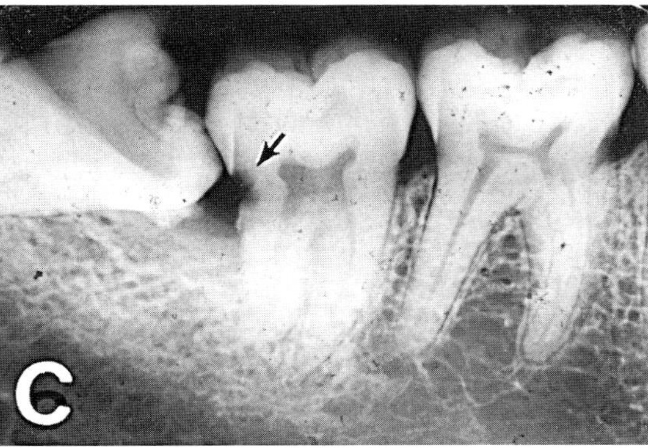

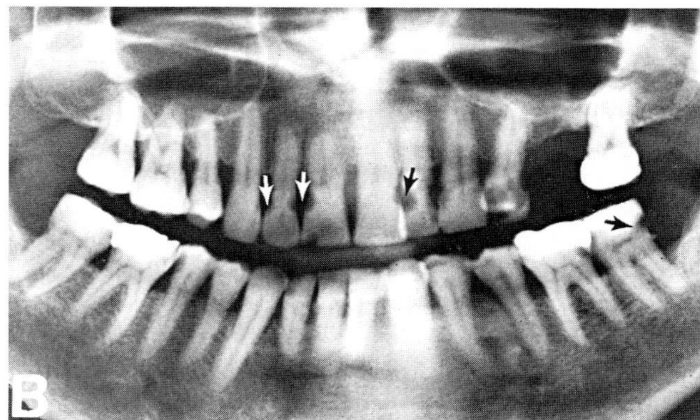

FIGURE 6–14.

Root (Cemental) Caries. A, Note cemental (root) caries on the distal surface of a lower second molar (white arrow). Also notice the root tip in the lower third molar area (black arrow). B, Note the characteristic cupped-out appearance of the carious lesions of cemental caries, as seen in the maxillary anterior teeth (arrows) and the distal surface of the lower left second molar (arrow). (From Langland OE, Langlais RP, Morris CR: Principles and Practice of Panoramic Radiology. Philadelphia:WB Saunders, 1982, p. 217.) C, Radiograph of cemental caries with a notched-out appearance as seen on the distal surface of a lower second molar. The impacted third molar should have been extracted earlier because it provided a food packing area distal to the second molar. (From Langland OE: Radiologic examination. In: Clark JW, ed., Clinical Dentistry. Hagerstown, MD:Harper & Row, 1976, p. 31.)

between the layers undermining the cementum. This gives the radiographic appearance of root caries described as "saucer-shaped" or "cupped-out." Root caries is usually located in the region of the proximal cementoenamel junction (Fig. 6–14). Although it does not usually involve the enamel, it may undermine the enamel by lateral extension of the root dentinal caries and may spread underneath the enamel.

Root caries may at times be misinterpreted as "cervical burnout," which is seen normally in the cervical region of the teeth as a radiolucent triangular area on the proximal surfaces of the posterior teeth and as a radiolucent band on the anterior teeth. Cervical burnout can be explained by the tissue density differences of the crown and the root of the tooth in the cervical region. The cervical area of the tooth is somewhat constricted as compared with the other portions of the tooth and is not covered by enamel or bone. Therefore, the x-radiation penetrates this region more readily than the rest of the tooth, resulting in a greater radiolucency in the cervical region. In many cases, an examination of the area by an explorer may be the only method of differentiating between root caries and cervical burnout. Also, root caries has a cupped-out or saucer-shape with a sharply outlined radiolucent appearance, rather than the wedge-shaped, more diffuse, lighter radiolucency seen in cervical burnout.

Recurrent or Secondary Caries (Figs. 6–15 and 6–16)

Recurrent or secondary caries develops at the margins or in the vicinity of a restoration and may indicate an unusual susceptibility to caries, poor oral hygiene, a deficient cavity preparation, a defective restoration, or a combination of these factors. Recurrent caries is defined as caries that occurs within the immediate vicinity of a restoration. It is usually due to a "leaky margin," which has been caused by inadequate extension for prevention of the cavity preparation, or

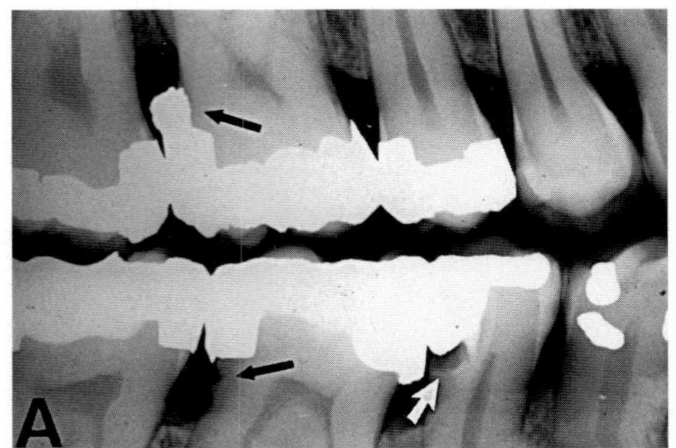

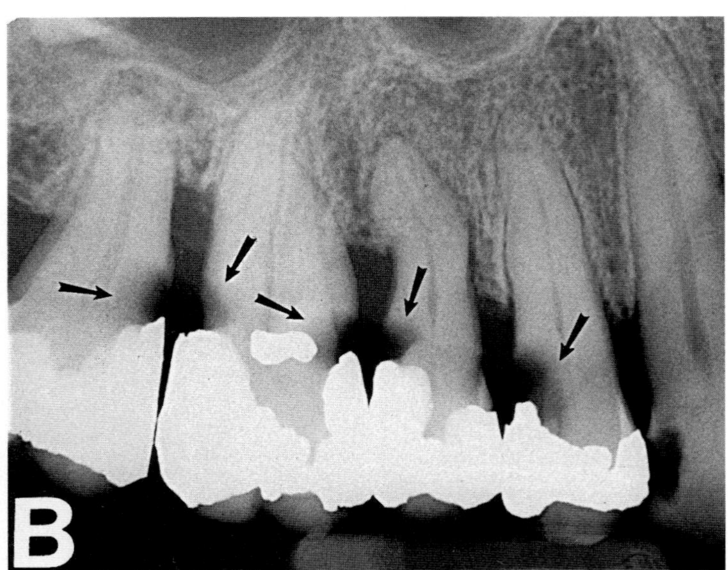

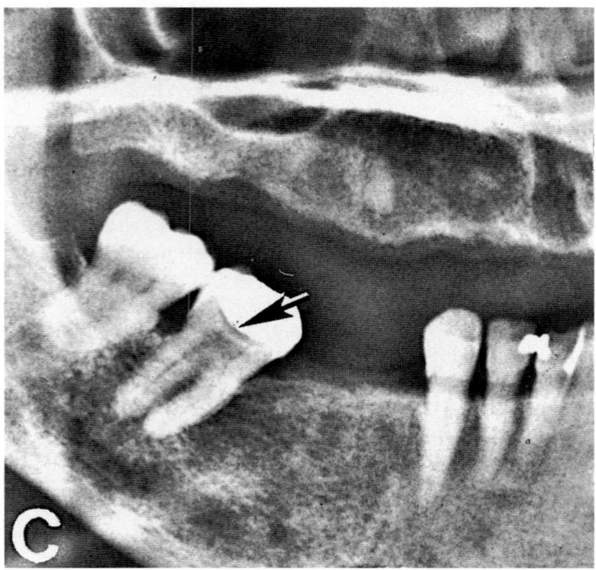

FIGURE 6–15.

Recurrent (Secondary) Caries. A, Note recurrent (secondary) caries of the distal surface of a lower second premolar (arrow) overhanging restoration of the distal surface of an upper first molar, and cemental caries of the distal surface of a lower first molar. B, Recurrent root caries in an elderly woman (arrows). C, Notice the radiolucent area under occlusal restoration in the lower second molar. This is most likely recurrent (secondary) caries (arrow), which was not removed at the time of the cavity preparation. The radiopaque band under the radiolucency has the radiographic appearance of sclerotic dentin. (A and C, From Langland OE, Langlais RP, Morris CR: Principles and Practice of Panoramic Radiology. Philadelphia:WB Saunders, 1982, p. 219.)

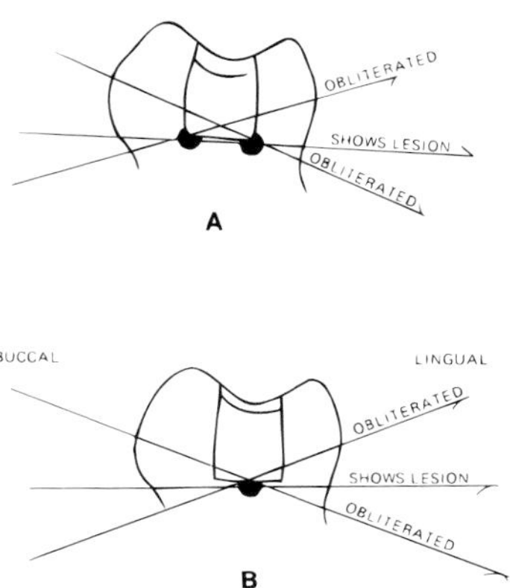

FIGURE 6–16.

Recurrent (Secondary) Caries: Diagram. Diagram illustrating how changes in vertical angulation may obliterate from radiographic view recurrent (secondary) caries on the interproximal surface of a tooth. A, Recurrent (secondary) caries at the corners of the proximal gingival portion of a class II restoration. B, Recurrent (secondary) caries under the proximal gingival portion of a class II restoration. (From Langland O: Radiologic examination. In: Clark JW, ed., Clinical Dentistry. Vol. 1. Philadelphia:Harper & Row, 1981, p. 33.)

it may result from poor adaptation of the restorative material to the cavity preparation. Recurrent caries is seen under the restoration as a dark, radiolucent area. Incomplete removal of dentinal caries prior to placing the restoration is also seen on the radiograph as a radiolucent area under the restoration (Fig. 6–15). Mjor (1981) reported that clinical studies, based on dentists' reports, show that 60% of all replacements of amalgam restorations are due to recurrent caries.

Recurrent or secondary caries is not always easy to detect radiographically because of variables such as (1) location of the caries lesion relative to the restoration and (2) the angulation of the x-ray beam in relation to the restoration and the carious lesion (Fig. 6–16).

Arrested Caries (Fig. 6–17)

Incipient and even more advanced carious lesions may become arrested if there is a significant shift in the oral environment from factors that cause caries to those that tend to slow down the caries process. Backer Dirks (1966) reported that clinical longitudinal studies suggest that incipient enamel caries can remain dormant for long periods of time and that some carious lesions may be reversed by remineralization. Most typically, the arrested incipient carious interproximal lesion is seen on teeth where the adjacent tooth has been extracted, so the local environmental conditions have changed completely. The incipient carious lesions may be discolored because of the uptake of dyes. Clinical exploration of the lesion reveals that it is the same hardness as normal enamel. Therefore, these lesions are defined as remineralized carious lesions. Another form of a large occlusal arrested caries is one in which a carious lesion becomes static or stops progressing for some reason. The appearance of the exposed dentin in the open cavity is yellow, brown, or black, has a polished surface, and is eburnated (hard). The carious lesion most likely becomes arrested because microorganisms cannot be retained on the polished surfaces of the lesion. The radiographic appearance of arrested caries is one in which the crown of the tooth is absent, with a dark radiolucent area on a roughened top surface of a destroyed tooth, as well as a white sclerotic line under the radiolucent area. This sclerotic white line represents sclerosis of dentinal tubules and secondary dentin formation commonly seen in arrested caries (Fig. 6–17).

Factors that Influence the Radiographic Interpretation of Caries

Radiographic Underestimation of Caries Size (Figs. 6–18 to 6–20)

A sufficient amount of calcium and phosphorus must be removed for the carious lesion to be seen on the radiograph. Early (1979) estimated that it takes approximately 50% of the calcium and phosphorus in a localized area of a tooth or bone to be absorbed before a radiolucency will be revealed on the radiograph. Therefore, the actual penetration of the carious lesion is not revealed on the radiograph (Fig. 6–18).

Silverstone (1982) reported that when a lesion is first detected on a radiograph and appears to be limited to the outer enamel, the lesion has already penetrated the dentin (see Fig. 6–3).

The radiograph underestimates the size of the carious lesion for another reason. It can be explained by the caries-to-normal tooth thickness ratio. The classic shape of the enamel caries lesion is V shaped, with the point of the V located nearest to the dentinoenamel junction. Therefore, the ratio of the thickness of the enamel to the size of the carious lesion becomes greater at the "V-point" of the carious lesion. At this point, the x-ray energy becomes reduced enough to

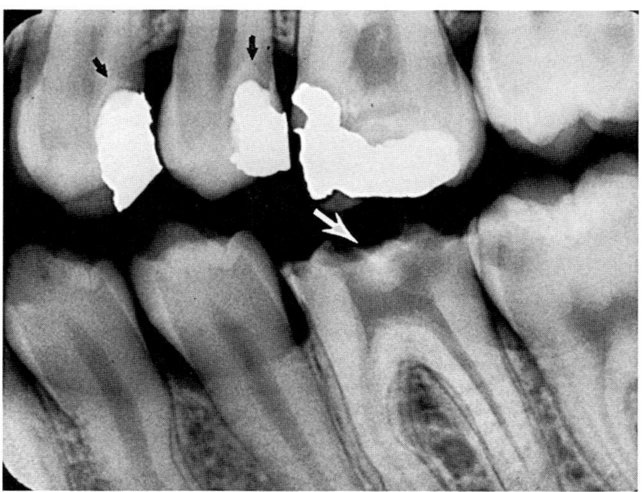

FIGURE 6–17.

Arrested Caries. Arrested caries in the lower first molar (white arrow). Clinically, the occlusal surface of the tooth has a black-brown polished appearance. Note the sclerotic dentin under the restorations in the maxillary premolars (black arrows).

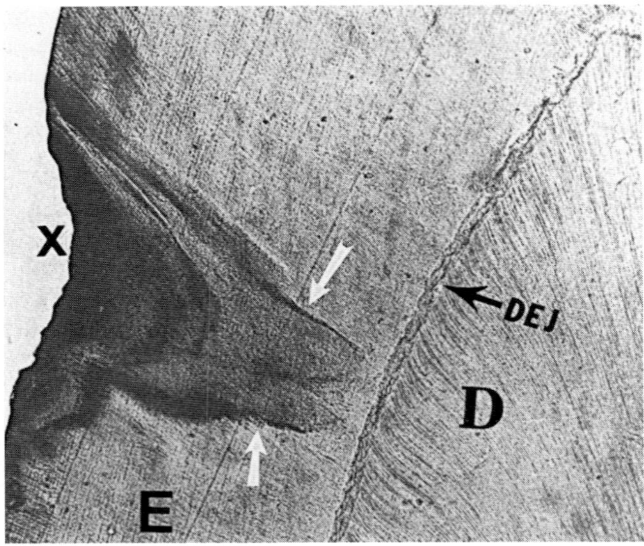

FIGURE 6–18.

Ground Section, Incipient Caries. Note the area of caries penetration at (X) where the outer ends of the enamel rods have broken away. The flame-shaped area of decalcification has almost reached the dentinoenamel junction (DEJ); however, the radiograph would reveal only a small, notchlike radiolucency. (From Black AD: G.V. Black's Operative Dentistry. Vol. I. 8th Ed. Chicago:Medico-Dental, 1948, p. 360.)

block out the registration of the radiolucent carious lesion in this region of the enamel. The carious lesion will then appear smaller on the radiograph than it actually should be.

When the carious lesion reaches the dentinoenamel junction, it spreads along the junction and progresses rapidly through the dentin to the pulp. This creates a smaller tooth structure to caries ratio, and the radiolucency of the carious lesion is seen again on the radiograph (Fig. 6–19). This creates a radiographic appearance of interproximal caries with a small opening on the enamel periphery, a band of normal enamel, and finally, carious dentin. This appearance could be misinterpreted as enamel caries only, and if the dentist decided to delay restorative treatment, it could cause the patient to undergo a root canal treatment or loss of a tooth.

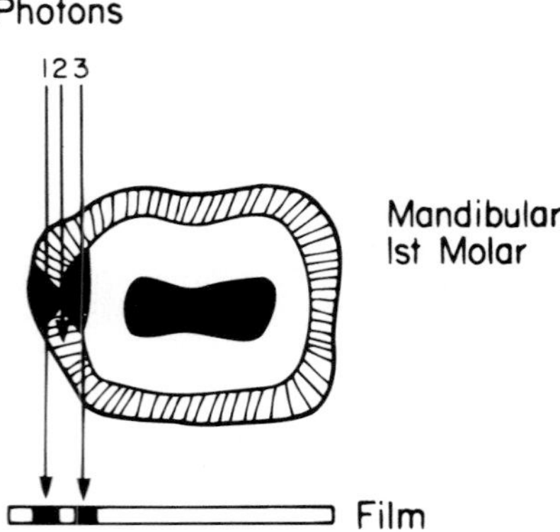

FIGURE 6–19.

Caries Diagram. Normal tooth structure to caries ratio phenomenon. The film records a radiopaque area for photon 2 because the normal tooth to carious tooth structure ratio is much greater in this area of the tooth, as compared with the tooth that photon 1 and 3 are penetrating. (Adapted from Wuehrman AH, Manson-Hing LR: Dental Radiology. 4th Ed. St. Louis:CV Mosby, 1977).

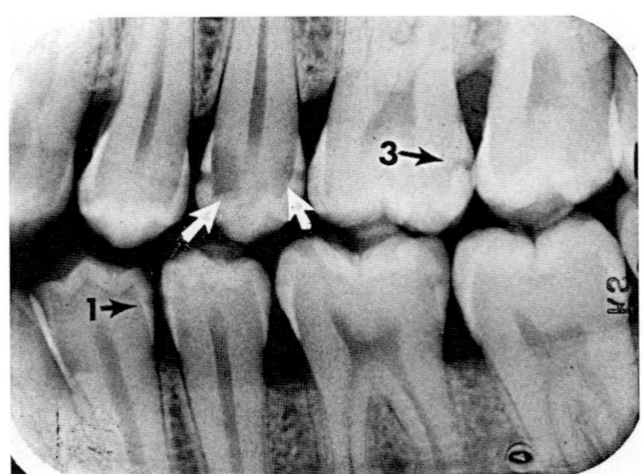

FIGURE 6–20.

Normal Tooth to Caries Ratio Radiograph. Normal tooth structure to carious tooth structure ratio phenomenon. Notice the apparent enamel carious lesion on the distal and mesial surface of the upper second premolar (white arrows). Closer observation, however, reveals that both lesions have penetrated the dentin. Note the class 3 caries, distal surface of the upper left first molar (arrow) and the class 1 lesion on the distal surface of the lower first premolar (arrow).

Cervical Burnout (Figs. 6–21 and 6–22)

The constricted cervical neck of the tooth, the area between the crown and the portion of the root covered with alveolar bone, absorbs less x-ray energy than the areas above and

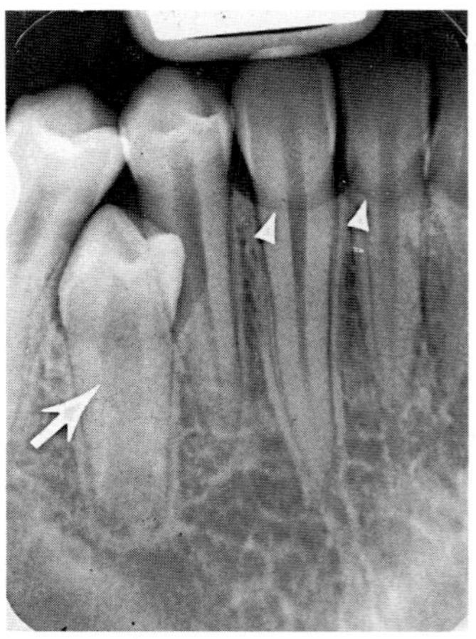

FIGURE 6–21.

Anterior Cervical Burnout. Cervical burnout (arrowheads) in the mandibular canine and lateral incisor cervical region. Note the dark radiolucent collar or band at the cervical neck of the teeth (white arrowheads). In addition, one sees an unerupted supernumerary premolar (white arrow). (From Langland OE, Langlais RP, Morris CR: Principles and Practice of Panoramic Radiology. Philadelphia:WB Saunders, 1982, p. 218.)

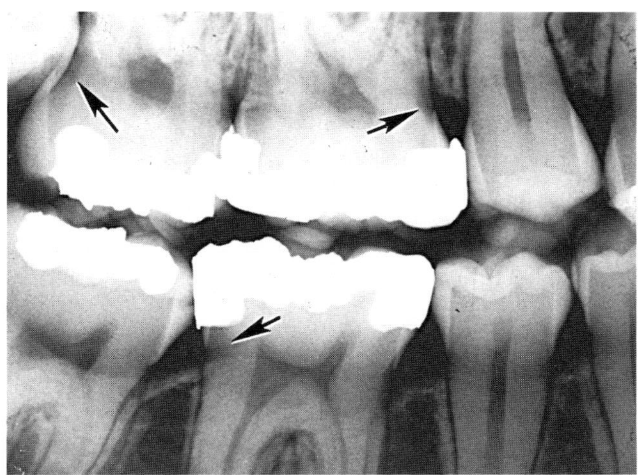

FIGURE 6–22.

Posterior Cervical Burnout. Cervical burnout in the maxillary first and second molars and the distal surface of the lower first molar (arrows). (From Langland OE, Langlais RP, Morris CR: Principles and Practice of Panoramic Radiology. Philadelphia:WB Saunders, 1982, p. 218.)

below it. This is because of the presence of enamel above and the alveolar bone covering the root of this tooth below the cervical neck. It results in a radiolucent band running across the cervical neck of anterior teeth (Fig. 6–21) and a triangular, wedge-shaped radiolucency at the interproximal cervical neck of the posterior teeth (Fig. 6–22). This is called cervical burnout because of the great density differences between the cervical neck of the tooth and the tissues above and below it. Other reasons for cervical burnout besides density tissue differences are anatomic differences such as the shape of the cementoenamel contour and various root configurations.

Cervical burnout should not be misinterpreted as cemental or root caries or recurrent caries under the proximal step of a class II restoration. Cemental caries will not occur unless the free margin of the gingiva has receded from its normal position. Cervical burnout is often seen when the alveolar bone is intact because cervical burnout radiolucencies depend partially on the presence of alveolar bone to provide the necessary contrast to be seen. However, the dentist should verify the presence of cemental caries by exploration, if one is in doubt.

Mach Band Effect (Figs. 6–23 and 6–24)

This visual illusion bears the name of Ernst Mach, who described the phenomenon in 1865, and results from lateral

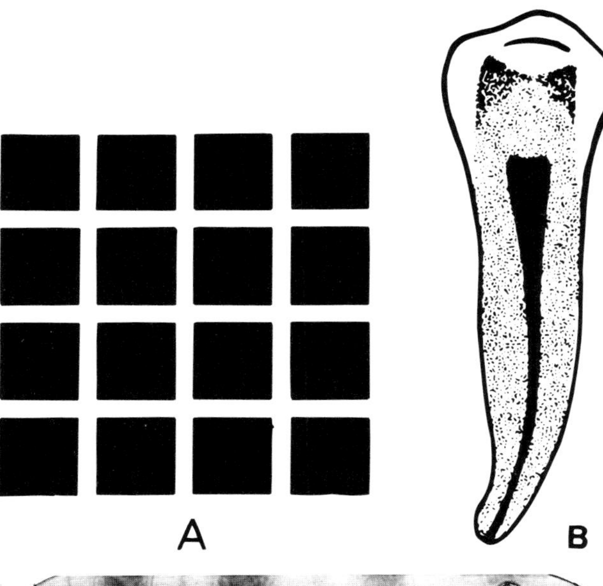

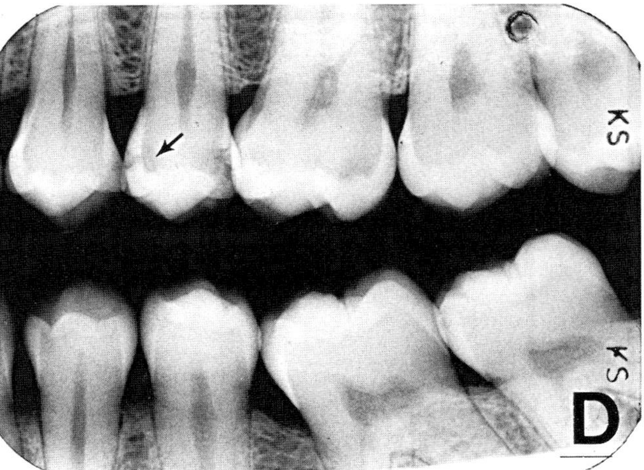

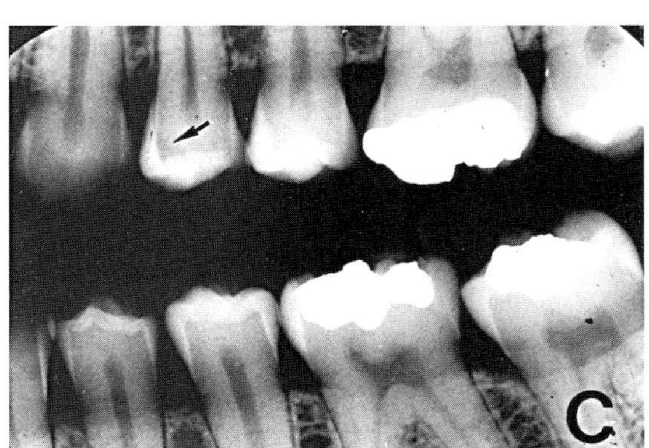

FIGURE 6–23.

Mach Band Effect. A, Notice dark areas produced at the white areas at the intersections of black squares when you stare at the center of the grid. B, Illustration of Mach band radiolucencies in dentinal peaks of mandibular premolar (A and B, From Berry HM: Cervical burnout and Mach band. J Am Dent Assoc 106:622, 1983. Copyright by the American Dental Association. Reprinted by permission.) C, Mach band radiolucent peak in the mesial surface of the upper first premolar. D, Actual carious lesion in the mesial surface of the upper second premolar (arrow).

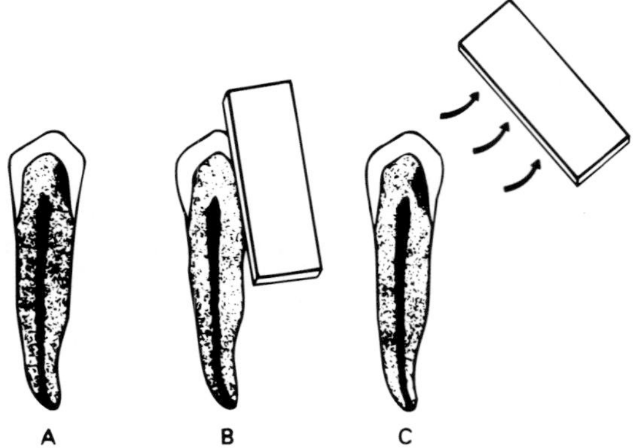

FIGURE 6–24.

Masking Technique for Mach Band Effect. In A, is it a Mach band or a carious lesion? In B, the opaque card covers the enamel, and the Mach-caused radiolucent area in the dentin disappears. (If actual caries were present, the radiolucent area would not disappear.) In C, when the card is snapped away, the Mach band reappears. (From Berry HM: Cervical burnout and Mach band. J Am Dent Assoc 106:622, 1983. Copyright by the American Dental Association. Reprinted by permission.)

neural inhibitory interactions within the eye of the beholder. Stimulation of retinal receptors by a bright light causes inhibition of the neural response of its adjacent (lateral) receptors, and the higher the degree of stimulation, the greater the inhibition (Fig. 6–23). Thus, when a uniformly dark shade meets a uniformly light shade (as when dentin meets enamel in a radiograph), the dark shade (dentin) appears even darker and the light shade (enamel) lighter as they approach the interface (dentinoenamel junction). This is edge enhancement phenomenon created in the eye and does not result from an actual density change in the film emulsion. A light shade that seems to become brighter is called positive Mach band, and a darker appearance of the dark shade is referred to as a negative Mach band.

In dental radiography, negative Mach bands may present some diagnostic dilemmas when they show fictitious radiolucent areas inside the dentinoenamel junction in incisors and canines and less frequently in premolars and to the least extent in molars.

The Mach band is also one reason for the darker appearance of dentinal peaks seen in radiographs of some premolars (more often mandibular than maxillary), where the dentin comes to a sharp peak in the corners bounded by the occlusal and proximal enamel surfaces. With lighter enamel on both sides of the dentinal peak, the dentin appears darker (Fig. 6–23B and C). Berry (1983) described a masking technique to facilitate differential interpretation between Mach band illusion and an actual carious lesion (Fig. 6–24).

Restorative Materials (Figs. 6–25 to 6–27)

Materials of relative high atomic weights, as amalgams, and gold, appear radiopaque on the radiograph and are not confused with caries, although silicates and plastics tend to be radiolucent and simulate dental caries (Fig. 6–25). Anterior composite restorations are radiopaque (Fig. 6–26). That silicate materials often require the use of a suitable radiopaque base assists the dentist in differentiating them from caries. Both zinc oxide-eugenol and zinc phosphate cements appear radiopaque. In addition, the typical anterior class III cavity preparations for silicates and plastics are U shaped and are different in outline form from the beginning carious lesion.

The older calcium hydroxide materials were radiolucent. The newer ones contain materials to render them radiopaque. Calcium hydroxide is ordinarily used as a subbase between a pulpal exposure or a near exposure and conventional base materials such as zinc phosphate cements. If the calcium hydroxide subbase used is radiolucent on the radiograph, it will be difficult to differentiate it from caries (Fig. 6–25).

A few clues are helpful in distinguishing caries from calcium hydroxide. When properly placed, only a thin line of calcium hydroxide will be used. If the radiolucency under the restorative material is more than a thin line, wider than a pencil line, it is probably caries rather than calcium hydroxide.

Observing the sharpness or unsharpness of the cavity preparation is also helpful. The border of the carious lesion in dentin is ordinarily poorly defined. If the border is sharp in outline, it is likely that the caries has been removed, and the dark line is probably calcium hydroxide (Fig. 6–27).

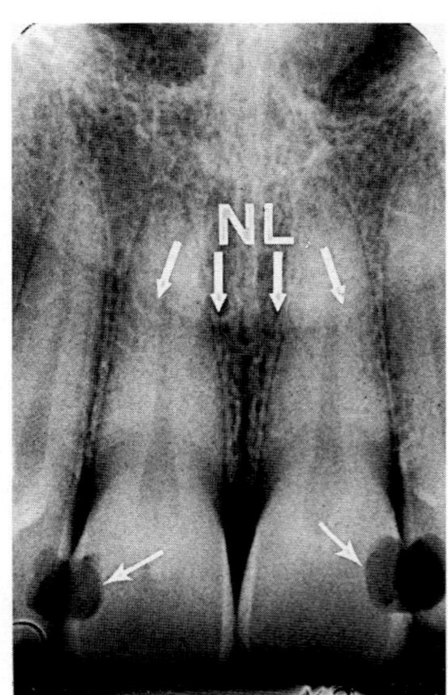

FIGURE 6–25.

Silicate Restorative Materials. Silicates are radiolucent and mimic caries. Conventional cavity preparation outlines aid in the differentiation of class III "tooth colored" filling materials from caries. The outline of the soft tissue of the nose is indicated by NL (arrows).

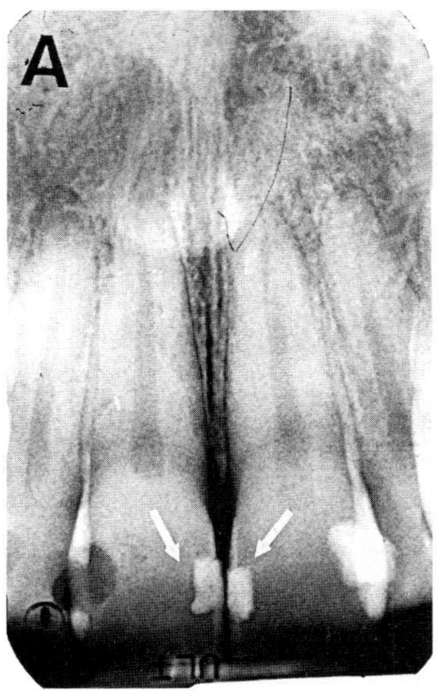

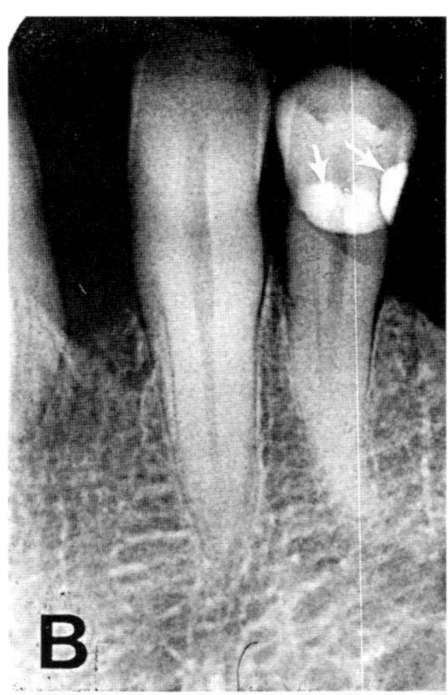

FIGURE 6–26.

Composite Restorative Materials. A, Composite restorations (arrows) on the mesial proximal surfaces of the maxillary central incisors are more radiopaque than silicate on the distal surface of the right maxillary central incisor. B, Composite restorations on the distal and facial surfaces of the lower first premolar (arrows).

Developmental Defects in Enamel (Figs. 6–28 to 6–30)

Developmental defects, particularly enamel hypoplasia, can simulate caries radiographically (Fig. 6–28). In the case of the hypoplastic pits, grooves, or fissures, the enamel surface tends to curve inward toward the defect. If a carious lesion is present, the contour of the enamel will be normal, but its periphery will be interrupted by an indentation filled with caries. Pits and fissures on the facial and lingual surfaces simulate caries, but are readily identified by clinical examination. Enamel hypoplasia occurring from deficiency or disease states usually is of the pitting variety. Because these pits tend to stain, caries is often suspected.

Caries is detected clinically if the explorer point sticks on removal from the defect. The lesion is termed an enamel developmental defect without caries involvement if the explorer does not stick.

Attrition is defined as the physiologic wearing away of teeth as a result of tooth-to-tooth contact, as in mastication, clenching, and bruxism. It generally occurs on the occlusal incisal and proximal surfaces of teeth. Attrition is associated with the elderly. Clinically, the earliest change occurs as a

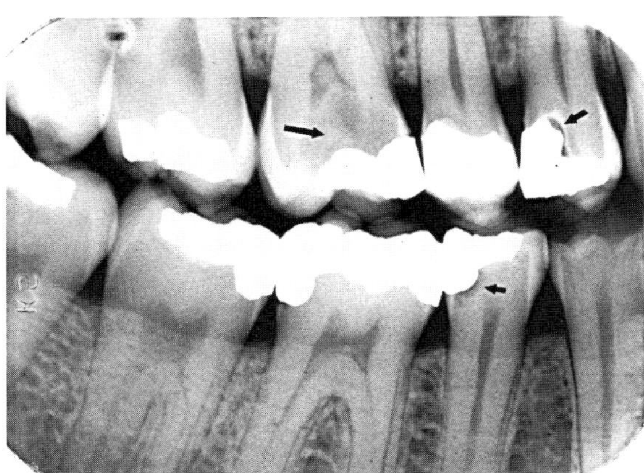

FIGURE 6–27.

Pulp Capping Materials (CaOH). The radiolucent area (arrow) under a DO restoration in the upper first premolar could be an older calcium hydroxide pulp capping material or caries. Usually, the radiolucency should be less than a pencil line if it is calcium hydroxide. Note the sclerotic dentin (radiopaque line) under the radiolucency. The newer pulp capping materials have $BaSO_4$ in them to make them radiopaque. Note that the recurrent caries under the DO restoration is in the lower second premolar and MO in the maxillary first molar (arrows).

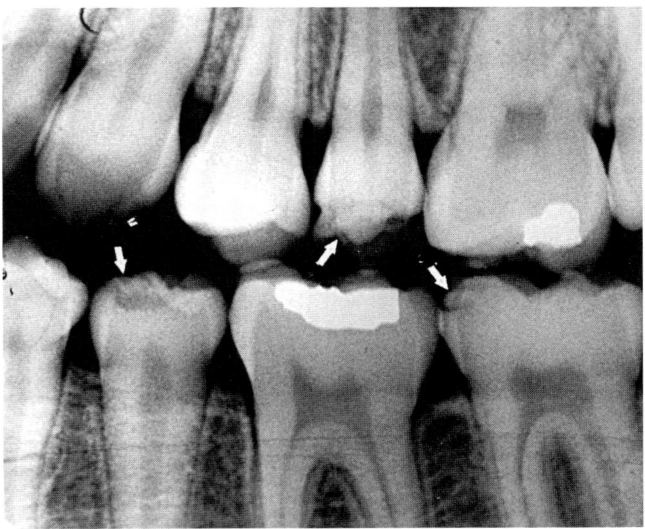

FIGURE 6–28.

Enamel Hypoplasia. Hypoplastic defects of the enamel mimic caries, as shown in the upper and lower second premolars and the mesial surface of the mandibular second molar (arrows).

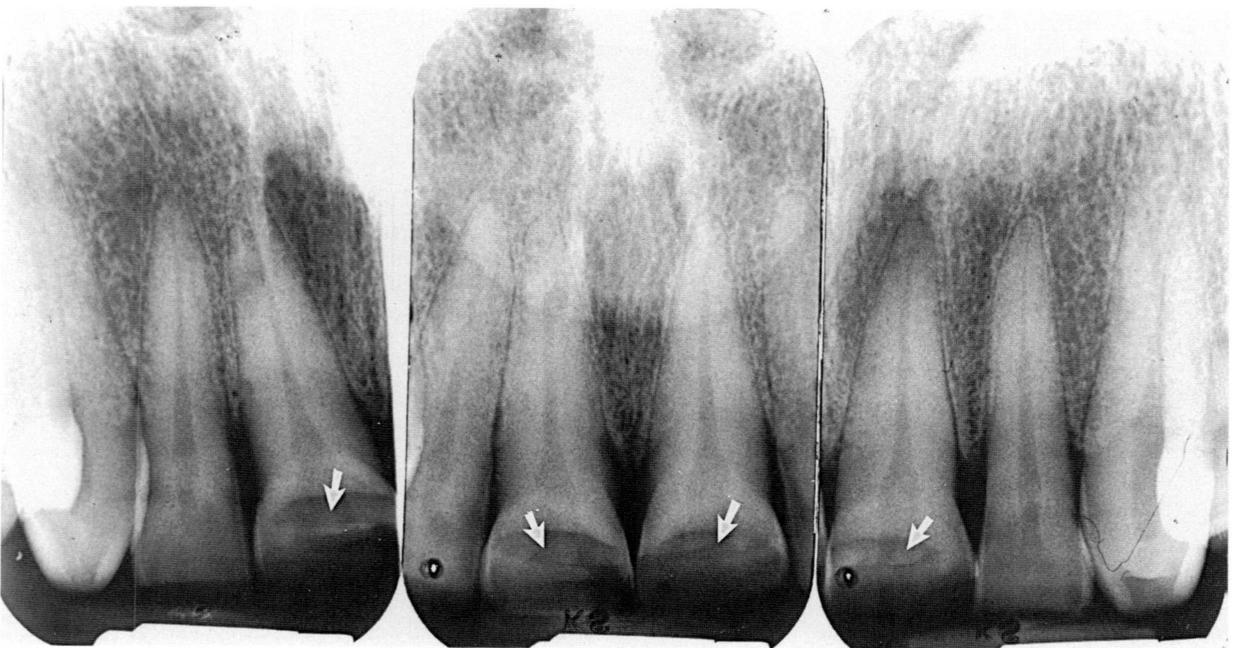

FIGURE 6–29.

Attrition. Severe attrition of the incisal surfaces of the lateral and central incisors mimics caries.

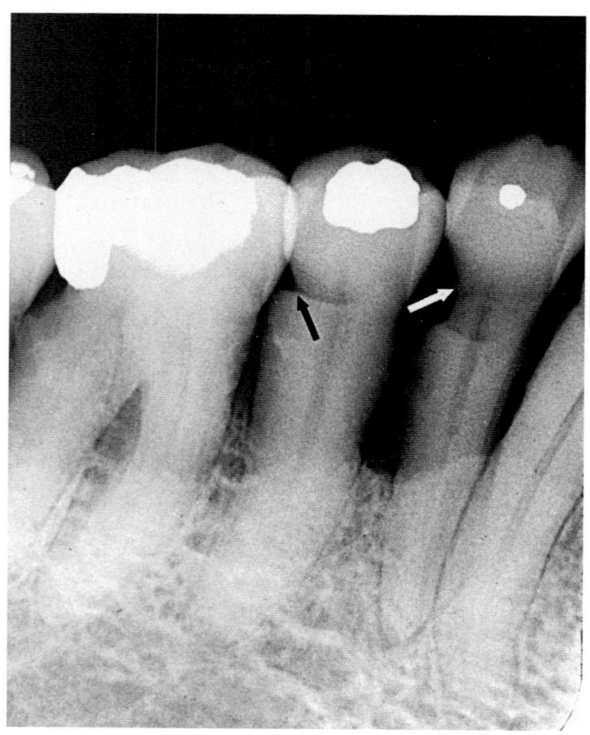

FIGURE 6–30.

Abrasion (Toothbrush). Toothbrush abrasion of the lower premolars (arrows).

small facet on a cusp or a ridge or a slight flattening of the incisal edge. Men are usually more prone to the wearing away of tooth surfaces than women, probably because of greater masticatory force in men. Variation also may be a result of differences in the coarseness of diet or of habits such as chewing tobacco or bruxism, either of which causes more rapid attrition of the teeth. When the enamel has been completely worn away and dentin exposed, a cavity in the tooth will appear. The attrition cavity on the occlusal surface of teeth may appear as dental caries on the radiograph (Fig. 6–29).

Abrasion is the abnormal wearing away of tooth substance by a mechanical process. This usually occurs on exposed root surfaces. The most common cause is the use of an abrasive dentifrice. Although modern dentifrices are not sufficiently abrasive to damage intact normal enamel, they can cause severe wear to cementum and dentin if the toothbrush is habitually used in a horizontal rather than a vertical direction. A V-shaped depression is created on the root side of the cementoenamel junction where there is some gingival recession. This V-shaped depression mimics carious lesions on the radiograph (Fig. 6–30). Other less common forms of abrasion may be related to the habit or the occupation of the patient such as holding bobby pins or nails between the teeth. The improper use of dental floss and toothpicks may also contribute to abrasive wearing away of the teeth.

Errors in Technique that Affect Caries Detection

Certain technical factors affect the ability of the dentist to detect carious lesions accurately. Some of the more important of these factors are discussed separately.

Common Errors in Exposure

The visual characteristics of radiographs, such as density and contrast, are important in the detection of caries.

Dark and Light Density Radiographs. The interpretation of dental caries is probably best done on films that have been slightly overexposed and therefore are a little darker than usual. Dark density films produce a dark carious area surrounded by a rather light density enamel that x-rays have difficulty penetrating. However, darker density films are not ordinarily satisfactory for the interpretation of other disease processes seen on the radiograph.

Peripheral Burnout. Overexposure of the peripheral surface of a tooth when low kilovoltages are used tends to burn out the enamel peripheral surface and thus can obliterate a carious lesion, especially a small or incipient enamel lesion. This phenomenon can be illustrated clinically. For instance, a space can be artificially widened between two teeth in proximal contact by increasing the exposure factors.

Long-Scale and Short-Scale Contrast. The desirable degree of contrast varies on the dental structures observed on the radiograph. The detection of carious lesions appears to be easier when kilovoltages in the range of 65 to 75 kVp are used. Kilovoltages above this level result in radiographs with a long-scale contrast in the radiograph that tends to impair the dentist's ability to observe the carious lesion. It is recommended that the bitewing radiograph be taken with a short-scale contrast technique between 65 and 75 kVp. It is more advantageous to expose radiographs for the detection of periapical and periodontal diseases with a higher kilovoltage technique. This produces a long-scale contrast radiograph, which is better for interpreting bony lesions.

Improper Angulation of X-Ray Beam

Improper angulation of the x-ray beam, both horizontal and vertical, frequently interferes with the detection of the interproximal carious lesions, particularly if they are small.

When the vertical angulation is increased more than it should be, the central x-ray is directed through the area of the carious lesion on the interproximal surface such that the carious lesion is superimposed on a great deal of sound tooth structure. This usually obliterates the lesion if it is small, so it cannot be seen on the radiograph.

Improper horizontal angulation can be defined as failure to project the x-ray beam accurately through the interproximal space or spaces of the teeth under observation. This faulty angulation results in superimposition of one adjacent tooth on another. Such improper angulation tends to hide the small interproximal carious lesion in the dense, superimposed enamel.

References

Backer Dirks O: Posteruptive changes in dental enamel. J Dent Res 45(Suppl 3):503, 1966.

Barmer DE: International comparative analysis of the findings in Yamanashi and in Onisi. In: Dental Care in Japan: Progressive Report on Yamanashi Survey of WHO/ICS. Tokyo:Ishiyaku, 1981.

Berry HM: Cervical burnout and Mach band: two shadows of doubt in radiologic interpretation of carious lesions. J Am Dent Assoc 106:622, 1983.

Bossert WA: The relation between the shape of the occlusal surface of molars and the prevalence of decay. J Dent Res 16:63, 1937.

Conference on the Declining Prevalence of Dental Caries. J Dent Res 61: Special Issue, 1982.

Dunning JM, Ferguson GW: Effect of bitewing roentgenograms on Navy dental examination findings. US Naval Med Bull 46:83, 1946.

Early PJ, Razzak MA, Dodee DB: Textbook of Nuclear Medicine Technology. 3rd Ed. St. Louis:CV Mosby, 1979, p. 379.

Fairbourn DR, Charbeneau GT, Loesche WJ: Effect of improved Dycal and IRM on bacteria in deep carious lesions. J Am Dent Assoc 100: 547, 1980.

Fitzgerald RJ: Gnotobiotic contribution to oral microbiology. J Dent Res 42:549, 1963.

Fitzgerald RJ, Keyes PH: Demonstration of the etiologic role of streptococci in experimental caries in the hamster. J Am Dent Assoc 61:9, 1960.

Fitzgerald RJ, Adams BO, Fitzgerald DB, Know KW: Cariogenicity of human plaque lactobacilli in gnotobiotic rats. J Dent Res 60:919, 1981.

Grondahl HG: Radiographic caries diagnosis and treatment decisions. Swed Dent J 3:109, 1979.

Hansen BF: Clinical and roentgenologic caries detection. Dentomaxillofac Radiol 9:34, 1980.

Haugejorden O: Study of the methods of radiologic diagnosis of dental caries in epidemiological investigations. Acta Odontol Scand (Suppl): 65, 1974.

Haugejorden O, Slack GL: The construction and use of diagnostic standards for radiographic caries incidence scores. Acta Odontol Scand 35:95, 1977.

Haugejorden O, Slack GL: A study of intra-examiner caries at different diagnostic levels. Acta Odontol Scand 33:169, 1975.

Ikeda T, Sandham HJ, Bradley EL Jr: Changes in streptococcus mutans and lactobacilli in relation to the initiation of dental caries in Negro children. Arch Oral Biol 18:556, 1973.

Loesche WJ, Straffon LH: Longitudinal investigation of the role of Streptococcus mutans in human fissure decay. Infect Immun 26:498, 1979.

Massler M, Pindborg JJ, Mohammed CA: A compilation of epidemiologic studies in dental caries. Am J Public Health 44:1357, 1954.

Mjor IA: Placement and replacement of restorations. Operative Dent 6:49, 1981.

Newbrun E: Cariology. 3rd Ed. Chicago:Quintessence, 1989a, p. 66.

Newbrun E: Cariology, 3rd Ed. Chicago:Quintessence, 1989b, p. 248.

Newbrun E, et al: Comparison of two screening tests for streptococcus mutants and evaluation of their suitability for mass screening and private practice. Commun Dent Oral Epidemiol 12:289, 1984.

Orland FJ, et al: The use of germ-free animal techniques in the study of experimental dental caries. I. Basic observations on rats reared free of all microorganisms. J Dent Res 33:147, 1954.

Orland FJ, et al: Experimental caries in germ-free rats inoculated with exterococci. J Am Dent Assoc 50:259, 1955.

Pitts NB: Monitoring of caries progression in permanent and primary posterior approximal enamel by bitewing radiography. Commun Dent Oral Epidemiol 11:228, 1983.

Schwartz M, Grondahl HG, Pliskin JS, Boffa JA: A longitudinal analysis from bitewing radiographs of the rate of progression of approximal carious lesions through human dental enamel. Arch Oral Biol 29:529, 1984.

Scott DB, Wyckoff RW: Studies of tooth surface structure by optical and electron microscopy. J Am Dent Assoc 39:276, 1949.

Silverstone LM: The relationship between the microscopic, histological and radiographic appearance of interproximal lesions in human teeth: an in vitro study using an artificial caries technique. In: Radiation exposure in pediatric dentistry. Pediatr Dent 3 (Special issue 2):414, 1982.

Sumney DL, Jordan HV, Englander HR: The prevalence of root surface caries in selected populations. J Periodontal 44:500, 1973.

Thylstrup A, Fejershov O: Textbook of Cariology. Copenhagen:Munksgaard, 1986, p. 1211.

Wagg BJ: ECSI: A new index for evaluating caries progression. Commun Dent Oral Epidemiol 2:219, 1974.

Zamir T, Fischer D, Fishel D, Sharav Y: A longitudinal radiographic study of the rate and spread of human approximal dental caries. Arch Oral Biol 21:523, 1976.

Suggested Readings

Aldous JA: Induced xerostomia and its relation to dental caries. J Dent Child 31:160, 1964.

Bahn SL: Drug-related dental destruction. Oral Surg 33:49, 1972.

Carlos JP, Gittelsohn AM: Longitudinal studies of the natural history of caries. II A life-table study of caries incidence in the permanent teeth. Arch Oral Biol 10:739, 1965.

Daniels TE, et al: The oral component of Sjogren's syndrome. Oral Surg 39:876, 1975.

Dreizen S, Daley TE, Diane JB, Brown LR: Oral complications of cancer radiotherapy. Postgrad Med 61:86, 1977.

Frank RM, Herdly J, Phillippe, E: Acquired dental defects and salivary gland lesions after irradiation from carcinoma. J Am Dent Assoc 70: 868, 1978.

Hager SP, Chilton NW, Mumma RD Jr: The problem of root caries. I. Literature review and clinical description. J Am Dent Assoc 86:137, 1973.

Jordan HV, Hammond, BF: Filamentous bacteria isolated from human root surface caries. Arch Oral Biol 17:1333, 1972.

Kermoil M, Walsh RF: Dental caries after radiotherapy of the oral regions. J Am Dent Assoc 91:838, 1975.

Keyes PH: The infections and transmissible nature of experimental dental caries: findings and implications. Arch Oral Biol 1:304, 1960.

Loesche WJ: Dental Caries: A Treatable Infection. Springfield, IL:Charles C Thomas, 1982.

Loesche WJ, Rowan J, Straffon LH, Loos PJ: Association of streptococcus mutans with human dental decay. Infect Immun 11:1252, 1975.

Mandel ID: Dental Caries. Am Sci 67:661, 1979.

Nesbitt WE, et al: Association of protein with the cell wall of streptococcus mutans. Infect Immun 28:118, 1980.

Onoce H, Sandham HJ: pH changes during culture of human dental plaque streptococci on mitis-salivarius agar. Arch Oral Biol 21:291, 1976.

Page L, Friend B: Level of the use of sugars in the U.S.. In: Sugars in Nutrition. New York:Sipple and McNutt, 1974, p. 93.

Shannon IL, Gibson WA, Terry JM: Caries experience in the U.S. Air Force. J Public Health Dent 26:206, 1960.

Shklaiv IL, Keene HJ, Collen P: The distribution of streptococcus mutans on the teeth of 2 groups of naval recruits. Arch Oral Biol 19:199, 1974.

Stephan RM: Clinical study of the etiology and control of rampant caries. In: 49th General Session of the International Association for Dental Research, 1971, Abstract 636, p. 211.

Stralfors A: Investigations into the bacterial chemistry of dental plaques. Odontol T 58:156, 1950.

Syed SA, Loesche WJ, Pape HL, Grenier E: Predominant cultivable flora isolated from human root surface plaque. Infect Immun 11:727, 1975.

van Houte J: Bacterial specificity in the etiology of dental caries. Int Dent J 30:305, 1980.

Chapter 7

Radiologic Diagnosis of Pulpal and Periapical Disease

PULPAL CAVITY

The pulp cavity is the central cavity within a tooth and is entirely enclosed by dentin except at the apical foramen. The pulp cavity may be divided into a coronal portion, the pulp chamber, and a radicular portion, the root canal. The roof of the pulp chamber refers to the dentin immediately bounding the pulp chamber, occlusally or incisally. The pulp horn is an accentuation of the roof of the pulp chamber directly under the cusp or developmental lobe. It refers more commonly to the prolongation of the pulp itself directly under a cusp.

The floor of the pulp chamber runs somewhat parallel to the roof and refers to the dentin bounding the pulp chamber near the cervix of the tooth, particularly that forming the furcation area in molar teeth.

Primary (Developmental) Dentin (Figs. 7–1 and 7–2)

The dentin of a young tooth is called primary (developmental) dentin and is formed during tooth development. In the young, the pulp horns are long, the pulp chamber is large, the root canals are wide, and the apical foramen is broad.

Physiologic (Functional) Secondary Dentin (Fig. 7–3)

The dentin formed physiologically after the root is fully developed is referred to as secondary (functional) dentin. The secondary dentin is deposited circumpulpally at a very slow rate throughout the life of the vital tooth. As the tooth matures, the tooth responds to stimuli associated with normal biologic function (mastication, small thermal changes, chemical irritants, and slight traumas) to deposit secondary dentin over the pulpal end of the tubules of primary dentin.

Continued formation of secondary dentin throughout life gradually reduces the size of the pulp chamber and root canals (Fig. 7–3A). Although dentin formation tends to occur on all surfaces with age, the formation of dentin on various walls of the pulp chamber is not uniform. More dentin is laid down on the floor and roof in the molars, making the chamber almost disklike in configuration (Fig. 7–3B).

Reparative (Irregular) Dentin (Figs. 7–4 and 7–5)

Dentin produced in response to the injury of primary odontoblasts has been known by a number of names: irregular secondary dentin, irritation dentin, adventitious dentin, tertiary dentin, and reparative dentin.

Anything that exposes dentin to the oral cavity has the potential for increased dentin formation at the base of the tubules in the underlying pulp. Causes of such dentin exposures include caries, periodontal disease, abrasion, erosion, attrition, cavity preparation, root planning, and cusp fractures.

Generally, the dentin that responds to surface dentin irritants is an irregular type of dentin—thus the term "irregular dentin." Compared with primary dentin, "reparative/irregular" dentin is less tubular and irregular, and the tubules have larger lumina. In some cases of reparative/irregular dentin, no tubules are formed.

The ability of the pulp to form irregular secondary (reparative) dentin is a fundamental defense mechanism. This is nature's way of "sealing off" cut or diseased dentinal tubules at the pulp surface. Thus, irregular secondary dentin formation makes it possible for the tooth to defend itself against the effects of attrition, dental caries, and other forms of trauma.

To briefly review this type of dentin, the most commonly applied term for irregularly formed dentin is reparative dentin, presumably because it forms so frequently in response to injury and appears to be a component of the reparative process. Reparative dentin occurs at the pulpal surface of primary or secondary dentin formation at sites corresponding to areas of irritation. For instance, when a carious lesion has invaded dentin, the pulp usually responds by depositing a layer of reparative dentin over the dentinal tubules of the primary or secondary dentin that communicates with the carious lesion. Also, when occlusal wear from attrition removes enamel and exposes the dentin to the oral environment, reparative dentin is deposited over the exposed tubules (Fig. 7–4).

How can reparative dentin be recognized? In most cases, the irritants responsible for the formation of reparative dentin will be recognized readily and include caries, restorations, attrition, abrasion, or fractures. Each of these result in dentin exposure and irritation to the underlying pulp. The second means of recognition is by carefully viewing the radiographs and focusing on regions of the pulp under the areas of dentin irritation and exposure (Fig. 7–5).

Constriction of part of the root canal occurs as an isolated deformity affecting one or several teeth. It results from trauma in most instances, although gross attrition may produce similar pulpal obliteration of root canals. Its only possible significance is that endodontic treatment may be difficult to perform if it becomes necessary.

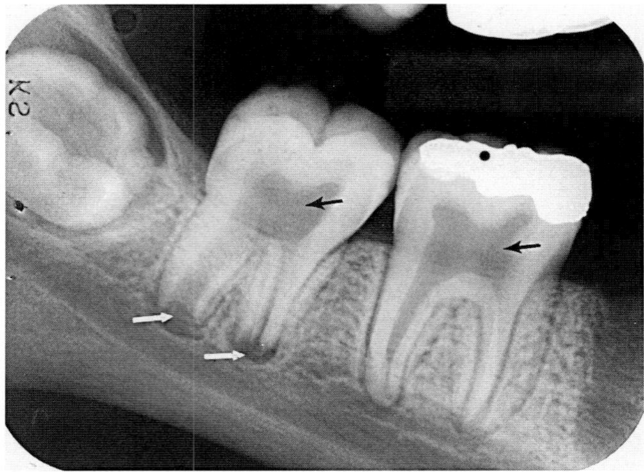

FIGURE 7–1.

Enlarged pulp. Enlarged pulp (black arrows) of teenager, with the apical foramen of the second molar not closed yet (white arrows).

Dentinal Sclerosis (Figs. 7–6 and 7–7)

Dentinal sclerosis is produced by milder or moderately irritating agents, such as slowly progressing chronic caries, the mild acute injury of cavity preparation, abrasion, erosion, attrition, and changes resulting from age. The formation of sclerotic dentin is minimal in rapidly advancing acute caries.

The term "transparent dentin" has been applied to sclerotic dentin because of the peculiar transparent appearance of the tooth structure when a ground section is viewed by transmitted light. Sclerotic dentin may be considered a defensive mechanism of the pulpodentinal complex because its formation alters the permeability of the dentinal tubules, blocking access of irritants to the pulp.

Dentinal sclerosis is the cumulative effect of several factors, including peritubular dentin formation by the dentinoblastic processes (physiologic sclerosis) and intratubular calcification (pathologic sclerosis).

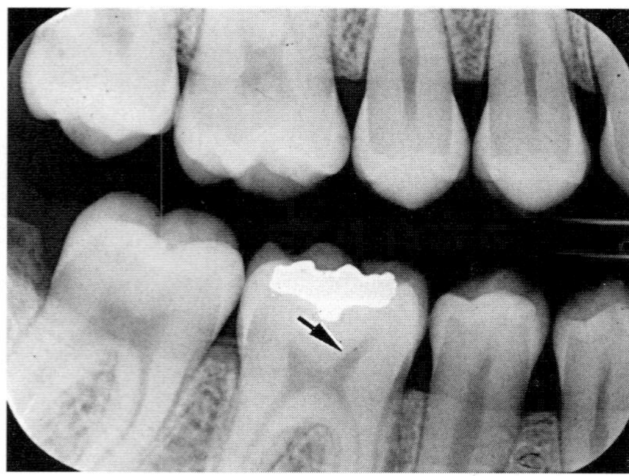

FIGURE 7–2.

Enlarged pulp of mandibular first molar. Notice the long narrow pulp horn of the mandibular first molar (arrow).

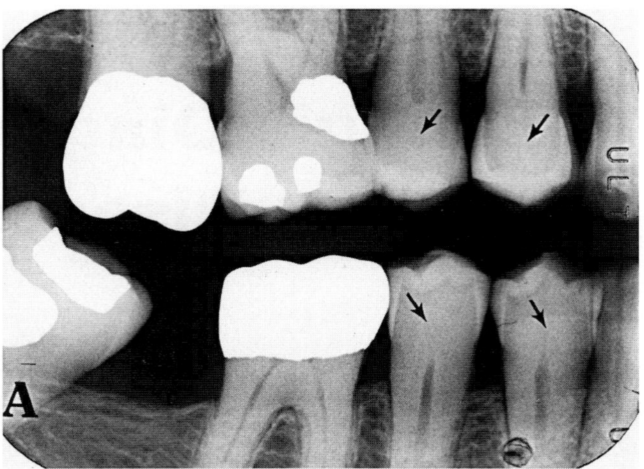

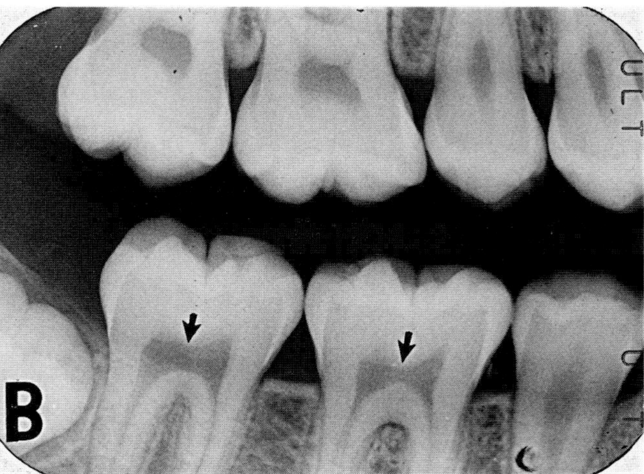

FIGURE 7–3.

Pulpal cavity. A, As a person grows older, physiologic secondary dentin is laid down as a response to stimuli associated with the normal aging process. See the amount of dentin laid down in the coronal portion of the premolars (arrows). B, Notice the disklike configuration of the pulp chambers of the mandibular molars because of the predominance of secondary dentin formation on the roof and floor of the chamber (arrows).

Peritubular dentin (physiologic sclerosis) is a calcified secretion of the dentinoblastic process. As a result of peritubular dentin formation and intratubular calcification (pathologic sclerosis), the dentinal tubules become narrower and ultimately close completely (sclerosis).

Intratubular calcification (pathologic sclerosis) is a physiochemical process caused by precipitation of mineral salt within the dentinal tubules and, therefore, is fundamentally different from peritubular dentin. This type of calcification is found in the translucent zone of carious dentin and in the dentin of severe attrition, erosion, and abrasion. One of the sources of the calcium salts of pathologic sclerosis is recrystallized calcium and phosphate ions that were dissolved previously during the demineralization of caries. In some areas of the dentin, the x-ray absorption of the sclerotic dentin

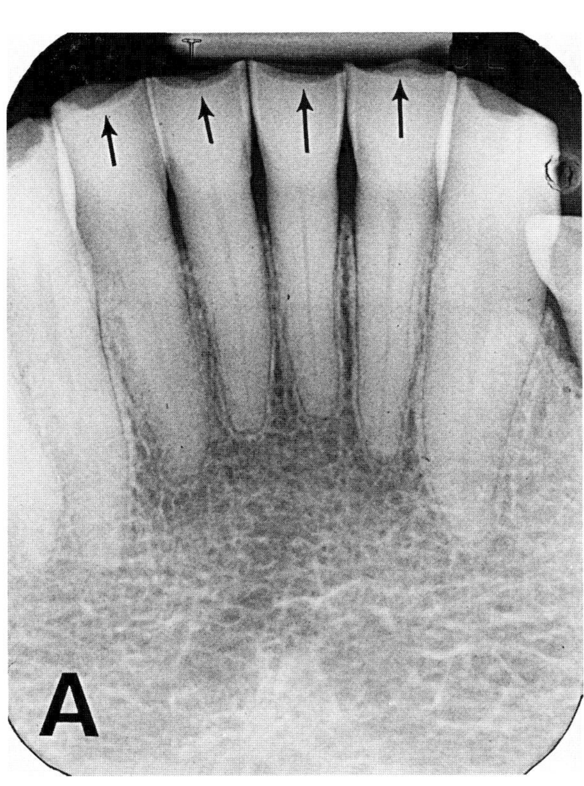

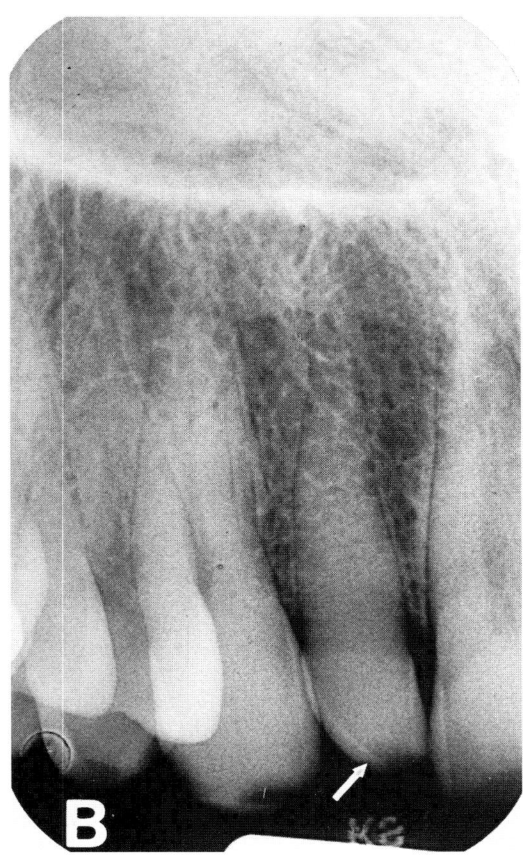

FIGURE 7–4.

Reparative/irregular dentin. A, When attrition removes enamel and exposes the dentin to the oral cavity, reparative dentin forms to reduce the size of the pulps. Notice the reduced size of the pulps of these mandibular incisor teeth from reparative dentin formation as a result of attrition. There is evidence of attrition of the incisal edges of the mandibular incisors (arrows). B, Notice the reduction of pulp in the "peg" lateral incisor (arrow).

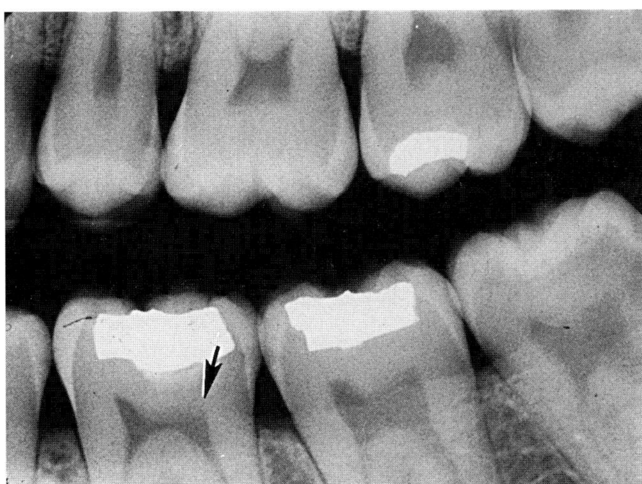

FIGURE 7–5.

Reparative/irregular dentin. Notice reduction of the distal horn of the pulp chamber of the mandibular first molar (arrow); most likely, it is deposition of reparative dentin in response to distal proximal caries in the tooth and occlusal cavity preparation.

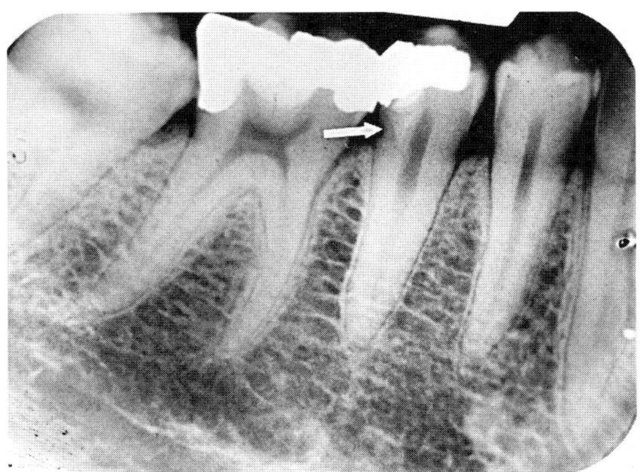

FIGURE 7–6.

Sclerotic dentin. Notice sclerotic dentin under the DO restoration of the lower second premolar (arrow).

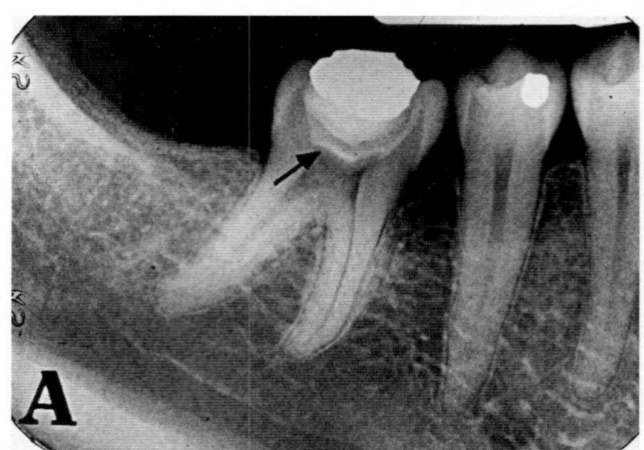

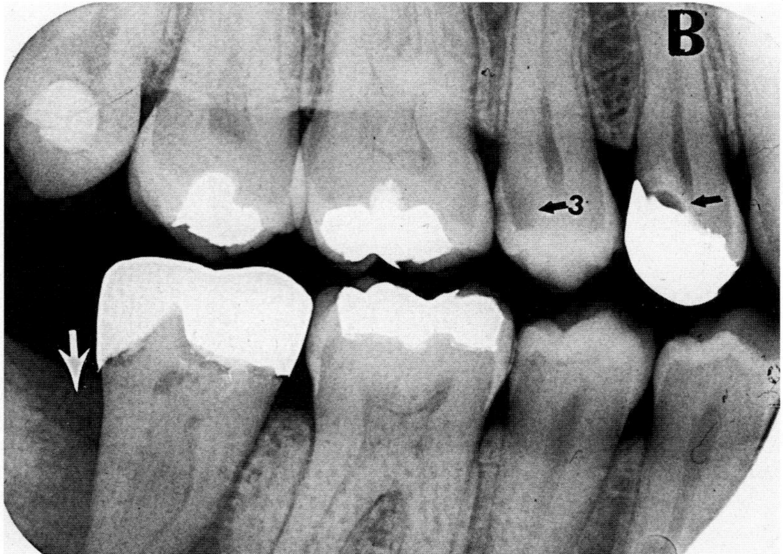

FIGURE 7–7.

Sclerotic dentin. A, Notice sclerotic dentin under the indirect pulp capping procedure in the lower first molar (arrow). B, Notice sclerotic dentin under the indirect pulp capping procedure in the maxillary first premolar (black arrow). Also, there is a class 3 caries in the distal upper second premolar (3, arrow). The lower second molar has a chronic apical abscess with a passageway for free drainage through PDL on this distal (white arrow).

will increase 10 to 25% compared with normal dentin and appear more radiopaque in the radiographs.

In the presence of recurrent caries beneath an amalgam restoration, zinc ions are released and are incorporated into the sclerotic dentin to contribute greatly to its radiopaque appearance. The calcium content of such sclerotic dentin may be diminished.

Dentinal Bridging

This is a layer or bridge of secondary dentin forming over exposed pulpal tissue as a response to vital pulp therapies such as indirect and direct pulp capping and pulpotomy procedures. Supposedly, this is radiographic evidence of success of a vital pulp procedure.

What causes the development of a dentinal bridge? Do the odontoblasts that are laterally disposed along the pulp cavity wall move up toward the area of exposed pulpal tissue and "close ranks," or do new odontoblasts form from the connective tissue cells of the pulp? Grossman (1974) believed the latter explanation was probably more plausible.

Mills (1953) showed that new odontoblasts develop from fibroblasts, are stimulated to activity, and form a calcific barrier or dentin bridge.

In evaluating the histologic sections of teeth with dentinal bridging, Mullaney and colleagues (1966) found some areas with considerable dentinoid bridging, whereas others in the same tooth showed the absence of complete bridging and sites of necrosis. These authors pointed out the fallacy of determining success on the basis of radiographs alone, which could not possibly show whether the dentin bridge had been complete. Therefore, the finding of a dentin bridge does not always indicate success by itself and negate the need for additional evaluation.

PULPAL OPACITIES OR CALCIFICATIONS

Pulp calcifications are found in healthy and aging pulps, and their incidence increases with age. They are found with such frequency that it is questionable whether they represent a pathologic state or merely an occurrence within the range of normal biologic variation.

A number of studies have been performed to determine the actual incidence of pulp calcifications, and the results of the investigations mostly are in agreement. Stones (1962) stated that pulpal calcifications are present in 66% of people 10 to 20 years of age and 90% of people older than 50 years. These figures refer to histologic investigation, not to radiographic identification.

Willman (1934) reported calcifications in 87% of 164 teeth selected at random. He pointed out that only 15% of the calcifications are large enough to be seen on the radiograph.

There is no apparent difference in frequency of occurrence either between sexes or among various teeth in the dental arch.

Calcifications in the pulp may appear as rough, circular, nodular areas (denticles, pulp stones) or diffuse, irregular, calcific deposits. The nodular type of pulp stone is classified by some as a false or true denticle. True denticles (pulp stones) are thought to be localized masses of calcified tissue that resemble dentin because of their tubular structure. They are seen rarely on the radiograph because they seldom get larger than 1 mm in diameter. False denticles (pulp stones) are composed of localized masses of calcified material, and they do not exhibit dentinal tubules. They appear to be composed of concentric layers or lamellae deposited around a central nidus. False denticles occur more commonly in pulp chambers and are generally much larger than true denticles. In fact, they occasionally may fill the entire pulp chamber.

Johnson and Bevelander (1956) concluded from their studies that a differentiation between "true" and "false" denticles should not be drawn because all denticles originally show no tubules and they subsequently may become surrounded by tissue containing dentinal tubules.

Diffuse calcifications generally are seen more commonly in the root canal but may be seen in the pulp chamber. This type of calcification usually is called "dystrophic calcification," which is a deposition of calcium salts in dead or degenerating tissue. It may result from local alkalinity of the destroyed tissue that attracts the salts.

Pulp stones within the pulp chamber may reach a considerable size and, although they may not block a canal orifice totally, they often make it difficult to locate the canal openings. These large pulp stones may be free or attached and usually are removed during access preparation. Calcifications may be a problem when in the pulp canal; however, they rarely form a barrier to instrument passage. The use of chelating agents has facilitated this operation greatly.

Ehlers-Danlos syndrome is a hereditary disorder of the connective tissue closely related to Marfans syndrome, osteogenesis imperfecta, and pseudoxanthoma elasticum. The main diagnostic features of Ehlers-Danlos syndrome are hyperelasticity of the skin, loose joints, and fragility of skin and blood vessels. Radiographically, in patients with Ehlers-Danlos syndrome, the teeth may have stunted and deformed roots and large pulp stones in the coronal part of the pulp chamber.

◆ *RADIOLOGY (Figs. 7–8 and 7–9)*

Calcifications of the pulp appear in the radiograph as radiopaque structures within the pulp chamber and root canal. There is no radiographic appearance common to all manifestations of calcifications in the pulp. Although pulp stones are usually in the chamber and diffuse calcifications within the radicular pulp, the reverse also may occur.

When the calcifications have reached a certain size, they can be recognized on the radiograph. It is very common to find several or many teeth with pupal calcification. The size of the pulpal calcifications of different teeth varies greatly.

Pulp stones are spherical or rounded and usually have a sharply defined margin. The nodular mass has the same radiographic density as dentin, and the pulp cavity gradually expands above and below the mass (Fig. 7–8).

The pulp stones seen most readily in the radiograph are those that have formed while the pulp chamber was still large early in life. If the pulp calcifications reach an appreciable size early in life, the pulp chamber is reduced in size and, therefore, there may be only slight or no alteration in the appearance of the pulp even many decades later. A radiolucent line separating the pulp stone from the pulpal wall may be seen, although when opaque bodies are present in molar teeth, they may appear to be attached to the floor of the pulp chamber because in some instances they actually may be.

Diffuse calcifications usually represent a single mass of calcified tissue with margins less sharply defined and less homogeneous than the pulp stone (denticle). The entire pulp tissue or only part of it may show these densities (Fig. 7–9). Many small irregular densities may occupy the pulp chamber alone or extend into the canal.

There are two conditions that may be confused with the single pulp stone (nodule). One is the enameloma, or "enamel pearl." A common site for the enamel pearl is at the cementoenamel junction, where often it is projected over the image of the pulp cavity and may be misinterpreted as a pulp stone. The two conditions can be differentiated with different projections; if the condition is an enamel pearl, it will move out of the pulp cavity image area in the second projection.

The other confusing radiographic appearance results from

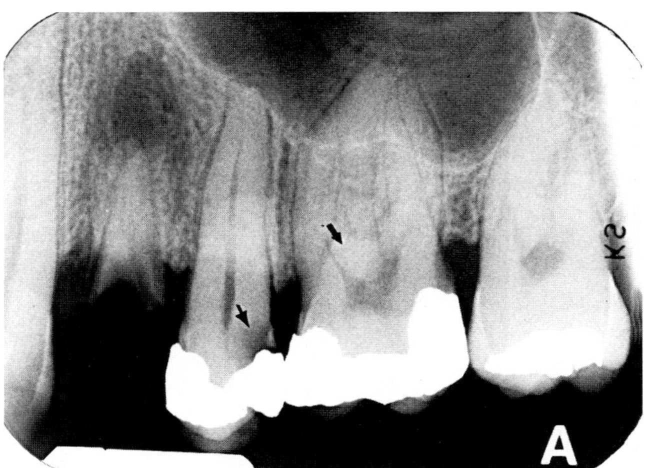

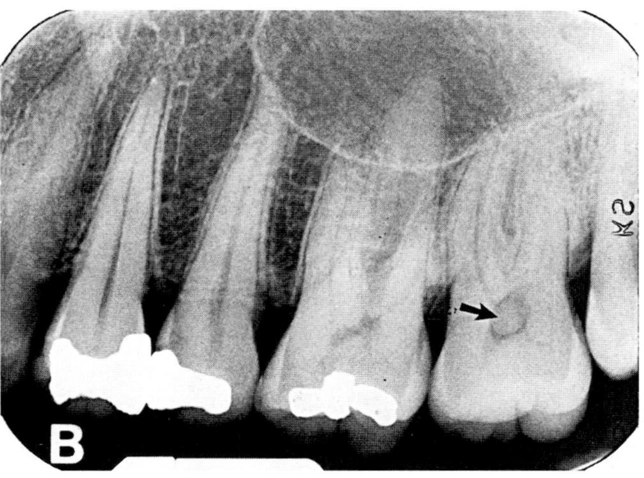

FIGURE 7–8.

Pulp stones. A, Pulp stones (denticles). There is a large pulp stone (denticle) in the pulp chamber of the maxillary first molar (arrow). See the recurrent caries under the DO restoration in the second premolar (arrow). B, Notice the pulp stone in the maxillary second molar.

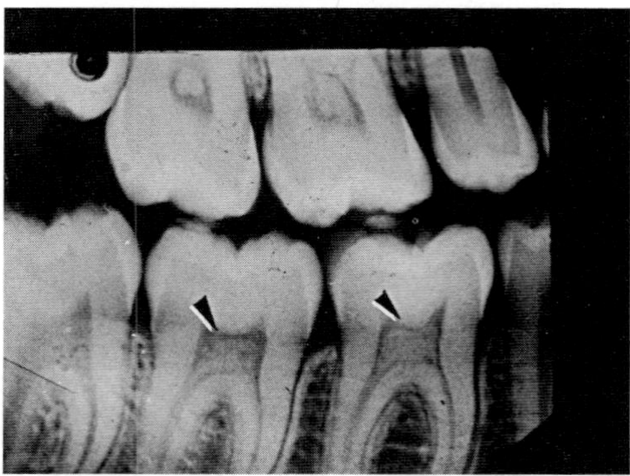

FIGURE 7–9.

Diffuse pulpal calcifications. The lower first and second molars have diffuse pulpal calcifications (arrowheads).

the projection of the two roots of a lower molar in such a manner that, at the bifurcation, the roots are superimposed partially over each other. When the adjacent portions of the roots overlay each other, it produces an image with increased density (whiteness), which is more or less rounded. This rounded white (radiopaque) area looks very much like a pulp stone; however, because it lies deep to the floor of the pulp chamber, it should not be mistaken for a pulp stone or nodule. A properly made radiograph eliminates this rounded, white image.

PULPAL ENLARGEMENT

Relative pulpal enlargement is a normal finding in newly erupted teeth. If only one tooth is affected, the clinician should suspect that an altered vitality has caused the tooth to stop developing. A clue to this situation is the blunderbuss or wide-open apex of the involved tooth. Endodontic treatment may consist of a pulpotomy initially to stimulate apex closure (apexification), followed by routine endodontic treatment. Because, normally, the pulp chamber gradually becomes smaller as a person grows older, the pulp can be considered abnormally large if its size does not conform to that for a given age or if it is abnormally large as compared with pulps of other teeth in the same patient.

In some instances, for reasons unknown, the pulp cavities undergo only a very slight reduction in size and remain abnormally large into adult life. Kronfeld and Boyle (1949) and others have discussed the individual reactions of pulps and have called attention to the fact that some show a weak defensive reaction by a failure to form secondary dentin. The factors that determine or regulate these individual variations are unknown. These teeth are susceptible to early pulpal involvement by caries and accidental mechanical exposure during routine operative procedures.

Pulpal enlargement may be present as developmental anomalies in teeth only, including taurodontism, regional odontodysplasia (ghost teeth), dentinogenesis imperfecta type III (shell teeth), and coronal dentinal dysplasia, type II (thistle-tube pulps). Generalized large pulps may be associated with metabolic diseases such as vitamin D-resistant rickets (familial hypophosphatemia), a defect in renal phosphate metabolism, and hypophosphatasia (low phosphatase rickets), an inborn error of metabolism with lowered phosphatase activity of the serum.

Witkop discussed the manifestations of genetic diseases in the human pulp in a comprehensive article in 1971.

◆ *RADIOLOGY (Fig. 7–10)*

The identification of enlarged pulps is of clinical significance because of the factors previously discussed. Panoramic radiographs are especially useful in classifying the condition as localized or generalized. The localized form is obvious when advanced. Minimal manifestations are best identified by comparing the tooth with its neighbors or with its opposite member on the other side of the arch. Generalized pulp enlargement may be suspected when the size of the pulp is unusual or inconsistent with the patient's age. This may be a clinical sign of systemic disease. A peculiarity of hypophosphatasia (low phosphatase rickets) is that the walls of the enlarged pulp spaces are parallel to each other, thus producing a characteristic picture.

In vitamin D-resistant rickets (familial hypophosphatemia), Archard and Witkop (1966), Gigliotti and associates (1971), and Finn (1973) reported that the primary teeth have large canals and a large pulp chamber, with pulp horns extending to the dentinoenamel junction.

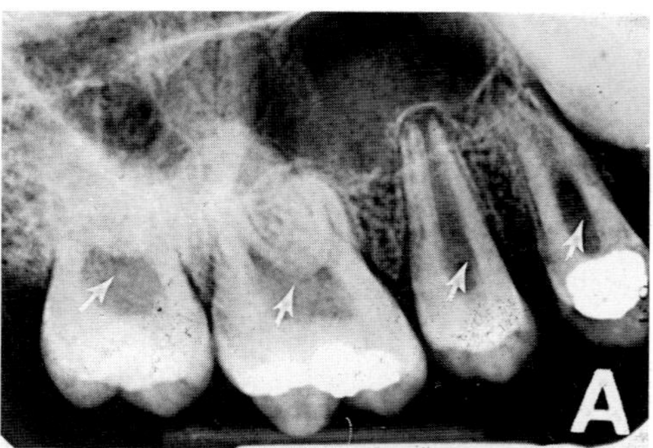

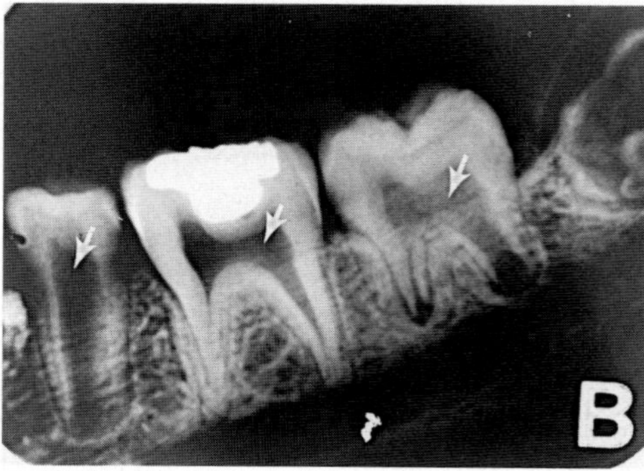

FIGURE 7–10.

Idiopathic pulpal enlargement. Fourteen-year-old boy with generalized abnormally large pulps (arrows). The cause is unknown because the patient had normal teeth otherwise, and results of his blood workup were normal. A, Right maxillary posteriors. B, Left mandibular molar.

PULP OBLITERATION

This phenomenon may be found in two forms: generalized and local pulp obliteration. In the absence of other tooth deformities, the generalized form is probably part of the aging process and usually is seen in older people. If only one tooth is involved, especially in a younger person, it usually is a sign of the altered vitality of the pulp. This may be seen after trauma to a tooth that did not fracture and may be analogous to internal resorption; however, in this case the stimulus, possibly anachoretic inflammation (noxious stimuli from blood), causes the injured pulp to lay down odontoblasts at an accelerated rate, thus attempting "self" or natural endodontia. Generalized pulp chamber obliteration in adults, along with a ground glass trabecular pattern and loss of the lamina dura, are suggestive of secondary hyperparathyroidism (renal osteodystrophy). Generalized pulpal obliteration also is seen in dentinogenesis imperfecta.

Naastrom and associates (1985) reported on the narrowing of the dental pulp studied radiologically in 51 patients with renal diseases. Two thirds of the patients had terminal uremia and were treated by renal transplantation or hemodialysis. The remaining patients were nonuremic and treated with immunosuppressants because of progressive renal diseases. There were significantly more patients with narrowing of the dental pulp chamber among the transplant recipients than among the other patients. Renal transplantation implies the use of higher doses of corticosteroids and cytotoxic medication. The amount of corticosteroids received and the pharmacokinetics seemed to be essential factors in the initiation of narrowing of the dental pulp chamber.

Jacobsen and Kerekes examined 122 traumatized teeth with radiographic evidence of abnormal hard tissue formation in the pulp cavity. The patients were 10 to 23 years of age (mean, 16 years) at the time of injury. Partial obliteration (pulp chamber not discernible, root canal significantly narrowed but clearly visible) had occurred in 36% of the teeth. Normal periradicular conditions were found in all teeth with partial obliterations. Sixty-four percent of the teeth were totally obliterated. Pathologic periapical changes indicating pulp necrosis as a sequel to the total obliteration were observed in 21% of these cases. The late development of pulpal necrosis was related significantly to teeth classified as severely impaired and to teeth with complete root formation at the time of injury.

◆ *RADIOLOGY (Figs. 7–11 to 7–13)*

The pulp chamber alone, the root canal alone, or the whole of the pulp cavity sometimes is partially or completely obliterated. This may be developmental or acquired. Congenital effacement of the root canal alone or in association with the pulp chamber usually results from dentinogenesis imperfecta and involves many or all of the teeth.

Acquired gross diminution of the pulp cavity, whether it is complete or partial, results from trauma in most instances, although gross attrition of the teeth may produce similar or less significant obliteration. There are times when trauma from orthodontic movement of teeth can cause pulpal obliteration and periapical abnormalities (Fig. 7–11). The maxillary central is the tooth injured most often from trauma, and it is also the tooth that shows obliteration of the pulp cavity most frequently (Fig. 7–12). Rarely, a posterior tooth shows the change. The whole pulp cavity may be replaced by tissue with a density equal to that of the normal dentin, or small remnants of the pulp may persist as a thin line of radiolucency in the root (Fig. 7–13).

If more than two teeth show the change in the pulp cavity, the possibility of a developmental anomaly should be considered.

HYPERCEMENTOSIS (Cementum Hyperplasia)

Cementum is formed on permanent teeth throughout life. Hypercementosis is the excessive formation of secondary cementum on the root surfaces. It is the abnormal increase in thickness of cementum, which may affect single teeth or the entire dentition.

The increased formation of cementum occurs mainly on the apical two thirds of the root, although in some instances the cementum formation is focal, occurring only on the apex of the tooth.

In a German population sample of 22,226 outpatients (average age, 42 years), Schehl (1966) reported that 1.7% showed radiographic evidence of hypercementosis. The mandibular first molars were affected most frequently by hypercementosis, followed by the mandibular and maxillary second premolars and mandibular first premolars. Mandibular teeth were affected 2.5 times more often than maxillary teeth.

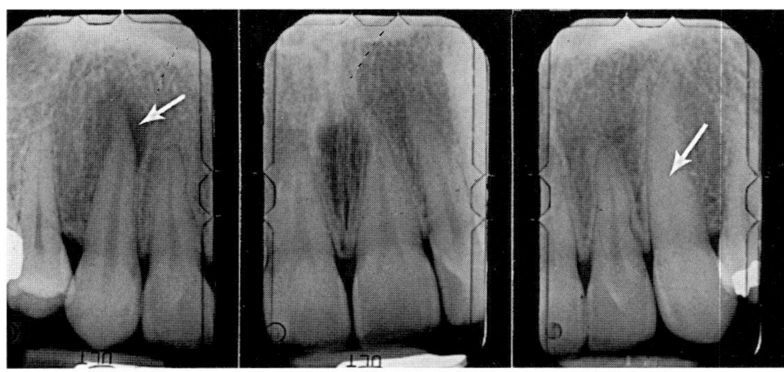

FIGURE 7–11.

Pulpal disturbances from orthodontic treatment. Patient with a history of previous orthodontic treatment showing periapical abnormalities associated with the maxillary right canine and pulpal obliteration in the maxillary left canine (arrows). This shows that pulpal tissue can respond to trauma by laying down reparative dentin, or, in other cases, the trauma may cause a necrotic response to the pulp, resulting in periapical disease.

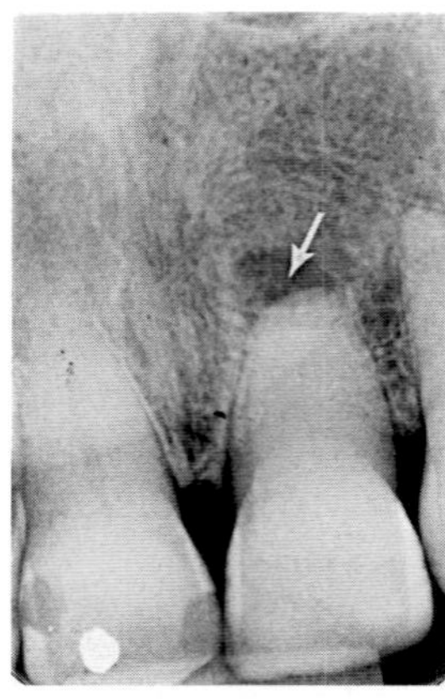

FIGURE 7–12.

Pulpal obliteration from trauma. Maxillary left central pulpal obliteration as a result of trauma (arrow). Notice that there is radiographic evidence of apical external resorption and periapical radiolucency.

The histologic study of teeth with hypercementosis shows that the cementum formed is usually osteocementum (acellular cementum).

Although some cases of hypercementosis are idiopathic, certain circumstances favor the association with hypercementosis, including the following: (1) supraeruption of a tooth because of the loss of an antagonist tooth, (2) inflammation at the apex of a tooth, (3) traumatic occlusion, and (4) systemic diseases such as Paget's disease, toxic goiter, acromegaly, and giantism.

Supraeruption of a tooth because of loss of an antagonist is accompanied by hypercementosis, apparently as a result of an inherent tendency for the maintenance of the normal width of the periodontal ligament.

Periapical inflammation resulting from pulpal infection sometimes stimulates excessive formation of cementum. The cementum is not laid down at the apex of the tooth directly adjacent to the area of inflammation. Instead, the cementum is laid down on the tooth surfaces some distance from the apex of the tooth, forming a collar-shaped hypercementosis.

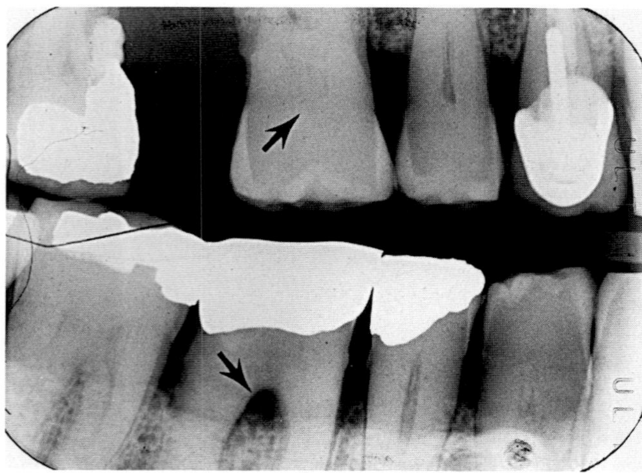

FIGURE 7–13.

Pulpal obliteration, localized. The pulp chamber and root canal are effaced by deposition of reparative dentin in the upper first molar (arrow). See furcation involvement of lower first molar (arrow).

The collar shape results from the fact that irritation from chronic apical periodontitis decreases with increasing distance from the apex. At a certain point, it acts as a stimulant for cementum formation, rather than as an inhibitor.

Rushton and Cooke (1959) stated that mild traumatic occlusions may cause hypercementosis. In rare cases, excessive occlusal trauma may lead to the formation of serrated hypercementosis (cemental spikes), which follows the course of Sharpey's fibers.

Paget's disease is a generalized disease of bone that is characterized by the formation of excessive amounts of secondary cementum on the tooth roots. Although the bone changes in Paget's disease are quite characteristic, generalized hypercementosis always should suggest the possibility that Paget's disease may be present.

Teeth with hypercementosis have no significant clinical signs or symptoms. The only practical clinical significance of hypercementosis is the difficulties that may be encountered in extracting such teeth. This may indicate the true biologic significance of hypercementosis, which probably is to anchor the tooth in the socket more securely.

◆ *RADIOLOGY (Figs. 7–14 to 7–16)*

Radiographically, hypercementosis is distinguished by the thickening and blunting of the roots of teeth. The tooth apices lose their typical ''pointed'' appearance and appear rounded (Fig. 7–14).

Hypercementosis is associated with low-grade chronic periapical infection (Fig. 7–15) and supraeruption of a tooth that has lost its antagonist. There are two types: (1) a nodular or bulbous enlargement near or at the root apex, and (2) a

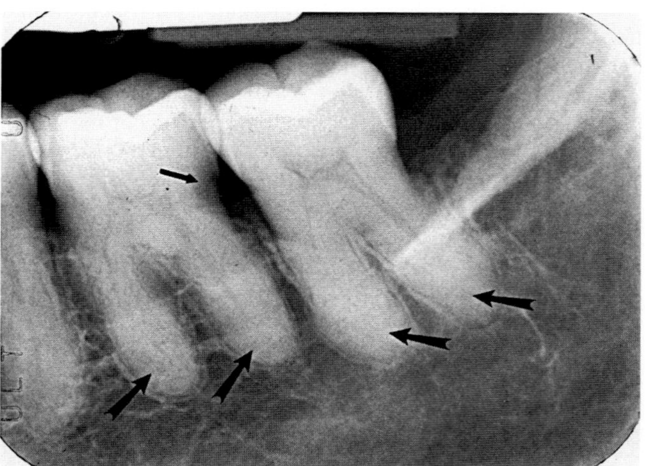

FIGURE 7–14.

Hypercementosis (dense cemental type). Hypercementosis with symmetric enlargement of entire roots of first and second molars (lower arrows). In this case, there is no difference in the radiodensity of the root dentin from primary or secondary cementum. Therefore, the radiographic diagnosis of hypercementosis is established by the shape or outline of the roots. Notice the area of possible root caries at the distal of the first molar (upper arrow). This should be checked with an explorer.

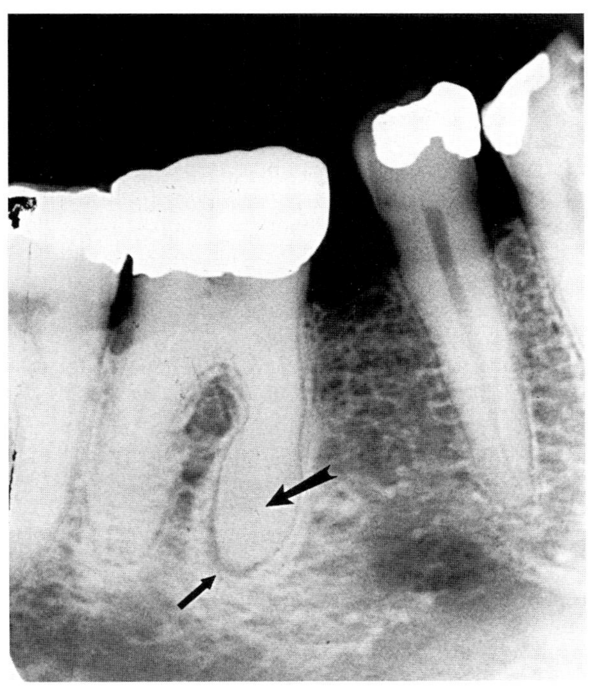

FIGURE 7–15.

Hypercementosis (low-grade chronic periapical infection). Nodular type of hypercementosis of first molar mesial root tip (large arrow). Probably caused by periapical inflammation (small arrow).

symmetric enlargement that involves all of the root surface. There are two symmetric enlargement types: (1) the secondary cementum is of the same density as the primary cementum and dentin (Fig. 7–16), and (2) the secondary cementum appears less dense and is clearly differentiated from the primary cementum and dentin (Fig. 7–16). In hypercementosis, the periodontal ligament space and lamina dura are continuous and surround the region of the hypercementosis; in periapical cemental dysplasia, the lesion is in the bone and not attached to the tooth.

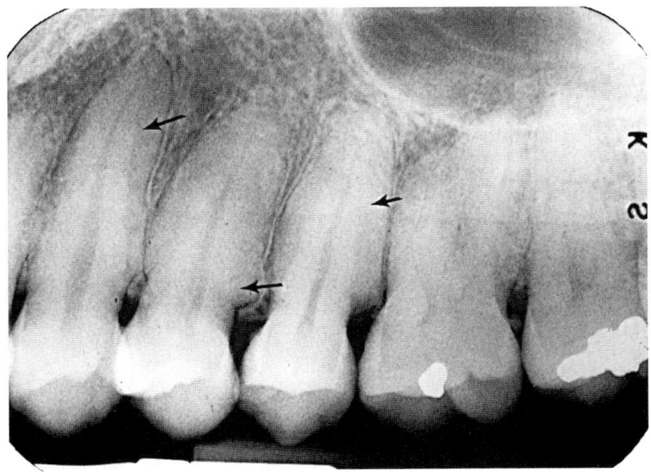

FIGURE 7–16.

Hypercementosis (transparent secondary cementum). Hypercementosis with deposition of transparent type of secondary cementum of roots of premolars. Notice the demarcation of transparent secondary cementum from actual roots of canine and premolars (arrows).

RESORPTION OF TEETH

Resorption is a condition when a physiologic or pathologic process results in a loss of substance from a tissue such as dentin, cementum, and alveolar bone.

Physiologic resorption is a normal process associated with the shedding of primary teeth. The roots of the primary teeth are removed gradually as the permanent teeth begin to erupt. Pathologic resorption is any resorption of teeth not associated with the shedding of primary teeth.

Root resorption affects the cementum or dentin of the root of a tooth. On the basis of the site of origin of the resorption, it may be referred to as internal and external, or root end resorption.

INTERNAL RESORPTION (Chronic Perforating Hyperplasia of the Pulp, Internal Granuloma, Odontoclastoma, Pink Tooth of Mummery)

Internal resorption is a process that begins centrally within the tooth. The term idiopathic resorption is used synonymously with internal resorption because the precise cause is unknown. Internal resorption is one of dentistry's great mysteries. Why does a normal tooth apparently resorb when thousands of them do not? Among the suggested causes are inflammatory processes, loss of vitality of the cementum, vascular changes in the pulp, accessory root canals, systemic disease, and trauma; however, several authors, Schroeder (1981), Seltzer and Bender (1975), Weine (1989), Burke (1976), and Dargent (1977), generally believe that trauma or persistent irreversible chronic pulpitis is probably the cause of internal resorption. It is thought that trauma or chronic pulpitis is responsible for the formation of dentinoblasts by activating undifferentiated embryonic connective tissue cells of the pulp. Dentinoblasts differentiate into multinucleated "clastic" cells and, when the growing granulation tissue compresses the wall of the pulp tissue or canal, the dentinoclasts cause a resorptive defect that is filled with hypervascular granulation tissue. Stafne and Slocumb (1949) stated that internal resorption usually is not associated with any systemic disease.

Bell (1829) was apparently the first to report internal resorption. He reported on a tooth extracted because of pain. The tooth was sectioned and showed a cavity within the dentin, despite normal surrounding dentin. He believed that this resorption of the dentin was caused by inflammation and the resultant pressure from the pus in the pulpal cavity.

If resorption occurs in the coronal portion of the tooth, a pink or red spot will appear in the crown where the hypervascular pulp shows through the translucent enamel. This condition is referred to as the "pink tooth of Mummery," after Mummery, who was the first to perform an extensive study of these "pink spots" in 1920. External resorption is asymptomatic, so if it occurs in the radicular pulp, it will be shown only on the radiograph.

Internal resorption has been found to exist more often than previously suspected. Andreasen reported there is a 2% incidence after luxation injuries, Allen and Gutman (1977) believed that it can follow vital root resection, and Cvek and associates (1976) stated that it can follow the application of calcium hydroxide after a pulpotomy.

When internal resorption is suspected, several radiographs taken from different horizontal angles may be necessary to examine the extent of the tooth loss and to determine the treatment plan.

Internal resorption is encountered more frequently in the permanent dentition, although it does occur in primary teeth more often than generally supposed. The root alone, the crown alone, or both root and crown may be involved. Any tooth may be affected, but the upper incisors are the most common sites. Usually only one tooth is affected, but there are cases in which several teeth show the condition at the same time.

The extent and rapidity of the resorptive process are unpredictable. Often the process is very slow and may continue over a period of many years.

Pain may become a factor when perforation of the crown or root occurs. Diagnosis is more difficult because of the possibility that the condition was initially external resorption that perforated the pulp canal.

When internal resorption of a tooth is found, removal of the altered pulp tissue is important. Spontaneous repair is extremely rare according to Hartness (1975) and Weisman and Rackley (1978). Therefore, it is important to start endodontic treatment early for all diagnosed cases of internal resorption. Chivian (1987) recommended three types of treatment for internal resorption: nonsurgical treatment, recalcification with calcium hydroxide, and surgical treatment.

If the resorptive defect does not perforate the canal wall, a nonsurgical approach is the treatment of choice, by sanitization, debridement, and obturation (see Fig. 7–19). If there is perforation of the canal wall apical to the epithelial attachment and the endodontic triad requirements of sanitization, debridement, and obturation can be met, the calcium hydroxide technique can be used. If there is perforation coronal to the epithelial attachment, uncontrollable bleeding, or extensive root destruction, a surgical approach is required. Extraction may be necessary in some cases (see Fig. 7–20).

◆ RADIOLOGY (Figs. 7–17 to 7–20)

The radiographic appearances are characteristic. The pulp chamber or root canal shows evidence of enlargement, which may be slight, considerable, or gross. The margins of the enlarged canal or chamber are usually sharp and clearly defined (Fig. 7–17B). The enlargement, of course, can only take place at the expense of the dentin, which is destroyed. The destruction may be situated symmetrically around the original site of initiation in the pulp, or it may be eccentric, so that it is located almost entirely on one side of the root.

The tooth substance that is destroyed in the root may assume any shape—rounded, oval, inverted pear, or irregular—but it is rarely possible to see the normal outline of the original canal, such as is possible when the resorption is external and superimposed by projection over the canal.

The dentin adjacent to the pulp is very resistant to resorption. Careful examination of radiographs often reveals evidence of a thin layer of unresorbed dentin adjacent to the pulp, and, in some instances, this dentin produces radiopaque lines that frame the pulp chamber and pulp canal with striking clearness.

When the root is involved, it may be necessary to differentiate the condition from external resorption, especially when the latter condition occupies a position on the facial or lingual aspect of the root. The margins of the two conditions usually differ, being smooth and even in internal resorption but irregular and scalloped in many cases of external resorption.

Supplemental radiographs from different horizontal angles, such as from mesial or distal projections, will aid in the diagnosis. If the resorption defect does not change position in comparison with the other multiple radiographs, it is within the confines of the root; therefore, it is internal resorption. Andreasen stated that labial and lingual external resorption superimposed over the canal can mimic internal resorption, but it will change position on multiple radiographs.

Gartner and colleagues (1976) simplified the diagnostic process by summarizing the radiographic appearance of external and internal resorption. The keys to the resorption criteria described by Gartner and associates (1976) are as follows: (1) In external resorption, the defect may be superimposed over the canal and the unaltered canal can be followed all the way to the apex. (2) In internal resorption, the canal or chamber shows an enlarged area and there is no outline of the canal within this enlarged area (Fig. 7–17A).

The radiologic differential diagnosis of internal resorption should take into consideration that dental caries sometimes looks very similar to internal resorption on the radiograph. If the internal resorption is in the root, then caries usually is not considered, but when the crown only is involved, caries must be included. The differences are that internal resorption appears to start within the tooth and destroys it concentrically, moving outward. In most cases, the enamel is not involved, so there is no evidence of an external orifice; however, caries may start on the facial or lingual aspects of the crown, and its orifice may not be apparent in radiographs. The difference in the sharpness of the margins of the radiolucent area suggests the nature of the lesion: With internal resorption, they are sharp and well defined; with caries, they are less sharp and ill defined. In most cases of caries, it is possible to identify a radiolucency in the enamel. With coronal caries, it is frequently possible to outline the margins of the pulp chamber, and the shape is normal. With internal resorption, the whole of the pulp is altered in shape and size.

Fischer and Guggenheimer (1977) observed internal and external root resorption in the same tooth. Also, Pomeranz (1983) reported a case of active external-internal root resorption. Frank (1981) described a category of resorption called "external-internal progressive resorption" (Fig. 7–18).

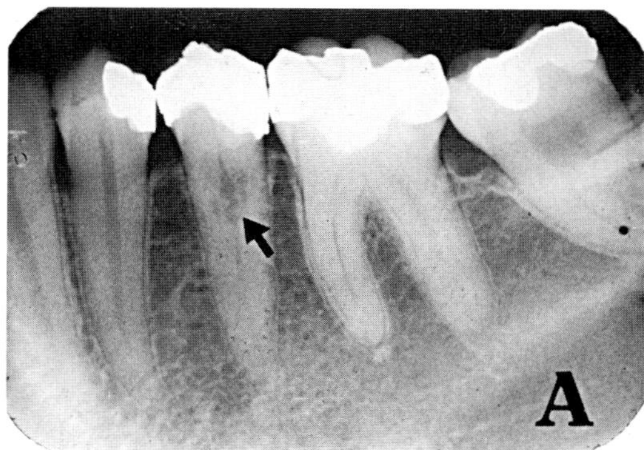

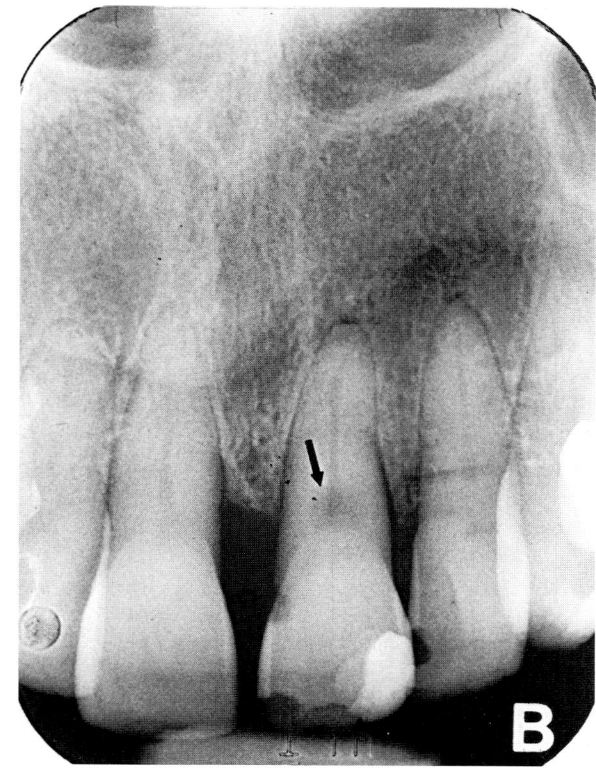

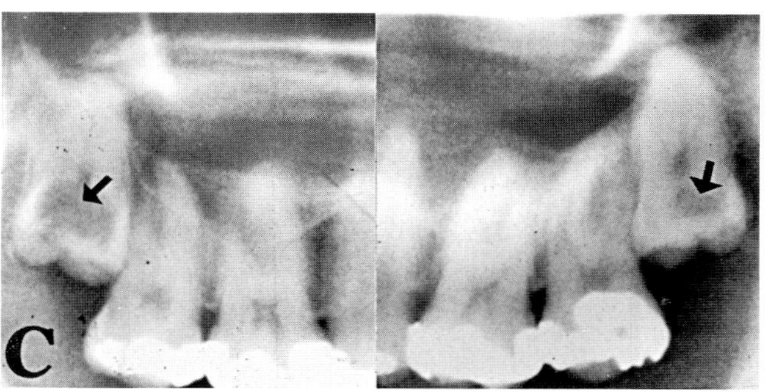

FIGURE 7–17.

Internal resorption. A, Irregular type of internal resorption of second premolar (arrow). (This is most likely internal resorption rather than external resorption because there is a slight widening of the canal in the affected area.) B, Internal resorption of upper left central incisor (arrow). C, Internal resorption of impacted third molars (arrows) in same patient. (Courtesy of B. Potter, Augusta, GA.)

EXTERNAL RESORPTION

External resorption is the loss of tooth material from the outer surface of the tooth, arising from a tissue reaction in the periodontal or pericoronal tissue. Although the cause of internal resorption is unknown, Shafer and colleagues (1983) stated many situations as causes of external resorption. They listed the following causes or situations in which external resorption may occur: periapical inflammation, reimplantation of teeth, tumors and cysts, excessive mechanical or occlusal forces, and impaction of teeth. Also, radiation therapy, luxation injuries, and periodontal disease are frequent causes of external resorption. When no cause can be determined for resorption of roots of erupted teeth, this is called idiopathic resorption.

External resorption may be found in patients with hypoparathyroidism, calcinosis, Gaucher's disease, hyperparathyroidism, Turner's syndrome, and Paget's disease. Morse (1974) reported that when external resorption occurs in a systemic disease, it usually is seen at the apices of several teeth and is bilateral.

External resorption is more prevalent than internal resorption; may be localized to the apical, middle, or cervical third of the roots of erupted teeth; and may be superficial or deep. Superficial external resorptions are shallow cavities with rounded contours; often the resorption begins at the apex and progresses in a coronal direction. Deep external resorption usually begins at the cervical part of the root and after several extensive ramifications that have a canalicular (resembling small, narrow tubular passages) structure. The enamel in the crown of the tooth may be resorbed, but this mainly affects impacted teeth.

Some degree of root resorption probably occurs in nearly all adults; however, it is minimal. Massler and Malone (1954) studied full mouth radiographs of 708 patients (age range, 12 and 49 years) and found that 100% of the patients examined showed some evidence of resorption of permanent teeth. There were no differences between resorption in male and female patients and no difference between the number of maxillary and mandibular teeth affected. Most resorptions were mild, and only 9% of patients had resorptions deeper than 2 mm. In a study in Switzerland, Hotz (1967) confirmed some of the results of Massler and Malone (1954) but showed a higher percentage (22.5%) of teeth with resorption and found more resorption among maxillary compared with mandibular teeth.

External resorption may have disturbing symptoms. In cases of significant external resorption, the teeth may be-

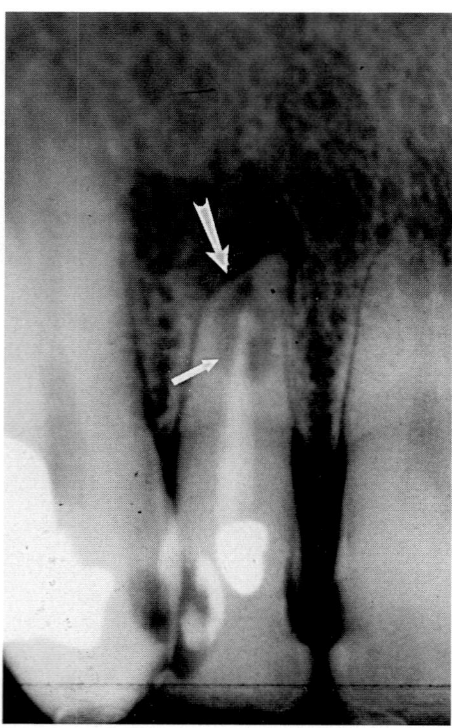

FIGURE 7–18.

External-internal progressive resorption. Case of previously endodontically treated maxillary lateral incisor with possible concurrent external root resorption of the apex and internal resorption of the root canal (arrows). (Courtesy of Drs. L. Archilla, R. Carlos, and F. Erales, Guatemala City, Guatemala.)

come loose; this often leads to the recognition of resorption. In external cervical resorption, the resorption process may result in complete undermining of the crown and its subsequent fracture. If the resorption (external or internal) becomes associated with pulp necrosis, the tooth may show a gray discoloration. External resorptions in teeth rarely cause pain. A tooth with extreme external deep resorption usually must be extracted because most often it is not a candidate for root canal therapy.

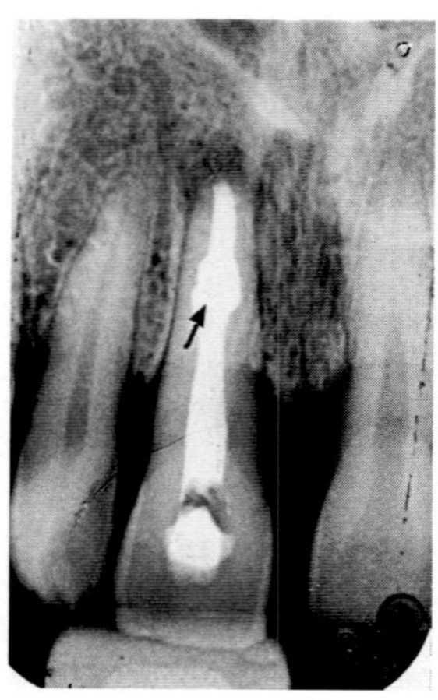

FIGURE 7–19.

Internal resorption. Completed root canal treatment of internal resorption of central incisor (arrow).

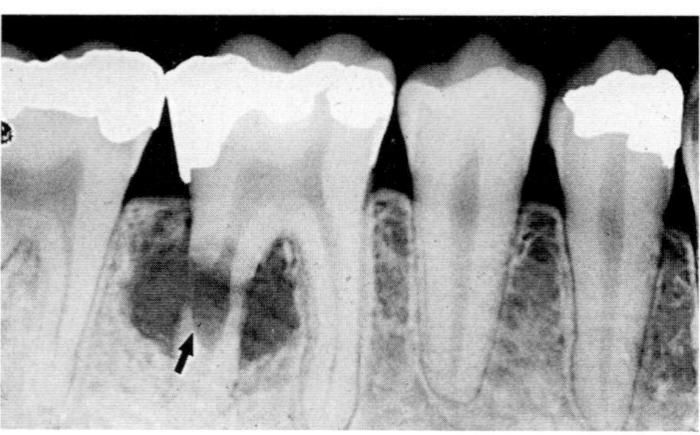

FIGURE 7–20.

Internal resorption. Severe internal resorption (see widened canal) that has resorbed through the tooth root and into the alveolar bone (arrow).

◆ RADIOLOGY (Figs. 7–21 to 7–28)

A radiographic examination is almost mandatory for the diagnosis of dental resorptions. In the early stages, external resorption may be difficult to diagnose on a single radiograph. Often, several exposures in different projections are necessary.

The most common site of external resorption is the apex, which is seen as a slightly or substantially shortened root. The conical shape of the normal apex is removed by resorption and replaced by a more or less blunt, and usually square, apex. It is important to observe the change in the root canal. In the radiograph, the normal root canal will fall short by a few millimeters from the end of the tooth. It also is not possible to see the actual foramen in most mature root apices. With external resorption, the end of the apex is removed so that it is usually possible to follow the canal to the extreme apex and see the foramen. When this can be seen, it is suggestive of external resorption.

Occasionally an apical granuloma arising as a result of pulpal infection or trauma will cause external resorption of the root apex if the periapical inflammatory lesion persists

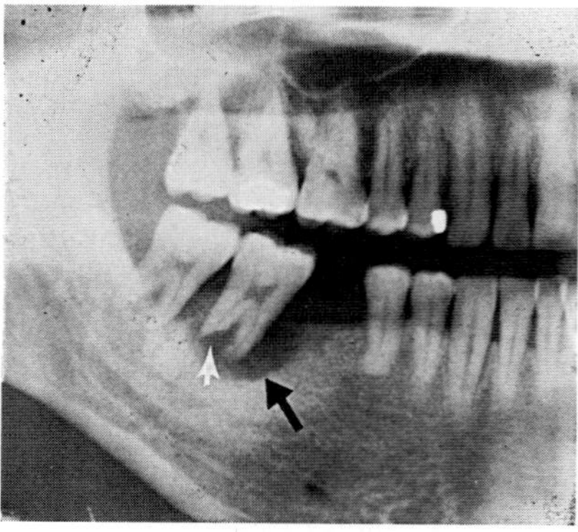

FIGURE 7–21.

External resorption. External resorption (white arrow) from periapical inflammation (black arrow) to lower right second molar. (From Langland OE, Langlais RP, Morris CR: Principles and Practice of Panoramic Radiology. Philadelphia:WB Saunders, 1982, p. 224.)

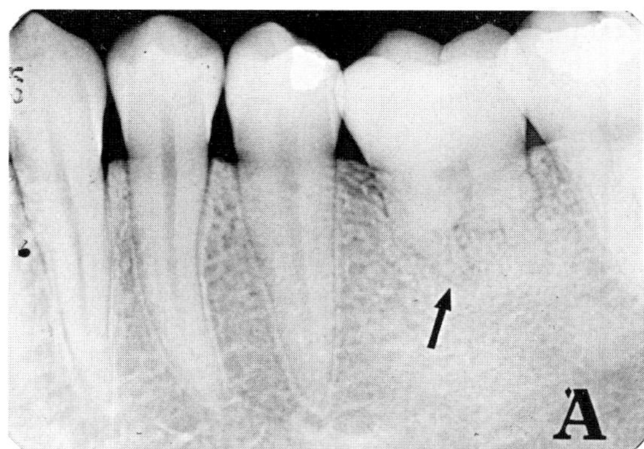

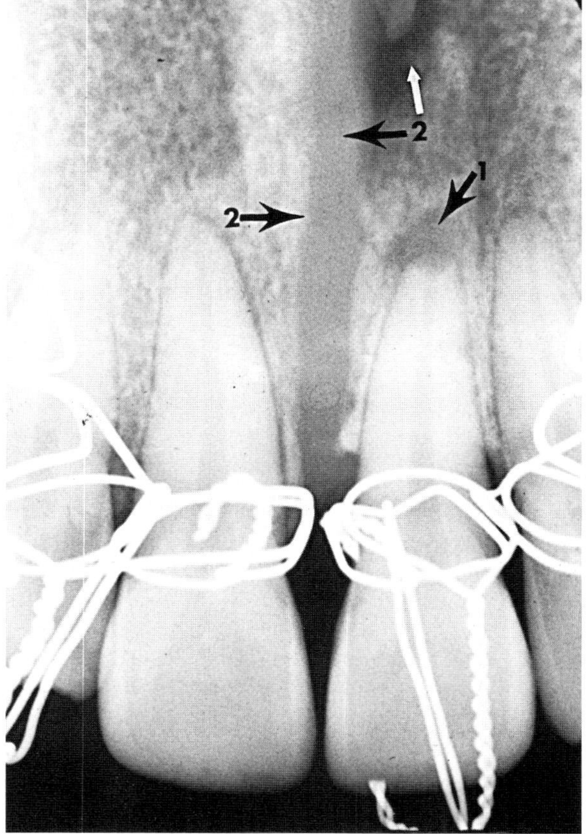

B

FIGURE 7–22.

External resorption. A, Transplanted third molar into first molar space with subsequent external resorption (arrow). B, Reimplanted central incisors. The maxillary centrals were transplanted and stabilized 90 minutes after they were completely exfoliated in an automobile accident. The left central is beginning to resorb at the apical end of the root (1, arrow). Notice the fractured maxilla (2, arrows).

for a fairly long period. The reason for the occasional occurrence is unknown. It is generally known that external resorption requires a rather high vascular region. Because apical granulomas are quite vascular, it is surprising that external resorption associated with periapical inflammation is not seen more often.

In cases in which periapical inflammation causes external root resorption, this condition appears as a slight raggedness or blunting of the root apex in the early stages, proceeding to severe loss of tooth substance (Fig. 7–21).

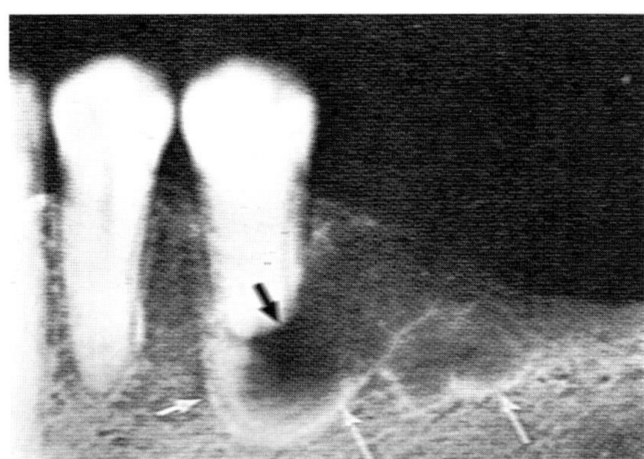

FIGURE 7–23.

External root resorption from tumors. Notice resorption of root of second premolar from pressure of maturing ameloblastoma (arrows) (confirmed by biopsy at surgery).

In a tooth in which a root canal has been filled and periapical inflammation persists, root resorption may occur and ultimately leave only the root canal filling projecting out of the shortened root (see Fig. 7–18).

It used to be thought that apical resorption was a contraindication for nonsurgical endodontic treatment; however, with the newer gutta-percha root canal techniques, even very severe cases of apical root resorption can be treated successfully with nonsurgical endodontic therapy. Apical closure techniques may be necessary when the resorption has enlarged the apical portion of the canal, making it impossible to use proper instrumentation and sealing.

Irregular external resorption of the apex usually is found after reimplantation or transplantation of a tooth. This procedure almost invariably results in severe resorption of the root. The implanted tooth acts only as a temporary scaffold and ultimately is resorbed and replaced by bone, producing ankylosis, or it may exhibit complete resorption of the root and eventually be exfoliated (Fig. 7–22A). Andreasen (1981) reviewed the frequency of progressive root resorption after reimplantation of avulsed permanent teeth and reported that it ranged from 80 to 96%.

In an intentional reimplantation of 1000 teeth, Deeb and associates (1965) reported that the greatest amount of resorption was found to be caused by the use of peroxide and

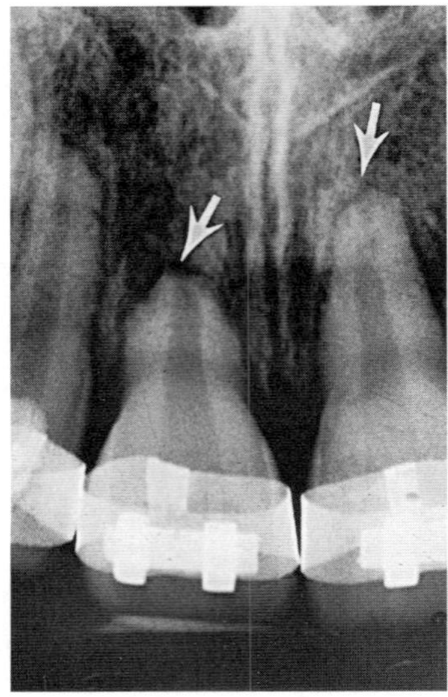

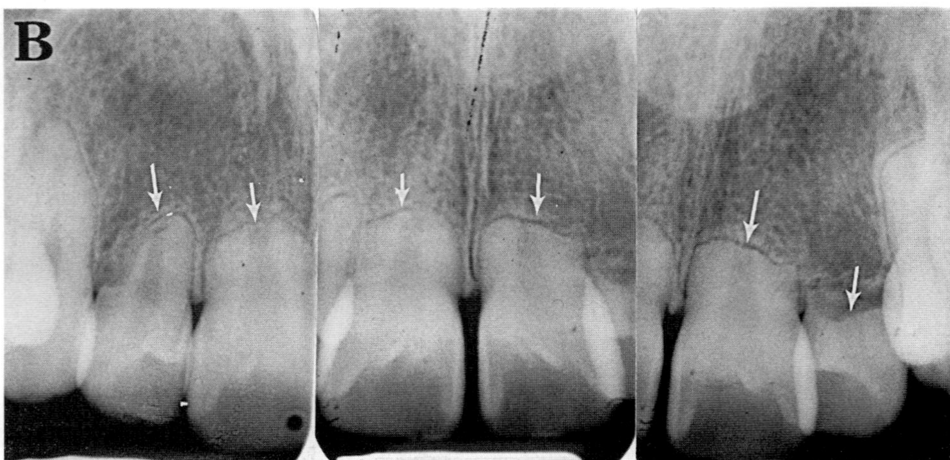

A

FIGURE 7–24.

External resorption. A, Excessive mechanical force applied to maxillary incisors by orthodontic appliances caused external root resorption (arrows). B, External resorption of maxillary incisors from excessive mechanical force from orthodontic appliances (arrows).

sodium hypochlorite for canal irrigation, the trauma of excessive manipulation, and curettement of the periodontal ligament. Fountain and Camp (1987) stated that the avulsed tooth must be reimplanted as soon as possible, preferably at the site the injury occurred (Fig. 7–22B). Obvious contamination with soil or foreign matter should be cleansed with physiologic saline or water. The periodontal ligament should not be removed or altered in any manner, and the pulp should not be removed. If a blood clot is present, it should be removed by irrigation rather than curettage. The tooth is repositioned with light finger pressure, and soft tissue lacerations should be sutured to arrest bleeding before the tooth is splinted.

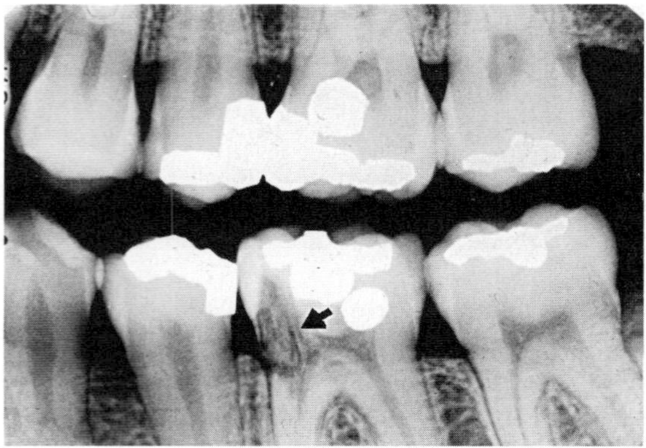

FIGURE 7–25.

External cervical resorption. Deep external resorption usually begins at the cervical part of the root and has a canalicular structure (arrow) (resembling small, narrow, tubular passages). (From Langland OE, Langlais RP, Morris CR: Principles and Practice of Panoramic Radiology. Philadelphia:WB Saunders, 1982, p. 226.)

Bjorvatin and colleagues (1989) reported that, in studies of beagle dogs, an application of 1% stannous fluoride (SnF_2) for 5 minutes, followed by 1% doxycycline hydrochloric acid before reimplantation of extracted teeth, greatly reduced subsequent root resorption.

Benign and malignant tumors may cause external root resorption; however, benign tumors are the ones that usually cause resorption, but most of the time they displace teeth. Usually there is connective tissue between the tumor and the tooth from which osteoclasts form. These cells appear to be responsible for the root resorption (Fig. 7–26).

Also, it is more common for cysts to displace a tooth rather than cause external resorption by pressure. Radicular cysts seem to cause resorption of the tooth root more than dentigerous, primordial or fissural cysts.

External root resorption may be associated with excessive mechanical forces such as that applied during orthodontic treatment (Fig. 7–24). Since the work of Ketcham, it has been recognized for many years that patients who have undergone orthodontic treatment frequently exhibit multiple areas of root resorption. In some patients, the resorption is mild and involves only a few teeth; in others, there may be loss of more than 50% of the root length in most of the teeth moved orthodontically.

Goldson and Hendrikson (1975) used a resorptive index in a study that permitted a quantitative assessment of the occurrence and degree of root resorption during orthodontic treatment. They reported that, 6 months after treatment, the highest incidence of root resorption was found in the mandibular central incisors (95%), maxillary central incisors (90%), and maxillary lateral incisors (87%). The lowest incidence was in the mandibular premolars (53%).

In their study of postorthodontic patients, Linge and Linge (1983) found that apical root resorption is a greater

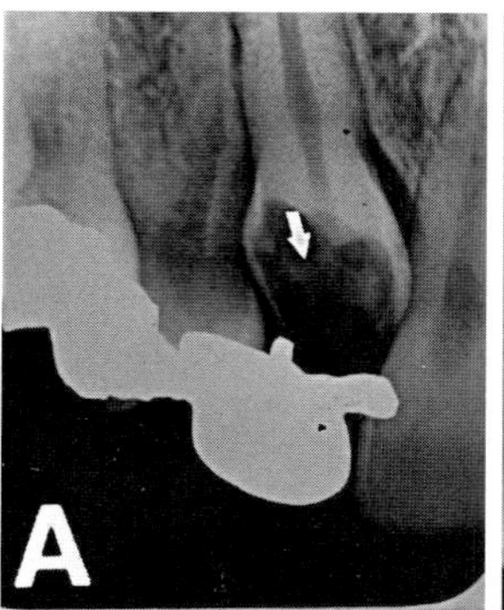

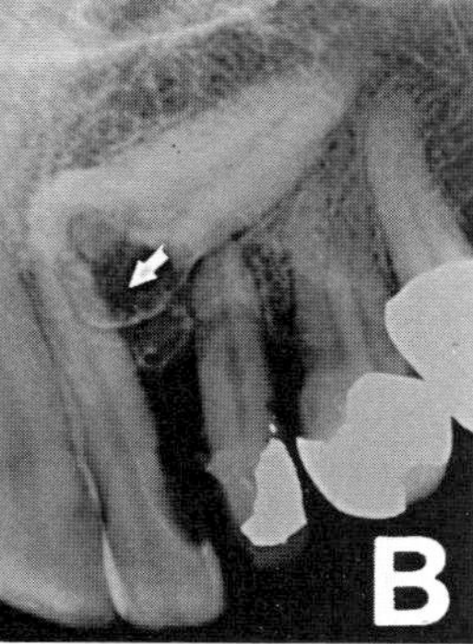

FIGURE 7–26.

External resorption. A, Impacted right canine with external resorption (arrow). B, Impacted left canine with external resorption (arrow).

risk when orthodontic treatment is started in a patient older than 11 years of age than in patients starting earlier. Root resorption associated with orthodontic treatment usually ceases at the completion of the active and retentive stages. The process may continue in some cases.

Cervical resorption is external resorption in the coronal third of the root near the cementoenamel junction (Fig. 7–25). It usually results from an inflammatory reaction in the periodontal ligament and may occur years after traumatic injury. Cvek and associates (1981) reported that it is seen primarily in reimplanted teeth and ankylosed teeth in infraposition, but it can occur in luxated (dislocated) teeth.

Cervical resorption can undermine the crown. Hammarstrom and Lindskog (1985) reported that extensive cervical external resorption may surround the pulp chamber and canal and not penetrate it. The odontoblastic layer and underlying predentin seem to act in concert as a barrier against resorption. Cervical resorption in advanced stages creates the classic ''pink spot'' and often is mistaken for internal resorption.

The upper incisors and lower premolars are affected most often by cervical external resorption. Scalloping is a term used to describe this type of external resorption. Each little excavation sometimes shows a thin band of dentin traversing the radiolucent area. The scalloped margins and the site should suggest cervical external resorption (Fig. 7–25).

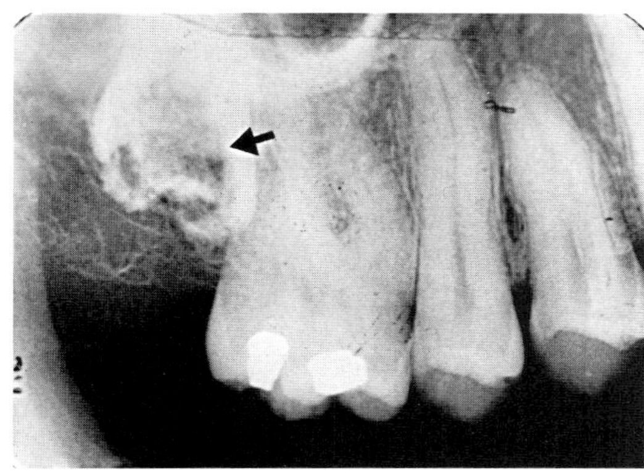

FIGURE 7–27.

External resorption, impacted maxillary third molar. External resorption of maxillary impacted third molar (arrow). (Second molar is missing.)

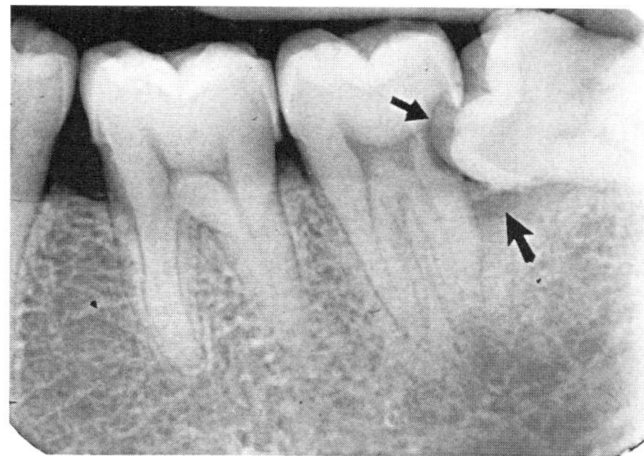

FIGURE 7–28.

External resorption, impacted third molar. External resorption of distal surface of mandibular second molar (small arrow) caused by inflammation (large arrow) and pressure from horizontally impacted third molar.

Teeth that are completely impacted or embedded may undergo resorption of the crown or both the crown and root. In a study of 226 embedded teeth in which resorption occurred, Stafne and Austin (1945) reported that 78% of the teeth were in the maxillary arch and 60% of these maxillary teeth were canines. This finding is unusual and significant because, although third molar impactions far outnumber maxillary canine impactions in incidence, the maxillary impacted canines undergo resorption more frequently than the impacted third molars. (Fig. 7–26).

The radiographic picture presented by external resorption of an impacted and embedded tooth usually is an irregular destruction of the crown that looks very much like caries; however, caries in the tooth would be unusual because the tooth has no communication with the oral cavity (Fig. 7–27).

Several authors (Goultschin and colleagues [1982], Halcomb and associates [1983], and Tasch and Kennon [1978]) reported that pressure from an impacted tooth can cause external root resorption. This is common in a horizontally or mesioangularly impacted third molar impinging on the roots of the second molar.

Nitzen and co-authors (1981) reported a 7.5% incidence of external resorption of impacted teeth in contact with roots of adjacent teeth. The incidence was highest in the younger age group (21 to 30 years), and male patients were twice as susceptible as female patients. They concluded that inflammation, in addition to pressure, may play a role in this type of resorption (Fig. 7–28).

PULPOPERIAPICAL DISEASE

(Periapical Pathoses of Pulpal Origin)

Diagnostic classifications of periapical disease usually are based on the patient's symptoms and clinical findings, rather than on a histopathologic basis. Mendoza and associates (1987), Morse and colleagues (1977), and Priebe and co-authors (1954) reported that there is little correlation between clinical signs and symptoms and the duration of periapical lesions and histopathologic findings. Therefore, because of these discrepancies in clinical and histopathologic findings, periapical lesions are classified into four main groups: acute apical periodontitis (AAP), acute apical abscess (AAA), chronic apical periodontitis (CAP), (apical granuloma, apical cyst, chronic apical abscess, and phoenix abscess), and apical condensing osteitis (ACO). Lesions with significant symptoms, such as pain or swelling, are designated as acute and those with mild or no symptoms are classified as chronic.

Acute Apical Periodontitis

AAP is an inflammatory response of the apical periodontal ligament to pulpal irritants via the root canal or from trauma. It is the first extension of pulpal inflammation into the periapical tissues. AAP is caused by irritants and contaminants from the pulp canals, including bacteria and their toxins, substances from necrotic pulps, and chemicals (such as irrigants or disinfecting medicaments). The cause of AAP also may be mechanical, such as a blow on the tooth, a high filling, or a foreign object wedged against the periodontal ligament.

In most cases, the pulp is irreversibly inflamed or necrotic; however, AAP may be associated with a vital tooth, such as occlusal trauma from irregular wear of teeth, or a recently inserted high restoration or from a foreign object wedged between the teeth. If AAP is associated with a vital tooth, thermal and electrical tests with careful examination are useful in ruling out pulpal involvement.

Weine (1989) reported that, in AAP, periapical hyperemia must take place first; if the irritant persists, the prolonged vasodilation in the narrow apical periodontal space is followed by an inflammatory exudate and leukocytic infiltration. The increased pressure may elevate the tooth slightly, stretching the periodontal ligament fibers. The nerve endings in this area are stimulated so that even slight pressure against the tooth will cause mild pain. The tooth becomes increasingly tender as long as the pulpal irritants persist in causing inflammation of the periapex. Application of pressure by a fingertip or tapping with an instrument will cause excruciating pain. Often, a localized sense of fullness accompanies the pain.

Walton and Torabinejad (1989) reported that the clinical features of AAP are slight to severe spontaneous pain, as well as pain from percussion. If the AAP is an extension of pulpitis, the most classic response is that heat causes intense pain, whereas cold relieves the pain; however, sensitivity to both heat and cold is not unusual. The tooth will be responsive to electricity. AAP induced by necrosis does not respond to vitality tests.

Grossman (1974) reported that treatment of AAP consists of determining the cause, and particularly whether the AAP is associated with a vital or pulpless tooth. Relieving the occlusion or removing the caries in some vital teeth generally eliminates the discomfort; however, AAP may be caused by irreversible pulpitis, which also responds to thermal and electrical tests. Therefore, careful evaluation of the signs and symptoms is necessary in these instances. The pain in irreversible pulpitis is usually continuous, spontaneous, and intermittent.

The treatment of a tooth with irreversible pulpitis and AAP requires a complete pulpectomy. According to Weine and associates (1975), the access cavity should be sealed to gain the best results.

◆ *RADIOLOGY (Fig. 7–29)*

On radiographs, AAP may exhibit a small periapical radiolucency or a slight thickening of the periodontal ligament (PDL) at the apex of the tooth, or it may appear normal. Most cases of AAP apical are associated with normal apical PDL spaces and intact lamina dura, and a slight widening of the apical PDL space usually indicates irreversible pulpitis or pupal necrosis (Fig. 7–29).

Acute Apical Abscess (Acute Alveolar Abscess, Acute Dentoalveolar Abscess, Acute Radicular Abscess)

An AAA is a painful localized collection of pus in the alveolar bone at the root apex of the tooth after the death of the pulp, with extension of the infection through the apical foramen into the periapical tissue.

The cause of AAA is an AAP with a necrotic pulp, which has advanced to an extensive acute suppurative inflammation stage. Although an acute abscess may result from trauma or chemical or mechanical irritation, the immediate cause is generally bacterial invasion of dead pulp tissue. The number and virulence of the bacteria passing from a contaminated, gangrenous pulp through the apical foramen may be sufficient to overwhelm the defenses of the periapical tissue; therefore, an AAA develops. At times, there is neither caries nor a restoration in the tooth, but there is a history of trauma. Therefore, an AAA is usually a severe inflammatory response to microbiologic irritants from a necrotic pulp, but

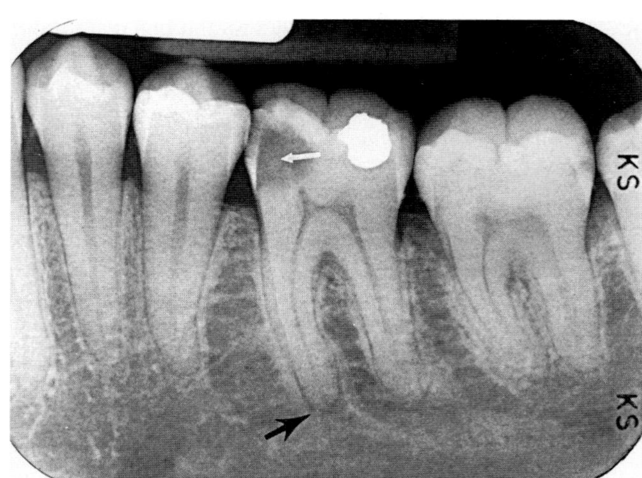

FIGURE 7–29.

Acute apical periodontitis. Notice thickening of the PDL space of the apex of the mandibular second molar mesial root (black arrow) with a large carious lesion on the mesial surface (white arrow). The tooth was nonvital and confirmed at root canal treatment to have a necrotic pulp.

it may be a severe response to nonbacterial irritants if the cause is trauma.

A tooth with an AAP will become increasingly tender, with advancement in time toward the next stage, the AAA. The intensity of the pain increases as pus formation adds to the periapical pressure. The pain becomes more intense and continuous, with the patient having a feeling of fullness in the area of pain. Unless drainage can be established, the exudative inflammatory response may spread diffusely, creating peripheral areas of cellulitis. The extent and distribution of the swelling are determined by the location of the apex, condition of the adjacent muscle attachments, and thickness of the cortical plate.

The soft vestibular tissues overlying the root end may become inflamed and painful to palpation. At this stage, if a pledget of cotton saturated with hydrogen peroxide is held against the mucous membrane at the apex of the affected tooth, the tissue will turn white. It is one of the earliest signs of an acute abscess and results from tissue breakdown. At this point, the patient may appear pale, irritable, and weakened from a loss of sleep, as well as from absorption of septic products into the bloodstream. In mild cases, there may be a slight increase in temperature (99° to 100° F), but in severe cases the temperature may reach several degrees above normal (102° to 103° F).

The affected tooth will not respond to electrical stimulation or cold, but heat may elicit pain. The tooth is tender to percussion and may be extremely mobile, with moderate to severe pain.

AAA should be differentiated from a periodontal abscess and acute pulpitis. A periodontal abscess is associated with a periodontal pocket and manifested by swelling; an accumulation of pus along the root surface of the tooth; and is manifested by swelling and slight pain. The swelling is usually opposite the midsection of the tooth and gingival border rather than opposite the root apex or above it.

A periodontal abscess generally is associated with vital rather than pulpless teeth. Also, hot mouth rinses relieve the pain from periodontal abscess but intensify the pain of AAA. Furthermore, there is almost always a periodontal pocket with the periodontal abscess, which may begin to exude a purulent exudate when probed.

AAA is differentiated from acute pulpitis by electrical stimulation and by the fact that, in acute pulpitis, the periapical tissue is not involved so that percussion, palpation, and mobility tests have negative results.

In the treatment of AAA, drainage is established at once. Whether drainage is by root canal, an incision, or both, depends on the case. Cold applications should be used externally and alternated with hot applications inside the mouth to bring about pointing the abscess within the mouth rather than externally on the face.

With establishment of drainage, the acute symptoms subside rapidly. When necessary, supportive treatment should consist of an anodyne when pain is present, a mild mouth wash, and much-needed sleep or rest. In severe cases, an antibiotic should be prescribed. When the acute symptoms have subsided, the tooth should be treated endodontically by conservative means. No special treatment of a fistula is necessary, if one is present.

◆ *RADIOLOGY (Fig. 7–30)*

Radiographically, the periapical tissue may appear normal because fulminating infections may not have had sufficient time to erode enough cortical bone to cause a radiolucency; however, some periapical change usually is present.

The AAA can be differentiated from a phoenix abscess (recrudescent abscess) because there will be a slight widening of the apical periodontal ligament space in AAA and a frank periapical lesion in a phoenix abscess (Figs. 7–30A and B). All other signs and symptoms will be identical in both. The main difference is that the phoenix abscess (recrudescent abscess) is preceded by a chronic condition. It is a chronic apical periodontitis that suddenly becomes symptomatic.

In the early stages of AAA it may be difficult to locate the tooth. When the infection has progressed far enough to produce apical periodontitis, a radiograph may help determine the tooth affected by disclosing caries, a leaky restoration, a thickened PDL space, or evidence of bone breakdown in the region of the root apex.

At times, differentiation of AAP and AAA may be difficult. The difference may be one of degree rather than kind because AAA represents an additional stage in the pulpoperiapical development, with breakdown of periapical tissue rather than simple inflammation of the periodontal ligament. The history, symptoms, and clinical tests will help differentiate these diseases.

Chronic Apical Periodontitis

(Apical Granuloma, Apical Cyst, Chronic Apical Abscess, and Phoenix Abscess)

This term implies longstanding asymptomatic inflammation around the apex. It results from pulp necrosis and usually is a sequela to AAP. Chronic apical periodontitis is a standoff between the host defensive mechanism and the irritating products from a necrotic pulp. The resultant periapical inflammation produced may be partially controlled by the body's defenses, by surgically induced drainage, or by antibiotic therapy. In the advanced form of chronic apical periodontitis, a dental granuloma, chronic apical abscess, or apical cyst develops. The dental granuloma in turn may evolve into an apical (radicular) cyst. If the odontogenic epithelial rests of Malassez (present in the periodontal ligament and frequently identified in dental granulomas) proliferate and the granuloma becomes cystic, an apical (radicular) cyst results. If bacteria are of sufficient virulence and number to counteract the host resistance in a dental granuloma or apical cyst, a phoenix abscess arises. As stated previously, a phoenix abscess is a chronic apical periodontitis that suddenly becomes symptomatic. All the signs and symptoms of the phoenix abscess are identical to those of AAA.

With a phoenix abscess, if the correct antibiotics are administered or the abscess is drained, it is aborted and the periapical lesion will regress into a dental granuloma or apical cyst again. If a sinus tract develops from an AAA or the phoenix abscess and it drains to the surface, the lesion becomes a chronic apical abscess.

The additional presence of a sinus tract indicates the production of frank pus. Symptoms are generally absent because

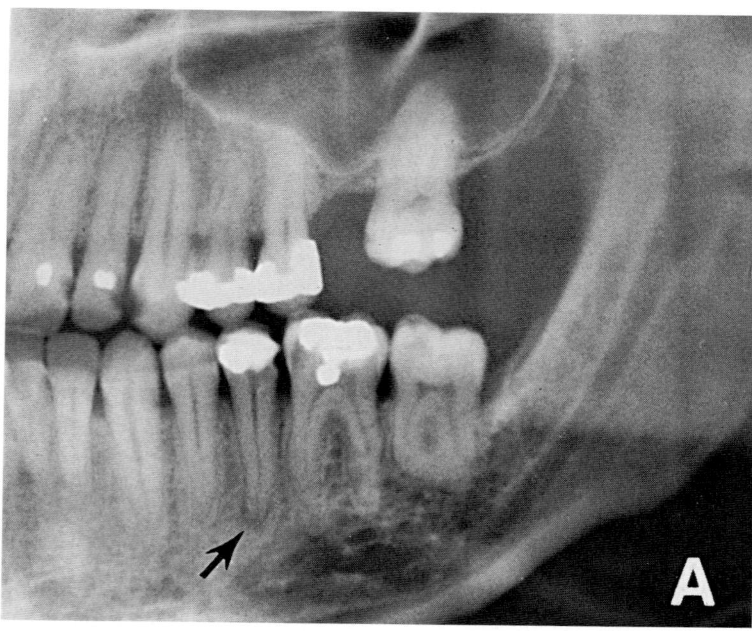

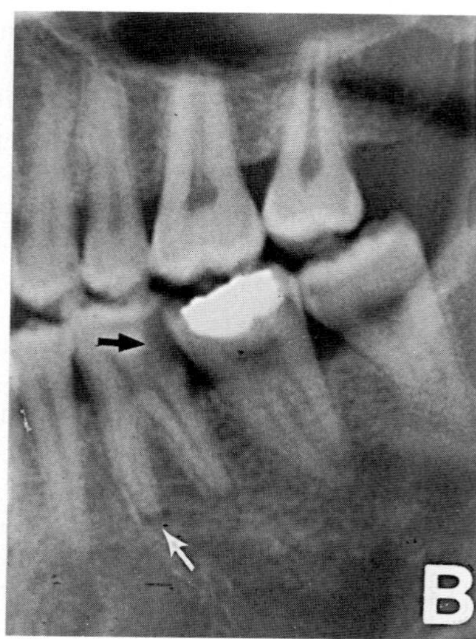

FIGURE 7–30.

Acute apical abscess. A, Notice the thickened PDL space of the apex of the root of the mandibular second premolar with a large restoration (arrow). The tooth was tender to percussion, mobile, and extremely painful. (From Langland OE, Langlais RP, Morris CR: Principles and Practice of Panoramic Radiology. Philadelphia:WB Saunders, 1982, p. 229.) B, Notice the thickened PDL of the mesial root of the lower first molar (white arrow) with a large distal carious lesion (black arrow). (From Langland OE, Langlais RP, Morris CR: Principles and Practice of Panoramic Radiology. Philadelphia:WB Saunders, 1982, p. 230.)

the pus drains through the sinus tract as quickly as it is produced. Epithelium may close the sinus tract opening (stoma). Pressure buildup by a continuous formation of pus will produce subacute (moderate) symptoms and cause the epithelium to balloon out (parulis, gumboil). The symptoms will subside when the epithelium ruptures.

Advanced chronic apical periodontitis is asymptomatic, but occasionally there may be tenderness to palpation and percussion. Also, because the pulps of the teeth are necrotic in advanced chronic apical periodontitis, they will not respond to electrical or thermal stimuli.

Histologically, Stern and co-workers (1981) reported that the apical granuloma consists of granulomatous tissue infiltrated by macrophages, histiocytes, lymphocytes, plasma cells, and occasional polymorphonuclear leukocytes. The apical cyst has a central cavity filled with an eosinophilic fluid or semisolid material and is lined incompletely by stratified squamous epithelium. The epithelium is surrounded by a connective tissue that contains all the cellular elements found in the apical granuloma. Thus, the apical cyst is an inflammatory lesion or, properly, a "cyst within a granuloma."

The chronic apical abscess is a longstanding, low-grade, inflammatory reaction of the periapical connective tissue to pulpal irritants and is characterized by formation of a parulis (gumboil) and active pus formation drawing through a sinus tract. It usually develops from a phoenix abscess (chronic apical periodontitis with symptoms) or an AAA that has found a pathway for drainage through the oral mucosa.

◆ *RADIOLOGY (Fig. 7–31)*

The radiograph of advanced chronic apical periodontitis shows a radiolucent periapical lesion of varying size, shape, and appearance. Radiographically, the lesions of chronic apical periodontitis may appear large or small, and they may be diffuse or well circumscribed. It is not possible for the clinician to make a positive diagnosis of chronic apical periodontitis by radiographic evidence only.

Priebe and associates found a lack of correlation between radiographic interpretation of periapical lesions and microscopic findings, which is partly in variance with the findings of Brynolf (1978), Kronfeld (1939), and Suzuki (1960). Therefore, to be safe, the term "advanced chronic apical periodontitis" should be used until the nature of the lesion is confirmed, whether it is an abscess, granuloma, or cyst.

An apical lesion can be diagnosed definitively only if the lesion is removed and studied under a microscope. It is possible, however, for the clinician to make a provisional diagnosis from the radiograph and clinical findings and to plan appropriate therapy for the tooth in question.

On the radiographic examination, a chronic apical abscess presents a diffuse area of radiolucency, whereas the apical granuloma has a more definitely limited or circumscribed area of radiolucency. The apical cyst shows an even more circumscribed radiolucency bounded by an unbroken line of sclerotic bone.

The lamina dura (alveolar bone proper) is applied to the thin layer of dense cortical bone that lines the normal tooth socket. The compact bone over the alveolar crest also is included as a portion of lamina dura. Because of its density, the lamina dura is shown in radiographs as a thin white line.

Persistent periapical inflammation results in resorption of the periapical lamina dura and will appear radiographically to have lost its continuity, its thickness, and varying degrees of its radiopacity. With few exceptions, it usually indicates that periapical disease is present (Fig. 7–31).

The absence of a break in the lamina dura, however, does not rule out an early periapical inflammatory lesion because the radiographic evidence lags behind the actual bone destruction. Early and colleagues (1979) estimated that at least a 30 to 60% mineral loss from bone must occur before this is visible on the radiograph.

It has been reported by Bender and Seltzer (1961), Ramadan and Mitchell (1961), and Shoha and associates (1974) that even though cancellous bone has been destroyed, the periapical radiograph will not show any change unless the lesion encroaches upon the junctional portion of the trabeculae with the inner portion of the cortical bone. Therefore, a lesion around the mesial root of the lower first molar would become more readily visible on the radiograph than the distal root because the mesial root usually is closer to the cortical plate.

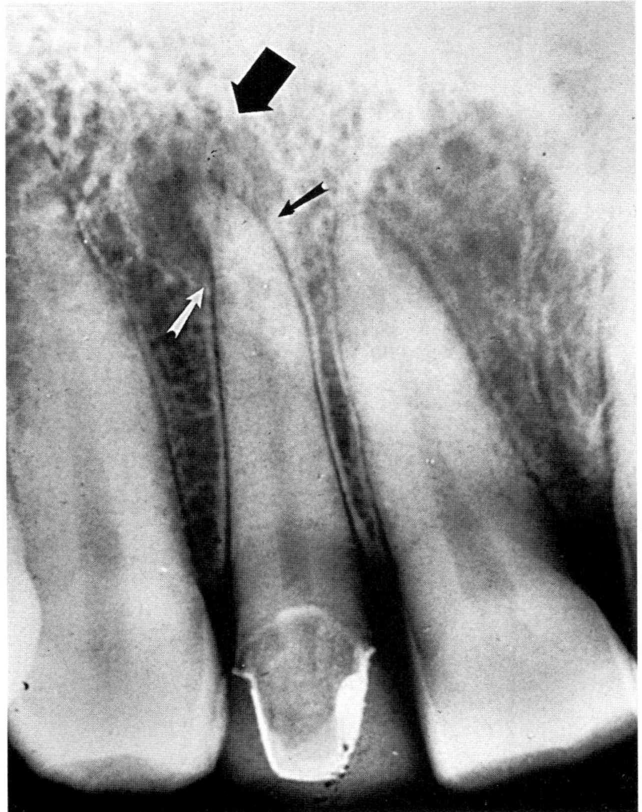

FIGURE 7–31.

Lamina dura discontinuity. See the loss of continuity of the lamina dura (small arrows) (white line surrounding the apex of a nonvital maxillary lateral incisor). This asymptomatic apical radiolucency is consistent with chronic apical periodontitis (large arrow).

Apical Granuloma (Periapical Granuloma, Dental Granuloma)

An apical granuloma is an advanced form of chronic apical periodontitis characterized by a growth of granulomatous tissue continuous with the periapical ligament, resulting from death of the pulp, with diffusion of mild infection or irritation of the periapical tissue, stimulating a productive cellular reaction. A massive invasion of infective or contaminated elements of the pulp canal will result in the formation of an AAA (recrudescent or phoenix abscess).

The term granuloma is a misnomer because the tissue referred to is composed principally of chronic inflammatory tissue; it is not a tumor, as is intimated; and it does not resemble the infectious or tuberculoid granuloma clinically or microscopically. The term ''apical or dental granuloma'' is in common usage and, until a more appropriate term is found, we will use it in our classification.

Basically, the apical granuloma may be viewed as a successful attempt by the periapical tissue to neutralize and confine the irritating toxic products that are escaping from the root canal. The continual discharge of chronic irritation products from the canal into the periapical tissue, however, is sufficient to maintain a chronic, low-grade defensive inflammatory reaction in these tissues. A requisite condition for the development of a granuloma is a continued mild irritation that is not severe enough to produce an abscess.

In 1981, McKinney clarified the difference between the terms ''granulation'' and ''granulomatous tissue.'' He pointed out that ''granulomatous'' refers to a specific type of inflammation, the outstanding feature of which is the presence of mononuclear phagocytic cells, such as monocytes, macrophages, and sometimes epithelioid cells (large fibroblasts and macrophages that have transformed into epithelium-like cells). McKinney (1981) also explained that granulomatous tissue generally has a distinctive pattern, an arrangement of cells with a central area of necrosis or fibroid material surrounded by a cellular reaction consisting mainly of mononuclear phagocytes and some lymphocytes. New collagen fibers and ground substance predominate toward the periphery of the lesion because fibrous healing already may have begun and the irritants are diluted and neutralized some distance from the apex. From this description, it would be best to consider the apical granuloma an example of granulomatous tissue.

Granulation tissue, in contrast to granulomatous tissue, is a tissue of healing and repair. It usually occurs after the injury and is characterized on microscopic examination by proliferating capillaries, many young fibroblasts, new collagen fibers, ground substance, and macrophages.

A granuloma often is thought to consist of granulation tissue only. Although it contains granulation tissue, its main constituent is chronic inflammatory tissue (granulomatous tissue). For this reason, the term granulomatous tissue is used in this chapter, rather than granulation tissue, in referring to a granuloma.

The diameter of granulomatous tissue of an apical granuloma may vary from the size of a pinhead to greater than a large pea. It consists of an outer, fibrous capsule that is continuous with the periodontal ligament and an inner portion composed of looser connective tissue and blood vessels. It is characterized by the presence of various chronic inflammatory cells (macrophages, lymphocytes, plasma cells, and occasional polymorphonuclear leukocytes). A wall of collagen fibers is laid down by the fibroblasts in an attempt to encapsulate the entire inflammatory complex, separating the granulomatous tissue from bone. Kronfeld (1939) stated that a "granuloma is not an area in which bacteria live, but an area in which they are destroyed."

Apical granuloma is the most common periapical radiolucency found in dental practice. Block and associates (1976) reported that, on microscopic evaluation of 230 pulpoperiapical radiolucent lesions treated by apicoectomy, 94% were granulomas and 6% were cysts. Smulson and Hagen (1989) reviewed nine biopsy studies; six were based on 200 or more cases. They found that the incidence of apical granulomas compared with apical cysts in these nine studies was from 84% to 51% apical granulomas. Lalonde (1970) and Natkin and associates (1984) reported that there appears to be a trend toward an increased incidence of cysts as the lesions become larger.

Bhaskar (1966) found that the incidence of apical granulomas was the same in both sexes, but they occurred in the maxilla approximately three times more frequently than in the mandible. The greatest incidence was in patients in the third decade of life.

Apical granulomas are asymptomatic, except in rare cases when they break down and undergo suppuration. In most cases, a granuloma generally is discovered on a radiograph, from which a tentative diagnosis is made. The involved tooth generally is not tender to percussion and is not loose. The tooth will not respond to thermal or electrical pulp tests. It may have a darker color than adjacent teeth because of blood pigments that have diffused into the empty dentinal tubules.

When a small apical granuloma is present, root canal therapy is usually the treatment of choice if the tooth is to be retained. Root canal treatment of an apical granuloma usually will result in resorption of the granulomatous/granulation tissue and repair with well-trabeculated bone. When a large area of radiolucency is found on a radiograph, root resection or periapical curettage may be indicated because the amount of destroyed bone may be too much for the reparative forces of the body to bring about a complete repair. Strindberg (1956) found a high incidence of endodontic failure in cases with large radiolucent areas.

◆ RADIOLOGY (Figs. 7–32 and 7–33)

Radiographically, the apical granuloma appears as a radiolucent, circular-to-ovoid area that encloses the root end and extends apically from it. Trabeculations of the alveolar bone may be seen superimposed over the lesion because the lesion has a grayish appearance and is not dark. In longstanding lesions, cancellous supporting (marrow) bone may become compact and radiopaque on the margin of the lesion (Figs. 7–32 and 7–33).

For a granuloma, the area of radiolucency is well defined, whereas that of a chronic abscess is generally diffuse. In some cases, however, the periapical tissue is in a transitional stage between an apical chronic abscess and an apical granuloma, and an exact diagnosis may be difficult. A well-defined radiolucency at the apex of an untreated, asymptomatic, nonvital tooth is an apical granuloma or apical cyst in approximately 90% of the cases.

Although an apical granuloma and apical cyst cannot be differentiated by radiologic features alone, Lalonde (1970) stated that, if the radiolucency is larger than 1.6 cm in diameter, it is most likely an apical cyst. Few granulomas ever

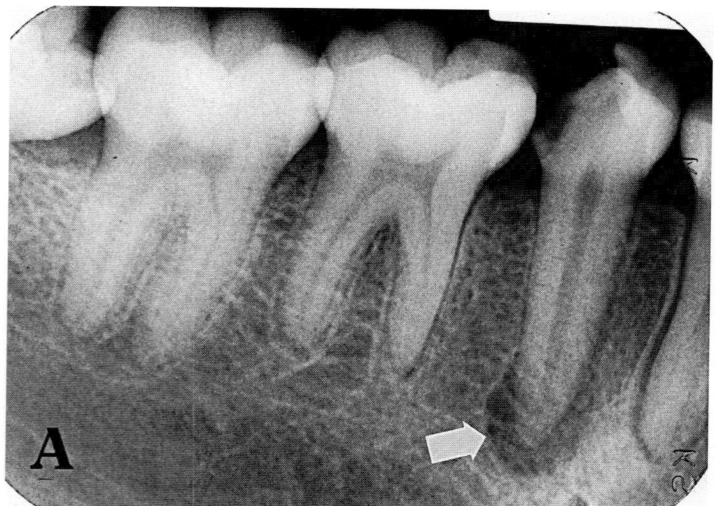

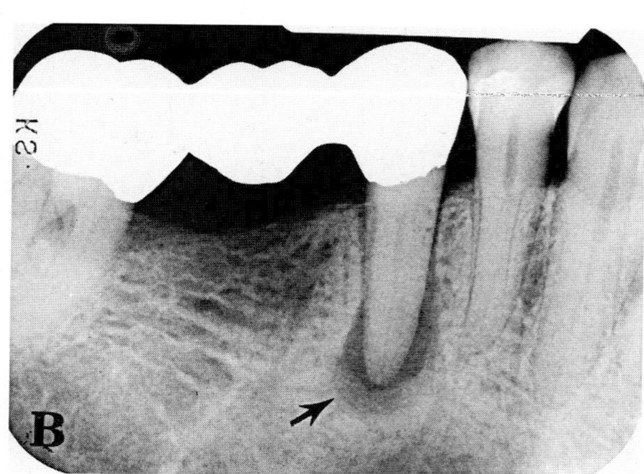

FIGURE 7–32.

Apical granuloma. A, Radiographic appearance of apical granuloma at apex of mandibular second premolar (arrow). Notice that bony trabeculations are superimposed over the lesion. B, Another radiographic appearance of apical granuloma at apex of second premolar (arrow).

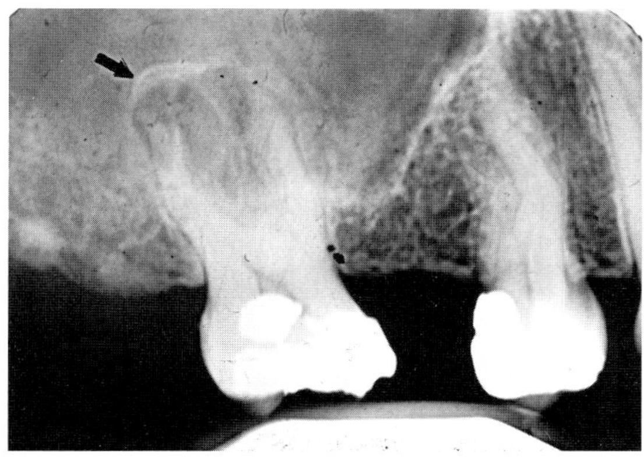

FIGURE 7–33.

Apical granuloma. Saclike structure (arrow) enucleated from the apical region of the lingual root of the maxillary second molar showed involvement of the maxillary sinus. Histologic examination showed tissue compatible with an apical granuloma with epithelium present along one margin that was typical of respiratory epithelium. (Courtesy of Dr. M. Kasle, Indianapolis, IN.)

become larger than 1.6 cm in diameter. Also, the cyst may cause the roots of adjacent teeth to spread apart because of the continued pressure of accumulated cystic fluid.

In practice, however, it usually is not necessary to differentiate between an apical granuloma and a cyst radiographically because both respond well to root canal therapy without surgical intervention. Also, the apical granuloma must be differentiated from the apical cementoma, which involves a vital tooth.

Apical Cyst (Radicular Cyst, Root End Cyst, Periapical Cyst, Alveolar Cyst)

The apical cyst is the second most common pathologic periapical radiolucency. The apical granuloma is the most common.

There seems to be intense disagreement as to the incidence of apical (radicular) cysts, which are granulomatous lesions with central epithelial-lined lumina. The incidence of apical cysts has been reported as follows in series of periapical radiolucencies: 6% (Block [1976]), 17% (Stockdale and Chandler [1988]), 42% (Bhaskar [1966]), 44% (Lalonde and Luebke [1968]), and 47% (Ross and Birch [1976]).

According to Browne (1961), approximately 75% of cysts occur in the maxilla and 25% in the mandible. He found that, in the maxilla, 62% of the cysts occurred with the incisors, and in the mandible, 48% of the cysts occurred with the molars.

In a large study, Bhaskar (1966) found that apical cysts were twice as common in male compared with female patients and occurred 10 times as frequently in the maxilla as the mandible. The greatest incidence was in the third decade of life.

In a histologic section, an apical cyst is seen as a granulomatous lesion with a central cavity filled with an eosinophilic fluid or semisolid material and is lined incompletely by stratified squamous epithelium. The epithelium is surrounded by connective tissue that contains all the cellular elements found in the apical granuloma. Thus, the apical cyst is an inflammatory lesion, or a "cyst within a granuloma."

Cysts expand slowly; the fluid formed within the cyst increases the interstitial pressure abutting the bone margins; and resorption results. Eventually, the lesion may become large.

Although the exact cause of apical cysts is unknown, there are several theories of how cysts form. Harris and Toller (1975) probably presented the most widely accepted view. They theorized that epithelial cell rests, in the vicinity of an inflammatory lesion, are stimulated to proliferate by pulpal inflammatory or necrotic irritants. The origin of the epithelium in the apical cyst is most frequently from the cell rests of Malassez, which are remnants of Hertwig's root sheath. Practically all apical cysts originate from a pre-existing apical granuloma, and their pathogenesis depends on an inflammatory response. Therefore, they are classified as inflammatory cysts; however, they also could be called odontogenic cysts because they originate from Hertwig's root sheath, which is a product of odontogenic epithelial layers (the inner and outer enamel epithelial layers). After root formation, disintegration of Hertwig's root sheath results in the persistence of epithelial rests in the periodontal ligament. These epithelial cells rests (called cell rests of Malassez) are present in practically all apical granulomas.

There are no symptoms associated with the development of an apical cyst, except those that may be incidental to chronic root canal infection. The pulp of a tooth with an apical cyst will not react to electrical or thermal stimuli. A cyst may grow large enough to become an obvious swelling. The pressure of the cyst may be sufficient to cause movement of the affected tooth because of the accumulation of fluid in the cystic cavity. In some cases, the root apices of the involved teeth become spread apart, so the crowns of the teeth are forced out of line. The teeth may become mobile. The swelling may develop on the buccal or lingual side of the alveolar process. It usually is covered with a normal-appearing mucous membrane. At first, the bone surrounding the cyst is bony hard to palpation, but later a crackling sound (crepitus) may be heard as the cortical bone becomes thinned. When the clinical swelling is rubbery and fluctuant, this is a sign that the apical cyst has completely resorbed the overlying bone. Larger cysts may involve a complete quadrant and some teeth are nonvital. If the cyst is filled with sterile fluid, neither the causative tooth nor the expanding cyst is painful. If the cyst becomes infected, the tooth and swelling have all the painful symptoms of an abscess.

On aspiration of a noninfected apical cyst, the fluid is light and straw colored, usually containing an abundance of shiny granules (cholesterol crystals).

A small apical cyst usually is treated by removal of necrotic pulpal irritants and complete obturation of the root canal system. The healing pattern is similar to that of the apical granuloma. Periodically, the radiolucent lesion should be examined radiographically to ensure that the lesion is regressing properly. Shah (1988) reported an 84.4% success rate for 132 teeth with periapical radiolucencies that were treated by root canal treatment alone without surgery. Many clinicians believe that when the lesion is large, healing is facilitated only by surgery; however, if the dominant periapical tissue is granulomatous, surgical intervention removes tissue already mobilized for healing and repair. Weine (1989) stated that large and small lesions have the capacity and potential for healing.

Most clinicians agree that nonsurgical treatment of periapical radiolucencies is correct because the root canal must be cleansed and filled in any case. Surgery should be initiated only if periapical healing has not occurred after a suitable observation period.

One of the most accepted theories explaining why apical cysts have the potential for healing without surgical intervention was presented by Seltzer and colleagues (1963) and Bender (1972). When the pressure of the irritating products of the necrotic pulp is eliminated by drainage or absorption of the fluid and the root canal is sealed, healing begins at the periphery of the cystic lesion and moves toward the center. Healing never starts from the center, as can be seen radiographically. Newly formed collagen fibers of repair are laid down, the blood supply to the epithelial lining of the apical cyst becomes impaired, and the epithelial cells die. The products from these degenerating epithelial cells are responsible for the inflammatory reaction that stimulates proliferation of granulation tissue, and, in turn, the granulation fills the cystic space.

Sometimes large apical cysts that have destroyed a great amount of bone are found. Grossman (1974) recommended that if the apical cyst is large, its removal by root resection and soft tissue curettement might endanger the vitality of an adjacent tooth or teeth because of interruption of the blood supply during curettement. Root canal treatment of the affected tooth, along with evacuation of the cyst contents, may be attempted. This is done by collapsing the cyst, inserting a rubber dam or gauze drain over a period of several weeks, and changing the drain weekly. When the cyst becomes smaller, root resection and curettement of soft tissue is performed in the usual manner without endangering the adjacent teeth.

Incomplete removal of the cyst lining after tooth extraction may result in the formation of a residual cyst or, in rare instances, a more aggressive type of pathosis.

◆ RADIOLOGY (Figs. 7–34 to 7–39)

The apical cyst is a cavity in bone that contains fluid. Consequently, the radiographic appearance is that of bone destruction, which is seen as a dark radiolucent area. The margins are sharp and clearly defined, and in uncomplicated cases a thin white line surrounds the margin of the cavity. This hyperostotic border indicates a reaction of the bone to the slowly expanding mass. The apical granuloma also may show an opaque border in some instances. Because the apical granuloma and apical cyst may have identical radiographic appearances, the cyst sometimes may be differentiated from the granuloma by virtue of its size. The apical granuloma is usually smaller than 1 cm in diameter, whereas the apical cyst may become as large as 10 cm (Figs. 7–34 and 7–35).

Studies by Lalonde (1970) showed that a well-defined periapical radiolucency at the apex of a tooth is more likely an apical cyst if the radiolucency is at least 1.6 cm in diameter. Strathers and Shear (1976) reported that 18% of radicular cysts showed external root resorption. An untreated cyst may enlarge slowly and cause expansion of the cortical plates. The larger apical cysts may involve two or more teeth (Fig. 7–36).

It is essential to take sequential posttreatment radiographs of the endodontically treated tooth with a possible apical cyst to be sure the radiolucency is regressing. The average

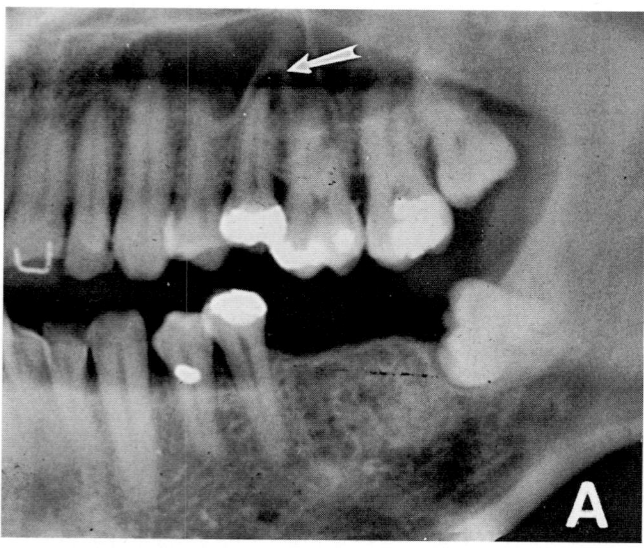

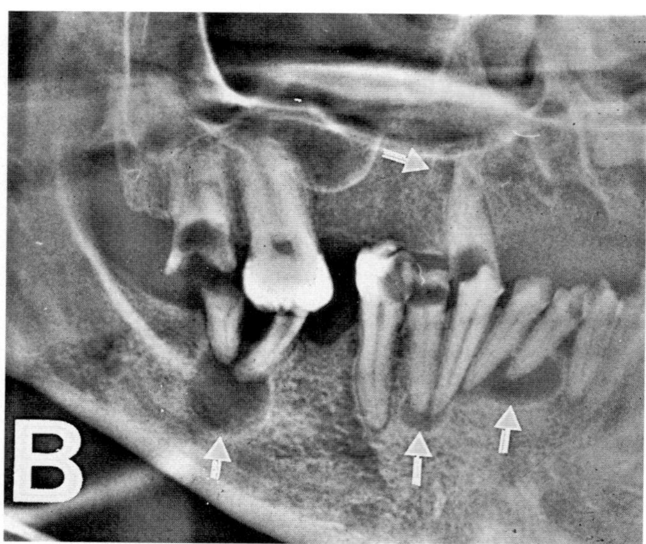

FIGURE 7–34.

Apical cyst. A, Classic appearance of an apical cyst of upper second premolar. The radiolucency is dark, circumscribed, sharply outlined, and bounded by a thin, even, white line that presumably represents reactive bone (arrow). B, Multiple cysts (arrows). (From Langland OE, Langlais RP, Morris CR: Principles and Practice of Panoramic Radiology. Philadelphia:WB Saunders, 1982, p. 235.)

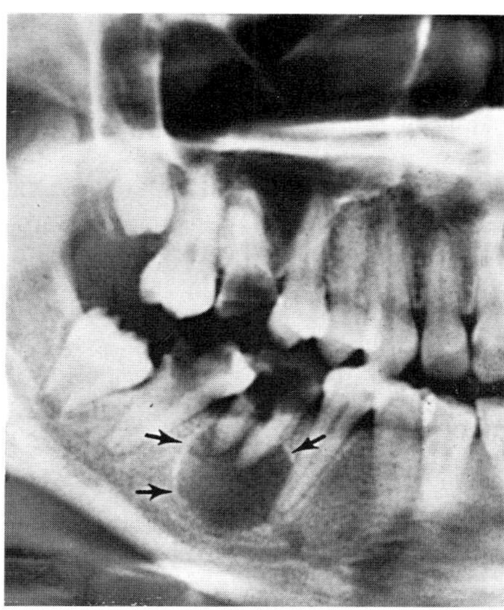

FIGURE 7–35.

Apical cyst. Apical cyst at retained root tips of mandibular first molar confirmed by microscopic examination (arrows).

healing time for cysts larger than 10 mm in diameter is 2.5 years. If repair does not occur, resection can be performed. Therefore, treatment of an apical cyst by nonsurgical intervention is possible on a theoretic basis, but there is no definite proof that healing will occur.

The incomplete surgical removal of the epithelial lining of some cysts, especially the large cysts, may result in the formation of a residual cyst. The term residual cyst can be applied to any cyst of the jaw that remains after a surgical procedure. A residual cyst is usually a radicular (apical) cyst that remains in the jaw after the associated tooth is extracted. Although on some occasions a dentigerous cyst may persist after removal of an unerupted tooth, most residual cysts were apical cysts before tooth removal.

The apical cyst should be differentiated from the nasopalatine (incisive foramen) cyst, globulomaxillary cyst, dentigerous cyst, traumatic bone cyst, apical cementoma, and mandibular infected buccal cyst. Usually the teeth associated with the above-mentioned cysts have a vital pulp and intact lamina dura, whereas the pulp of the tooth associated with an apical cyst is nonvital and the lamina dura is not intact.

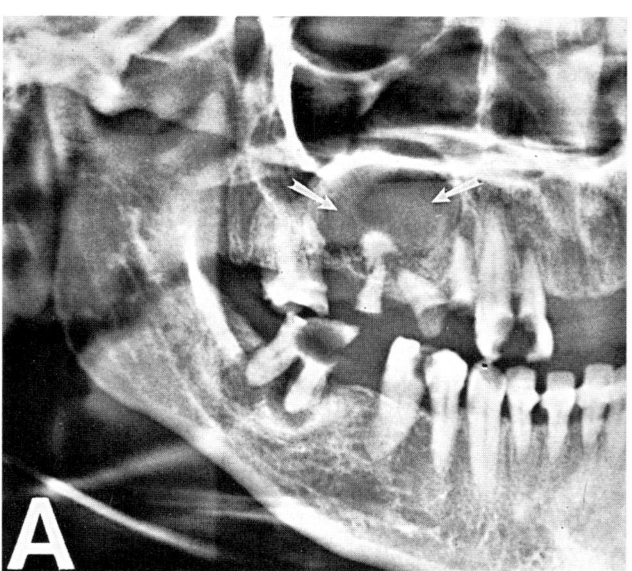

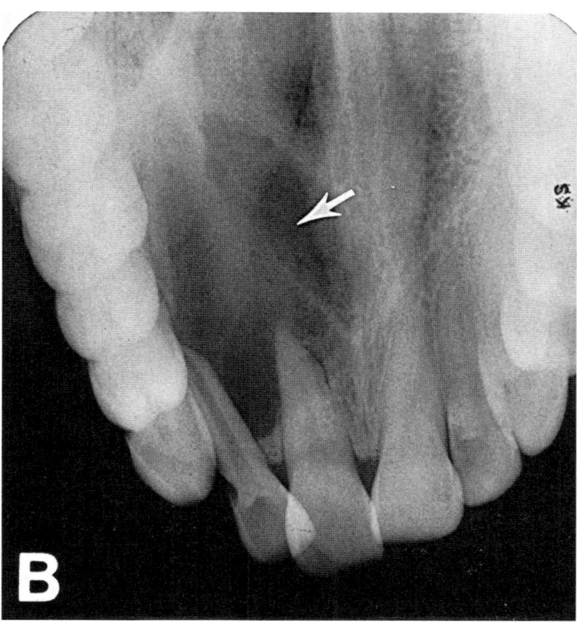

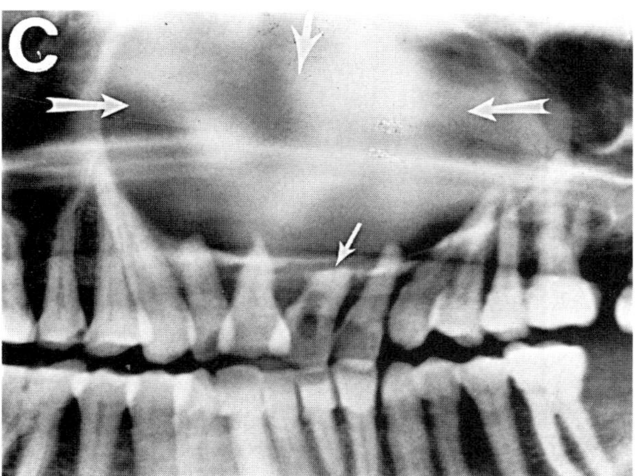

FIGURE 7–36.

Apical cyst. A, Panoramic radiograph of confirmed large apical cyst associated with root tips of maxillary first premolar and first molar. The cyst was encroaching on the maxillary sinus (arrows). (From Langland OE, Langlais RP, Morris CR: Principles and Practice of Panoramic Radiology. Philadelphia: WB Saunders, 1982, p. 235.) B, Occlusal radiograph of large apical cyst associated with central and lateral incisor (arrow). (Courtesy of Drs. L. Archilla, F. Erales, R. Carlos, Guatemala City, Guatemala.) C, Large apical cyst (large arrows) in maxilla associated with left central incisor (small arrow) in a 68-year-old man. (Courtesy of Dr. E. Romero, Monterrey, Mexico.)

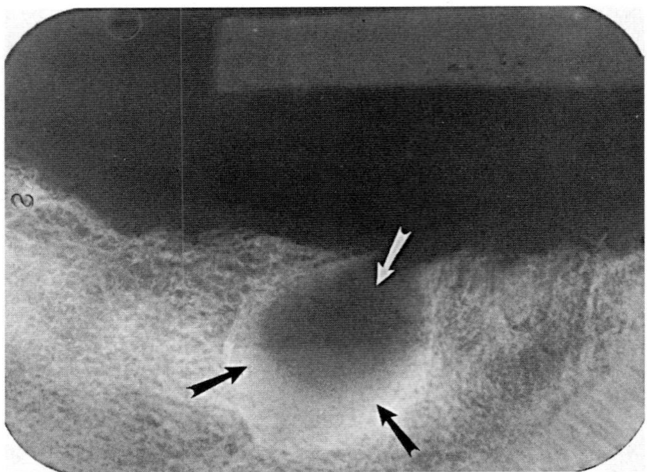

FIGURE 7–37.

Residual cyst. Residual cyst in mandibular bone after extraction of the mandibular second molar (arrows).

When a radiolucency is present on the lateral portion of a root rather than at the apex of an nonvital tooth, it is usually an indication that a significant lateral canal is present or that the apical foramen exits on the lateral portion of the root rather than on the apical portion. When surgery is performed in these cases, the portion of the root contacting the inflamed area must be examined to locate the canal. If the canal can be located, a reverse filling is placed.

The lateral periodontal cyst is uncommon and is thought to originate from postfunctional dental lamina rests. The teeth usually are vital, and the radiograph discloses a radiolucent area in apposition to the lateral surface of a tooth root. The lesion is small, seldom larger than 1 cm in diameter, and may or may not be well circumscribed. In a study of 39 cases by Wysocki and associates (1980), 67% of cases were in the mandibular premolar/canine/incisor region.

A periapical granuloma, cyst, or abscess may end in the formation of dense scar tissue rather than bone in the lesion defect. Although there is scant literature concerning the periapical scar, Wood and associates (1980) estimated that 2 to 5% of all periapical radiolucent lesions are periapical scars.

When a tooth has been treated successfully by nonsurgical endodontic techniques and the inciting irritants have been removed, the granuloma or cyst usually resolves itself and no longer can be seen on the radiograph. Sometimes the granulation tissue produces more and more collagen fibers, and eventually dense tissue scar results, which remains as a permanent radiolucency on the radiograph (Fig. 7–38).

The periapical scar usually is a well-circumscribed radiolucency that resembles a granuloma or cyst. It is frequently smaller than the cyst or granuloma. Over the years, the size of the radiolucency will remain constant or may even diminish.

A surgical or fibrous healing defect forms occasionally when large amounts of faciolingual cortical bone, along with the periosteum, have been destroyed by a surgical procedure. Wood and colleagues (1980) estimated that approximately 45% of all periapical radiolucencies treated surgically require 1 to 10 years for complete resolution, and another 45% take longer than 10 years.

The healing or surgical defect is especially prevalent in the anterior portion of the maxilla after an apicoectomy or root resection has been performed and a large portion of the lingual and labial cortical bone has been destroyed. There will be a deficiency in the bone-forming elements required to repair the defect. The bone defect is filled with dense fibrous connective tissue, and it should not be interpreted as an area of infection. If the bone surrounding the defect and root apex is normal, this usually indicates that no form of irritation is present. It does not indicate that the root resection or apicoectomy was a failure. The defect may never repair itself fully, but most become smaller as time passes. If the radiolucency increases in size, it must be considered a recurrence of the original pathologic process or a new lesion.

Radiographically, the healing or surgical defect radiolucency appears as a cystlike, well-defined, round or ovoid lesion within the bone (Fig. 7–39). It usually is not larger than 1 cm in diameter and is frequently smaller. The healing defect is completely asymptomatic.

The surgical (fibrous healing) defect can be confused with the periapical scar. If the radiolucency moves from the apex when the x-ray beam is shifted in sequential radiographs, the radiolucency is most likely a surgical defect. The periapical scar will not move from the tooth apex when the angle of the x-ray beam is shifted.

If the radiolucency is caused by a surgical defect, it will show a reduction in size as it is examined periodically, especially during the first 6 months after surgery.

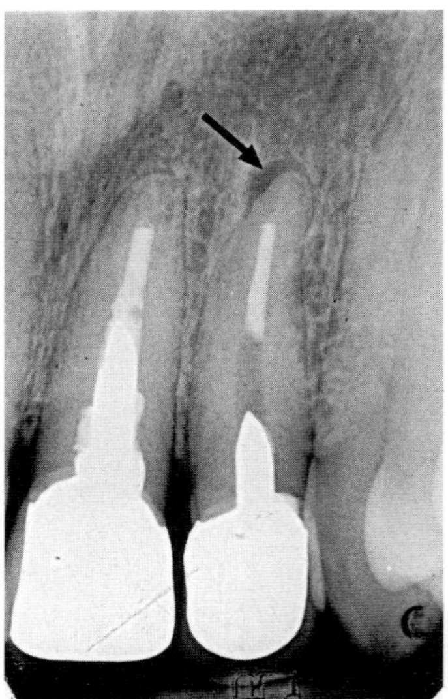

FIGURE 7–38.

Apical scar. The maxillary lateral incisor was treated endodontically for post and core crown. The tooth has remained asymptomatic since the root canal was completed. The reduced size of the periapical radiolucency has remained constant for a number of years. It is assumed to be a periapical scar (arrow).

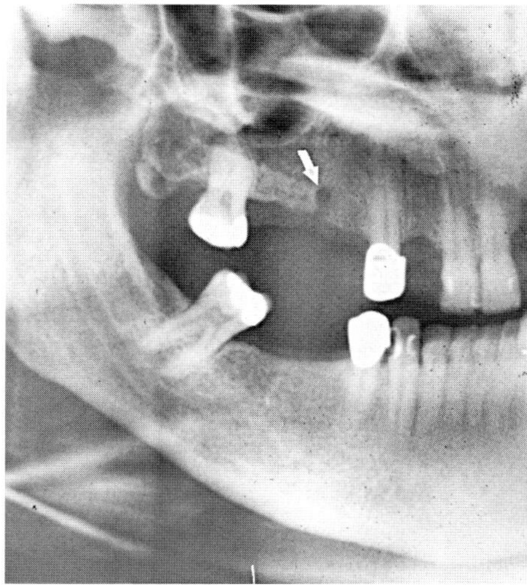

A

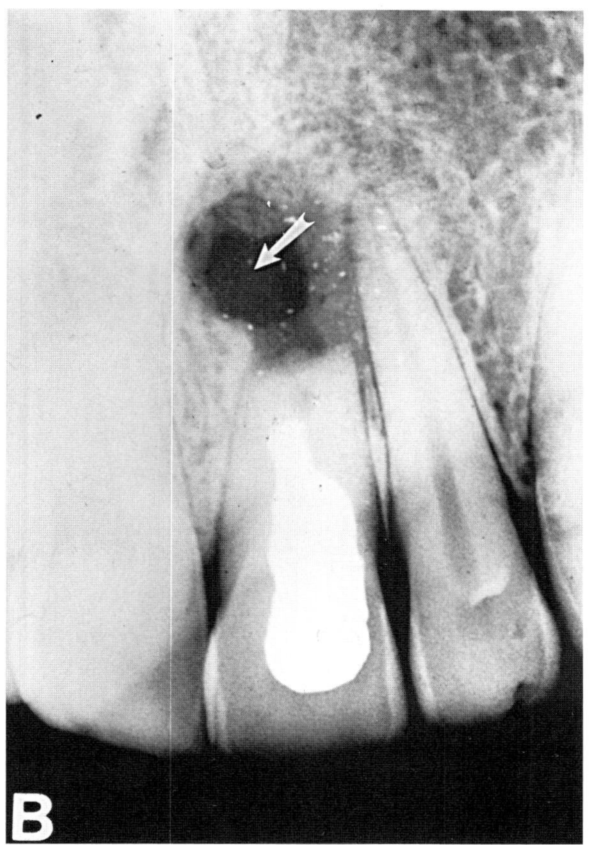

FIGURE 7–39.

Fibrous healing defect. A, The surgical treatment of a periapical lesion caused a fibrous healing defect probably because portions of the buccolingual cortical bone and periosteum were destroyed during the surgical procedure (notice arrow in edentulous ridge of maxillary arch). B, Fibrous healing defect after apicoectomy of central incisor (arrow).

Chronic Apical Abscess (Suppurative Apical Periodontitis, Chronic Alveolar Abscess, Chronic Dentoalveolar Abscess, Subacute Periapical Abscess)

The chronic apical abscess is a longstanding, low-grade inflammatory reaction to irritating products from a necrotic pulp. It is characterized by the formation of an abscess (pus) at the periapical region of a tooth.

If the chronic infection is untreated, the chronic abscess frequently forms a sinus tract, permitting the pus to drain to the surface of the oral mucosa or the skin of the face. At the sinus tract stoma (mouth), a small proliferation of granulomatous tissue often forms on the mucosal surface and is referred to as a parulis or ''gumboil.'' The gumboil or parulis frequently is observed in conjunction with infection of primary or permanent teeth. Sometimes the chronic apical abscess may drain through the periodontium into the sulcus and mimic a periodontal pocket (see Fig. 7–41). Where an open cavity is present in the tooth, drainage may occur by the root canal. When no fistula is present and the toxic products are absorbed through blood and lymph channels, the condition sometimes is referred to as a ''blind abscess.''

A chronic apical abscess may occur as a natural developmental sequence of the death of the pulp with extension of the infective process periapically, in which the virulence and number of bacterial organisms are low and the host resistance is high. Grossman (1974) stated that the microorganisms most commonly recovered from a pulpless tooth with a chronic abscess are primarily alpha streptococci of low virulence. Also, the chronic apical abscess may result from an AAA that has found drainage through a sinus through the oral mucosa. Sometimes a chronic apical abscess may occur after unsatisfactory root canal therapy.

Mild painful symptoms occur when the sinus tract stoma becomes blocked either by a clot of drainage material or the growth of mucosal epithelium over the stoma (mouth). During this mild symptomatic phase, the term subacute periapical abscess is used. It is during this mild phase of the chronic apical abscess cycle that drainage ceases, the periapical pressure increases, and the tooth becomes mildly tender to percussion. The pressure causes the tissue to swell again, and the inflammation spreads to the soft tissue adjacent to the sinus tract stoma (mouth). A parulis (gumboil) develops over the mucosa, and a circumscribed red swelling may develop in the gingiva.

The opening may be reopened when pressure from the contained pus overcomes the resistance of the undermined layer of soft tissue. Therefore, there is a delicate interplay for dominance of one phase of the chronic apical abscess over the other, depending on whether the abscess is draining adequately.

When there is proper drainage of the chronic apical abscess, it is asymptomatic. It may be detected during routine radiographic examination, or because of the sinus tract. The tissues seldom swell. The radiograph will show a diffuse area of bone radiolucency (Figs. 7–40 and 7–41).

When the patient is questioned regarding the possible

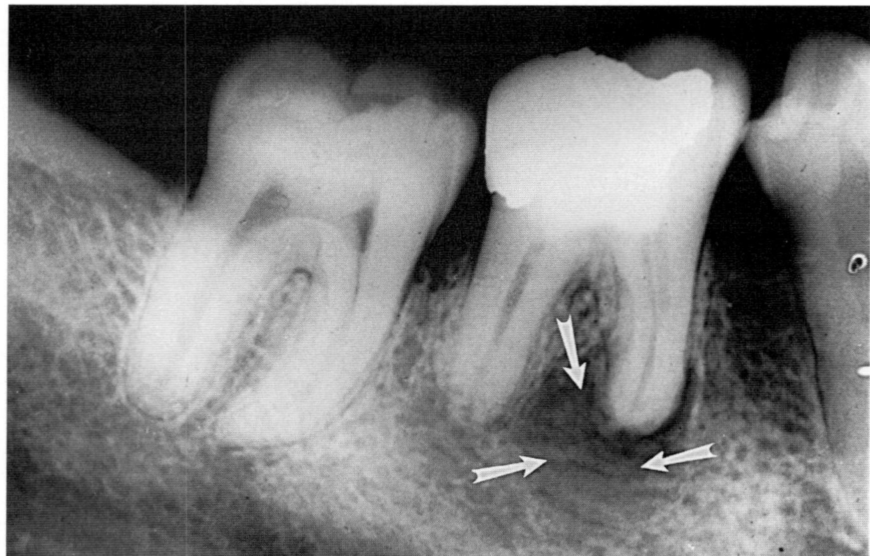

FIGURE 7–40.

Chronic apical abscess. Notice the diffuse area of radiolucency of the mesial root of the lower first molar (arrows). The granuloma and cyst have a more definite circumscribed area of radiolucency than the apical abscess.

cause of the abscess, he or she may remember a sudden, sharp pain that eased after awhile, with the tooth being comfortable since then, or the patient may recall a traumatic injury that happened months or years previously. On clinical examination of the teeth, one may discover a discolored tooth or the presence of caries, a restoration, or a crown under which the pulp has died without causing any symptoms. The tooth may be slightly loose or tender to percussion. On palpation, the apical soft tissue may be slightly swollen and tender. Often a parulis is found. The tooth shows no reaction to the electric pulp test.

The microscopic picture varies, but, depending on the stage of infection, it basically consists of a central area of necrosis containing a dense accumulation of disintegrating polymorphonuclear leukocytes surrounded by variable leukocytes and occasional lymphocytes. Surrounding the abscess or necrotic center is granulomatous tissue. Actually it is an abscess within a granuloma. Fibroblasts may be seen at the periphery, beginning to form a capsule. Baumgartner and associates (1984) reported that the additional microscopic feature of the chronic apical abscess is the sinus tract, which may be lined partially or totally by epithelium surrounded by inflamed connective tissue.

The chronic apical abscess heals spontaneously after adequate root canal treatment. Once the infection in the root canal is eliminated and the canal is filled, repair of the periapical tissues generally will occur. If a fistula is present, it will close up or disappear without any special treatment as soon as the root canal is rendered sterile.

◆ *RADIOLOGY (Figs. 7–40 and 7–41)*

Radiographically, the chronic apical abscess presents a diffuse area of radiolucency at the apex of a tooth. Often the radiolucency is represented by an area of lesser density than the granuloma or cyst (Figs. 7–40 and 7–41).

When a fistula is present, it may be near the root apex of the tooth or it may be some distance from it. The insertion of a gutta percha cone into the fistula often will indicate which tooth is involved. At times the fistula stoma (opening) is located several teeth from the involved tooth.

The most usual route of the fistulous tract is through the facial or lingual alveolar bone, where there is usually formation of a parulis and active pus formation draining through the stoma of a sinus tract. Sometimes the pus may drain through the periodontal ligament space (Fig. 7–41).

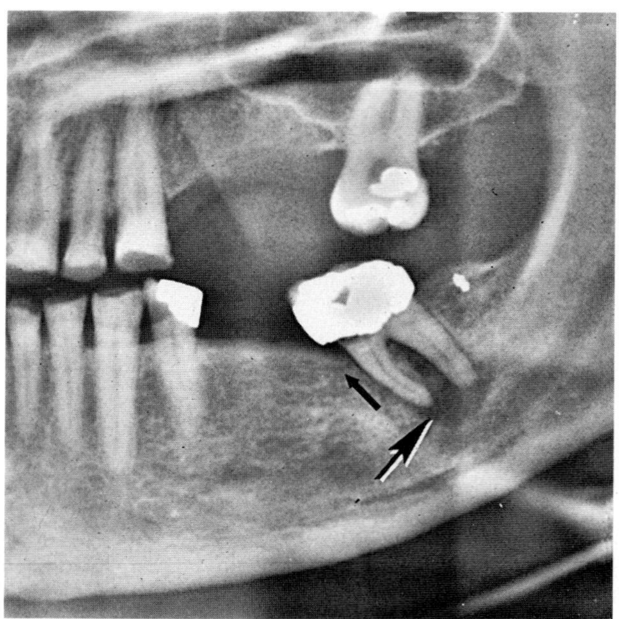

FIGURE 7–41.

Chronic apical abscess. Chronic apical abscess with passageway established through the PDL space on mesial root of lower second molar for free drainage of pus to surface (arrow). (From Langland OE, Langlais RP, Morris CR: Principles and Practice of Panoramic Radiology. Philadelphia: WB Saunders, 1982, p. 246.)

Phoenix Abscess (Recrudescent Abscess)

There are abscesses that have developed in a previously existing asymptomatic periapical radiolucent lesion, for instance, a granuloma, cyst, or scar. The phoenix abscess is an acute periapical exacerbation that arises from a previously existing chronic granulomatous lesion. It develops when the granulomatous tissue becomes contaminated or infected by elements from the root canal. It has this name because the phoenix was the bird from Egyptian mythology that arose every 500 years from its own ashes in the desert and then consumed itself in fire. Therefore, it is an appropriate name for this abscess. Recrudescence is defined as the recurrence of symptoms after a temporary abatement.

A phoenix abscess is advanced chronic apical periodontitis without a sinus tract that suddenly becomes symptomatic. The symptoms are identical to those of an AAA. The main difference is that a phoenix abscess is preceded by a chronic condition. The diagnosis is based on the acute symptoms and a radiograph that shows a large periapical radiolucency.

A phoenix abscess may develop spontaneously or almost immediately after initiation of endodontic treatment on a tooth diagnosed as having chronic apical periodontitis without a sinus tract. During biomechanical preparation of the root canal, bacteria or other irritants may be forced inadvertently through the apical foramen and may upset the dynamic equilibrium of a chronic apical periodontitis. The development of a phoenix abscess depends on various factors: the number and virulence of the invading organisms, resistance of the host, and type and timing of the treatment instituted. The treatment is the same as for the AAA, which is the removal of the underlying cause (necrotic pulp), release of pressure (drainage where possible), and then routine root canal therapy.

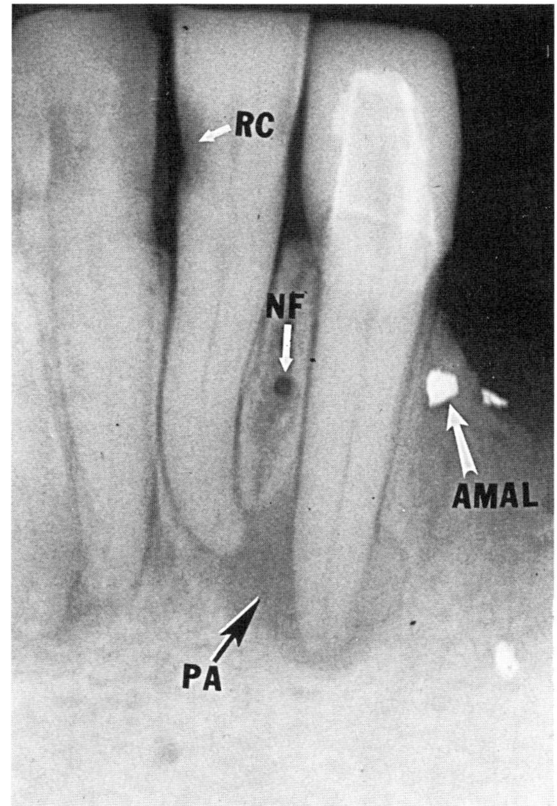

FIGURE 7–42.

Phoenix (recrudescent) abscess. Definite periapical radiolucency of mandibular central and lateral with a porcelain crown. The tooth has all the acute symptoms of an acute apical abscess (PA). Notice the root caries (RC), nutrient foramen (NF), and amalgam (AMAL) debris or tattoo. (From Langland OE, Langlais RP, Morris CR: Principles and Practice of Panoramic Radiology. Philadelphia:WB Saunders, 1982, p. 234.)

◆ *RADIOLOGY (Fig. 7–42)*

Diagnosis of a phoenix abscess is based on the acute symptoms plus radiographic examination, which shows a large periapical radiolucency. Sometimes the radiolucency will be so diffuse as to fade indistinctly into normal bone, or else it may be well demarcated from bone like the radiolucency of a cyst or granuloma (Fig. 7–42).

Apical Condensing Osteitis (Focal Sclerosing Osteomyelitis)

This is a mild inflammatory productive response of periapical bone to a low-grade longstanding pulpal irritation. It is characterized by an increase in the density of the periapical bone, not because of a greater concentration of minerals (hypercalcification) but because of osteoblastic activity. There is more bone tissue in a given space because the bony trabeculae increase in thickness to such a degree that the marrow spaces are eliminated or reduced to small tags of fibrous tissue.

Condensing osteitis (focal sclerosing osteomyelitis) is a variant of chronic apical periodontitis and represents a diffuse increase in trabecular bone in response to a persistent irritant. Although the terms osteomyelitis and osteitis often are used interchangeably, osteitis actually describes the more localized condition and osteomyelitis describes the more active diffuse condition. Differing responses to treatment also aid in the delineation of the two diseases: osteitis may be managed readily, whereas osteomyelitis often is difficult to treat.

The irritants in condensing osteitis come from pulp inflammation or necrosis. Condensing osteitis usually is found in patients younger than 20 years of age around the apices of mandibular teeth with large carious lesions and chronically inflamed pulps; however, condensing osteitis may occur around the apex of any tooth. Basically, it is a reaction of bone to a mild bacterial bone infection in people who have a high degree of tissue resistance and tissue reactivity. In such instances, the tissues react to the infection by proliferation, rather than destruction. Therefore, the infection acts as a stimulus rather than an irritant.

Depending on the cause (pulpitis or pulpal necrosis),

condensing osteitis can be asymptomatic or may be associated with pain and discomfort. Usually there are no signs or symptoms of disease other than mild pain associated with an infected pulp.

The pulp tissue of these teeth with condensing osteitis usually does not respond to electrical or thermal stimuli. Also, these teeth generally will not be sensitive to palpation or percussion.

Boyne (1960) found 38 cases of condensing osteitis sclerotic areas in a review of 927 full mouth radiographs of patients between 22 and 56 years of age, an incidence of 4%. This incidence is somewhat higher than previously supposed.

Histologically, there is an increase in irregularly arranged trabecular bone. If interstitial soft tissue is present, it is generally fibrotic and infiltrated only by small numbers of lymphocytes.

Hedin and Polhagen (1971) reported that root canal therapy, when indicated, may result in complete resolution of condensing osteitis. Therefore, a return to the normal trabecular pattern may occur after root canal therapy.

◆ RADIOLOGY (Figs. 7–43 to 7–48)

Radiographically, apical condensing osteitis appears as a pathognomonic, well-circumscribed radiopaque mass of sclerotic bone surrounding and extending below the apex of one or both roots (Figs. 7–43 and 7–44). Usually there is a radiolucency immediately adjacent to the apical end of the involved tooth. The entire root outline is always visible, which is an important feature in differentiating it from benign cementoblastoma.

The lesions vary greatly in size and shape. The margins of the affected area may be well defined or poorly defined, or trail off gradually into normal bone. A critical study of sclerotic bone in condensing osteitis determines that the separate trabeculae are thicker and denser than normal. Eventually the bone spaces are obliterated or lost to view from the superimposition of the many enlarged trabeculae. The result is a bony structure with greatly reduced marrow spaces and thick trabeculae.

It will be observed that the dense tissue lies outside the periodontal ligament space and lamina dura. This contrasts with the appearance of hypercementosis.

The sclerotic bone constituting the osteitis is not attached to the tooth and remains after the tooth is removed. It sometimes is not remodeled and, in many cases, may be seen several years later. The condensed sclerotic bone remaining in the normal bone often is confused with a nonpathologic entity known as enostosis or osteosclerosis.

Osteosclerosis (enostosis, bone whorls, bone islands, focal osteopetrosis) is a general term meaning "an increased bone formation resulting in reduced marrow spaces and increased radiopacity." It sometimes is used interchangeably with condensing osteitis, but it is best to limit osteosclerosis to abnormally dense areas in the bone resulting from trauma, stress, or some other noninflammatory cause and to use condensing osteitis when the origin is thought to be infection or inflammation resulting from a low-grade periapical or periodontal infection.

Radiographically, osteosclerosis presents as a more or less rounded or, less commonly, irregularly shaped area of increased density in which it is unusual to see bone structure (Fig. 7–45). Varying in size from a few millimeters to 1 cm

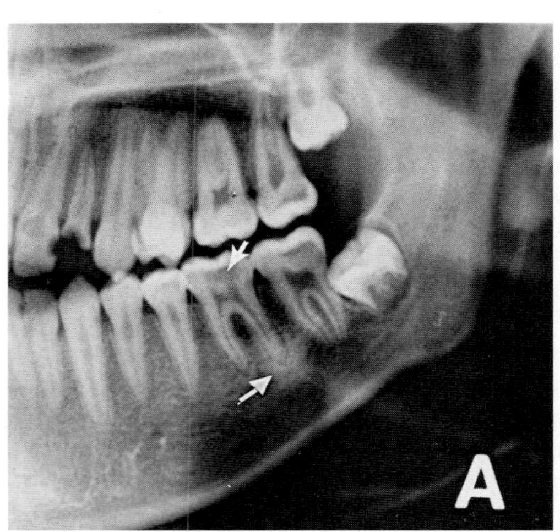

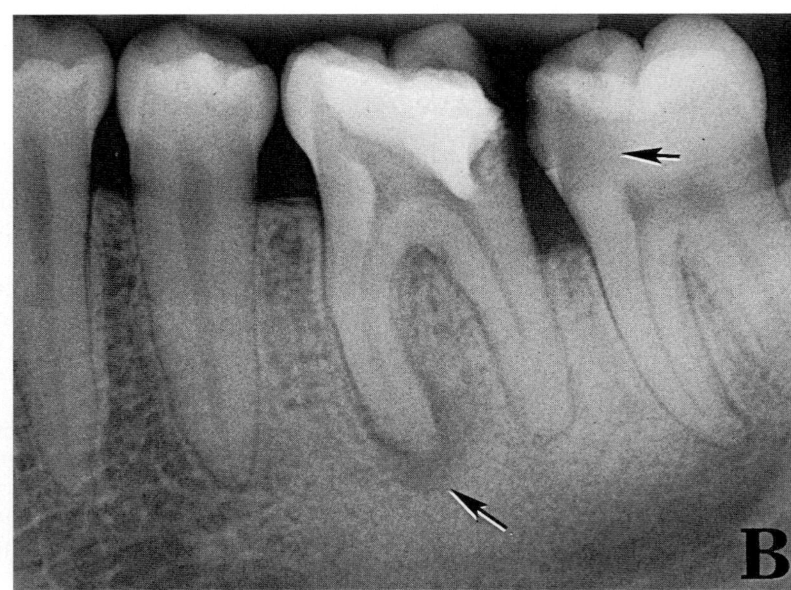

FIGURE 7–43.

Apical condensing osteitis. A, Teenager with large carious lesion (upper arrow) of mandibular first molar, which proved to have a nonvital pulp. Notice the area of condensing osteitis at distal root tip (lower arrow). B, Condensing osteitis (lower arrow) of mandibular first molar with large temporary restoration. The second molar has a class 4 carious lesion (upper arrow).

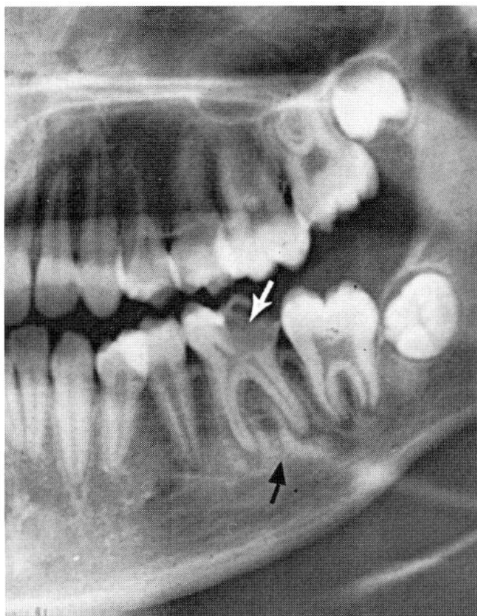

FIGURE 7–44.

Apical condensing osteitis. Young teenager with condensing osteitis of nonvital carious first molar (arrows). (From Langland OE, Langlais RP, Morris CR: Principles and Practice of Panoramic Radiology. Philadelphia:WB Saunders, 1982, p. 235.)

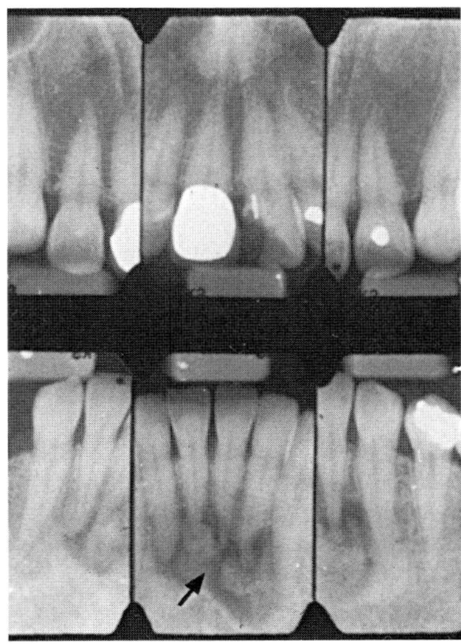

FIGURE 7–46.

Apical cementoma (periapical cemental dysplasia). Third or mature cementoblastic stage of apical cementoma of vital mandibular incisors (arrow). (Courtesy of Drs. L. Archilla, F. Erales, and R. Carlos, Guatemala City, Guatemala.)

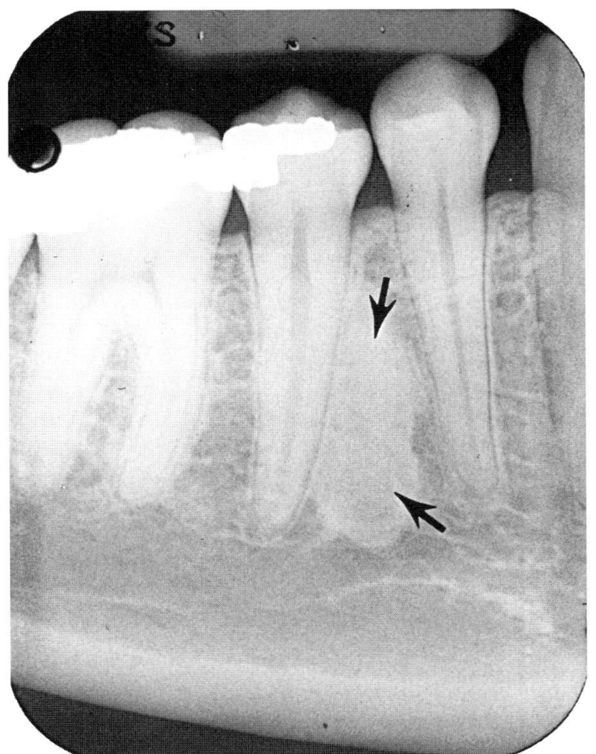

FIGURE 7–45.

Osteosclerosis. Notice condensed bone at mesial side of root of mandibular second premolar (arrows). The radiopaque area is not attached to premolar. It is thought to have a noninflammatory cause (trauma or stress) or possibly a developmental origin, such as enostosis.

or more, it is usually present some distance below the roots of the mandibular teeth or above them in the maxilla. Superimposition of osteosclerosis on the root of a tooth suggests the condition may be condensing osteitis; however, condensing osteitis is associated with a nonvital tooth, whereas osteosclerosis usually is not. The margins of the dense bone may be sharp or indistinct, although it is always possible to identify the boundaries. More than one area of osteosclerosis is often present in the same jaw. Osteosclerosis rarely is seen in the maxilla, but it is very common in the mandible, where it appears to have a slight predilection for the region below the premolars and canine.

Osteosclerosis and condensing osteitis can be confused with apical cementoma and benign cementoblastoma. In condensing osteitis, the entire root outline is nearly always visible, an important feature in distinguishing it from a benign cementoblastoma, in which the roots appear continuous with a radiopaque mass.

The apical cementoma should not be confused with condensing osteitis or any of the periapical radiolucencies related to pulpal disease. The apical cementoma is asymptomatic; the pulp of the involved teeth usually is vital, and the lesion most frequently affects the mandibular incisors in middle-aged African-American women (Fig. 46).

Apical cementomas (periapical cemental dysplasia) are benign lesions that contain cementumlike tissue and originate from cellular elements of the periodontal ligament space. They are nonexpansile radiolucencies in the early or immature stage. There may be single or multiple lesions. Bone expansion is absent, and pain is not a feature. No treatment is required. As the lesion matures, increasing amounts of cementumlike material are laid down in the lesion. In the mature stage, the radiographic appearance of the apical

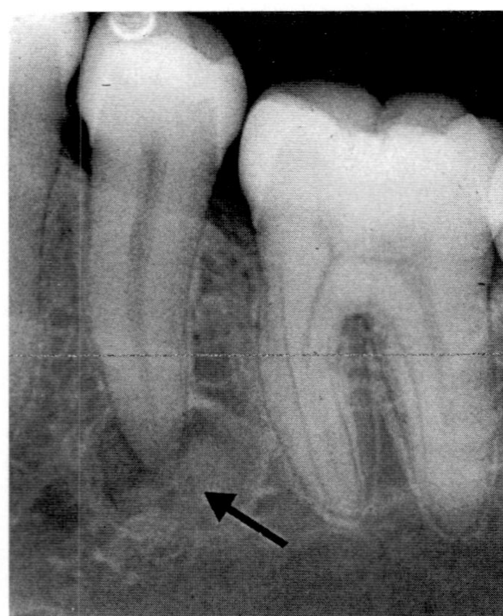

FIGURE 7–47.

Apical cementomas (periapical cemental dysplasia). Target or halo-effect radiographic appearance of apical cementoma of vital mandibular premolar (arrow).

cementoma is a well-defined radiopacity usually bordered by a thin radiolucent line or band (Fig. 7–47). It is the radiographic feature of the radiolucent band separating the calcified mass from the bone that distinguishes the apical cementomas from osteosclerosis and condensing osteitis.

Condensing osteitis usually is seen in young adults with large carious lesions in nonvital mandibular molars. After the teeth with apical cementomas are extracted, the radiopaque apical cementomas are retained in the alveolar bone. These remaining radiopaque lesions of the apical cementoma could be confused with remaining radiopaque areas of condensing osteitis, osteosclerosis, or root tips.

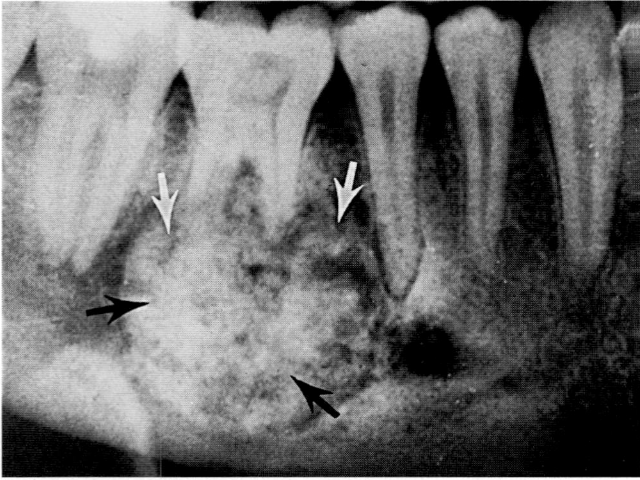

FIGURE 7–48.

Benign cementoblastoma (true cementoma). In an 18-year-old man, the outer periphery of the lesion is well delineated by a thin radiolucent line. The mesial root apex appears to be continuous or fused to the radiopaque mass (arrows).

Benign cementoblastoma (true cementoma) is a rare neoplasm of functional cementoblasts that forms a large mass of cementum or cementumlike tissue on the tooth root. Approximately 50% of reported cases were associated with mandibular first molars and in patients younger than 20 years of age. Cases usually are asymptomatic, and the tooth is vital. Because a tooth with condensing osteitis usually is nonvital, this symptom generally will distinguish the benign cementoblastoma from condensing osteitis.

Radiographically, the mature benign cementoblastoma appears as a tumor mass attached to a tooth root and as a well-circumscribed dense radiopaque mass often surrounded by a thin, uniform line. The outline of the affected root generally is obliterated because of resorption of the root and fusion of the mass to the tooth (Fig. 7–48). The lesion grows slowly and may cause expansion of the cortical plates of bone. The treatment is usually tooth extraction because of the tendency for expansion of the jaw. In distinguishing this lesion from condensing osteitis radiographically, the important feature is that the entire root outline is visible in condensing osteitis and the roots appear continuous with the radiopaque mass in benign cementoblastoma.

References

Pulp Cavity

Bergenholtz G, Reit C: Reactions of the dental pulp to microbial provocation of calcium hydroxide treated dentin. Scand J Dent Res 88:187, 1980.

Grossman LI: Endodontic Practice. 5th Ed. Philadelphia:Lea & Febiger, 1974, p. 104.

Miller WA, Massler M: Permeability and starving of active and arrested lesions in dentin. Br Dent J 112:187, 1962.

Mills JS: A calcific barrier or dentin bridge. Aust Dent J 57:241, 1953.

Mullaney TC, Lawson BF, Mitchell DF: Pharmacologic treatment of pulpitis: a continuing investigation. Oral Surg 21:479, 1966.

Pulpal Opacities or Calcifications

Johnson PL, Bevelander G: Histogenesis and histochemistry of pulpal calcification. J Dent Res 35:714, 1956.

Stones HH: Oral and Dental Diseases. 4th Ed. Baltimore:Williams and Wilkins, 1962, p. 343.

Willman W: Calcifications in the pulp. Bur 34:73, 1934.

Pulpal Enlargement

Archard HO, Witkop CJ Jr: Hereditary hypophosphatemia (vitamin D-resistant rickets) presenting primary dental manifestations. Oral Surg 22: 184, 1966.

Finn SB: Clinical Pedodontics. Philadelphia:WB Saunders, 1973.

Gigliotti R, Harrison JH, Reveley RA, Drabkowski AJ: Familial vitamin D-refractory rickets. J Am Dent Assoc 82:383, 1971.

Kronfeld R, Boyle PE: Histopathology of the Teeth and Their Surrounding Structures. 3rd Ed. Philadelphia:Lea & Febiger, 1949, p. 71.

Witkop CJ Jr: Manifestations of genetic diseases in the human pulp. Oral Surg 32:278, 1971.

Pulp Obliteration

Jacobsen I, Kerekes K: Long-term prognosis of traumatized permanent anterior teeth showing calcifying processes in the pulp cavity. Scand J Dent Res 85:588, 1977.

Naastrom K, Forsberg B, Petersson A, Westesson PL: Narrowing of the dental pulp chamber in patients with renal diseases. Oral Surg 59:242, 1985.

Hypercementosis

Rushton MA, Cooke BED: Oral Histopathology. Edinburgh:E & S Livingstone, 1959.

Schehl S: Rontgenologisch-statistische Untersuchungen uber Hyperzementosen. Wiss Z Ernst-Moritz-Arndt-Univ Greifswald 15:279, 1966.

Internal Resorption

Allen AL, Gutman JL: Internal root resorption after vital root resection. J Endod 3:438, 1977.

Andreasen JO: Luxation of permanent teeth due to trauma: a clinical and radiographic follow-up study of 189 injured teeth. Scand J Dent Res 78:273, 1970.

Andreasen JO, ed: Traumatic Injuries of the Teeth. 2nd Ed. Philadelphia: WB Saunders, 1981.

Bell T: The Anatomy, Physiology and Disease of the Teeth. Philadelphia: Carey and Lea, 1829, p. 171.

Burke JH: Reversal of external root resorption. J Endod 2:87, 1976.

Chivian N: Root Resorption. In: Cohen LS, Burns RC, eds. Pathways of the Pulp. 4th Ed. St. Louis:CV Mosby, 1987, p. 514.

Cvek M, Hollander L, Nord CE: Treatment of non-vital incisors with calcium hydroxide: VI. A clinical, microbiological, radiological evaluation of treatment in one sitting of teeth with mature and immature roots. Odontol Rev 27:93, 1976.

Dargent P: A study of root resorption. Actual Odontoslomatol 117:47, 1977.

Fischer WG, Guggenheimer J: Concurrent external and internal resorption. Oral Surg 43:161, 1977.

Frank AL: External-internal progressive resorption and its nonsurgical correction. J Endod 7:473, 1981.

Gartner AH, et al: Differential diagnosis of internal and external resorption. J Endont 1:329, 1976.

Hartness JD: Fractured root and internal resorption, repair and formation of callus. J Endod 1:73, 1975.

Mummery JH: The pathology of "pink spots" on teeth. Br Dent J 41:301, 1920.

Pomeranz H: A very active case of idiopathic external root resorption. Oral Surg 55:521, 1983.

Schroeder A: Endodontics: Science and Practice. Chicago:Quintessence Publishing, 1981.

Seltzer S, Bender IB: The Dental Pulp. 2nd Ed. Philadelphia:JB Lippincott, 1975.

Stafne EC, Slocumb CH: Idiopathic resorption of teeth. Am J Orthod 30: 41, 1949.

Weine FS: Endodontic Therapy. 4th Ed. St. Louis:CV Mosby, 1989, p. 150.

Weisman MI, Rackley RH: Recalcification of internal resorption: a rare case. J Ga Dent Assoc 41:15, 1978.

External Resorption

Andreasen JO, ed: Traumatic Injuries of Teeth. 2nd Ed. Philadelphia:WB Saunders, 1981.

Bjorvatin K, Selvig K, Klinge B: Effect of tetracycline and SuF_2 on root resorption in reimplanted incisors in dogs. Scand J Dent Res 97:477, 1989.

Cvek M: Endodontic treatment of traumatized teeth. In: Andreasen JO, ed. Traumatic Injuries of the Teeth. 2nd Ed. Philadelphia:WB Saunders, 1981.

Deeb G, Prietto PP, McKenna RC: Reimplantation of luxated teeth in humans. J South Calif Dent Assoc 33:194, 1965.

Fountain SB, Camp JH: Traumatic injuries. In: Cohen S, Burns RC, eds. Pathways of the Pulp. 4th Ed. St. Louis:CV Mosby, 1987, p. 494.

Goldson C, Hendrikson CO: Root resorption during Begg treatment: longitudinal roentgenologic study. Am J Orthod 68:55, 1975.

Goultschin J, Nitgan D, Azaz B: Root resorption: review and discussion. Oral Surg 54:586, 1982.

Halcomb JB, Dodds RN, England MC: Endodontic treatment modalities for external root resorption associated with impacted mandibular third molars. J Endod 9:335, 1983.

Hammarstrom L, Lindskog S: General morphologic aspects of resorption of teeth and alveolar bone. Int Endod J 18:293, 1985.

Hotz R: Wurzel resorptionen an bleibenden Zahnen. Dtsh Zahn-Mund Kieferheilk 18:217, 1967.

Ketcham AH: A preliminary report of an investigation of apical root resorption of vital permanent teeth. Int J Orthod 13:92, 1927.

Ketcham AH: A progress report of an investigation of apical root resorption of vital permanent teeth. Int J Orthod 15:310, 1929.

Linge BO, Linge L: Apical root resorption in upper anterior teeth. Eur J Orthod 5:173, 1983.

Massler M, Malone JA: Root resorption in human permanent teeth. Am J Orthod 40:619, 1954.

Morse DR: Clinical Endodontology. Springfield, IL:Charles C Thomas, 1974.

Nitzen D, Kerman T, Marmany Y: Does an impacted tooth cause root resorption of the adjacent one? Oral Surg 51:221, 1981.

Shafer WG, Hine MK, Levy BM: A Textbook of Oral Pathology. Philadelphia:WB Saunders, 1983, p. 328.

Stafne EC, Austin LT: Resorption of embedded teeth. J Am Dent Assoc 32:1003, 1945.

Tasch EG, Kennon S: Implications of related impacted third molars. J Ky Dent Assoc 30:13, 1978.

Pulpoperiapical Disease

Mendoza M, Reeder A, Meyers W, Marguard J: An ultrastructural investigation of the human apical pulp in irreversible pulpitis: II. Vasculature and connective tissue. J Endod 13:318, 1987.

Morse D, Seltzer S, Sinai I, Biron G: Endodontic classification. J Am Dent Assoc 94:685, 1977.

Priebe WA, et al: The value of the roentgenographic film in the differential diagnosis of periapical lesions. Oral Surg 7:979, 1954.

Acute Apical Periodontitis

Grossman CI: Endodontic Practice. Philadelphia:Lea & Febiger, 1974, p. 68.

Walton RE, Torabinejad M: Principles and Practice of Endodontics. Philadelphia:WB Saunders, 1989, p. 41.

Weine, et al: Endodontic emergency dilemma: leave the tooth open or keep closed. Oral Surg 40:531, 1975.

Weine FS: Endodontic Therapy. 4th Ed. St. Louis:CV Mosby, 1989, p. 160.

Chronic Apical Periodontitis

Bender IB, Seltzer S: Roentgenographic and direct observation of experimental lesions in bone. J Am Dent Assoc 62:152, 708, 1961.

Brynolf I: Radiography of the periapical region as a diagnostic aid. I. Diagnosis of marginal changes. Dent Radiogr Photogr 51:21, 1978.

Early PJ, Razzak MA, Dodee DB: Textbook of Nuclear Medicine Technology. 3rd Ed. St. Louis:CV Mosby, 1979, p. 379.

Kronfeld R: Histopathology of the Teeth. 2nd Ed. Philadelphia:Lea & Febiger, 1939, p. 209.

Priebe WA, Lazansky JP, Wuehrmann AH: The value of the roentgenographic film in the differential diagnosis of periapical lesions. Oral Surg 7:979, 1954.

Ramadan AE, Mitchell DF: Roentgenographic study of experimental bone destruction. Oral Surg 15:934, 1961.

Shoha N, Dawson J, Richards AG: Radiographic interpretation of experimentally produced bony lesions. Oral Surg 38:294, 1974.

Stern M, et al: Antibody producing cells in human periapical granuloma and cysts. J Endod 7:447, 1981.

Syzuki A: Histologic and radiographic study of periapical lesions. Shikwa Gakuho 60:37, 1960.

Apical Granuloma

Bhaskar SN: Periapical lesion: types, incidence, and clinical features. Oral Surg 21:657, 1966.

Block RM, Bushell A, Rodrigues H, Langeland K: A histopathologic, histobacteriologic and radiographic study of periapical endodontic surgical specimens. Oral Surg 42:657, 1976.

Kronfeld R: Histopathology of the Teeth. 2nd Ed. Philadelphia:Lea & Febiger, 1939, p. 209.

Lalonde ER: A new rationale for the management of periapical granulomas and cysts: an evaluation of histopathological and radiologic findings. J Am Dent Assoc 80:1056, 1970.

McKinney RV: Clarification of the terms granulomatous and granulation tissue [letter to the editor]. J Oral Pathol 10:307, 1981.

Natkin E, Oswald RJ, Carnes LI: The relationship of lesion size to diagnosis, incidence, and treatment of periapical cysts and granulomas. Oral Surg 57:82, 1984.

Smulson MH, Hagen JC: Pulpoperiapical pathology and immunologic considerations. In: Weine F, ed. Endodontic Therapy. 4th Ed. St. Louis: CV Mosby, 1989, p. 173.

Strindberg LZ: The dependence of the results of pulp therapy on certain factors. Acta Odont Scand 14(Suppl 21):100, 1956.

Apical Cyst

Bender IB: A commentary on General Bhaskar's hypothesis. Oral Surg 34: 469, 1972.

Bhaskar SN: Periapical lesions: types, incidence, and clinical features. Oral Surg 21:657, 1966.

Block RM, Bushnell A, Rodrigues H, Langeland K: A histopathologic, histobacteriologic, and radiographic study of periapical surgical specimens. Oral Surg 42:655, 1976.

Browne WG: Periodontal cysts: an analysis of over 500 cysts. Oral Surg 14:1103, 1961.

Grossman LI: Endodontic Practice. 8th Ed. Philadelphia:Lea & Febiger, 1974.

Harris M, Toller P: The pathogenesis of dental cysts. Br Med Bull 31:159, 1975.

Lalonde ER: A new estimate for the management of periapical granulomas and cysts: an evaluation of histopathological and radiographic findings. J Am Dent Assoc 80:1057, 1970.

Lalonde ER, Luebke RG: The frequency and distribution of periapical cysts and granulomas. Oral Surg 25:861, 1968.

Ross PN, Birch BS: A clinical histopathologic study of conservative endodontic failures. J Dent Res (special issue B) 1976, abstract 271.

Seltzer S, Bender IB, Ziontz M: The dynamics of pulp inflammation correlations between diagnostic data and actual histologic findings in the pulp. Oral Surg 16:846, 1963.

Shah N: Nonsurgical management of periapical lesions. Oral Surg 66:367, 1988.

Stockdale CR, Chandler NP: The nature of the periapical lesion: a review of 1108 cases. J Dent 16:123, 1988.

Strathers R, Shear M: Root resorption by ameloblastoma and cysts of the jaws. Int J Oral Surg 5:128, 1976.

Weine FS: Endodontic Therapy. 4th Ed. St. Louis:CV Mosby, 1989, p. 171.

Wood NK, Goaz PW, Jacobs MC: Periapical Radiolucencies, Differential Diagnosis of Oral Lesions. 2nd Ed. St. Louis:CV Mosby, 1980, p. 321.

Wysocki GP, Brannon RB, Gardner DG, Sapp P: Histogenesis of the lateral periodontal cyst and the gingival cyst of the adult. Oral Surg 50:327, 1980.

Chronic Apical Abscess

Baumgartner J, et al: Microscopic examination of oral sinus tracts and their associated periapical lesions. J Endod 10:146, 1984.

Grossman LI: Endodontic Practice. 8th Ed. Philadelphia:Lea & Febiger, 1974, p. 82.

Apical Condensing Osteitis

Boyne PJ: Incidence of osteosclerotic areas in the mandible and maxilla. J Oral Surg 18:486, 1960.

Hedin M, Polhagen L: Follow-up study of periradicular bone condensation. Scand J Dent Res 79:436, 1971.

Suggested Readings

Pulp Cavity

Bergenholtz G, Reit C: Reactions of the dental pulp to microbial provocation of calcium hydroxide treated dentin. Scand J Dent Res 88:187, 1980.

Miller WA, Massler M: Permeability and starving of active and arrested lesions in dentin. Br Dent J 112:187, 1962.

Pulpal Opacities or Calcifications

Barabas GM, Barabas AP: The Ehlers-Danlos syndrome: a report of the oral and hematological findings in nine cases. Br Dent J 123:473, 1967.

Benjamin B, Werner H: Syndrome of cutaneous fragility and hyperelasticity and articular hyperlaxity. Am J Dis Child 65:247, 1943.

Danlos H: Un cas de cutis laxa avec tumeurs par contusion chronique des condes et des genoux. Bull Soc Franc Dermat Et Syph 19:70, 1908.

Ehler E: Cutus laxa, Nelgung zu Hemorrhagien in der Haut, Lockerung mehrerer Artiikulationen. Derm Ztschr 8:173, 1901.

Freeman JJ: Ehlers-Danlos syndrome. Am J Dis Child 79:1049, 1950.

Gorlin RJ, Pindborg JJ: Syndromes of the Head and Neck. New York: McGraw-Hill, 1964, p. 197.

Jacobsen I, Kerekes K: Long-term prognosis of traumatized permanent anterior teeth showing calcifying processes in the pulp cavity. Scand J Dent Res 85:588, 1977.

McKusick VA: Heritable Disorders of Connective Tissues. 2nd Ed. St. Louis:CV Mosby, 1960.

Sundell JR, Stanley HR, White CC: The relationship of coronal pulp stone formation to experimental procedures. Oral Surg 25:579, 1968.

Pulpal Enlargement

Hintze H, Wengel A, Kruhoffer F: Dental hypersensitivity due to hypophosphatemia. Dentomaxillofac Radiol 19:81, 1990.

Pulp Obliteration

Andreasen JO, ed: Traumatic Injuries of the Teeth. Copenhagen:Munksgaard, 1972, p. 172.

Webman MS, Hirsch SA, Webman H, Stanley HR: Obliterated pulp cavities in the Sanfilippo syndrome (mucopolysaccharidosis III). Oral Surg 1977, p. 734.

Internal Resorption

Pindborg JJ: Resorptions. In: Pathology of Dental Hard Tissues. Philadelphia:WB Saunders, 1970, p. 327.

Schweitzer G: Interne granulome de zahapulpa and ihre resorbierende wirkung im innera des zahnkorpers die ''Rosa-Flechen'' (Pink Spots) Krankhert de zahne. Duetsche Zahartliche Wochenschrift 34:177, 247, 1931.

Tamse A, Littner MM, Keffe I: Roentgenographic features of external root resorption. Quint Int B(1) 115, 1982.

External Resorption

Alexander SA, Swerdloff M: Collagen activity of the p.l. and hydroxyproline context during human deciduous root resorption. J Periodontol Res 15:434, 1980.

Alexander SA, Swerdloff M: Mucopolysaccharidase activity during human deciduous root resorption. Arch Oral Biol 24:735, 1979.

Becks H, Cowden RC: Root resorptions and their relation to pathologic bone formation: Part II. Classification, degrees, prognosis and frequency. Am J Orthodont Oral Surg 28:513, 1942.

Goon W, Cohen S, Boner RF: External cervical root resorption following bleaching. J Endod 12:414, 1986.

Harrington GW, Nathin E: External resorption associated with bleaching of pulpless teeth. J Endod 5:344, 1979.

Kerr DA, Courtney RM, Binker EJ: Multiple idiopathic root resorption. Oral Surg 29:552, 1970.

Lado EA, Stanley HR, Weisman MI: Cervical resorption in bleached teeth. Oral Surg 55:78, 1983.

Latcham NL: Postbleaching cervical resorption. J Endod 12:262, 1986.

Pindborg JJ: Resorptions. In: Pathology of Hard Dental Tissues. Philadelphia:WB Saunders, 1970, p. 327.

Chronic Apical Periodontitis

Brynolf I: A histological and roentgenological study of the periapical region of human upper incisors. Odont Revy 18(suppl 11):458, 1967.

Apical Granuloma

Barlocco JC, Poladian JA: Una tecnica diagnostica de quistes y granuloma periapicales. AJ: Odontol Bonaerense 22, 1979.

Grossman LI: Endodontic Practice. 8th Ed. Philadelphia:Lea & Febiger, 1974, p. 87.

Grossman LI: Bacteriologic status of periapical tissue in 150 cases of infected pulpless teeth. J Dent Res 38:101, 1959.

Morse D, Patnik J, Schacterle G: Electrophoretic differentiation of radicular cysts and granulomas. Oral Surg 35:249, 1973.

Stockdale CR, Chandler NP: The nature of the periapical lesion: a review of 1108 cases. J Dent 16:123, 1988.

Apical Cyst

Arwill R, Persson G, Thilander H: The microscopic appearance of the periapical tissue in cases classified as ''uncertain'' or ''unsuccessful'' after apicectomy. Odont Revy 25:27, 1974.

Natkin E, Oswald RS, Carnes CI: The relationship of lesion size to diagnosis, incidence, and treatment of apical cysts and granulomas. Oral Surg 57:82, 1984.

Chapter 8

Radiologic Diagnosis of Periodontal Disease

PERIODONTAL DISEASE

Periodontal disease encompasses all diseases of the periodontium Table 8–1). Initially it is confined to the gingiva and is termed gingival disease; later the supporting structures become involved and the condition is termed periodontal disease.

The most common periodontal diseases are microbiologic infections associated with local accumulation of dental plaques, subgingival pathogens, periodontal flora, and calculus. There are other periodontal diseases of the gingiva and periodontal attachment apparatus that are not infectious but are caused by traumatic, cystic, granulomatous, neoplastic, or degenerative processes.

The most common periodontal diseases are gingivitis and periodontitis. Gingivitis is an inflammatory process of the gingiva in which the junctional gingiva remains attached at its original level. In gingivitis, the most apical portion of the junctional epithelium is on the enamel, at or near the cementoenamel junction (CEJ). Periodontitis is characterized by gingival inflammation, periodontal pocket formation, destruction of the periodontal ligament and alveolar bone, and gradual loosening of the teeth. It is associated with apical migration of the junctional epithelium onto the root surface.

Hoag and Pawlak (1990) reported that the incidence of periodontitis is approximately one in four adults. The incidence of periodontal disease with pocket formation is approximately 40% in people 50 years of age. In general, male patients have a higher incidence and severity of periodontal disease than female patients. Periodontal disease is related universally to level of education and income.

Periodontitis occurs in different forms and has been classified by Page and Schroeder (1982). They identified prepubertal, juvenile, rapidly progressive, and adult periodontitis.

Prepubertal periodontitis, juvenile periodontitis, and rapidly progressive periodontitis are aggressive forms that affect people at relatively young ages and have been grouped under the term "early-onset periodontitis."

Although the early-onset aggressive forms of periodontitis are relatively rare, they are significant. During the first 3 decades of life, periodontitis presents especially difficult diagnostic and treatment challenges. It can be extremely complex and costly to treat and is highly destructive, resulting in the loss of many or all of the teeth in young patients.

PREPUBERTAL PERIODONTITIS

Prepubertal periodontitis is an unusual disease that results in resorption of the periodontal tissues in young children during or shortly after the eruption of the primary teeth. The disease leads to early loss of the primary teeth and may affect the permanent teeth as well.

Prepubertal periodontal disease is rare and has a genetic basis. Prepubertal periodontitis seems to be more common in female than male patients. In some families, susceptibility seems to have a maternal pattern of inheritance, whereas others have no apparent pattern of transmission. Prepubertal periodontitis may be followed by severe periodontitis of the permanent teeth or by a normal permanent dentition. Page and colleagues (1983) reported that abnormalities in peripheral blood leukocyte chemotaxis were found in all children with prepubertal periodontitis whom they studied. Prepubertal periodontitis is infectious; however, almost all affected children manifest serum antibodies reactive with putative periodontal pathogens. Species implicated include Capnocytophaga sputigena, Eikenella corrodens, and Bacteroides intermedius.

The disease occurs in generalized and localized forms that differ greatly in their features and progression.

In generalized prepubertal periodontitis, there is extreme, fiery-red inflammation of the marginal and attached gingiva around all teeth, spontaneous hemorrhage, gingival proliferation, cleft formation, and recession. In time, the clefts extend, and the tissues may recede completely to the root apex. Alveolar bone destruction proceeds at an alarming rate.

In the generalized form of the disease, there are profound defects of peripheral blood neutrophils and monocytes. Phagocytic cells have a defective adherence receptor and cannot exit the blood vessels. The leukocyte defect is thought to be transmitted as an autosomal recessive trait. This disease often is associated with frequent infectious upper respiratory tract infections and otitis media. The generalized form of prepubertal periodontitis seems to be refractory to antibiotic therapy. Page and colleagues (1983) reported that one case of the generalized disease was controlled by extraction of the uncorrectable teeth combined with meticulous plaque control.

In children with localized prepubertal periodontitis, signs of inflammation may be absent or confined to the marginal gingiva and may be overlooked. Periodontitis is evident only with the periodontal probe and observation of alveolar bone destruction on radiographs. The rate of tissue destruction is

TABLE 8–1
Summary of Periodontal Diseases, Their Characteristics, and Associated Microbes

Type of Disease	Characteristics	Associated Microbes
Adult periodontitis	Affects patients 35 years of age or older; microbial deposits; no systemic illness	Bacteroides gingivalis, Bacteroides intermedius, Eikenella corrodens, Fusobacterium nucleatum, Wolinella recta, Peptostreptococcus micros, spirochetes
Juvenile periodontitis	Circumpubertal; neutrophil dysfunction; affects first molars and incisors in teenagers	Actinobacillus actinomycetemcomitans, capnocytophaga sp
Prepubertal periodontitis	Generalized; neutrophil dysfunction affects deciduous dentition; affects young children	A. actinomycetemcomitans, S. sputigena, E. corrodens, B. intermedius
Rapid progressive periodontitis	Affects young adults; rapid, progressive, neutrophil dysfunction	B. gingivalis, W. recta; E. corrodens, Bacteroides forsythus, B. intermedius, A. actinomycetemcomitans
Refractory destructive periodontitis	Does not respond to conventional therapy (form of rapidly progressive periodontitis)	B. gingivalis, B. intermedius, A. actinomycetemcomitans
Gingivitis	Isolated or generalized; endemic; redness, bleeding on probing	Streptococcus sp, actinomyces sp, spirochetes
ANUG	Necrosed papilla; gingival pain (seems to be related to stress factors, lack of adequate nutrition and sleep.)	Fusospirochetes

ANUG = acute necrotizing ulcerative gingivitis.
(From Greenstein G: Advances in periodontal disease diagnosis. Int J Periodont Rest Dent 10:351, 1990.)

slower than with the generalized form. The cause of this local condition is not fully known, but a defect in the patient's ability to resist the effect of the plaque microorganisms is suspected. In the localized form, the leukocyte defects involve the neutrophils or monocytes. Either one may be abnormal, but not both. Neutrophils are considered an important first line of defense in the gingiva. Also, abnormal formation or maintenance of cementum in this disease creates a defective periodontal attachment that lowers the resistance of periodontal tissues to microbial infection and allows rapid tissue destruction. This localized form of prepubertal periodontitis responds well to curettage of the affected sites, improved tooth brushing, and systemic administration of antibiotics. The drug of choice is penicillin or erythromycin in a dosage of 250 mg four times a day for 3 weeks.

In a position paper in 1987, the American Academy of Periodontology suggested that patients affected with periodontitis of the primary dentition, who have systemic diseases such as neutropenia, agranulocytosis, aplastic anemia, hypophosphatasia, or Papillon-Lefèvre syndrome, should be differentiated from patients with prepubertal periodontitis.

◆ *RADIOLOGY (Fig. 8–1)*

In prepubertal periodontitis, the onset of alveolar bone destruction occurs in children immediately after eruption of the primary teeth. The disease occurs in generalized and localized forms that differ greatly in their features and progression. In generalized prepubertal periodontitis, alveolar bone destruction and root resorption are extremely rapid, and the primary teeth may be lost by the time the patient is 2 to 3 years of age. All primary teeth are affected; the permanent teeth may be affected or they may be normal. In children with localized prepubertal periodontitis, the signs of inflammation may be absent or confined to marginal gingiva with radiographic evidence of alveolar bone destruction, which may be less rapid than in the generalized form. Only some teeth are affected; the pattern has not yet been determined.

In generalized and localized forms of prepubertal periodontics, open furcation of the primary molar can be seen. Sometimes the primary molar roots are almost totally resorbed and the tooth buds of the permanent teeth may become exposed. Prepubertal periodontitis may be followed by severe alveolar bone destruction of the bone supporting the permanent teeth, or the disease may become dormant and the alveolar bony support of the permanent dentition may become normal.

JUVENILE PERIODONTITIS (Periodontosis)

Juvenile periodontitis refers to an uncommon form of periodontitis in teenagers and young adults. It is characterized by rapid alveolar bone destruction with minimal signs of gingival inflammation. It is classified into localized (LJP) and generalized (GJP) forms based on its distribution in the dentition. Hormund and Frandsen (1979) described more than 150 cases of juvenile periodontitis and distinguished localized from generalized periodontitis. They proposed that these two forms of juvenile periodontitis are discrete, with the localized variety often seen in younger patients. The localized form is self-limiting, whereas the generalized form may continue to include severe destruction of the entire periodontium.

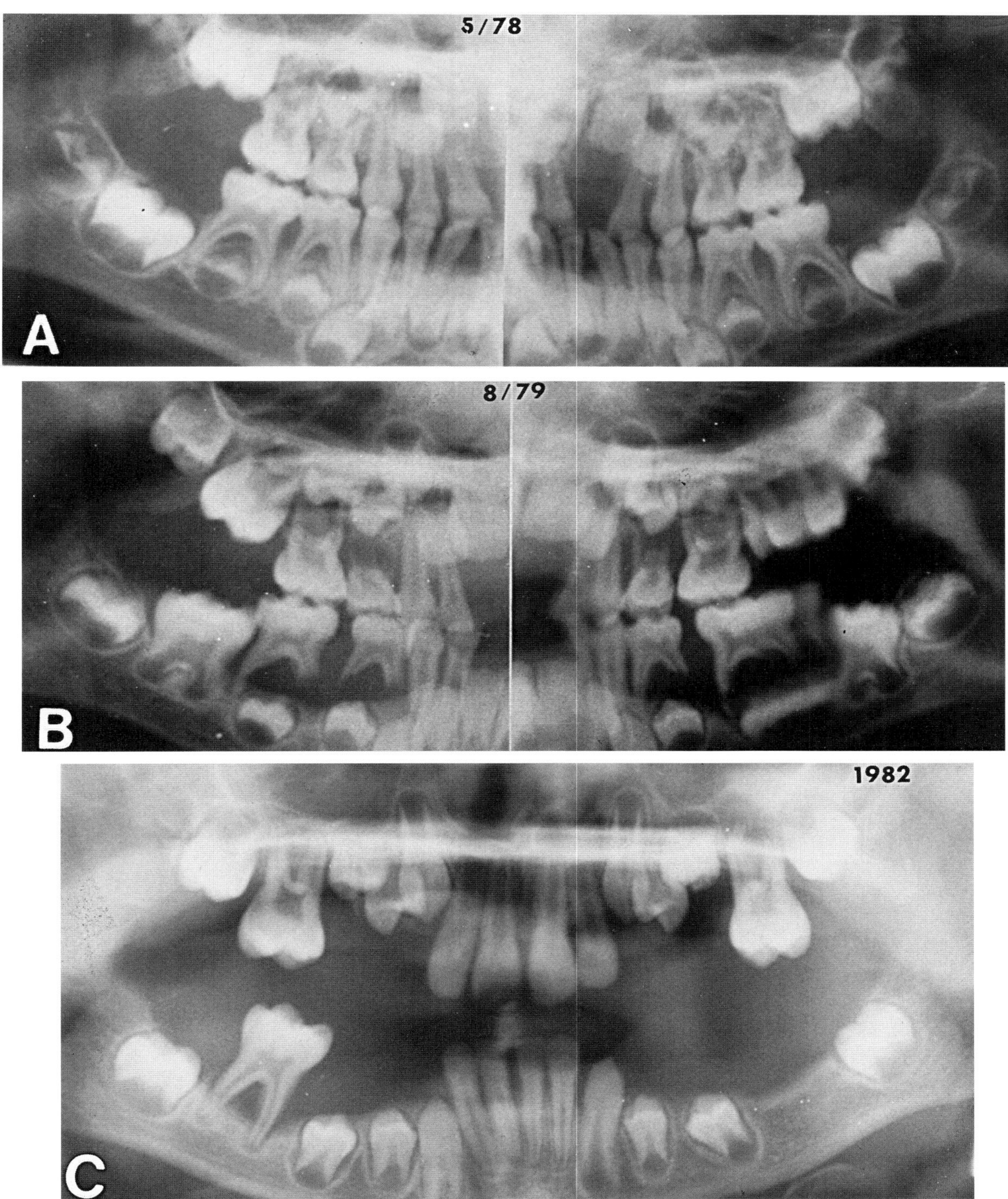

FIGURE 8–1.

Generalized prepubertal periodontitis. Case in a 5-year-old patient, showing the extent of alveolar bone and tooth root destruction over a 15-month period. A, Radiographs taken May 1978. B, Radiographs taken August 1979. The molar roots are almost totally destroyed, and the permanent tooth buds are beginning to be exposed. C, Same patient, at 8 years of age. After removal of primary molars and institution of more thorough toothbrushing, the tissues improved, although inflammation persisted around some teeth. The permanent first molars erupted and appeared normal at first; however, alveolar bone destruction caused extraction of one mandibular permanent first molar, and the remaining permanent first molars have a guarded prognosis. (From Page RC, et al: Prepubertal periodontitis: definition of a clinical disease entity. J Periodontol 54:266, 1983.)

Localized Juvenile Periodontitis

Saxby (1984) reported that the overall prevalence of LJP is 0.1%, with a prevalence of 0.8% in black people, 0.2% in Asians, and 0.02% in white people. Hoag and Pawlak stated that the incidence is less than 1% in developed nations and approximately 5% in underdeveloped nations.

Although male and female patients are affected by this disease, the incidence is higher in female patients. The primary teeth are not affected. Members of the same family frequently have the disease, and it has a genetic basis consistent with an autosomal recessive or an X-linked dominant genetic trait.

The onset of LJP occurs during the circumpubertal period (Fig. 8–2). LJP is characterized by pocket formation, connective tissue, and alveolar bone loss mainly affecting the first molars and incisors and may be bilaterally symmetric. During the early phases, the disease frequently is not recognized because the gingiva appears to be healthy.

Clinically, patients with LJP rarely show calculus or plaque formation and often exhibit little or no gingivitis; however, bleeding on deep probing almost always occurs in the sites where pocket depth, attachment loss, and radiographic bone loss are seen on the radiograph, suggesting that there is inflammation deep in the tissue. Although probing depths may extend 10 to 12 mm, the gingival tissue may show no inflammation clinically, and microbial plaque may not be clinically apparent. If the pockets have been present for several years, however, plaque, calculus, and gingival inflammation will be more evident.

Van Dyke and associates (1985) reported the neutrophil chemotactic disorders (reduced migration of neutrophil to a chemotactic agent) also are found in approximately 70% of patients with LJP. The defects in chemotaxis also are found in siblings without disease in families with LJP, suggesting that the reduced neutrophil function precedes the disease and may be related to the increased susceptibility of patients to LJP.

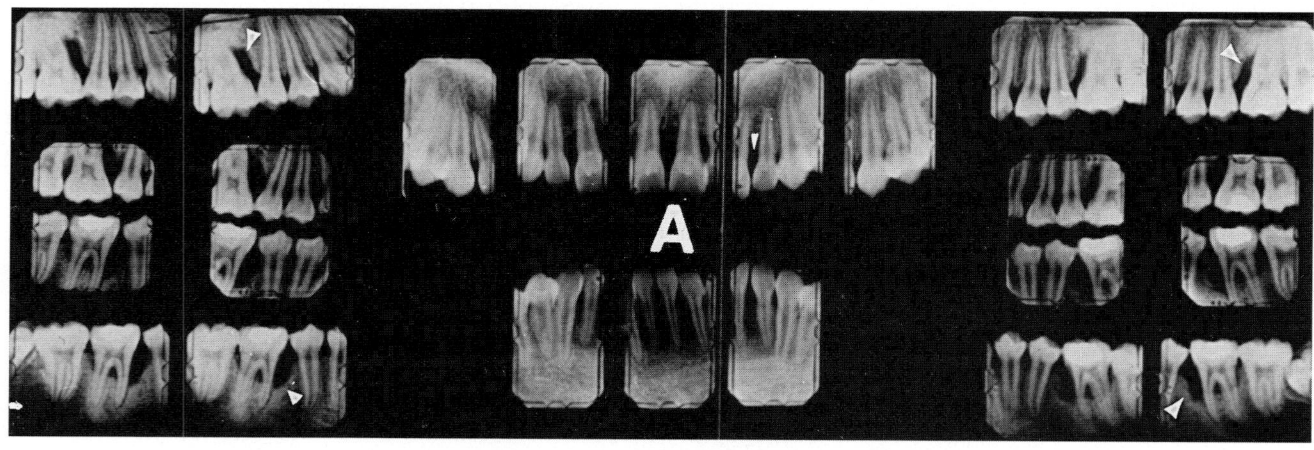

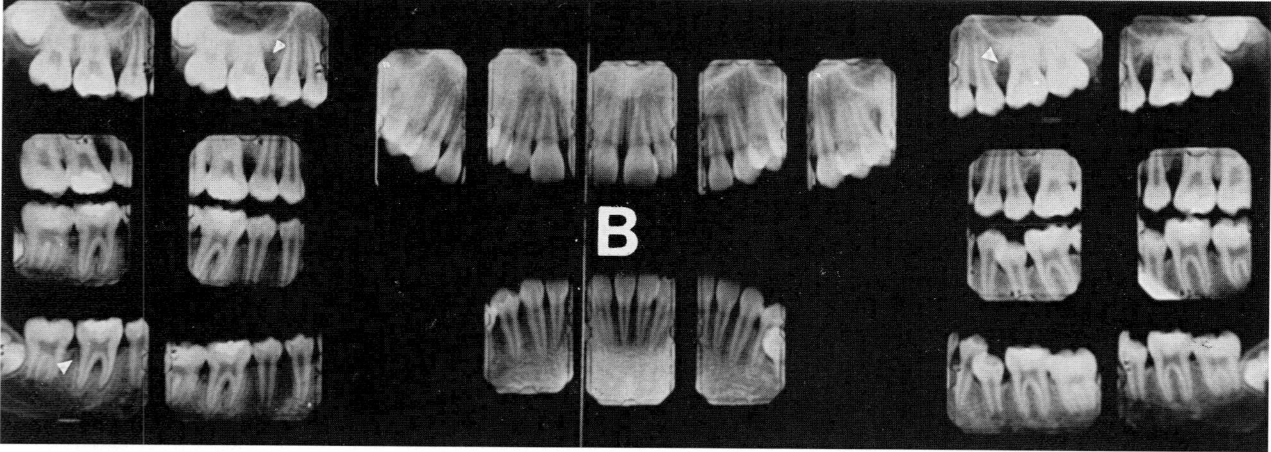

FIGURE 8–2.

Localized juvenile periodontitis. A, A 14-year-old boy, with severe bone resorption characteristic of juvenile periodontitis that can be observed around the first molars and maxillary incisors (arrowheads). B, Twelve-year-old sister of boy in panel A, with typical bone destruction of juvenile periodontitis around maxillary first molars and mandibular right first molar (arrowheads). (From Page RC, et al: Family studies of juvenile periodontitis. J Periodontol 56:602, 1985.)

The definitive etiologic factors for LJP are not known, but most people think that the principal cause is bacterial, with the possibility of an altered host response.

Although the pocket flora is sparse, with only a very thin layer of adherent microbial plaque on the root surface in LJP, there are increased proportions of gram-negative anaerotic rods (organisms of healthy gingival sulci are predominantly gram positive), including large numbers of Actinobacillus actinomycetemcomitans and capnocytophaga. Most patients with LJP manifest high serum-antibody titers specific for antigenic determinants of these bacteria. These data provided strong support for the idea that LJP is caused by these bacteria. A. actinomycetemcomitans is a leukotoxin producer, and C. sputigena produces an antineutrophil factor.

The immune response in LJP is much more intense than in adult periodontitis, resulting in much more destruction of the periodontal tissues.

The reason for the onset of LJP at puberty is obscure, but it may be related to elevated levels of certain hormones in the blood and gingival fluid that may serve as growth factors for infecting bacteria, or it may be associated with changes in the host-response mechanism. Immediately after onset, the lesions slow down or eventually they may cease entirely.

The prognosis for maintaining the health of LJP-affected teeth and periodontal tissues on a long-term basis varies from questionable to hopeless, depending on the extent of the bone destruction and the etiologic factors; however, if the disease is treated early enough with plaque control and pocket elimination, the teeth can be preserved for many years.

The treatment of choice is to open a soft tissue flap around the affected teeth, plane the tooth roots thoroughly, remove any granulation tissue, and suture the flap back into place. Krill and Fry (1987) recommended the systemic administration of tetracycline at a standard dose (250 mg, one tablet every 6 hours) for 1 to 3 weeks. The periodontopathic organisms in LJP are particularly sensitive to tetracycline. After healing, meticulous plaque control, including interproximal brushing, is essential. The routine extraction of all teeth involved by this condition cannot be justified because the success ratio is high enough to warrant periodontal treatment of these teeth in many patients.

◆ *RADIOLOGY (Fig. 8–2)*

In LJP, the affected first molars and incisors show angular or vertical alveolar bone loss. The reasons for the extreme site specificity are not understood. An arch-shaped pattern of bone loss extends from the distal aspect of the second premolar to the mesial aspect of the second molar. Bilateral bone loss is common. The bone loss may involve furcations but often does not. The bone destruction may decrease after an initial period of rapid destruction.

Generalized Juvenile Periodontitis

GJP occurs in older teenagers and young adults. The mean age of patients with GJP is slightly greater than that of patients with LJP. Its prevalence is unknown but probably is much less than that of LJP. It may represent two or more types of periodontal disease in juveniles, including early-onset adult periodontitis and cases of LJP that progressed to a more generalized form. GJP usually is not associated with overt systemic disease such as Papillon-Lefèvre syndrome, hypophosphatasia, cyclic neutropenia, and agranulocytosis. Hormand and Frandsen (1979) stated that the two entities, LJP and GJP, seem clinically and radiographically distinct and evidence is accumulating that they are associated with different bacteria: A. actinomycetemcomitans in LJP and Bacteroides gingivalis and others in GJP.

In GJP there is severe gingival inflammation, with extensive plaque and calculus formation and associated gingival inflammation. The gingival inflammation differentiates it from LJP. The gingiva is described as "angry looking" in GJP, with suppurative pockets and generalized bone loss affecting most teeth. The bone loss is generalized horizontal and vertical. The patient with GJP usually has a neutrophil chemotactic disorder, and often the prognosis is poor for long-term retention of the teeth. The bacteria involved do not seem to be responsive to antibiotic therapy.

◆ *RADIOLOGY*

In GJP, alveolar bone loss occurs around all the teeth. The tooth and bone loss are generalized and vertical. Often the prognosis for long-term retention of teeth is poor. Both the primary and permanent dentition may be affected. This condition affects older teenagers and young adults—a slightly older age group than patients with LJP.

RAPIDLY PROGRESSIVE PERIODONTITIS

Page and colleagues (1983) were the first to describe rapidly progressive periodontitis as a distinct clinical condition with a specific diagnosis. This form of periodontitis is seen most often in young adults in their 20s, but it can occur in patients as old as approximately 35 years of age. This disease may be related to the generalized form of juvenile periodontitis. Disease progression is highly episodic, with exacerbations of acute inflammation followed by periods of remission.

The clinical characteristics of the acute phases of the disease include highly inflamed gingiva that bleeds easily, proliferation of marginal gingiva producing a mulberrylike surface, and exudation. Destruction is very rapid, with loss of much of the alveolar bone within a few weeks or months. This phase may be accompanied by general malaise, weight loss, and depression, although these symptoms are not seen in all patients. The amounts of microbial plaque vary greatly, and pus may or may not be seen within the pockets.

The dormant phase is characterized by normal gingival tissues, even though the bone destruction may have been extreme, and deep periodontal pockets (greater than 10 mm) still may persist. The extreme bone destruction may cease completely. The quiescent or dormant phase may be permanent or temporary.

According to Tanner and associates (1979), most patients with rapidly progressive periodontitis have serum antibodies for various species of gram-negative anaerobic asaccharolytic rods, especially actinobacillus, bacteroides, and possibly capnocytophagia.

Most patients with this condition manifest neutrophil or monocyte chemotaxis, and their compromised defense systems may account partly for the symptoms.

Several systemic diseases are associated with rapid periodontal tissue destruction or related to rapid progressive periodontitis, including diabetes mellitus, Down's syndrome, Crohn's disease, neutropenia, agranulocytosis, ''lazy leukocytic'' syndrome, and Chédiak-Higashi syndrome.

Most patients with rapidly progressive periodontitis not associated with a known systemic disease respond favorably to treatment by scaling, open and closed curettage, and antibiotic therapy (systemic administration of 250 mg tetracycline four times a day for 1 or 2 weeks). This must be followed by careful monitoring and careful plaque control. A small number of patients, however, do not respond to any form of periodontal therapy, and the teeth are lost. Unfortunately, before treatment, it is not possible to determine which patients will respond to therapy and which will not (this is called refractory destructive periodontitis).

◆ *RADIOLOGY (Figs. 8–3)*

In rapidly progressive periodontitis, there is radiographic evidence of severe and rapid bone destruction, after which the destruction process may cease spontaneously or slow down significantly. During the active phase, destruction of the alveolar bone, periodontal ligament, and sometimes the tooth roots can occur with astounding speed. The quiescent phase is characterized by clinically normal gingiva with very advanced bone loss and deep periodontal pockets. The quiescent period may be permanent, it may persist for an indefinite period, or the disease activity may return.

ADULT PERIODONTITIS (Slowly Progressing Periodontitis)

Periodontitis occurs when the periodontal ligament attachment and alveolar bony support of the tooth have been lost. This is associated with apical migration of the junctional epithelium onto the root surface; hence, by definition, periodontitis occurs when the junctional epithelium migrates apical to the CEJ. The attachment loss and periodontal pocket depths may be found on any root surface of single-rooted or multirooted teeth and in furcations of multirooted teeth.

Adult periodontitis is the most common form of periodontitis. It may have an early onset but is not common in teenagers and young adults. A significant increase in prevalence occurs in the third and fourth decades of life. Therefore, the disease usually begins after a patient reaches 35 years of age. The prevalence of adult periodontitis depends on the criteria used to define the disease. For example, in a 1985 to 1986 study of the employed United States population, Miller (1987) showed that, at all ages, 75% of this population showed attachment loss at one or more sites. In this study, 8% of adults had severe periodontal disease, which was defined as one or more sites with 6 mm or greater attachment loss. A 1981 study of adults in the United States, by Brown and associates (1989), showed that approximately 65% of the people between 19 and 65 years of age had a maximum pocket depth of 3 mm or less; maximum pocket depths between 4 and 6 mm occurred in 28% of people, and 8% had one or more pockets deeper than 6 mm.

Therefore, it can be seen that most of the adult population has at least moderate periodontitis, whereas a smaller but significant portion of the population has the severe form of periodontal disease.

The subgingival plaque in adult periodontitis tends to be very complex, and the organisms most often found include several species of gram-negative, anaerobic rods (some of which are mobile) and spirochetes. No single organism has been identified as the principal pathogen in adult periodontitis, but most likely it is caused by several organisms. Therefore, almost all patients with adult periodontitis have serum antibodies to the putative (commonly accepted) periodontal pathogens (B. gingivalis, B. intermedius, and others).

In adult periodontitis, putative periodontal pathogens such as B. gingivalis are virulent and can cause direct extensive tissue damage. They also can trigger host-mediated indirect destruction of local periodontal tissues. Many of these are immunologic responses to the bacterial substances, resulting in destruction of the soft and hard tissues of the periodontium.

No serum, neutrophil, or monocyte abnormalities have been identified. Goodson and colleagues (1982), Lindke and associates (1983), and Socransky and co-authors (1984) reported that adult periodontitis appears to be site specific and episodic, undergoing cycles of active destruction and remission.

Clinical features of adult periodontitis include varying degrees of proliferation of marginal gingiva, although some inflammation may be present. The disease is generalized and usually affects many teeth. It is associated with the development of periodontal pockets and loss of attachment apical to the CEJ. The teeth with more advanced disease show furcation involvement in multirooted teeth and several mobile teeth, which may exhibit ''pathologic migration,'' with spaces developing between the teeth as they migrate out of their original position. The pockets may bleed on probing, and the exudate from the pockets is hemorrhagic, suppurative, or clear and watery.

In most cases of untreated adult periodontitis, the amount of plaque and especially calculus is usually commensurate with the amount of pocket formation and bone loss. Open interdental contacts, defective restoration margins, and malposed teeth are observed frequently. Periodontal abscesses also are seen in areas of severe periodontal pocket formation.

Various classification schemes have been applied to periodontitis in otherwise healthy adults. The American Academy of Periodontics has recommended the following classification when reporting cases to third parties for reimbursement:

Gingivitis: An inflammation of the gingiva characterized clinically by changes in color, gingival form, position, surface appearance, and the presence of bleeding or exudate. Shallow pockets are seen, and there is no bone loss.

Slight periodontitis: Progression of gingival inflammation into the deeper periodontal tissues and the alveolar bony

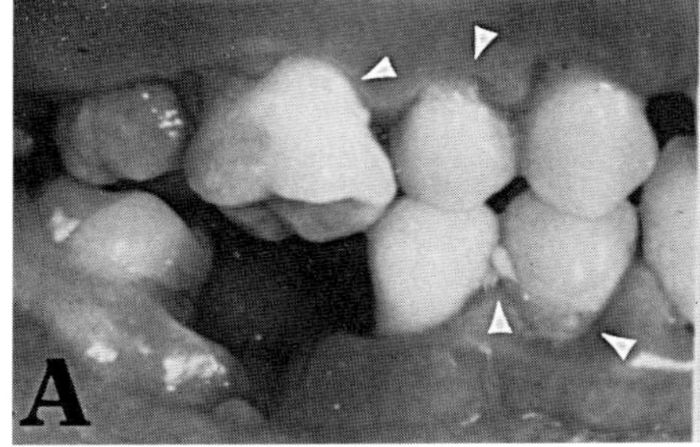
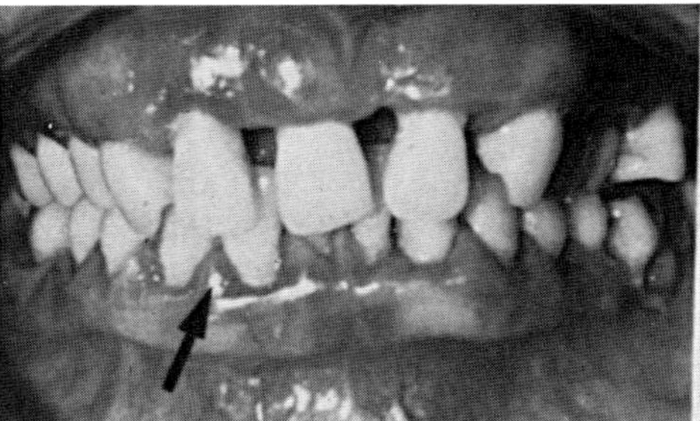
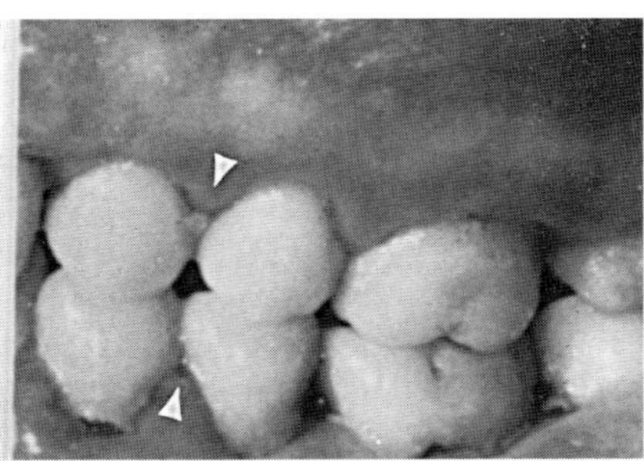
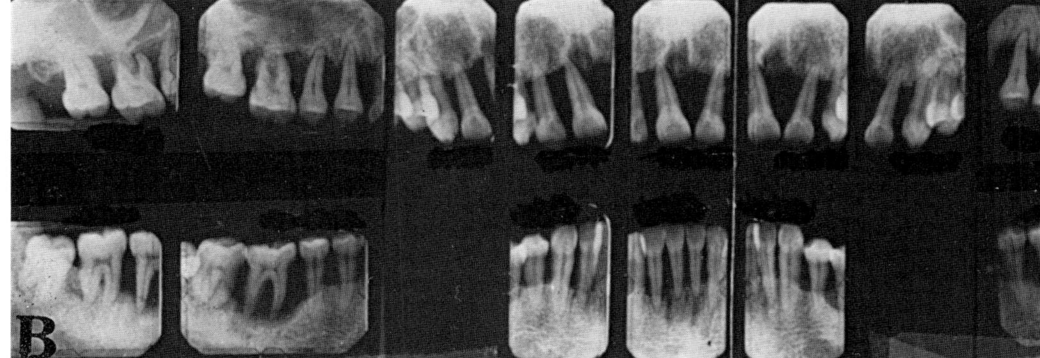
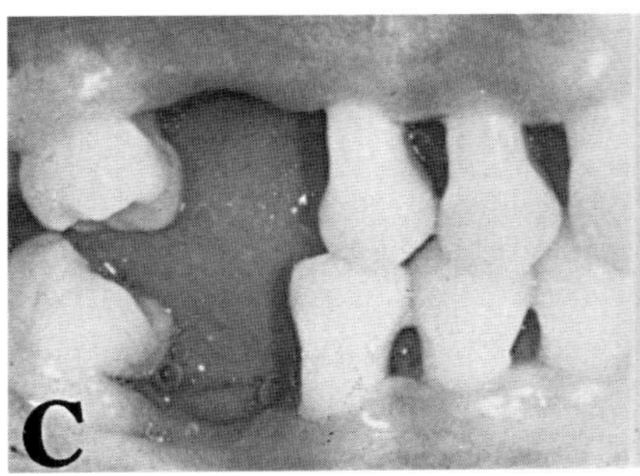
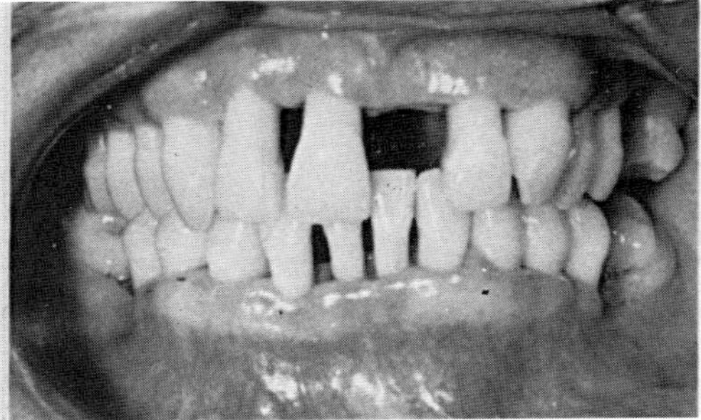
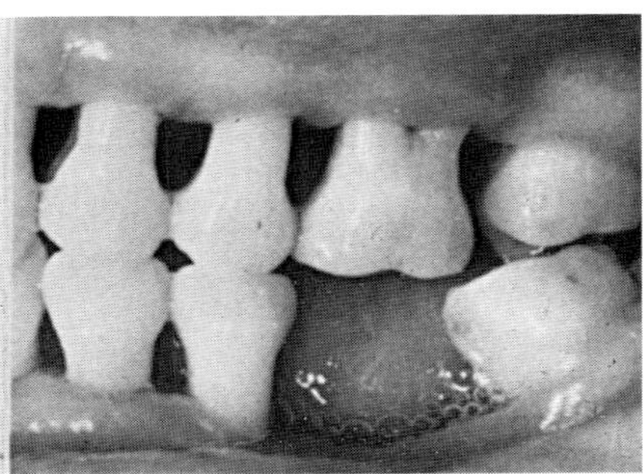

FIGURE 8–3.

Rapidly progressive periodontitis (acute phase). Case in a 26-year-old Chinese female immigrant from Formosa. A, Notice the masses of microbial plaque on all the teeth, especially near the gingival margins (arrowheads), and the extremely acute inflammation affecting the marginal and attached gingiva. In many areas, the gingival tissue margins manifest a mulberrylike surface, resulting from proliferation (arrow, middle figure). One central incisor has been extracted, and the remaining incisors are extremely loose and drifting. Pus could be expressed from many of the sockets. B, Radiographs of patient show that almost all of the bone has been resorbed from around all the teeth except the lower second molars and one third molar. Destruction extends beyond the root apices of the first molars. Notice the large vascular channels in the remaining bone between the mandibular central and lateral incisors. C, After debridement, repositioning of some teeth, and temporary splinting, the inflammation resolved completely and the teeth began to tighten. Notice the extent of recession resulting from reduction in inflammatory edema. (From Page RC, et al: Rapidly progressive periodontitis. J Periodontol 54:204, 1983).

crest with slight bone loss. There are moderate soft tissue pockets and satisfactory topography, which refers to the number of bony walls surrounding the teeth and contours of the bony defects.

Moderate periodontitis: A more advanced stage of slight periodontitis. There is increased destruction of periodontal structures, with a noticeable loss of bony support, sometimes accompanied by increased tooth mobility. There may be furcation involvement in multirooted teeth. The soft tissue pockets are moderate to deep, the bone loss is moderate to severe, and the topography is unsatisfactory.

Advanced periodontitis: Shows deep soft tissue pockets, a major loss of alveolar bone support, advanced mobility patterns, and, most likely, furcation involvement of multirooted teeth.

Removal of microbial deposits and calculus from the root surfaces by root planing and curettage, with or without opening flaps, and the elimination of pockets are effective means of treatment, but antibiotic administration may be less effective than in early-onset forms of periodontitis. When identified, systemic causes also are treated, but local therapy usually is necessary to control the bacteria that initiate inflammation. In adult periodontitis, the overall goal of treatment is eliminating or at least minimizing the inflammatory process in the gingiva. In general, the prognosis for retaining the periodontal health of teeth affected by periodontal disease is based on the control the therapist and patient have over the etiologic factors. The cause of adult periodontitis is related primarily to the microorganisms and their products found in supra and subgingival plaque.

In most patients, the single most important factor in determining prognosis is whether an adequate level of plaque control can be established over a long time period. In addition, the prognosis is based on which teeth still have an adequate level of periodontal support. This support is necessary because periodontal health depends on adequate occlusal function as well as gingival health.

◆ *RADIOLOGY (Figs. 8–4 and 8–5)*

Characteristic radiographic changes are seen in adult periodontitis. On intraoral radiographs taken with the paralleling technique, early lesions of the interdental bone may appear fuzzy, and the alveolar bone shows a decrease in density. Later, cuplike radiolucent lesions develop interproximally, and bone loss is seen at the crest of the interproximal alveolar process. Alveolar bone loss is indicated when the crest of the interdental alveolar bone is more than 2 to 3 mm apical to the CEJ.

If the bone loss involves most of the teeth at the same rate, generalized horizontal bone loss will be seen. If the interdental alveolar bone progresses more rapidly at one site than another, vertical bone loss is observed.

Bone loss also can be seen between roots (furcations) of multirooted teeth. The prognosis is poor if the bone loss extends to the apex of the tooth, as seen in advanced cases of periodontitis. A thickened or widened periodontal ligament space may indicate infectious periodontitis, occlusal traumatism, or tooth mobility.

THE ROLE OF THE RADIOGRAPH IN PERIODONTAL DISEASE

The radiograph is an essential part of the initial examination and diagnosis of periodontal disease in establishing the prognosis and assessing the outcome of treatment. Radiographs give a two-dimensional representation of three-dimensional anatomic structures. The radiographic image is a superimposition of the bone and tooth structures over each other because the image lacks the third dimension of depth. Therefore, it must be remembered that the radiograph is not a substitute for the clinical examination; however, it is an important diagnostic aid.

To reduce some limitations of radiography, the intraoral radiograph must be taken with the long-cone paralleling technique. This provides a radiograph for diagnosis that approaches anatomic accuracy. Also, in the interpretation of intraoral radiographs for periodontal disease, it is important that a high kilovoltage (80 to 90 kVp) technique be used because it produces a radiograph with long-scale contrast that has proved to be better in the interpretation of bony lesions.

A radiograph gives the dentist crucial information regarding the untreated periodontal patient in dental practice but does not provide data concerning the activity or rate of periodontal destruction at the time of the examination.

Sequential radiographic examinations performed after occurrence of bone destruction can detect disease activity retrospectively because radiographic examinations can be compared; however, this is a relatively crude measurement of periodontal destruction.

Early and associates (1979) estimated that, for interpretation of radiographs, a 30 to 50% change in bone mineral is needed before the dentist is reasonably certain bone loss has

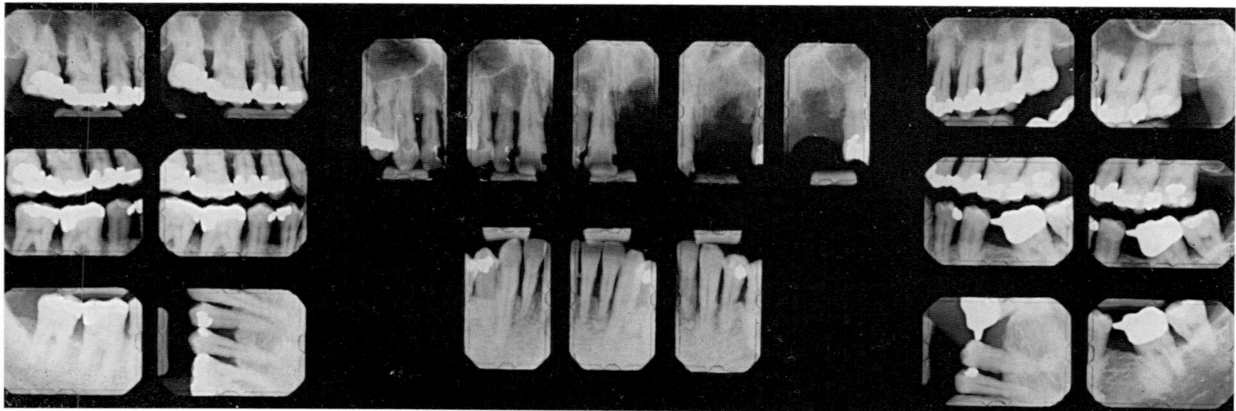

FIGURE 8–4.

Advanced adult periodontitis, CMX. In a 55-year-old man, generalized horizontal bone destruction is seen.

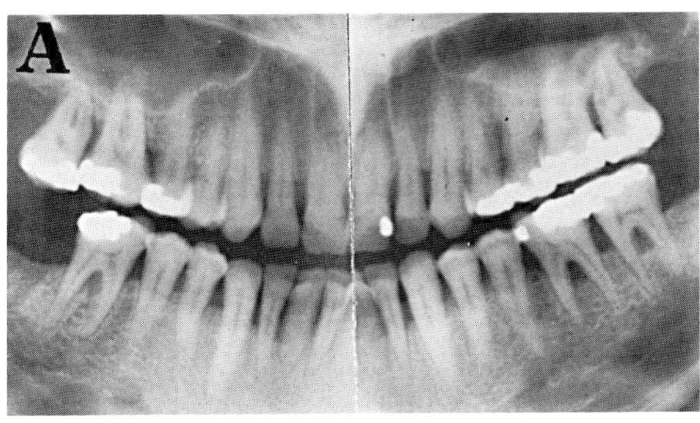

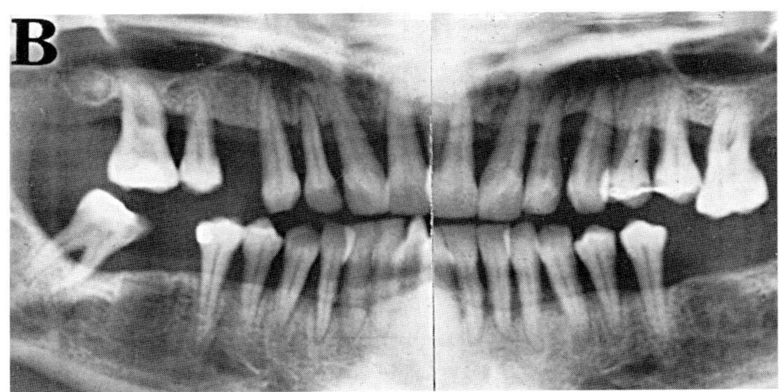

FIGURE 8–5.

Advanced adult periodontitis. Panoramic radiographs. A, Moderate to severe horizontal bone loss in a 50-year-old woman with furcation involvement of lower molars. B, Severe bone loss in a 54-year-old man.

occurred. Therefore, small amounts of alveolar bone loss are difficult to see when dental radiographs are compared.

Fortunately, Jeffcoat and colleagues (1984, 1987), Webber (1982), and McHenry and associates (1987) reported that digital substraction radiography can detect small osseous changes by substracting all unchanged bony structures from a set of dental radiographs, leaving only the area of change in the resultant substraction radiograph. Digital substraction radiography can detect lesions with less than 5% bone loss with a specificity of 96% and 91%.

In the future, perhaps the digital substraction radiograph will be used routinely by the dentist to detect small osseous changes (loss or gain) in the alveolar bone supporting the teeth.

Limitations

Although the radiograph has an important role in the diagnosis of periodontal disease, it is misunderstood. Before interpreting radiographs of a patient with periodontal disease, the dentist must realize that radiographs have certain limitations or restrictions. Some of the important limitations are listed below.

Presence or Absence of Periodontal Pockets (Figs. 8–6 and 8–7)

Because the periodontal pocket is a pathologically deepened gingival sulcus, the only reliable method of locating periodontal pockets and evaluating their extent is by careful probing of the gingival margin along each tooth surface. The periodontal pocket is composed of soft tissue, so it will not show up on the radiograph; however, if a radiopaque material such as gutta percha root canal points or Hirschfeld calibrated points is inserted into the pocket, the base of the pocket can be recorded in most instances on the radiograph.

Early Bone Loss in Periodontal Disease

In a study by Pauls and Trott (1966), interseptal bony defects smaller than 3 mm could not be seen on radiographs. The sensitivity of radiographs in measuring early bone destruction in periodontal disease is only fair. In their studies, Ramadan and Mitchell (1962) reported that when periodontal bone destruction first is seen on the radiograph, it usually has progressed beyond its earliest stage. Therefore, the very earliest signs of periodontal disease must be detected clinically. Also, the status of bone on facial and lingual aspects of the teeth is difficult to evaluate because the dense tooth structures are superimposed over the bone.

Early Furcation Involvement (Fig. 8–8)

Furcation involvement is detected by clinical examination, which includes careful probing with specialized probes. Radiographs are helpful, but they usually show less bone loss than actually present. Variations in x-ray beam alignment will obliterate the presence or extent of furcation involvement. Often the facial and lingual aspects of the alveolar

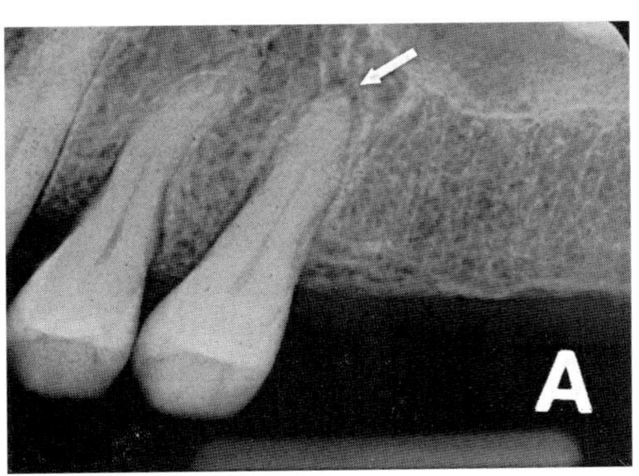

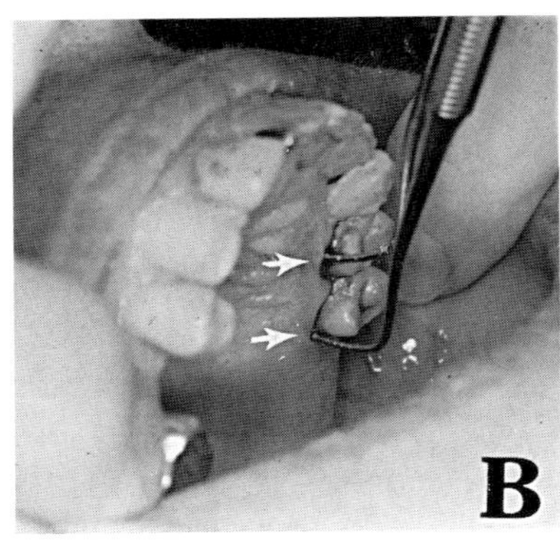

FIGURE 8–6.

Absence of periodontal pockets on radiograph. A, Radiograph of a patient with 10-mm pockets on lingual surfaces of maxillary premolars (arrow). B, Actual probing of pockets in panel A showing 10-mm pockets on lingual surface of premolars (arrows).

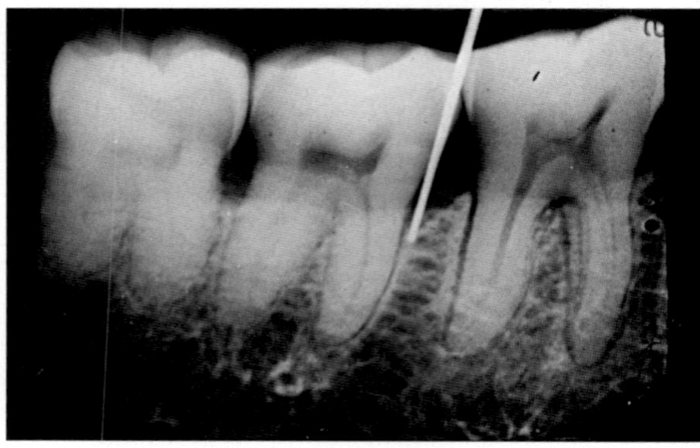

FIGURE 8–7.

Use of silver points. Silver points were used to assess the bottom of periodontal pockets. (Courtesy of Dr. R. H. Watkins, Phoenix, AZ.)

bone will be superimposed over the furcation. The furcation area of a tooth should be examined clinically, even if the radiograph shows only a very small radiolucency or a diminished radiodensity at the furcation. Also, if a great amount of bone loss is seen on one side of a multirooted tooth on a radiograph, most likely the furcation also has been invaded.

Calculus

Radiographs may be useful in detecting subgingival calculus. The ability to detect calculus radiographically will depend on its degree of mineralization and on angulation factors of the x-ray beam. The radiograph shows heavy calculus deposits and calculus spurs or spicules interproximally and sometimes even on the facial and lingual surfaces; however, it cannot be relied on for the thorough detection of calculus.

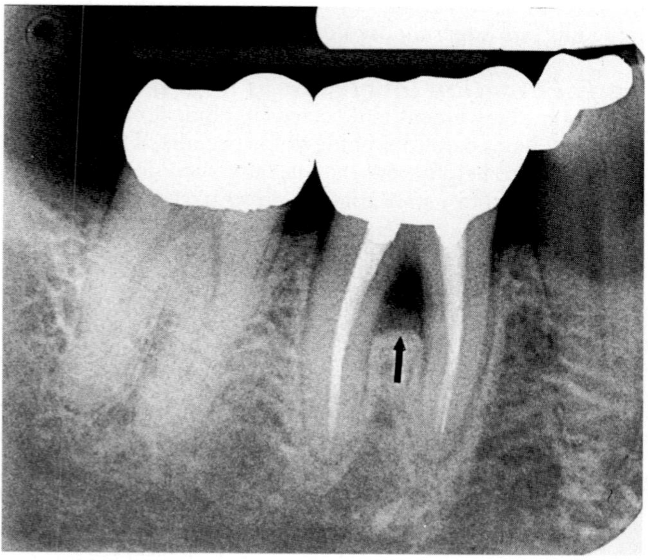

FIGURE 8–8.

Furcation involvement. Radiograph showing a furcation involvement (arrow) that extends through the entire furcation.

Mobility

The most common clinical sign of trauma to the periodontium is increased tooth mobility. The final stage of accommodation of the periodontal structures to increased forces results in widening of the periodontal ligament, which leads to increased mobility. Other causes of increased tooth mobility and thickening of the periodontal ligament include advanced bone loss, inflammation of the periodontal ligament, orthodontic treatment, and systemic causes such as pregnancy and scleroderma.

The radiographic signs of trauma from occlusion include the following: (1) the increased width of the periodontal ligament space, often with thickening of the lamina dura along the lateral aspect of the root, in the apical region, and in furcation areas; (2) vertical or angular destruction of the interseptal bone; (3) radiographic radiolucency and condensation of the alveolar bone, and (4) root resorption.

Widening of the periodontal ligament space and thickening of the lamina dura do not necessarily indicate destructive changes. They could indicate a favorable response of the periodontal ligament and alveolar bone to increased occlusal forces.

Morphologic Characteristics of Bone Deformities

The presence of osseous defects or bone deformities may be suggested on the radiograph, but careful probing and surgical exposure are necessary to determine the shape and dimensions.

Because the radiograph lacks depth, it will not record the true picture of the bone deformities accurately, such as showing the number of remaining walls of an infrabony pocket. Hausmann reported that it is not possible to determine from a radiograph the number of walls of an infrabony pocket defect with a combination of horizontal crestal bone loss on one side of the intercrestal bone and vertical crestal bone loss on the other side.

Benefits of the Radiograph in Diagnosis of Periodontal Disease

Despite its limitations, the periodontal examination is incomplete without accurate radiographs, which can show most bone lesions in periodontal disease when viewed under good lighting conditions. The remainder of this chapter will be devoted to the benefits of the radiograph in the diagnosis of periodontal disease.

Radiographic Changes in Periodontitis

Although the radiograph is not sensitive enough to detect the earliest signs of periodontal disease, it is still an essential part of the clinical examination. Glickman (1972) listed the following sequence of early radiographic changes that occur in periodontitis:

1. Crestal irregularities.
2. Triangulation.
3. Interdental septal bone changes.

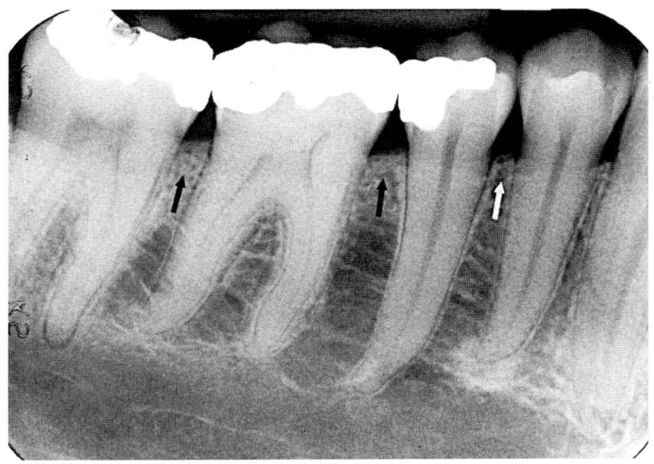

FIGURE 8–9.

Crestal irregularities. Normal interdental crestal septal bone. Normally the interproximal alveolar crest appears as a well-defined radiopaque line (arrows) in the radiograph approximately 1 to 1.5 mm from the cementoenamel junction (white arrow). Indistinct, interrupted lamina dura at the alveolar crest (black arrows).

Crestal Irregularities (Fig. 8–9). One of the first radiographic signs of periodontal disease is the indistinctness and interruption in the continuity of the lamina dura seen along the mesial or distal aspect of the interdental alveolar crest. This bone resorption at the interdental septal crest results from the extension of the inflammation into the interdental bone and associated widening of the vessel channels and a reduction in calcified tissue per unit of bone at the septal margin. Polymorphonuclear neutrophils usually are the defense cells found in acute inflammation and are replaced gradually by macrophages in chronic inflammation. Leukocytes can be activated by products of the dental plaque to produce a substance known as the osteoclast-activating factor. Osteoclasts and macrophages (mononuclear phagocytes), which are increased in chronic inflammatory periodontal disease, are capable of resorbing bone by first removing the minerals and then digesting the exposed collagen.

Triangulation (Fig. 8–10). Triangulation is a wedge-shaped radiolucent area formed at the mesial or distal aspect of the crest of the interalveolar bone. The apex of the wedge is pointed in the direction of the root. It is produced by resorption of the bone of the lateral aspect of the crest of the interalveolar bone in combination with widening of the periodontal ligament space.

Interseptal Alveolar Bone Changes (Figs. 8–11 and 8–12). The height of the bone is reduced as the interseptal alveolar bone is destroyed by periodontal disease. Fingerlike radiolucent projections can be seen extending from the crest of the interalveolar bone into the septal alveolar bone (Fig. 8–11). These result from the inflammation extending down into the interseptal alveolar bone, which causes increased bone resorption along the enosteal margins of the medullary spaces. When the tooth loses all its alveolar bone support and seems to "hang in air" on the radiograph, it is called the "terminal stage of chronic destructive periodontitis" (Fig. 8–12).

Evaluation of Bone Loss (Figs. 8–13 to 8–15)

The radiograph is an indirect method of detecting bone loss in periodontal disease. It shows the amount of bone remaining rather than the amount lost. The amount of bone loss is estimated by subtracting the present bone level from the physiologic bone level (which is related to the age of the

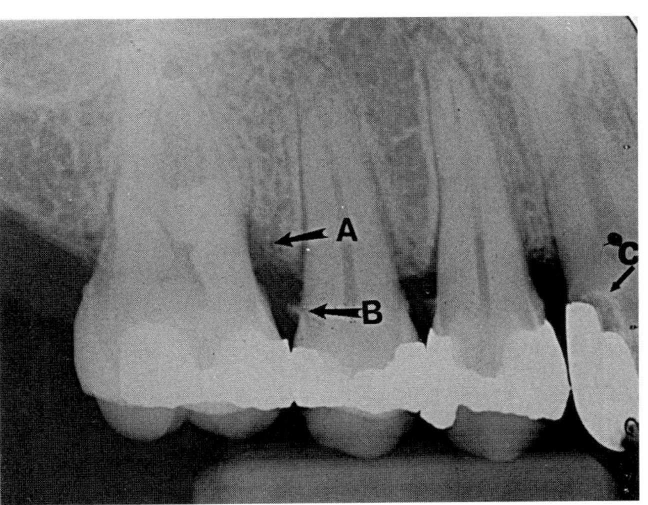

FIGURE 8–10.

Triangulation. Notice the triangular-shaped bone destruction between the second premolar and first molar at A and a calculus spur at B. See sclerotic dentin under restoration in canine. (From Langland OE, Langlais RP, Morris CR: Principles and Practice of Panoramic Radiology. Philadelphia:WB Saunders, 1982, p. 238.)

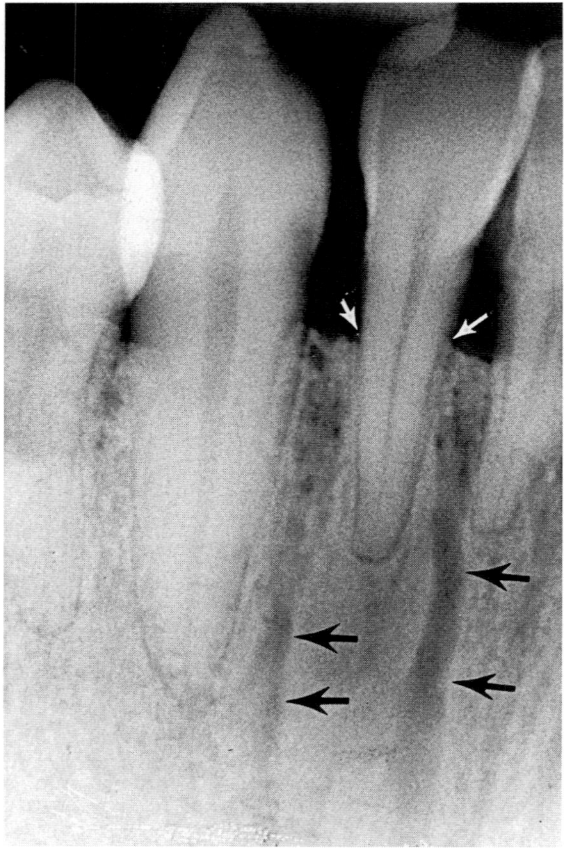

FIGURE 8–11.

Interseptal alveolar bone changes. Fingerlike radiolucent projections in interseptal alveolar bone (black arrows). These are widened nutrient canals. Notice the advanced horizontal bone loss (white arrows).

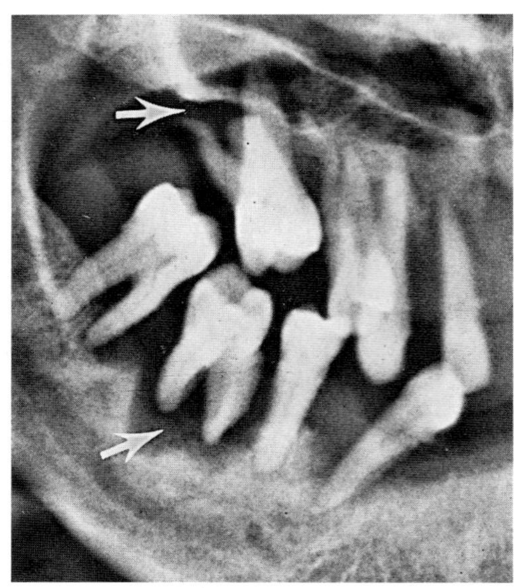

FIGURE 8–12.

Terminal stage of adult periodontitis. Panoramic radiograph of several teeth "hanging in air" (arrows) because of terminal adult periodontitis.

patient). The bone loss is considered localized if it occurs in isolated areas (Fig. 8–13), and generalized bone loss is seen uniformly throughout both arches (Fig. 8–14). Generalized advanced bone loss throughout both arches has a poor prognosis.

Periodontal and periapical conditions can mimic each other radiographically; therefore, pulp testing and periodontal probing must be used along with the radiograph. If bone loss exists around one tooth in an otherwise periodontally healthy patient and the pulp test has negative results, then the bone loss must be of endodontic origin. When bone loss exists in periodontally susceptible patients and the pulp tests have normal results, the lesions are of periodontal origin. True combined endodontic-periodontic lesions are usually of periodontal origin. The lesion is formed when pulpal and periodontal pathoses develop independently and unite (Fig. 8–15).

If the alveolar bone loss from periodontitis is severe in the posterior maxillary molar region, the radiograph is useful in determining the approximation of the coronal bone level to the floor of the maxillary sinus. This is especially important if bone surgery is contemplated in this region.

Direction or Pattern of Bone Loss (Figs. 8–16 and 8–17). In addition to altering the bone height, periodontal disease alters the morphologic features of the bone. The most common pattern of bone loss in periodontal disease is horizontal (Fig. 8–16). In this pattern, the bone is reduced in

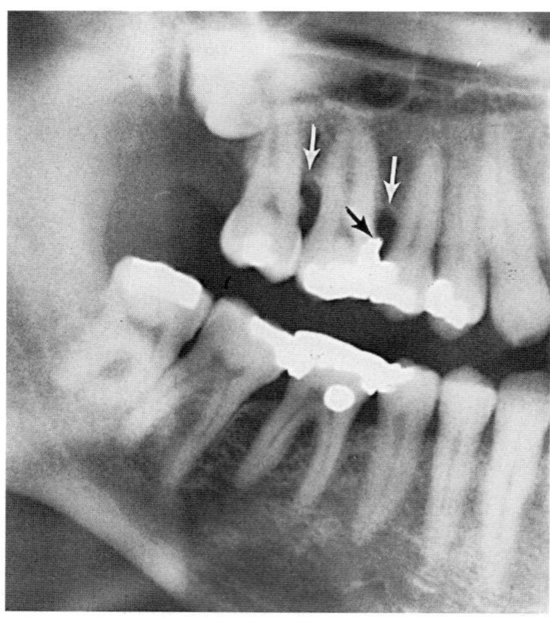

FIGURE 8–13.

Localized bone loss. Localized horizontal bone loss (arrows) between maxillary molars and mesial overhanging restoration in maxillary first molar. (From Langland OE, Langlais RP, Morris CR: Principles and Practice of Panoramic Radiology. Philadelphia:WB Saunders, 1982, p. 243.)

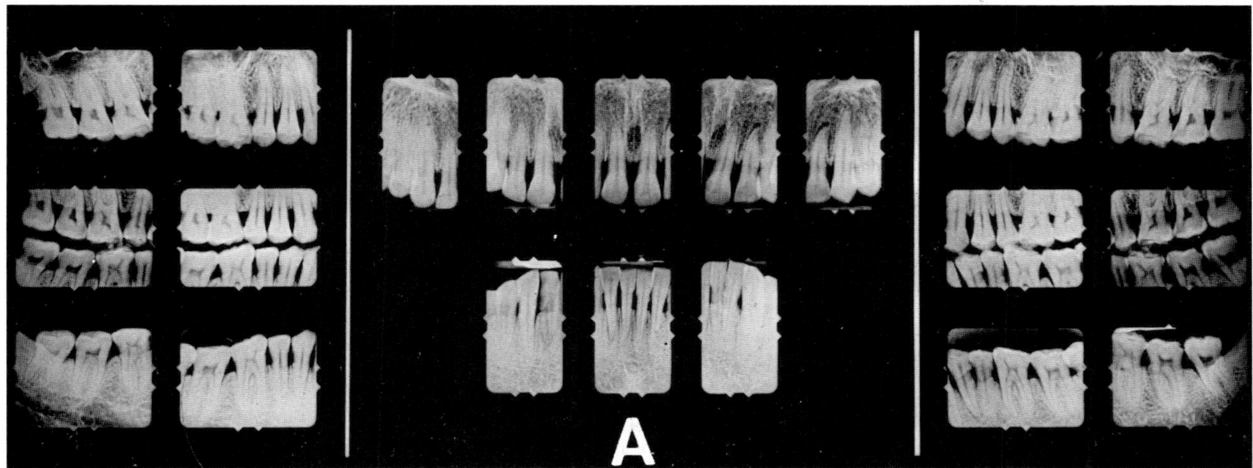

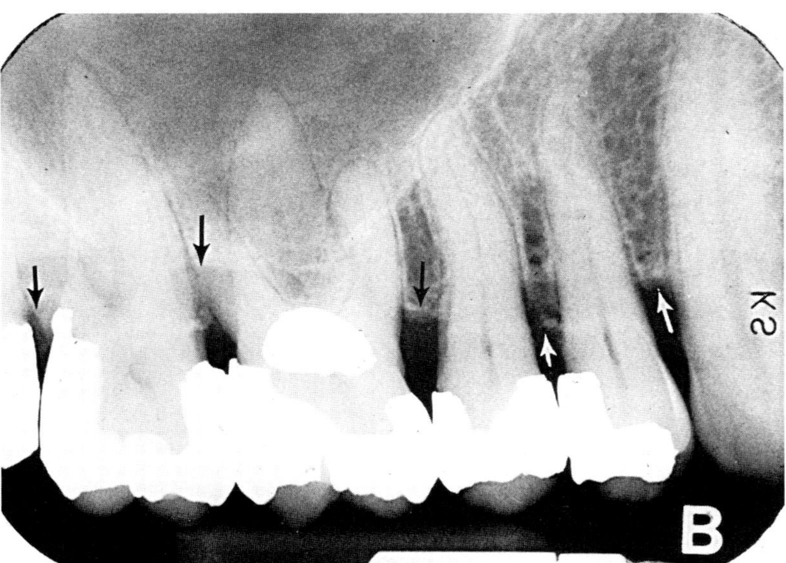

FIGURE 8–14.

Generalized bone loss. A, Complete radiographic mouth survey of patient with moderate generalized horizontal bone loss. (From Langland OE: Radiologic examination. In: Clark JW, ed. Clinical Dentistry. Hagerstown, MD:Harper & Row, 1976.) B, Generalized bone loss in maxillary right quadrant.

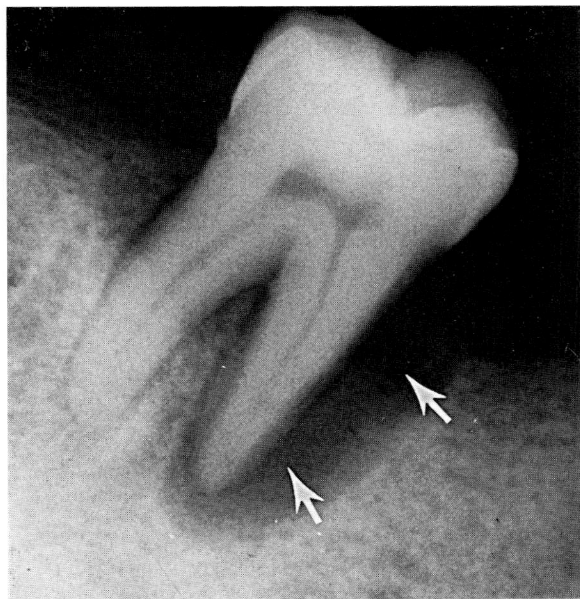

FIGURE 8–15.

Combined periodontal-endodontic pathoses. Periapical radiograph of nonvital mesial root of periodontally involved second molar (arrows). (From Langland OE, Langlais RP, Morris CR: Principles and Practice of Panoramic Radiology. Philadelphia:WB Saunders, 1982, p. 246.)

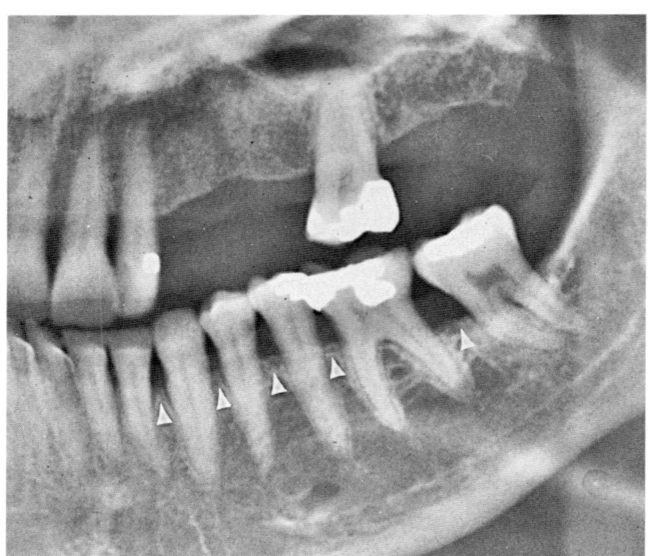

FIGURE 8–16.

Horizontal bone loss. Generalized horizontal bone loss in lower posterior quadrant (arrowheads). (From Langland OE, Langlais RP, Morris CR: Principles and Practice of Panoramic Radiology. Philadelphia:WB Saunders, 1982, p. 248.)

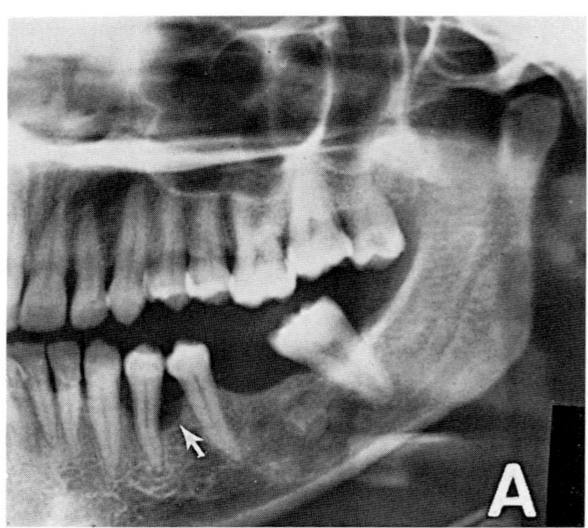

FIGURE 8–17.

Vertical bone loss. A, Vertical bone loss between mandibular premolars (arrow). (From Langland OE, Langlais RP, Morris CR: Principles and Practice of Panoramic Radiology. Philadelphia:WB Saunders, 1982, p. 243.) B, Vertical bone loss between first and second premolars (large white arrow). This is the classic angular (vertical) bone deformity seen in LJP (arrows). (From Langland OE: Radiologic examination. In: Clark JW, ed. Clinical Dentistry. Hagerstown, MD:Harper & Row, 1976.)

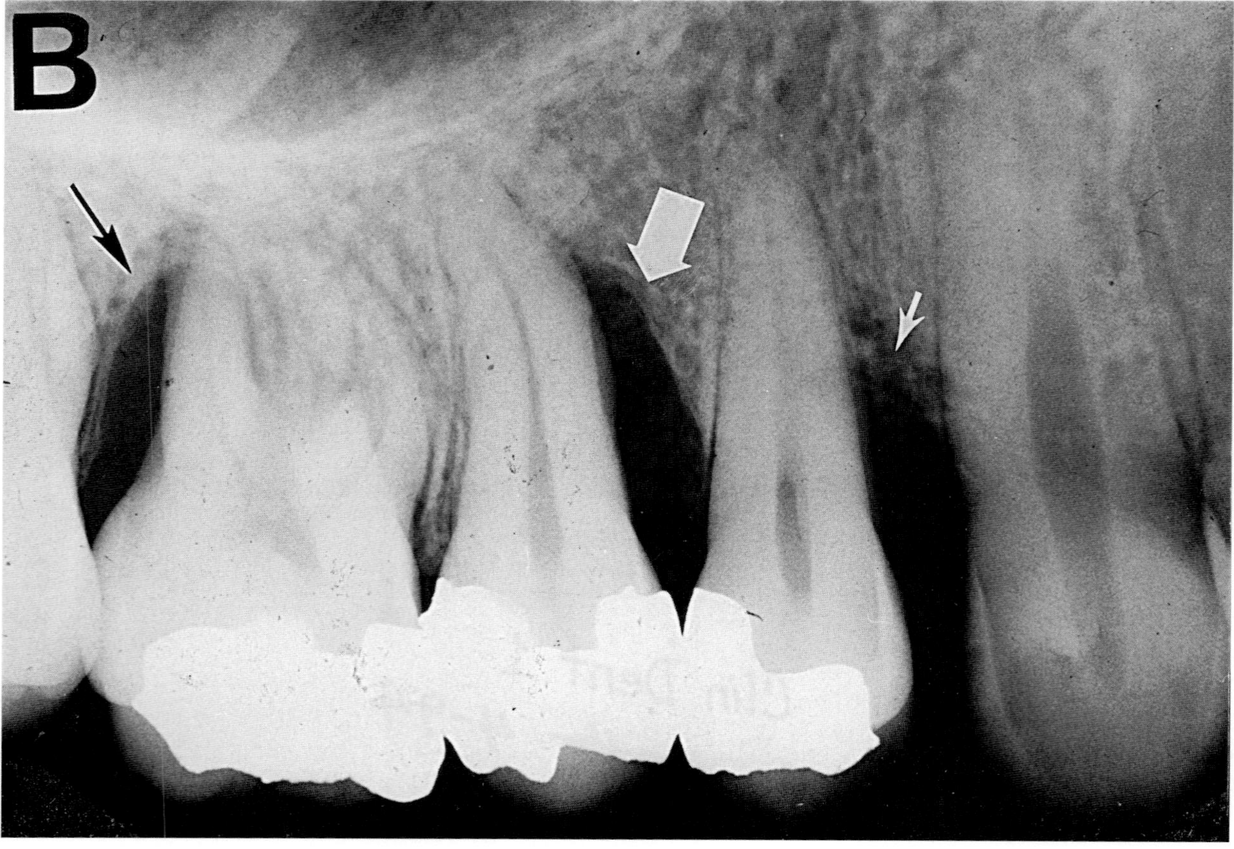

height and the bone margin is roughly perpendicular to the tooth surface. All surfaces of the bone around the same tooth may be affected but not necessarily to the same degree. Vertical or angular bony defects occur in an oblique direction (Fig. 8–17). They have a hollowed-out trough in the bone, with the base of the osseous deformity located apical to the surrounding bone.

In most cases, angular or vertical bone defects have accompanying infrabony pockets. Vertical defects occurring between the teeth generally can be seen on the radiograph. Those that appear on the facial and lingual or palatal surfaces usually are not seen on the radiograph. Surgical exposure is the only sure way to determine the presence of vertical osseous defects. The most common location of vertical defects, when seen on the radiograph, is on the distal surface of molar teeth. Nielsen and associates (1980) reported that angular defects increase with age, and approximately 60% of people with angular defects have only one defect.

Generally, alveolar crestal periodontal ligament fibers create an effective barrier to the spreading inflammation. This is one reason why the supporting bone usually is invaded before the periodontal ligament; however, in certain circumstances and in occlusal trauma particularly, the crestal periodontal ligament fibers are weakened and the pathway of least resistance sometimes is modified to follow directly into the periodontal ligament. This results in resorption of the periapical fibers and lamina dura before the supporting alveolar bone. This separates the coronal portion of the supporting alveolar bone from the periodontal ligament and tooth, resulting in a resorption pattern that is angular or vertical, and the pockets are of the infrabony type.

In LJP the classic pattern of bone destruction is angular or vertical, and it occurs first around the permanent first molars and incisors.

Evaluation of Alveolar Bone Height (Figs. 8–18 to 8–21). Although bone loss occurs on all surfaces of the root, the density of the tooth roots obscures the radiographic image of the bone level on the facial and lingual surfaces.

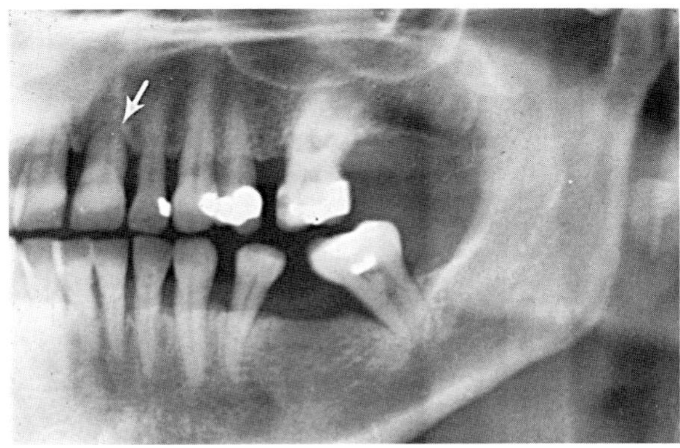

FIGURE 8–18.

Amount of bone loss. Notice horizontal line across the root of a maxillary central incisor, indicating height of lingual bone (arrow). (From Langland OE, Langlais RP, Morris CR: Principles and Practice of Panoramic Radiology. Philadelphia: WB Saunders, 1982, p. 241.)

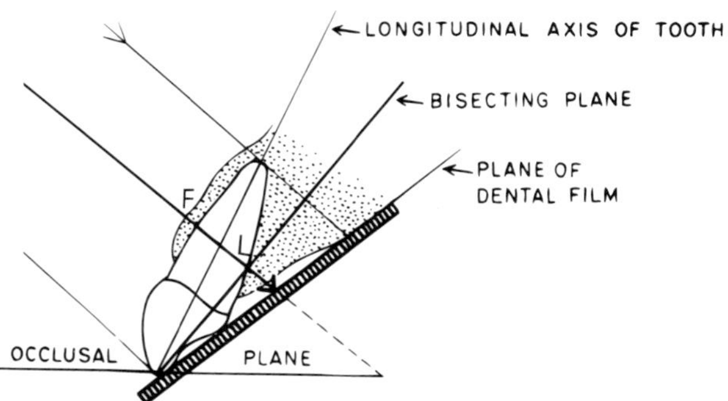

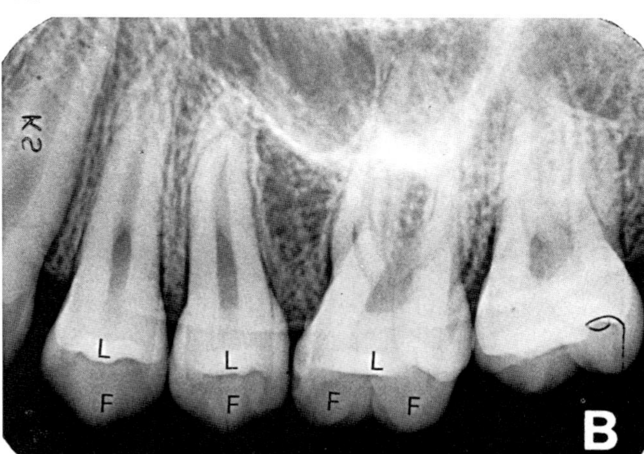

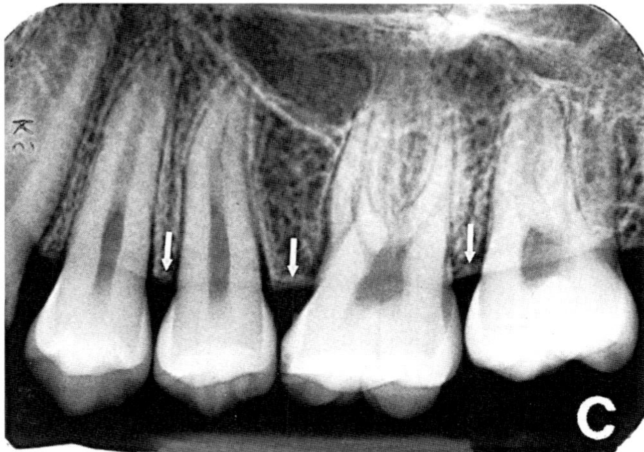

FIGURE 8–19.

Bisecting angle technique. Bisecting angle technique and assessment of coronal interdental septal bone height. A, In the bisecting angle technique, the facial (F) portion of the interdental alveolar bone is projected more coronally than the lingual portion of the interdental alveolar crest. B, Periapical radiograph taken with bisecting angle technique. The facial septal bone projected more coronally past the height of the lingual bone, filling the interproximal space with interseptal bone. The facial (F) cusps also are projected more coronally than the lingual (L) cusps of the teeth. C, Paralleling technique used to take periapical radiograph of the same patient in panel B. Notice the anatomic accuracy of the projection of interdental septal bone with the paralleling technique (arrows) compared with the bisecting angle radiograph in panel B.

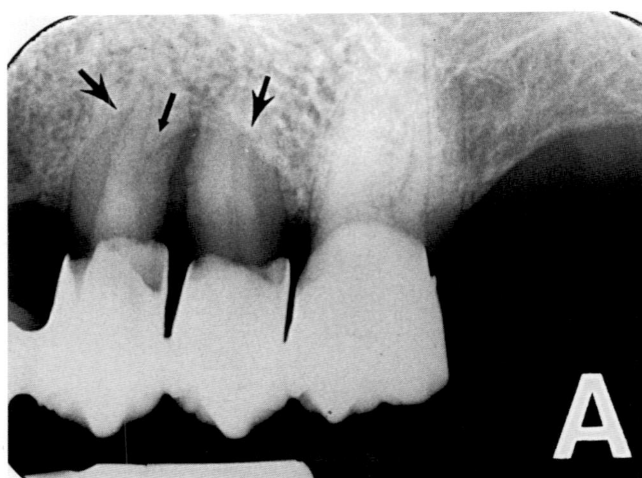

FIGURE 8–20.

Evaluation of bone height. A, Severe bone loss on the lingual surfaces of the maxillary premolars (arrows). B, Severe bone loss on the lingual surface (confirmed at surgery) of the second and third molars (arrows) outlines the height of bone on the lingual surface.

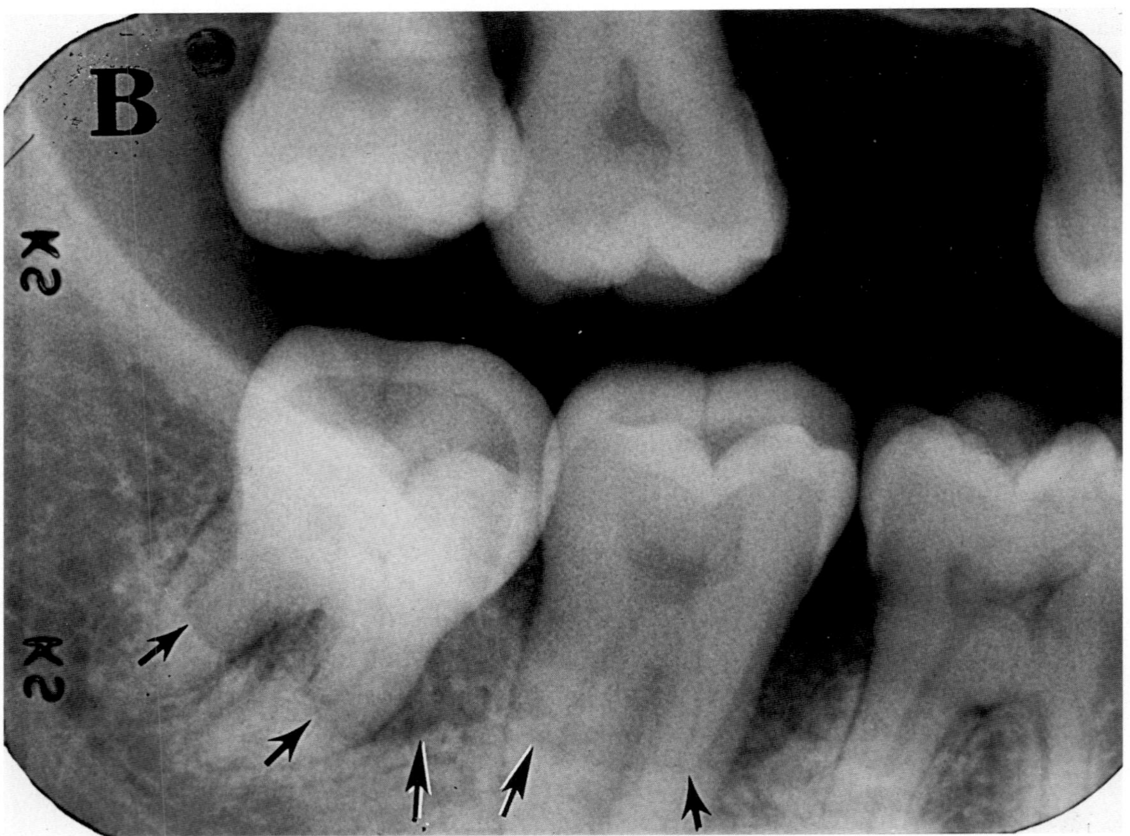

When the conditions are right, two different procedures can be used to roughly estimate the true height of the facial or lingual marginal bone:

1. As the lamina dura is traced from the apex of a tooth coronally on the radiograph, it will lose its opacity at some point. This provides a rough estimate of the true height of the interseptal bone. Any amount of bone cast coronally from this point is the facial marginal bone. Ordinarily, the difference from the point of initial loss of lamina dura opacity to the maximum height of the bone is approximately equal to the distance between the facial and lingual/palatal cusp tips. The difference between the bone (and cusp) levels ordinarily is caused by vertical angulation that has cast the facial bone coronally more than the lingual/palatal bone. In most cases, if the distance between the point of maximum lamina dura opacity and the observable bone height is greater than the distance between the cusp tips, the facial bone is probably higher than the lingual bone. The converse of this also is true (Fig. 8–20).
2. There is a second procedure for evaluating bone height. Starting at the apex of the tooth, the trabecular

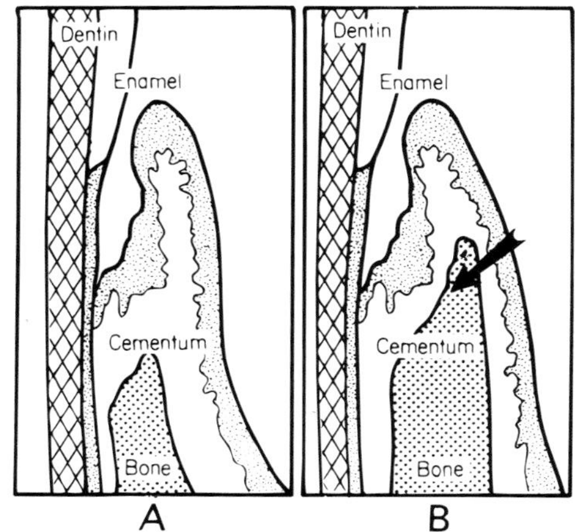

FIGURE 8–21.

Suprabony and infrabony pockets. A, Suprabony pocket: the bottom of the periodontal soft tissue pocket is coronal to the adjacent alveolar crest. B, Infrabony pocket: the bottom of the periodontal soft tissue pocket is apical to the adjacent alveolar bony crest. The bony defect is a vertical bone defect (arrow). The soft tissue pocket lies between the cementum of the tooth surface and the alveolar bone. (From Glickman I: Clinical Periodontology. 2nd Ed. Philadelphia:WB Saunders, 1958.)

bone is examined coronally until it terminates at some level on the tooth root. It will give an appearance of a radiopaque horizontal line running across the root. The portion of the root between the line and enamel will look bare or denuded (Fig. 8–18 and 8–21). This horizontal line usually represents the lingual bone level and will join the terminal point of maximum lamina dura opacity described in the first procedure.

Evaluation of Bone Deformities (Figs. 8–22 and 8–23)

There are different types of bone defects produced by periodontal disease. The accurate radiograph usually will show a bony defect in the interseptal bone, but its exact form can be determined only by careful probing and direct vision during surgical exposure. In most instances, angular or vertical bone defects have accompanying infrabony pockets. The bone of the pocket is apical to the level of the alveolar bone in infrabony pockets, and the pocket wall lies between the tooth and bone. Infrabony pockets most often occur interproximally but may be located on the facial and lingual surfaces. The bone destruction pattern is vertical (angular) (Fig. 8–21). As suggested by Goldman and Cohen (1958), infrabony pockets can be classified according to the number of bony walls associated with the pocket. Infrabony pockets may be classified as one-, two-, three-, or four-wall defects (Figs. 8–22 and 8–23).

One-Wall Infrabony Pocket or Defect (Figs. 8–23 and 8–24). In the one-wall angular defect, one bony wall of the interseptal bone remains after the mesial or the distal portion of the interseptal bone has been destroyed. It is called the "hemiseptum defect" and is identical to vertical or angular bony deformities (Figs. 8–17 and 8–23). Sometimes the one-wall defect will take the form of a ramp when the facial or lingual cortical bone is destroyed (Fig. 8–24). This defect is called "ramping." When one-wall bony defects are seen

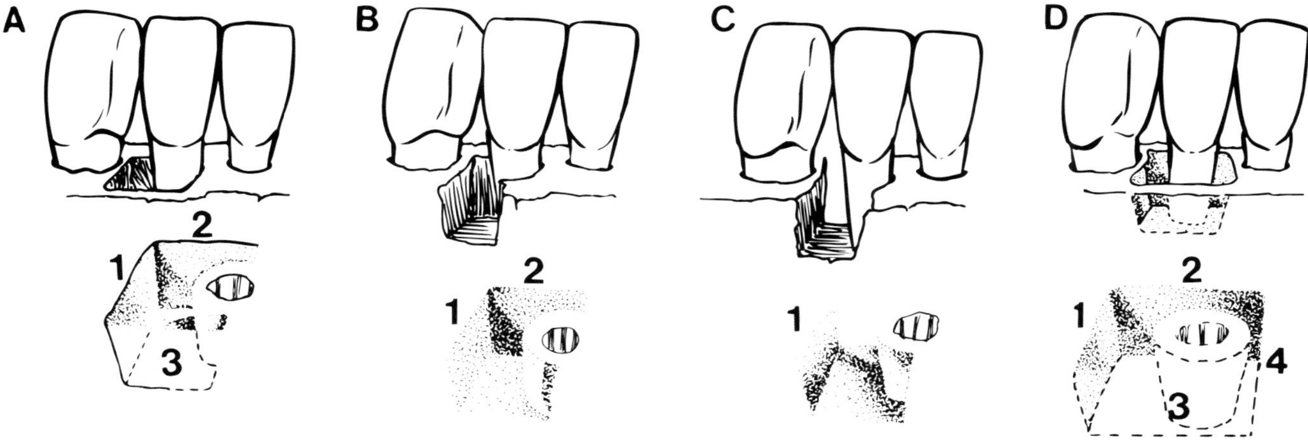

FIGURE 8–22.

Infrabony defects. A, Three-wall bony infrabony defect. (Three alveolar bony walls surround the defect, sometimes called an intrabony defect.) B, Two-wall infrabony defect. Another type of two-wall bony defect is the osseous crater, in which the facial and lingual walls are intact, but the interdental alveolar crestal bone has been resorbed, forming a crater in the bone. C, One-wall infrabony defect or "hemiseptum defect," in which only one wall of the interdental bony septum remains after the facial and lingual walls have been resorbed. Ramping is another form of a one-wall defect in which, for instance, the interdental septal bone may slope toward the destroyed facial or lingual wall, forming a ramplike appearance. D, Four-wall infrabony defect completely surrounding the tooth. (From Carranza F: Glickman's Periodontology. 5th Ed. Philadelphia:WB Saunders, 1979, p. 228.)

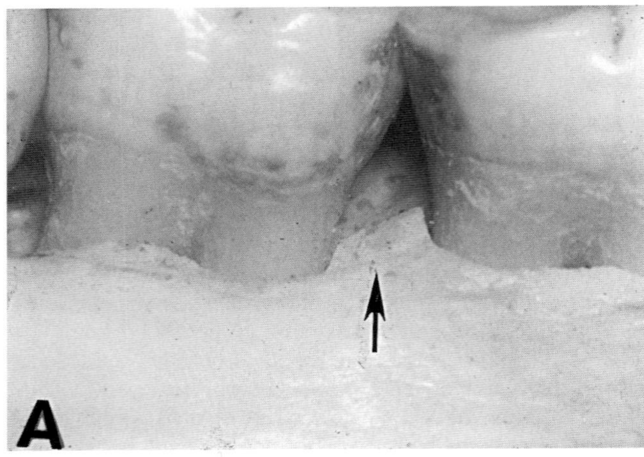

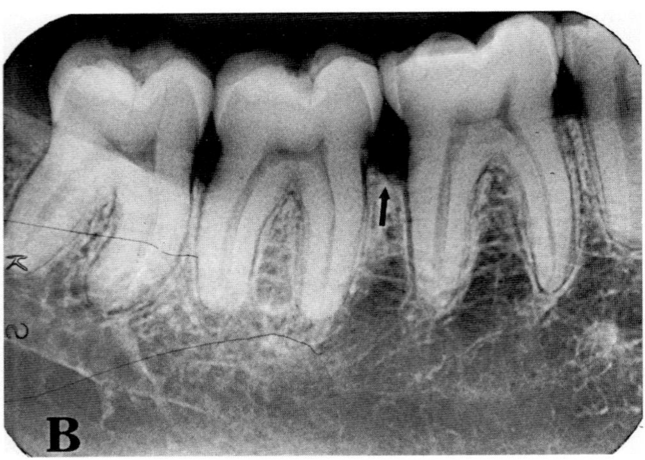

FIGURE 8–23.

One-wall hemiseptum defect. A, One-wall hemiseptum defect between mandibular first and second molars of dry specimen (arrow). (Courtesy of Dr. R. H. Watkins, Phoenix, AZ.) B, Radiograph of specimen like that in A, showing a one-wall hemiseptum defect between the first and second molars (arrow).

on the radiograph, usually the facial bone is less distinct than the lingual bone and is positioned more coronally if it is still present and has not been resorbed.

Two-Wall Infrabony Pocket (Defect) (Figs. 8–25 and 8–26). An osseous crater is a concavity in the crest of the interdental bone confined within the facial and lingual walls (Fig. 8–25; see Fig. 3–17). It is a two-wall infrabony pocket deformity. Manson and Nicholson (1974) found that the craters constitute approximately one-third of all defects (35.2%) and two thirds (62.0%) of all mandibular defects; they also were twice as common in the posterior segments compared with the anterior segments. A less common two-wall defect occurs when the facial or lingual cortical plate of bone is missing (Figs. 8–22B and 8–26). When the remaining facial or lingual wall is very thin or if a high-contrast low-kilovolt peak technique is used, this defect may not be seen on the radiograph. The remaining thin bony wall will be ''burnt-out'' and erased from the radiograph.

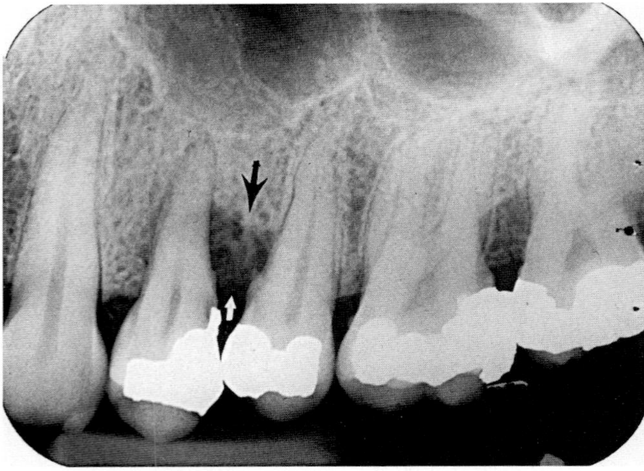

FIGURE 8–24.

One-wall defect with a ramplike appearance. The defect has formed a ramplike appearance (arrows) because the interdental septal bone slopes down from the facial/lingual wall crest of bone toward the crest of the destroyed facial/lingual bone. Thorough probing of the area will confirm whether the facial or lingual wall is destroyed.

Three-Wall Infrabony Pocket or Defect (Intrabony Pocket) (Fig. 8–27). The three-wall defect is an infrabony defect surrounded by bony walls on three sides, with the tooth root forming the fourth wall. The infrabony defect is not a circumferential defect because there is an osseous wall on each side of the root; however, the defect may extend around the root and stop on the buccal or lingual aspect instead of the interproximal surface. Defects with three bony walls occur most often in the mandibular molar region but can occur wherever bone is thick enough to have cancellous bone between the alveolar bone and cortical plate (Fig. 8–27).

Four-Wall Infrabony Pocket (Defect) (Fig. 8–28). The circumferential defect is the four-wall defect that completely surrounds the root of the tooth (Fig. 8–28).

Furcation Involvement (Figs. 8–8 and 8–29)

Glickman (1950) defined furcation as a ''commonly occurring condition in which the bifurcation and trifurcation of multirooted teeth are denuded by periodontal disease.'' The denuded bifurcation or trifurcation may be seen or may be concealed by the wall of alveolar bone. The amount of tissue destruction can be evaluated by exploration with a blunt instrument with a simultaneous blast of warm air. The tooth may or may not be mobile and usually is symptom free. Usually the bifurcation or trifurcation involvement will not be seen until the bone has resorbed apically to the furcation area (Fig. 8–8). Trifurcation involvement of the maxillary molars is not as sharply defined on the radiograph as the mandibular molar bifurcation involvement because the

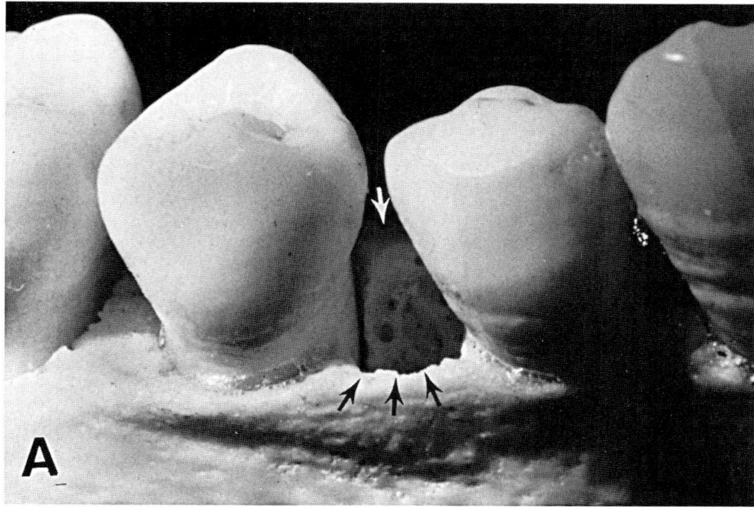

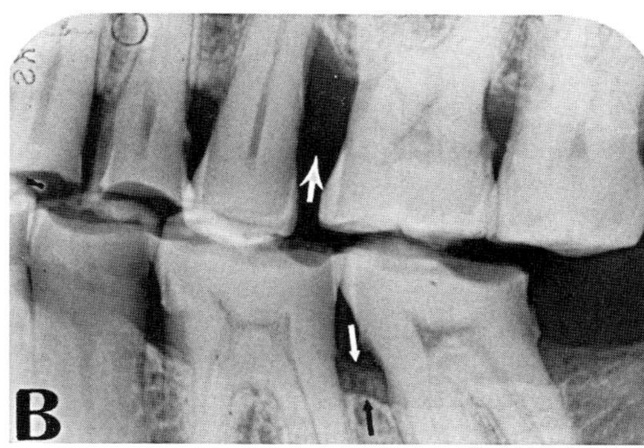

FIGURE 8–25.

Osseous crater. A, Osseous crater between two molars in a dry specimen (arrows). B, Crater deformity between lower first and second molars (arrows). Open contact between the second premolar and the first molar has produced a food packing area (arrow). (See Fig. 3–17 for another radiograph of crater formation.)

opaque palatal root of the maxillary molar is superimposed over the trifurcation area, which attenuates the radiolucency (Figs. 8–29D; see Fig. 8–32).

If there is a slight thickening of the periodontal ligament (PDL) space in the furcation area, the area should be investigated clinically because it is a general rule that bone loss is always greater than the radiograph shows. Also, if there is severe bone loss on the mesial or distal surface of a multirooted tooth, furcation involvement should be suspected.

Types of Etiologic Factors

The primary cause of inflammatory periodontal diseases is the accumulation and growth of bacterial plaque on the teeth near the gingival margin or in the sulcus or pocket; however, the periodontal tissue response to the bacteria is influenced by local, immune, and systemic factors.

Local factors are found in the immediate environment of the periodontal tissues and can be divided into irritating and functional factors. Local irritating factors are separated into

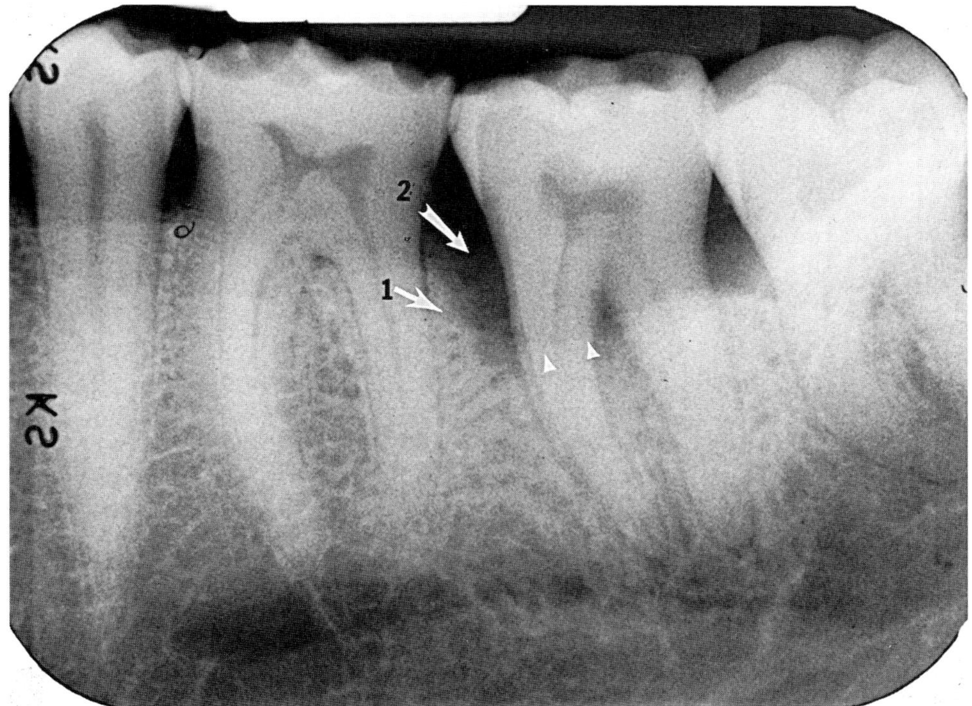

FIGURE 8–26.

Two-wall infrabony pocket (defect). This was confirmed by exposure at surgery. Mesial (1) and facial (2) walls were intact, with furcation involvement. Notice the horizontal bone line across the molar roots (arrowheads) depicting the height of the lingual alveolar bone.

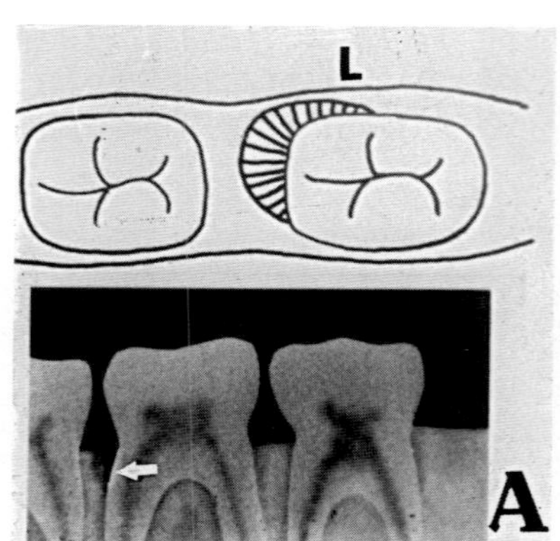

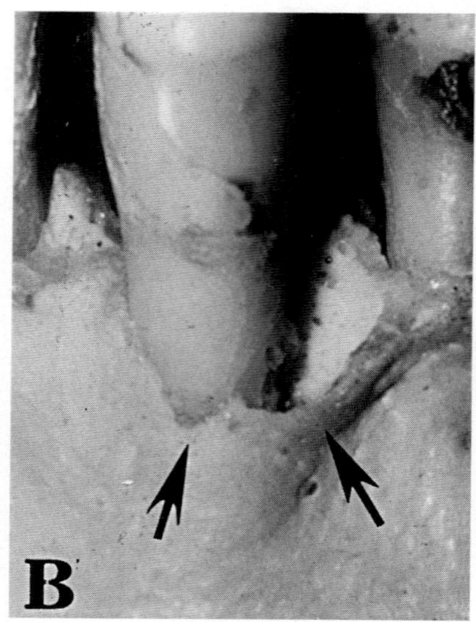

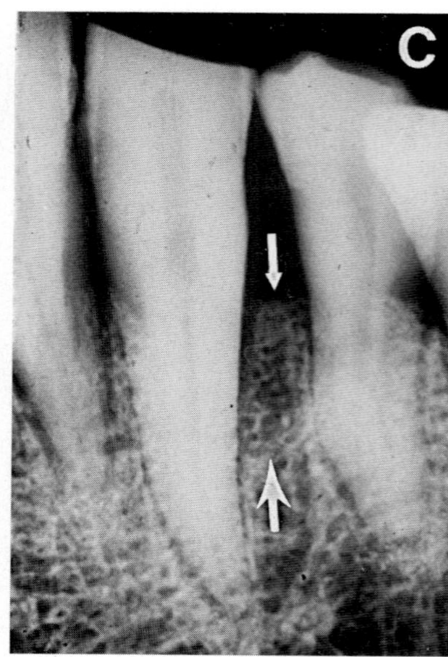

FIGURE 8–27.

Three-wall infrabony pocket defect (intrabony defect). A, Diagram of infrabony pocket defect within the facial, mesial proximal, and lingual (L) walls of alveolar bone. The radiograph of this type of three-wall defect (below diagram) may show only a wedge-shaped radiolucency of mesial interdental septal bone adjacent to the tooth (arrow). The lingual defect would be hidden by the superimposed tooth root unless, of course, the furcation of the molar was severely involved. B, A three-wall (infrabony) defect of a mandibular canine in a dry specimen within the lingual, distal proximal, and facial alveolar bone (arrows). C, Radiograph of the three-wall defect in panel B. Although there is a radiolucency on the distal surface of the canine (arrows), the three-wall defect is difficult to see on the radiograph because the facial bone is so thin and it is superimposed partially over the canine. (Courtesy of Dr. R. H. Watkins, Phoenix, AZ.)

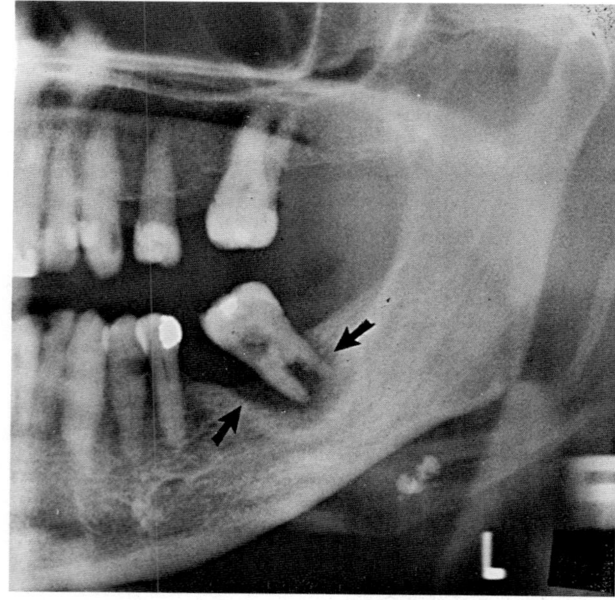

FIGURE 8–28.

Four-wall infrabony pocket. A four-wall infrabony pocket around a lower second molar with mesial proximal, distal proximal, facial, and lingual walls still remaining (arrows).

local initiating and local predisposing factors. Bacterial plaque is the local initiating factor because it causes gingival inflammation when it accumulates on the teeth adjacent to the gingiva. Local predisposing factors such as overhanging restorations, calculus, and food retention areas create a dentogingival environment that favors the accumulation of bacterial plaque. Local functional factors such as bruxism and occlusal trauma create occlusal forces that cause destruction of the periodontal ligament and alveolar bone but do not affect the inflammatory process directly.

Detection of Local Predisposing Factors

Several local predisposing factors may be detected on the radiograph: calculus deposits, faulty restorations, and food packing areas. The radiograph plays no role in determining the cause of the predisposing factors in periodontal disease; it only detects them.

Calculus (Fig. 8–30). Calculus is a bacterial plaque that has been mineralized. It can form on all tooth surfaces and dental prostheses. Calculus is classified into two groups, according to its location and source: supragingival (salivary) and subgingival (serumal).

Supragingival calculus is usually light in color and chalky in consistency. The mineral source is primarily the saliva.

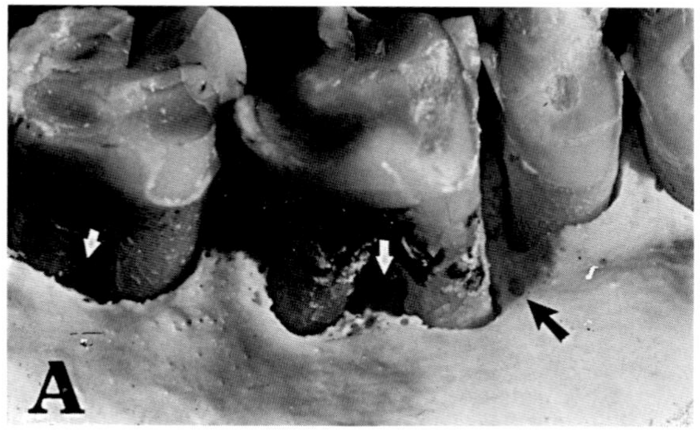

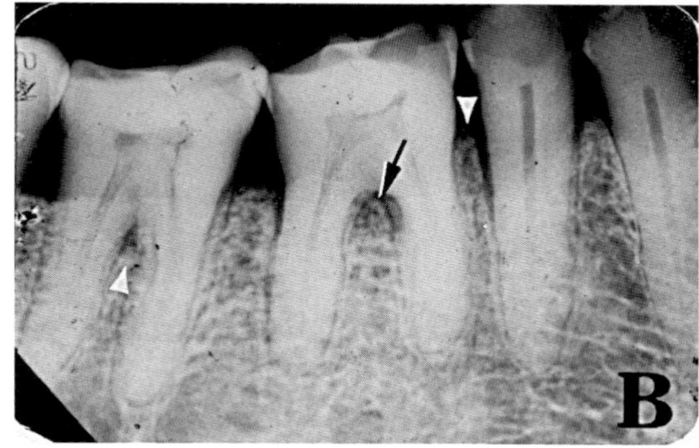

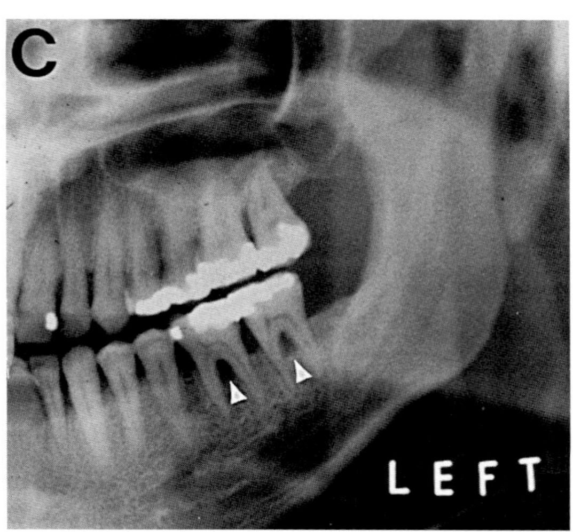

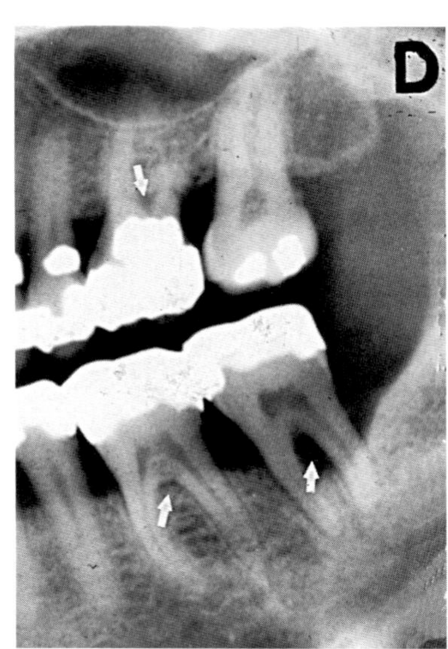

FIGURE 8–29.

Furcation involvement. A, Furcation involvement of first and second molars (white arrows) of a dry specimen (Class II type because they are not complete furcations). There is a two-wall infrabony defect (crater) on the mesial surface of the first molar, with lingual and mesial proximal walls remaining (black arrow). B, Radiograph of dry specimen in panel A. Furcation involvement appears as slight radiolucency (black arrow); notice osseous crater radiolucency between the first molar and second premolar (white arrowheads). (A and B, Courtesy of Dr. R. H. Watkins, Phoenix, AZ.) C, Class III through-and-through furcation involvement of mandibular first and second molars (arrowheads). D, Class III through-and-through trifurcation involvement of a maxillary first molar (upper arrow). The radiolucency is not as dark as the radiolucency of mandibular molar Class III furcation involvement because of the superimposition of the palatal root over the furca. Notice furca involvement of mandibular first and second molars (lower arrows). (From Langland OE, Langlais RP, Morris CR: Principles and Practice of Panoramic Radiology. Philadelphia:WB Saunders, 1982, p. 240.)

The calcified deposits form on the clinical crowns above the free gingival margin. Subgingival calculus is normally darker in color and more dense; it is found on the tooth surface below the free margin of the gingiva and extends into the periodontal pocket. The main source of mineralization is usually blood serum, so it is referred to as serumal calculus.

The primary etiologic role of calculus in periodontal tissue is that it acts as a holding mechanism for nonmineralized bacterial plaque and keeps the bacterial plaque in direct contact with the tissue.

Calculus Detection (Figs. 8–31 to 8–33). The radiograph shows heavy calculus deposits interproximally and sometimes even on the facial and lingual surfaces. The ability to diagnose and detect calculus radiographically depends on its degree of mineralization and the angulation factors of the x-ray beam. Sometimes the detection of calculus spicules is useful in diagnosing and monitoring periodontal disease (Figs. 8–31 to 8–33).

Faulty Restorations (Figs. 8–34 and 8–35). Inadequate dental restorations and prostheses are common causes of gingival inflammation and periodontal destruction. Some problems with restorations and prostheses include the following: (1) overhanging margins of dental restorations (Fig. 8–34); (2) open interproximal contacts of dental resto-

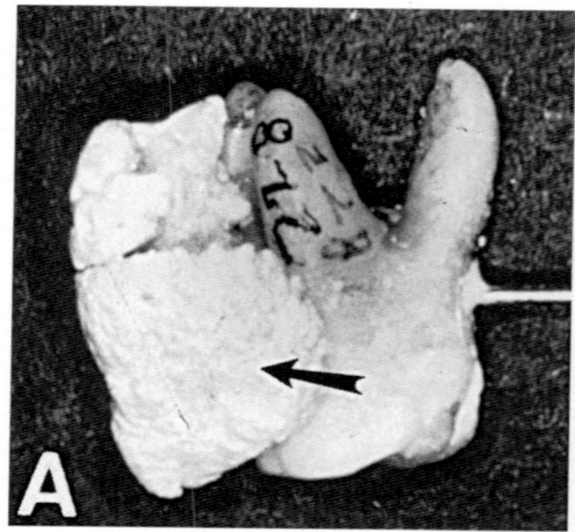

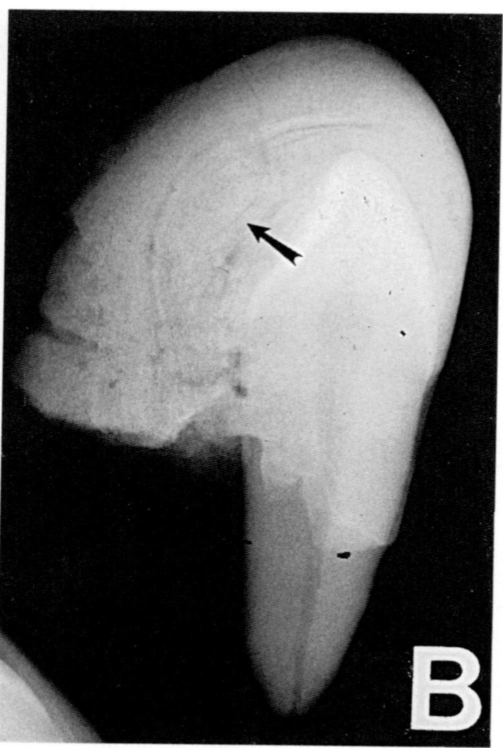

FIGURE 8–30.

Gross amounts of calculus. A, Gross calculus deposits on the buccal crown and roots of an extracted maxillary first molar (arrow). B, Radiograph of extracted lower canine with gross amounts of supragingival calculus (arrow). Calculus is formed from mineral salts of salivary glands and is found in abundance on the lingual surfaces of lower anterior teeth opposite the ducts of the submandibular glands and on buccal surfaces of the maxillary molars.

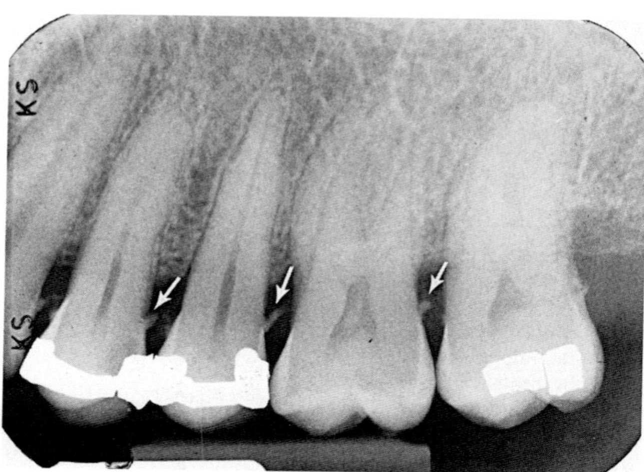

FIGURE 8–31.

Spurlike calculus. Figure shows this between all interproximal surfaces of premolars and molars (arrows).

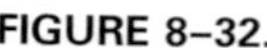

FIGURE 8–32.

Veneer type of calculus with a smooth contour (arrows). On the distal surface of the second premolar, clinically the deposit has a glossy, veneerlike appearance. There is trifurcation involvement of the first molar. Notice the spur-type calculus (second molar).

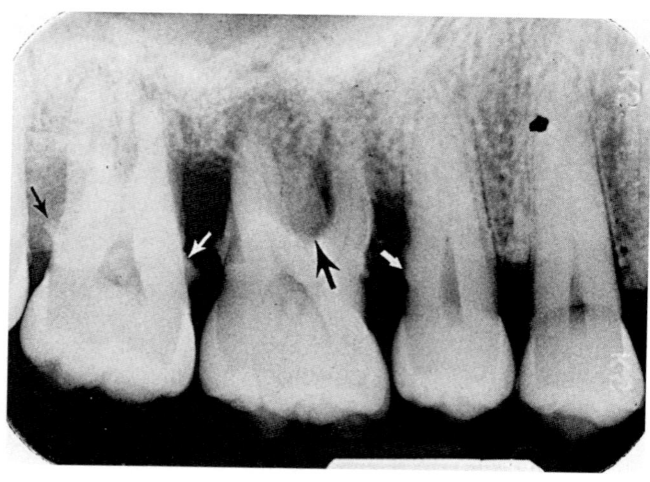

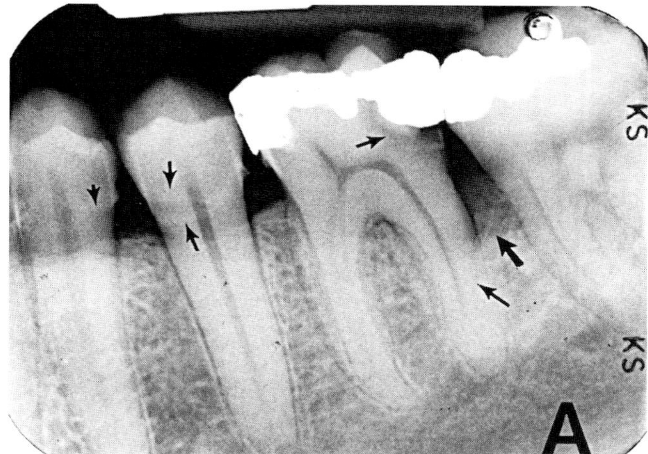

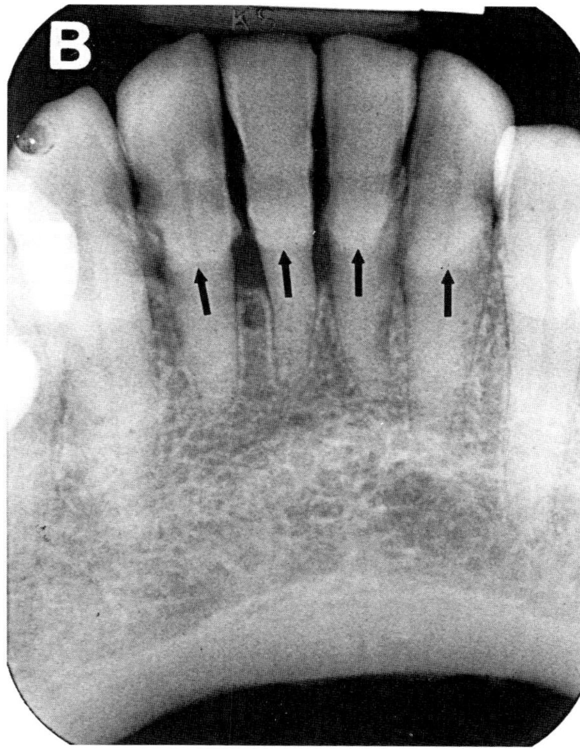

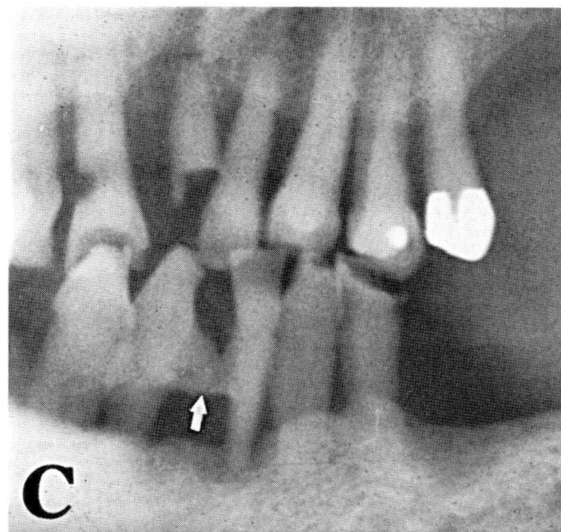

FIGURE 8–33.

Calculus. A, Ringlike calculus encircling premolars (arrows). Notice the lingual alveolar bone horizontal line across the distal root of the first molar and recurrent caries on the distal surface of the first molar. Also, there is a ramping defect between the first and second molars (large arrow). B, Archlike large masses of calculus at level of gingiva will form radiopaque areas on the tooth (arrows). C, Calculus bridge between two lower incisors (arrow). (From Langland OE, Langlais RP, Morris CR: Principles and Practice of Panoramic Radiology. Philadelphia:WB Saunders, 1982, p. 249.)

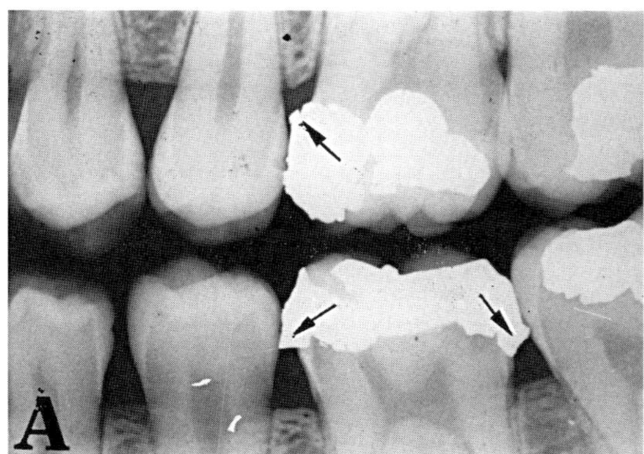

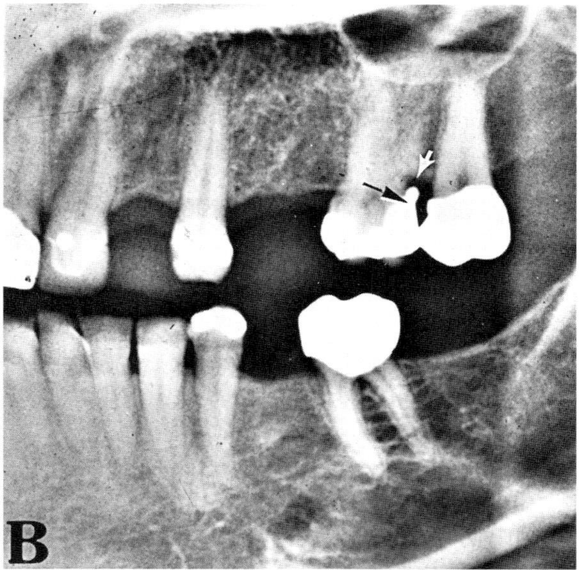

FIGURE 8–34.

Overhanging restorations. A, There are overhanging restorations on the mesial and distal surfaces of the lower first molar (arrows) and mesial surface of the upper first molar. Recurrent caries is under an MOD restoration in a lower first molar. (From Langland OE, Langlais RP, Morris CR: Principles and Practice of Panoramic Radiology. Philadelphia:WB Saunders, 1982, p. 219.) B, There is an overhanging restoration on the distal surface of an upper second molar (black arrow). Notice caries under overhang (white arrow). (From Langland OE, Langlais RP, Morris CR: Principles and Practice of Panoramic Radiology. Philadelphia:WB Saunders, 1982, p. 250.)

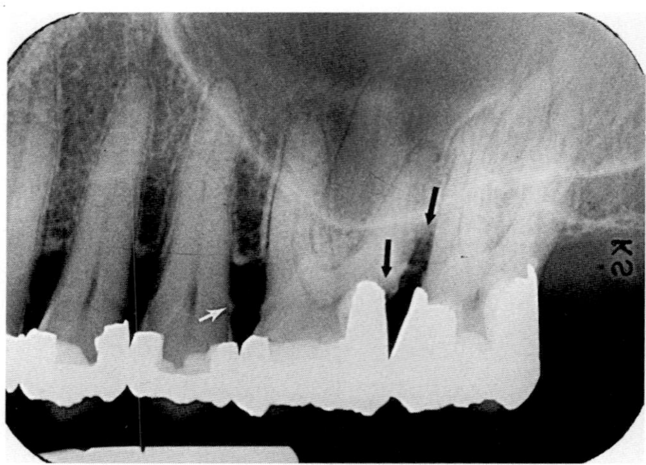

FIGURE 8–35.

Imperfectly formed embrasure of disto-occlusal restoration. This is seen in a maxillary first molar. Notice the loss of coronal height of bone in interdental septal area between first and second molars (black arrows) and veneer-type of calculus on the distal surface of the second premolar (white arrow).

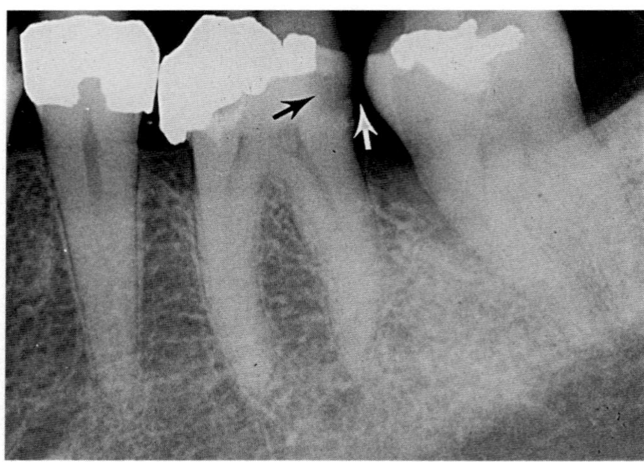

FIGURE 8–37.

Loose contact. Loose contact from interproximal caries (arrow) on the distal aspect of a first molar, resulting in a food packing area and periodontal bone destruction (arrows). (From Langland OE, Langlais RP, Morris CR: Principles and Practice of Panoramic Radiology. Philadelphia:WB Saunders, 1982, p. 251.)

rations (see Fig. 8–38); (3) deficient margins of crowns, jackets, and synthetic porcelain restorations; (4) fixed and removable prostheses that were adapted improperly; (5) overcontoured restorations and pontics, creating excessive buccolingual contours and inadequate interproximal embrasure spaces (Fig. 8–35); and (6) clasps of partial dentures that retain plaque on the gingiva or exert excessive occlusal forces.

Food Packing Areas (Figs. 8–36 to 8–38). Hirschfeld (1930) defined food impaction as the forceful wedging of food through occlusal pressure into the interproximal spaces. Food impaction is a very common cause of gingival and periodontal disease. The absence of tooth contact or presence of an unsatisfactory proximal relationship is conducive to food impaction. As the teeth wear down and the flattened surfaces replace normal convexities, the wedging effect of the opposing cusp into the interproximal space is exaggerated and food impaction results (Fig. 8–36). Cusps that tend to forcibly wedge food interproximally are known as "plunger cusps." Some factors leading to food impaction include the following: (1) wear from attrition, opening contact points (Fig. 8–36); (2) loss of occlusal support by extraction of adjacent teeth, which will open contacts by shifting the teeth (Fig. 8–38); (3) opening of the contact areas by caries (Fig. 8–37); (4) supraeruption of teeth, opening up

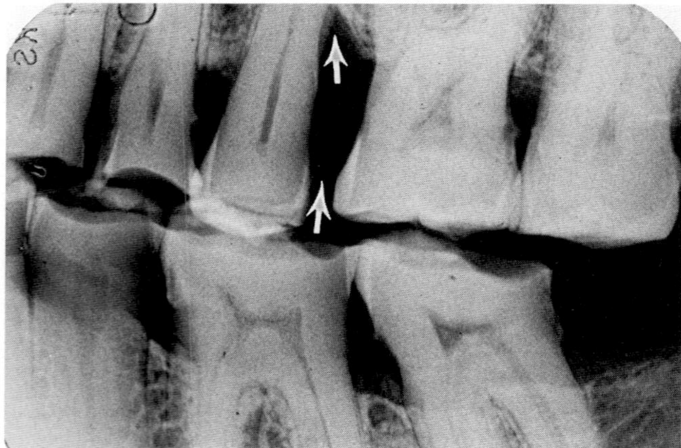

FIGURE 8–36.

Severe attrition causing loose contact. Severe attrition has caused a loose contact (arrows) and food packing area between the second premolar and first molar, with resultant periodontal destruction of the alveolar bone.

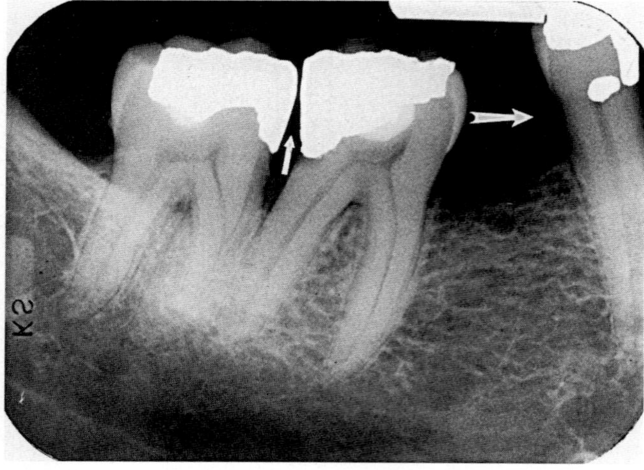

FIGURE 8–38.

Food packing area. A food packing area between the second and third molars resulting from open contact caused by a failure to replace the missing first molar.

contact points when opposing teeth are not replaced; (5) partially impacted teeth, producing food-lodging areas around the impaction; and (6) improperly constructed restorations.

Periodontal Occlusal Trauma

Periodontal occlusal trauma gives rise to a degenerative lesion that develops when occlusal forces exceed the adaptive capacity of the supporting periodontal tissues. Clinically, it is characterized by breakdown of the periodontal ligament fibers, bone resorption, widening of the periodontal ligament space, and loosening of the teeth.

There are primary and secondary types of occlusal trauma. Primary occlusal trauma results when increases in the magnitude or the duration of the occlusal forces or a change in the direction of forces becomes excessive in the presence of normal tissue support. Secondary occlusal trauma develops when the normal forces of occlusion become severe because of the excessive loss of periodontal support rather than an increase in occlusal forces.

Etiologic factors in occlusal trauma include the following: (1) bruxism, clenching, and biting habits; (2) faulty dental restorations and prosthetic appliances; (3) tipping forces from occlusal interferences, such as centric prematurities and balancing side contacts; (4) drifting and extrusion of teeth after extraction; and (5) periodontal disease.

Although the etiologic factors mentioned above have the potential to cause occlusal trauma, they do not always result in degenerative periodontal changes. For instance, young adults have centric prematurities, but only a small percentage of the age group show clinical evidence of periodontal occlusal trauma. Also, some patients with bruxism cause severe wearing of the occlusal surfaces of the teeth rather than showing clinical evidence of periodontal occlusal trauma.

◆ *RADIOLOGY (Occlusal Trauma) (Fig. 8–39)*

The most common clinical sign of trauma to the periodontium is increased tooth mobility. The increased forces on the periodontal fibers result in widening of the periodontal ligament, which leads to increased tooth mobility.

The radiographic signs of trauma from occlusion include the following: (1) an increased width of the periodontal ligament space (Fig. 8–39), often with thickening of the lamina dura along the lateral aspect of the root and in bifurcation areas; (2) "vertical" rather than "horizontal" destruction of the interdental septum; (3) alveolar bone radiolucency or condensation; and (4) root resorption.

Root Morphologic Characteristics and Crown-Root Ratio (Figs. 8–40 and 8–41)

The prognosis is poor in patients with short, tapered roots and relatively large crowns (Fig. 8–40). Kay and associates (1954) reported that the periodontium is more susceptible to injury from occlusal forces when there is a disproportionate crown-root ratio and reduced surface available for periodontal support.

When the crown-root ratio becomes great because of periodontal bone destruction to the alveolar support of the tooth, the tooth is under a severe amount of leverage. The clinical crown is the tooth above the bone, and the clinical root is the root in bone (Fig. 8–40). A clinical crown to clinical root ratio of 1:3 is favorable.

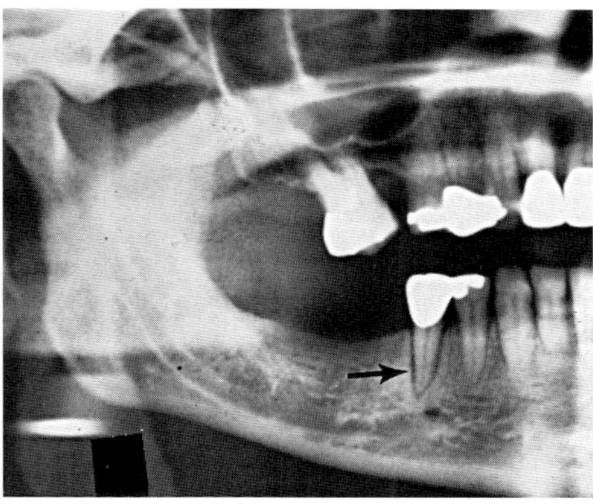

FIGURE 8–39.

Thickened periodontal ligament space. Thickened periodontal ligament space of second premolar. Tooth was extremely mobile. (From Langland OE, Langlais RP, Morris CR: Principles and Practice of Panoramic Radiology. Philadelphia: WB Saunders, 1982, p. 252.)

Activity of Destructive Process (Fig. 8–42)

With several standardized radiographs, the activity of the destructive process of bone in periodontal disease can be evaluated roughly. The interseptal bone resorption is active if the interseptal alveolar bone crests are uneven and irregu-

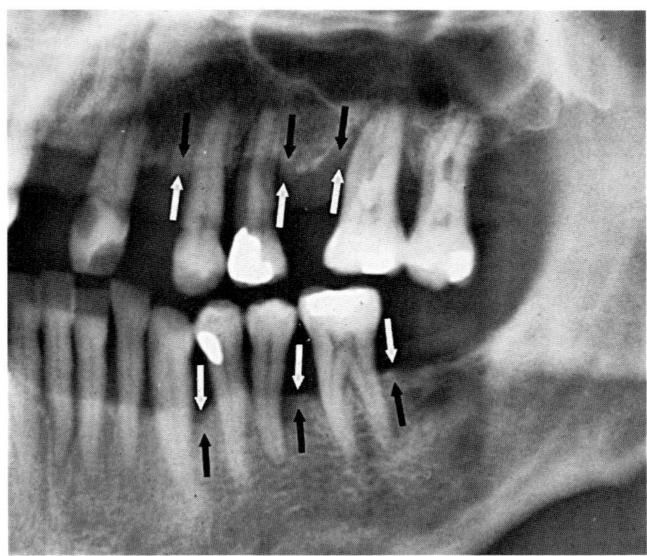

FIGURE 8–40.

Unfavorable clinical crown-clinical root ratios. The long roots preserved a favorable crown-to-root ratio for more years than usual (arrows). (From Langland OE, Langlais RP, Morris CR: Principles and Practice of Panoramic Radiology. Philadelphia:WB Saunders, 1982, p. 241.)

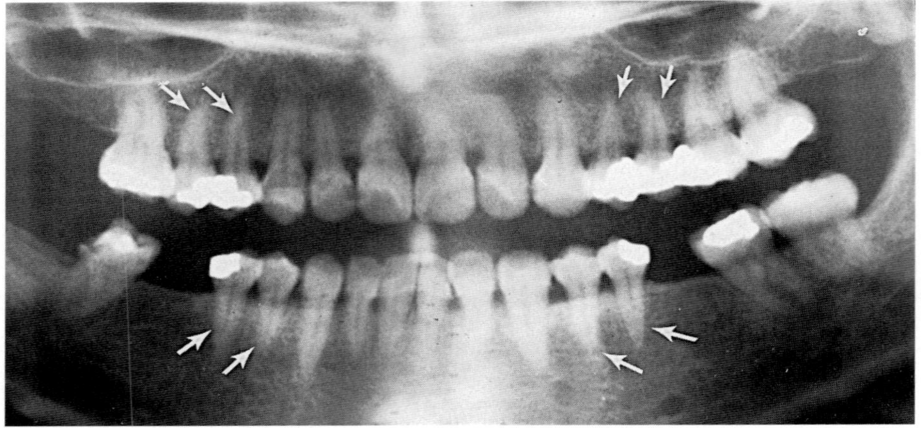

FIGURE 8–41.

Spiked roots. Notice spiked roots (arrows) of all premolars. (From Langland OE, Langlais RP, Morris CR: Principles and Practice of Panoramic Radiology. Philadelphia: WB Saunders, 1982, p. 242.)

lar and there is steady progressive bone loss of the alveolar crests (Fig. 8–42A).

The destructive bone activity is stabilized if there is a smooth, condensed alveolar crest surface and the bone loss has been minimal over a period of years (Fig. 8–42B).

Radiographic Evaluation of Therapy

Radiographic changes must be correlated closely with clinical measurements for accurate assessment of the existence of periodontal destruction. Reproducibility of radiographs is important before and after treatment to show changes, especially in the alveolar bone crest. Of course, the radiographs must be projected, exposed, and processed accurately.

Conventional intraoral radiographs provide only a two-dimensional image of the alveolar bone. The image lacks depth and does not show changes in facial and lingual bony areas superimposed over the tooth roots. Under the most ideal circumstances, when two radiographs of the same location are taken with identical geometric relations of the beam of x-radiation angulation and placement of the film, Hausmann and associates (1986) reported a difference in alveolar crest levels of approximately 0.6 mm. Digital substraction radiography addresses this problem. It has been shown by Hausmann and colleagues (1986) that bony defects can be detected with substraction radiography when only 1 to 5% of the mineral is lost or there is less than 0.5 mm of bone loss along the tooth root.

In assessing bony dimensions and contours when im-

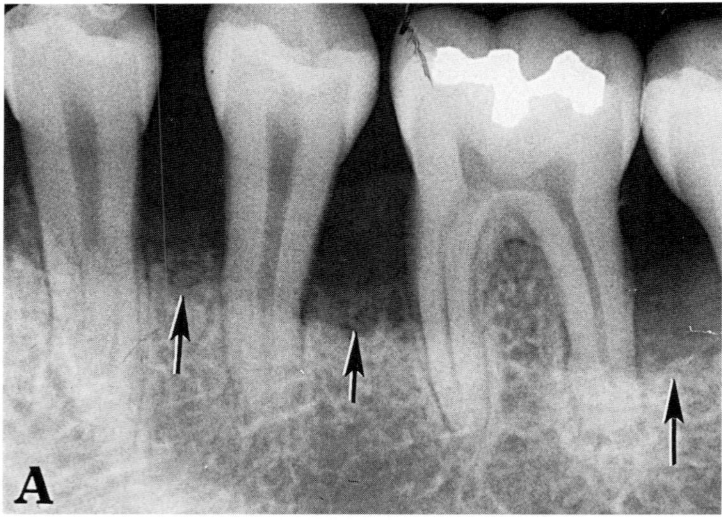

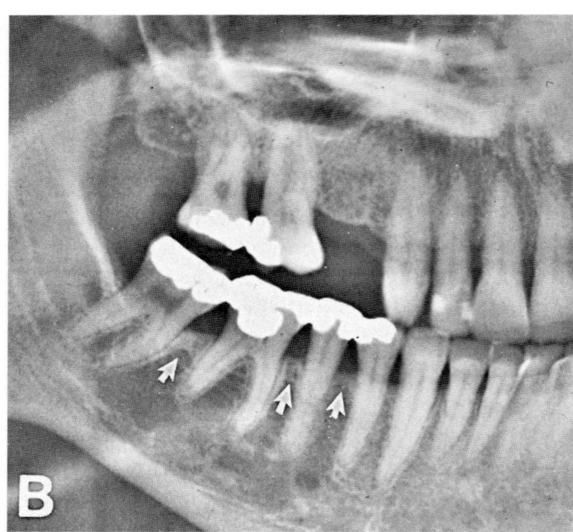

FIGURE 8–42.

Destructive process. A, Radiograph that appears to show an actively destructive process (arrows). (From Langland OE, Langlais RP, Morris CR: Principles and Practice of Panoramic Radiology. Philadelphia:WB Saunders, 1982, p. 247.) B, Radiograph of a patient with static or slowly destructive periodontal disease. The crests of interseptal alveolar bone between the first and second premolars and molars are smooth and radiopaque (arrows). (From Langland OE, Langlais RP, Morris CR: Principles and Practice of Panoramic Radiology. Philadelphia:WB Saunders, 1982, p. 248.)

plants are to be considered, tomography and computed tomography scans of the mandible and maxilla are important diagnostic aids.

If there is inadequate bone available for the use of implants, especially in partially edentulous patients, the treatment plan should be altered to emphasize the preservation of the remaining periodontally involved teeth. If implants can be used, the emphasis on the preservation of periodontally involved teeth is less important.

References

Radiologic Diagnosis of Periodontal Disease

Hoag PM, Pawlak EA: Essentials of Periodontics. 4th Ed. St. Louis:CV Mosby, 1990, pp. 69, 88.

Page RC, Schroeder HE: Periodontitis in Man and Other Animals. Basel: S Karger, 1982, p. 330.

Prepubertal Periodontitis

Page RC, et al: Prepubertal periodontitis: I. Definition of a clinical disease entity. J Periodontol 54:257, 1983.

Juvenile Periodontitis

Hoag PM, Pawlak EA: Essentials of Periodontitis. 4th Ed. St. Louis:CV Mosby, 1990, p. 87.

Hormand J, Frandsen A: Juvenile periodontitis: localization of bone loss in relation to age, sex and teeth. J Clin Periodontol 6:407, 1979.

Krill DB, Fry HR: Treatment of localized juvenile periodontitis (periodontosis). J Periodontol 58:1, 1987.

Saxby M: Prevalence of juvenile periodontitis in a British school population. Community Dent Oral Epidemiol 12:185, 1984.

Van Dyke TE, et al: Neutrophil chemotaxis in families with localized juvenile periodontitis. J Periodontol 20:503, 1985.

Rapidly Progressive Periodontitis

Page RC, et al: Rapidly progressive periodontitis: a distinct clinical condition. J Periodontol 54:198, 1983.

Tanner ACR, et al: A study of bacteria associated with advancing periodontitis in man. J Clin Periodontol 6:278, 1979.

Adult Periodontitis

Brown LJ, et al: Periodontal disease in the U.S. in 1981: prevalence, severity, extent and role in tooth mortality. J Periodontol 60:363, 1989.

Goodson JM, et al: Patterns of progression and regression of advanced destructive periodontal disease. J Clin Periodontol 9:472, 1982.

Lindke J, Haffayee AD, Socransky SS: Progression of periodontal disease in adult subjects in the absence of periodontal therapy. J Clin Periodontol 10:433, 1983.

Miller AJ: NIH publication no. 88–2868, Aug 1987.

Socransky SS, et al: New concept of destructive periodontal disease. J Clin Periodontol 11:21, 1984.

The Role of the Radiograph in Diagnosis of Periodontal Disease

Early PJ, et al: Textbook of Nuclear Medicine Technology. 3rd Ed. St. Louis:CV Mosby, 1979, p. 379.

Glickman I: Bifurcation involvement in periodontal disease. J Am Dent Assoc 40:528, 1950.

Glickman I: Clinical Periodontology. 4th Ed. Philadelphia:WB Saunders, 1972, p. 499.

Goldman HM, Cohen DW: The infrabony pocket: classification and treatment. J Periodontol 29:272, 1958.

Hausmann E: Radiographic examination. In: Genco RJ, Goldman HM, Cohen DW, eds. Contemporary Periodontics. St. Louis:CV Mosby, 1990, p. 334.

Hausmann E, et al: Progression of untreated periodontitis as assessed by subtraction radiography. J Periodont Res 6:716, 1986.

Hirschfeld I: Food impaction. J Am Dent Assoc 17:1504, 1930.

Jeffcoat MK: A new method for comparison of bone loss measurement on nonstandardized radiographs. J Periodont Res 19:434, 1984.

Jeffcoat MK, et al: Extraoral control of geometry for digital substraction radiology. J Periodont Res 22:398, 1987.

Kay S, Forseher BK, Sackett LM: Tooth root length-volume relationships: an aid to periodontal prognosis. I. Anterior teeth. Oral Surg 7:735, 1954.

Mason JD, Nicholson K: The distribution of bone defects in chronic periodontitis. J Periodontol 45:88, 1974.

McHenry K, et al: Methodical aspects and quantitative adjuncts to computerized substraction radiology. J Periodontal Res 22:125, 1987.

Nielsen JJ, Glavina L, Karring T: Interproximal periodontal infrabony defects: prevalence, localization and etiological factors. J Clin Periodontol 7:187, 1980.

Pauls V, Trott JR: A radiological study of experimentally produced lesions of bone. Dent Pract 16:254, 1966.

Ramadan A-BE, Mitchell DF: A roentgenographic study of experimental bone destruction. Oral Surg 15:934, 1962.

Webber RL, et al: X-ray image subtraction as the basis for assessment of periodontal changes. J Periodont Res 17:509, 1982.

Suggested Readings

Radiologic Diagnosis of Periodontal Disease

Page RC, et al: Prepubertal periodontitis: I. Definition of a clinical disease entity. J Periodontol 54:257, 1983.

Prepubertal Periodontitis

Lavine WS, et al: Impaired neutrophils chemotaxis in patients with juvenile and rapidly progressing periodontitis. J Periodont Res 14:10, 1979.

Adult Periodontitis

Loe H, et al: Natural history of periodontal disease in man: rapid, moderate and no loss of attachment in Sri Lankan laborers 14 to 46 years of age. J Clin Periodontol 13:431, 1986.

The Role of the Radiograph in Diagnosis of Periodontal Disease

Animo J, Tammisalo EH: Comparison of radiographic and clinical signs of early periodontal disease. Scand J Dent 81:548, 1973.

Baer PN, Benjamin S: Periodontal disease in children and adolescents. Philadelphia:JB Lippincott, 1974.

Barr JH, Stephens RB: Dental Radiology. Philadelphia:WB Saunders, 1980, p. 298.

Bassiouny MA, Grant AA: Radiographic assessment of proximal infrabony pocket topography. J Periodontol 47:440, 1976.

Baumhammers A, Ceravola FJ: An improved diagnostic point to aid in radiographic interpretation. J Periodontol 48:52, 1977.

Bender IB, Seltzer S: Roentgenographic and direct observation of experimental lesions in bone: I. J Am Dent Assoc 62:152, 1961.

Bender IB, Seltzer S: Roentgenographic and direct observation of experimental lesions in bone: II. J Am Dent Assoc 62:708, 1961.

Bjorn H, Holmberg K: Radiographic determination of periodontal bone destruction in epidemiological research. Odontol Revy 17:232, 1966.

Bower RC: Furcation morphology relative to periodontal treatment: furcation entrance architecture. J Periodontol 50:23, 1979.

Brown IS, Owings JR Jr: A reproducible method for evaluating radiographic changes in periodontal defects. J Periodont Res 8:389, 1973.

Butler JH: A familial pattern of juvenile periodontitis (periodontosis). J Periodontol 40:51, 1969.

Easley JR: Methods of determining alveolar osseous form. J Periodontol 38:112, 1967.

Everett FG, Fixott HC: Use of an incorporated grid in the interpretation of dental roentgenograms. Oral Surg 16:1061, 1963.

Grondahl HG, Johnson E, Lindahl B: Diagnosis of marginal bone destruction with orthopantomography and intraoral full mouth radiography. Sven Tandlak Tidskr 64:439, 1971.

Gutmann JL: Prevalence, location, and patency of accessory canals in the furcation region of permanent molars. J Periodontol 419:21, 1978.
Heins PJ, Canter SR: The furca involvement: a classification of deformities. J Periodontol 6:84, 1968.
Hirschfeld L: A calibrated silver point for periodontal diagnosis and recording. J Periodontol 24:94, 1953.
Larato DC: Intrabony defects in the dry human skull. J Periodontol 41:496, 1970.
Larato DC: Furcation involvements: incidence and distribution. J Periodontol 41:4919, 1970.
Larato DC: Some anatomical factors related to furcation involvements. J Periodontol 46:608, 1975.
Mason JD: Bone morphology and bone loss in periodontal disease. J Clin Periodontol 3:14, 1976.
Mason JD, Lehner T: Clinical features of juvenile periodontitis (periodontosis). J Periodontol 45:636, 1974.
Miller SC: Precocious advanced alveolar atrophy. J Periodontol 19:146, 1948.
Newman MG, Sanz M: Oral microbiology with emphasis on etiology. In: Perspectives on Antimicrobial Therapeutics. Littleton, MA, PSG, 1987.
Orban B, Weinmann JP: Diffuse atrophy of the alveolar bone (periodontosis). J Periodontol 13:31, 1952.
Patur B, Glickman I: Roentgenographic evaluation of alveolar bone changes in periodontal disease. Dent Clin North Am 48:47, 1960.

Chapter 9

Circumscribed Radiolucencies

VARIATIONS IN TRABECULAR PATTERNS AND BONE MARROW SPACES

The panoramic radiograph frequently produces variations in trabecular patterns and marrow spaces that are often not reproducible on intraoral films. If some doubt still exists after several radiographs have been taken, the area should undergo biopsy or should be followed by periodic radiographic examination.

◆ *RADIOLOGY (Fig. 9–1)*

These variations may mimic cystlike radiolucent lesions. Some aspect of the area may not seem to fit any particular pattern; a normal variation may be suspected in this situation, especially in the absence of symptoms or clinical findings. These variations are often seen in the mandibular canine-premolar area on panoramic films and may not be duplicated on standard films. The reason for the frequency of this location is the presence of the mandibular fossa in this area. This may produce an area of decreased density with the trabecular pattern in the buccal cortex still apparent. The sclerosis at the margin may represent a tangential effect of the beam along the margin through the depth of the fossa, similar to that seen in salivary gland depressions, but less so because no resorption of the lingual cortex occurs in this instance.

EARLY STAGE TOOTH CRYPTS

If early stage tooth crypts are not recognized, the clinician may perceive the developing tooth bud as a pathologic condition. Early stage tooth crypts may be seen from birth to late adolescence.

◆ *RADIOLOGY (Fig. 9–2)*

The uncalcified crypt usually consists of a bilateral, well-corticated, solitary radiolucency of the approximate diameter of the crown of the developing tooth. In the permanent teeth, especially the premolars, the uncalcified crypt may resemble a small central lesion or radiolucency of pulpal origin, particularly when the radiolucency occurs at the bifurcation of a primary molar. In the permanent molars, the uncalcified crypts are located just under the crest of the ridge and may strongly resemble primordial cysts or large marrow spaces. As the cusp tips begin to calcify, circumflex or inverted V-shaped radiopacities appear.

MEDIAL SIGMOID DEPRESSION

The medial sigmoid depression was first observed on a panoramic radiograph by Steven Bricker and was first reported by Langlais and co-authors in 1983. It consists of an anatomic depression on the medial side of the upper ramus just below and anterior to the greatest depth of the sigmoid notch of the ramus. According to Wood and Goaz (1991), the depression is defined by the temporal crest and the crest of the mandibular neck. In anatomic specimens, the overall incidence was 66%. Among these, about half were described as slight and half as typical. In addition, 55% were bilateral and 45% were unilateral. The incidence on radiographs was lower, at 10%. Of these, 4% were bilateral and 6% were unilateral. The only significance of these depressions is to recognize them as anatomic, an important consideration when the depression is unilateral. The medial sigmoid depression does not require treatment.

◆ *RADIOLOGY (Figs. 9–3 and 9–4)*

The medial sigmoid depression consists of a small round, ovoid, or triangular radiolucency on the medial aspect of the ramus, just below and anterior to the greatest depth of the sigmoid notch. This depression has only been reported on panoramic radiographs, although we have observed it on a periapical radiograph and on some lateral jaw views. The diagnosis is most certain when the depression is bilateral. The radiolucent area is well defined but usually lacks a cortical margin. It is usually less than 5 mm in diameter. Its radiographic appearance is considered pathognomonic. The most important condition to rule out in the differential diagnosis is the parotid salivary gland depression.

SUBMANDIBULAR SALIVARY GLAND DEPRESSION (Developmental lingual mandibular salivary gland depression posterior variant, developmental bone defect of the mandible, lingual mandibular bone concavity or depression, Stafne's cyst, static bone cyst, latent bone cyst)

This first type of salivary gland depression was first recognized by Stafne in 1942, in a report of 35 cases in the posterior mandible. According to Chen and Ohba (1981), some 300 cases had been reported by 1978. In a study of 6300 dried mandibles, Mann and Keenleyside (1992) found an incidence of 115 cases (1.8%), whereas the incidence in radiographs of live patients is 5 to 10 times lower.

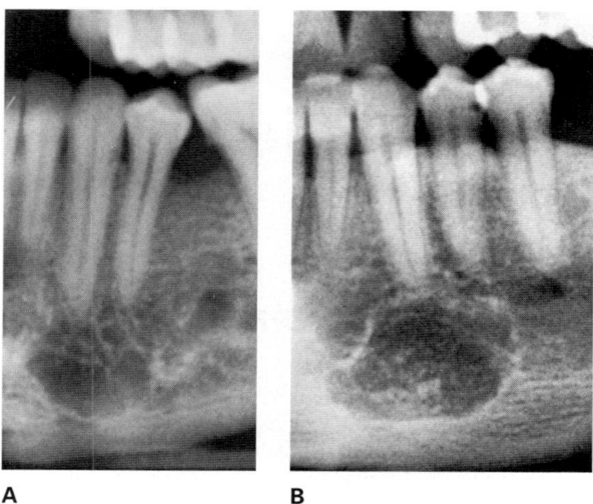

FIGURE 9–1.

Variations in trabecular patterns and marrow spaces: mandibular canine area. A, Sclerotic margin is partially absent. B, A distinct sclerotic rim is present.

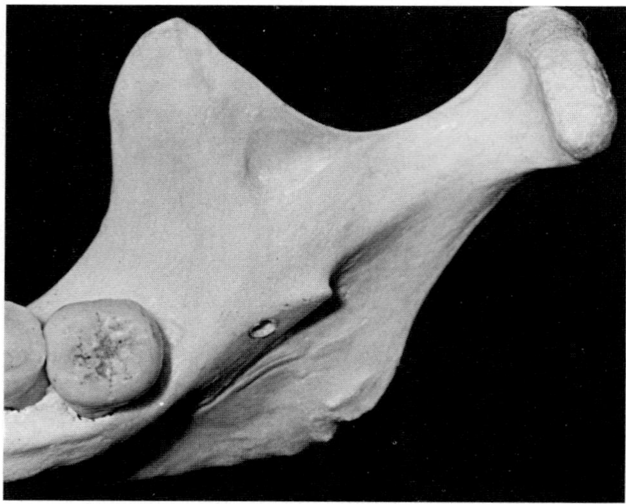

FIGURE 9–3.

Medial sigmoid depression. Gross appearance on a dried mandible.

Pathologic Characteristics

Most authors believe that these depressions develop to accommodate submandibular salivary gland tissue that lies in close proximity to the lingual side of the mandible. These depressions are considered developmental rather than congenital. In 1960, Seward demonstrated an intimate relationship between a submandibular gland lobule and a salivary gland depression by using sialography. In 1976, Langlais and co-workers studied 469 dried mandibles and found that earlier, smaller lesions consisted of shallow areas of cortical erosion, whereas larger lesions were deeper, having penetrated the cortex into the medullary space. Deeper lesions had well-defined walls, whereas the base was usually roughened, suggesting a resorptive process. Although most investigators believe that the depressions usually contain salivary gland tissue, Lello and Makek (1985) have reviewed other theories. According to Chen and Ohba (1981), who reviewed 74 cases that had been surgically explored, the reported contents consisted of salivary gland tissue in most cases. Other tissues found in these depressions included fat, lymphatic tissue, and muscle; rarely, pleomorphic adenoma and hemolymphangioma were reported, and in 8 cases, an empty cavity was found.

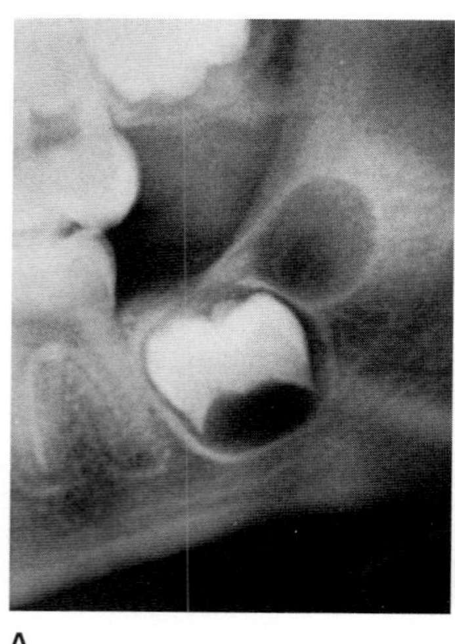

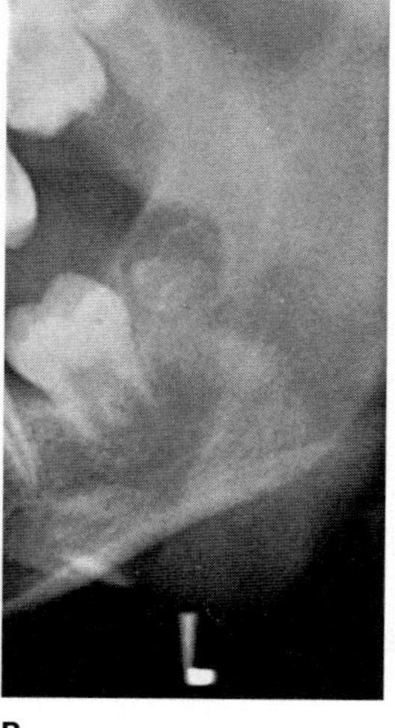

FIGURE 9–2.

Early stage tooth crypts. A, Entirely radiolucent. B, Radiolucent with circumflex radiopacities.

Clinical Features

In a review of 23,000 panoramic radiographs, Chen and Ohba (1981) found an incidence of 0.1%. Other reported incidences vary from 0.1 to 0.4%, as reported by Johnson (1970) in a series of 2486 older patients who were military veterans. In a series of 7 studies reviewed by Chen and Ohba (1981), 54,736 patients had an average incidence of 0.23%. Higher incidences of 0.9% ,1.3%, and 1.8% have been reported by Harvey and Noble (1968), by Langlais and co-workers (1976), and by Mann and Keenleyside (1992), respectively, who made their observations on dried mandibles. We believe that only 10 to 50% of all defects in patients are sufficiently advanced to be detectable at the time of the radiologic examination. Most cases occur in men in the fourth or fifth decade of life. Mann and Keenleyside (1992) noted 11 of 115 cases in female specimens (9.5%). Hansson (1980) reported a case of mandibular salivary gland depression developing in an 11-year-old boy (see Fig. 9–8).

Treatment/Prognosis

Submandibular salivary gland depressions are not usually treated. In most studies, including a case reported by Wolf and colleagues (1986), a 5- to 8-year period occurs between the time the defect is first seen and the time when it achieves its mature presentation. Thereafter, the depressions tend to remain more stable.

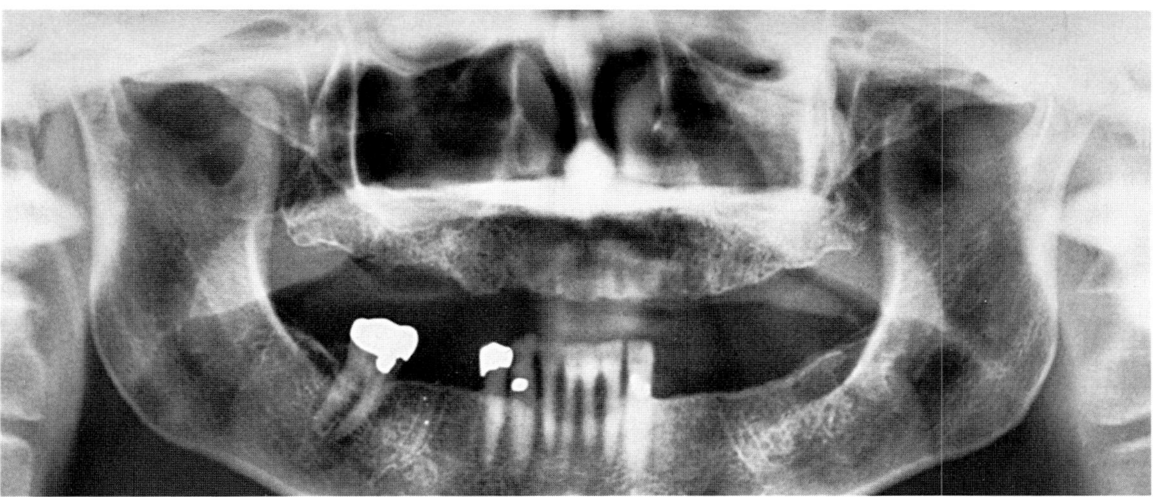

FIGURE 9–4.

Medial sigmoid depression. This depression is bilateral in the coronoid process areas.

◆ *RADIOLOGY (Figs. 9–5 to 9–12)*

Location

The submandibular salivary gland depression occurs mainly in the second molar-angle region. A significant diagnostic feature is that all depressions lie between the inferior alveolar canal and the lower cortical margin of the mandible and may encroach on either of these structures. The submandibular salivary gland depression rarely occurs bilaterally. Gorab and co-workers (1986) reported a rare case of two separate and distinct depressions on the same side of the mandible. D'Eramo and Poidmore (1986) also reported a case of several depressions occurring unilaterally. Chen and Ohba (1981) analyzed 135 cases with regard to location. The depressions were below the inferior alveolar canal in 27%, contacting the inferior margin of the canal only in 35%, overlapping the inferior wall of the canal in 28%, overlapping the inferior and superior walls of the canal in 7%, and associated with displacement or deviation of the canal in 4%. With respect to the inferior border of the mandible, 17% were above the cortex, 30% were in contact with the superior margin of the cortex, 41% partially obliterated the cortical plate, and 11% produced saucerization of the entire thickness of the cortex. Because most studies use panoramic radiographs, it must be remembered that lingual objects are projected upward, so some lesions may appear higher than they really are. For this reason, the observations of Chen and Ohba (1981) are important, because the observation of resorption of the cortex of the inferior alveolar canal and the inferior cortex of the mandible does not depend on projection geometry.

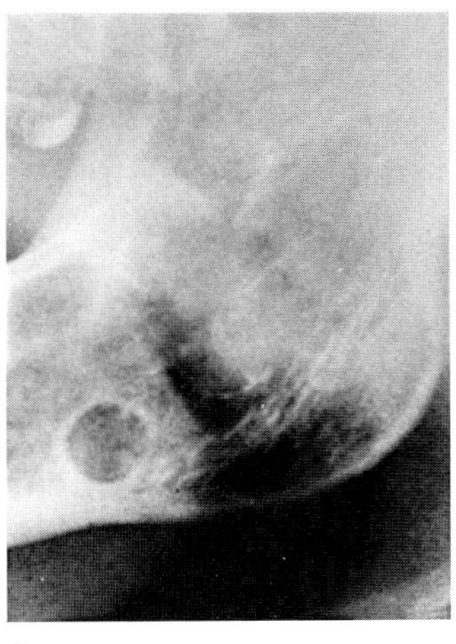

A

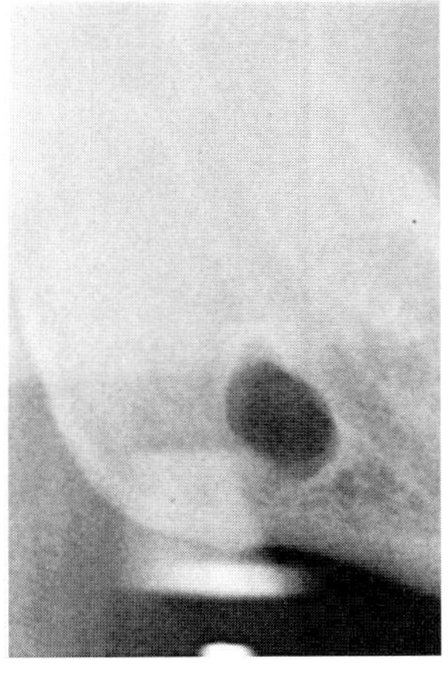

B

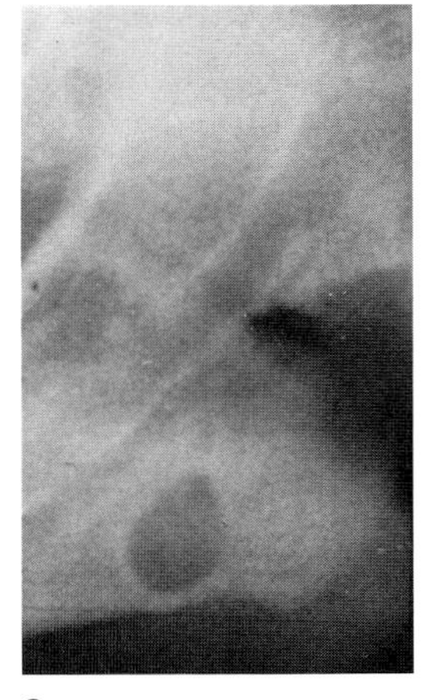

C

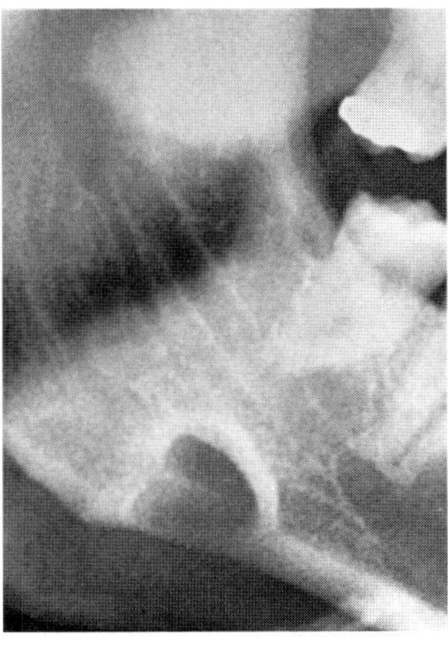

D

FIGURE 9–5.

Submandibular salivary gland depression: various shapes. A, Round; B, ovoid; C, triangular; D, heart-shaped. (A, Courtesy of Dr. B. Pass, Dalhousie University, Halifax, Nova Scotia, Canada; D, Courtesy of Dr. B.Scarfe, Louisville University, Louisville, KY.)

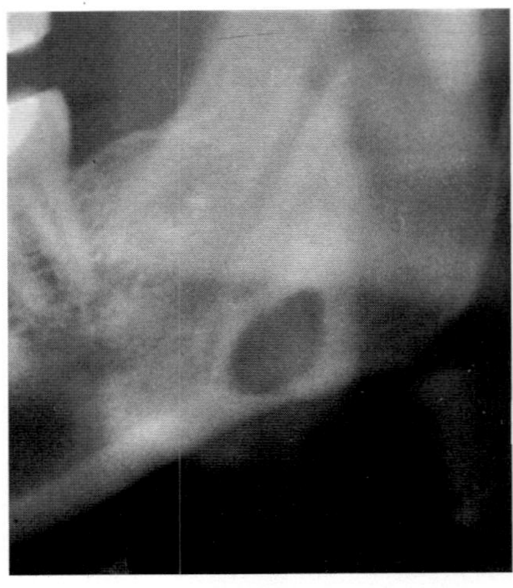

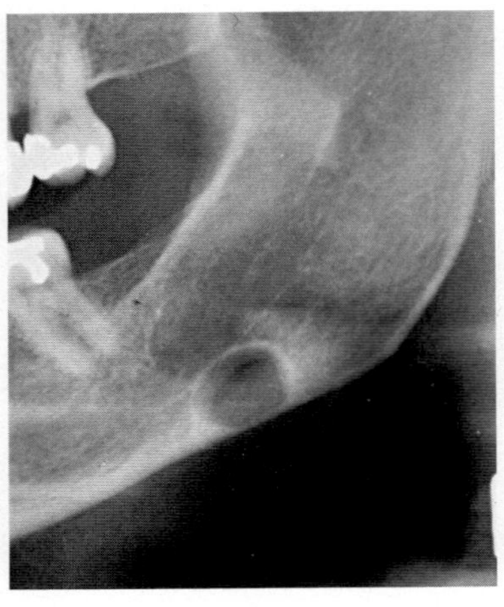

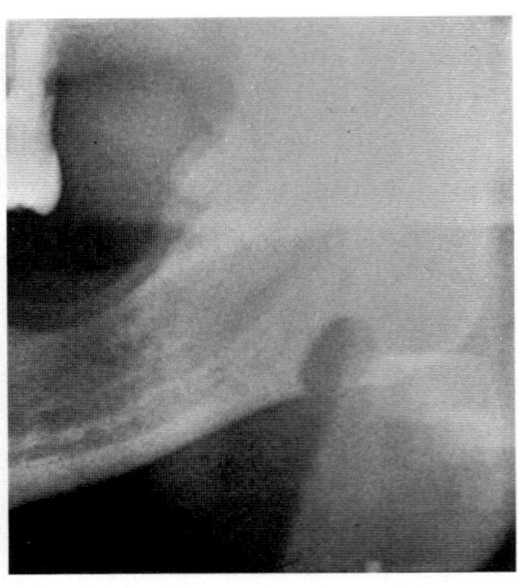

A B C

FIGURE 9–6.

Submandibular salivary gland depression: relation to the inferior cortex of the mandible. A, Partially eroded; B, almost completely eroded; C saucerization. (A, Courtesy of Dr. J. Preece, University of Texas Health Science Center at San Antonio, San Antonio, TX.)

Specific Radiologic Features

The depressions appear radiolucent and may or may not contain trabeculae from the adjacent thinned lingual cortex and normal buccal cortex. In the series of 24 cases analyzed by Chen and Ohba (1981), only 2 lesions measured less than 1 cm in diameter (7 and 9 mm), and most were in the range of 1.0 to 1.7 cm in diameter. The height ranged from about 0.5 to 1.2 cm. The largest lesion was 3.5 × 2.0 cm. The shape is usually ovoid, sometimes round, and rarely triangular. The margin may appear punched out with no evidence of cortication, or a part of the margin may appear corticated especially at the anterior and superior portions, or the margin may be entirely corticated. In all instances, Uemura and colleagues (1976) observed that the corticated margin is much thicker and denser than that produced by epithelium-lined cysts. These investigators also noted that, in posteroanterior views, the laterally located margins appear thick and sclerotic, whereas the medially placed margins are more obscure. On occlusal views, Uemura and co-workers (1976) observed a half-ovoid sclerotic border with the convexity toward the buccal side and an opening on the lingual side of the lingual cortex.

Sialography

Reports involving correlations with sialography either confirm the findings of Seward or show no relationship whatsoever. However, extension of the mandible during the radiographic procedure could pull the salivary gland lobule away from the defect, thus giving the impression that no relationship exists. In the stereosialographic study of seven cases, Oikarinen and colleagues (1974) found a proximity of salivary gland tissue to the defect in six of seven cases.

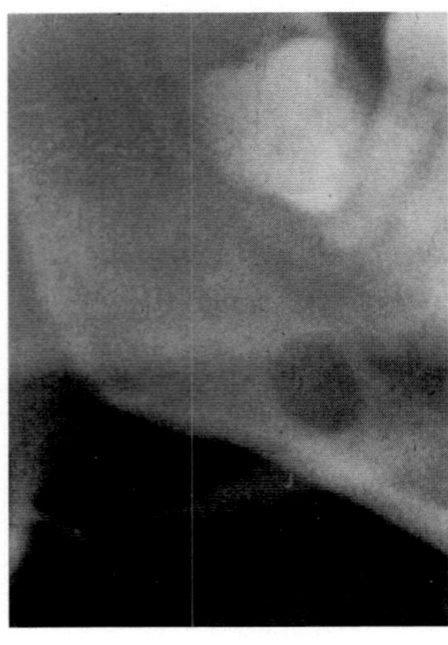

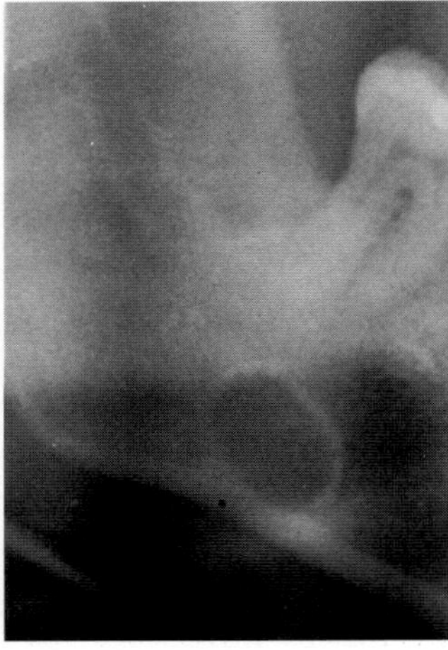

A B

FIGURE 9–7.

Submandibular salivary gland depression: enlargement over 3 years. A, At age 54; B, at age 57. (Courtesy of Drs. F. Sammis and C. Portales, San Antonio, TX.)

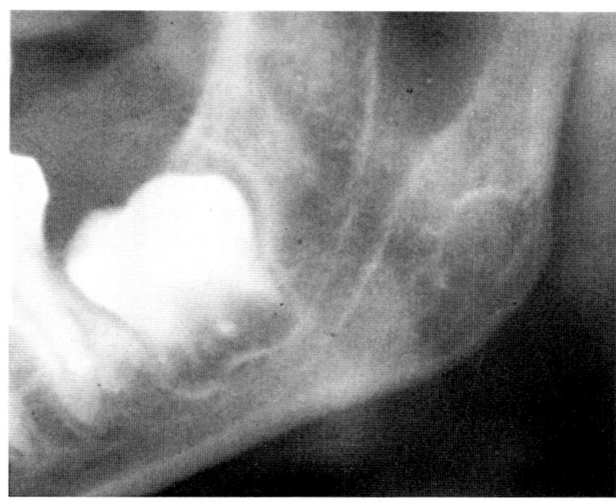

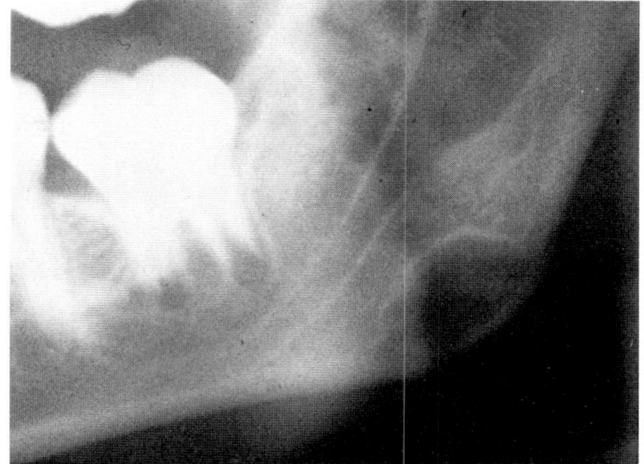

A B

FIGURE 9–8.

Submandibular salivary gland depression in a child. A, At age 11; B, at age 12½. At age 14, a typical salivary gland depression had developed. (From Hansson LG: Development of a lingual mandibular bone cavity in an 11-year-old boy. J Oral Surg 49:376, 1980.)

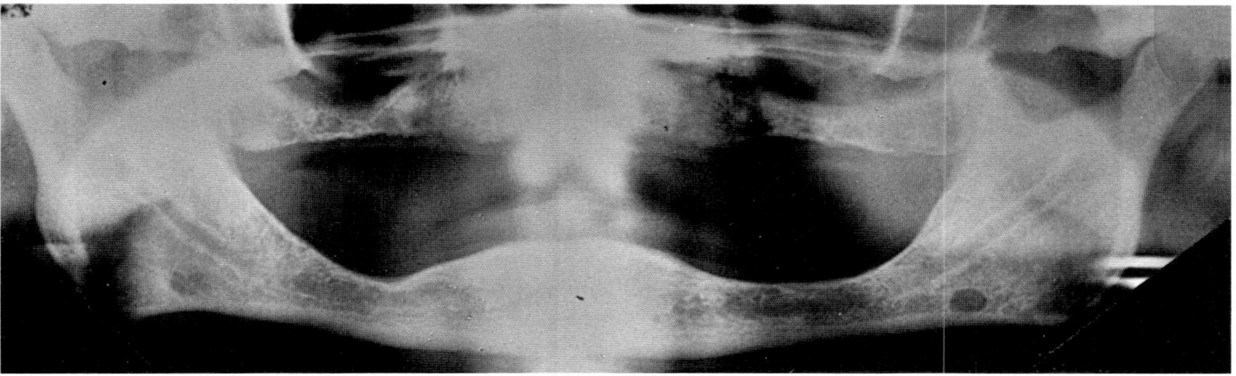

FIGURE 9–9.

Submandibular salivary gland depression: bilateral.

FIGURE 9–10.

Submandibular salivary gland depression: double lesions. A, Panoramic radiograph. B, Tomogram of the same lesion demonstrating lingual location. (Courtesy of Dr. S. Prapanpoch, Bangkok, Thailand.)

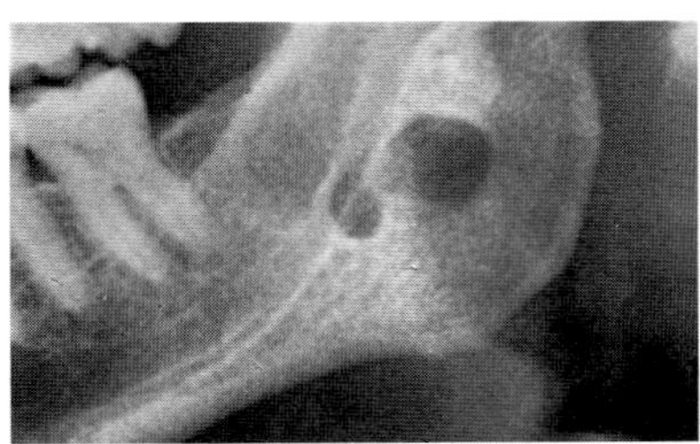

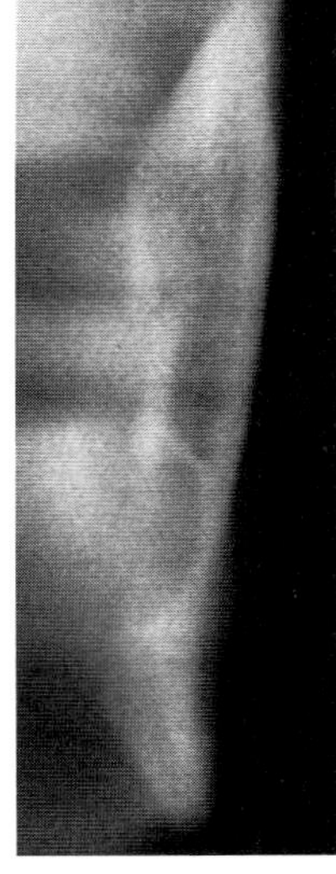

A B

SUBLINGUAL SALIVARY GLAND DEPRESSION (Developmental lingual mandibular salivary gland depression, anterior variant)

These salivary gland depressions were first reported by Richard and Ziskind in 1957. Sublingual salivary gland depressions are much less common than submandibular salivary gland depressions. According to Strom and Fjellstrom, 12 cases had been reported by 1987.

Pathologic Characteristics

Anterior salivary gland depressions may develop to accommodate sublingual salivary gland tissue that lies in close proximity to the lingual cortex of the mandible in the canine region. In 1963, Gaughran demonstrated nodules of sublingual salivary gland tissue extending through slits in the mylohyoid muscle. He termed these nodules ''boutons'' or buttons and the slits ''boutonnières'' or buttonholes. The study

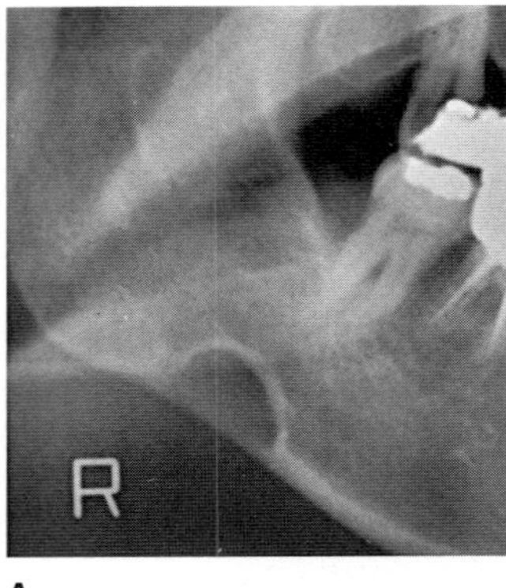

A

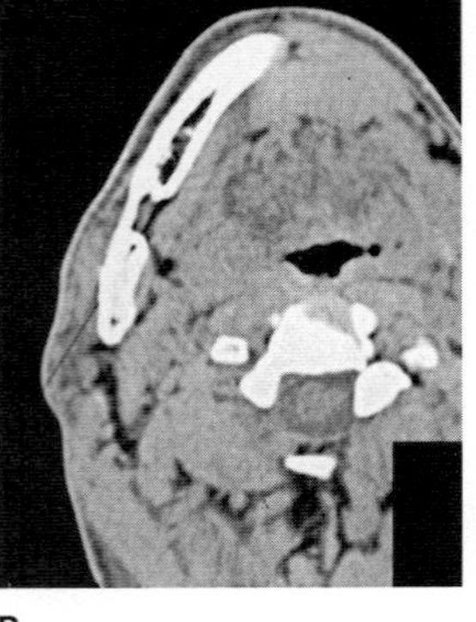

B

FIGURE 9–11.

Submandibular salivary gland depression. A, Panoramic radiograph. B, Axial computed tomographic image of the same lesion. (Courtesy of Drs. M. Araki and K. Hashimoto, Nihon University School of Dentistry, Tokyo, Japan.)

consisted of 324 cadaver half-heads from 162 individuals. Among this number, 36% were found to have distinct masses of tissue resting on the inferior surface of the mylohyoid muscle. These buttons were usually located in the anterior one half or two thirds of the anteroposterior extent of the mylohyoid muscle nestled in the cleft between the muscle and the body of the mandible. Gaughran (1963) found that most of these buttons consisted of inframylohyoid processes of the sublingual gland, although about 5% consisted exclusively of fat herniations and 1% consisted of fascia only without extensions of salivary gland or fat. These boutons were located on the left side in 38%, the right side in 43%, and bilaterally in 19% of the cases. In 1985, Nathan and Luchansky studied 150 cadavers and found an incidence of mylohyoid boutonnières of 42%. Among these, 73% were unilateral and 27% were bilateral. The herniated tissue in most cases consisted of sublingual salivary gland tissue and in few cases consisted of fatty tissue covered by mylohyoid fascia. In the same report, 12 clinical cases of sublingual salivary gland depression underwent biopsy, and 9 contained sublingual salivary gland tissue, 1 had submaxillary salivary gland tissue, 1 was fibrous connective tissue, and in 1 case

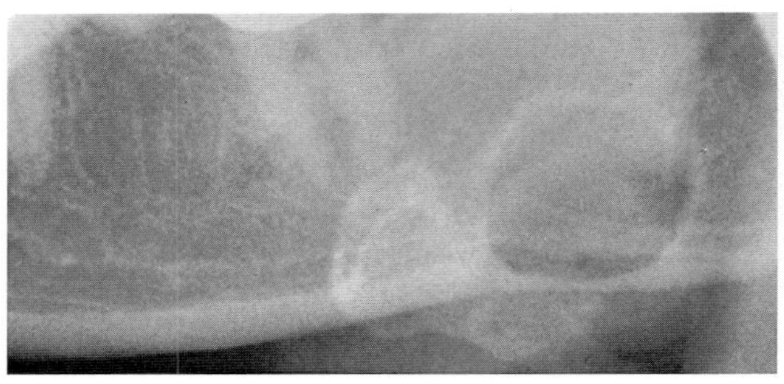

A

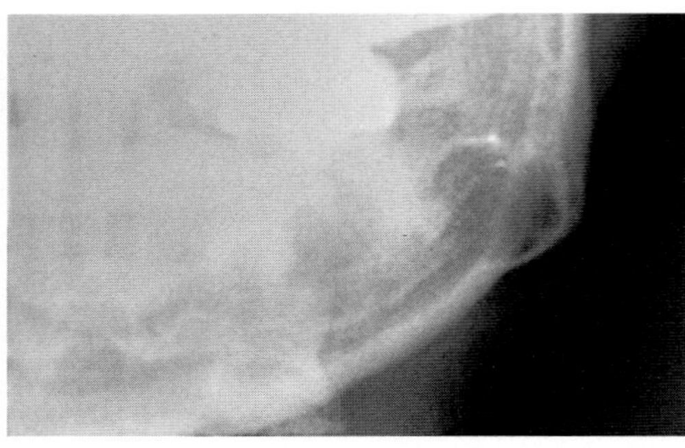

B

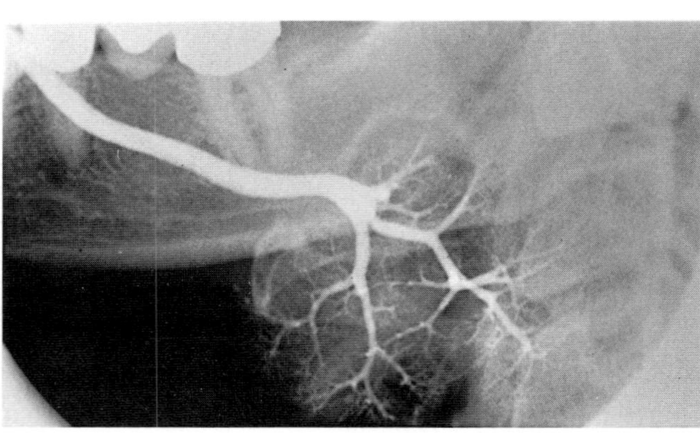

C

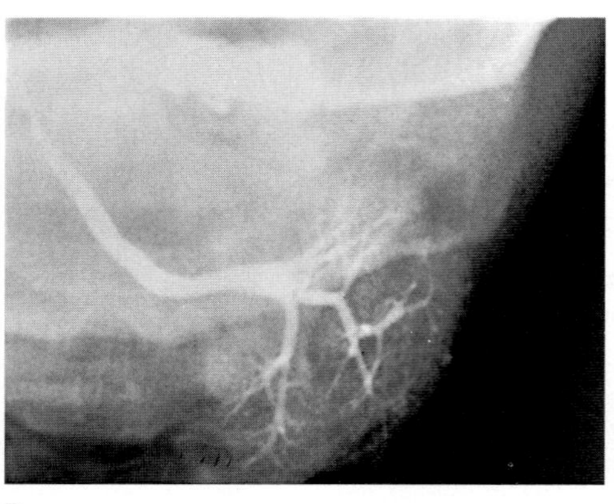

D

FIGURE 9–12.

Submandibular salivary gland depression. A and B, Lateral and anteroposterior views. C and D, Sialogram indicates filling of the defect. (Courtesy of Dr. T. Razmus, West Virginia University, Morgantown, WV.)

nothing was found. The exact nature of the bone defect is still in question. In his report of a classic-appearing sublingual salivary gland depression, Connor observed that the cortical plate in the bone concavity was intact at surgery. Miller and Winnick (1971), however, found a defect in the cortical bone at surgery, and Strom and Fjellstrom (1987) found that the lingual cortex was absent on blunt dissection. Hayashi and colleagues (1984) found a similar defect in the lingual cortex.

Clinical Features

In the series reviewed by Hayashi and co-authors (1984), the average age was 43 years, and the range was from 20 to 56 years. Among the 12 reported cases, 66% occurred in men. The condition is asymptomatic and is discovered when radiographs are taken for other purposes.

Treatment/Prognosis

Although radiographs are sometimes highly suggestive of the diagnosis, the radiologic appearance of the sublingual salivary gland depression appears to be more variable than that of the submaxillary salivary gland depression. Therefore, in the opinion of the present authors, surgical exploration may be required to establish the diagnosis. We are unaware whether the bone returns to a normal appearance after removal of the herniated tissue.

◆ *RADIOLOGY (Figs. 9–13 and 9–14)*

The most important features that suggest the diagnosis are an association with a vital anterior mandibular tooth and the location, often a canine, sometimes the incisors, and rarely the second premolar. The lesions average about 1.2 cm in diameter. Within the radiolucent area, trabeculations from the intact buccal cortex and variable portions of the lingual cortex can be seen. In intraoral radiographs, trabeculations represent cortical structure and are not trabeculations within the medullary cavity. A feature that helps to suggest the diagnosis, when present, is the tendency of this lesion to involve the apical region of an adjacent tooth and to extend upward onto the apical third of the root. Another diagnostic feature, when present, is cortication of the margin, up to 3 mm in thickness. In other instances, the lesion appears punched out, without evidence of cortication at the margin. A bilateral case has not yet been reported. We are not aware of a successful sialogram being performed to confirm the diagnosis.

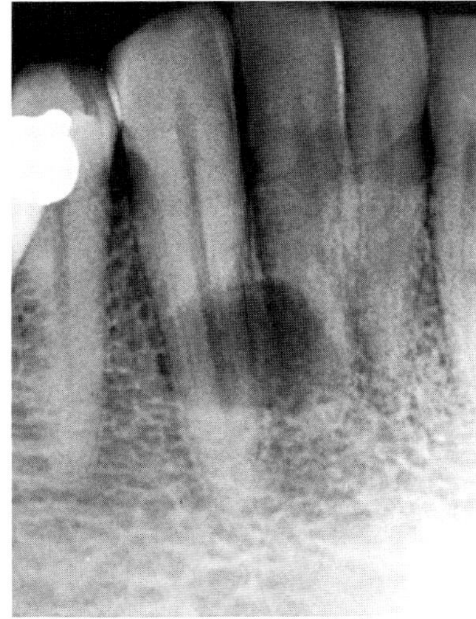

FIGURE 9–13.

Sublingual salivary gland depression: typical location without a sclerotic margin.

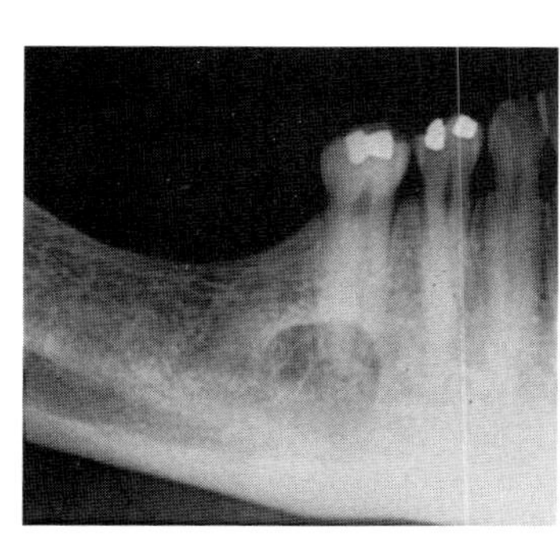

A

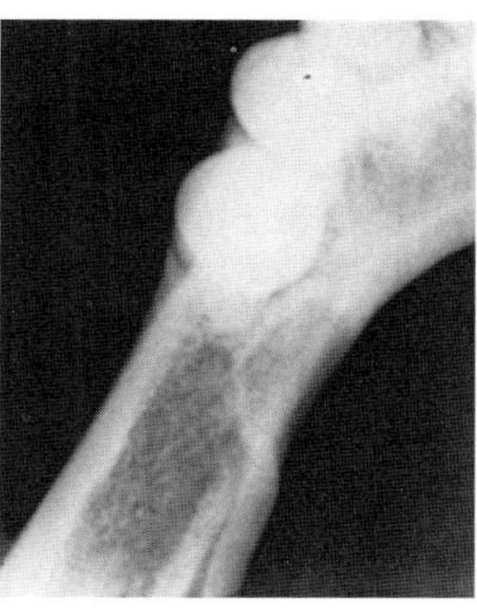

B

FIGURE 9–14.

Sublingual salivary gland depression. A and B, A more posterior location. (Courtesy of Dr. D. Barnett, University of Oregon Health Sciences Center, Portland, OR.)

PAROTID SALIVARY GLAND DEPRESSION (Developmental parotid salivary gland depression)

The parotid salivary gland depression was first recognized by Wolf in 1985, in a report of 5 cases occurring in Finnish men. Retrospectively, a report of ectopically placed parotid gland tissue in the mandible was reported by Slavin in 1950, although his case differs from those of Wolf. Since Wolf's original report, one further case has been reported by Barker (1988), and an anatomic study by Mann and Keenleyside (1992) has demonstrated the defect on the lingual side of the upper posterior ramus in 2 dried specimens. Among 6300 human mandibles studied, Mann and Keenleyside (1992) found an incidence of 2 cases; the incidence was similar to that of the sublingual salivary gland depression, of which 3 cases were noted by them. By comparison, these same authors noted an incidence of 115 submandibular salivary gland depressions. Since studying these reports, we have collected a further 6 cases.

Pathologic Features

As yet, no case has been vivisected, nor has any anatomic study been presented confirming the presence of parotid salivary gland tissue. To date, evidence for the theory is as follows: (1) the lesions bear a strong resemblance to submandibular and sublingual salivary gland depressions radiologically; (2) stereoradiography and anatomic studies on dried mandibles have shown that the defects are on the lingual side of the ramus; (3) studies of dried specimens indicate the depressions resemble those reported in the submandibular gland; (4) Barker (1988) has shown sialographic evidence suggesting a possible association with the parotid gland. We believe that these depressions are caused by the deep lobe of the parotid gland.

Other ectopically placed parotid gland depressions are possible. In 1950, Slavin reported on a case in the upper body of the mandible just distal to the second molar. The lesion resembled a small dentigerous cyst associated with an impacted third molar; however, at surgery the radiolucent area proved to be unrelated to the third molar and was a depression on the lingual aspect of the mandible, above the level of the inferior alveolar canal in the third molar region. The depression contained extremely adherent material that was histologically proved to consist of normal parotid gland.

Clinical Features

The six reported cases of parotid salivary gland depression are all in men. The ages range from 36 to 60 years, and the average is 48 years. All cases have been asymptomatic and were discovered on routine radiographic examination. The two cases found on dried specimens were also from male mandibles, within a similar age range.

Treatment/Prognosis

To date, none of the six patients have been treated. All cases have been followed for a minimum of 1 year up to over 6 years, and none of the depressions have been reported to have changed.

◆ *RADIOLOGY (Figs. 9–15 to 9–17)*

All six reported clinical cases and the two cases from dried specimens have occurred within precise anatomic boundaries. All are located on the medial aspect of the upper ramus. They are level with or above the mandibular foramen and may extend superiorly to the base of the condylar neck. Additionally, many of the defects are aligned along the posterior margin of the ramus in a manner identical to that of submandibular salivary gland depressions in relation to the inferior cortex. The depressions are round when small and are oval when larger. The most common shape has been ovoid. In one case, the posterior margin of the cortex of the ramus was resorbed, creating a saucerization of the cortex similar to those seen in submandibular defects. In five of the six reported cases, the margins were smooth, with a relatively thick margin of sclerotic bone and an appearance similar to that of submandibular salivary gland depression. In one instance, the lesion appeared punched out, with no sclerotic margin. The size ranged from 0.5 × 0.5 cm to 1.5 × 0.7 cm. The average size was 1.0 × 0.5 cm.

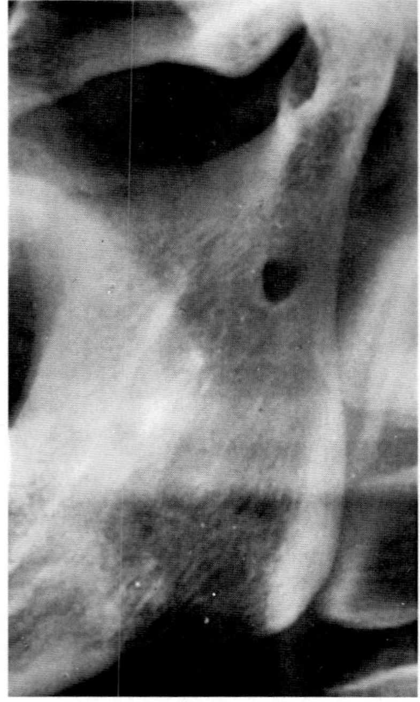
A

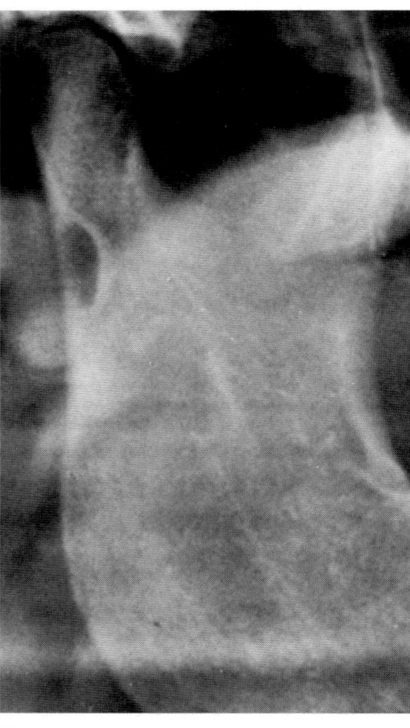
B

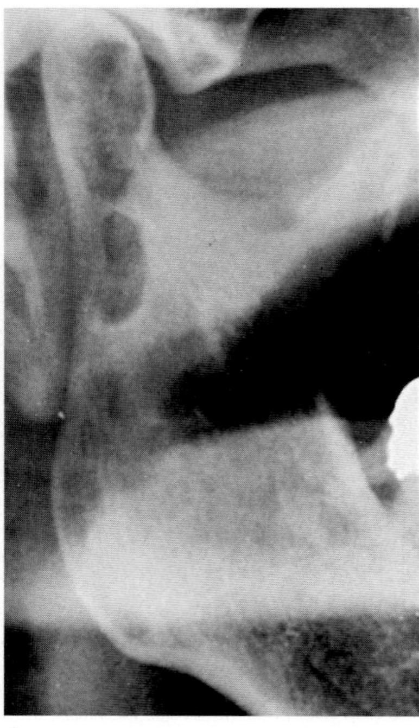
C

FIGURE 9–15.

Parotid salivary gland depression. A, B, and C, Varying presentations as originally described by Wolf. (From Wolf J: Bone defects in mandibular ramus resembling developmental bone cavity. Proc Finn Dent Soc 81:215, 1985.)

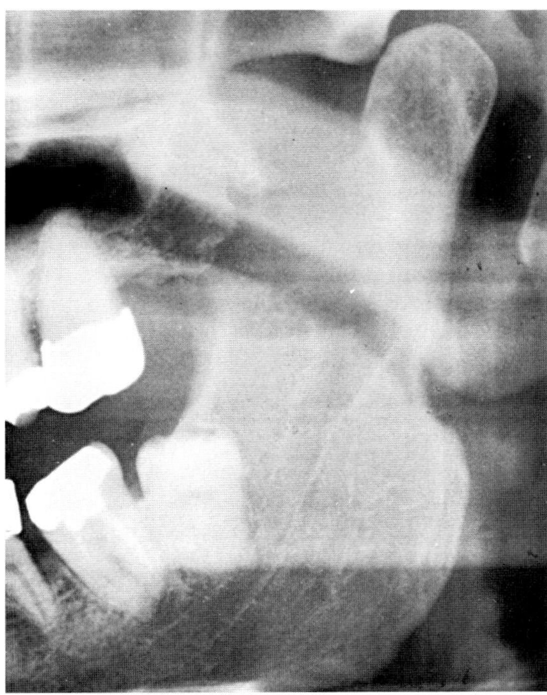

A

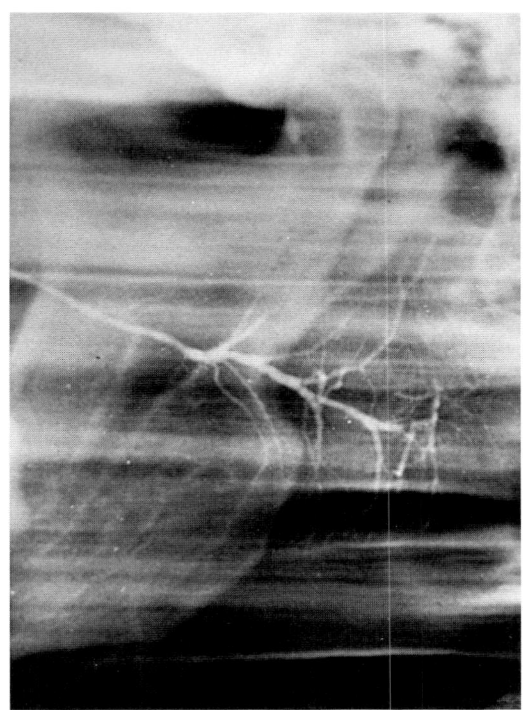

B

FIGURE 9–16.

Parotid salivary gland depression. A, Wolf's fifth original case. B, Wolf's sialogram of the same case. (From Wolf J: Bone defects in mandibular ramus resembling developmental bone cavity. Proc Finn Dent Soc 81:215, 1985.)

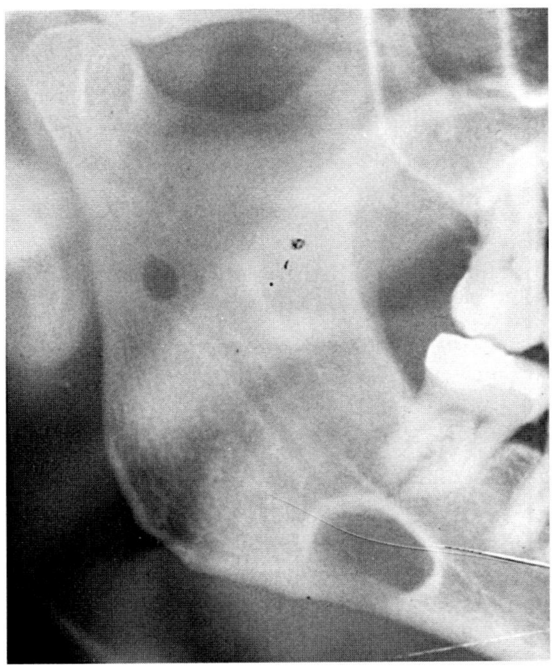

FIGURE 9–17.

Parotid and submandibular salivary gland depressions. Unusual simultaneous occurrence of both defects.

POSTEXTRACTION SOCKET

Generally, postextraction sockets are easily recognized. They are usually apparent on the radiograph for 6 to 12 months, after which they become indistinguishable from the surrounding alveolar bone.

◆ *RADIOLOGY (Fig. 9–18)*

As the socket heals, the cortical outline of the roots disappears first. The area fills with bone trabeculae and marrow spaces and becomes indistinguishable from the surrounding bone.

HEMATOPOIETIC BONE MARROW DEFECT (Focal osteoporotic bone marrow defect of the jaws)

The hematopoietic bone marrow defect was first reported by Standish and Shafer in 1962. Crawford and Weathers (1970) pointed out that hematopoietic bone marrow is present in all bones in childhood and is gradually replaced by fatty marrow in adulthood. The sternum, ribs, vertebrae, proximal ends of the humerus and femur, ileum, and diploe of the skull are the main locations of hematopoietic bone marrow in adults. Standish and Shafer (1962) further stated

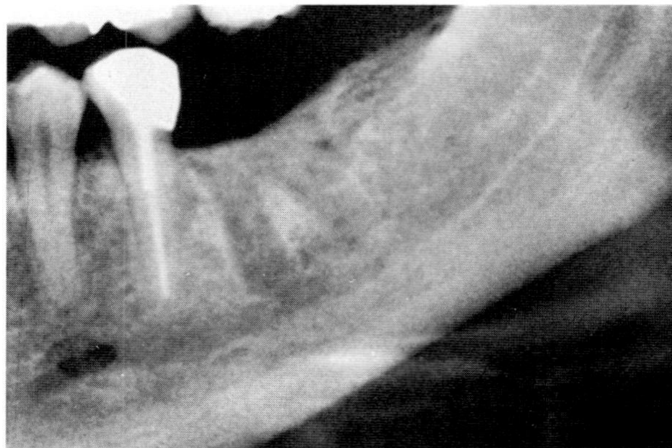

FIGURE 9–18.

Extraction socket: recent with some healing. Note the absent areas of lamina dura and the more opacified appearance of socket areas because of the presence of distinct trabeculae.

that hematopoietic bone marrow occurs in the angle of the mandible and in the maxillary tuberosity. Fatty marrow may be replaced by red marrow when the demand for blood cell formation increases. Histologically, the defect contains normal red marrow, fatty marrow, or both, with a few elongated, thin trabeculae of bone scattered throughout the lesion. The focal osteoporotic bone marrow defect is much more common in females. Standish and Shafer (1962) reported a ratio of 15:3 females over males (83%), whereas Crawford and Weathers (1970) found a ratio of 12:5 (71%). The average age is about 42 years, with cases reported from 20 to 79 years. Because this lesion has no pathognomonic features, biopsy is recommended. Resolution may occur following biopsy. Standish and Shafer (1962) stated that these lesions are almost always asymptomatic and only discovered on routine roentgenologic examination.

◆ *RADIOLOGY (Fig. 9–19)*

The mandibular molar region is the most common site. In the series of Standish and Shafer (1962), 89% occurred in this location, whereas Crawford and Weathers (1970) found this to be the favored location in 71% of their cases. They also noted that 23% of the lesions occurred in the maxillary tuberosity. The mandibular premolar area may also be affected, and the lesion is usually in an edentulous area or at the site of previous surgery or injury. Barker and associates (1974) found that some lesions occurred bilaterally. In some instances, all teeth are present. The lesion is rarely larger than 1.5 cm in diameter. The appearance of the periphery of the defect is greatly variable, although a thin, slightly wavy sclerotic line is usually present at some part of the margin. At times, the lesion is ill defined, with margins that are difficult to identify. In other cases, focal areas of thicker sclerotic bone may be seen at the margin. Most authors report faint, elongated, bony trabeculae or flecks of radiopaque material within the lesions. Rarely, one sees a small mass of condensed bone within the lesion. Once the lesion is present, it is our impression that the defect does not increase or decrease in size over time.

FIBROUS HEALING DEFECT (Surgical defect, apical scar, fibrous union)

These defects consist of small cavities within the jaws that are filled with fibrous connective tissue. The mechanism by which they occur is not fully understood. They are found under one of two circumstances, both of which involve surgical manipulation of the tissue. First is destruction of the buccal and lingual cortical plates with the accompanying periosteum. In this circumstance, there is a loss of the periosteal supply of fibroblasts with osteoblastic potential. Prior apicoectomy, inflammation, large lesion size, difficult tooth extraction, or injury may contribute to this functional failure

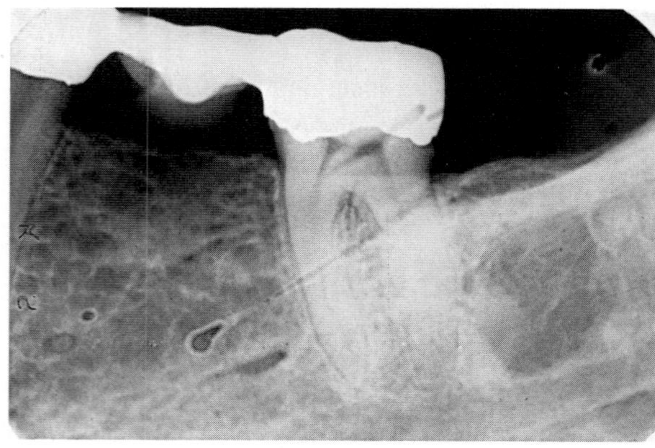

A

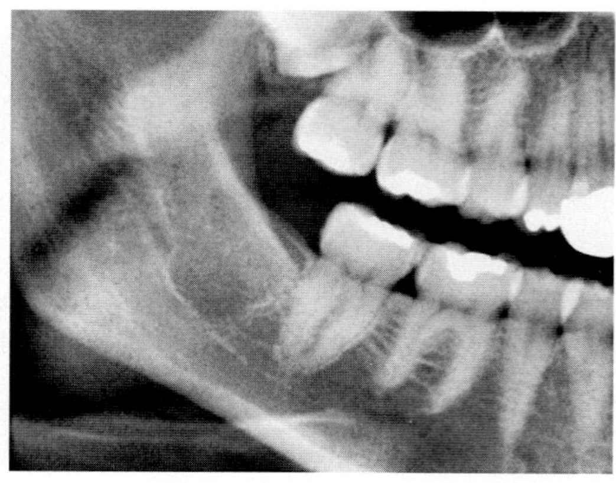

B

FIGURE 9–19.

Hematopoietic bone marrow defect. A, Thin, wavy sclerotic margin; a few faint and some elongated trabeculae are seen within the lesion. B, Thin sclerotic line at margin and tiny flecks of bone within. (A, Courtesy of Dr. G. Kaugars, Medical College of Virginia School of Dentistry, Richmond, VA.)

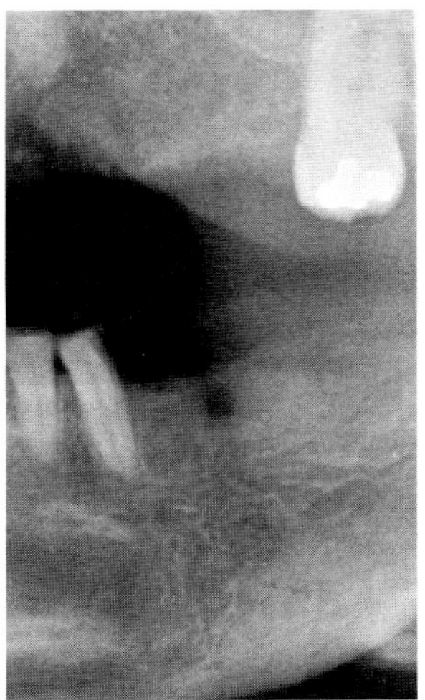

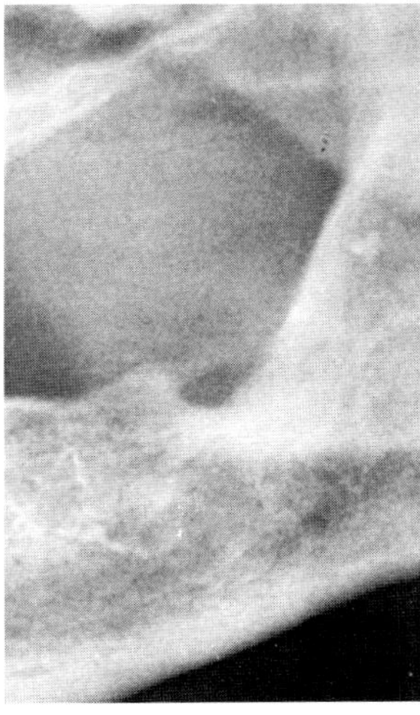

A B

FIGURE 9–20.

Fibrous healing defect. A and B, Small mandibular lesions.

of the periosteum. Second is a lack of fixation of the bony margins at the sites of fracture or along orthognathic surgical margins. In this instance, fibrous union occurs between the bony fragments. The reason for nonossification is not clear; however, insufficient immobilization promotes nonossification. These defects are almost invariably asymptomatic and are found when the jaws are radiographed for other reasons. We found no report about sex or age predilection, although most lesions are seen in adults.

◆ *RADIOLOGY (Figs. 9–20 to 9–25)*

Fibrous healing defects occur at the sites of previous injury. The size of fibrous defects tends to remain static over time. Most defects resulting from apicoectomy or difficult extraction are rarely larger than 5 mm in diameter, although defects may be up to several centimeters in diameter when large lesions or severe injuries have occurred. In edentulous regions, a fibrous defect may disappear in time because of resorption of the adjacent alveolar bone. During this process, the crest of the ridge may appear saucerized or indented in the area of the lesion.

Our impression is that postextraction fibrous healing defects occur most frequently in the maxillary premolar and anterior regions, although they may be found anywhere in the jaws. They are usually densely radiolucent with no evidence of trabeculation within the lesion, and they have a punched out appearance with a well-defined margin. The margin is most often nonsclerotic; however, some defects have a thick condensation of bone completely surrounding the area, whereas others are cystlike in appearance, with a thin, sclerotic margin. The defects are often circular or ovoid. Postfracture or fibrous healing defects occurring at surgical margins appear as longitudinal radiolucent bands at those sites. In some instances, these radiolucent bands may be interrupted by focal areas of osseous union or bridging.

A unique variant of fibrous healing defect may occur at the apices of endodontically treated teeth without apicoectomy. A radiolucency remains at the apex of the treated tooth and greatly resembles a persistence of the original pathologic process. In this instance, the fibrous healing defect is usually less than 1 or 2 mm in diameter, does not tend to enlarge or diminish in size over time, and may be surrounded by an area of condensed bone.

Fibrous healing defects may also be accompanied by focal areas of osseous healing defects. These areas are similar in appearance to idiopathic osteosclerosis, except these lesions are seen in association with previous known injury or surgery. At times, osseous healing defects occur without an adjacent area of fibrous healing. In this circumstance, the diagnosis may not be obvious without an adequate history.

MYOSPHERULOSIS (Paraffinoma)

This lesion was first reported in 1969 by McClatchie and colleagues, who coined the term myospherulosis. They reported on 7 African patients with soft tissue swellings of

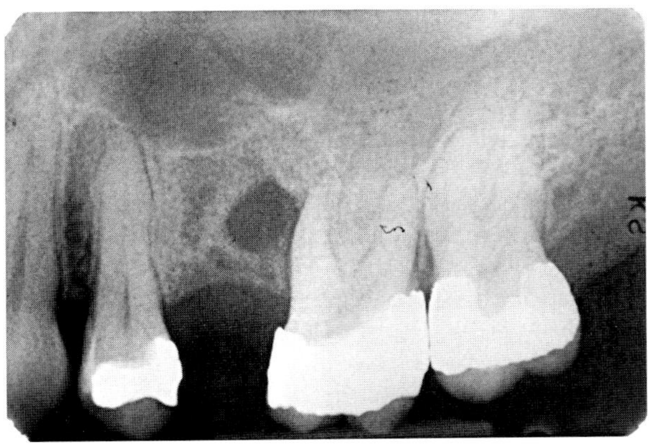

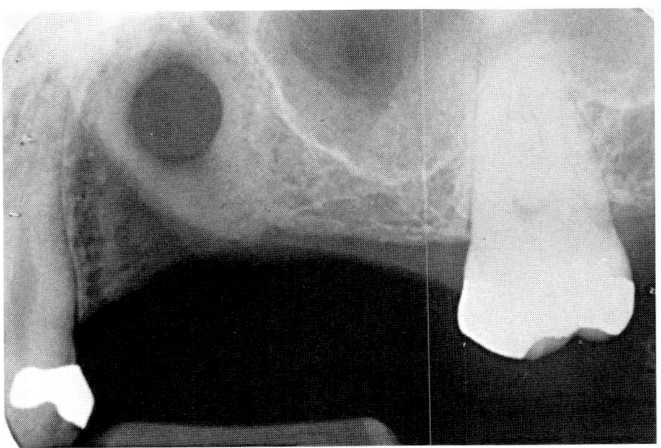

A B

FIGURE 9–21.

Fibrous healing defect. A and B, Maxillary lesions.

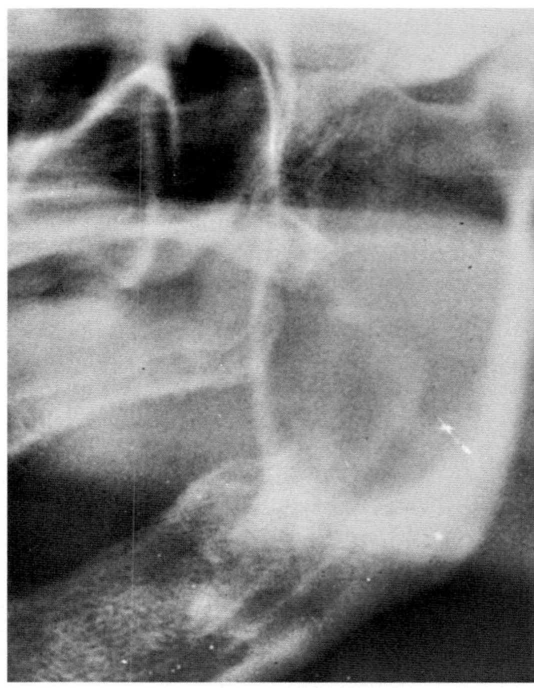

A

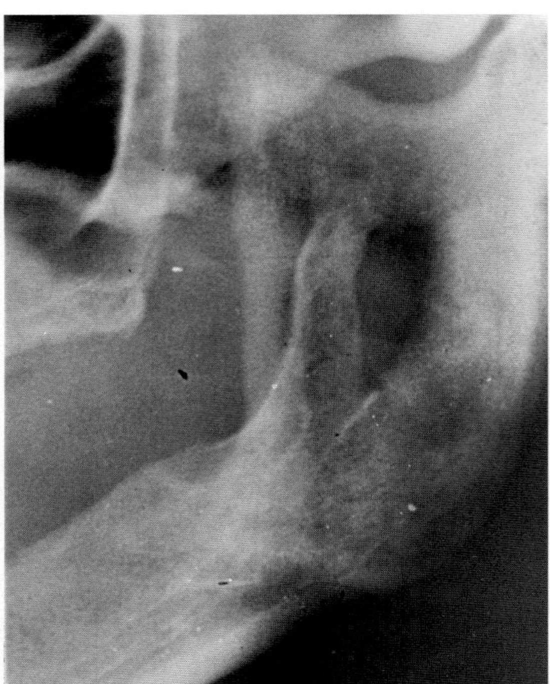

B

FIGURE 9–22.

Fibrous healing defect after removal of a primordial cyst. A, Preoperatively; B, 5 years postoperatively. (Courtesy of Drs. F. Sammis and C. Portales, San Antonio, TX.)

the arms, legs, gluteal region, and scapula. The first case occurring in the jaws was reported by Dunlap and Barker in 1980. Several cases have since been reported by Belfiglio and colleagues (1986) and by Lynch and co-authors (1984), who reviewed the literature and found 52 cases in all jaw locations including 6 cases of their own. These investigators stated that myospherulosis is an inflammatory granulomatous lesion resulting from the action of lipid substances on extravasated erythrocytes. Most lesions result from the use of petrolatum-based antibiotic ointments in extraction sites. The patient may become symptomatic within several months or within 1 or 2 years, and in one case the patient remained asymptomatic for 7 years. Patients have either asymptomatic swelling, or the lesions in the jaws are found on routine radiographic examination. On surgical exploration, a black, greasy, tarlike substance is found. Lynch and colleagues (1984) advised against the use of petrolatum-based antibiotics at the sites of surgical wounds in the oral cavity.

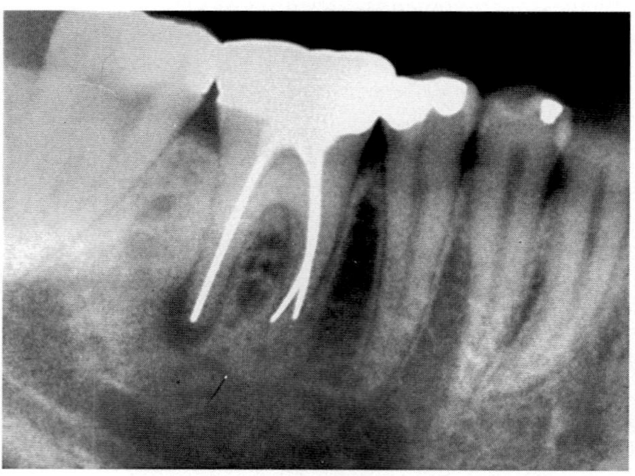

FIGURE 9–23.

Fibrous healing defect. Postendodontic defect: the tooth is asymptomatic, and the periapical radiolucent area does not change in size over time.

◆ *RADIOLOGY (Figs. 9–26 and 9–27)*

From the descriptions of Lynch and colleagues (1984) and from the case of Gibilisco (1985), it appears that petrolatum produces a persistent radiolucent lesion in an area previously occupied by a tooth. The most common location appears to be the mandibular third molar area. In most instances, the radiolucency is well defined and just beneath the crest of the ridge. It is ovoid or circular, with a thin sclerotic rim similar to that of a cyst, but it may be slightly irregular or focally absent in areas. One may see a discontinuity of the sclerotic rim at the crest of the ridge. In the case of Dunlap and Barker (1980), the lesion in the maxillary canine area was well defined, but with only a hint of a sclerotic rim 6 years after surgery. The lesions are confined to alveolar bone and rarely exceed 1.5 cm in diameter. More than one lesion may be present in the same patient. From the cases of Lynch and colleagues (1984), it would appear that earlier lesions

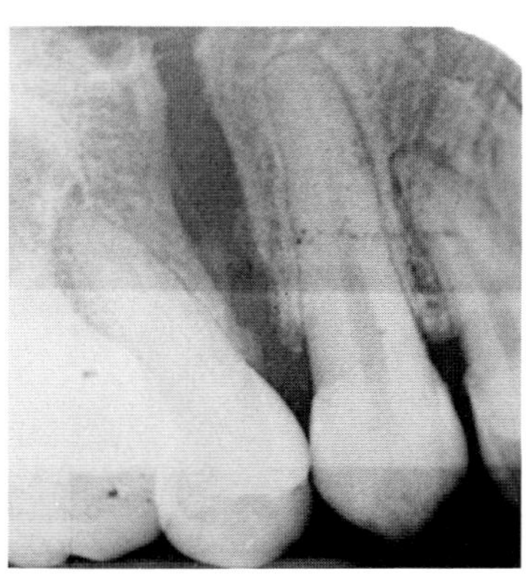
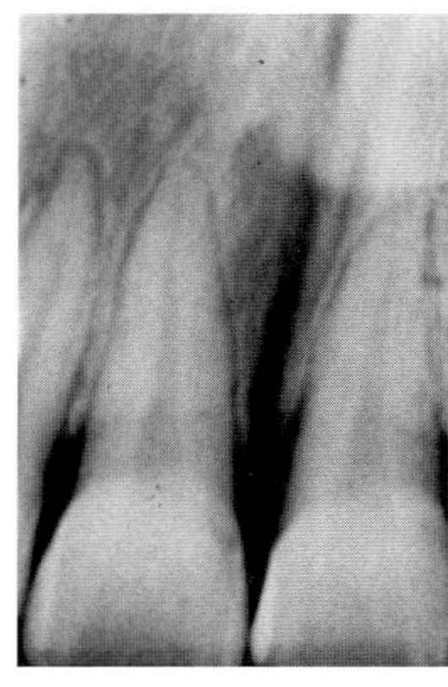
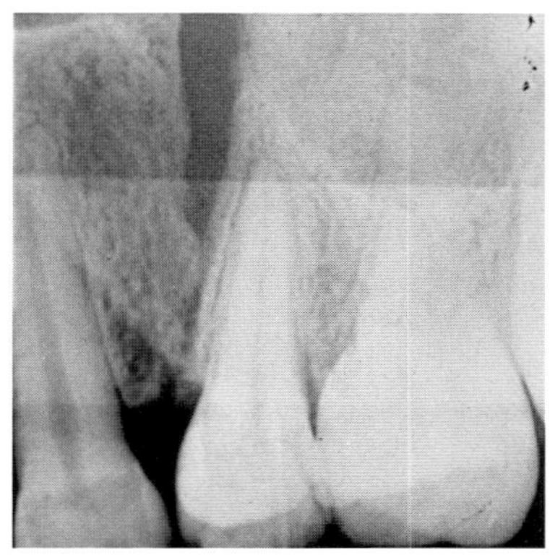

A B C

FIGURE 9–24.

Fibrous union at surgical margins. A, B, and C, One year after osteotomy; clinically, the entire segment was mobile.

occurring within several months do not develop this characteristic appearance; such lesions are more poorly defined and appear inflammatory.

PRIMORDIAL CYST (Odontogenic keratocyst)

The oceans, the World Health Organization (WHO), and a variety of conflicting reports appear to have divided North American thinking from that of the rest of the world concerning this cyst. On the American side, it is postulated that the primordial cyst arises from a developing tooth that undergoes cystic degeneration before calcification; in some cases the epithelial lining is nonkeratinized, in other instances the lining is orthokeratinized, and in further examples the epithelium exhibits the typical appearance of an odontogenic keratocyst with a parakeratinized, corrugated surface. The WHO classifies the primordial cyst as a synonym for odontogenic keratocyst with a parakeratinized corrugated surface. Robinson (1975), of the University of Missouri, stated that there is no justification for the use of these two terms as synonyms. Brannon (1976), in his clinicopathologic study of 312 odontogenic keratocysts, found that only 44% of all odontogenic keratocysts satisfied his criteria for classification as primordial cysts. For the time being, and as radiologists, we discuss the odontogenic keratocyst separately in Chapter 13; here the primordial cyst is presented from the North American perspective.

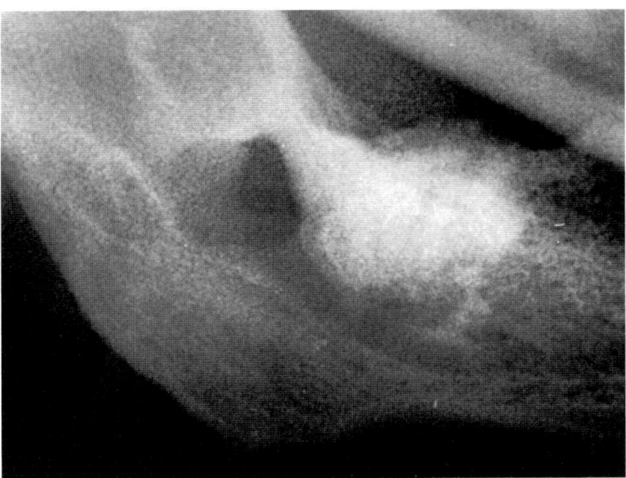

FIGURE 9–25.

Fibrous and osseous healing defects. Both conditions have occurred simultaneously after removal of an impacted third molar and a dentigerous cyst.

Primordial cysts are seen with equal frequency among males and females. They are often detected in young adults, but may be found at older ages because of a perceived lack of need for radiographic examination. This is because many primordial cysts are odontogenic keratocysts, which enlarge at the expense of the medullary space with little expansion. The most common locations are in the mandibular third molar regions and at the sites of supernumerary teeth, such as the mandibular premolars and maxillary mesiodens. By definition, the primordial cyst develops instead of a tooth.

◆ *RADIOLOGY (Fig. 9–28)*

In North America, the diagnosis of primordial cyst is clinical because several histopathologic diagnoses are possible. The diagnosis is made when the history and clinical findings suggest that a cyst has developed in place of a tooth. In the earlier lesion, and in the younger patient, the primordial cyst is usually a round or oval radiolucency with a well-defined sclerotic margin. The primordial cyst may also exhibit all the radiographic features of the odontogenic keratocyst. Because many reports on the primordial cyst do not separate it from the odontogenic keratocyst, it is difficult to ascribe separate features to the three histologic subtypes. It appears, however, that even the nonkeratocyst subtypes may achieve a fairly large size, with a smooth, well-corticated outline and a radiolucent lumen. The cyst may occupy the entire width of the mandible or a large portion of the ramus. Mild expansion may be present. Evidence of perforation is a variable feature,

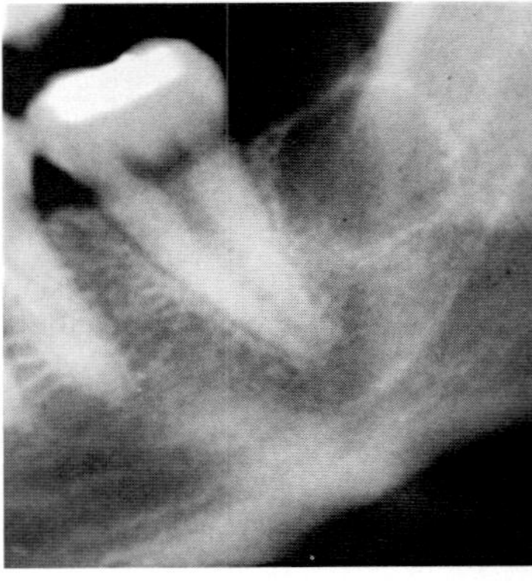

A

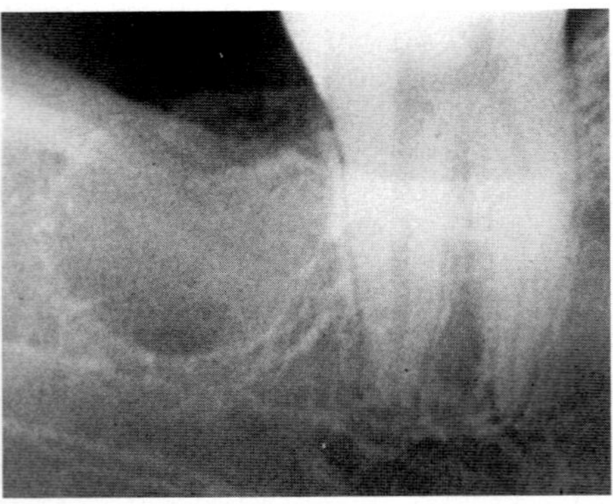

B

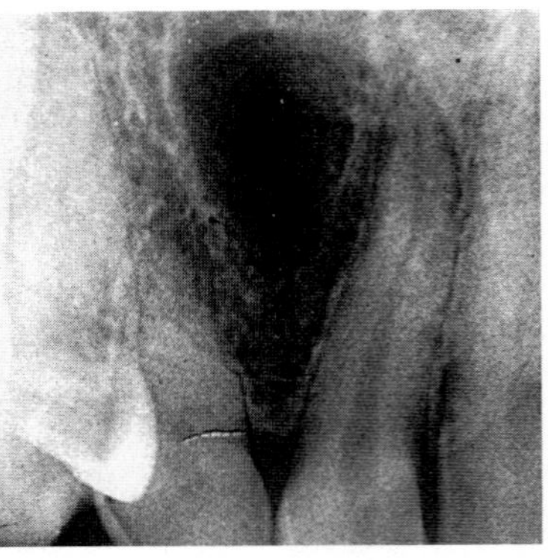

C

Figure 9–26.

Myospherulosis. A, Thick and slightly irregular sclerotic margin; B, thin and slightly irregular sclerotic margin; C, 4 years postoperatively. (A, From Lynch DP, Newland JR, McClendon JL: Myospherulosis of the oral hard and soft tissues. J Oral Maxillofac Surg 42:349, 1984; B and C, from Dunlap CL, Barker BF: Myospherulosis of the jaws. Oral Surg Oral Med Oral Pathol 50:238, 1980.)

however, depending on the histologic subtype. According to Struthers and Shear (1976), root resorption of adjacent teeth is rare, although displacement of teeth may occur with some frequency. We believe that, in time, the primordial cyst may no longer be considered a separate histopathologic entity, just as the globulomaxillary cyst, median palatal cyst, anterior median maxillary cyst, and median mandibular cyst have all been described as variations of other specific cyst types.

RESIDUAL CYST

The residual cyst is the first of 3 radiologically distinct cysts, each with a variety of possible specific histopathologic diagnoses. The other 2 are the globulomaxillary cyst and the median mandibular cyst. Shafer and colleagues (1983), as well as Shear (1985), have stated that the term ''residual cyst'' is frequently applied to an apical periodontal cyst, which remains after or develops subsequent to extraction of an infected tooth. However, Shafer and associates (1983) also stated that the term can be applied to any cyst of the jaw that remains following surgery. In a series of 289 jaw cysts examined by Main (1970), Shafer and co-workers (1983) found that 68% of these lesions were apical periodontal cysts and 8% were residual cysts, which they defined as apical periodontal cysts remaining after tooth extraction. Martinelli and colleagues (1976) have reported a case of squamous cell carcinoma arising in a mandibular residual cyst in a 60-year-old edentulous woman. Residual cysts should be excised, sent for histopathologic examination, and followed radiographically for recurrence. The recurrence rate is low.

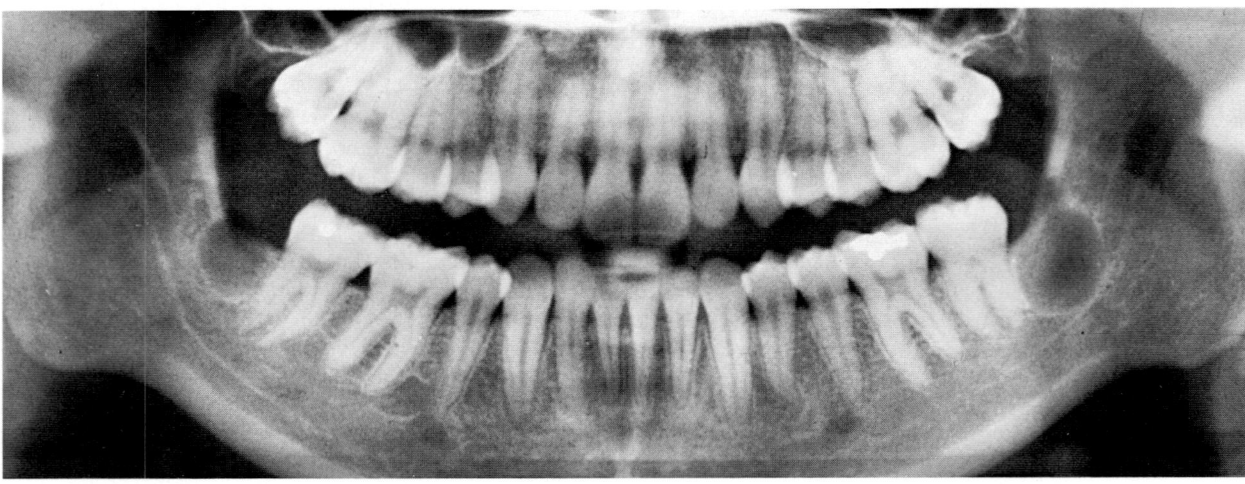

FIGURE 9–27.

Myospherulosis occurring bilaterally. (From Lynch DP, Newland JR, McClendon JL: Myospherulosis of the oral hard and soft tissues. J Oral Maxillofac Surg 42:349, 1984.)

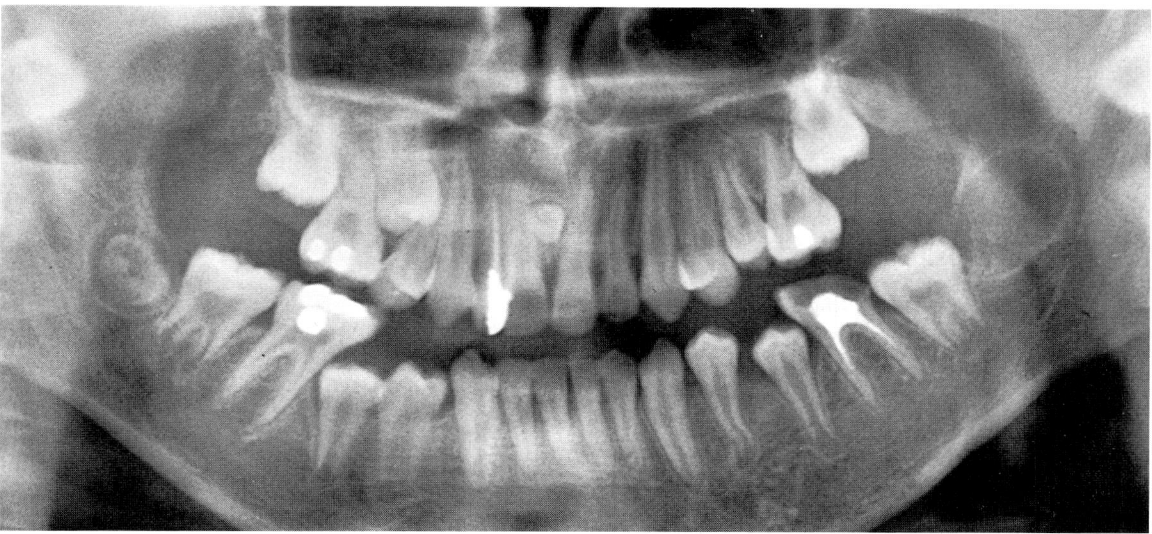

FIGURE 9–28.

Primordial cyst. This cyst has developed instead of the mandibular left third molar. (Courtesy of Drs. M. Araki and K. Hashimoto, Nihon University School of Dentistry, Tokyo, Japan.)

◆ *RADIOLOGY (Fig. 9–29)*

The residual cyst is a well-defined radiolucency with a distinct sclerotic margin in an edentulous area. The sclerotic margin may be fine and thin, or it may be thicker and diffusely sclerotic, especially when residual infection is present. In many instances, the residual cyst is less than 1 cm in diameter, with some lesions achieving a size of several centimeters in diameter. Expansion occurs infrequently. On rare occasions, the cyst may be large and expansile and may occupy a large portion of the jaw. In the occlusal view, it is helpful to study the expanded cortex for a hydraulic effect in which there is an even thickness of subperiosteal new bone that meets the mandible at equal angles on either side of the expanded margin. The borders of the cyst may be scalloped. The lumen may be uniformly radiolucent, it may contain trabeculations, or it may have a cloudy appearance. The location of the residual cyst may help to suggest the final histologic diagnosis. For example, a small residual cyst in the mandibular canine region may consist of a lateral periodontal cyst; a small or large residual cyst in the angle-ramus area may turn out to be a dentigerous cyst; whereas in the maxillary canine-premolar region, the histologic diagnosis may be apical periodontal cyst.

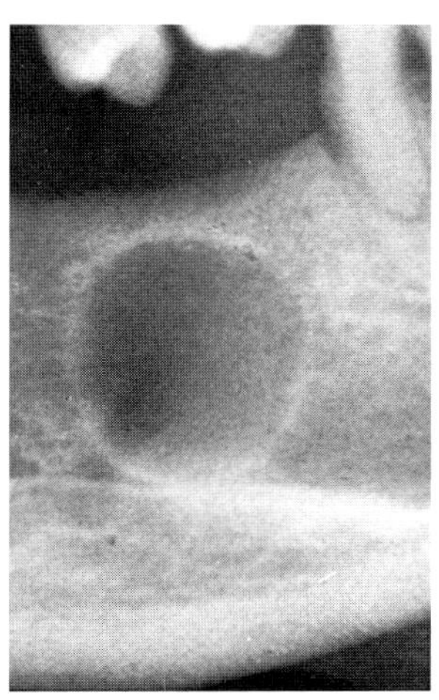

A

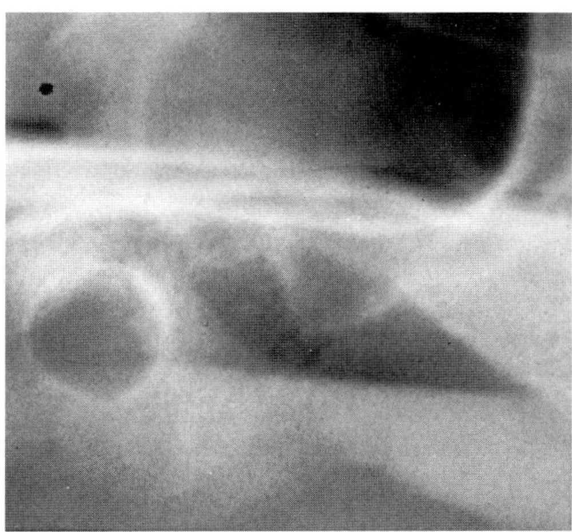

B

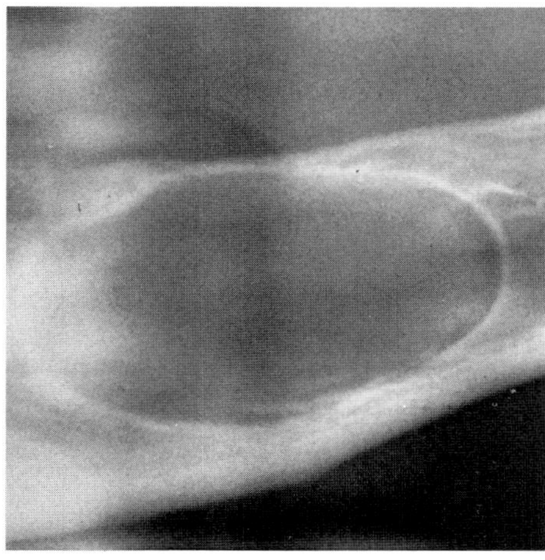

C

FIGURE 9–29.

Residual cyst. Originally, all were radicular cysts. A, Small mandibular cyst; B, small maxillary cyst; C, large mandibular cyst.

SURGICAL CILIATED CYST OF THE MAXILLA (Postoperative maxillary cyst)

The surgical ciliated cyst of the maxilla was first reported by Kubo in 1927 in Japan. Without knowledge of this original Japanese report, Gregory and Shafer first introduced the cyst to the Western literature in 1958, with a report of four cases. Ohba and colleagues (1980) stated that the surgical ciliated cyst of the maxilla is much more common in Japan than in the Americas or Europe. Basu and colleagues (1988) believe that the lesion is not rare outside Japan, but that it is perhaps underdiagnosed.

Pathologic Characteristics

In a series of 23 cases, Basu and colleagues (1988) found that all patients had previous surgical entry into the maxillary sinus during a Caldwell-Luc operation. Gregory and Shafer (1958) believe that the cystic lining is derived from the epithelial lining of the maxillary sinus because of its histologic similarity, characterized as pseudostratified ciliated columnar epithelium. Iinuma (1972) stated that these cysts may arise when infected sinus mucosa is implanted during a sinus operation.

Clinical Features

Ohba and colleagues (1980) reported that the lesion tends to develop between the ages of 30 and 40 in patients who had undergone sinus surgery some 10 to 20 years earlier. Basu and colleagues (1988) found that the mean period of prior sinus surgery was 20 years, with a range of 7 to 39 years. In a review of 71 cases in Japan, Kaneshiro and colleagues (1981) found that 75% occurred between the ages of 30 and 49, with no cases before the age of 20 or after 70 years. The surgery was performed in the second and third decades in 87% of cases. In the series of 23 cases reported by Basu and colleagues (1988), there was a 1.3:1 female-to-male ratio. According to Kaneshiro and colleagues (1981), typical findings consisted of facial swelling (71%), pain (65%), discomfort (7%), and paresthesia (2%), and 13 were asymptomatic. Intraorally, there was gingival swelling from the gingiva to the mucobuccal fold in 84% of the cases, fluctuation (fluid in cavity) in 43% of the cases, and purulent discharge in 21% of the cases. In the series of 23 cases reported by Basu and colleagues (1988), only one case was discovered as a result of routine radiography; all the other patients had signs and symptoms. It is important to suspect this cyst of the maxilla in patients complaining of pain or other vague neurologic symptoms with a history of a Caldwell-Luc procedure many years previously.

Treatment/Prognosis

Kaneshiro and colleagues (1981) stated that smaller lesions may be enucleated and packed with a dressing. In this instance, epithelialization usually occurs within 2 weeks, leaving a depression on the buccal aspect of the maxilla. Larger lesions may be treated by marsupialization with complete resolution within 6 months.

♦ *RADIOLOGY (Figs. 9–30 to 9–32)*

Ohba and colleagues (1980) have discussed the radiology of these cysts, which may have one of the following appearances. First, it may consist of a small radiolucency less than 1 cm in diameter, entirely within the maxilla and not encroaching on the antrum. This small lesion is usually round or oval, is well demarcated by a thin sclerotic border, and may have a radiolucent or even slightly cloudy lumen. Second, the moderate-size cyst may enlarge to involve more of the maxilla and may expand into the maxillary sinus. The pencil-like line of the maxillary sinus floor, or more frequently, the anterior wall, becomes more continuous, curved, and thickened as it bulges up into the antrum. In this region, the margin acquires a smooth, domed appearance. In larger lesions within the maxilla and antrum, this bony margin may be lost radiographically as it blends with other structures in the upper reaches of the antrum. Third, the cyst may appear to involve the maxilla minimally, with most of its bulk entirely within the maxillary sinus. In this instance, the floor or anterior wall of the antrum may or may not be apparent in the panoramic radiograph, and the entire sinus often appears cloudy. Ohba and colleagues (1980) stressed the following: (1) the sclerotic cystic margin, although usually present (70%), may be excessively thinned and may appear absent, possibly because of exposure technique; (2) the best plain view used to study this cyst is Waters' projection; (3) in a review of 63 patients using panoramic radiographs, 32% were located at the junction of the anterior wall of the antrum and the alveolar bone; 25% were located in the alveolar bone alone; and 81% were unilocular. This cyst may occur bilaterally, especially in Japanese persons who have lived in Japan.

Contrast studies

Gregory and Shafer (1958) have recommended the use of radiopaque contrast material to outline the cyst. They suggest injecting either the antrum to outline the cyst or injecting into the cyst to show its relationship with the antrum. Basu and colleagues (1988) showed that most of their cases were distinct from the antrum when this procedure was performed. Uemura and Hashida (1985) recommended the use of injected contrast material along with frontal tomography to identify the presence and extent of this cyst. With computed tomography (CT), the extent of this cyst can be determined without the need for contrast medium. In almost all reported cases, the radiologic workup, along with special procedures, was the key to the diagnosis.

NEURAL SHEATH TUMORS (Neurilemmoma/schwannoma, neurofibroma, neurofibromatosis)

In their 1985 review of the literature, Murphy and Giunta found 27 cases of central neurilemmoma. Prescott and White (1970) presented one of the most extensive reviews of central neurofibromas and found 16 cases. Shapiro and colleagues (1984) published a complete report on intraosseous findings in multiple neurofibromatosis.

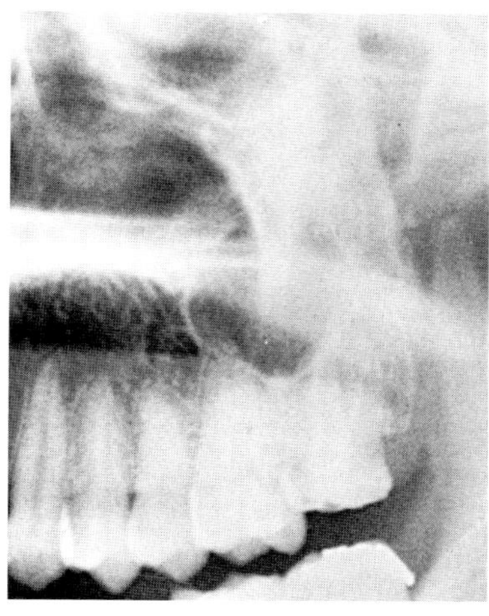

A

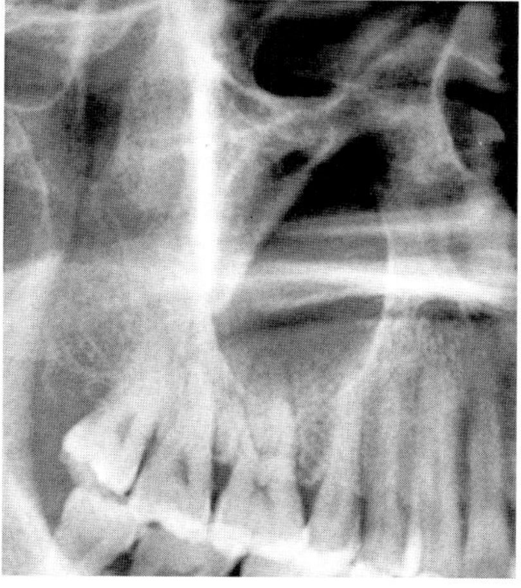

B

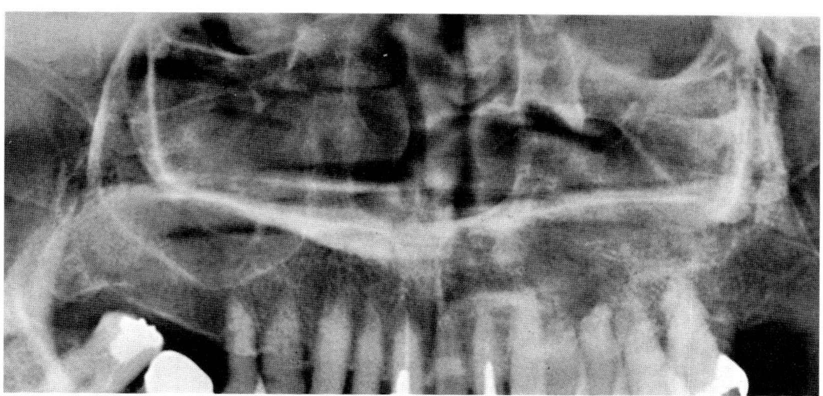

C

FIGURE 9–30.

Surgical ciliated cyst of the maxilla. A, First type, confined mostly to the maxilla. B, Second type, in the maxilla with expansion into the sinus. C, Third type, involving the entire left antrum with loss of the sinus floor outline. (Courtesy of Drs. M. Araki, K. Hashimoto, and K. Honda, Nihon University School of Dentistry, Tokyo, Japan.)

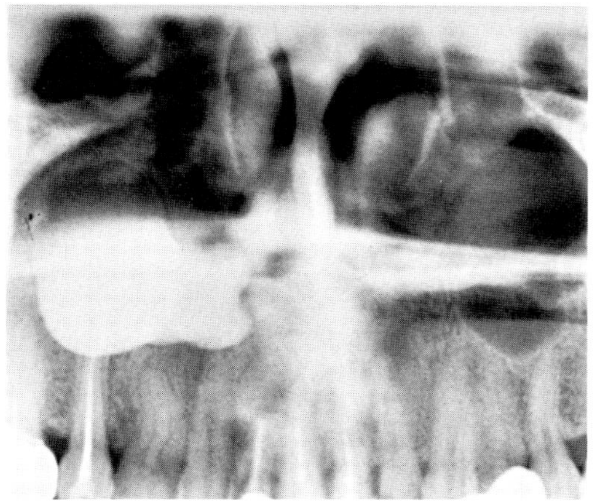

FIGURE 9–31.

Surgical ciliated cyst of the maxilla. The cyst has had contrast medium injected into the cyst lumen. (Courtesy of Drs. M. Araki and K. Hashimoto, Nihon University School of Dentistry, Tokyo, Japan.)

Pathologic Characteristics

As described by Shafer and colleagues (1983), the microscopic picture of neurilemmoma is characterized by the presence of Antoni-A and Antoni-B tissue. Antoni-A nuclei sometimes form Verocay bodies; Antoni-B is a random arrangement of tissue with microcysts. The tumor is encapsulated. The neurofibroma is not a typical neural sheath tumor. According to Shafer and co-workers (1983), it is composed of delicate spindle cells with thin, wavy nuclei intermingled with neurons in an irregular pattern plus delicate intertwining connective tissue fibrils. Melanocytes may be present, and mast cells are common. A capsule is absent.

Clinical Features

In a 1977 search for intrabony neural sheath tumors, Ellis and colleagues found 28 previously reported cases and added 7 new cases. Among these data, these investigators could find only 3 cases of intraosseous multiple neurofibromatosis. Thus, central benign neural sheath tumors are rare in the jaws, and because of the commonality among these lesions, they are treated as a group rather than individually. Central neural sheath tumors may arise in bone, within the inferior alveolar canal or subperiosteally. In their collapsed data, Ellis and colleagues (1977) found that neural sheath tumors are seen more commonly in females, with a ratio of 2:1 over

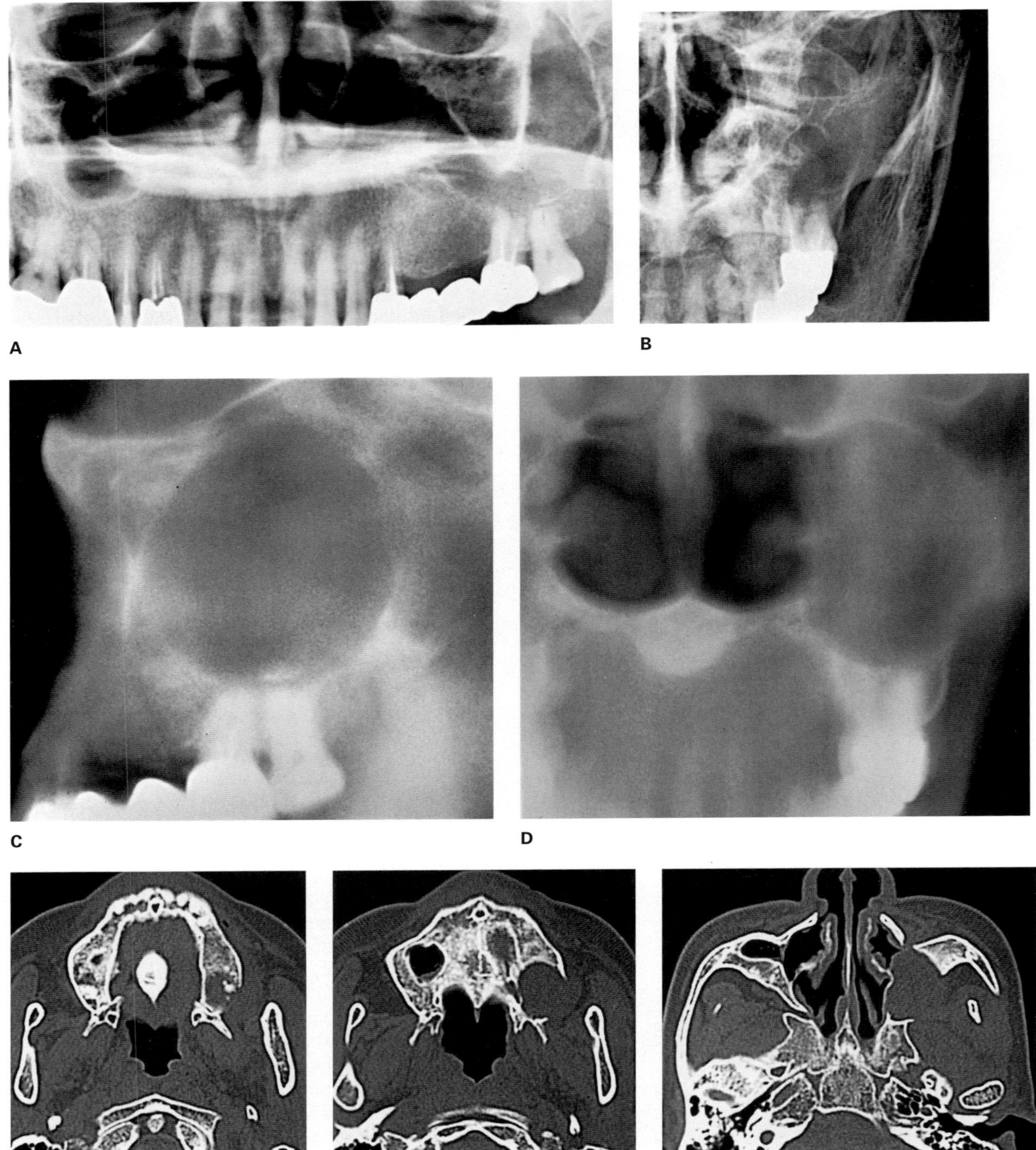

FIGURE 9–32.

Postoperative maxillary cyst: radiologic workup of the second type, involving both the maxilla and the antrum. A, Panoramic radiograph demonstrates the cyst in left maxilla expanding into the antrum. B, A posteroanterior view shows expansion of the lateral wall of the antrum, which appears intact. C and D, The lateral and anteroposterior tomographic views demonstrate erosion of the lateral wall of the nasal fossa and possible perforation of the lateral wall of the sinus. E, F, and G, axial computed tomographic images of the cyst at the level of a torus palatinus; sinus floor with perforation of the buccal cortex of the maxilla; upper antrum at the level of the condyle and coronoid process with perforation of the posterolateral sinus wall. (Courtesy of Drs. M. Araki, K. Hashimoto, and K. Honda, Nihon University School of Dentistry, Tokyo, Japan.)

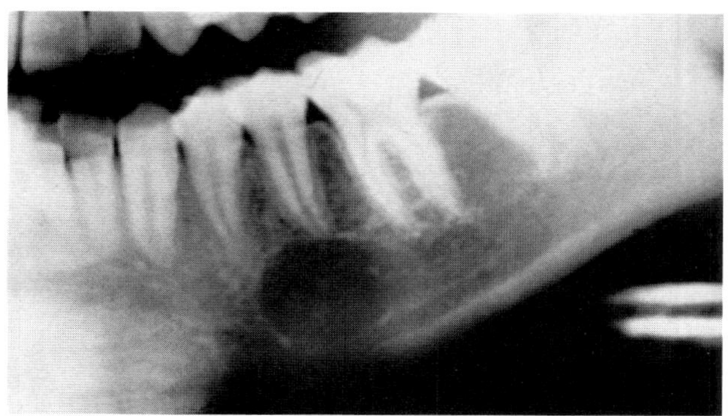

FIGURE 9–33.

Neurilemmoma. The lesion has a cystic appearance because of its circular shape and thin, regular, sclerotic margin. (Courtesy of Dr. H. Schwartz, Southern California Permanente Medical Group, Los Angeles, CA.)

males. The average age was 29 years. Among the 25 cases reviewed, 8 occurred in children aged 12 years and under. The age spread was from 2 to 72 years. As noted by Ellis and colleagues (1977), swelling and jaw expansion are the most common presenting signs and, pain, a burning sensation, and paresthesia are frequent complaints. In the series of Ellis and co-workers (1977), at least one of these signs or symptoms was present in 32 of 35 patients. The other 3 were asymptomatic; the lesion was found on routine radiologic examination.

Treatment/Prognosis

The neurofibroma recurs much more frequently than the neurilemmoma. This is perhaps because the neurilemmoma is well encapsulated and the neurofibroma is not.

◆ *RADIOLOGY (Figs. 9–33 and 9–34)*

As stated by Ellis and co-workers (1977), the posterior mandible is the preferred site of occurrence of neurogenic tumors of the jaws. Among the 35 reported cases, 32 were in the mandible and 3 were in the maxilla. Three of the 32 mandibular cases were in an anterior location. Ord and Rennie (1981) reported a case of neurilemmoma in the maxilla. The lesions are usually radiolucent, and a few may have varying degrees of radiopaque material within the lesion. Some lesions may be large at diagnosis. Smaller lesions are 1 or 2 cm in diameter; they tend to enlarge, however, as evidenced by the frequency of swelling as a presenting sign. The lesion may occupy the entire body or ramus of the mandible. Most lesions are well defined, and a sclerotic rim of varying thicknesses, even within the same lesion, is invariably present. In some instances, the sclerotic rim is absent focally, especially toward the crest of the ridge or in areas of cortical thinning or perforation. In the series of 16 central neurofibromas reviewed by Prescott and White (1970), 14 exhibited expansion of the cortex and 8 had cortical perforation. The inferior cortex of the mandible as well as the anterior and posterior cortices of the ramus may be eroded. This erosion tends to be focal rather than generalized. Even well-defined margins are often irregular, and this irregularity may involve all of the margin or be limited to part of the margin within a given lesion. This irregularity is described as scalloped by some, and in 8 of 35 cases reviewed by Ellis and colleagues (1977), the pattern was described as multilocular. These investigators also found 4 cases in which the borders of the lesion were poorly defined; all 4 of these cases were neurofibromas, and both cases that were followed up recurred.

Rarely, the lesion arises in the inferior alveolar canal and causes this structure to be expanded. In reviewing the literature and the descriptions of other textbook authors, it is our impression that the neurofibroma specifically has the great-

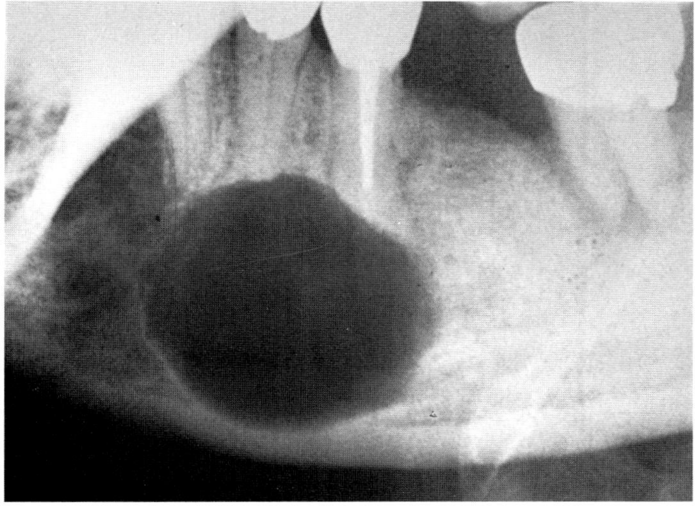

A

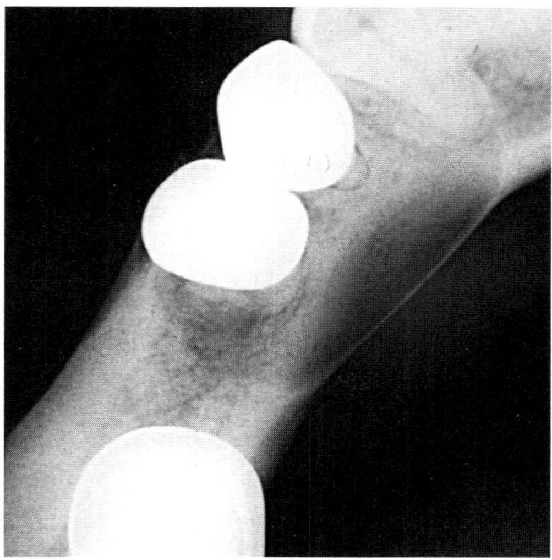

B

FIGURE 9–34.

Neurilemmoma. The lesion has a typical irregular outline, sclerotic margin of varying thicknesses, and expansion of the lingual cortex. A, Lateral jaw view; B, occlusal view. (Courtesy of Drs. M. Araki and K. Hashimoto, Nihon University School of Dentistry, Tokyo, Japan.)

est tendency to appear in this manner. In such cases, the inferior alveolar canal may become ovoid, or it may become widened with undulating margins. One such case, a neurilemmoma, was reported by Shimura and colleagues (1973). It was 5 cm wide × 6 cm long, extending from the mandibular foramen to the distal root of the first molar, and appeared continuous with the mandibular canal anteriorly. The lesion had an undulating outline. In addition, as described by Worth (1983), some neural sheath tumors arise subperiosteally, causing saucerization of the bone. These tumors are radiolucent and may or may not have a cortical outline. As the indentation deepens, the lesion becomes darker and with a greater tendency for a corticated outline. Subperiosteal lesions are usually circular, and the periosteum may lay down a layer of bone on the superficial aspect of the tumor, thus giving the superficial aspect an expanded appearance in the occlusal radiograph. One such neurofibroma was reported by Schneider and colleagues (1979); the central portion of the lesion was described as mottled, and at surgery, the lesion appeared to be covered with bone. Other findings include displacement of teeth, especially developing teeth in children. Root resorption has been reported, but is infrequent.

TRAUMATIC NEUROMA (Neuroma, amputation neuroma)

Traumatic neuroma was first reported by Cahn in 1939, in the region of the mental foramen. Most intrabony neuromas are seen in the mandible and result from injury to the inferior alveolar nerve. This injury may be caused by a jaw fracture, by extraction of an impacted tooth, by surgical removal of a lesion, or by orthognathic surgery. The neuroma usually develops when the regenerating nerve cannot reach its distal end because of obstruction by scar tissue or discontinuity of the canal. As stated by Shklar and Meyer (1963), spontaneous neuromas are exceedingly rare in the jaws. Histologically, the lesion consists of a tangled, irregular mass of nerve axons and sheaths, seen in longitudinal and cross-sections. Neuromas are usually painful and almost always elicit a painful response when palpated. As pointed out by Robinson and Slavkin (1965), however, in their review of amputation neuromas, these lesions are not always painful; additionally, extraosseous traumatic neuromas may follow routine extractions. These may be extremely small, only 1 or 2 mm in diameter. They are located much more readily by obtaining a painful response to palpation of the area than by actually feeling them. On excision of traumatic neuromas, healing is usually uneventful.

◆ *RADIOLOGY*

Traumatic neuromas, although rare, often involve the inferior alveolar canal. The canal is enlarged and may assume the same undulating outline as described for neural sheath tumors, especially when some blockage, such as bone fill at the site of a previous tumor, prevents the regenerating nerve tissue from reaching its distal end. Thus, radiographic evidence of such blockage is helpful in separating the traumatic neuroma from the nerve sheath tumors. The traumatic neuroma may also involve other areas of bone, but because there have been so few cases, it is difficult to describe distinctive features.

References

Medial Sigmoid Depression

Langlais RP, Glass BJ, Bricker SL, Miles DA: Medial sigmoid depression: a panoramic pseudoforamen in the upper ramus. Oral Surg Oral Med Oral Pathol 55:635, 1983.

Wood NK, Goaz P: Differential Diagnosis of Oral Lesions. 4th Ed. Philadelphia:Mosby-Year Book, 1991, p. 293.

Submandibular Salivary Gland Depression

Chen CY, Ohba T: An analysis of radiological findings of Stafne's idiopathic bone cavity. Dentomaxillofac Radiol 10:81, 1981.

D'Eramo EM, Poidmore SJ: Developmental submandibular gland defect of the mandible: review of the literature and report of a case. Oral Surg Oral Med Oral Pathol 61:213, 1986.

Gorab DN, Brahney C, Aria A: Unusual presentation of a Stafne bone cyst. Oral Surg Oral Med Oral Pathol 61:213, 1986.

Hansson LG: Development of a lingual mandibular bone cavity in an 11 year old boy. J Oral Surg 49:376, 1980.

Harvey W, Noble HW: Defects on the lingual surface of the mandible near the angle. Br J Oral Surg 6:75, 1968.

Johnson CC: Analysis of panoramic survey. J Am Dent Assoc 81:151, 1970.

Langlais RP, Cottone JA, Kasle M: Anterior and posterior lingual depressions of the mandible. J Oral Surg 34:502, 1976.

Lello GF, Makek M: Stafne's mandibular lingual cortical defect. J Oral Maxillofac Surg 13:172, 1985.

Mann RW, Keenleyside A: Developmental lingual defects on the mandibular ramus. Oral Surg Oral Med Oral Pathol 74:124, 1992.

Oikarinen JV, Wolf J, Julku M: A stereosialographic study of developmental mandibular bone defects. Int J Oral Surg 4:51, 1974.

Seward GR: Salivary gland inclusions in the mandible. Br Dent J 108:321, 1960.

Stafne EC: Bone cavities situated near the angle of the mandible. J Am Dent Assoc 29:1969, 1942.

Uemura S, Fujishita M, Fuchihata H: Radiographic interpretation of so-called developmental defects of the mandible. Oral Surg Oral Med Oral Pathol 41:120, 1976.

Wolf J: Bone defects in mandibular ramus resembling developmental bone cavity. Proc Finn Dent Soc 81:215, 1985.

Wolf J, Mattila K, Ankkuriniemi O: Development of a Stafne mandibular bone cavity. Oral Surg Oral Med Oral Pathol 61:519, 1986.

Sublingual Salivary Gland Depression

Connor MS: Anterior lingual mandibular bone concavity. Oral Surg Oral Med Oral Pathol 48:413, 1979.

Gaughran GR: Mylohyoid boutonniere and sublingual bouton. J Anat (Lond) 97:565, 1963.

Hayashi Y, Kimura Y, Nagumo M: Anterior lingual bone concavity. Oral Surg Oral Med Oral Pathol 57:139, 1984.

Langlais RP, Cottone J, Kasle M: Anterior and posterior lingual depressions of the mandible. J Oral Surg 34:502, 1976.

Miller AS, Winnick M: Salivary gland inclusion in the anterior mandible. Oral Surg Oral Med Oral Pathol 31:790, 1971.

Nathan H, Luchansky E: Sublingual gland herniation through the mylohyoid muscle. Oral Surg Oral Med Oral Pathol 59:21, 1985.

Richard EL, Ziskind J: Aberrant salivary gland tissue in the mandible. Oral Surg Oral Med Oral Pathol 10:1086, 1957.

Strom C, Fjellstrom CA: An unusual case of lingual mandibular depression. Oral Surg Oral Med Oral Pathol 64:159, 1987.

Parotid Salivary Gland Depression

Barker GR: A radiolucency of the ascending ramus of the mandible associated with invested parotid salivary gland material and analogous with Stafne bone cavity. Br J Oral Maxillofac Surg 26:81, 1988.

Mann RW, Keenleyside A: A developmental lingual defects on the mandibular ramus. Oral Surg Oral Med Oral Pathol 74:124, 1992.

Slavin MS: Ectopically laced salivary gland in the mandible. Oral Surg Oral Med Oral Pathol 3:1372, 1950.
Wolf J: Bone defects in mandibular ramus resembling developmental bone cavity (Stafne). Proc Finn Dent Soc 81:25, 1985.

Hematopoietic Bone Marrow Defect

Barker BF, Jensen JL, Howell FV: Focal osteoporotic bone marrow defects of the jaws: an analysis of 197 new cases. Oral Surg Oral Med Oral Pathol 38:404, 1974.
Crawford BE, Weathers DR: Osteoporotic marrow defects of the jaws. J Oral Surg 28:600, 1970.
Standish SM, Shafer, WG: Focal osteoporotic bone marrow defect of the jaws. J Oral Surg Anesth Hosp Dent Serv 20:123, 1962.

Myospherulosis

Belfiglio EH, Wonderlich ST, Fox LJ: Myospherulosis of the alveolus secondary to the use of Terra-Cortril and Gelfoam. Oral Surg Oral Med Oral Pathol 61:12, 1986.
Dunlap CL, Barker BF: Myospherulosis of the jaws. Oral Surg Oral Med Oral Pathol 50:238, 1980.
Gibilisco JA: Stafne's Oral Radiographic Diagnosis. 5th Ed. Philadelphia: WB Saunders, 1985 p. 178.
Lynch DP, Newland JR, McClendon, JL: Myospherulosis of the oral hard and soft tissues. J Oral Maxillofac Surg 42:349, 1984.
McClatchie MD, Warambo MW, Bremner AD: Myospherulosis, a previously unreported disease? Am J Clin Pathol 51:699, 1969.

Primordial Cyst

Brannon RB: The odontogenic keratocyst: a clinicopathologic study of 312 cases. Part 1. Clinical features. Oral Surg Oral Med Oral Pathol 42:54, 1976.
Robinson HBG: Primordial cyst versus keratocyst. Oral Surg Oral Med Oral Pathol 39:362, 1975.
Struthers P, Shear M: Root resorption produced by the enlargement of ameloblastomas and cysts of the jaws. Int J Oral Surg 5:128, 1976.

Residual Cyst

Main DMG: Epithelial jaw cysts: a clinicopathological reappraisal. Br J Oral Surg 8:114, 1970.
Martinelli C, Melhado R, Callestini EA: Squamous-cell carcinoma in residual mandibular cyst. Oral Surg Oral Med Oral Pathol 44:274, 1976.
Shafer WG, Hine MK, Levy BM, Tomich CE: In: A Textbook of Oral Pathology. 4th Ed. Philadelphia:WB Saunders, 1983, p. 265.
Shear M: Cysts of the jaws: recent advances. J Oral Pathol 14:43, 1985.

Surgical Ciliated Cyst of the Maxilla

Basu MK, Rout PG, Rippin JW, Smith JJ: The post-operative maxillary cyst: experience with 23 cases. Int J Maxillofac Surg 17:282, 1988.
Gregory GT, Shafer WG: Surgical ciliated cyst of the maxilla: report of cases. Oral Surg Oral Med Oral Pathol 16:251, 1958.
Iinuma T: X-ray diagnosis of the postoperative cysts of the maxilla. (In Japanese.) Otol Tokyo 44:459, 1972.
Kaneshiro S, et al: The post-operative maxillary cyst: report of 71 cases. J Oral Surg 39:191, 1981.
Kubo I: A malar cyst appearing after radical operation of maxillary sinusitis. (In Japanese.) Dai Nippon Jibi (Otol Tokyo) 33:896, 1927.
Ohba T, Yang RC, Chen CY: Pantomographic findings of post-operative maxillary cyst. (In Japanese.) Otol Tokyo 51:319, 1979.
Ohba T, Yang RC, Chen CY, Uneoka M: Postoperative maxillary cyst. Int J Oral Surg 9:840, 1980.
Uemura S, Hashida T: Radiologic interpretation of fissural cysts and postoperative maxillary cyst. Oral Radiol 1:69, 1985.

Neural Sheath Tumors

Ellis GL, Abrams AM, Melrose RJ: Intraosseous benign neural sheath neoplasms of the jaws. Oral Surg Oral Med Oral Pathol 44:731, 1977.
Murphy J, Giunta JL: Atypical central neurilemmoma of the mandible. Oral Surg Oral Med Oral Pathol 59:275, 1985.
Ord RA, Rennie JS: Central neurilemmoma of the maxilla. Int J Oral Surg 10:137, 1981.
Prescott GH, White RE: Solitary central neurofibroma of the mandible. J Oral Surg 28:305, 1970.
Schneider L, Mesa M, Weisinger E, Weimer P: Solitary intramandibular neurofibroma: report of a case. J Oral Med 34:37, 1979.
Shafer WG, Hine MK, Levy BM, Tomich CE: A Textbook of Oral Pathology. 4th Ed. Philadelphia:WB Saunders, 1983, p. 208.
Shapiro SD, et al: Neurofibromatosis: oral and radiographic manifestations. Oral Surg Oral Med Oral Pathol 58:493, 1984.
Shimura K, Allen EC, Kinoshita Y, Takaesu T: Central neurilemmoma in the mandible. J Oral Surg 31:363, 1973.
Worth HM: Principles and Practice of Oral Radiographic Interpretation. Chicago:Yearbook Medical Publishers, 1983, p. 512.

Traumatic Neuroma

Cahn L: Traumatic neuroma. Am J Orthod Oral Surg 25:190, 1939.
Robinson M, Slavkin H: Dental amputation neuromas. J Am Dent Assoc 70:662, 1965.
Shklar G, Meyer I: Neurogenic tumors of the mouth and jaws. Oral Surg Oral Med Oral Pathol 16:1075, 1963.

Chapter 10

Interradicular Radiolucencies

ANTERIOR MEDIAN MAXILLARY CLEFT

The anterior median maxillary cleft first was described by Gier and Fast in 1967 and refers to a lack of fusion in the the anterior median maxillary suture. The true nature of this condition is not fully understood, but it is not considered to be genetically induced or related to the other forms of cleft palate. It may develop in association with or cause a midline diastema. In either instance, there is usually a low frenal attachment. In edentulous patients, the condition is not apparent clinically; however, a low frenal attachment still may be present clinically. It is treated with a combination of surgical and orthodontic therapy and sometimes by the judicious placement of esthetic restorations.

◆ *RADIOLOGY (Fig. 10–1)*

When teeth are present, a small or large midline diastema invariably is present between the maxillary incisors. A V-shaped defect can be seen in the crestal bone between the maxillary incisors, which may extend to the apical region. The margins of the V-shaped cleft may consist of alveolar bone only, with little or no evidence of a cortical margin, or there may be a distinct band of sclerotic bone at the margin. This latter appearance may result from excessive tension on the periosteum caused by frenal pull.

In edentulous patients, the cleft often mimics a tooth socket after a recent extraction. This is especially true when there is a fine cortical lining along the V-shaped margin. Even when no lamina dura-like cortical margin is present, the condition may resemble a recent extraction socket in which pre-existing periodontitis caused loss of the lamina dura, or the lamina dura has disappeared, as occurs in the earliest stages of healing. In edentulous cases, the most important clue of the diagnosis is the midline location of the V-shaped cleft.

LATERAL (DEVELOPMENTAL) PERIODONTAL CYST (Lateral periodontal cyst)

The definitive histologic characteristics of the lateral developmental periodontal cyst first were described by Shear and Pindborg in 1975. Since the 1980 report of Wysocki and coauthors, all previous theories concerning the histogenesis and varying histopathologic and clinical findings have been repudiated but not universally accepted.

Pathologic Characteristics

Wysocki and colleagues (1980) postulated that islands of odontogenic epithelium within the gingival connective tissue represent rests of the dental lamina. These rests give rise to intraosseous and extraosseous variants of the same cystic entity. The extraosseous variant is the gingival cyst of the adult; the intraosseous cyst may be unilocular, in which case it is termed a lateral developmental periodontal cyst, or it may be multilocular and called a botryoid odontogenic cyst. The latter will be discussed in the chapter on multilocular lesions. All have the same basic histologic appearance, consisting of a thin lining of epithelial cells with areas of focal thickening representing the characteristic epithelial plaques. Within the connective tissue beneath the epithelial lining, islands of clear cell rests of the dental lamina are seen occasionally. The botryoid odontogenic cyst is simply a multifocal variant of the lateral developmental periodontal cyst; it is multifocal radiographically, grossly, and microscopically.

Clinical Features

In their review of lateral developmental periodontal cysts, Ross and colleagues (1986) reported a preponderance of cases in male patients. Most cases occur in people between the ages of 40 and 70 years, but they may be found in patients at any age and of any race. The cyst usually causes no symptoms and is found during routine radiologic examination. On close inspection, a very slight buccal expansion sometimes can be palpated; if the cyst is large enough, the overlying expanded bone is yielding on palpation. Periodontal disease is not a factor in the development of this cyst, but it may be present coincidentally.

Treatment/Prognosis

The cyst should be excised, and there is no tendency for recurrence. Baker and colleagues (1979) reported a case of well-differentiated squamous cell carcinoma arising in a lateral developmental periodontal cyst in the mandible of a 22-year-old man. The lesion was 3 mm in diameter and located between the first and second mandibular premolars. This particular lesion was painful and prompted the patient's visit. Over a period of several years, the patient required six surgical procedures to resect the tumor and reconstruct the mandible.

◆ *RADIOLOGY (Figs. 10–2 and 10–3)*

Location

Fantasia (1979) found 72% of cases in the mandible and 28% in the maxilla. In the series of 46 cases, the most common location was the premolar-canine area (76% of cases). It also may be found rarely in other areas. DiFiore and Hartwell (1987) reported a case between the mandibular central inci-

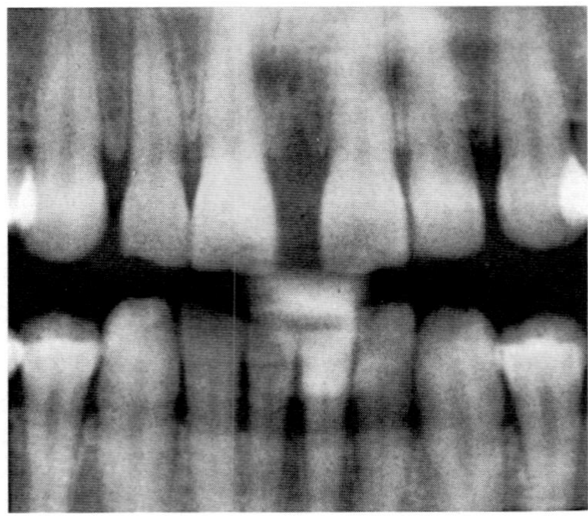

A

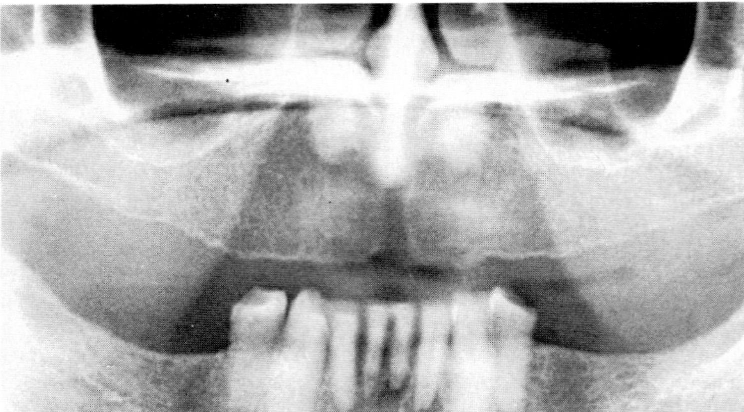

B

FIGURE 10–1.

Anterior median maxillary cleft. A, Dentate patient with a V-shaped defect and midline diastema. B, Edentulous patient with a socketlike lesion.

sors, and Smith (1978) described a case associated with an unerupted, impacted mandibular second premolar.

Radiologic Features

The lateral developmental periodontal cyst has specific radiomorphologic characteristics. Because it has a limited growth potential, it usually is a small, round, well-corticated radiolucency. It is located within the alveolar bone between the involved teeth, midway between the cervical and apical portions of the root. The lesion is usually small, very seldom more than 1 cm in diameter. The buccal cortical plate may or may not reveal moderate bulging or expansion and, in rare instances, perforation may be seen in the occlusal radiograph. Resorption of the adjacent lamina dura may occur. There is little tendency to move the adjacent teeth, but slight displacement may occur with larger lesions (1 to 1.5 cm in diameter). When a lesion is larger than 1.5 cm, the botryoid variant should be suspected, even if the lesion does not appear multilocular radiologically. The adjacent teeth are vital unless infected coincidentally. Periodontal disease is usually absent.

GINGIVAL CYST OF THE ADULT

Shear discussed gingival cysts in adults in his 1985 review of cysts of the jaws. Buchner and Hansen (1979) published a series of 33 cases, with 27 meeting the histologic criteria for true gingival cysts of the adult. In their report on the histogenesis of these cysts, Wysocki and colleagues (1980) examined 10 additional cases. As with the lateral developmental periodontal cyst, Shear (1985) found that 75% of gingival cysts occur in the canine/premolar region of the mandible. In the series of Wysocki and co-workers (1980), patients' ages ranged from 41 to 75 years (mean, 51 years). Gingival cysts are excised, and recurrence is not expected.

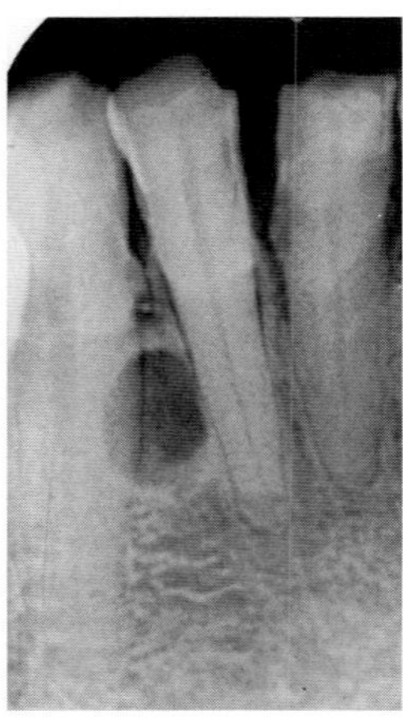

A

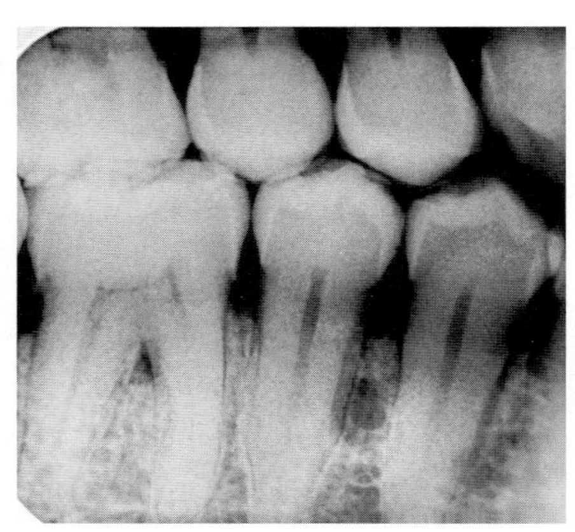

B

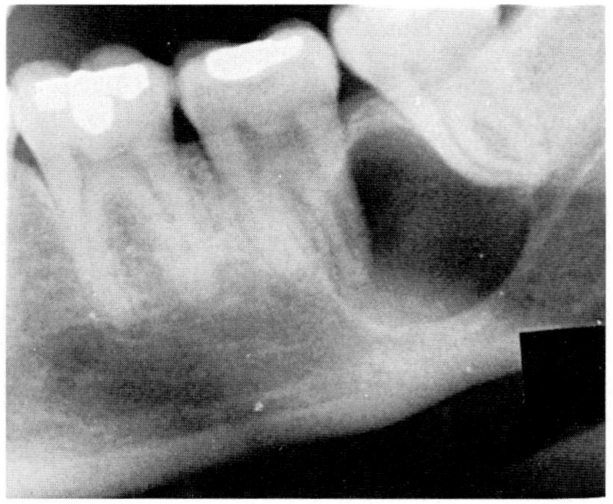

C

FIGURE 10–2.

Lateral developmental periodontal cyst. Small lesions: A, Mesial to canine. B, Between premolars. Large lesion: C, Mesial to third molar.

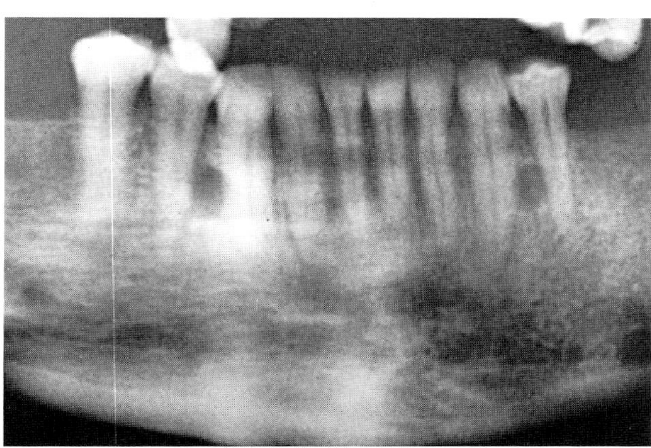

FIGURE 10–3.

Lateral developmental periodontal cyst. Rare bilateral occurrence. (From Farman AG, Nortjé CJ, Wood RE: Oral and Maxillofacial Diagnostic Imaging. Philadelphia: Mosby, 1993, p. 221.)

◆ *RADIOLOGY (Figs. 10–4 and 10–5)*

When the gingival cyst is small, there are no radiologic changes in the underlying bone. In a small number of cases, a gingival cyst of the adult may erode the outer cortex of the mandible, especially on the buccal side. Once this erosion is several millimeters deep, the cyst begins to appear on radiographs. It is located in the alveolar bone midway between the cervical area and apex of the adjacent teeth. The authors believe that this lesion is much less radiolucent than the lateral periodontal cyst, it may show some trabeculation within the luminal area, and a distinct cortical outline may be absent, especially in more shallow erosions. A second appearance of the gingival cyst is seen when the lesion is high up on the gingiva near the interdental papilla. In this instance, saucerization of the intercrestal bone is seen. The curved appearance of the intercrestal bone is unlike the changes produced by periodontitis.

There are usually three features that help to differentiate this lesion from the lateral developmental periodontal cyst:

1. Clinically, there may be a small gingival nodule that yields readily on palpation; the expansion of the lateral periodontal cyst tends to be bony hard and only slightly yielding.
2. On aspiration or needle biopsy, the gingival cyst is penetrated easily by the needle tip; some pressure must be exerted on the needle to enter the lateral periodontal cyst.
3. In the occlusal view of the gingival cyst, a depression in the outer cortical bone is observed; in the lateral periodontal cyst, the outer cortex is intact or expanded.

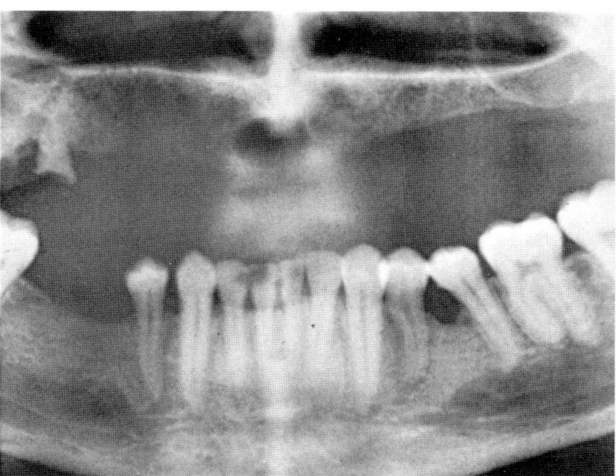

FIGURE 10–5.

Gingival cyst of the adult. Underlying bone has eroded, with dense zone of sclerosis immediately subadjacent; second premolar root is displaced distally. There is an unrelated incisive canal cyst in maxillary midline.

LATERAL (INFLAMMATORY) PERIODONTAL CYST (Inflammatory periodontal cyst, inflammatory collateral cyst)

The lateral (inflammatory) periodontal cyst first was reported in 1970 by Main, who termed it an inflammatory collateral cyst. According to Shear (1983), this cyst probably originates from epithelial rests in the periodontal ligament that proliferate as a result of inflammation in a periodontal pocket. Shear (1983) stated that this cyst is distinct from a

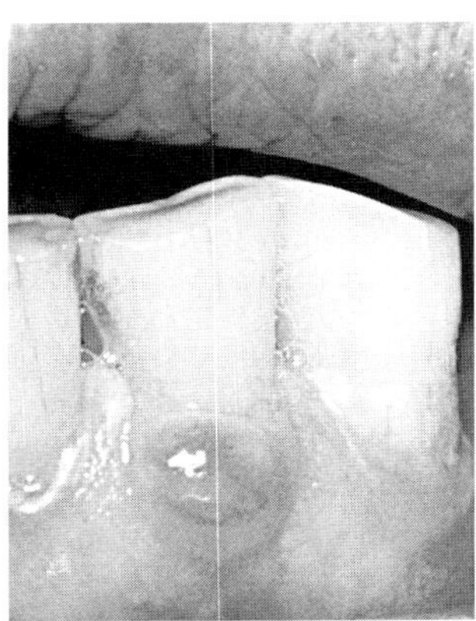

A

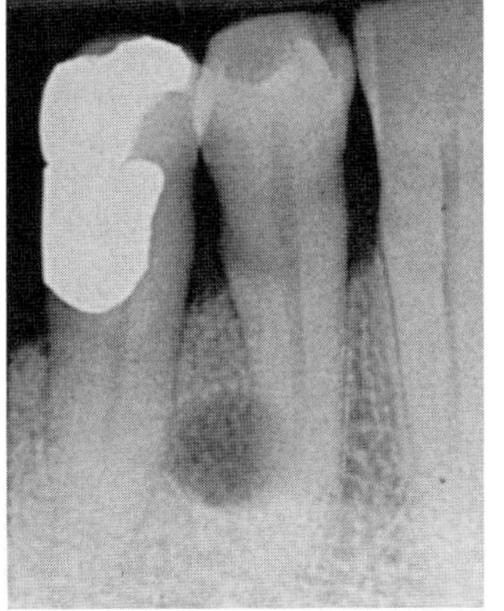

B

FIGURE 10–4.

Gingival cyst of the adult. A, Clinical appearance. B, Saucerization of cortex produces radiolucent lesion appearing punched-out, with trabeculae within. (Courtesy of Dr. T. Weaver, Commander USN [DC], National Naval Dental Hospital, Bethesda, MD.)

radicular cyst associated with a lateral accessory root canal of a nonvital tooth, a lateral developmental periodontal cyst, and the inflammatory paradental cyst. Craig (1976) first described the inflammatory paradental cyst and believed it was the same clinicopathologic entity as the lateral (inflammatory) periodontal cyst. Shear (1983) maintains the lateral (inflammatory) periodontal cyst is a separate clinicopathologic entity. Many pathologists in the United States do not recognize the lateral (inflammatory) periodontal cyst or inflammatory paradental cyst as distinct clinicopathologic entities.

According to Shear (1983), the lateral (inflammatory) periodontal cyst is rare, possibly because drainage occurs from a periodontal pocket before the cyst can form. When these cysts do arise, the tooth is vital unless coincidentally nonvital. A small number of patients have mild pain. Treatment consists of enucleation, along with the appropriate periodontal therapy. Recurrence is not expected.

◆ *RADIOLOGY (Fig. 10–6)*

There is very little descriptive information regarding the lateral (inflammatory) periodontal cyst. Presumably the cyst can occur anywhere in association with a periodontal pocket. Thus, there is radiologic evidence of a cystic lesion on the lateral aspect of the root of a tooth, along with a periodontal pocket. This cyst tends to remain small, approximately 1 cm or less in diameter. It is round or oval and abuts against the tooth root. Often it is high up in the alveolar bone, near the crest of the ridge. The margin consists of a diffuse area of reactive sclerotic bone, or it may be punched-out. In some areas, the margin may consist of thin wisps of noncontinuous sclerotic bone. On close examination, there may be slight irregularities at the host bone interface, representing areas of lysis by the inflammation. The cystic margin may extend across the breadth of the root, indicating extension of the lesion around the buccal or lingual side. The cervical margin of the cyst may be adjacent to a radiologically visible periodontal defect in the alveolar bone.

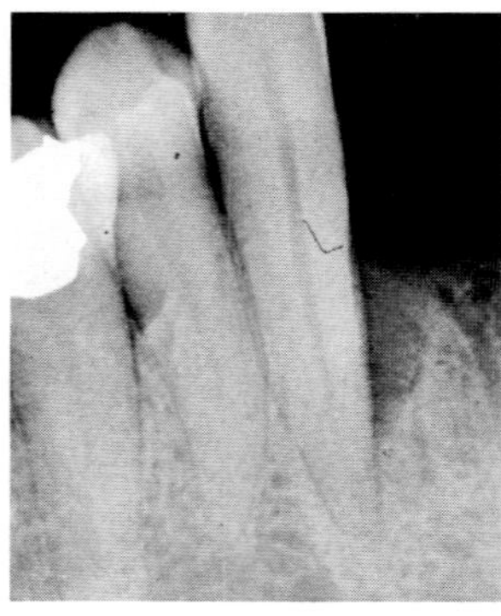

A

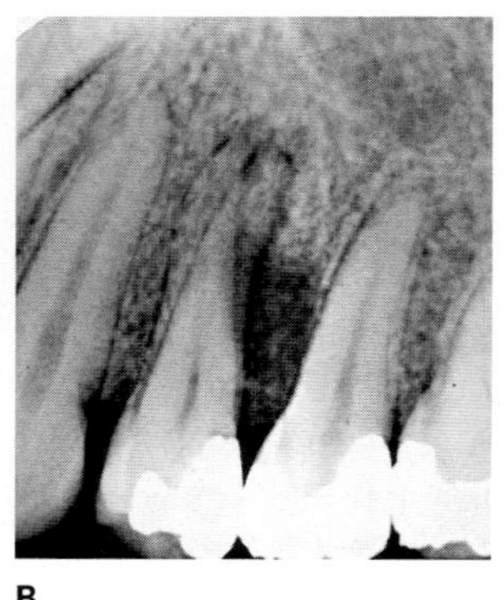

B

FIGURE 10–6.

Lateral (inflammatory) periodontal cyst. A, Diffuse condensation of reactive sclerotic bone at margin. B, Destruction of the lamina dura on both sides of cyst and spread of infection to apex of first premolar.

LATERAL RADICULAR CYST

The lateral radicular cyst is a variant of the apical radicular cyst associated with a nonvital pulp. This condition is discussed in some detail in Chapter 7 on "Pulpal and Periapical Disease." It may occur to one side of the apex of the tooth idiopathically or because of a lateral accessory canal. In either case, the tooth requires endodontic therapy or extraction.

◆ *RADIOLOGY (Fig. 10–7)*

The radiologic features are similar to those of an apical radicular cyst. The lesion tends to remain smaller than 1 cm in diameter. Rarely it may occupy the entire mandible. The appearance of this cyst can retrogress back and forth between a granulomatous histologic picture to that of a cystic lesion. Thus, the sclerotic margin may be absent or present in most cysts, depending on the degree of inflammation at examination. A diffuse zone of reactive bone also may be seen at the margins of the cyst.

INCISIVE CANAL CYST (Median anterior maxillary cyst, nasopalatine duct cyst, median palatal cyst)

The incisive canal cyst is the most common developmental cyst in the jaws. Stafne and colleagues (1936) reported that this cyst may be found in 1 of 100 people. In studies by Chamda and Shear (1980) and Meyer (1931), incidences of 1.3% and 1.5% were found, respectively; however, Killey and Kay (1977) found only two incisive canal cysts in a series of 2394 dry skulls. The incisive canal cyst develops from epithelial remnants of the nasopalatine duct contents. This cyst has intraosseous and extraosseous variants. The extraosseous cyst is termed a cyst of the incisive papilla and is discussed separately in this chapter. The incisive canal cyst includes the median palatal cyst and anterior median

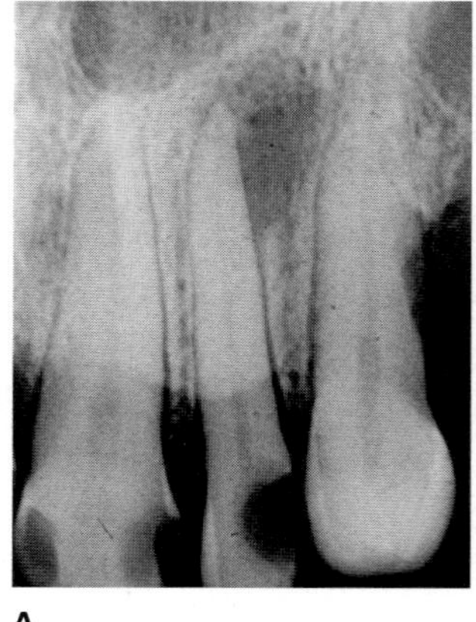

A

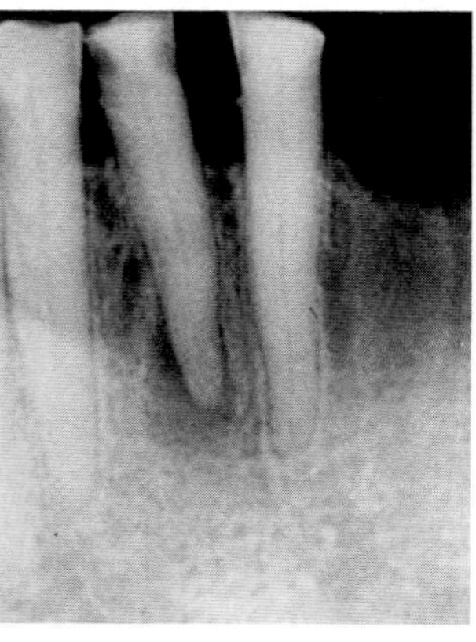

B

FIGURE 10–7.

Lateral radicular cyst. A and B, Distinction between granuloma, cyst, and abscess cannot be made on basis of radiograph.

maxillary cyst, although these once were thought to represent separate entities. Nortjé and Farman (1978) reported one of the largest series of biopsy-proven incisive canal cysts in living patients. Among their 51 cases, they reported a male-to-female ratio of 2.3:1 for Africans living in Africa, whereas other races had an equal distribution among sexes. They also observed that these cysts may occur in people of any age, but they are rare in the first decade of life. The most common signs were palatal swelling (88%), anterior tooth displacement (78%), sublabial swelling (18%), and low-grade pain (24%). Most patients complained of a transient salty taste. The adjacent teeth were vital. Smaller lesions are treated by surgical enucleation, and marsupialization has worked well for larger cysts. In their series of 51 cases treated with these two methods, Nortjé and Farman (1978) reported no recurrences.

◆ *RADIOLOGY (Figs. 10–8 to 10–10)*

In the radiologic diagnosis of this cyst, the first step is to determine whether the maxillary midline radiolucency represents a normal incisive foramen or incisive canal cyst. In a study of 2000 skulls, Roper-Hall (1938) found that the normal incisive foramen was 5 mm wide and 7 mm deep anteroposteriorly. Chamda and Shear (1980) examined 970 African skulls and found the dimensions to be 6 mm wide and up to 10 mm deep anteroposteriorly. These measurements are useful norms when there are no other signs and symptoms. The incisive foramen, although radiolucent, lacks a corticated outline. Thus, when a corticated radiolucency is observed in the maxillary midline, even when the lesion is small, an incisive canal cyst should be suspected.

According to Uemura and Hashida (1985), the most characteristic radiographic sign of the incisive canal cyst is a partial lack of a cortical margin at the most inferior and superior aspects of some lesions. These authors stated that the diameter of the canal and tangential x-ray effect cause this variation. If the canal is narrow with respect to the diameter of the cyst, the cystic margin probably will be continuous because the x-ray beam will have tangential points on the bone, which forms the corticated margin of the cyst; however, when the incisive canal is wide, there will be no tangential points within the bone encompassing the corticated margin, and the incisive canal cyst will lack a corticated margin at the superior and inferior aspects within the area overlying the incisive canal. With these findings, the most likely diagnosis is incisive canal cyst.

Smaller lesions are round or ovoid; however, the most unique appearance is a heart shape, which is caused by the superimposition of the anterior nasal spine over the superior portion of the lesion. The central incisors may be displaced; according to Nortjé and Farman (1978), resorption of the adjacent roots is rare, although Uemura and Hashida (1985) reported that resorption and displacement may be seen. Campbell and colleagues (1973) described a large heart-shaped incisive canal cyst in a 15-year-old African-American boy with tooth displacement and resorption of the apical portion of the roots. Nortjé and Farman (1978) pointed out that some cysts are much higher up, beyond the apices of the central incisors. They also observed that very large incisive canal cysts (3 cm in diameter) may develop in Africans younger than 20 years of age. In such patients, expansion and extreme thinning of the buccal cortex have been observed. Occasionally the incisive canal cyst develops asymmetrically and enlarges more to one side. In some instances, the incisive canal cyst may reach a certain size and then remain static for many years. A long-standing cyst is indicated by a much thicker and more densely sclerotic cortical outline than that of the usual incisive canal cyst. Some incisive canal cysts have no sclerotic margin; this finding usually results from infection, most likely originating in the nasal mucosa and spreading to the cyst wall. Other common sources of infection include the dental pulp and periodontal disease.

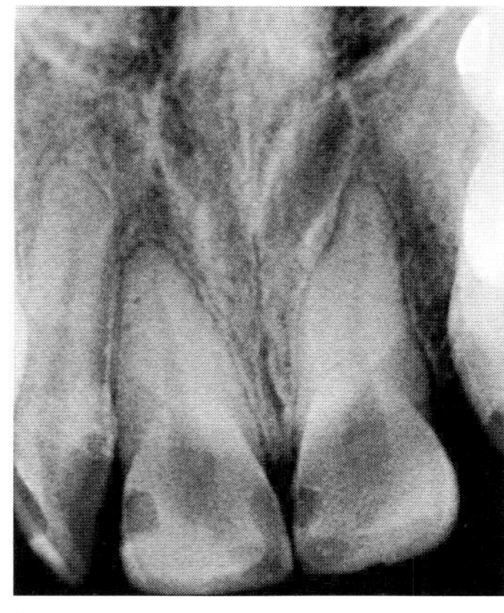

A

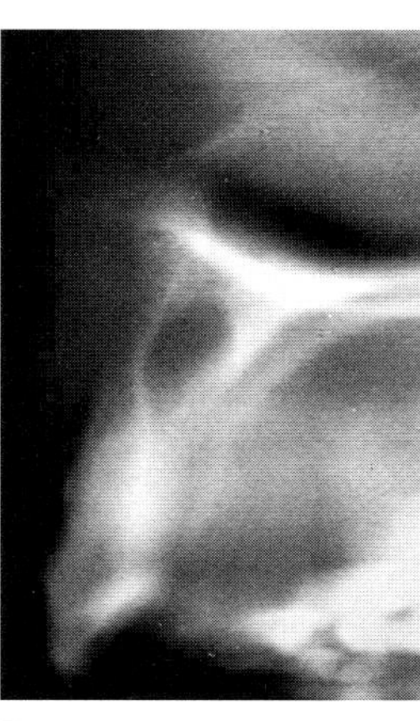

B

FIGURE 10–9.

Incisive canal cyst. Absent superior and inferior margins. A, Periapical view. B, Tomographic view of same case. (Courtesy of Drs. Alvaro Castro Delgado and Gabriel Castro Delgado, Universidad Haveriana, Santa Fé de Bogotá, Columbia.)

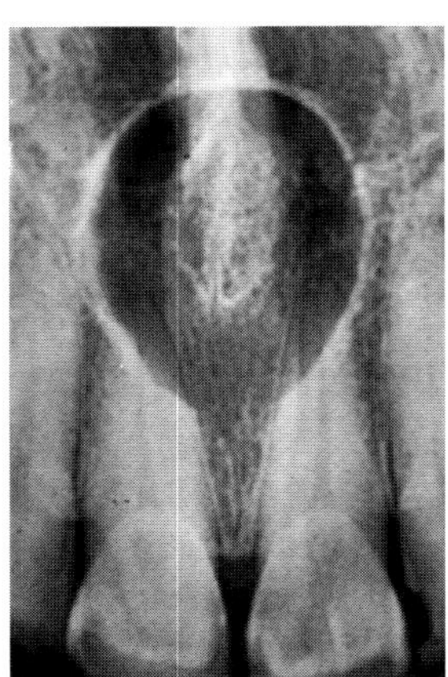

A

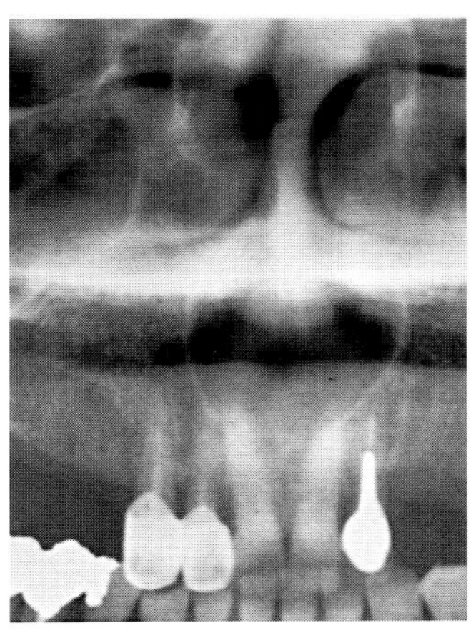

B

FIGURE 10–8.

Incisive canal cyst. A, Occlusal view. (Courtesy of Dr. S. Matteson, University of Texas Health Science Center, San Antonio, TX.) B, Panoramic view. (Courtesy of Drs. M. Araki and K. Hashimoto, Nihon University School of Dentistry, Tokyo, Japan.)

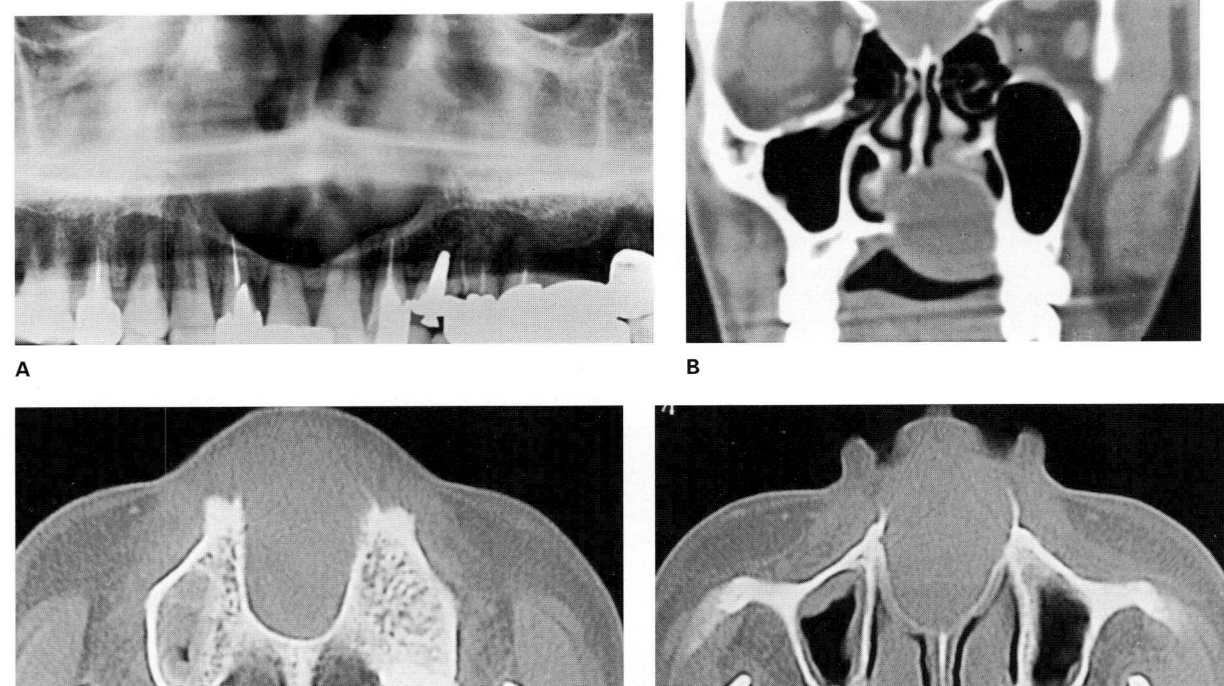

FIGURE 10–10.

Incisive canal cyst. Case in a 49-year-old man. A, Panoramic view shows few details. B, Coronal CT image. C and D, Axial CT images indicate erosion of hard palate and extension into nasal cavity, including nasal septum. Labial sclerotic margin is absent with bone window. (Courtesy of Drs. M. Araki, K. Hashimoto, and K. Honda, Nihon University School of Dentistry, Tokyo, Japan.)

CYST OF THE INCISIVE PAPILLA (Cyst of the palatine papilla)

The cyst of the incisive papilla is the soft tissue variant of the incisive canal cyst. In such instances, the incisive papilla appears enlarged and may be painful because of secondary infection or trauma from the mandibular incisor teeth. This cyst is usually smaller than 1 cm and occupies the natural depression in the maxilla on the palatal side at the incisive foramen. When it is enucleated, it usually does not recur.

◆ *RADIOLOGY (Fig. 10–11)*

We could not find radiographic features peculiar to this cyst. This is not surprising because it is entirely within soft tissue. The extent of the cyst may be estimated by injecting radiopaque dye into the lumen and subsequently taking a periapical radiograph with the paralleling technique.

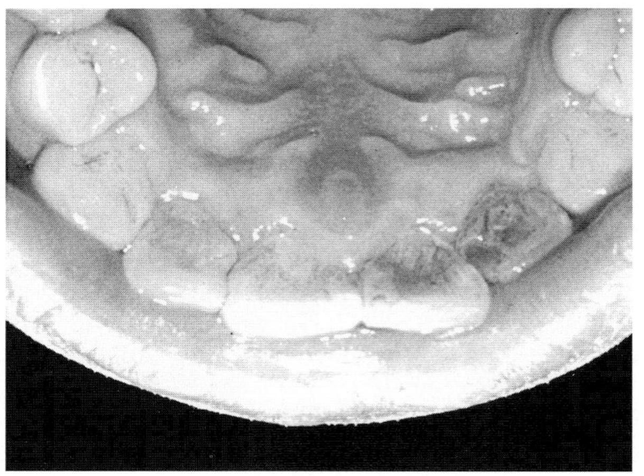

FIGURE 10–11.

Cyst of the incisive papilla. Soft tissue cyst was traumatized by mandibular incisor teeth and became infected. Radiograph appeared normal.

NASOLABIAL CYST (Nasoalveolar cyst, Klestadt's cyst)

Most authors, including Christ (1970) and Shear (1985), believed that this is a true developmental cyst. It probably arises from the lower anterior part of the nasolacrimal duct, which is lined by pseudostratified columnar epithelium, the same type of epithelial lining found in the nasolabial cyst. In his review of jaw cysts, Shear (1985) reported a wide age distribution, ranging from 12 to 75 years. Seventy-nine percent of cases occur in female patients. In the series of eight cases reported by Chinellato and Damante (1984), seven occurred in female patients. Clinical evidence of this cyst includes the "canine fossa sign," characterized by the following features:

1. Loss of the nasolabial fold on the affected side.
2. Elevation of the ala on the affected side.
3. Deformation of the naris on the affected side.
4. A diminished depth of the mucobuccal fold on the affected side.

Intraorally, swelling is observed in the mucobuccal fold in the region of the canine fossa. Straw-colored fluid may be obtained on aspiration. Patients usually have no symptoms. These cysts are excised, and recurrence is unlikely.

◆ *RADIOLOGY (Figs. 10–12 to 10–14)*

Contrary to popular belief, these cysts may be studied with occlusal radiographs and other imaging modalities. Chinellato and Damante (1984) reviewed the radiologic features of eight nasoalveolar cysts. Normally the corticated margins corresponding to the lateral and anterior limits of the nasal fossa are thin and convex in a lateral direction. When a nasolabial cyst is present, there is expansion and sometimes thickening of this line, with the convexity reversed toward the medial or nasal fossa because of pressure from the adjacent soft tissue cyst. Pressure of the cyst on the periosteal surface of the maxilla results in rarefaction,

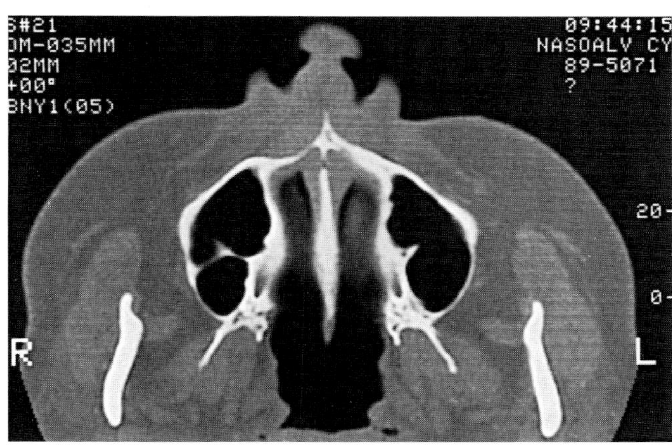

FIGURE 10–13.

Nasolabial cyst. Axial CT image shows reverse architecture and buttress formation at the nasal wall on the right side. (Courtesy of Professor H. Fuchihata, Osaka University School of Dentistry, Osaka, Japan.)

which produces a diffuse area of diminished density immediately beneath the cyst. There is an increased distance between the apices of adjacent teeth and the margin of the nasal fossa on the affected side when compared with the normal side. Only one case had no observable change. Seward (1962) made similar observations, emphasizing the appearance of the lateral wall of the nasal fossa in the occlusal view.

The extent of the cyst may be determined by injecting radiopaque contrast material into the lumen and subsequently taking radiographs, preferably two different views at right angles to each other so that all three dimensions (height, width, and depth) can be observed.

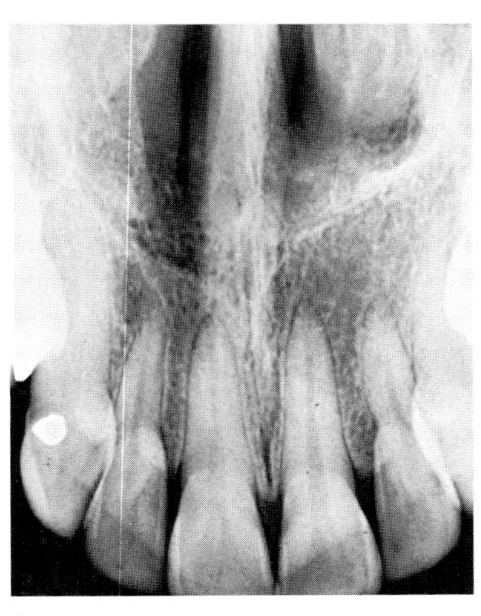

A

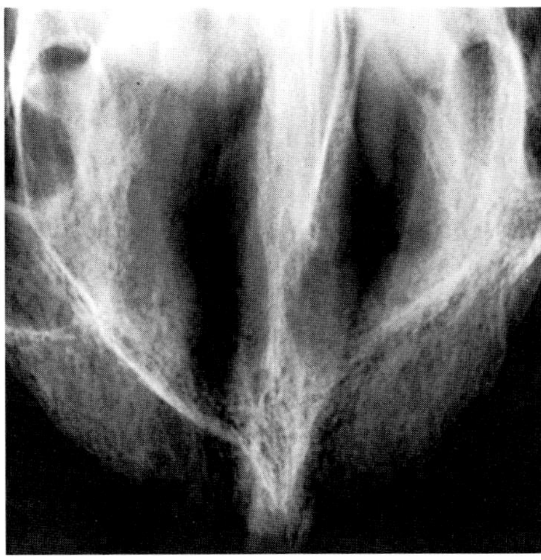

B

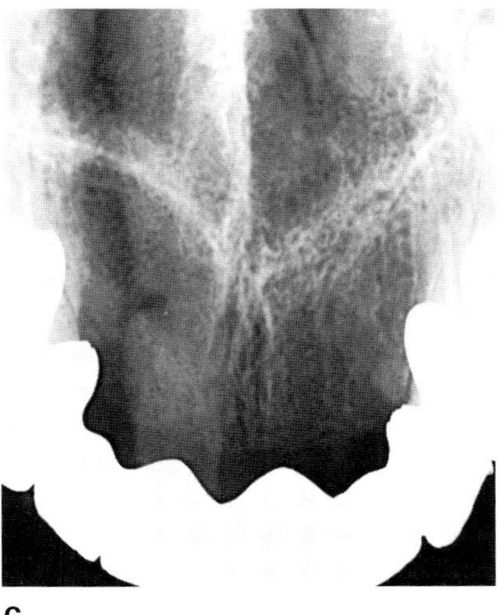

C

FIGURE 10–12.

Nasolabial cyst. A, Reverse architecture of wall of nasal fossa and increased distance between this line and apices of adjacent teeth. B, Reverse architecture and thinning of nasal fossa wall. C, Wall of nasal fossa is diffusely sclerotic and appears as a straight line. (From Chinellato LEM, Damante JH: Contribution of radiographs in the diagnosis of nasoalveolar cyst. Oral Surg Oral Med Oral Pathol 58:729, 1984.)

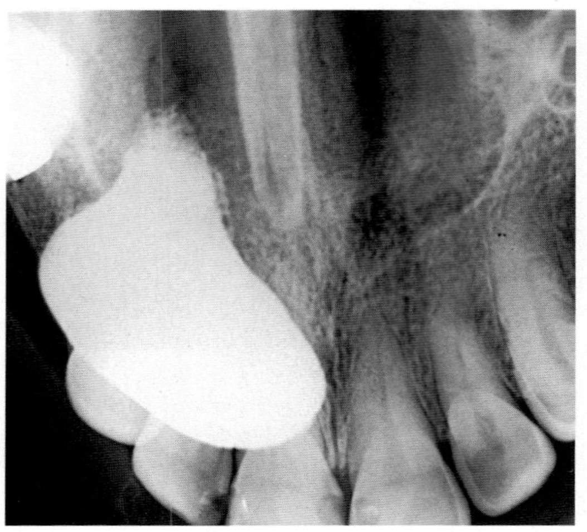

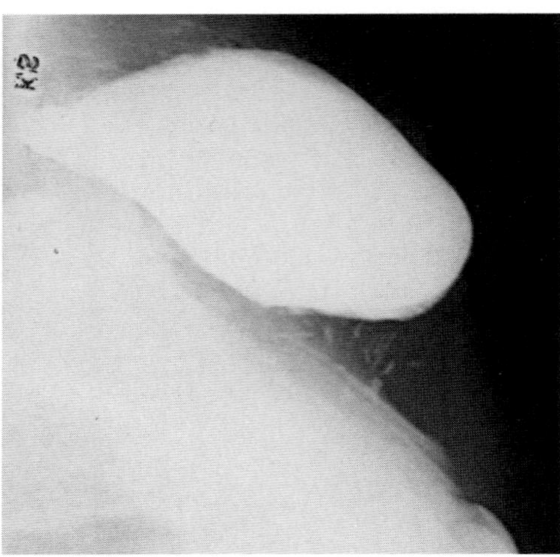

A B

FIGURE 10–14.

Nasolabial cyst. Injected cysts in different patients. A, Occlusal view. B, Lateral Miller right-angle view. (Courtesy of Professor L. Alfaro, University of Chile School of Dentistry, Pathology Referral Center, Santiago, Chile.)

Cohen and Hertzanu (1985) emphasized the huge growth potential of some nasolabial cysts when they are not excised. They also stressed the utility of coronal and axial computed tomography (CT) images and a soft tissue window. In addition, these authors described a huge case approximately the size of a lemon. The CT scans showed erosion of the maxilla and penetration into the maxillary sinus and nasal fossa.

GLOBULOMAXILLARY CYST
(Globulomaxillary lesion)

The globulomaxillary cyst is one of three radiologically distinct ''cysts'' that may have a variety of histopathologic diagnoses. The other two cystic conditions are the residual cyst and median mandibular cyst. The clinical term globulomaxillary lesion might be more appropriate. In 1937, Thoma originated the fissural concept for the development of the globulomaxillary cyst. In Wysocki's 1981 review of this report, he found that Thoma's original cases appeared to be consistent with a diagnosis of radicular cyst. Others, including Christ (1970), have proposed an odontogenic origin of the globulomaxillary cyst; Little and Jacobsen (1973) suggested a dual origin, indicating that it may arise from odontogenic or nonodontogenic epithelium. In 1981, Wysocki examined 10,000 consecutive biopsy specimens at the University of Western Ontario. In 37 cases, the clinical diagnosis was globulomaxillary cyst. On examination of the radiographs and histopathologic features of these 37 cases, he found the following: radicular cyst, 25 cases (68%); periapical granuloma, 6 cases (16%); lateral (developmental) periodontal cyst, 4 cases (11%); odontogenic keratocyst, 3 cases (8%); central giant cell granuloma, 3 cases (8%); calcifying odontogenic cyst, 1 case (3%); and odontogenic myxoma, 1 case (3%). Wysocki (1981) concluded that fissural inclusion is a misconception and the globulomaxillary cyst should be deleted from the classification of orofacial fissural cysts. Several other cases of adenomatoid odontogenic tumor masquerading as a globulomaxillary cyst have been reported by Glickman and colleagues (1983) and Khan and co-workers (1977); Tiacher and Azaz (1977) reported two lesions resembling globulomaxillary cysts: one was an odontogenic myxoma and the other a radicular cyst in association with a nonvital lateral incisor.

◆ *RADIOLOGY (Figs. 10–15 and 10–16)*

The globulomaxillary lesion has radiodistinct features, probably resulting from the location rather than the pathologic process. It is located uniquely between the maxillary lateral incisor and canine teeth and consists of a well-defined radiolucency, usually with a round, ovoid, or, more classically,

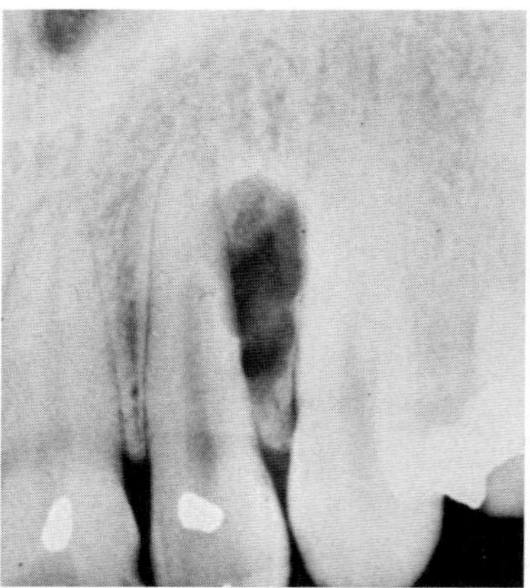

FIGURE 10–15.

Globulomaxillary lesion. This lesion was signed out as a globulomaxillary cyst. (Courtesy of Professor Gunilla Tronje, Karolinska Institutet, Stockholm, Sweden.)

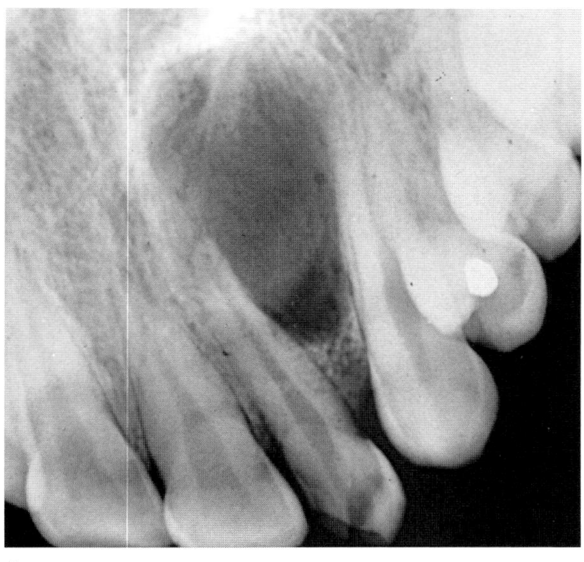

A

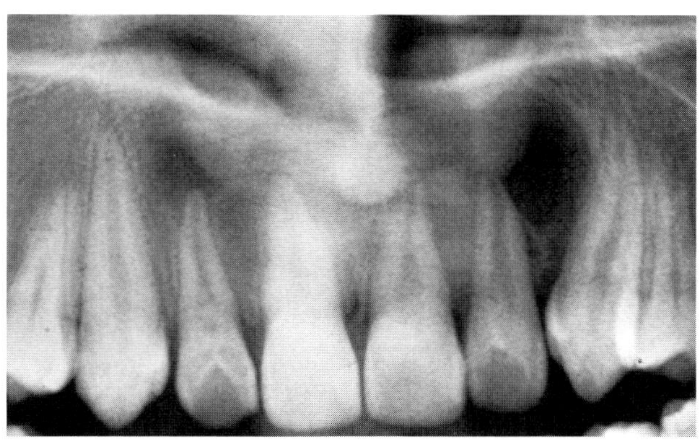

B

FIGURE 10–16.

Globulomaxillary lesion. Sequelae of nonvital lateral incisors. A, Classic pear-shaped appearance. B, Bilateral lesions. Right lesion is located periapically, whereas the left is globulomaxillary.

pearlike shape. The margins may be well corticated. This lesion rarely exceeds 1.5 cm in diameter but often causes divergence of the roots of the adjacent lateral and canine teeth. In some instances the lamina dura may be resorbed. The rarer, larger lesions may appear to encroach upon the nasal fossa. A dens-in-dente may be observed within the coronal portion of the lateral incisor, and deep caries, large restorations, incomplete endodontic treatment, and signs of trauma such as fracture of a cusp tip may be found in an adjacent tooth. The globulomaxillary lesion must be diagnosed clinically and radiologically, with additional endodontic and sometimes histopathologic evaluation needed to determine the final diagnosis.

MEDIAN MANDIBULAR CYST

The median mandibular cyst is one of the three radiologically distinct lesions that may have a variety of specific histopathologic diagnoses. The other two are the globulomaxillary cyst and residual cyst. The term median mandibular cyst still may be used because all of the re-reviewed cases of this entity were cystic; however, the current authors recommend reservation of the term for clinical use when a cystic lesion is suspected in this specific location. Studies by Richany and associates (1956) and Ten Cate (1980) led many investigators to question the validity of the theory of epithelial entrapment between the mandibular symphysis during development. Currently, most authors do not accept the existence of the median mandibular cyst as a distinct histopathologic entity. In 1977, Soskolne and Shteyer proposed that the median mandibular cyst consists of one of three basic cyst types: (1) inflammatory cyst arising adjacent to a lateral accessory root canal, (2) odontogenic keratocyst, and (3) lateral (developmental) periodontal cyst. In his 1988 review of the literature, Gardner critically analyzed all reports of median mandibular cysts and found 20 cases. His interpretations of the histopathologic findings were as follows: radicular cyst, 12 cases; odontogenic keratocyst, 2 cases; and residual cyst, lateral (developmental) periodontal cyst, lateral (inflammatory) periodontal cyst, residual or radicular cyst, radicular or odontogenic keratocyst, and developmental odontogenic cyst with pseudostratified ciliated columnar epithelium with mucous cells, 1 case each. Gardner (1988) emphasized the importance of recognizing that cilia and mucous cells may be found in odontogenic cysts. Treatment should include enucleation when appropriate, but endodontic therapy may be the only treatment required in some cases.

◆ *RADIOLOGY (Figs. 10–17 and 10–18)*

Some median mandibular cysts are small and confined to the area between the central incisors. Other slightly larger lesions, such as the two reported by Buchner and Ramon (1974), may cause divergence of the roots of the mandibular central incisors. Occasionally, as with the case of Lacourt and Dones (1976), a huge lesion is reported, extending from second molar to second molar bilaterally; none of the mandibular teeth, except the second and third molars, responded to the electric pulp test. In his review of this large cystlike lesion, Gardner (1988) interpreted this lesion as a radicular cyst. He stated that, in this case, one must look for radiologic signs of a nonvital mandibular central incisor, such as a deep carious lesion, deep or large restoration, fractured cusp, or even a fractured maxillary central or lateral incisor, indicating possible trauma to the mandibular incisors.

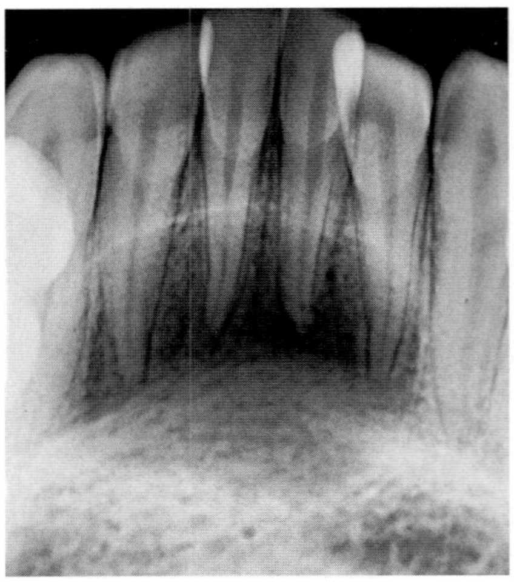

A

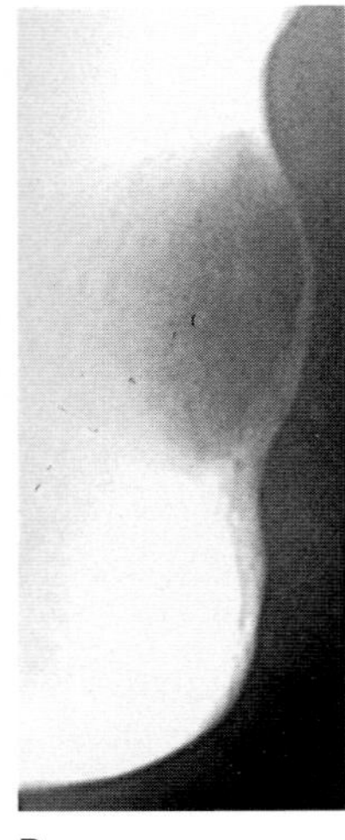

B

FIGURE 10–17.

Median mandibular cyst. A, No obvious tooth with nonvital pulp can be seen. B, Expanded buccal cortex shows typical cystic morphologic characteristics; lesion was signed out as a median mandibular cyst. (Courtesy of Professor L. Alfaro, University of Chile School of Dentistry, Santiago, Chile.)

TRAUMATIC CYST (Solitary bone cyst, hemorrhagic bone cyst, extravasation cyst, simple bone cyst, unicameral cyst)

The traumatic cyst is one of several pseudocysts of the jaws; the others are aneurysmal bone cyst and Stafne's cyst (submandibular salivary gland depression). The lesion is common, and approximately 250 cases have been reported.

Pathologic Characteristics

The traumatic cyst has an empty cavity. Sometimes it contains a small amount of fluid, and when the walls are curetted, the pathologist identifies connective tissue and viable bone fragments. The cause and pathogenesis of this lesion remain a mystery, and the role of trauma is questioned by many.

Clinical Features

Traumatic cysts are common, with many large series being reported, including 22 cases by Morris and colleagues (1970), 30 cases by Beasley (1970), and 66 cases by Hansen and co-authors (1974). Huebner and Turlington (1971) reviewed the literature and analyzed 150 reported cases. In 1987, Kaugars and Cale critically reviewed the literature, finding 94 cases that met their criteria; with 67 new cases of their own, their sample consisted of 161 traumatic cysts. Although many authors reported a male-to-female ratio of 2:1, Kaugars and Cale (1987) found an equal sex distribution. This finding leads one to question the role of trauma because one may expect men to experience more facial trauma than women. They found that the incidence of prior trauma was equivalent to that in the general population. The average patient age was 18 years. In the series reported by Hansen and colleagues (1974), 58% of patients were 20 years or younger, whereas Beasley (1976) found that 65% were 20 years or younger. Kaugars and Cale (1987) stated that 27% of the patients in their series were older than 30 years, and in this group there was a much higher percentage of female African-Americans. They also found a slight predilection for African-American people compared with other racial groups. Kaugars and Cale (1987) discovered that 60% of the reported cases were symptomatic, but in their own series only 26% of the cases were accompanied by symptoms. They believe the lower percentage is more accurate because cases with unusual features are more likely to be published. In a 16-year-old girl, Freedman and Beigleman (1985) reported a huge traumatic cyst extending from the second premolar to the sigmoid notch in the ramus; although there was extensive cortical erosion and expansion, the patient had no symptoms.

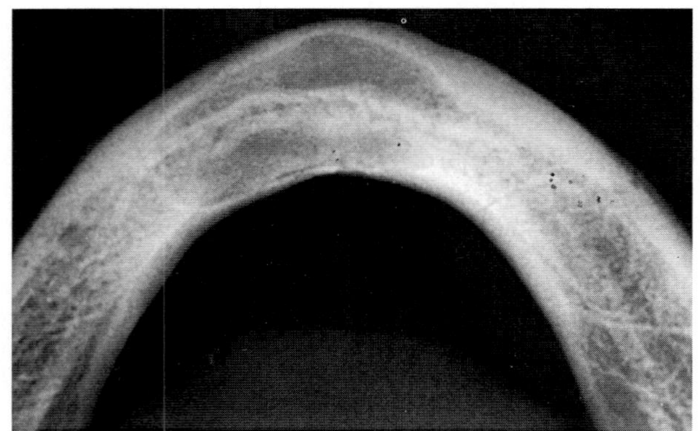

FIGURE 10–18.

Median mandibular cyst. Occlusal view. Case was a residual cyst.

Treatment/Prognosis

Treatment usually consists of surgical exploration and curettage of the bony walls. Kaugars and Cale (1987) believed it was not necessary to treat teeth whose apices were within the cavity. Curettage usually results in uneventful resolution. Some traumatic cysts may resolve spontaneously, without surgical intervention. Szerlip (1966) reported a patient with bilateral traumatic cysts that resolved in 4 years. Kaugars and Cale (1987) did not recommend observation of lesions that appear to be traumatic cysts because of the possibility of an erroneous diagnosis or, in rare instances, the occurrence of pathologic fracture because the cyst was not treated. Several reported cases of traumatic cyst involve fractures, including the case of Baird and Askew (1958). Although recurrence is rare, Kaugars and Cale (1987) found that lesions were more likely to recur in female patients, those with multiple lesions, or patients who had a bluish discoloration of the bone at surgery, which results from the thinness of the overlying bone and transmission of the blue portion of the color spectrum by the fluid within the cavity. With such thin bone, it may not be so much a question of recurrence, but a lack of resolution when such a degree of bone destruction has occurred. Precious and McFadden (1984) injected autogenic blood into one large cyst that had not resolved with curettage. This second procedure produced rapid bony filling and healing within 3 months.

Traumatic cysts have been reported in association with florid osseous dysplasia. These will be discussed with florid osseous dysplasia in the chapter titled "Generalized Radiopacities."

◆ RADIOLOGY (Figs. 10–19 and 10–24)

Uemura and Hashida (1985) stated that the traumatic cyst is an asymptomatic lesion discovered by routine panoramic radiographs. All of their 15 cases were found in this manner. In addition, the authors stated that this cyst has been detected more frequently in Japan with the increased use of rotational panoramic radiography.

Location

In their review of the literature, Kaugars and Cale (1987) found that 95% of cases occurred in the mandible; of their own cases, 98.5% were mandibular lesions. Huebner and Turlington (1971) reported that, of the 150 traumatic jaw cysts they reviewed, 96% occurred in the mandible and 4% in the maxilla. Among the mandibular lesions, most occur in the region of the premolars and molars and a few extend into the ramus. One unique feature of this cyst is that it may occur in or cross the midline. Huebner and Turlington (1971) reported that 24% occurred in the symphysis area; in their series of 22 cases, Morris and colleagues (1970) stated that 23% crossed the midline. Kaugars and Cale (1987) found that 27% of cases were anterior to the distal surface of the canines, and 20% of these crossed the midline. Bilateral traumatic cysts have been reported by Patrikiou and colleagues (1981) and Pogrel (1978).

Radiologic Features

The classic description of the traumatic cyst, as well as its most diagnostic feature, is that it lies above the inferior alveolar canal and squeezes up between the roots of teeth, producing a scalloped or wavy superior outline; approximately 70% of cases will have this feature. The lamina dura of the adjacent root sockets is said to be unaffected, although resorption is seen in many cases. Uemura and Hashida (1985) found that the lamina dura was absent in all but two of their cases and observed a return of the lamina dura 3 months after surgery. There is rarely any resorption or displacement of the roots of adjacent teeth; these teeth usually are vital.

Uemura and Hashida (1985) indicated an important feature sometimes seen on periapical radiographs—a double contour characterized as fine white lines superimposed on the roots or inter-radicular septa of bone. They consider these findings pathognomonic of any condition that may destroy alveolar bone buccal and lingual to the adjacent teeth without appreciable root resorption. This finding is seen in traumatic cysts and odontogenic myxoma.

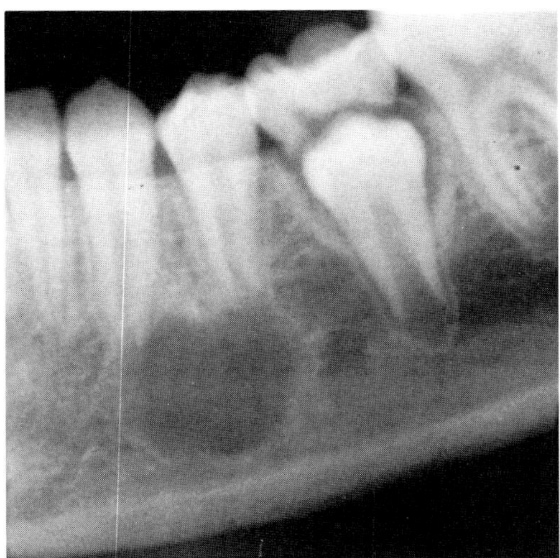
A

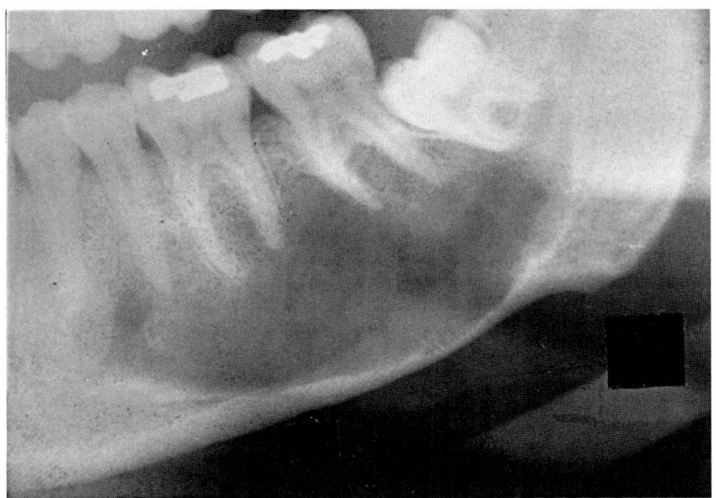
B

FIGURE 10–19.

Traumatic cyst. A, Early lesion does not extend between roots of teeth. (Courtesy of Dr. J. Preece, University of Texas Health Science Center, San Antonio, TX.) B, Large lesion extending between roots, with erosion and expansion of inferior cortex. (Courtesy of Dr. G. Moyer, National Naval Dental Center, Bethesda, MD.)

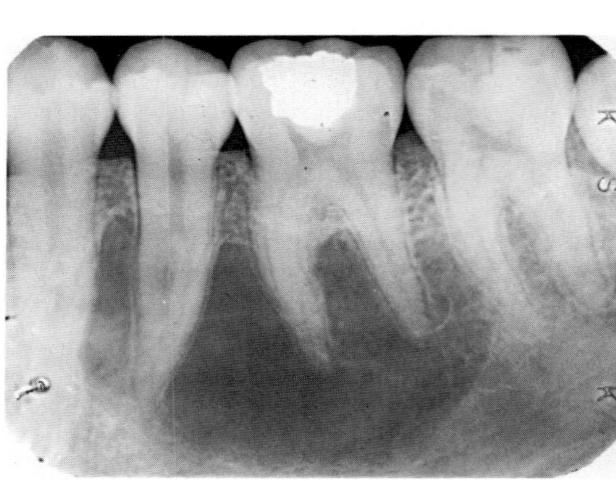

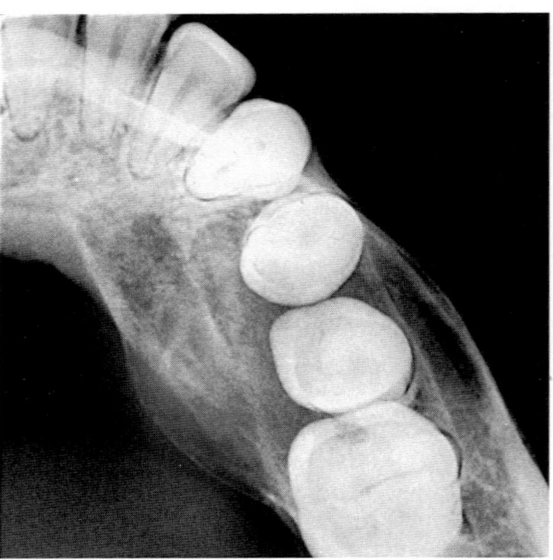

A B

FIGURE 10–20.

Traumatic cyst. A, Lamina dura is relatively intact. B, Expansion of lingual cortex and endosteal erosion of buccal cortex.

Mild expansion and thinning of the cortex may occur often, and the buccal or lingual cortical plates usually are affected. The occlusal view is useful in detecting this expansion. In the review of the literature by Kaugars and Cale (1987), expansion was observed in 44% of the cases. Rarely, there is expansion of the inferior cortex, and it may be thinned significantly by larger lesions. The inferior alveolar canal may appear to be displaced inferiorly, or its cortical outline may be resorbed completely. In this instance, the surgeon will find the neurovascular bundle hanging within the defect like a clothesline.

The lesions may be small and confined to one or two teeth, or they may fill the entire length of the body of the mandible and extend into the ramus or cross the midline. Approximately 50% will be greater than 3 cm in diameter when detected and roughly 25% each will be between 2 and 3 cm and 1 and 2 cm in diameter; few cases smaller than 1 cm are seen. Approximately 64% of the cases will have a cone shape at one end; the remainder are distributed equally between irregular, ovoid, or round shapes. Smaller lesions appear unilocular, whereas large ones may have a scalloped outline. In 27% of the lesions reported by Morris and colleagues (1970), at least half or more of the margin of the defect was well defined by a delicate sclerotic rim. In the remaining cases, lesser amounts of cortication were apparent at the margins, and in some there was no apparent cortication. In 69% of the cases studied by Uemura and Hashida (1985), a well-corticated but fine margin was seen. Thus,

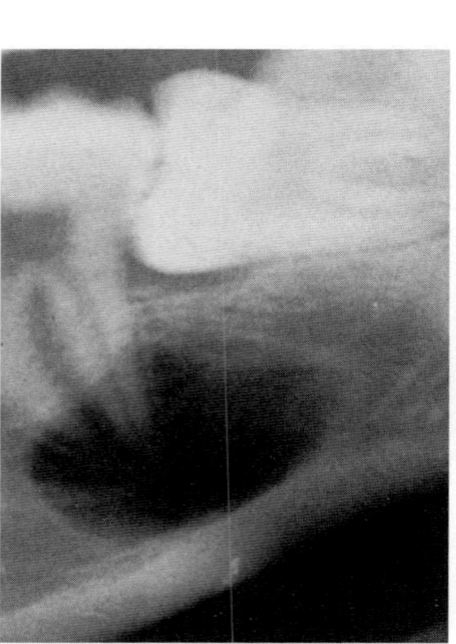

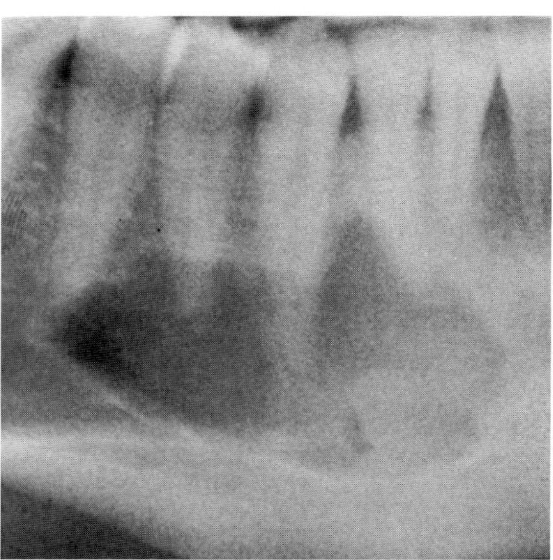

A B

FIGURE 10–21.

Traumatic cyst. Linear margin forms straight plane at interface, with normal bone imparting V-shaped leading edge. A, Posterior view. B, Anterior view.

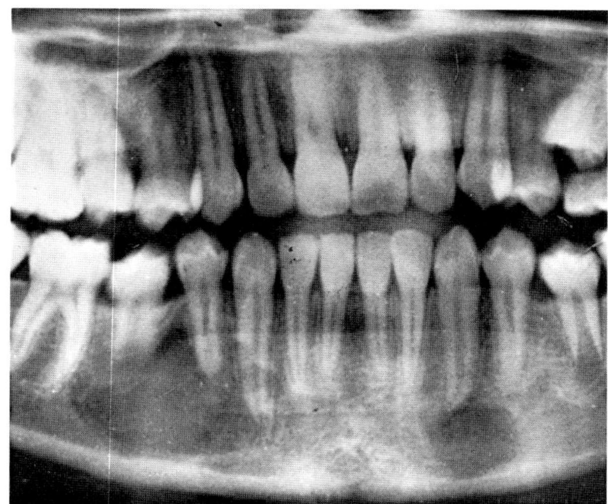

FIGURE 10–22.

Traumatic cyst. Bilateral lesions in mandible.

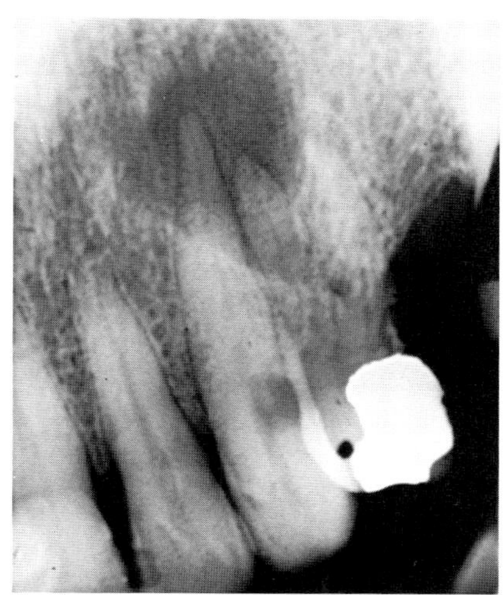

FIGURE 10–23.

Traumatic cyst. Case in an unusual maxillary location. The margin has a linear appearance. (Courtesy of Dr. L. Otis, University of California at San Francisco, San Francisco, CA.)

the margin may be thin, condensed, and intact; it may consist of irregular, discontinuous, almost interwoven areas of sclerotic bone; it may appear essentially punched-out; or there may be varying combinations of these three patterns.

To our knowledge, the following new features of traumatic cyst have never been reported: First, is the finding that nearly all lesions are broader anteroposteriorly than superoinferiorly. The second is a tendency for the radiograph to be overexposed in the area of the lesion, a phenomenon that becomes more characteristic as lesions become larger. This probably is because the traumatic cyst often does not contain anything but air, whereas similar radiolucent lesions contain cystic fluid or tumor, with both attenuating the beam of radiation so that the radiograph will not be overexposed. Third, the leading margin forms a very straight plane at the interface, with normal bone and an adjacent similar plane forming a "V" or cone shape; this V-shape may be seen anteriorly or posteriorly, and infrequently the tip of the cone is directed toward the teeth. This feature is highly characteristic because

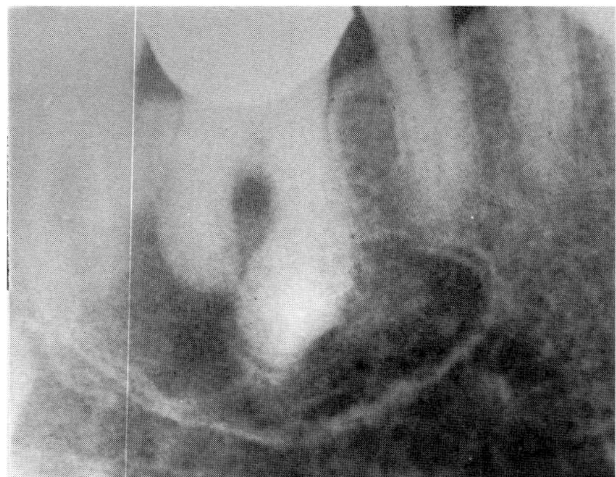

A

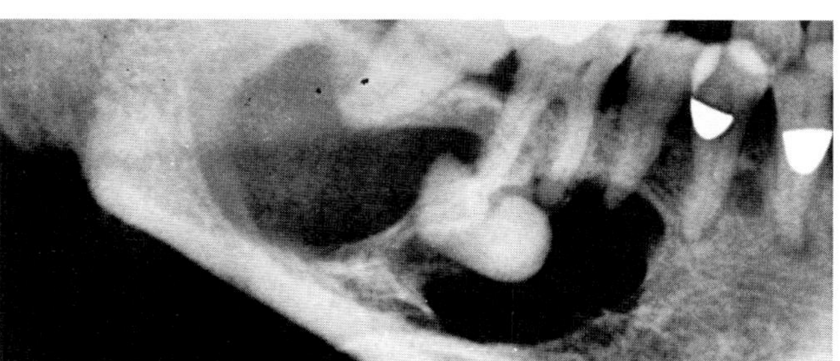

B

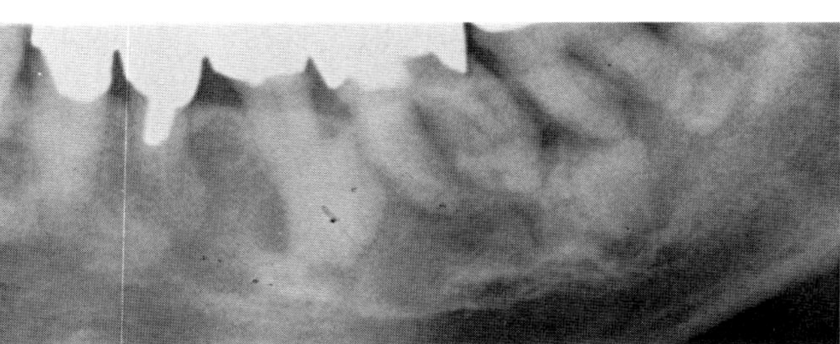

C

FIGURE 10–24.

Traumatic cyst. Association with cemental lesions. A, Hypercementosis. B, Periapical cemental dysplasia. C, Florid cemento-osseous dysplasia. (Courtesy of M. Araki, K. Hashimoto, and K. Honda, Nihon University, School of Dentistry, Tokyo, Japan.)

we know of no other jaw lesion manifesting in this way except nonossifying fibroma, which is very rare. Fourth, evidence of trauma, consisting mainly of nondisplaced or incomplete fractures of the mandible, may be seen in approximately 15 to 25% of cases; other less reliable signs of trauma include a recent extraction socket, orthodontic appliances, surgical wires, and location in an edentulous area. The fractures are fine lines that sometimes extend up into the alveolar bone between teeth adjacent to the cystic lesion; the fracture line may branch within the body of the mandible and extend to the inferior cortex of the mandible. Displacement of the fracture segments does not occur, and the fracture rarely is on the side opposite the cyst. Once we noticed a thin fragment of dense bone within the central part of a cyst, resembling the "fallen trabecula" sign seen exclusively in bones with traumatic cyst and pathologic fracture; however, we found no jaw fractures in our case with an apparent "fallen trabecula" sign.

The relationship of traumatic cyst to cemental lesions has been reviewed, and we have included several illustrations in this chapter. Additional details appear in the discussions on hypercementosis, periapical cemental dysplasia, and florid cemento-osseous dysplasia.

Radiologic Features of the Skeleton

Traumatic cyst of the jaws is the same lesion as the simple, solitary or unicameral bone cyst found in other parts of the skeleton. The simple bone cyst occurs in the same age group; however, the male-to-female ratio is 2.5:1. Edeiken (1981) outlined the following features: Seventy-five percent occur in the humerus or femur, usually in the metaphysis close to the epiphyseal plate. The simple bone cyst is seen as an oval radiolucency whose long axis is parallel to that of the bone. It is bounded by a thin sclerotic border, may erode the inner cortex, and may cause slight expansion. A periosteal reaction almost invariably is absent unless pathologic fracture has occurred. Pathologic fracture frequently occurs if the cyst is not treated, and it results in the "fallen trabecula" sign. When discovered, these cysts usually are 2 to 3 cm long, but may fill the entire length of the involved bone.

SQUAMOUS ODONTOGENIC TUMOR

(Benign epithelial odontogenic tumor)

Squamous odontogenic tumor first was reported in 1975 by Pullon and associates. According to Leider and colleagues (1989), 29 cases have been reported, including 3 of their own.

Pathologic Characteristics

Because many of these lesions seem to arise within the alveolar bone, between the roots of teeth, they may result from the proliferation of the epithelial rests of Malassez. The lesion is characterized by islands of stratified squamous epithelium in a fibrous connective tissue stroma. Some islands may show a single cell layer thickness of cuboidal or flattened epithelial cells and vacuolization or microcyst formation inside the islands. Sometimes laminated calcific structures or connective tissue may be within the islands.

Clinical Features

In 1982, Goldblatt and colleagues reviewed the literature and presented five new cases. The patients' ages ranged from 11 to 67 years; when the most recent cases are included, 65% occurred in patients between 19 and 31 years of age. According to Leider and colleagues (1989), the average age is 36 years. There may be a predilection for African-Americans. In the 1986 review by Mills and associates, there was an even distribution between male and female patients. Leider and colleagues (1989) reported the only cases of squamous odontogenic tumor occurring in siblings. The lesions developed when the patients were 25, 26, and 29 years of age; there were two brothers and a sister. The patients were African-American, and multiple sites were involved. Goldblatt and co-workers (1982) stated that the most common sign is tooth mobility, which occurred in 50% of patients; 25% complained of tooth pain or tenderness, particularly with percussion. In the case of Anneroth and Hansen (1982), there was thermal sensitivity, and a painless swelling also was observed.

Treatment/Prognosis

Cases usually are treated by local excision after extraction of the involved teeth. Maxillary lesions appear to be more destructive; thus, more extensive surgical excision is required. Currently, no lesions have recurred, except the first case of Pullon and colleagues (1975), which did not return once generalized extraction and alveoloplasty were performed.

◆ *RADIOLOGY (Figs. 10–25 to 10–27)*

Location

Goldblatt and colleagues (1982) found that 60% of the 16 cases they studied were in the maxilla; of these, all but one were in the lateral-canine region. They also reported that 50% of the cases had mandibular involvement, with the most common location being the premolar-molar region. Approximately 25 to 30% of the cases have had multiple sites of involvement.

Radiologic Features

As Goldblatt and colleagues (1982) indicated, one of the most strikingly constant features of the squamous odontogenic tumor is its presentation as a triangular or semicircular radiolucency within the alveolar bone between the roots of several teeth. In most reports for which radiographs were published, the authors observed three additional features concerning mandibular lesions: (1) one or both of the adjacent roots often are displaced, (2) the crestal bone tends to be destroyed, and (3) most cases appear to have a sclerotic rim; it may be thin and wispy, but more frequently it is thick and condensed or more diffuse. The mandibular lesions rarely seem to spread more than 1 cm beyond the apices of the involved teeth, but in some cases they appear to spread from tooth to tooth.

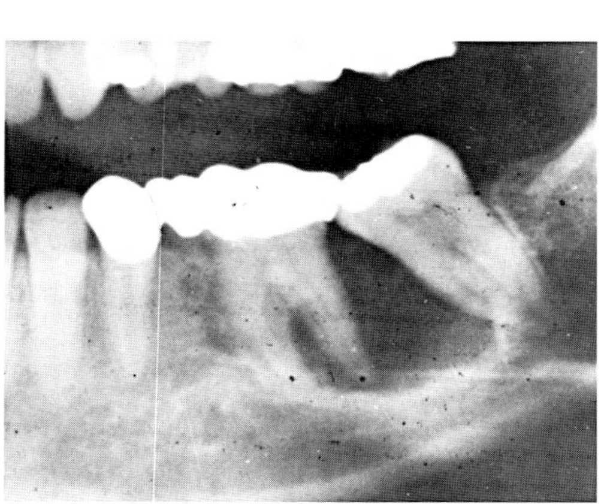

A

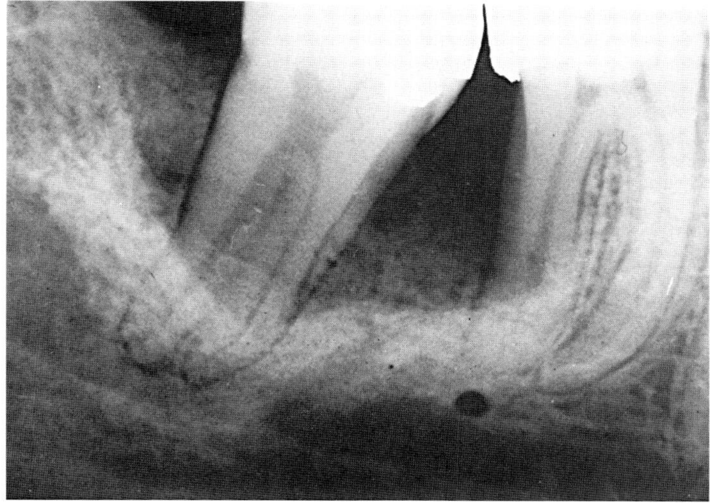

B

FIGURE 10–25.

Squamous odontogenic tumor. A and B, Displacement of an adjacent tooth and loss of crestal bone in the lesional area, which is triangular and has a prominent diffuse sclerotic margin. (From Goldblatt LI, Brannon RB, Ellis GL: Squamous odontogenic tumor: report of five cases and review of literature. Oral Surg Oral Med Oral Pathol 54:187, 1982.)

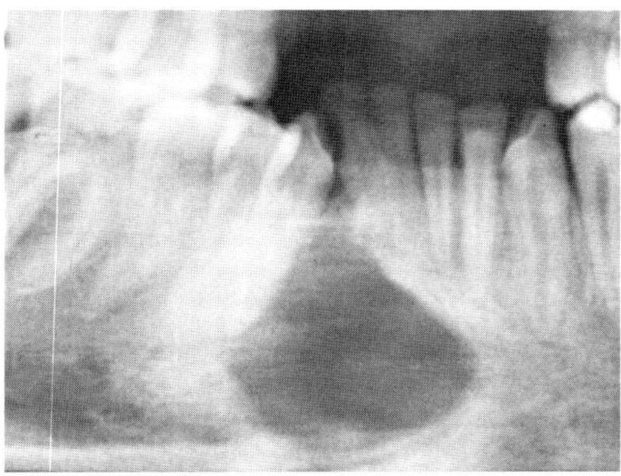

FIGURE 10–26.

Squamous odontogenic tumor. Lesion is in mandibular canine-lateral area: it is triangular, and there is displacement of adjacent teeth, destruction of associated crestal bone, and a diffuse sclerotic margin.

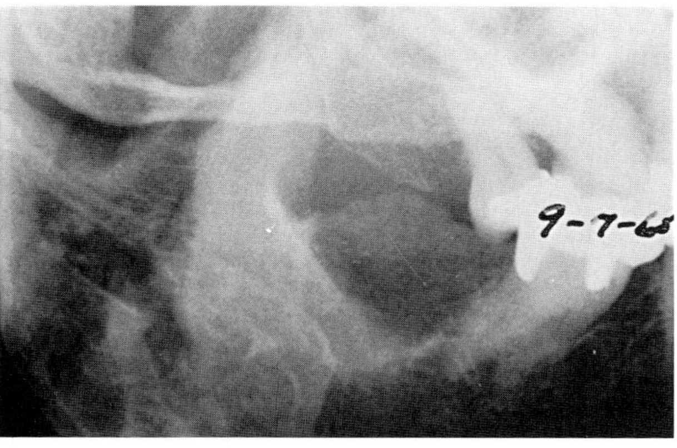

FIGURE 10–27.

Squamous odontogenic tumor. After tooth removal, marginal sclerosis is diminished; soft tissue mass overlies the lesion, with destruction of crestal part of ridge. (From Goldblatt LI, Brannon RB, Ellis GL: Squamous odontogenic tumor: report of five cases and review of literature. Oral Surg Oral Med Oral Pathol 54:187, 1982.)

Maxillary Lesions

Goldblatt and colleagues (1982) emphasized the more destructive nature of lesions in the maxilla, where there is a tendency to perforate through the cortices and extend to involve the palate, maxillary sinuses, nasal floor, and nasal spine. Hopper and colleagues (1980) reported such a case with multiple sites of involvement. One of the cases reported by Pullon and colleagues (1975) consisted of a large pericoronal radiolucency about the crown of an unerupted maxillary canine. There was displacement of the adjacent teeth, and no sclerotic rim appeared to be present at any part of the periphery of the lesion. In one of three cases occurring in the maxilla reported by Doyle and colleagues (1977), the large lesion extending from the maxillary canine to the second molar had a soap bubble appearance. Because maxillary and mandibular lesions are histologically identical, one must assume that the more aggressive nature of the maxillary lesions is a function of location, much as it is with maxillary ameloblastoma and other locally aggressive benign lesions.

References

Anterior Median Maxillary Cleft

Gier RE, Fast TB: Median maxillary anterior alveolar cleft. Oral Surg Oral Med Oral Pathol 24:496, 1967.

Lateral (Developmental) Periodontal Cyst

Baker RD, et al: Squamous cell carcinoma arising in a lateral periodontal cyst. Oral Surg Oral Med Oral Pathol 47:495, 1979.

DiFiore PM, Hartwell GR: Median mandibular lateral periodontal cyst. Oral Surg Oral Med Oral Pathol 63:545, 1987.

Fantasia JE: Lateral periodontal cyst. Oral Surg Oral Med Oral Pathol 48: 237, 1979.

Ross VA, Craig RM, Vizuete JR: A radiolucent lesion adjacent to the roots of the mandibular right first and second premolars. J Am Dent Assoc 112:235, 1986.

Shear M, Pindborg JJ: Microscopic view of the lateral periodontal cyst. Scand J Dent Res 83:103, 1975.

Smith BJ: A lateral periodontal cyst associated with an unerupted premolar. Ann Dent 37:100, 1978.

Wysocki GP, Brannon RB, Gardner DG, Sapp P: Histogenesis of the lateral periodontal cyst and the gingival cyst of the adult. Oral Surg Oral Med Oral Pathol 50:327, 1980.

Gingival Cyst of the Adult

Buchner A, Hansen LS: The histomorphologic spectrum of the gingival cyst in the adult. Oral Surg Oral Med Oral Pathol 48:532, 1979.

Shear M: Cysts of the jaws: recent advances. J Oral Pathol 14:43, 1985.

Wysocki GP, Brannon RB, Gardner DG, Sapp P: Histogenesis of the lateral periodontal cyst and gingival cyst of the adult. Oral Surg Oral Med Oral Pathol 50:327, 1980.

Lateral (Inflammatory) Periodontal Cyst

Craig GT: The paradental cyst: a specific inflammatory odontogenic cyst. Br Dent J 141:9, 1976.

Main DMG: Epithelial jaw cysts: a clinicopathologic reappraisal. Br J Oral Surg 8:114, 1970.

Shear M: Cysts of the Oral Regions. 2nd Ed. Bristol:Wright PSG, 1983, p. 138.

Incisive Canal Cyst

Campbell JJ, Baden E, Williams AC: Nasopalatine cyst of unusual size: report of a case. J Oral Surg 31:776, 1973.

Chamda RA, Shear M: Dimensions of the incisive fossae on dry skulls and radiographs. Int J Oral Surg 9:452, 1980.

Killey HC, Kay LW: Benign Cystic Lesions of the Jaws. 3rd Ed. Edinburgh: Churchill Livingstone, 1977, p. 107.

Meyer AW: Median anterior maxillary cysts. J Am Dent Assoc 18:1851, 1931.

Nortjé CJ, Farman AG: Nasopalatine duct cyst: an aggressive condition in adolescent Negroes from South Africa. Int J Oral Surg 7:65, 1978.

Roper-Hall HT: Cysts of developmental origin in the premaxillary region with special reference to their diagnosis. Br Dent J 65:405, 1938.

Stafne EC, Austin LT, Gardner B: Median anterior maxillary cysts. J Am Dent Assoc 23:801, 1936.

Uemura S, Hashida T: Radiologic interpretation of fissural cysts and postoperative maxillary cyst and simple bone cyst. Oral Radiol 1:69, 1985.

Nasolabial Cyst

Chinellato LEM, Damante JH: Contribution of radiographs in the diagnosis of nasoalveolar cyst. Oral Surg Oral Med Oral Pathol 58:729, 1984.

Christ TF: The globulomaxillary cyst: an embryologic misconception. Oral Surg Oral Med Oral Pathol 30:515, 1970.

Cohen MA, Hertzanu Y: Huge growth potential of the nasolabial cyst. Oral Surg Oral Med Oral Pathol 59:441, 1985.

Seward GR: Nasolabial cysts and their radiology. Dent Pract 12:154, 1962.

Shear M: Cysts of the jaws: recent advances. J Oral Pathol 14:43, 1985.

Globulomaxillary Cyst

Christ TF: The globulomaxillary cyst: an embryonic misconception. Oral Surg Oral Med Oral Pathol 30:515, 1970.

Glickman R, et al: An adenomatoid odontogenic tumor simulating a globulomaxillary cyst. J Oral Med 38:26, 1983.

Khan YM, Kwee H, Schneider LC, Saber I: Adenomatoid odontogenic tumor resembling a globulomaxillary cyst: light and electron microscope studies. J Oral Surg 35:739, 1977.

Little JW, Jacobsen J: Origin of the globulomaxillary cyst. J Oral Surg 31: 188, 1973.

Taicher S, Azaz B: Lesions resembling globulomaxillary cyst. Oral Surg Oral Med Oral Pathol 44:25, 1977.

Thoma K: Facial cleft or fissural cysts. Int J Orthod 23:83, 1937.

Wysocki GP: The differential diagnosis of globulomaxillary radiolucencies. Oral Surg Oral Med Oral Pathol 51:281, 1981.

Median Mandibular Cyst

Buchner A, Ramon Y: Median mandibular cyst: a rare lesion of debatable origin. Oral Surg Oral Med Oral Pathol 37:431, 1974.

Gardner DG: An evaluation of reported cases of median mandibular cysts. Oral Surg Oral Med Oral Pathol 65:208, 1988.

Lacourt L, Dones MA: Median mandibular cyst: report of a case. J Oral Surg 34:739, 1976.

Richany SF, Bast TH, Anson BJ: The development of the first bronchial arch in man and the fate of Meckel's cartilage. Q Bull Northwest Univ Med School 30:331, 1956.

Soskolne WA, Shteyer A: Median mandibular cyst. Oral Surg Oral Med Oral Pathol 44:84, 1977.

Ten Cate AR: Oral Histology: Development, Structure, and Function. St. Louis:CV Mosby, 1980, p. 22.

Traumatic Cyst

Baird WO, Askew PA: Traumatic mandibular bone cyst involved in line of fracture. Oral Surg Oral Med Oral Pathol 11:1351, 1958.

Beasley JD: Traumatic cysts of the jaws: report of 30 cases. J Am Dent Assoc 92:145, 1976.

Edeiken J: Roentgen Diagnosis of Diseases of Bone. 3rd Ed. Baltimore: Williams & Wilkins, 1981, p. 105.

Freedman GL, Beigleman MB: The traumatic bone cyst: a new dimension. Oral Surg Oral Med Oral Pathol 59:616, 1985.

Hansen LS, Sapone J, Sproat RC: Traumatic bone cysts of the jaws: report of 66 cases. Oral Surg Oral Med Oral Pathol 37:899, 1974.

Heubner GR, Turlington EG: So-called traumatic bone cysts of the jaws. Oral Surg Oral Med Oral Pathol 31:354, 1971.

Kaugars GE, Cale AE: Traumatic bone cyst. Oral Surg Oral Med Oral Pathol 63:318, 1987.

Morris CR, Steed DL, Jacoby JJ: Traumatic bone cysts. J Oral Surg 28: 188, 1970.

Patrikiou A, Seperiadon-Mavro-Poulou TH, Zarnbelis G: Bilateral traumatic bone cyst of the mandible. Oral Surg Oral Med Oral Pathol 51: 131, 1981.

Pogrel MA: Bilateral solitary bone cysts: report of a case. J Oral Surg 36: 55, 1978.

Precious DS, McFadden LR: Treatment of traumatic bone cyst of the mandible by infection of autogenic blood. Oral Surg Oral Med Oral Pathol 58:137, 1984.

Szerlip L: Traumatic bone cysts. Oral Surg Oral Med Oral Pathol 21:201, 1966.

Uemura S, Hashida T: Radiologic interpretation of fissural cysts and postoperative maxillary cyst and simple bone cyst. Oral Radiol 1:69, 1985.

Squamous Odontogenic Tumor

Anneroth G, Hansen LS: Variations in keratinizing odontogenic cysts and tumors. Oral Surg Oral Med Oral Pathol 54:530, 1982.

Doyle JL, Grodjesk JE, Dolinsky HB, Rafel SS: Squamous odontogenic tumor: report of three cases. J Oral Surg 35:994, 1977.

Goldblatt LI, Brannon RB, Ellis GL: Squamous odontogenic tumor: report of five cases and review of literature. Oral Surg Oral Med Oral Pathol 54:187, 1982.

Hopper TL, Sadeghi EM, Pricco DF: Squamous odontogenic tumor: report of a case with multiple lesions. Oral Surg Oral Med Oral Pathol 50: 404, 1980.

Leider AS, Jonker LA, Cook HE: Multicentric familial squamous odontogenic tumor. Oral Surg Oral Med Oral Pathol 68:175, 1989.

Mills WP, Danila MA, Beuttenmuller EA, Kandelka BM: Squamous odontogenic tumor: report of a case with lesions in three quadrants. Oral Surg Oral Med Oral Pathol 61:557, 1986.

Pullon PA, et al: Squamous odontogenic tumor: report of 6 cases of a previously undescribed lesion. Oral Surg Oral Med Oral Pathol 40:616, 1975.

Chapter 11

Pericoronal Radiolucencies Without Opacities

NORMAL FOLLICULAR SPACE

(Follicular sac)

A pericoronal radiolucency usually is seen around the crowns of normally erupting teeth. Radiographs are valuable in distinguishing this entity from the dentigerous cyst. Histologically, a normal follicular sac may be identical to a dentigerous cyst; thus, it cannot be diagnosed accurately without radiographs.

◆ *RADIOLOGY (Fig. 11–1)*

In its widest dimension, a normal follicular space generally measures up to 3 mm on panoramic radiographs and 2.5 mm on intraoral radiographs. Greater magnification usually is associated with panoramic images, although the amount varies from one machine to another. Conklin and Stafne (1949) concluded that cystic transformation of the follicular sac occurs once this space exceeds 2.5 mm on the periapical radiograph. They found this to be true in 80% of the cases. There are exceptions to this measurement in some anatomic locations such as the permanent maxillary canines, which may have a larger follicular space. Other patients have generalized follicular space enlargement. In marginal cases in younger patients, it is important to evaluate the degree of root formation. If the follicular space appears enlarged and root formation is complete, as indicated by closure of the apex, then the eruptive potential of the tooth is diminished greatly and cystic transformation of the follicular sac probably has occurred. In such cases, additional observation has little value and treatment should be initiated. If a normal follicular space is found radiologically and the pathologist diagnoses dentigerous cyst, follicular cyst, or odontogenic cyst histologically, the final definitive diagnosis is normal follicular space; however, if any other histopathologic diagnosis is received, such as odontogenic keratocyst, calcifying odontogenic cyst, or inflammatory paradental cyst, the histologic diagnosis must be considered final.

OSTEITIS UNDERLYING PERICORONITIS

This condition is somewhat analogous to the periapical abscess and may represent a middle stage between pericoronitis, in which no bony changes are seen, and the inflammatory paradental cyst. Most available information deals with pericoronitis, with few data on the underlying osteitis. Pericoronitis is an inflammation of the soft tissue surrounding the crown of a partly erupted or impacted tooth. Weinberg and colleagues (1986) tried to determine the organisms that cause the condition. Streptococcus viridans and Staphylococcus aureus coagulase positive, spirochetes, and fusobacteria have been isolated. Nitzan and colleagues (1985) performed aerobic and anaerobic cultures and found normal oral microbiota; however, in direct smears of the exudate with Giemsa staining, the predominant organisms were fusobacteria and spirochetes. Bean and King (1971) studied stress in their sample of 137 patients with pericoronitis and found an incidence of 70%. The following stresses were reported most frequently: fatigue, school examinations, financial worries, and menstruation. In their series of 245 cases of pericoronitis, 81% occurred in people between the ages of 20 and 29 years; cases are rare in those younger than 20 years or older than 40 years. There was no sex predilection.

The condition often is painful and may be associated with trismus and cellulitis. The inflamed and swollen operculum sometimes is traumatized by the maxillary third molar, usually the palatal cusp tip. The operculum often is red, and necrotic edges may be seen occasionally. When the pericoronitis is chronic, an underlying lytic osteitis develops, thus contributing to the symptoms of halitosis and pain. The bony defect acts as a reservoir for purulent material and food debris and greatly contributes to the chronicity of the overlying pericoronitis. In some instances, there is regional lymphadenopathy, especially in the neck near the angle of the mandible, as well as other constitutional symptoms such as fever and malaise. Treatment usually is provided in two phases. First, the inflamed operculum may be irrigated with saline and the maxillary third molar reduced or extracted. When fever is evident, antibiotics are prescribed. The second phase usually involves surgical removal of the underlying tooth. Because the inflammatory paradental cyst has not developed at this stage, no unusual soft tissue mass is attached to the extracted tooth. Curettage of the flame-shaped osteolytic defect should yield granulation tissue with foci of odontogenic epithelium. Additional studies are necessary to elucidate the nature of this tissue.

◆ *RADIOLOGY (Fig. 11–2)*

Location

In the series of 245 cases of pericoronitis analyzed by Nitzan and co-workers (1985), 95% occurred in association with a lower third molar. The teeth were partially erupted in 88% of the cases; also, 67% were vertically impacted, with only 12% mesioangular and 14% distoangular impactions.

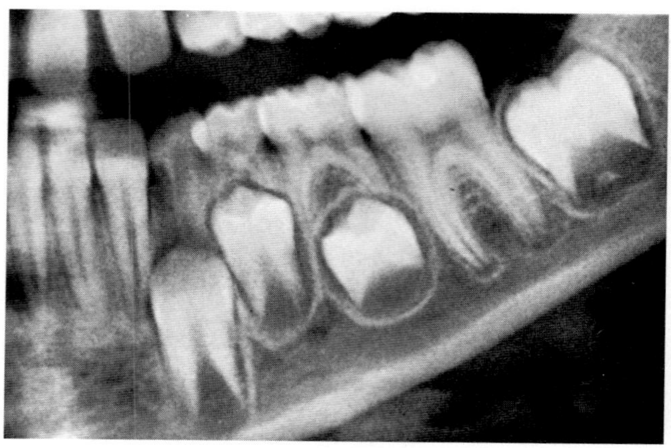

A

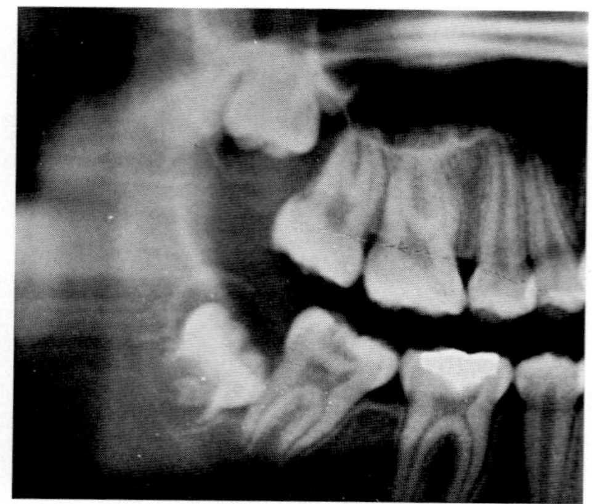

B

FIGURE 11–1.

Normal follicular space. A, Typical follicular spaces in a 7-year-old child. B, Large but normal third molar follicular spaces.

Radiologic Features

Radiologic changes are not expected in acute pericoronitis. Nitzan and colleagues (1985) stated that the alveolar bone distal to the third molar, which forms the basis of a periodontal pocket, did not show resorption in any of their 245 cases. We agree that when only the soft tissue is involved, radiologic features are absent, other than those pertaining to tooth position.

In some instances of pericoronitis, osteitis is present and usually occurs in the bone surrounding the distal portion of an impacted lower third molar. A small, characteristic, flame-shaped radiolucent area may be seen just distal to the affected tooth. The flame-shaped area may lack a sclerotic rim. In chronic low-grade cases, one may see a relatively thick sclerotic rim lined by an adjacent diffuse zone of reactive bone delineating the flame-shaped area. This condensed bone generally is more diffuse and less well defined than the cortical lining of the normal follicular space and thicker than that in the inflammatory paradental cyst. Marginal sclerosis may be partially present in some cases. The area of rarefaction rarely exceeds 3 mm in diameter.

INFLAMMATORY PARADENTAL CYST

(Paradental cyst, buccal cyst, mandibular infected buccal cyst, inflammatory collateral cyst, inflammatory lateral periodontal cyst, Craig's cyst)

The inflammatory paradental cyst (IPC) first was described by Craig in 1976 in a report of 49 cases. He suggested the term paradental cyst. In 1970, Main described the inflammatory collateral cyst, now referred to as lateral (inflammatory)

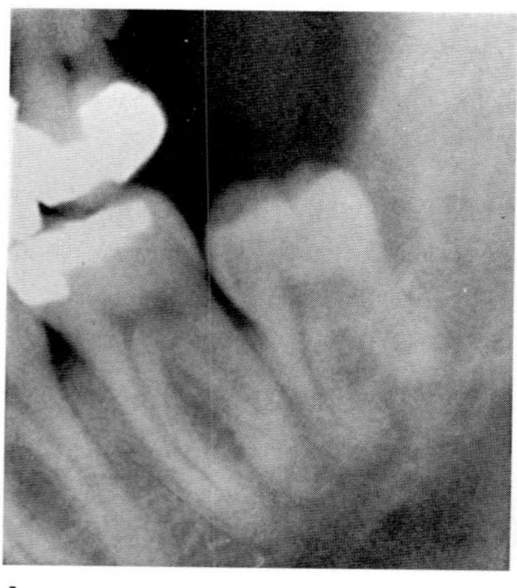

A

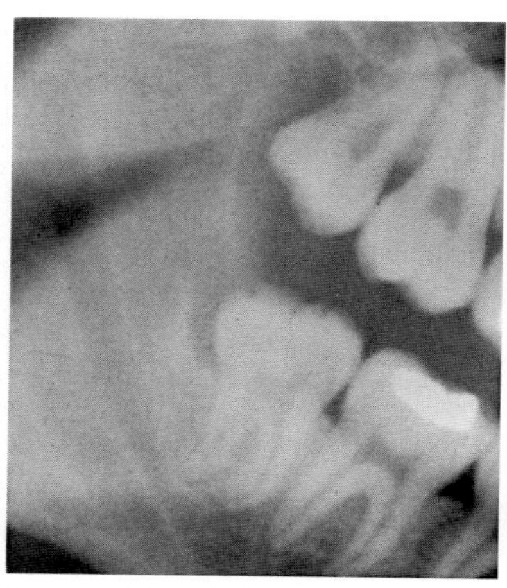

B

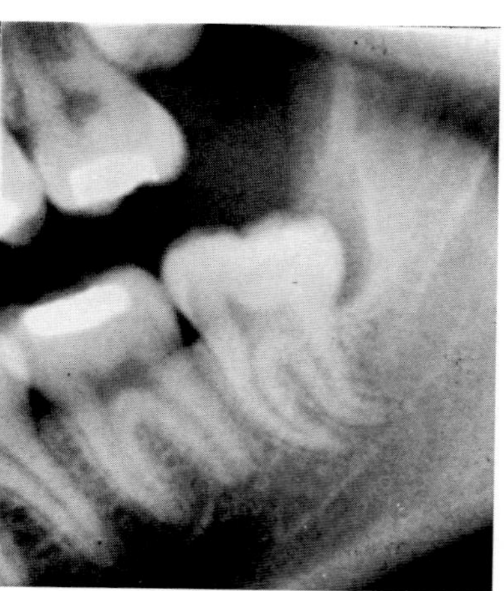

C

FIGURE 11–2.

Osteitis underlying pericoronitis. A, Flame-shaped radiolucency with no sclerotic margin. B, Sclerotic margin focally absent. C, Thick sclerotic margin with an adjacent more diffuse zone of reactive bone. There is soft tissue swelling above the occlusal of the third molar.

periodontal cyst, and may have included some cases of IPC. Shear (1983) recognized the IPC and inflammatory collateral cyst as distinct and separate pathologic entities. In 1983, Stoneman and Worth described the infected buccal cyst-molar area occurring in the mandibular first and second molar regions, whereas Ackermann and colleagues (1987) found that the condition occurred uniquely in association with mandibular third molars with a history of pericoronitis. A more complete understanding of this cyst did not develop until Vedtofte and Praetorius published an article in 1989 that suggested the term inflammatory paradental cyst. In their review of 1985 odontogenic cysts, Ackermann and colleagues (1987) found that IPC had an incidence of 3%. Other cysts included radicular cyst (62%), dentigerous cyst (19%), odontogenic keratocyst (12%), lateral periodontal cyst (2%), eruption cyst (1%), calcifying odontogenic cyst (0.5%), and gingival cyst (0.5%). These authors asserted that the IPC probably is much more common; either it is not recognized or is reported as a dentigerous cyst.

Pathologic Characteristics

Most believe that the IPC is an odontogenic cyst of inflammatory origin, somewhat analogous to the apical periodontal cyst resulting from infected pulp. In IPC, the source of inflammation is the infected operculum around an erupting tooth, usually a mandibular molar, or pericoronitis, most often involving a mandibular third molar. The majority of investigators think this cyst arises from inflammatory stimulation of the reduced enamel epithelium of the dental follicle around the erupting tooth. Another potential source of the cystic lining might be the epithelial rests of Malassez. Ackermann and colleagues (1987) indicated that, although the dentigerous cyst and IPC result from dilatation of the dental follicle, their histogenesis is different. In the dentigerous cyst, expansion of the follicle is the primary event, whereas the IPC is based on inflammatory bone destruction, with subsequent expansion of the follicle. They also found that the two cysts are histologically distinct: dentigerous cysts seldom are lined with thick proliferating odontogenic epithelium, as in the IPC; the dentigerous cyst occurs in many sites, whereas the IPC appears almost uniquely in the mandibular molar region.

Ackermann and colleagues (1987) and Vedtofte and Praetorius (1989) found that, histologically, the IPC was identical to the apical periodontal cyst. The lining consists of spongiotic, proliferating, nonkeratinized, stratified squamous epithelium of varying thicknesses. The wall is composed of dense, mature, fibrovascular connective tissue with an intense chronic or mixed inflammatory cell infiltrate. Some cases have had large foamy histiocytes and cholesterol clefts, as well as hyaline bodies in the epithelium and dystrophic calcification in the wall. The cyst lining may be continuous with the reduced enamel epithelium or in continuity with the gingival epithelium. In all 50 cases reported by Ackerman and colleagues (1987), the connective tissue of the cyst wall was clearly continuous with the follicle of the tooth, being firmly attached to the neck and cervical root surface of the tooth.

Grossly, the IPC is attached to the cementoenamel junction (CEJ) of the tooth and extends for variable distances along the root surface. Enamel spurs have been observed along the buccal aspect of some affected teeth, especially first molars, extending from the CEJ into the furcation area of the root. Craig (1976) believed that the enamel spurs were related to the pathogenesis and possibly the buccal location of most of his cases.

Clinical Features

Some studies have shown a preponderance of cases in male patients, especially those reported by Craig (1976) (83%) and Ackermann and colleagues (1987) (70%). This is difficult to explain because there are no known differences between male and female patients with respect to impaction, pericoronitis, and infected opercula. Vedtofte and Praetorius (1989), however, found an almost equal sex distribution in their series of 29 IPCs. Ackermann and co-workers (1987) reported that the IPC was more common in white versus black people living in Africa. They believed this was not surprising because the frequency of third molar impaction and partial eruption is higher in white people. According to different sources, patients' ages range from 4 to 62 years. As Vedtofte and Praetorius (1989) indicated, age depends on the location of the cyst. For cases in the mandibular first molar, the mean patient age was 8 years; the second molar, 13 years; and the third molar, 24 years. In cases involving the first and second mandibular molars, symptoms usually developed within 1 year of the expected eruption time, whereas this time lapse was more variable for third molars. For first and second molars, the most common symptoms were pain, swelling, and pus discharge from a periodontal defect. Vedtofte and Praetorius (1989) observed a communication from the periodontal pocket to the cyst on the buccal or distal aspects of all mandibular first and second molars. In third molars, almost all associated teeth are impacted or partially erupted and there is a history of one or more episodes of pericoronitis in almost every case. Halitosis, acute pain, swelling, and trismus commonly occur in such cases.

Treatment/Prognosis

Third molars usually are treated by cystectomy, along with tooth extraction. In the series reported by Stoneman and Worth (1986), most cases involved the mandibular first molar in children 4 to 8 years of age, and treatment usually consisted of extraction of the involved teeth, along with cyst removal. With better recognition of the radiomorphologic characteristics of this cyst, Vedtofte and Praetorius (1989) suggested that cystectomy alone has been successful in these areas. In 11 of 13 cases in which the tooth was preserved, normal healing occurred. The follow-up period was 1 to 3 years in seven cases, 3 to 6 years in five cases, and 5 years in one case. A periodontal defect occurred in one patient with an unsuccessful case and necessitated reoperation after 1 year; in another patient, a distobuccal IPC recurred 1 year later to the distal, causing displacement of the second molar and necessitating reoperation.

◆ RADIOLOGY (Figs. 11–3 to 11–6)

Location

In the series of Vedtofte and Praetorius (1989), 27 cases (93%) occurred in the mandible and 2 in the maxilla. One of the maxillary cases developed between the canine and lateral incisor, producing a ''globulomaxillary lesion,'' as defined by us; the second was located on the buccal aspect of the maxillary second molar. In the mandible, 56% were associated with a third molar, 26% with a second molar, and 19% with a first molar. Bilateral IPCs were found in two patients, one each involving the mandibular first and second molars. Packota and colleagues (1990) reported a case of bilateral IPC associated with the mandibular first molars. Ackermann and colleagues (1987) found three cases with bilateral involvement in mandibular third molars. They also analyzed the location of the IPC with respect to the involved tooth and discovered that the distal and distobuccal locations were seen most often in third molars. In the series of Stoneman and Worth (1983), a buccal location was observed frequently in first molars, although buccal and distal locations are possible for first and second molars. Mesial lesions have been reported rarely.

Radiologic Features

In cases affecting first molars, Packota and colleagues (1990) described especially notable definitive radiologic features that may apply to second and third molars.

In panoramic or periapical radiographs, the following may be seen:

1. Loss or attenuation of the lamina dura surrounding the root apices or in the furcation region of the affected tooth, or a radiolucency within the furcation.
2. Attenuation of the cortical boundary of the crypt of the developing second molar.
3. Variable presence of a radiopaque inferior margin of the cyst.
4. Buccolingual tilting of the crown of the affected tooth.
5. Distal displacement of the crypt of the second molar.

Occlusal radiographs may show the following:

1. A radiolucency with borders of varying degrees of definition and cortication, located buccal to the involved tooth.
2. A continuous or discontinuous buccal periosteal reaction; it may be composed of a single layer of new bone, several laminations, or a relatively homogeneous bony protuberance.
3. Displacement of the root apices of the involved tooth into the lingual cortex.

The cyst usually is 1 to 2 cm in diameter and typically consists of a well-defined radiolucency buccal or distal to the involved tooth. The cystic margin consists of a thin sclerotic rim, although this feature is variable and sometimes is discontinuous or only faintly apparent. This variability results from the intense inflammatory component within the connective tissue wall of the cyst that lies against the bony margin. Cystic pressure causes an even, thin, distinct sclerotic margin; acute inflammation may prompt a breakdown of the margin, whereas chronic low-grade inflammation may stimulate a diffuse sclerotic zone of reactive bone at the margin. In the IPC, there is a combination of cystic and reactive inflammatory changes at the margin. Depending on the position of the tooth, the IPC may be buccal to the coronal portion of the tooth, extend distally to involve one side

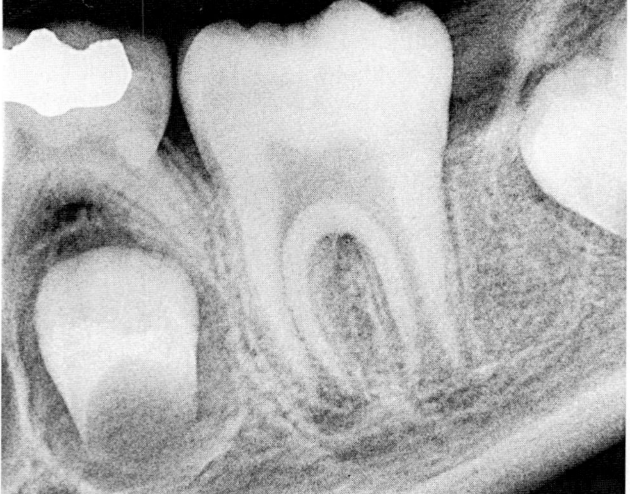

A

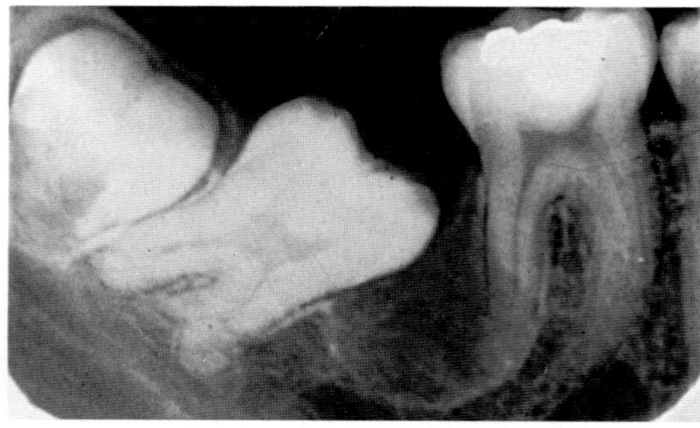

B

FIGURE 11–3.

Inflammatory paradental cyst: distal to mandibular first molar. A, Faint, slightly diffuse sclerotic margin, disruption of follicular margin, and distal displacement of second molar. (From Packota GV, Hall JM, Lanigan DT, Cohen MA: Paradental cysts on mandibular first molars in children: report of five cases. Dentomaxillofac Radiol 19:126, 1990.) B, Erosion into oral cavity at crest of ridge; distal displacement of second molar.

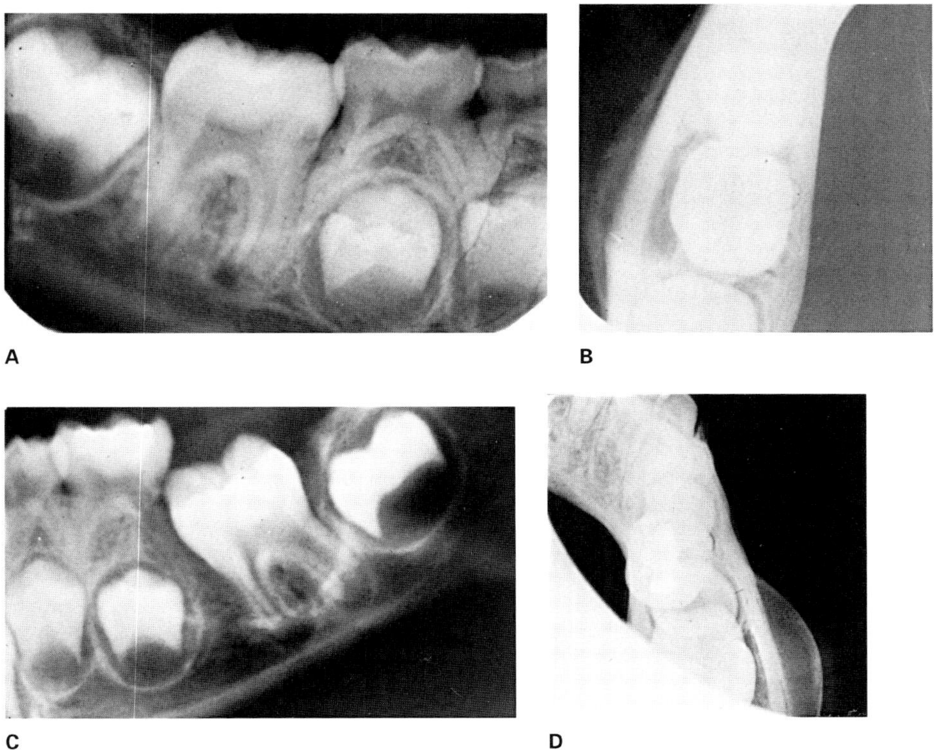

FIGURE 11–4.

Inflammatory paradental cyst: buccal of mandibular first molar. A and B, Case 1: Panel A shows subtle sclerotic margin, but occlusal view demonstrates periosteal reaction, buccal rarefaction, and lingual shifting of first molar roots. C and D, Case 2: There is a more apparent sclerotic margin and single layer of subperiosteal new bone on buccal. (C and D, From Packota GV, Hall JM, Lanigan DT, Cohen MA: Paradental cysts on mandibular first molars in children: report of five cases. Dentomaxillofac Radiol 19:126, 1990.)

of the root, progress inferiorly to involve one or more apices, or, rarely, appear to surround the involved tooth completely. Thus, the IPC may have a crescent or quarter-circle shape at the crest of the ridge and a more round or ovoid shape as it extends deeper into the bone along the distal root surface. Discontinuity of the crestal alveolar bone may be observed. Expansion is not a feature, although some cases have a periosteal reaction. When the IPC is in a distal or distobuccal

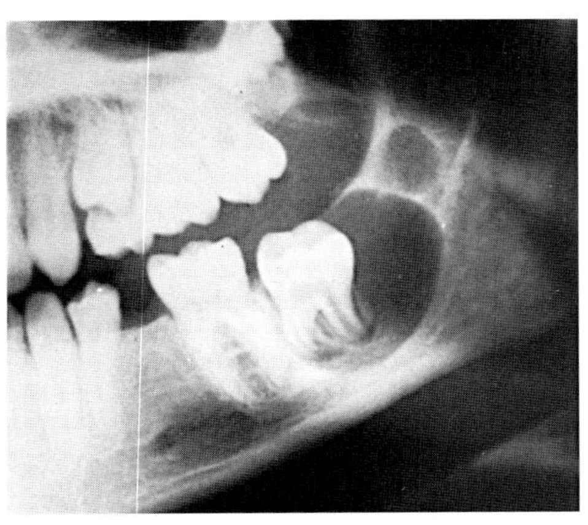

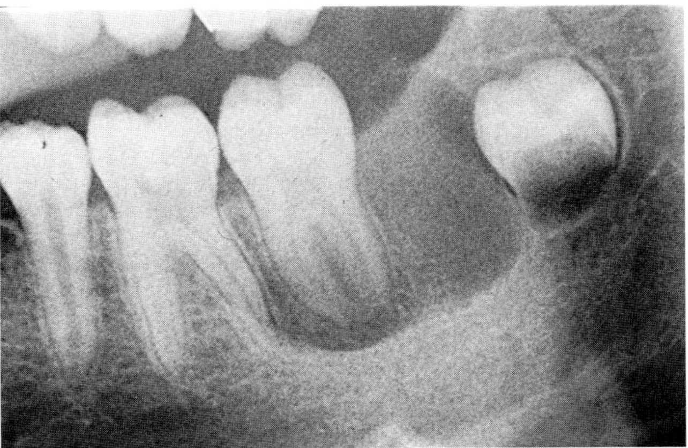

FIGURE 11–5.

Inflammatory paradental cyst: second molar. A, Displacement of crypt of third molar. B, Displacement of developing third molar and resorption of cortical margin of crypt.

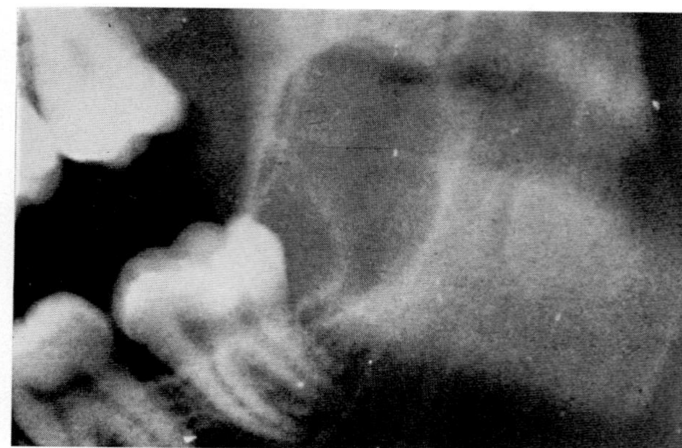

A B

FIGURE 11–6.

Inflammatory paradental cyst: third molar. A, Typical appearance and size. B, Largest size. Figure shows flame-shaped outline of original lesion and extension into ramus of second cystic lacuna.

position, it is observed easily; this is the common presentation in third molars. For first and second molars, a buccal position may be seen. In this instance, a radiolucent lesion may be found readily; often there is only a thin sclerotic rim traversing the roots of the teeth and it could be missed easily. Because of this, Packota and colleagues (1990) recommended the occlusal radiograph, which is highly diagnostic.

Relationship to Teeth

First and second molars usually are partially erupted and are not impacted. Root formation typically is incomplete. Although third molars may be impacted, they normally are partially erupted. Invariably, root formation is complete in cases involving third molars. When the cyst develops distal to a first or second molar, the tooth distal to the involved tooth may be displaced, but less than it would be with some dentigerous cysts. Because the cyst does not exceed 1 or 2 cm, tooth displacement is limited. In such instances, one is tempted to diagnose a dentigerous cyst of the displaced erupting tooth. To avoid this circumstance, the following features may help one to differentiate IPCs from dentigerous cysts:

1. There is a clinical ability to enter the cystic cavity relatively easily by probing distal to the involved tooth.
2. Radiographic evidence of discontinuity of the crestal bone is found, especially just distal to the involved tooth.
3. The most severe bone destruction is seen along the distal root of the involved tooth.
4. The IPC may have a more diffuse sclerotic margin with focally absent areas, especially toward the crestal portion of the cyst.
5. There is radiologic evidence of a connection between the cyst lumen and oral cavity, usually through a periodontal defect just distal to the involved tooth.
6. Although the sclerotic margin of the tooth crypt of the displaced tooth may be resorbed, there is no evidence of an increased follicular sac space.
7. Resorption of any portion of the involved teeth, either the host tooth or displaced tooth, is not a feature; however, dentigerous cysts may be associated with tooth resorption.

DENTIGEROUS CYST (Follicular cyst, eruption cyst)

The dentigerous cyst is the most common pathologic pericoronal radiolucency in the jaws. According to Ackermann and colleagues (1987), it is the second most common jaw cyst, with the radicular cyst being seen most often. There are three primary variants of the dentigerous cyst, based on the location of the cyst with respect to the erupting tooth: (1) the eruption cyst, (2) circumferential dentigerous cyst, and (3) lateral dentigerous cyst. An additional variant is termed the "inflammatory dentigerous cyst." Multiple dentigerous cysts have occurred in association with the Maroteaux-Lamy syndrome.

The dentigerous cyst and its variants arise from the reduced enamel epithelium about the crown of an unerupted or impacted tooth. It also may develop in association with an odontoma.

Pathologic Characteristics

It generally is believed that this cyst results from passive hemodynamic pooling of fluid beneath the follicle as a result of impeded eruption. The bone-resorbing potential of the follicular sac has been studied by Cahill and Mark (1980) and explains why these cysts may become very large.

Clinical Features

Patients have dentigerous cysts during the years when teeth are erupting. Thus, most of these cysts occur in patients younger than 20 years of age. Cabini and colleagues (1970) found a male-to-female sex ratio of 2:1 in their review of cysts of the jaws. Shear (1985) reported that dentigerous cysts occur more frequently in white than black people living in Africa. In addition, Africans have a lower incidence of impacted teeth, thus lending credibility to theories implicating impacted teeth in the pathogenesis of dentigerous cysts.

The **eruption cyst** is a variant of the follicular cyst that is close to the alveolar crest. Clinically, one may see a bluish, domelike bump on the gingiva, which is the crestal portion of the cyst that has eroded through the alveolar ridge and is expanding into the soft tissue. The bluish color results from the refractory properties of the cystic fluid as seen through the soft tissue, or it may be caused by blood within the cyst due to trauma from an opposing tooth.

The **"circumferential" dentigerous cyst** occurs when the associated tooth erupts or is erupting through the superior wall of the cyst as though through a hole in a doughnut. In a lateral view, the cyst appears on both sides of the crown and ultimately may surround the roots of the erupting or erupted tooth.

The **"lateral" dentigerous cyst** often is seen alongside the involved tooth. Somehow the cyst is displaced to one side of the crown as the involved tooth attempts to erupt, causing the lateral position of the cyst.

The **inflammatory dentigerous cyst** arises from the spread of periapical inflammation from an overlying nonvital primary tooth. This possibility first was reported by Shaw and colleagues (1980), who suggested the term inflammatory follicular cyst. They found that the most common sequel to untreated periapical inflammation in a primary tooth was intrafollicular penetration of inflammatory elements of the underlying permanent tooth. Subsequent proliferation of the reduced enamel epithelium is stimulated by the inflammatory process. In such cysts, the epithelial lining consists of hyperplastic, arcading, stratified squamous epithelium in close association with a dense, chronic, inflammatory infiltrate within the connective tissue wall. In their series, all 13 cases involved premolars, mainly in the mandible.

Multiple dentigerous cysts have been reported in association with mucopolysaccharidosis type VI, also known as the Maroteaux-Lamy syndrome. Roberts and colleagues (1984) reported a case in a 6-year-old boy. Their patient had dentigerous cysts in each quadrant, associated with the erupting first permanent molars, with displacement of the associated tooth and adjacent developing teeth. The cystic fluid was similar to that in people without mucopolysaccharide storage disorders. In patients with mucopolysaccharidosis, it is important to differentiate dentigerous cysts from enlarged follicles filled with dense collagenous connective tissue. Cystic lesions cause more bone destruction and displacement of the involved tooth and adjacent teeth; however, it is said that connective tissue lesions are limited primarily to the crown of the unerupted tooth and rarely cause tooth displacement.

Treatment/Prognosis

Ramzy and co-workers (1985) claimed that fine-needle aspiration and subsequent histologic examination yield diagnostic features of dentigerous cysts. For the clinician who is planning treatment, clinical observation of the straw-colored fluid, which is usually clear and sometimes blood tinged, probably is the most useful part of the aspiration procedure. The cyst usually is treated by enucleation, and sometimes the involved tooth is removed. Orthodontic traction of the involved tooth may follow cystectomy when extraction is not desired. In larger lesions, marsupialization may be used to shrink the lesion and is followed later by enucleation and removal of the involved tooth, usually a third molar. Lapier (1985) has discussed this treatment. Complete resolution may take 3 months to 1 year (for larger lesions).

◆ RADIOLOGY (Figs. 11–7 to 11–17)

The dentigerous cyst classically consists of a well-corticated pericoronal radiolucency, which exceeds 3 mm when measured from the edge of the crown to the periphery of the lesion on panoramic radiographs and 2.5 mm on periapical radiographs. The cystic cavity often originates from the cervical region of the tooth.

Location

According to Cabini and colleagues (1970), most jaw cysts of various types occur in the maxilla (59% of cases); however, the dentigerous cyst develops more often in the lower jaw (56% of cases). Shear (1985) reported that maxillary third molars have a comparatively low frequency of dentigerous cyst formation compared with impacted mandibular third molars; however, maxillary canines have a higher risk of dentigerous cysts than do mandibular canines, and mandibular second premolars, if unerupted, are particularly susceptible to cyst formation. According to Gibilisco (1985), the following teeth are involved most often (in descending order of frequency): third molars, canines, and second premolars.

Radiologic Features

The dentigerous cyst may become large enough to fill the body or ramus completely. Buttress formation may be seen at the expanded cortex, with a thin but intact cortical outline in larger cysts. Also, if a right-angle view such as an occlusal radiograph can be obtained, a hydraulic effect may be seen in association with the expanded cortex. Although most lesions are unicystic, some are multilocular. The locules tend to be very large, with the septa forming only partial cavities. It must be remembered that a single cystic wall and sac is enucleated from such lesions; thus, the locules represent simple bosselation of the bone beneath the advancing cystic margin. The margin of most dentigerous cysts is well corticated unless infection is present. It is thin and smoothly curved, with little tendency toward scalloping or discontinuity. The cortex often is expanded, usually toward the buccal only and rarely the lingual only. Buccal and lingual expansion by the same lesion is extremely rare. The expanded margin is thin, smooth, and of uniform thickness.

When radiopaque foci are seen within the lumen of the lesion, the radiopaque material may represent a complex or compound odontoma, supernumerary tooth, or paramolar that may be in various stages of development. These entities also may give rise to dentigerous cysts.

The inflammatory dentigerous cyst may be suspected when a mandibular premolar is involved and when the over-

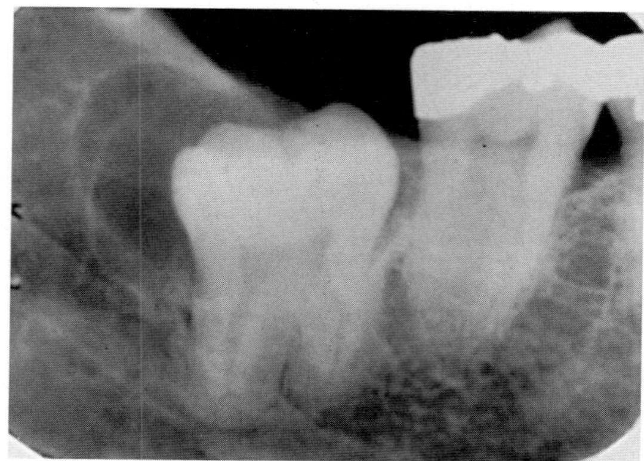

A

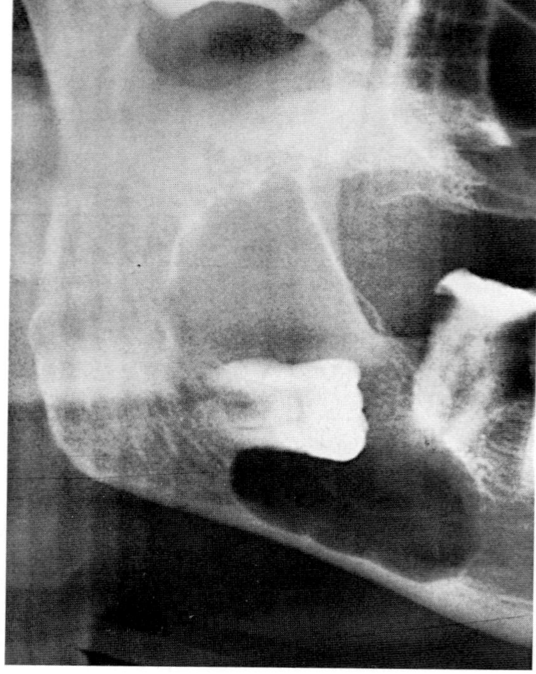

B

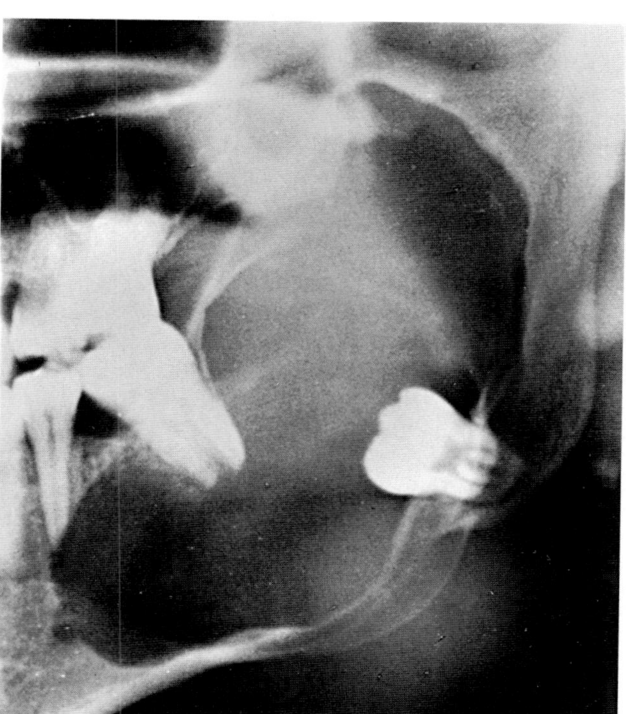

C

FIGURE 11–7.

Dentigerous cyst: mandibular third molar. A, Small cyst with early loculus formation. B, Larger cyst with displacement of third molar, scalloping at margin in ramus, and endosteal scalloping of inferior cortex. C, Large cyst with hydraulic effect at expanded cortex near angle, displacement of third molar, and resorption of apex of second premolar.

lying primary molar appears to be nonvital. There also may be evidence of failed pulpal therapy. In such instances, the roots of the primary molars may not be as resorbed as those of the contralateral twin. The most important feature indicating inflammation is loss of the thin sclerotic cystic margin. The margin may appear punched-out, or areas of reactive sclerosis may be present at the host bone interface.

Various sequelae such as ameloblastoma, epidermoid carcinoma, or mucoepidermoid carcinoma may develop from a dentigerous cyst. In these instances, the cyst may acquire the characteristic radiographic appearance of the new lesion, or it may retain the features of a dentigerous cyst. These sequelae are discussed in sections on mural ameloblastoma and mucoepidermoid carcinoma.

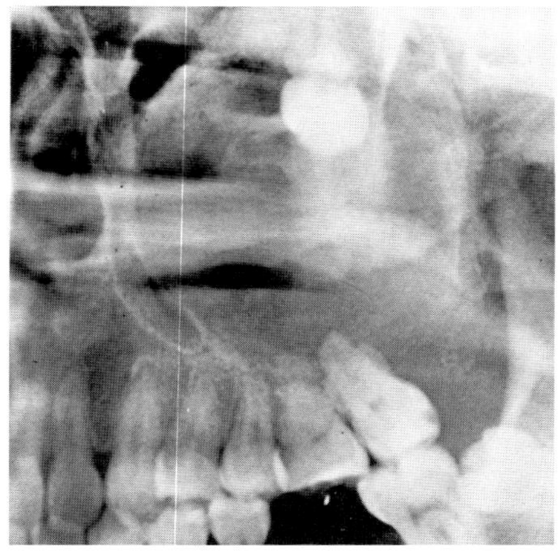

A

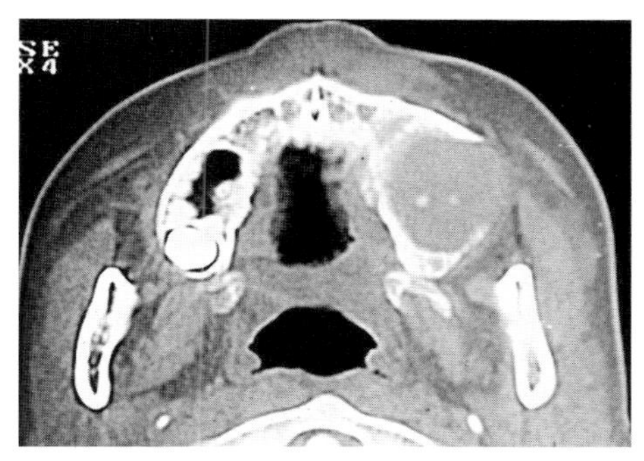

B

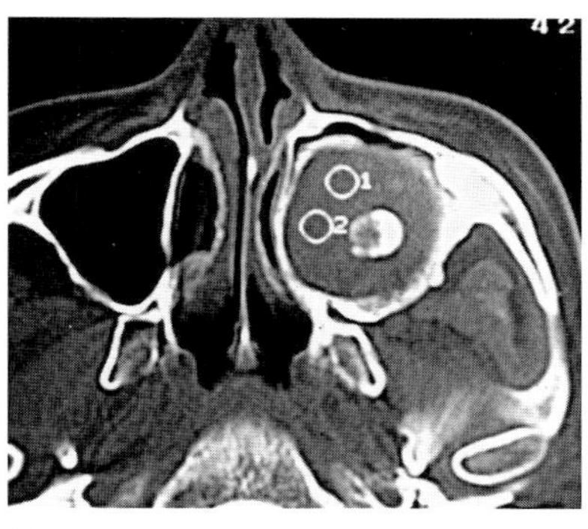

C

FIGURE 11–8.

Dentigerous cyst: maxillary third molar. A, Figure shows superior expansion of sinus floor, absent sinus wall, premolar-molar region, and superior displacement of third molar into the antrum. B, Axial CT scan shows apices of several root tips and buttress formation at lateral wall of maxilla. C, Circle #1 = 0.4 Hounsfield units and #2 = −1.0. Values approach zero, which is the value of water, suggesting serous cystic fluid. (Courtesy of Drs. M. Araki, K. Hashimoto, and K. Honda, Nihon University School of Dentistry, Department of Radiology, Tokyo, Japan.)

Relationship to Teeth

Teeth are an integral part of the dentigerous cyst because the cyst consists of an enlarged follicular sac attached to the cervical area of a developing or erupting tooth that may be displaced, unerupted, or impacted. Shear (1985) also observed that dentigerous cysts appear to have a greater tendency than other jaw cysts to resorb the roots of adjacent teeth, which may result from the ability of the dental follicle to resorb the roots of the deciduous predecessors.

The term eruption cyst is used when a dentigerous cyst breaks through the crestal alveolar bone. The involved tooth may have incompletely formed roots, and thus eruptive potential. If the cyst is incised or bursts spontaneously, the involved tooth may erupt. If apex closure has occurred, then the eruptive potential may be considered nil.

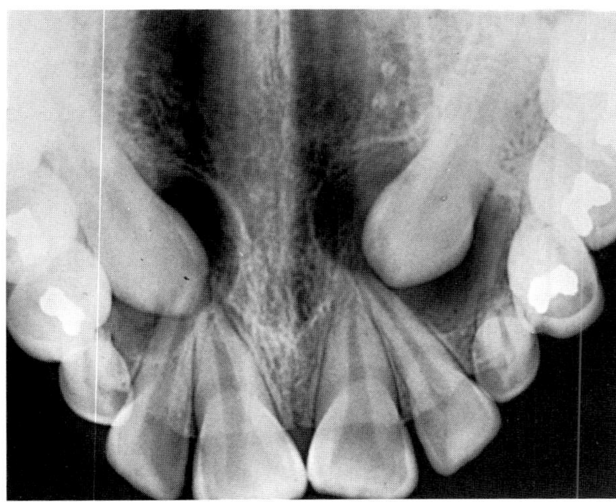

FIGURE 11–9.

Dentigerous cyst: maxillary canine. Small bilateral cysts. Canines will not erupt because root formation is complete. (Courtesy of Professor L. Alfaro, University of Chile, Pathology Referral Center, Santiago, Chile.)

As explained by Shafer and co-authors (1983), the circumferential dentigerous cyst surrounds the entire crown but not the occlusal surface, so the tooth may erupt through the cyst as "through the hole in a doughnut." The cyst remains around the roots of the erupted or erupting tooth, looking much like an apical periodontal cyst.

The lateral dentigerous cyst (LDC) occurs on one side of the involved tooth, which invariably is impacted or displaced, and the cyst may vary from small (1 cm) to medium sized (2 cm). When the LDC is distal to a nearly erupted vertically impacted mandibular third molar, it greatly resembles the inflammatory paradental cyst (IPC), with the following differences:

1. The IPC usually is accompanied by a partially erupted third molar with associated pericoronitis clinically; the LDC is associated most often with an unerupted tooth.
2. The IPC may have a characteristic semilunar, crescent, or flame shape when it is small, whereas the smaller LDC is more symmetric and round, taking on a ovoid semicircular shape, with its bisected diameter at the distal surface of the tooth.
3. The IPC rarely grows larger than several centimeters, whereas the LDC may occupy the entire hemimandible.
4. At times, the sclerotic margin of the IPC may appear thickened, with or without evidence of additional sclerosis within the marginal bone; the sclerotic margin of the LDC usually is thin, sharp, well defined, and without evidence of reactive bone formation.

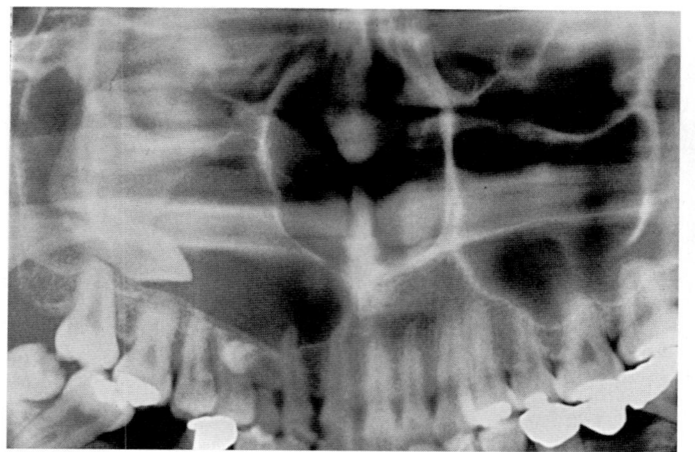
A

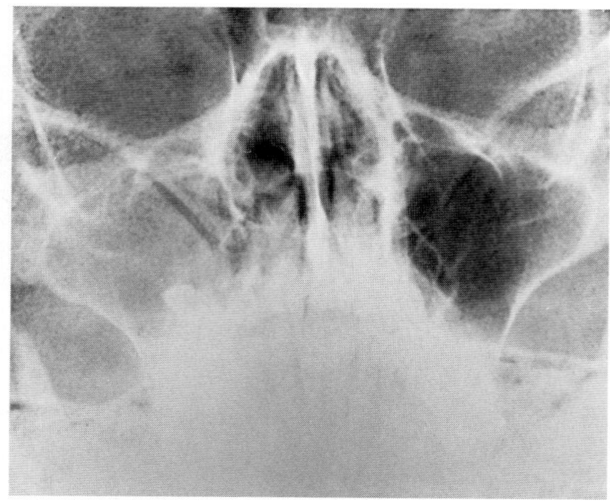
B

C

D

FIGURE 11–10.

Dentigerous cyst: maxillary canine. A, Cyst occupies right maxillary sinus, with displacement of canine into antrum. B, Waters' view: cloudiness of right antrum. C and D, Axial and coronal CT images: lateral expansion of sinus wall, displaced canine tooth, and faint superior bony margins of cyst in antrum. (Courtesy of Professor H. Fuchihata, Dean, Osaka University School of Dentistry, Osaka, Japan.)

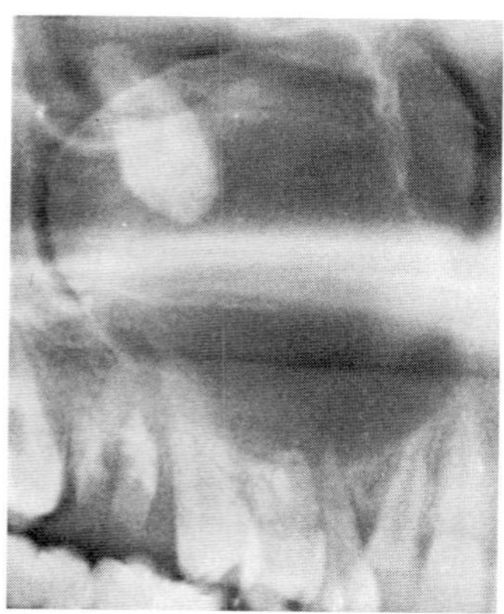
A

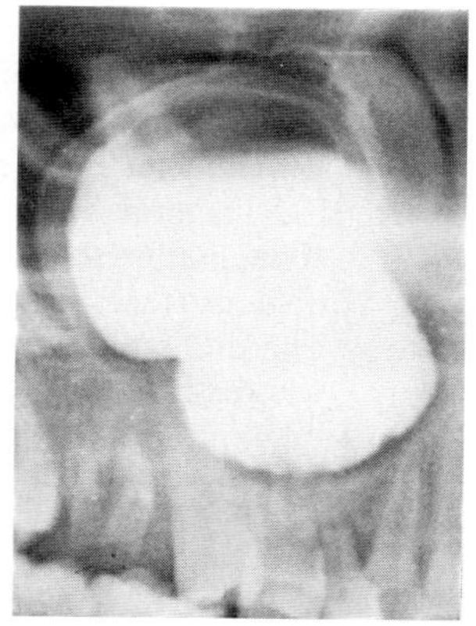
B

FIGURE 11–11.

Dentigerous cyst: maxillary canine. A, Panoramic radiograph shows lesion. B, Injection of contrast fluid confirms its cystic nature and extent, and the thickness of the lining. (Courtesy of Drs. Lilian and Israel Chilvarquer, Sao Paulo, Brazil.)

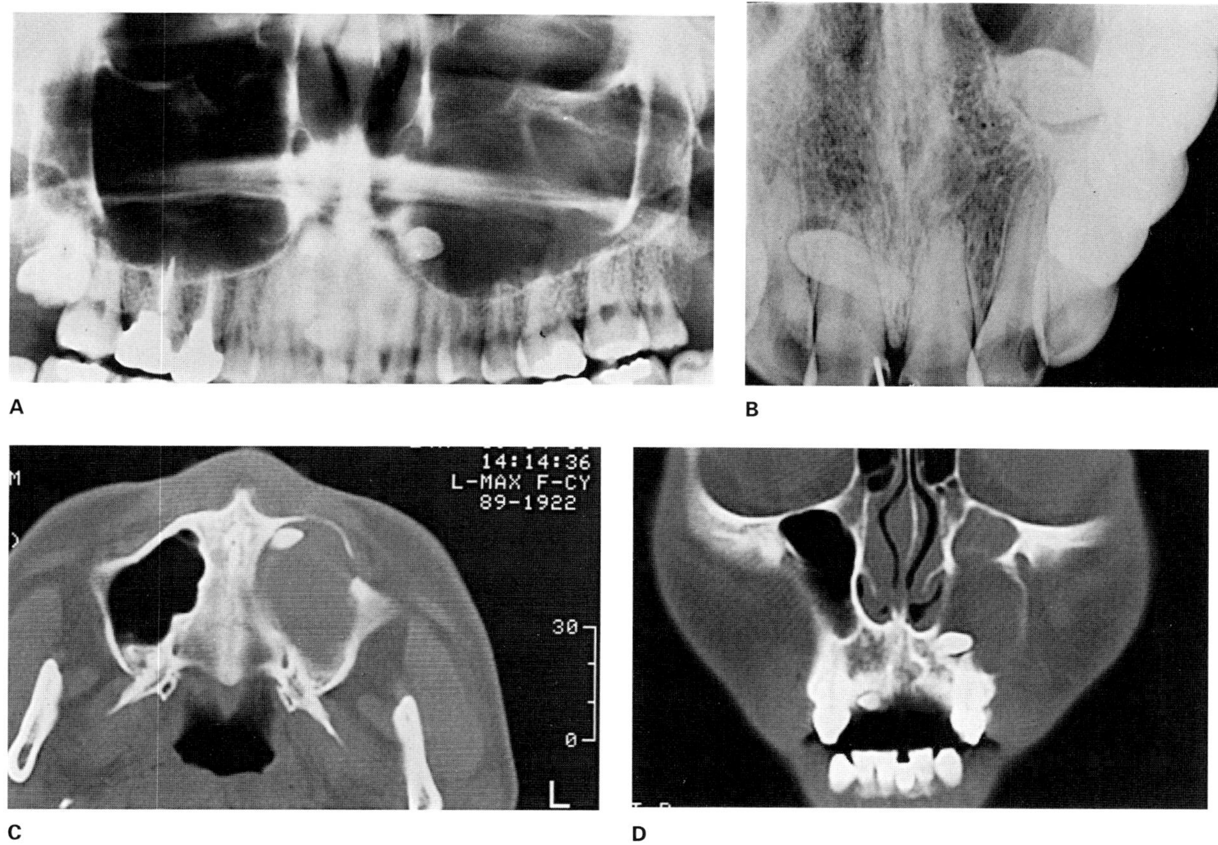

FIGURE 11–12.

Dentigerous cyst: supernumerary tooth. A, Bilateral mesiodens. Cyst is not apparent. B, Displacement of left mesiodens into sinus. Smooth sharp outline of left sinus floor in premolar area suggests the presence of a large cyst within. C, Axial CT scan showing buttress formation at expanded lateral wall of sinus. D, Erosion of lateral sinus wall and nasal wall beneath inferior turbinate. (Courtesy of Professor H. Fuchihata, Dean, Osaka University School of Dentistry, Osaka, Japan.)

Involvement of the Antrum

When maxillary lesions occur in the antrum region, the cyst may expand into, completely fill, and enlarge the maxillary sinus. The involved tooth often may be found within the antrum, having been displaced upward by the developing cyst. In such instances, the Waters' view may show expansion and thinning of the antral wall, antral opacification within the area occupied by the cyst, and expansion of the floor of the orbit, lateral wall of the nose, and hard palate. The normal antral wall, especially on periapical views, looks like the continuous but slightly irregular line made by an artist's pencil on coarse, kraft-type drawing paper. When cystic involvement of the antrum occurs, this line becomes very sharp, thickened, and denser and loses its wavy outline. When the antrum is involved, the cystic lumen can be injected with water-soluble contrast material, after the cystic fluid is aspirated. This procedure helps delineate the extent of the cyst. Chuong (1984) reported a case involving the maxillary sinus and discussed the utility of computed tomography (CT) imaging in determining its extent.

ORTHOKERATINIZED ODONTOGENIC KERATOCYST (Odontogenic keratocyst: orthokeratinized variant)

The orthokeratinized odontogenic keratocyst first was reported by Wright in 1981. In a review of 450 odontogenic keratocysts, he found that 60 of these cases contained a thin layer of luminal orthokeratin (without cell nuclei), whereas the remainder were parakeratinized (with cell nuclei). This cyst is classified as a pericoronal radiolucency because Wright (1981) reported that 72% (43 cases) of his 60 cases were pericoronal radiolucencies associated with an impacted tooth and resembling a dentigerous cyst. The cyst is characterized by a thin, uniform epithelial lining with orthokeratinization and a subjacent granular cell layer. The basal cells usually are cuboidal or flattened. On additional investigation of the clinical features, Wright (1981) found a distinctively different pattern from that of the parakeratinized archtypical variant.

The male-to-female ratio of patients was 3.2:1. All but

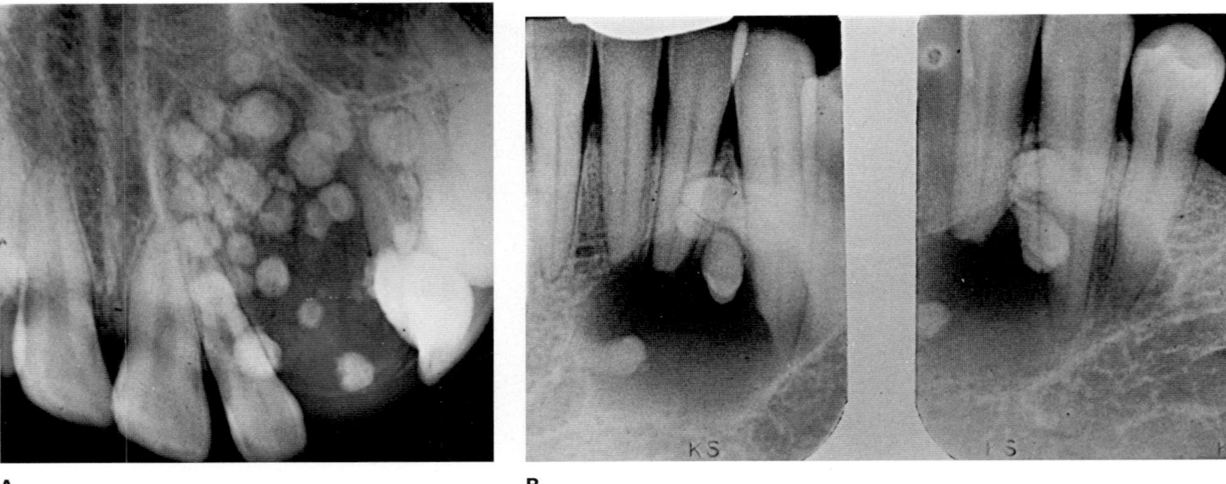

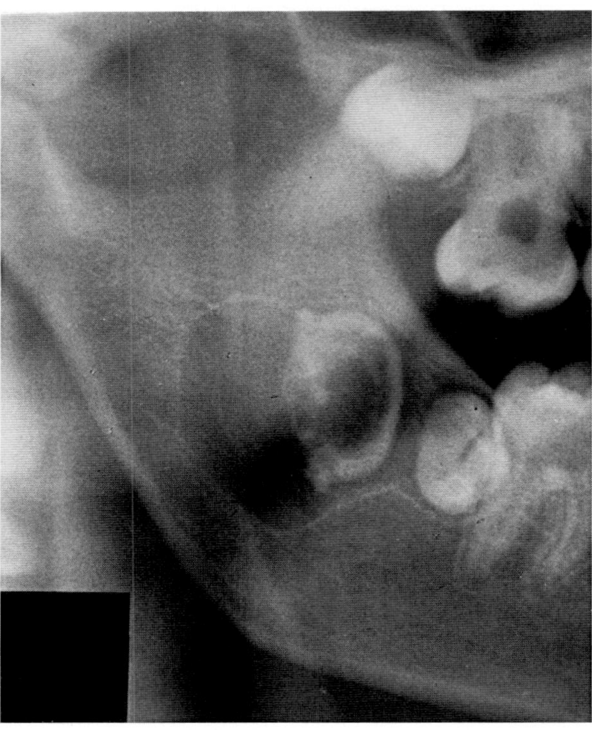

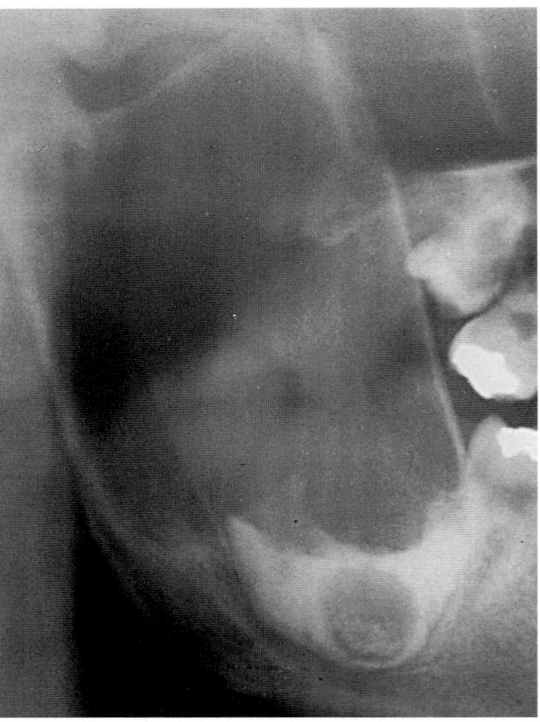

FIGURE 11–13.

Dentigerous cyst: associated with odontoma. A, Predominance of compound odontoma component; separation of odontomatous masses suggests cyst. (Courtesy of Dr. P. Dhiravarangkura, Chulalonghorn University School of Dentistry, Bangkok, Thailand.) B, Predominance of cystic component. (Courtesy of Dr. G. Terezhalmy, Dean, Case Western School of Dentistry, Cleveland, OH.) C, Associated with developing complex odontoma. D, Large cyst and complex odontoma. (C and D, Courtesy of Dr. H. Schwartz, Kaiser Permanente Medical Group, Los Angeles, CA.)

one of the patients were white, with the exception being African-American. Patients' ages ranged from 15 to 73 years (mean, 35 years). Forty-two percent had no symptoms, and cases were discovered during routine radiographic examination. There was pain in 13 cases (22%), swelling in 8 cases (13%), and clinical evidence of infection in 5 cases (8%). Although not specifically mentioned in all cases, the basal cell nevus-bifid rib syndrome was not observed in any of the 19 patients examined for the syndrome. Among 24 patients observed on a follow-up basis for 6 months to 8 years, there

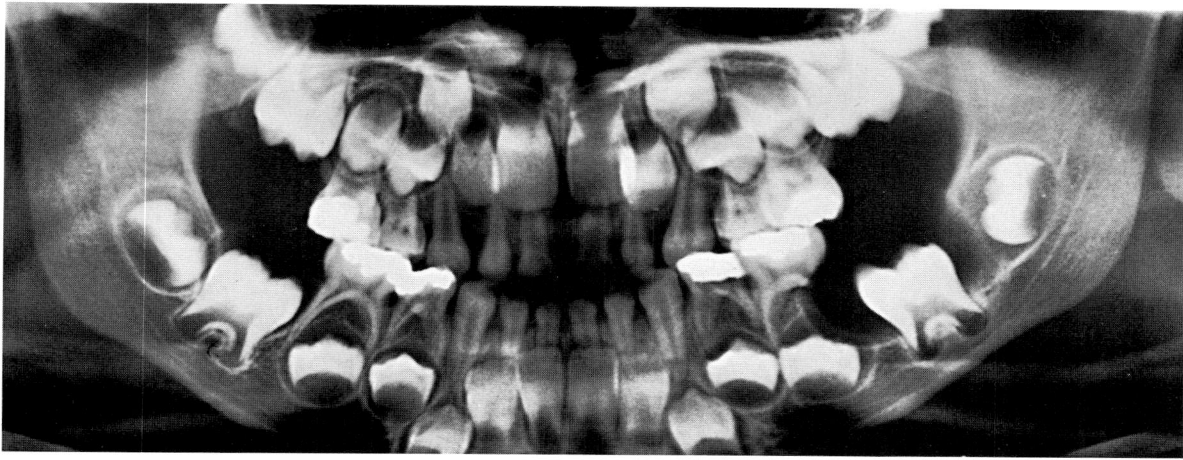

FIGURE 11–14.

Eruption cyst. Mandibular left first molar. Resorption of cortical walls of adjacent dental follicles and ectopic resorption of distal root of primary second molar.

was only one recurrence. This was in a 34-year-old woman, who had an extensive maxillary anterior cyst around an impacted central incisor; the cyst extended posteriorly to the second premolar and superiorly into the floor of the nose and antrum.

◆ *RADIOLOGY (Fig. 11–18)*

Location

Wright (1981) found that almost twice as many cases occurred in the mandible (38 cases) as the maxilla (20 cases). In both jaws, most lesions (67%) were posterior to the second premolar region. A few cases were seen in the premolar area, and 18% were observed in the anterior regions. A small number of cases involved several areas.

Radiologic Features

The size of the lesions varied from less than 1 cm in diameter to 7 cm in length. In 72% of cases, the diameter ranged from 1 to 3 cm. Most cases were solitary radiolucencies, and only one was described specifically as multilocular. Wright (1981) found that 72% consisted of a pericoronal radiolucency about an impacted tooth. Expansion of the cortex was observed in three cases (5%). In the two radiographs shown by Wright (1981), there was displacement of the involved tooth and resorption of adjacent teeth. This does not imply that these features were seen frequently, however; root resorption generally is not a feature of the classic odontogenic keratocyst.

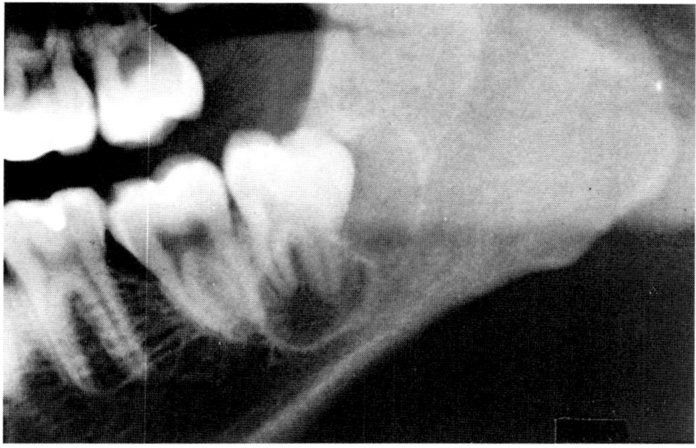

FIGURE 11–15.

Circumferential dentigerous cyst. Tooth appears to have partially erupted through cyst.

UNICYSTIC AMELOBLASTOMA (Mural ameloblastoma, cytogenic ameloblastoma, cystic variant of ameloblastoma, cystic ameloblastoma, intracystic ameloblastoma)

The unicystic ameloblastoma arises from the wall of a cyst. According to Shteyer and colleagues (1978), this variant represents 5% of all ameloblastomas. In their review, Wood and Goaz (1991) stated that as many as 30% of ameloblastomas may form in a cyst wall. Reviews of unicystic ameloblastoma were presented by Eversole and colleagues (1984), Shteyer and co-authors (1978), and Leider and co-workers (1985). In 1977, Robinson and Martinez suggested that unicystic ameloblastoma should be considered a distinct entity because of its significantly improved prognosis compared with that of conventional ameloblastomas. According to Wood and Goaz (1991), the unicystic ameloblastoma ranks next to the dentigerous cyst as the most frequently occurring pathologic pericoronal radiolucency.

Pathologic Characteristics

Most authors believe that the unicystic ameloblastoma arises from the wall of a pre-existing cyst rather than from cystic degeneration of a solid tumor. According to Wood and Goaz (1991), the dentigerous cyst is the most common cyst associ-

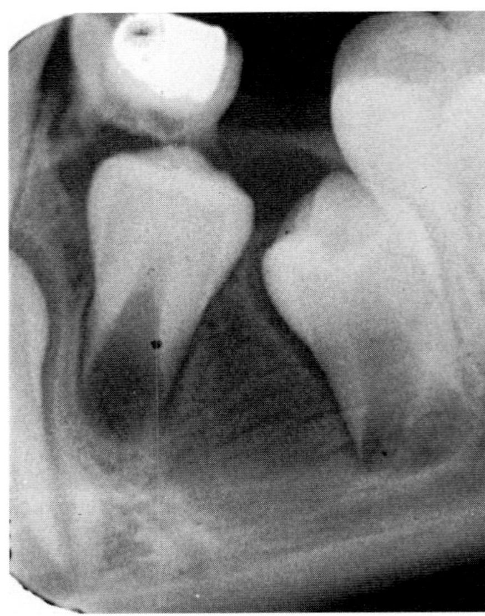

A

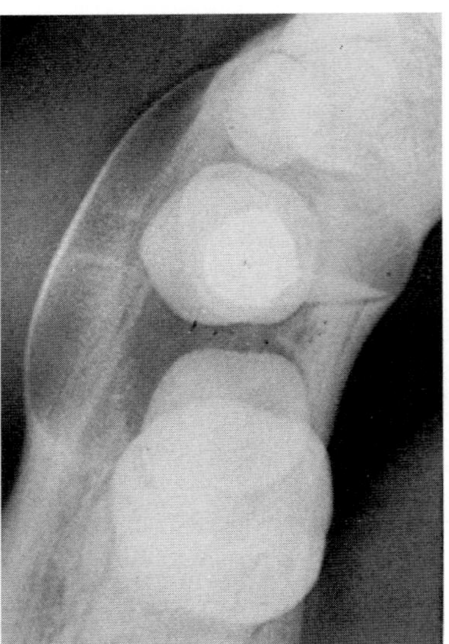

B

FIGURE 11–16.

Inflammatory dentigerous cyst. A, Large restoration in first primary molar and loss of sclerotic cystic margin. B, Expansion of cortex with hydraulic (cystic) effect, fistulous tract on buccal, and lingual shifting of the apex of developing first premolar. (Courtesy of Dr. D. Barnett, Oregon Health Sciences Center, School of Dentistry, Portland, OR.)

ated with the ameloblastoma (85%), with the remainder consisting of residual, radicular, globulomaxillary, and primordial types. Shortly after induction, the neoplasm (ameloblastoma) begins as a mural (within wall lining) nodule. Ultimately, the nodule grows and fills the entire cystic lumen. At some point, the tumor tissue infiltrates beyond the connective tissue capsule of the cyst wall and invades between the trabeculae of the medullary spaces in the adjacent bone. Once this happens, the unicystic ameloblastoma behaves similarly to the conventional ameloblastoma, especially with regard to appearance and recurrence.

Clinical Features

In their series of 31 cases, Eversole and colleagues (1984) reported the typical demographics of the unicystic ameloblastoma. They reported a male-to-female ratio of 1.5:1, average patient age of 27 years, and median age of 22 years.

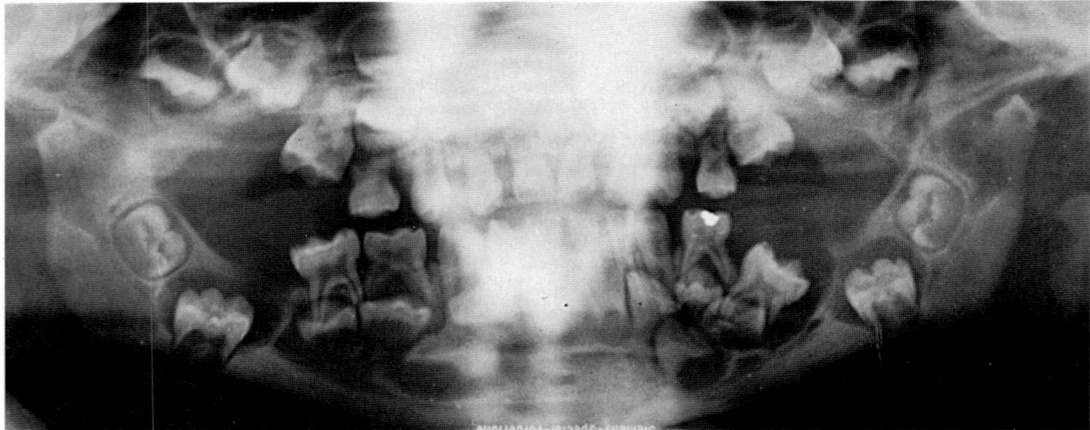

FIGURE 11–17.

Multiple dentigerous cysts: Maroteaux-Lamy syndrome. Involvement of at least one tooth in each quadrant. (From Roberts M, et al: Occurrence of multiple dentigerous cysts in a patient with the Maroteaux-Lamy syndrome [mucopolysaccharidosis, type VI]. Oral Surg Oral Med Oral Pathol 58:169, 1984.)

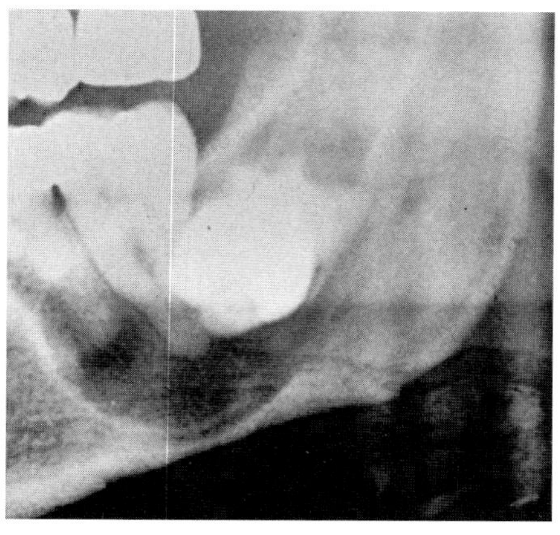
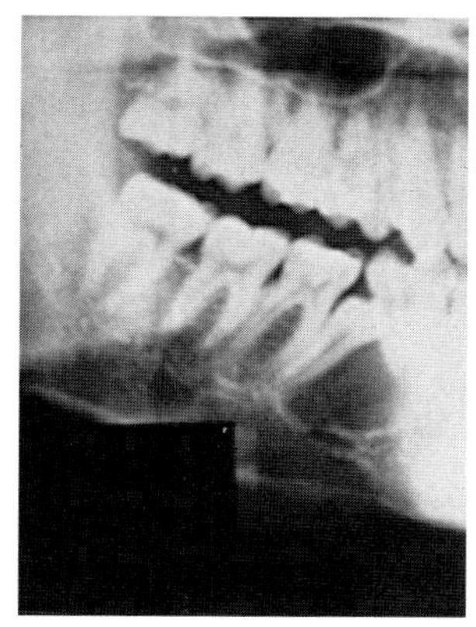
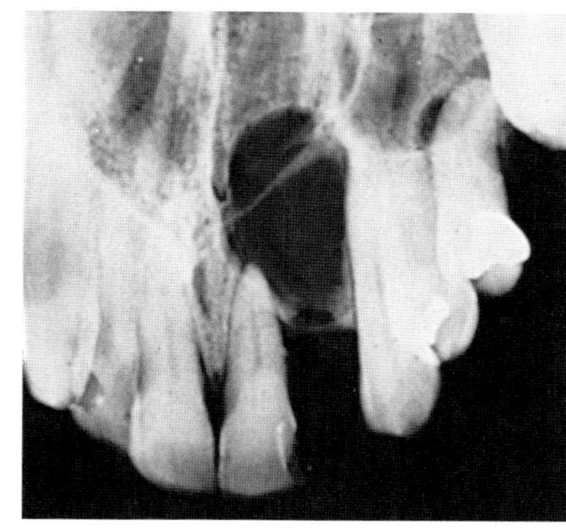

A B C

FIGURE 11–18.

Orthokeratinized odontogenic keratocyst. A, Case resembling ordinary dentigerous cyst. (Courtesy of Dr. G. Kaugars, Medical College of Virginia School of Dentistry, Richmond, VA.) B, Similar to other cystic lesions occurring in this area, principally lateral periodontal cyst, botryoid lateral periodontal cyst, primordial cyst, and odontogenic keratocyst. C, Case resembling many cystic lesions occurring in this location, such as apical periodontal cyst, residual cyst, incisive canal cyst, odontogenic keratocyst, and Gorlin cyst. (B and C, From Wright J: The odontogenic keratocyst: orthokeratinized variant. Oral Surg Oral Med Oral Pathol 51:609, 1981.)

Most mural ameloblastomas are discovered as asymptomatic swellings when they are large; the remainder are found serendipitously on routine dental radiographs.

Treatment/Prognosis

It is difficult to suspect a unicystic ameloblastoma clinically. Usually it appears to be a small or large dentigerous cyst. Careful attention to the radiologic details and the manner in which the cystic wall separates from the underlying bone at surgery may improve the prognosis. Areas where the cystic lining adheres to the bone may represent foci of capsular penetration and bone infiltration. Depending on the number and extent of such areas, more or less aggressive surgery will have to be planned.

In their review of unicystic ameloblastomas, Shteyer and colleagues (1978) found that the following forms of surgery were mentioned for 62 cases: enucleation (50 cases), resection (10 cases), and marsupialization plus enucleation (2 cases). Only three cases had recurrences (5%). In their series, Eversole and colleagues (1984) reported that 22 cases with available follow-up information were treated by enucleation or curettage; 4 of these (18%) recurred, with a follow-up period of 2 to 25 years. Leider and colleagues (1985) found a 25% recurrence rate. For unicystic ameloblastoma, Gardner and colleagues (1987) recommended yearly radiographic follow-up for at least 10 years.

◆ *RADIOLOGY (Figs. 11–19 to 11–22)*

The term unicystic ameloblastoma is synonymous with mural ameloblastoma. It refers to a specific diagnosis separable from ameloblastoma and should not be used to describe a suspected classic ameloblastoma that is unilocular.

Location

Eversole and colleagues (1984) reported the location of 31 cases: All were in the mandible. All 46 cases studied by Gardner and Corio (1984) also were in the mandible. Maxillary unicystic ameloblastomas are very rare, with the first case being reported by Gardner and colleagues in 1987. Of mandibular unicystic ameloblastomas, 77% were in the molar-ramus region, 10% in the premolar area, and 13% in the symphysis.

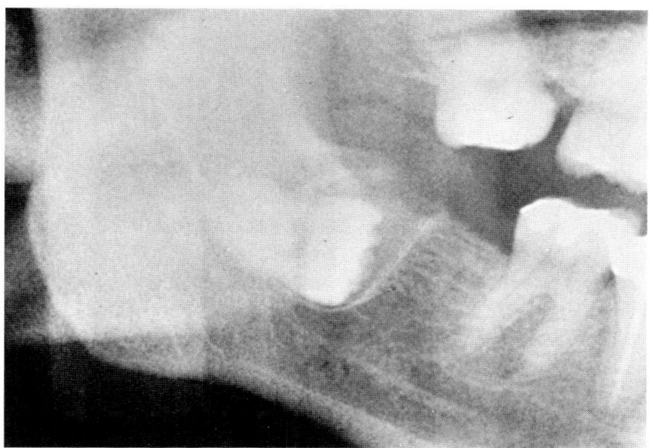

FIGURE 11–19.

Mural ameloblastoma. Case superficially resembles an early dentigerous cyst. The perforation of the sclerotic margin and the soft tissue mass at the crest of the ridge suggest ameloblastomatous change. The trauma to the mass by the upper molar caused the patient's pain. (Courtesy of Dr. J. McDowell, Colorado University School of Dentistry, Denver, CO.)

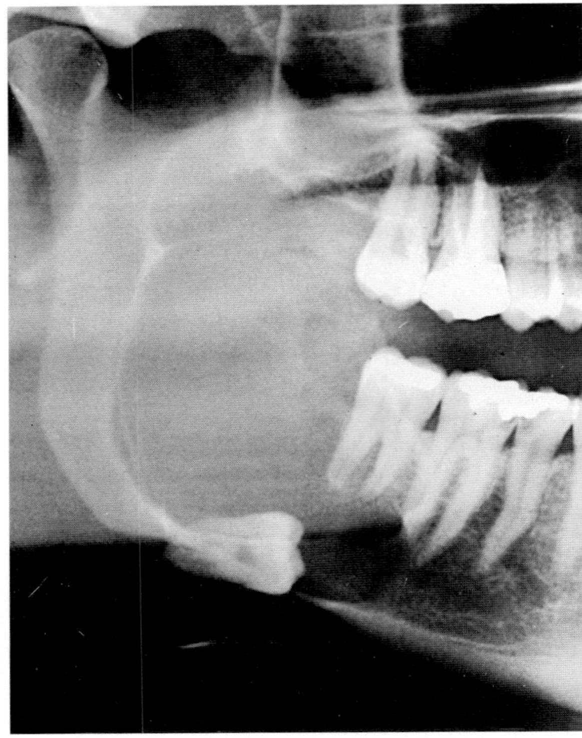

A

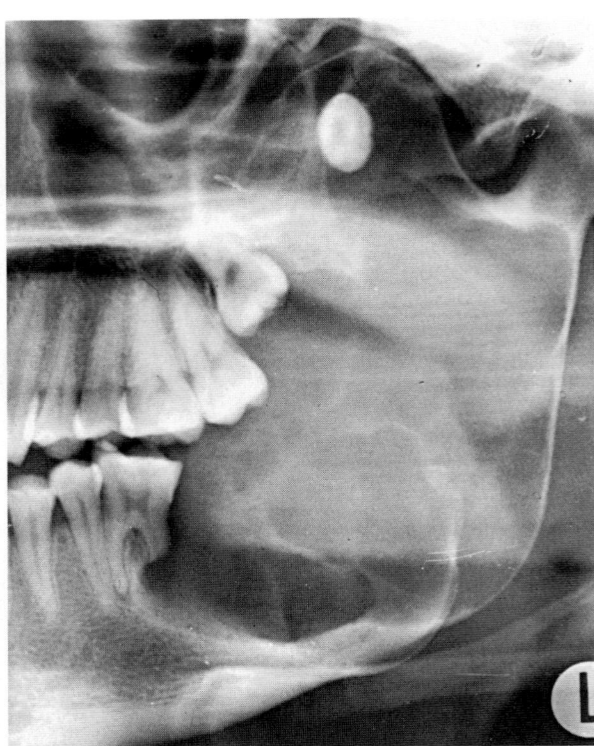

B

FIGURE 11–20.

Mural ameloblastoma. Large lesions. A, Inferior displacement of third molar, slight loculation within, and loss of anterior wall of the ramus. (Courtesy of Gunilla Tronje, Karolinska Institutet, Stockholm, Sweden.) B, Superior displacement of third molar, faint locules, loss of anterior wall of ramus and retromolar pad area, and knife edge resorption of distal root of first molar. (Courtesy of Dr. P. Dhiravarangkura, Cholalonghorn University, Bangkok, Thailand.)

Radiologic Features

The typical presentation of mural ameloblastoma is as follows:

1. There is a pericoronal radiolucency associated with an unerupted mandibular third molar.
2. The associated third molar is displaced distally, superiorly (into the ramus), inferiorly, or mesially; the mandibular second molar also may be displaced.
3. The adjacent erupted second or first molar may show a knife edge pattern of root resorption of the apical one third of the distal root or both roots.
4. There may be evidence of one or several locules, although these are few and tend to remain faint or poorly opacified; internal septa may be absent.
5. Thinning of the sclerotic margin or a cloudiness within the lumen signals ameloblastomatous change.
6. Expansion is often present, which tends to be greatest on the buccal, but lingual expansion also is possible.
7. There may be perforation at the anterior margin of the ramus or at the retromolar pad area.
8. On CT scans, two distinctly different CT numbers can be obtained from the luminal material—one representing cystic fluid, which is often less than 30 Hounsfield units if infection, blood, or keratin is absent; and a CT number similar to that of epithelium, representing the ameloblastomatous tissue proliferating in the cyst wall and invading bone.
9. On axial CT scans, most dentigerous cysts typically expand in only one direction, usually the buccal, because the bone is thinner at this site. With more extensive ameloblastomatous change, expansion may be toward the buccal and lingual, as is typical of garden-variety ameloblastomas. Small locules at the margin of the lesion are suggestive of ameloblastomatous change.

Other Features

Eversole and colleagues (1984) reported that 52% of cases were associated with an impacted third molar and 48% did not involve teeth. Among those associated with an impacted tooth, three radiologic patterns were observed:

1. A small unilocular pericoronal radiolucency less than 2 cm in diameter. In most cases the tooth was displaced.
2. A large unilocular expansile radiolucency extending to the coronoid process. In many of their illustrations there was a slight hint of one or several septa, sometimes with loss of the superior or anterior wall.

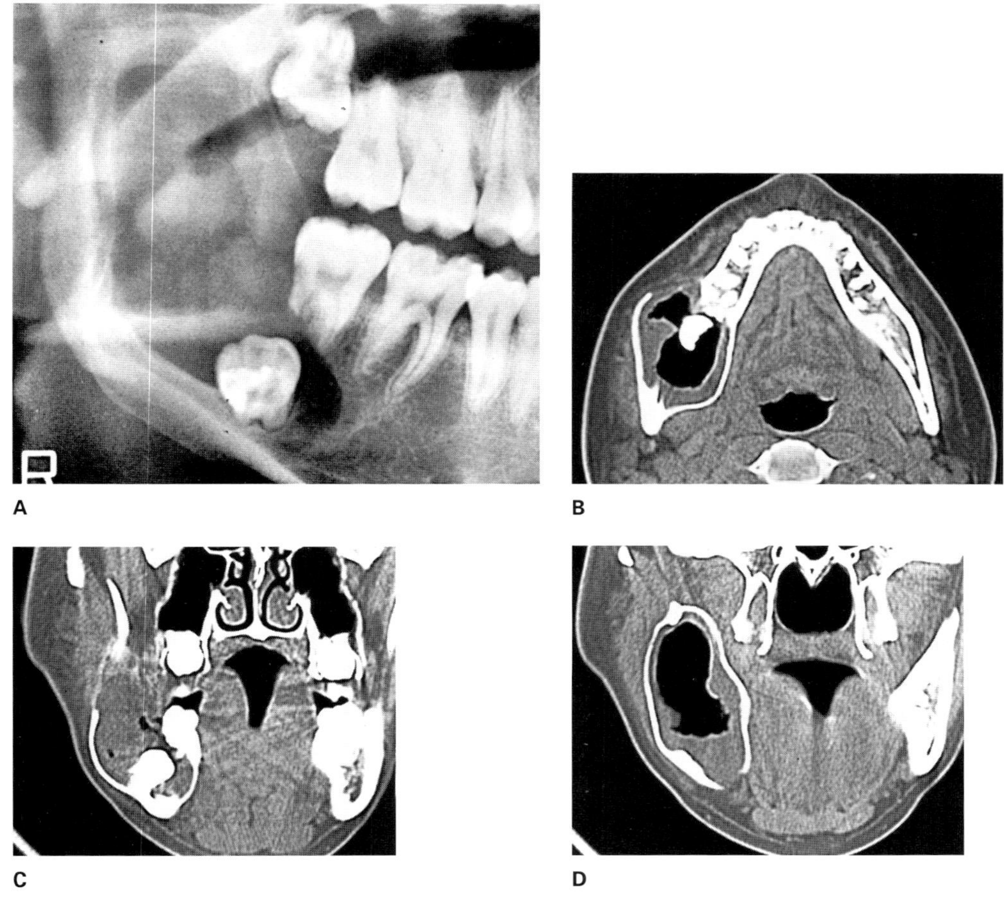

FIGURE 11–21.

Mural ameloblastoma. A, Typical appearance, with cloudiness in lumen resulting from ameloblastomatous proliferation. B, Axial CT scan showing buccal and lingual expansion of cortex with perforation laterally. C, Coronal CT scan of second molar region showing buccal and lingual expansion with perforation of cortex in areas adjacent to solid intraluminal soft tissue density. D, Coronal CT scan of ramus area showing buccal and lingual expansion. The luminal area in Band D is black because the cystic fluid has been aspirated. (Courtesy of Drs. M. Araki, K. Hashimoto, and K. Honda, Nihon University School of Dentistry, Tokyo, Japan.)

3. An expansile radiolucency with scalloped margins or microlocules.

The unicystic ameloblastomas not associated with teeth showed the following patterns:

1. An expansile periapical radiolucency with root resorption and an occasional tendency for the roots to project into the lesion.
2. A pear-shaped radiolucency interposed between contiguous teeth, causing divergence of the roots.
3. A periapical multilocular radiolucency with root resorption.

Rapidis and co-authors (1982) recommended injection of radiopaque contrast solution into the lesion. A cystic cavity can be seen readily, as well as mural nodules. Although this procedure may be helpful, CT soft tissue windows should provide even more information.

The rare maxillary unicystic ameloblastoma reported by Gardner and colleagues (1987) occurred in a 12-year-old boy. The lesion was in the second molar area, and the developing third molar was displaced superiorly and anteriorly to the floor of the orbit. On CT scans, there was involvement of the whole maxillary sinus and extension into the nasal fossa and ethmoid air cells. Histologically, the lesional tissue had not penetrated through the cyst capsule; thus, recurrence was not expected.

AMELOBLASTIC FIBROMA (Fibrous adamantinoma, soft mixed odontogenic tumor, soft mixed odontoma, fibroadamantoblastoma)

The ameloblastic fibroma first was described by Kruse in 1891. In a review of 709 odontogenic tumors, Regezi and co-authors (1978) and Zallen and colleagues (1982) found

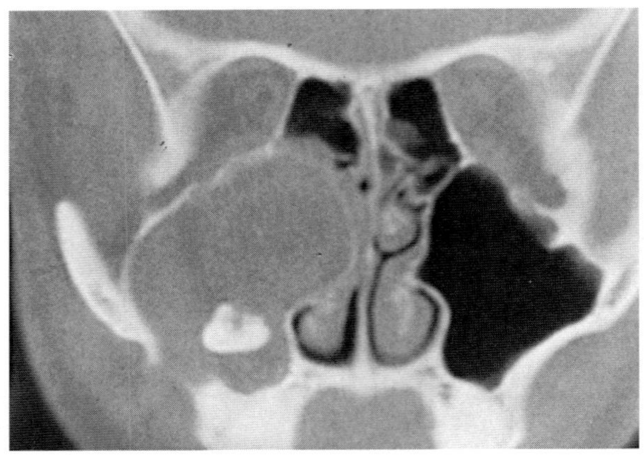

FIGURE 11–22.

Mural ameloblastoma. In a 21-year-old American man of African origin, a rare maxillary case involves the antrum, with perforation of the lateral wall and expansion into the middle part of the nasal cavity. (Courtesy of Dr. H. Schwartz, Kaiser Permanente Medical Group, Los Angeles, CA.)

that ameloblastic fibromas accounted for 2% of these lesions. This lesion is classified as a true mixed neoplasm of odontogenic origin.

Pathologic Characteristics

Histologically, it consists of buds, cords, and nests of ameloblastlike epithelium, from which a central stellate reticulum may develop. The mesenchymal element resembles primitive dental papillalike connective tissue. The presence of this connective tissue distinguishes this lesion from ameloblastoma. Eversole and colleagues (1981) postulated that the ameloblastic fibroma may differentiate into an ameloblastic fibro-odontoma, which in turn may become an odontoma. Farman and colleagues (1986) recently found electron microscopic evidence suggesting that inductive stimuli directed toward tooth formation were present in an ameloblastic fibroma. Slootweg (1981) postulated that if there is a continuum from ameloblastic fibroma through ameloblastic fibro-odontoma to odontoma, the ameloblastic fibroma would be the least differentiated lesion and occur in the youngest group, ameloblastic fibro-odontoma would be seen in an intermediate age group, and odontoma would be observed in the oldest group. Also, all three lesions should occur in similar locations at these age intervals. Slootweg (1981) found that this continuum, with respect to age and location, did not occur with ameloblastic fibroma, although it was observed with ameloblastic fibro-odontoma and odontoma. Therefore, he concluded that the ameloblastic fibroma is a separate entity and probably consists of an embryonal neoplasm. Although the ameloblastic fibro-odontoma probably represents an immature odontoma, both may be hamartomas.

Clinical Features

Slootweg (1981) reported a male-to-female ratio of 1.1:1, whereas that stated by Eversole and colleagues (1981) was 1.6:1. Slootweg (1981) found a mean patient age of 15 years, with 40% of cases occurring in children younger than 10 years. According to Zallen and colleagues (1982), this neoplasm may be seen in patients between 1.5 and 42 years of age, although there are several reports of this tumor in infants, including the case of Shira and Bhaskar (1963) in a 6-month-old baby. In the 24 cases studied by Trodahl (1972), swelling was the initial sign in more than 50% of the patients. Other findings include discharge, pain, tenderness, and failure of teeth to erupt.

Treatment/Prognosis

Simple enucleation produces excellent results in most cases. Carr and associates (1970) emphasized a maturation of the connective tissue component in recurrent lesions with a much greater predominance of epithelial components. In their extensive review of the literature, Zallen and associates (1982) found 82 cases with follow-up and 18 of these recurred (22%). In the case reported by Carr and associates (1970), recurrence was detected 4.5 years later. Blankestijn and colleagues (1986) recommended a 10-year postoperative follow-up for patients with ameloblastic fibroma.

According to Reichart and Zobl (1978), the ameloblastic fibroma may undergo malignant transformation into ameloblastic fibrosarcoma. In 1978, they found 23 cases of ameloblastic fibrosarcoma in the literature. In their case, a 16-year-old adolescent had fibrosarcoma in a region treated 4 years previously for ameloblastic fibroma. In 1988, Wood and colleagues found 43 cases of ameloblastic fibrosarcoma in the literature and added a new case. Although their case developed de novo, they found that more than half the reported cases arose from a previously existing benign ameloblastic fibroma. Among cases that underwent malignant transformation, a history of multiple surgical procedures was a prominent feature. The average patient age was 26 years, and the male-to-female ratio was 1.6:1. The mandible was involved in 73% of the cases and the maxilla in 27%. Ameloblastic fibrosarcoma tends to recur, especially when treated by curettage or local excision. Metastases also have been reported.

◆ *RADIOLOGY (Figs. 11–23 to 11–26)*

The findings of Trodahl (1972) shed some light on the value of routine radiologic examinations in the dental office because 17% of their cases were detected as incidental radiologic findings. As with many odontogenic lesions, the radiologic characteristics of this tumor have been described poorly. The following is a summary:

1. In patients younger than 20 years, cases are found in the posterior mandible.
2. An impacted tooth usually is present, but not always.
3. This tumor is large and expansile, resembling a dentigerous cyst because an unerupted tooth is involved.
4. The relationship of the lesion to the tooth is not cystic radiologically.

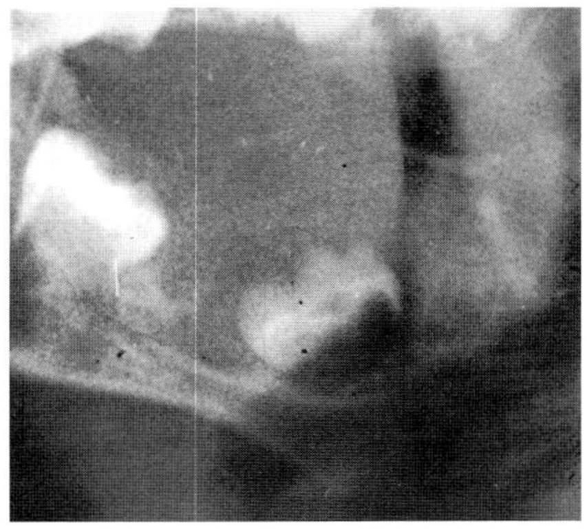
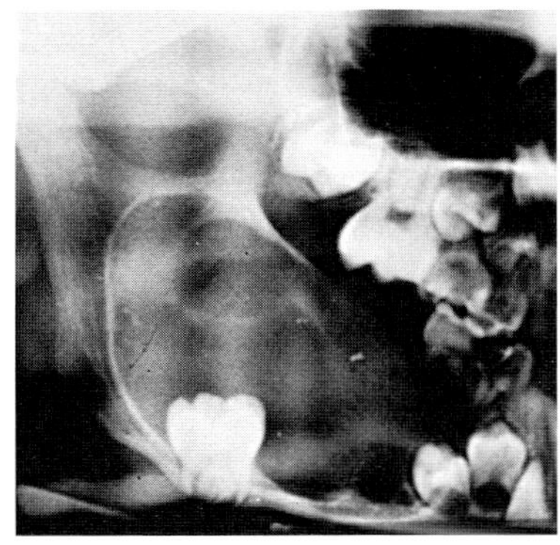
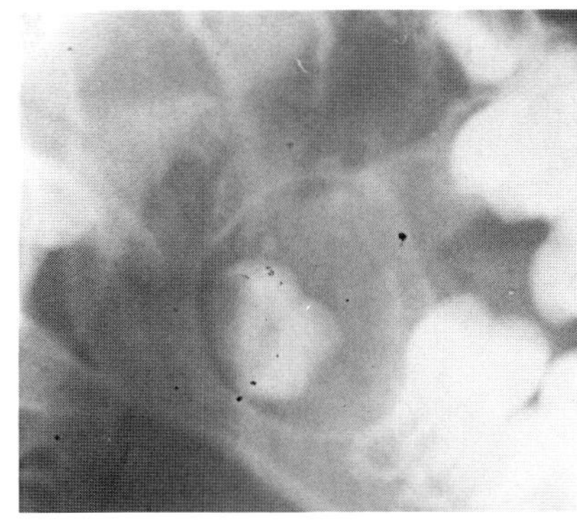

A B C

FIGURE 11–23.

Ameloblastic fibroma. A, Case in a 15-month-old girl. (Courtesy of Dr. M. E. Parker, University of the Western Cape, Tygerberg, South Africa.) B, Case in a 6-year-old boy. (Courtesy of Dr. J. J. Joubert, Stellenbosch University School of Dentistry, Tygerberg, South Africa.) C, Case in a 12-year-old child. In each case, the tooth is fully contained within the lesion and is displaced toward the margin of the lesion, which extends apically beyond the cervical part of the developing tooth.

Location

Slootweg (1981) found 54 cases for which location was specified. Almost all of the cases occurred in the posterior or molar region of the jaws, with 73% in the posterior mandible and 15% in the posterior maxilla. In the anterior areas, only one case was detected in the anterior maxilla and five in the anterior mandible. Three of four cases reported by Nilsen and Magnussen (1979) were in the posterior maxilla, and the other was in the anterior mandible. In Trodhal's (1972) series, 88% were in the mandible, of which 63% occurred in the molar region.

Radiologic Features

Although the lesion may be small, it often causes expansion of the cortex, and many cases are large when discovered. The margins usually appear distinct and well corticated in plain radiographs, but a disappearing margin sometimes is seen. When the CT window is adjusted for bone, a very thin layer of subperiosteal new bone often will be found in the same areas appearing to be burnt out or perforated in plain radiographs. This may be a characteristic feature of ameloblastic fibroma on CT scans, and its presence may explain the low recurrence rate of this tumor. In one instance we observed a very thick solid cortical reaction.

In their review of the literature, Blankestijn and colleagues (1986) found that 65% were described as multilocular. Nilsen and Magnussen (1979) observed this appearance in two of their four cases, and other authors had similar findings. In such instances, Worth (1963) stated that the lesion resembles an ameloblastoma. In contrast to the amelo-

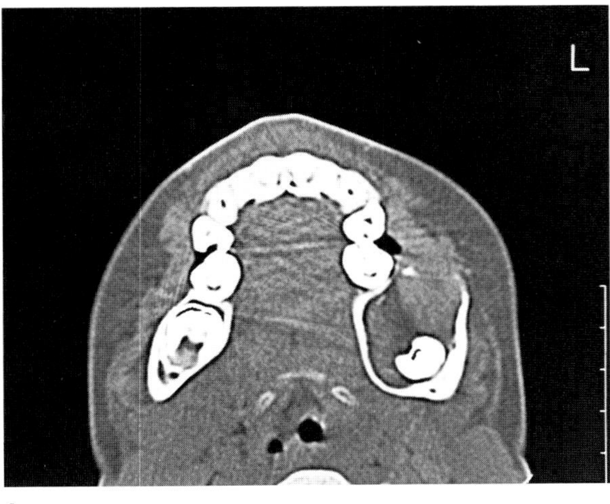

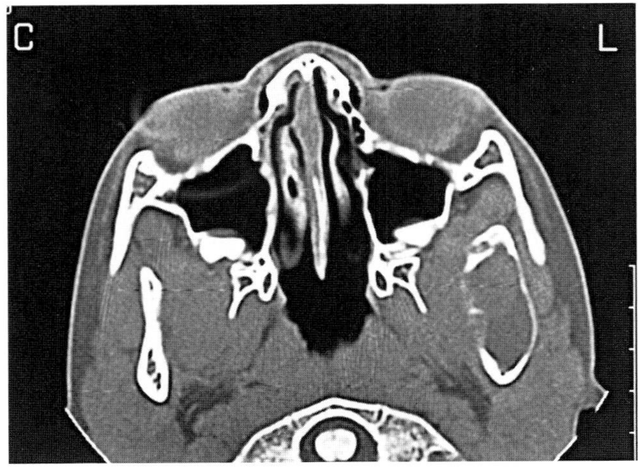

A B

FIGURE 11–24.

Ameloblastic fibroma. Case in a 6-year-old boy. A, Buccal and lingual expansion, with perforation of cortex. B, Extension into ramus showing expansion and thinning of cortex, with diffuse loss of density on lingual side. (Courtesy of Dr. L. Skoczylas, Warren, MI.)

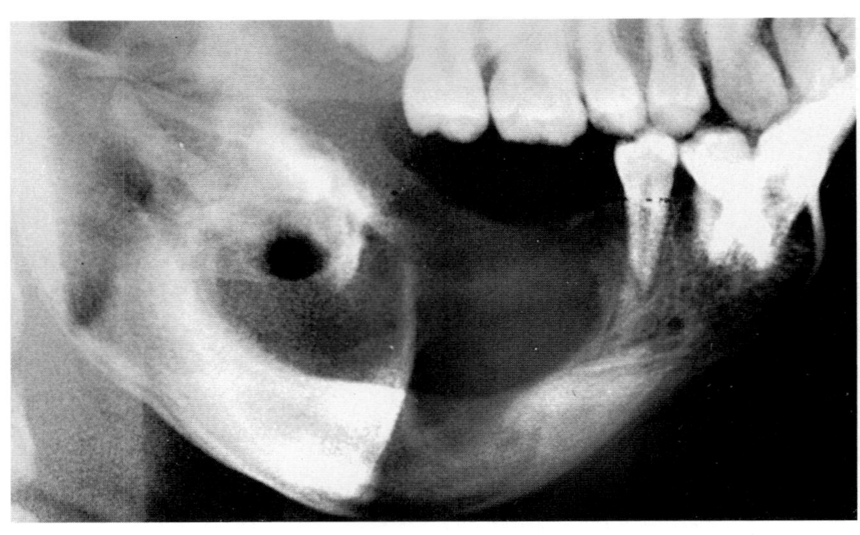
A

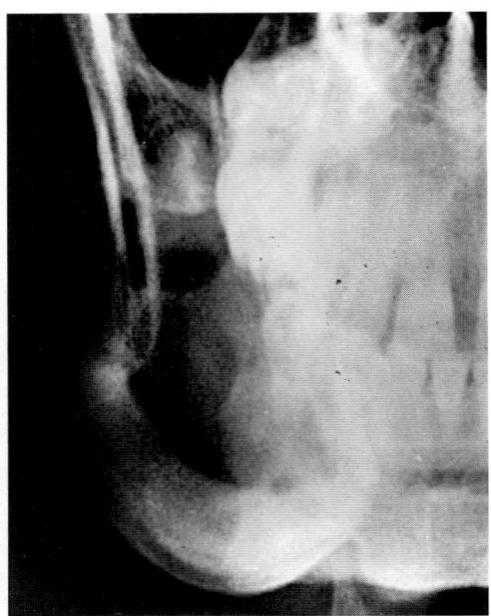
B

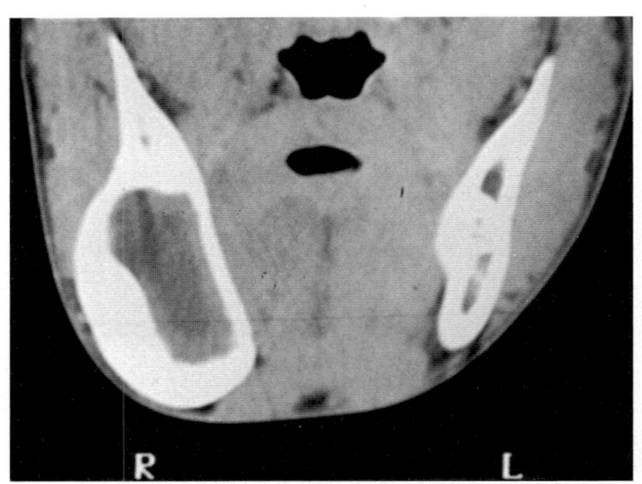

C

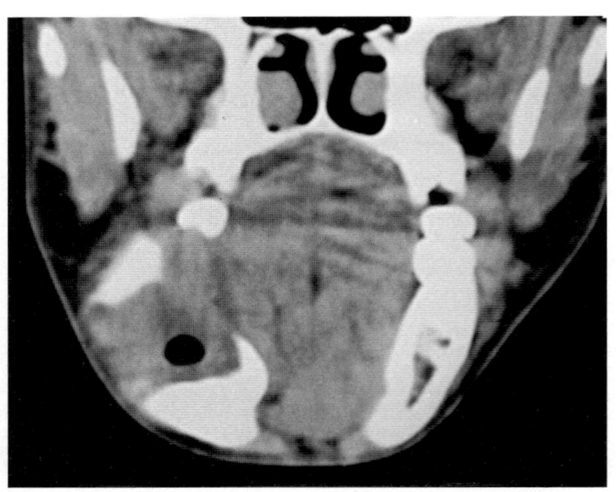
D

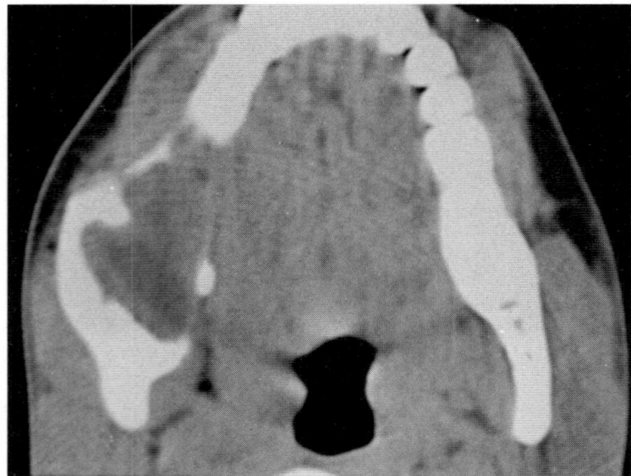
E

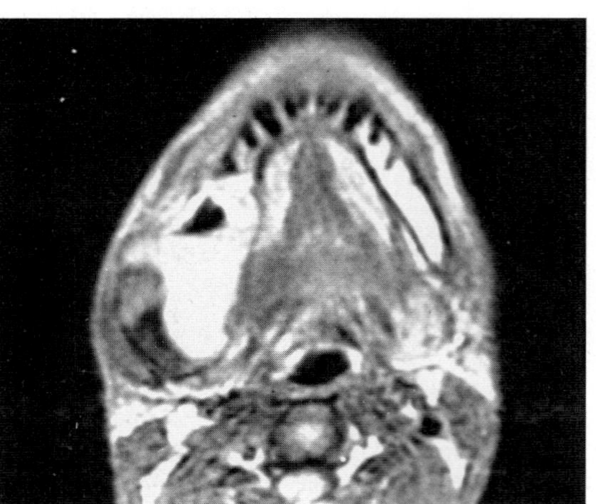
F

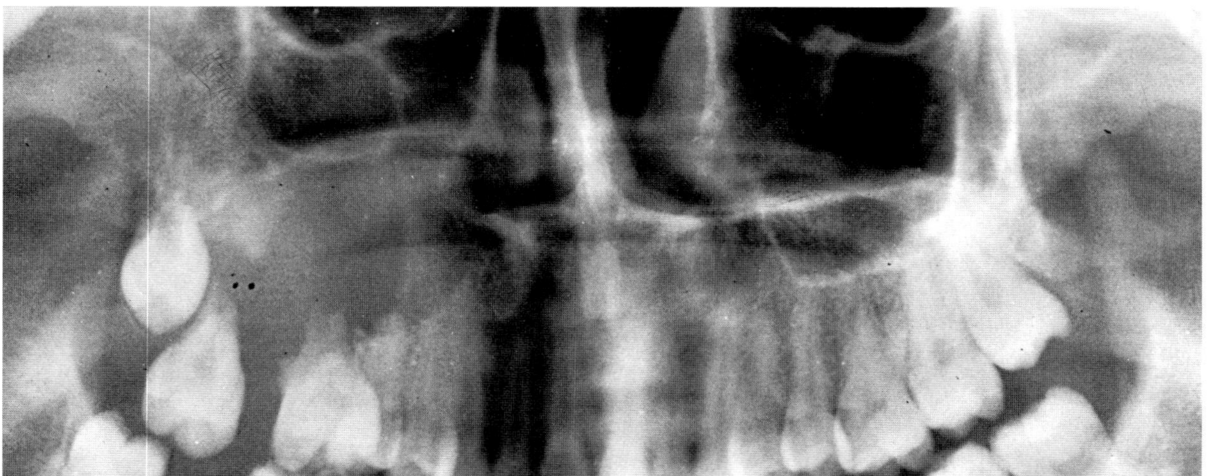

FIGURE 11–26.

Ameloblastic fibrosarcoma. Case in right maxilla in an 18-year-old Thai. (Courtesy of Dr. P. Dhiravarangkura, Chulalonghorn University School of Dentistry, Bangkok, Thailand.)

blastoma and mural ameloblastoma, the ameloblastic fibroma may not be as likely to destroy areas of expanded cortex completely. This lesion also may resemble a lateral periodontal cyst.

Relationship to Teeth

In most reported series, including those of Trodahl (1972) and Nilsen and Magnussen (1979), as well as individual case reports that we reviewed, ameloblastic fibromas were associated with an impacted or unerupted tooth or teeth. The involved teeth usually are displaced. Although the displaced teeth appear within the lesion, they are usually at the edge of it, just inside the radiolucent area. When the tooth is examined closely, there is no evidence of the lesion originating from or attaching at the cervical portion of the tooth, as would be seen in a dentigerous cyst. A right-angle view, such as an occlusal radiograph, would show that there is no hydraulic effect in the expanded cortex, as might be seen in a dentigerous cyst. Further, dentigerous cysts and ameloblastomas have a great tendency to resorb the roots of erupted teeth in the region of the lesion. We found no mention of root resorption in association with ameloblastic fibroma. Although solitary lesions not associated with impacted or unerupted teeth do occur, their radiologic features have not been well described.

MELANOTIC NEUROECTODERMAL TUMOR OF INFANCY (Pigmented ameloblastoma, melanoameloblastoma, melanotic ameloblastoma, retinal anlage tumor, melanotic progonoma, pigmented adamantinoma, congenital pigmented epulis)

Most investigators believe this tumor has a neural crest origin. Borello and Gorlin (1966) provided its current name. Histologically, Shafer and co-authors (1983) described the lesion as a nonencapsulated infiltrating tumor mass of cells arranged in alveoluslike spaces lined by cuboidal cells. Within the spaces are small, round, neuroblastlike cells with little cytoplasm and deeply staining nuclei. Almost all cases were seen in infants younger than 6 months, although they may occur in children as old as 1 year of age. Stowens and Lin (1974) reported an equal sex distribution in their review of 77 cases.

The child's mother usually notices a small to moderately large dome-shaped swelling on the anterior gingiva. The tumor is treated by curettage or even enucleation. When incised, the lesion appears bluish-black. A few cases have recurred, including two cases reported by Tiecke and Bernier (1956). Steinberg and colleagues (1988) estimated a recurrence rate of 10 to 15% and indicated that some so-called

FIGURE 11–25.

Ameloblastic fibroma. A and B, Plain radiographs show radiolucent lesion with solid, thick cortical expansion and focal circular area of perforation. C and D, CT images show that the cortex is thickened and intact in ramus (C), and there are apparent multiple perforations in body of mandible with selected window (D). E and F, Axial CT and magnetic resonance contrast study on same plane indicates area of increased signal in region corresponding to lesional tissue. On close scrutiny of axial CT scan (E) at a slightly different window, a very thin, almost imperceptible, layer of subperiosteal bone is seen. Magnetic resonance contrast study shows that the lesional tissue is confined to the area within the thin line of bone.

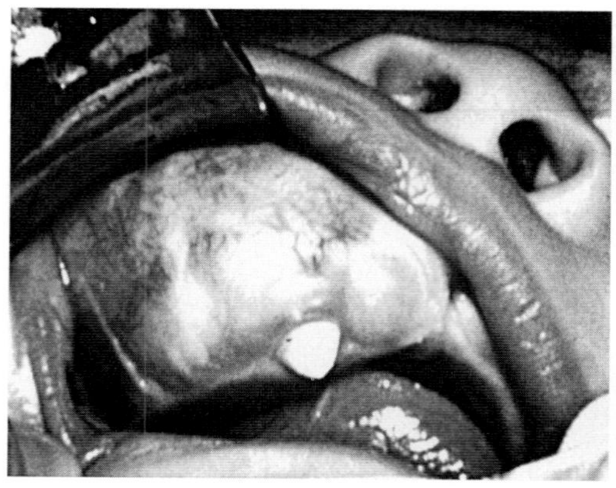

A

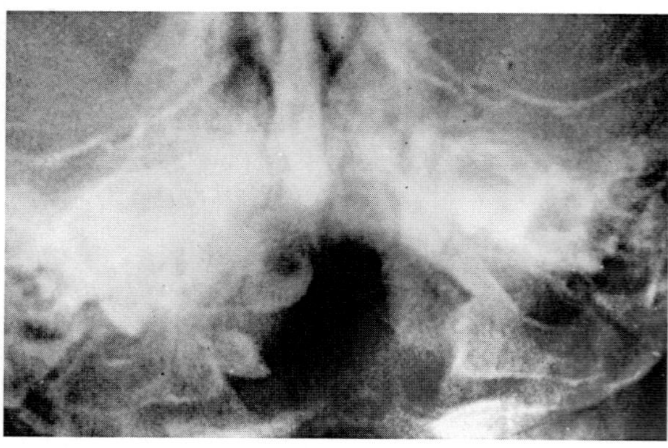

B

FIGURE 11–27.

Melanotic ectodermal tumor of infancy. Case in a 5-month-old infant. A, On excision, the internal aspect was a dark blue-black color. B, Several floating teeth displaced by mass.

recurrences are actually additional foci of tumor that enlarge after the first surgery. In their case, at least four separate foci of tumor were observed. The original tumor was excised, with a second tumor developing 6 weeks later in an adjacent location. At the second surgery, they found two additional nests of tumor all interconnected by a thin process of deeply pigmented cells within the bony trabeculae. Steinberg and colleagues (1988) recommended preoperative CT scans and careful identification of pigmented processes at the surgical margins, which may lead to additional nests of tumor cells along the crest of the infant's edentulous ridge.

Dehner and colleagues (1979) reported a histologically benign case; the recurrent lesion metastasized to regional lymph nodes, and then widespread dissemination of the lesion occurred. They termed this as malignant melanotic neuralectodermal tumor of infancy. The clinical course of this very rare variant was very similar to that of the malignant ameloblastoma.

◆ RADIOLOGY (Fig. 11–27)

According to Worth (1963), the radiologic features are specific, especially when the age group is taken into account. A developing primary anterior tooth is seen in a satellite position to an adjacent infiltrating, locally destructive tumor involving the developing alveolar crest. The maxilla is affected more commonly than the mandible, and the anterior region involving the lateral-canine area is the most common location. Some lesions may extend to the midline. The lesion is destructive and does not form bone. Although the margins may be well defined, they are very rarely corticated. The margins also may appear irregular and infiltrative, with a wide zone of transition. In addition, the lamina dura about the developing adjacent teeth invariably is destroyed. The expanded cortex may be intact or destroyed completely. The lesion produces saucerization of the superficial portion of the developing alveolar crest. Worth (1963) reported that the lesion is usually ovoid or rounded, and it may enlarge to several centimeters in diameter. Deeper involvement to the nose or maxillary sinus is not a usual feature. According to Shafer and co-authors (1983), similar lesions have been reported in the palate, skull, shoulder, mediastinum, brain, skin, epididymis, and uterus.

References

Normal Follicular Space

Conklin WW, Stafne EC: A study of odontogenic epithelium in the dental follicle. J Am Dent Assoc 39:143, 1949.

Osteitis Underlying Pericoronitis

Bean LR, King DR: Pericoronitis: its nature and etiology. J Am Dent Assoc 83:1074, 1971.

Nitzan DW, Tal O, Sela MN, Shteyer A: Pericoronitis: a reappraisal of its clinical and microbiologic aspects. J Oral Maxillofac Surg 43:510, 1985.

Weinberg A, Nitzan DW, Shteyer A, Sela MN: Inflammatory cells and bacteria in pericoronal exudates from acute pericoronitis. Int J Oral Maxillofac Surg 15:606, 1986.

Inflammatory Paradental Cyst

Ackermann G, Cohen MA, Altini M: The paradental cyst: a clinicopathologic study of 50 cases. Oral Surg Oral Med Oral Pathol 64:308, 1987.

Craig GT: The paradental cyst: a specific inflammatory odontogenic cyst. Br Dent J 141:9, 1976.

Main DMG: Epithelial jaw cyst: a clinicopathological reappraisal. Br J Oral Surg 8:114, 1970.

Packota GV, Hall JM, Lanigan DT, Cohen MA: Paradental cysts on mandibular first molars in children: report of five cases. Dentomaxillofac Radiol 19:126, 1990.

Shear M: Cysts of the Oral Regions. 2nd Ed. London:John Wright PSG, 1983, p. 61.

Stoneman DW, Worth HM: The mandibular infected buccal cyst: molar area. Dent Radiogr Photogr 56:1, 1983.

Vedtofte P, Praetorius F: The inflammatory paradental cyst. Oral Surg Oral Med Oral Pathol 68:182, 1989.

Dentigerous Cyst

Ackermann G, Cohen MA, Altini M: The paradental cyst: a clinicopathologic study of 50 cases. Oral Surg Oral Med Oral Pathol 64:308, 1987.

Cabini RL, Barros RE, Albano H: Cysts of the jaws: a statistical analysis. J Oral Surg 28:485, 1970.

Cahill DR, Mark SC: Tooth eruption: evidence for the central role of the dental follicle. J Oral Pathol 9:189, 1980.

Chuong R: Dentigerous cyst involving the maxillary sinus. J Am Dent Assoc 109:58, 1984.
Gibilisco JA: Stafne's Oral Radiographic Diagnosis. 5th Ed. Philadelphia: WB Saunders, 1985, p. 161.
Lapier G: The use of marsupialization in resorbing a dentigerous cystic lesion. Can Dent Assoc J 51:569, 1985.
Ramzy I, Aufdemorte T, Duncan DL: Diagnosis of radiolucent lesions of the jaw by fine needle aspiration biopsy. Acta Cytol (Baltimore) 29: 419, 1985.
Roberts MW, et al: Occurrence of multiple dentigerous cysts in a patient with the Maroteaux-Lamy syndrome (mucopolysaccharidosis, type VI). Oral Surg Oral Med Oral Pathol 58:169, 1984.
Shafer WG, Hine MK, Levy BM: A Textbook of Oral Pathology. 4th Ed. Philadelphia:WB Saunders, 1983, p. 260.
Shaw W, Smith M, Hill F: Inflammatory follicular cysts. ASDC J Dent Child 47:97, 1980.
Shear M: Cysts of the jaws: recent advances. J Oral Pathol 14:43, 1985.

Orthokeratinized Odontogenic Keratocyst

Wright JM: The odontogenic keratocyst: orthokeratinized variant. Oral Surg Oral Med Oral Pathol 51:609, 1981.

Unicystic Ameloblastoma

Eversole CR, Leider AS, Strub D: Radiologic characteristics of cystogenic ameloblastoma. Oral Surg Oral Med Oral Pathol 57:572, 1984.
Gardner DG, Corio RL: Plexiform unicystic ameloblastoma: a variant of ameloblastoma with low recurrence rate after enucleation. Cancer 53: 1730, 1984.
Gardner DG, Morton TH, Warsham JC: Plexiform unicystic ameloblastoma of the maxilla. Oral Surg Oral Med Oral Pathol 63:221, 1987.
Leider AS, Eversole LR, Barkin ME: Cystic ameloblastoma: a clinicopathologic analysis. Oral Surg Oral Med Oral Pathol 60:624, 1985.
Rapidis AD, et al: Mural (intracystic) ameloblastoma. Int J Oral Surg 11: 166, 1982.
Robinson L, Martinez MG: Unicystic ameloblastoma: a prognostically distinct entity. Cancer 40:2278, 1977.
Shteyer A, Lustmann J, Lewin-Epstein J: The mural ameloblastoma: a review of the literature. J Oral Surg 36:866, 1978.
Wood NK, Goaz PW: Differential diagnosis of oral lesions. 4th Ed. St. Louis:Mosby-Year Book, 1991, p. 347.

Ameloblastic Fibroma

Blankestijn J, Panders AK, Wymenga JP: Ameloblastic fibroma of the mandible. Br J Oral Maxillofac Surg 24:417, 1986.
Carr RF, et al: Recurrent ameloblastic fibroma. Oral Surg Oral Med Oral Pathol 29:85, 1970.
Eversole LR, Tomich CE, Cheurick HM: Histogenesis of odontogenic tumors. Oral Surg Oral Med Oral Pathol 32:569, 1981.
Farman AG, Gould AR, Merrell E: Epithelium-connective tissue junction in follicular ameloblastoma and ameloblastic fibroma: an ultrastructural analysis. Int J Oral Maxillofac Surg 15:176, 1986.
Kruse A: Uber die entwicklung cystichen geschwulste in unterkiefer. Arch F Pathol Anat 124:137, 1891.
Nilsen R, Magnusson BC: Ameloblastic fibroma. Int J Oral Surg 8:370, 1979.
Regezi JA, Kerr DA, Courtney RM: Odontogenic tumors: analysis of 706 cases. J Oral Surg 36:771, 1978.
Reichart PA, Zobl H: Transformation of ameloblastic fibroma to fibrosarcoma: report of a case. Int J Oral Surg 7:503, 1978.
Shira RB, Bhaskar SN: Oral pathology conference no. 7, Walter Reed Army Medical Center. Oral Surg Oral Med Oral Pathol 16:1377, 1963.
Slootweg PJ: An analysis of the interrelationship of the mixed odontogenic tumors: ameloblastic fibroma, ameloblastic fibro-odontoma and the odontomas. Oral Surg Oral Med Oral Pathol 51:266, 1981.
Trodahl JN: Ameloblastic fibroma. Oral Surg Oral Med Oral Pathol 33: 547, 1972.
Wood RM, Markle TL, Barker BF, Hiatt WR: Ameloblastic fibrosarcoma. Oral Surg Oral Med Oral Pathol 66:74, 1988.
Worth HM: Principles and Practice of Oral Radiologic Interpretation. Chicago:Yearbook Medical Publishers, 1963, p. 488.
Zallen RD, Preskar MH, McClary SH: Ameloblastic fibroma. J Oral Maxillofac Surg 57:513, 1982.

Melanotic Neuroectodermal Tumor of Infancy

Borello ED, Gorlin RJ: Melanotic neuroectodermal tumor of infancy: a neoplasm of neural crest origin. Cancer 19:196, 1966.
Dehner LP, et al: Malignant melanotic neuroectodermal tumor of infancy. Cancer 43:1389, 1979.
Shafer WG, Hine MK, Levy BM: A Textbook of Oral Pathology. 4th Ed. Philadelphia:WB Saunders, 1983, p. 210.
Steinberg B, Shuler C, Wilson S: Melanotic neuroectodermal tumor of infancy: evidence for multicentricity. Oral Surg Oral Med Oral Pathol 66:666, 1988.
Stowens D, Lin T-H: Melanotic progonoma of the brain. Hum Pathol 5: 105, 1974.
Tiecke RW, Bernier JL: Melanotic ameloblastoma. Oral Surg Oral Med Oral Pathol 9:1197, 1956.
Worth HM: Principles and Practice of the Oral Radiologic Interpretation. Chicago:Yearbook Medical Publishers, 1963, p. 494.

Chapter 12

Pericoronal Radiolucencies with Opacities

CALCIFYING ODONTOGENIC CYST

(Keratinizing and/or calcifying epithelial odontogenic cyst, Gorlin cyst, cystic keratinizing tumor, calcifying ghost cell odontogenic tumor, cystic calcifying odontogenic tumor)

For this discussion, we prefer the term calcifying odontogenic lesion (COL) because some cases are cysts, some are tumors, and others contain elements of both, which has led to confusion about their nature and clinical features. Although most believe that the COL first was reported as a calcifying odontogenic cyst (COC) in 1962 by Gorlin and co-authors, it may have been described first by Rykwind in 1932. In their analysis of 706 odontogenic tumors, Regezi and colleagues (1978) observed that the COC accounted for 2% of the sample. According to Wright and associates (1984), approximately 83 cases have been reported in the literature.

Pathologic Characteristics

Many authors now accept the classification developed by Praetorius and co-workers (1981) in an analysis of 16 cases, and much of this discussion is based on their findings. They divided these lesions into four subtypes, all of which are characterized histologically by varying presentations of the three main tissue components: odontogenic epithelium, ghost cells, and dental hard tissue. Type 1A, the simple unicystic type, consists of the typical Gorlin cyst, with or without dentinoid. Type 1B, the odontoma-producing type, has all the features of Type 1A, but the dental hard tissue consists of compound or complex odontomas and an additional component may be composed of ameloblastic fibroma within the cyst wall and invading surrounding bone. Type 1C, the ameloblastomatous proliferating type, is characterized by vivid ameloblastomatous proliferation, both luminal and mural, and the dental hard tissue consists of vivid formation of dentinoid in relation to the islands of epithelium in the connective tissue wall. Type 2 has been termed dentinogenic ghost cell tumor and is neoplastic in nature. The epithelial component consists of numerous ameloblastomatous-like proliferations in a fibrous connective tissue stroma; the ghost cells are seen in varying amounts within the epithelial islands; and the dental hard tissue is composed of varying amounts of dentinoid in intimate contact with the epithelium The growth pattern is similar to that of an ameloblastoma.

Clinical Features

Although Type 1A can occur in any age group, four of five patients reported by Praetorius and associates (1981) were older than 45 years. In the group with Type 1B, the ages of seven patients ranged from 11 to 32 years; however, five of the seven were younger than 20 years, the same age group in which odontomas and ameloblastic fibromas are found. In their review of 15 COCs, Kaugars and colleagues (1989) found that five cases (33%) were associated with odontomas, and all occurred in adolescents. These accounted for 1% of their series of 351 odontomas. In the cases reported by Praetorius and colleagues (1981), Type 1C was found in only one patient, who was 47 years old. Type 2 occurred in a 52-year-old man and a 63-year-old woman. Because Praetorius and colleagues (1981) did not fully discuss all of the clinical and radiologic differences for each subtype, some clinical features must be explained in a general way.

Almost everyone reported an equal sex distribution, including Altini and Farman (1975) and Nagao and colleagues (1983). The COC often is diagnosed in the second decade of life, although it may occur at any time. The COC usually is a painless, slow-growing swelling. This was found in 22 of 23 of the cases reported by Nagao and colleagues (1983).

Treatment/Prognosis

Twenty-two of the 23 cases reported by Nagao and colleagues (1983) were treated by enucleation and none recurred; however, because recurrence is reported in some cases, the subtypes classified by Praetorius are useful. Recurrence is rare in Type 1 cases. The neoplastic tumor in Type 2 cases tends to recur, and Praetorius and associates (1981) found recurrence in one of their two cases and cited several other examples from the literature. Wright and colleagues (1984) reviewed the literature regarding recurrence of COCs and found only four reported recurrences and added a new case. They stressed the importance of age with respect to recurrence because all recurrences were in patients older than 60 years. They also found that recurrences were discovered at least 5 years after the initial therapy. Their case, a Type 1B (odontoma-producing type) lesion, occurred in a 6-year-old child, and the recurrent lesion was Type 1A (classic Gorlin cyst) and developed when the child was 11 years old.

In rare instances, malignant transformation of COCs has been reported, including a case by Ikemura and co-workers (1985) in a 48-year-old woman. The lesion occurred in the maxilla, and the patient died 20 months later of intracranial extension. No metastases were detected. Ikemura and colleagues (1985) found two other cases of malignant transformation in the literature. The first was a maxillary lesion in a 57-year-old Japanese man, in whom malignant transformation occurred in a recurrent lesion, 1 year after the original enucleation of the COC. The second was published by Witto (Seeliger and Reyneke, 1978) but was not described in detail. The malignant odontogenic ghost cell tumor is discussed further in Chapter 14, "Poorly Defined Radiolucencies."

◆ RADIOLOGY (Figs. 12–1 to 12–5)

Seeliger and Reyneke (1978) demonstrated the importance of multiple radiographic views. In their case, affecting the anterior maxilla of a 14-year-old African girl, the description was of a Type 1B lesion with a compound odontoma. The intraoral occlusal radiograph showed excellent details concerning the smooth regular margins, expansion, adjacent root displacement, and odontoma-like nature of the radiopaque material; however, the panoramic radiograph provided the best view of the adjacent unerupted and displaced canine tooth and its location.

Location

The reviews of Altini and Farman (1975), Regezi and colleagues (1978), and Nagao and co-authors (1983) mentioned location. These findings are confusing and contradictory. Since the classification of Praetorius and colleagues (1981) was published, additional work is needed to correlate subtypes with location. In our analysis of the literature, we concluded that the COL can be found anywhere in the jaws, with approximately an equal propensity to occur in the maxilla or mandible, anteriorly or posteriorly. Seeliger and Reyneke (1978) stated that the COC developed on the right side in 70% of the cases they reviewed.

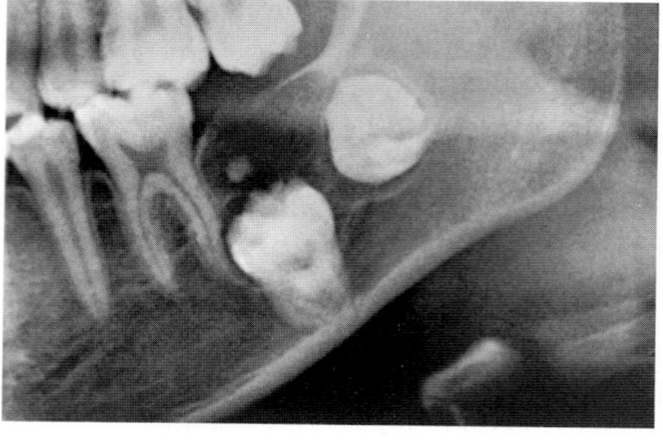

FIGURE 12–2.

Calcifying odontogenic cyst: Small lesion showing rare involvement with a molar. (Courtesy of Professor H. Fuchihata, Dean, Osaka School of Dentistry, Osaka, Japan.)

Radiologic Features

In the series reported by Praetorius and colleagues (1981), the most common radiologic appearance was of a cystic radiolucency, which was found in 9 of the 14 cases (64%) in which the radiologic features were described. Three cases (21%) specifically resembled dentigerous cysts. In the series of 23 cases reported by Nagao and colleagues (1983), all but one showed a radiolucency in some aspect of the lesion. The one exception was associated with an odontoma (Type 1B) in which a complex odontoma occupied the entire lesion. Twenty cases (87%) were unilocular; however, 3 cases were

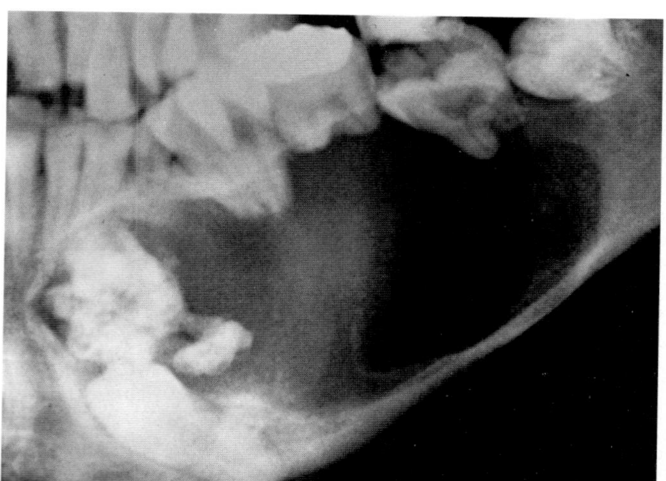

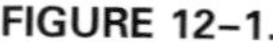

A

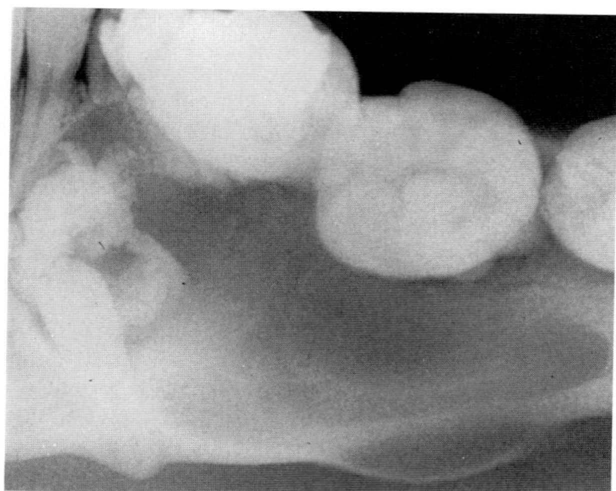

B

FIGURE 12–1.

Calcifying odontogenic cyst: A, Many typical features are present: involvement of nonmolar tooth, occlusal clustering of calcified material, and root tip resorption. The thin white line crossing premolar and molar teeth represents the expanded margin. B, Hydraulic effect at expanded margin, suggesting a cystic lesion (Courtesy of Drs. M. Araki, K. Hashimoto, and K. Honda, Nihon School of Dentistry, Tokyo, Japan.)

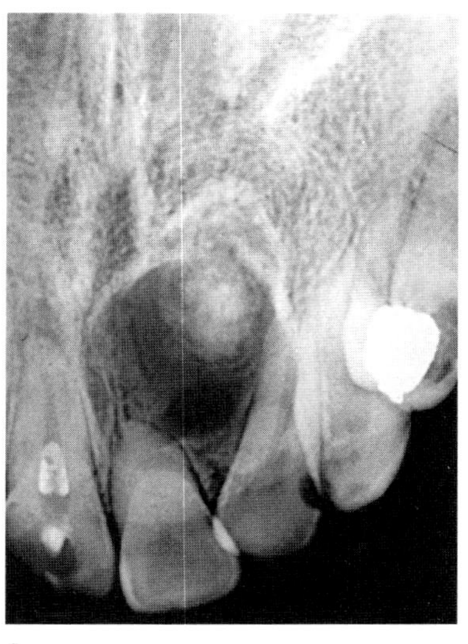
A

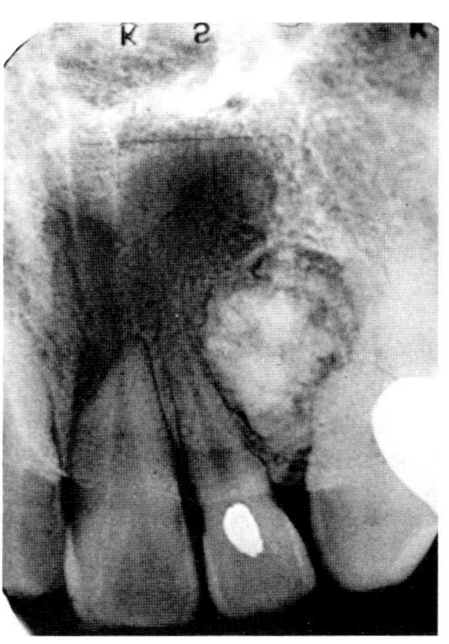
B

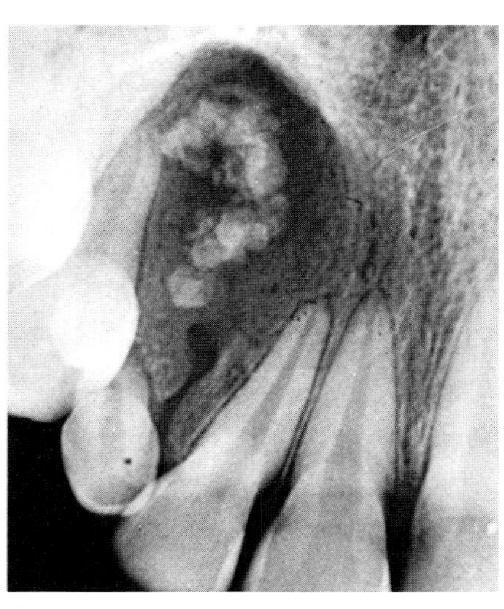
C

FIGURE 12–3.

Calcifying odontogenic cyst: Case in the anterior maxilla. A, B, and C, There is no impacted tooth, and calcified material tends to cluster and locate near the margin. (A, Courtesy of Professor T. Noikura, Kagoshima University, First Department of Oral Surgery, Kagoshima, Japan. B, Courtesy of Drs. M. Araki and K. Hashimoto, Nihon University, Tokyo, Japan. C, From Seeliger JE, Reyneke JP: The calcifying odontogenic cyst: report of a case. J Oral Surg 36:469, 1978.)

multilocular. In 19 cases, expansion was observed (83%), and perforation was identified in 8 of 18 cases (44%) in which perforation was mentioned. Expansion and perforation are rare features of the garden variety odontoma. Nagao and colleagues (1983) stressed that the growth pattern of some COCs resembles that of the ameloblastoma. In some instances, the COC develops in an edentulous area. As Shear (1983, 1985) mentioned, this lesion may have a regular outline, with well-demarcated margins, or the outline may be irregular, with poorly defined margins. There may be varying admixtures of focally thickened, thinned, and absent sclerotic margins.

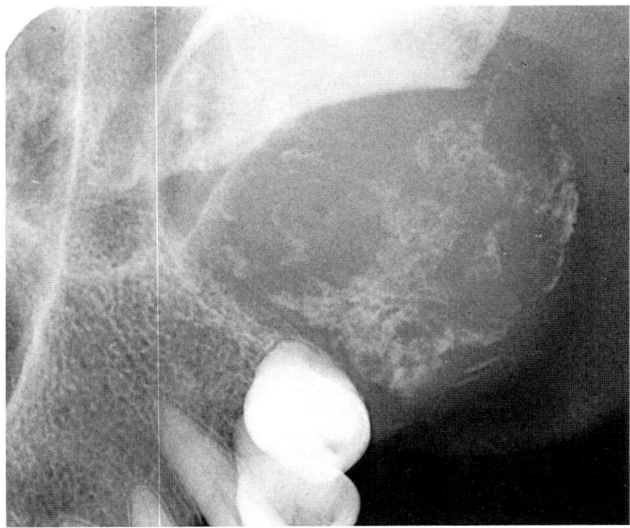
A

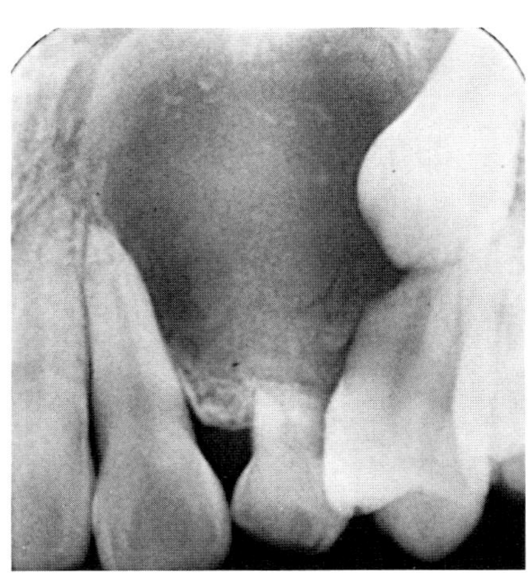
B

FIGURE 12–4.

Calcifying odontogenic cyst: A, In a 54-year-old woman, there are focal interruptions of margin at crestal area. Round washer-like shapes occur in some odontomas. (Courtesy of Dr. E. Romero, Monterrey, Mexico.) B, In a 23-year-old Japanese woman, the lesion greatly resembles the adenomatoid odontogenic tumor. (Courtesy of Professor T. Noikura, First Oral Surgery Department, Kagoshima University, Kagoshima, Japan.)

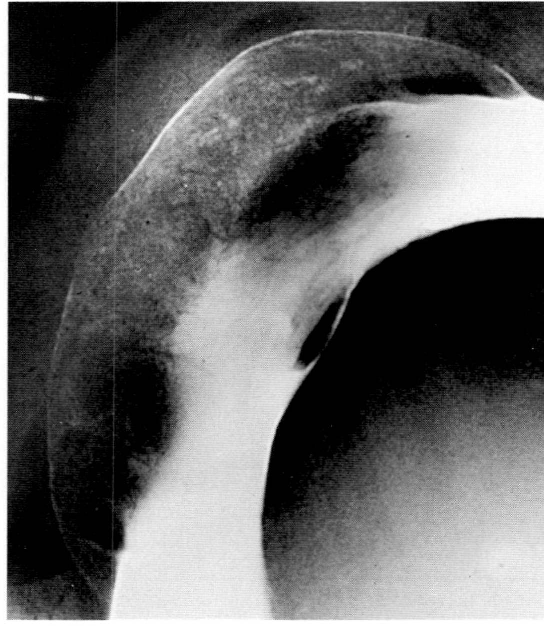

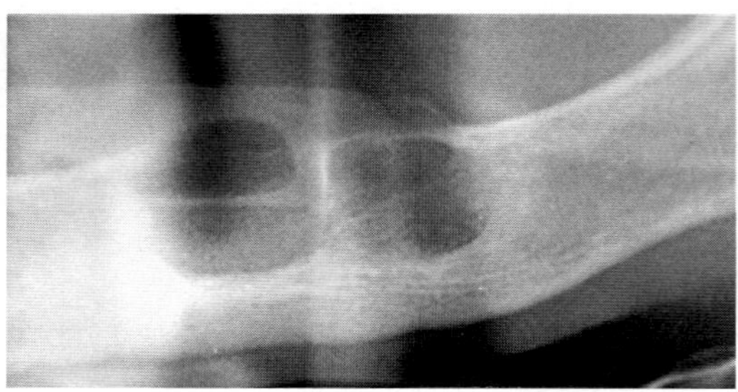

A B

FIGURE 12–5.

Calcifying odontogenic cyst: Cases in edentulous areas. A, In a 42-year-old woman with associated ameloblastic fibro-odontoma, the expanded cortex varies from thick to thin, to focally absent and is slightly wavy, suggesting a tumorlike lesion. (From Farman AG, Nortjé CJ, Wood RE: Oral and Maxillofacial Diagnostic Imaging. Philadelphia:Mosby, 1993, p. 211.) B, In a 79-year-old man, a rare multilocular lesion is a recurrence 3 years after surgery. (Courtesy of Professor G. Tronje, Karolinska Institutet, Stockholm, Sweden.)

Radiopaque Flecks. As implied by the name, calcification is a characteristic of this lesion. In an analysis of 70 cases, Friedman and colleagues (1985) found radiopacities in only 15 of 70 cases (21%); Altini and Farman (1975) reported an incidence of 39%, whereas Nagao and colleagues (1983) detected radiopaque foci in 19 of 23 cases (83%). The latter group observed that these calcifications resembled tooth-like structures in some instances, whereas in other cases the radiopaque foci were rather faint, dispersed, and almost unidentifiable. A cystic or hydraulic effect, in which the expanded bone meets the cortex at an almost equal obtuse angle on both sides, and the presence of radiopaque foci should help suggest the diagnosis. Five additional radiologic signs may be useful: (1) the radiopaque foci often are clustered around the occlusal or incisal surface of an impacted tooth; (2) the radiopaque material may appear clustered toward an edge of the lesion; (3) the radiopaque foci resemble a compound or complex odontoma; (4) the impacted tooth is not a permanent molar; and (5) the expanded bone appears perforated.

Relationship to Teeth

As with the calcifying epithelial odontogenic tumor (CEOT), we observed a common pattern in which the radiopaque foci appeared to be clustered around the crown of an unerupted tooth, particularly the occlusal surface. Also, the largest aggregations are seen at the occlusal, with smaller mineralized flecks toward the central or peripheral parts of the lesion. Nagao and colleagues (1983) reported that odontomas occurred in 5 of 21 cases (24%), whereas 11 of 23 cases (48%) were associated with an unerupted tooth. They found no instance in which the COC was associated with an unerupted molar, although we have illustrated such a case. In the series of Altini and Farman (1975), resorption of an adjacent root was described in 9% of the cases, whereas Friedman and colleagues (1975) found resorption in 14% of the lesions. Nagao and colleagues (1983) reported root resorption in 50% of the cases for which this was specified. Displacement of erupted and unerupted teeth has been mentioned.

CALCIFYING EPITHELIAL ODONTOGENIC TUMOR (Pindborg tumor)

The CEOT first was discussed by Pindborg in 1955 in an abstract and more definitively in 1958 in a report of three cases. Approximately 20 years later, Franklin and Pindborg (1976) found 113 cases in the literature and presented an extensive review. They reported that the CEOT represents 1% of all odontogenic tumors, including odontomas. In most series, the ameloblastoma occurs 10 to 12 times more frequently than the CEOT.

Pathologic Characteristics

Most investigators believe the CEOT has an odontogenic epithelial origin, either from the stratum intermedium of the enamel organ or oral epithelium. Others believe the cells are derived from the reduced enamel epithelium of a closely related embedded tooth. Histologically, the CEOT consists of sheets of polyhedral cells with prominent intercellular bridges. Within the sheets of epithelial cells are round or ovoid areas filled with a homogeneous eosinophilic substance. This is believed to consist of amyloid and becomes mineralized, forming a pattern of concentric rings of calcification, described by Pindborg (1958) as Liesegang's concentric banded rings. Histologically, these are very smooth and rounded. It is possible that the calcified areas occur in the oldest part of the tumor and tend to form a conglomerate, which appears as radiopaque flecks on the radiograph.

Lesions Associated with Calcified Epithelial Odontogenic Tumor

Mural CEOTs have been reported rarely. In 1968, Jones and colleagues discussed possible association of the CEOT with a dentigerous cyst; other reports include those of Ismail and Al-Talabani (1986) and Ficarra and colleagues (1987). These three lesions resembled dentigerous cysts in association with a maxillary molar, maxillary canine, and a mandibular first molar. Two of the cases were in 37- and 50-year-old women. In 1983, Damm and colleagues coined the term ''combined epithelial odontogenic tumor'' to describe a lesion characterized by the simultaneous occurrence of adenomatoid odontogenic tumor (AOT) and CEOT. Other reports include those of Siar and Ng (1987) and Takeda and Kudo (1986). Damm and colleagues (1983) and Siar and Ng (1987) stressed that the combined epithelial odontogenic tumor behaves much more like the AOT component. Three of the four cases occurred in teenagers, and none recurred. Franklin and Pindborg (1976) also found a case of CEOT associated with an odontoma.

Clinical Features

In the series of 113 cases reviewed by Franklin and Pindborg (1976), the mean patient age was 40 years, with a range from 8 to 92 years. The sex distribution was almost even between men and women. Seventy-three percent of the patients were white. Most patients have a painless mass that has increased slowly. In a few cases, pain has been reported and, rarely, nasal stuffiness, epistaxis, headaches, and proptosis. An infrequent extraosseous variant occurs as an epulis-like growth on the gingiva, especially in the anterior region. This lesion has been reviewed in Chapter 19, ''Soft Tissue Opacities.''

Treatment/Prognosis

Although the CEOT often is compared with the ameloblastoma, it appears that its biologic behavior is less aggressive; it grows more slowly; it may be treated more conservatively in some instances; and a lower recurrence rate may be expected with adequate treatment. Based on their review, Franklin and Pindborg (1976) recommended marginal resection, with a rim of apparently normal tissue, as the treatment of choice; they also stated that wide resection or hemisection of either jaw seems to be unwarranted in most cases. Follow-up information was available for 79 of their 113 cases (70%). The follow-up period ranged from a few months to more than 30 years. Among this group, the recurrence rate was 20%. The initial treatment was conservative for most lesions that subsequently recurred, consisting of curettage, enucleation, or simple excision. Shafer and colleagues (1983) stated a recurrence rate of 14%.

Franklin and Pindborg (1976) reported that Shafer suggested, in an oral communication, that there is a malignant variant of the CEOT. Recently, Basu and colleagues (1984) described a malignant CEOT with local tissue invasion and lymph node metastasis.

◆ *RADIOLOGY (Figs. 12–6 to 12–10)*

The most characteristic presentation of CEOT is as a radiolucency associated with an impacted or unerupted mandibular first or second molar that may be displaced, causing a bulge in the inferior cortex. Within the radiolucency, calcified material is seen and may be clustered at the occlusal surface of the involved tooth; in the occlusal view, a hydraulic effect is notably absent.

Location

In the series of Franklin and Pindborg (1976), twice as many lesions occurred in the mandible as in the maxilla. The most frequent location was the molar-premolar area, with the molar area being affected three times more frequently than the premolar region. The other regions of the jaws were affected approximately equally.

Radiologic Features

According to Franklin and Pindborg (1976), the most common radiographic presentation was that of a dentigerous cyst. The lesion may be well or poorly defined. In some areas, a thick or thin sclerotic margin may be present, along with expansion and thinning of the cortex. A honeycomb pattern sometimes is evident in part of the lesion, with the locules appearing small, round, and somewhat corticated. Although the angle area of the mandible may be involved, the lesions tend to extend more into the body of the mandible than toward the ramus.

Radiopaque Flecks. The calcified material consists of tiny separate pinpoint areas of calcification. The radiopaque material tends to coalesce, with roughened or, usually, smooth outlines and sometimes linear streaks that crisscross, causing some areas to appear much more mineralized than others. Occasionally these streaks resemble driven snow and are suggestive of CEOT. The calcified bodies often appear round or oval; these may cluster at the coronal portion of the impacted tooth, with the largest, most radiopaque material at the occlusal surface. We believe the ''driven snow'' or ''linear streaking'' of the radiopaque flecks is an indication of the vector of growth of the tumor, with the progenitor end of the streaks at the occlusal surface of the displaced tooth. This is especially prone to occur when the vector of growth

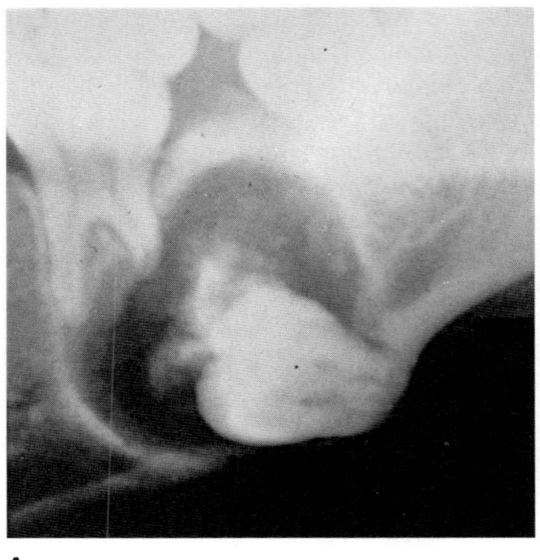

A

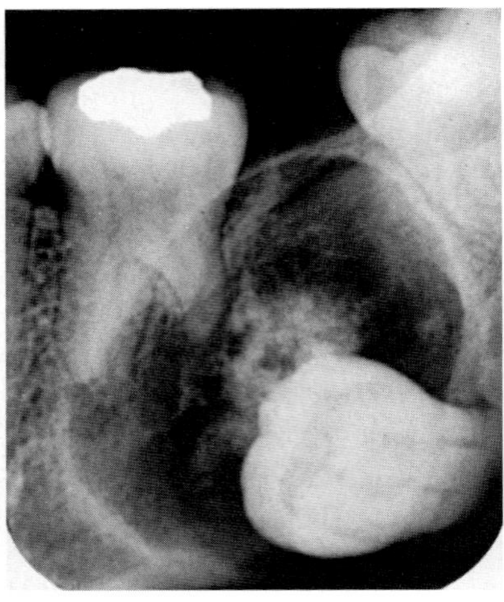

B

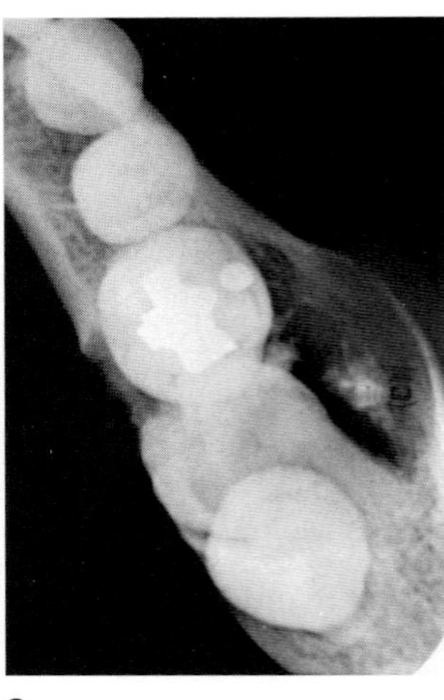

C

FIGURE 12–6.

Calcifying epithelial odontogenic tumor: Case in a 27-year-old woman. A, B, and C, Classic presentation, with displaced molar indentation in the inferior cortex of the mandible. (Courtesy of Professor T. Noikura, First Oral Surgery Department, Kagoshima University, Kagoshima, Japan.)

occurs in the same direction as the displaced tooth. Occlusal clustering is associated with Gorlin cyst and CEOT. In CEOT, the mineralized material may continue to aggregate about the impacted tooth as to render it completely obscured to all but the keenest of observers. The mineralized material also may locate at the margin of the lesion.

Relationship to Teeth

Franklin and Pindborg (1976) found that 52% of cases were associated undoubtedly with an unerupted or embedded tooth or teeth. In an additional 10% of the cases, there was a possibility that a tooth once had been present at the CEOT site. In 34%, no tooth was associated or none was mentioned. Although the lesion often resembles a dentigerous cyst, there are three features associated with teeth that greatly assist in the diagnosis of CEOT: It first is suspected when the embedded tooth is a rarely impacted one, such as a first or second molar. Second, a mandibular unerupted tooth may be displaced inferiorly, with its apex penetrating the inferior cortex, causing a protuberance in this area. The third feature is apical extension of the occlusal clustering to obscure the embedded tooth. Erupted teeth may be displaced, and root resorption may be seen in adjacent teeth, although this feature has not been emphasized strongly in the literature. In one lesion, Goaz and White (1987) described severe, knife edge resorption of two erupted premolar roots; we observed similar root re-

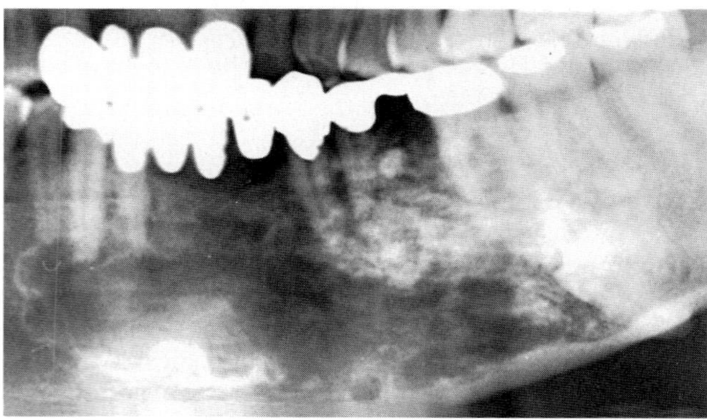

FIGURE 12–7.

Calcifying epithelial odontogenic tumor: In a 42-year-old man, case shows a honeycombed multilocular pattern, and the streaked appearance of the calcified material resembles driven snow. (Courtesy of Drs. A. and G. Castro Delgado, Universidad Javeriana, Santa Fé de Bogota, Columbia.)

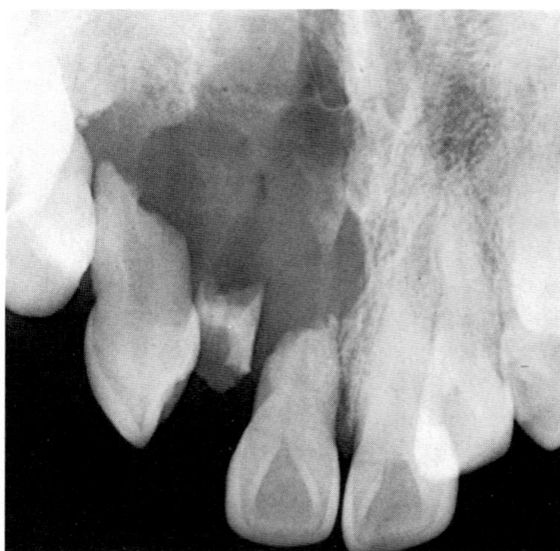

FIGURE 12–8.

Calcifying epithelial odontogenic tumor: Case in a 49-year-old woman, showing an aggressive, locally destructive pattern, with scalloped margins, a few internal septa, and resorption of the adjacent roots. (Courtesy of Drs. M. Araki and K. Hashimoto, Nihon University School of Dentistry, Tokyo, Japan.)

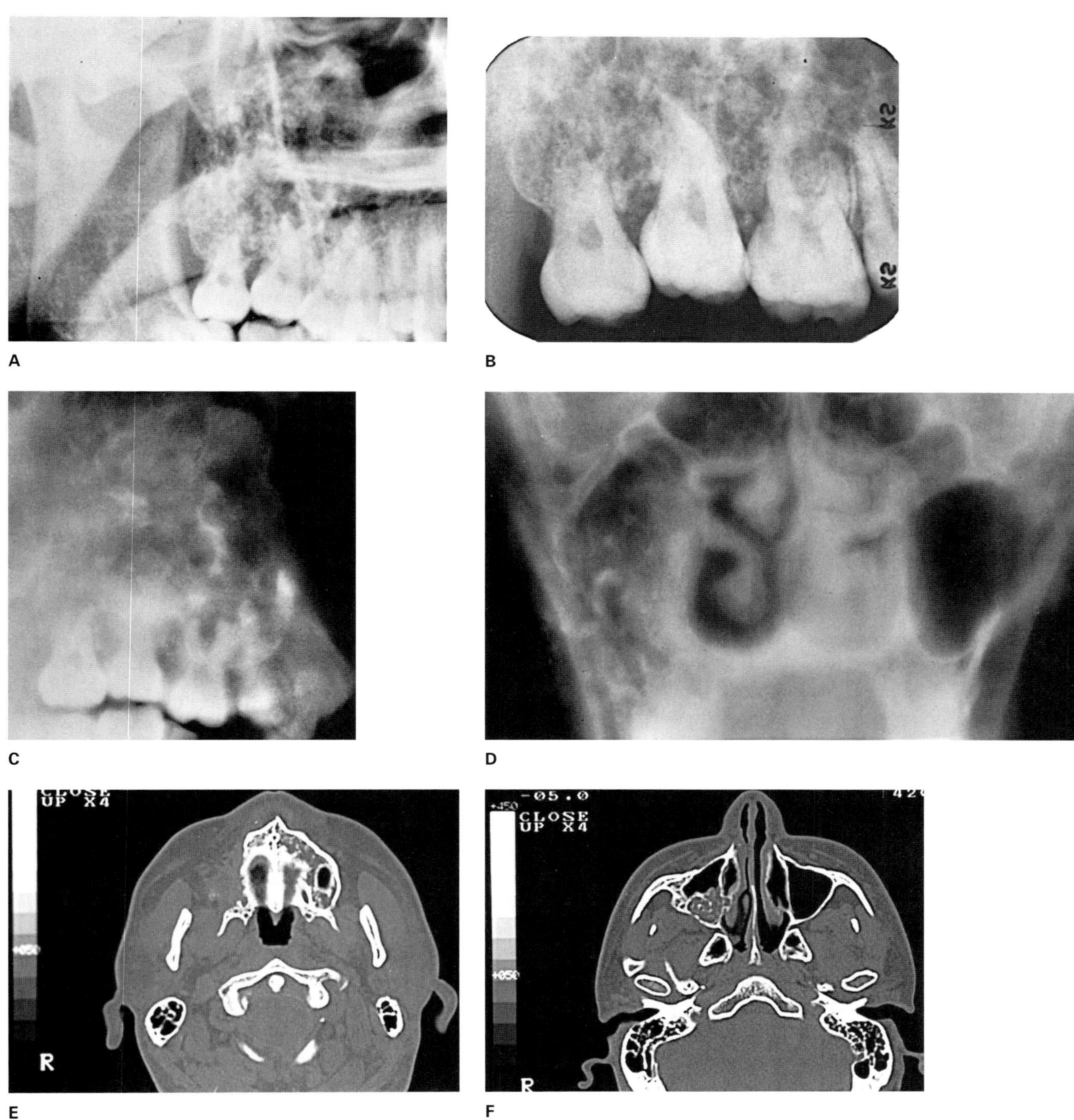

FIGURE 12–9.

Calcifying epithelial odontogenic tumor: Lesion in the right maxilla of a 27-year-old man. A and B, Calcified flecks and extension into maxillary sinus. C and D, Tomograms showing a honeycomb pattern. The inflammatory problem in the left side of the nose was unrelated. E and F, CT images showing destruction of the maxilla and extension to the upper antrum and nasal cavity. (Courtesy of Drs. M. Araki, K. Hashimoto, and K. Honda, Nihon University School of Dentistry, Tokyo, Japan.)

sorption in a few of our cases. Smith and colleagues (1977) also reported this finding in one case, in association with the roots of a mandibular second molar.

Because the Pindborg tumor often may resemble a Gorlin cyst radiologically, the following features are important in distinguishing the Pindborg tumor from the Gorlin cyst:

1. The Gorlin cyst rarely is associated with an unerupted molar, as occurs with the Pindborg tumor.

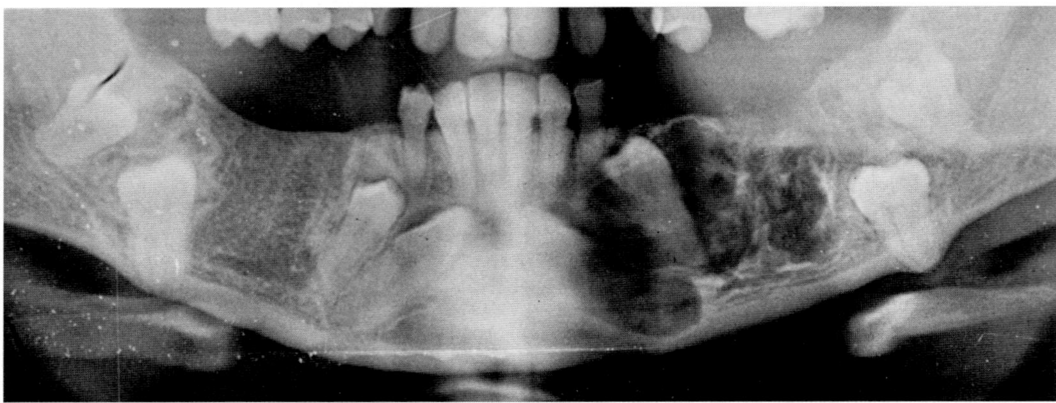

FIGURE 12–10.

Calcifying epithelial odontogenic tumor: Bilateral case in a 42-year-old American woman of African origin, who had asymptomatic swelling in the left mandible that had started 1 year previously. There is notching of the inferior cortex caused by displaced molars. (Courtesy of Dr. R. Arm, Temple University, Philadelphia, PA, and Drs. C. Fisher and E. Reichert, Wilmington, DE.)

2. The Gorlin cyst may show a hydraulic effect at the expanded cortex in an occlusal view, whereas the Pindborg tumor may have a more irregular, tumorlike pattern of expanded cortex.
3. The Gorlin cyst rarely has locules, whereas the Pindborg tumor often shows this feature, especially small honeycomb locules at the margins.
4. In the Gorlin cyst, the mineralized material may resemble an odontoma; in the CEOT it may look like driven snow.

Because the Pindborg tumor may recur, radiographic follow-up is recommended for at least 10 years after surgery.

ADENOMATOID ODONTOGENIC TUMOR

(Adenoameloblastoma, ameloblastic adenomatoid tumor, odontogenic adenomatoid tumor, pseudoadenoma adamantinum)

Stafne often is credited for recognizing the adenomatoid odontogenic tumor (AOT) as a separate entity in 1948; however, according to Miles and colleagues (1991), the lesion first was described by Dreibaldt in 1907. In a review of 706 odontogenic tumors by Regezi and colleagues (1978), this lesion accounted for 3% of cases. Ajagbe and colleagues (1985) found that it represented 7% of odontogenic tumors in their African population and 22% of all odontogenic tumors in patients younger than 20 years. In 1981, Stroncek and colleagues reviewed the literature and summarized the findings in the 168 reported cases. There are several large series of cases, including 111 cases reported by Giansanti and colleagues (1970), 20 cases by Courtney and Kerr (1975), and 13 cases by Ajagbe and colleagues (1985). We estimate that approximately 185 cases have been reported. The lesion is more common than the reported cases would indicate.

Pathologic Characteristics

Although the pathogenesis is not understood, most believe this lesion has an odontogenic origin, perhaps from primitive epithelium of the enamel. Histologically, the tumor is surrounded by a thick capsule, and the lesional tissue is composed of ductlike structures, often containing eosinophilic material resembling amyloid in a connective tissue stroma. According to the review of Stroncek and colleagues (1981), two other epithelial patterns are seen: strands of cells forming a trabecular configuration or solid nodules of epithelial cells with minimal connective tissue stroma. Rosettelike structures often are found within these nodules. Varying amounts of calcification are present, and, according to Stroncek and colleagues (1981), this has been regarded as dystrophic calcification, enamel, dentin, or cementum. It is believed that the AOT may be seen in one of two stages of development: (1) the early radiolucent stage, with histologic evidence of calcification only; or (2) the mature stage, characterized by calcification within the lesion.

Clinical Features

Although the AOT is uncommon, it is not rare, and it is very typical in its presentation. Stroncek and colleagues (1981) found that the lesion is most common in the second decade of life. Giansanti and colleagues (1970) reported that 70% occurred during the second decade of life, whereas Courtney and Kerr (1975) found that 80% were seen during this time. Stroncek and associates (1981) reported that the mean age was 18 years, whereas Ajagbe and co-authors (1985) stated that it was 15 years. Most authors report a greater number of female patients, with a ratio of 2:1 over male patients. For the few cases in patients older than 30 years, Giansanti and colleagues (1970) pointed out that the sex distribution was equal. In the 13 cases reported by Ajagbe and co-workers (1985), there was an almost even sex distribution, with a female-to-male ratio of 1.2:1. According to Giansanti and colleagues (1970), growth is slow but progressive. In their

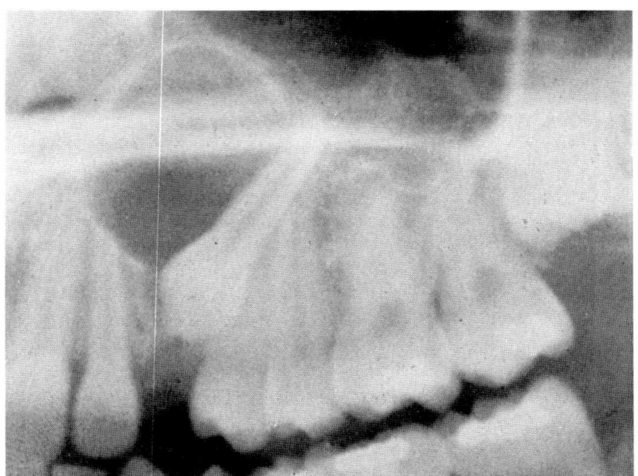

FIGURE 12–11.

Adenomatoid odontogenic tumor: Case in a 15-year-old girl with AOT in the early stages, with no calcified flecks. The sclerotic margin is thicker than most cysts.

series, the mean duration of the lesion was 12 months. Only 5% were present longer than 3 years. According to Stroncek and associates (1981), the lesion is often asymptomatic and "discovered only after radiographic examination." The most frequent complaint was swelling and, very rarely, pain. Although many are associated with an unerupted tooth (usually the canine), noneruption of teeth was not noticed by patients in most reports. Clinically, Ajagbe and colleagues (1985) found that some lesions felt spongy, like a cyst, on palpation, whereas others felt firm or hard, like a fibro-osseous lesion.

Treatment/Prognosis

Cases usually are treated by simple enucleation because the lesion shells out quite nicely. In the series of 168 cases reviewed by Stroncek and co-authors (1981), none recurred.

◆ *RADIOLOGY (Figs. 12–11 to 12–14)*

The AOT typically is seen as a pericoronal radiolucency in the maxillary canine region in 13- or 14-year-old girls. The mandibular canine and premolar areas are also frequent sites, and there are often radiopaque flecks of mineralized material within the lesion. Courtney and Kerr (1975) stated that there are few conditions that occur in such a narrow age range and at such a restrictive site. When these demographic factors are present, along with typical radiologic findings, the radiologic diagnosis is almost certain.

Location

Giansanti and colleagues (1970) reported the location of 106 cases; 65% were in the maxilla and 35% in the mandible. Of the maxillary lesions, 80% occurred in the anterior region, 14% in the premolar region, and a few in the molar area. Of the mandibular lesions, 69% were found in the anterior region, 27% in the premolar region, and a few in the molar region.

Radiologic Features

The size of the lesion ranges from 1.5 to 3 cm, and very large lesions exceeding 7 cm have been reported. There is often a well-corticated nonscalloped outer margin, and sometimes it may be very thick; however, this feature may be absent in parts of the lesion. In a right-angle view, only

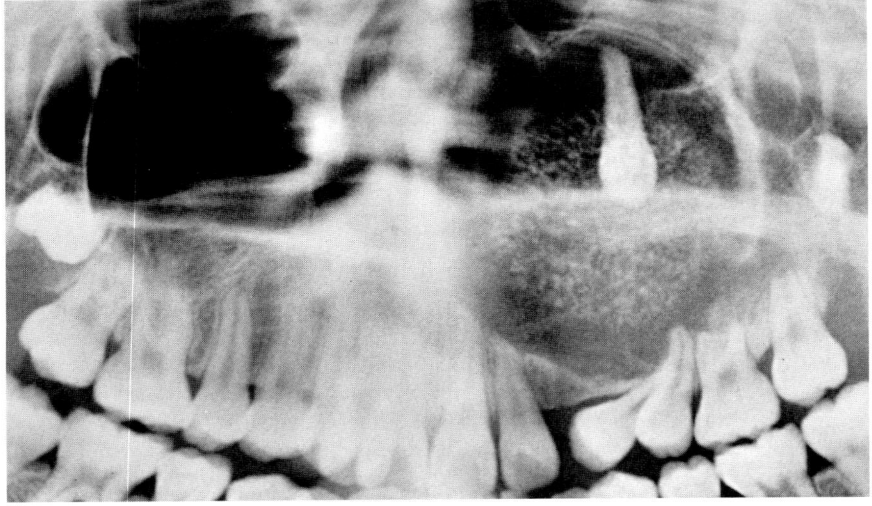

A

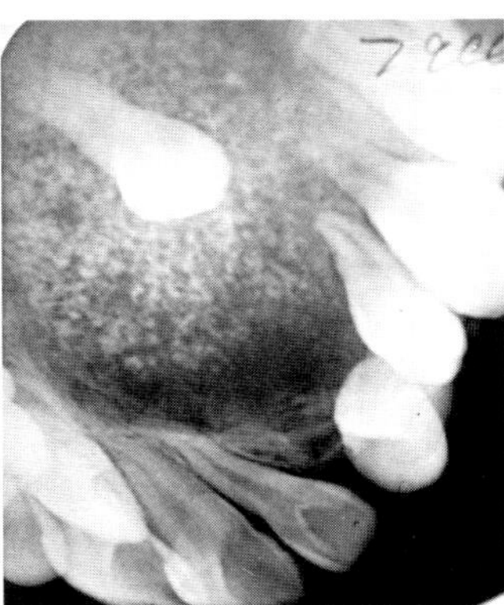

B

FIGURE 12–12.

Adenomatoid odontogenic tumor: Case in an 11-year-old girl. Classic presentation in mature stage. A, Notice the peripheral radiolucent band free of calcific material, which represents a thick capsular space. B, Radiopaque flecks may group together to form many different small patterns resembling a snowflake, footprint, handprint, pawprint, doughnut, semicircles, or groups of dots. (Courtesy of Drs. M. Araki, K. Hashimoto, and K. Honda, Nihon School of Dentistry, Tokyo, Japan.)

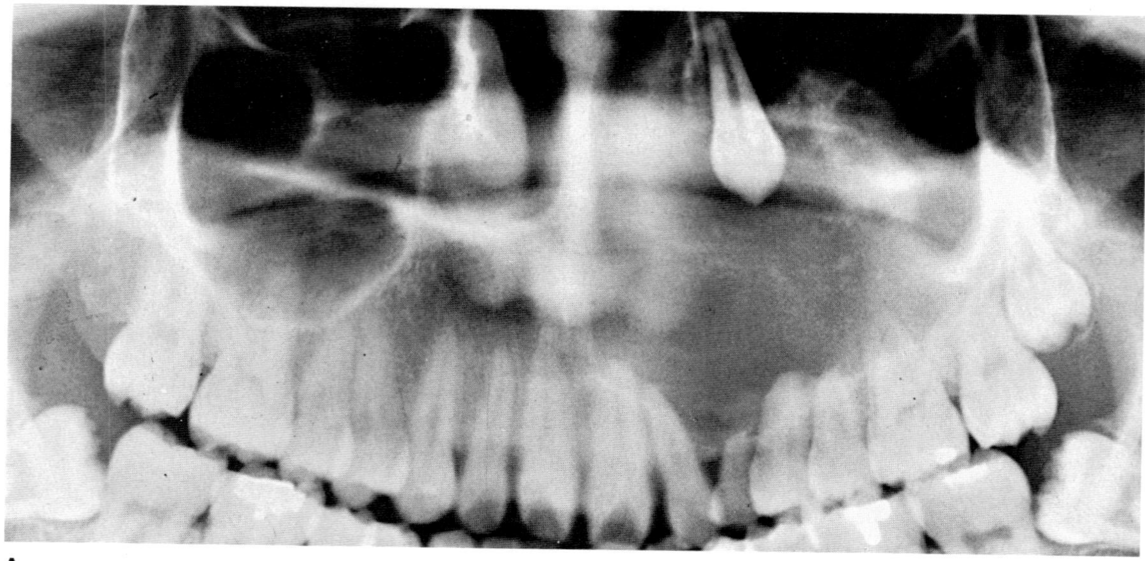

A

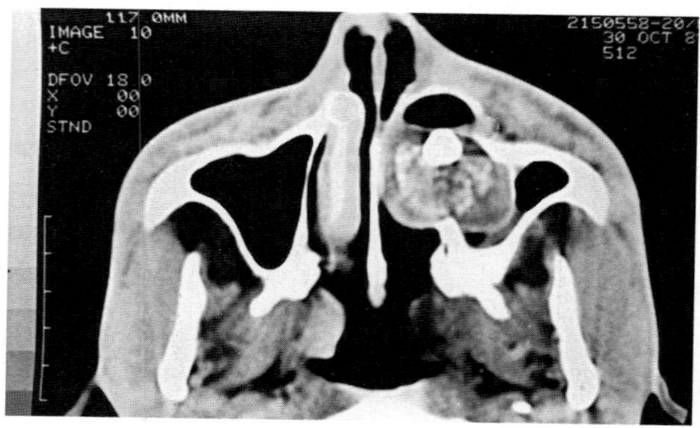

B

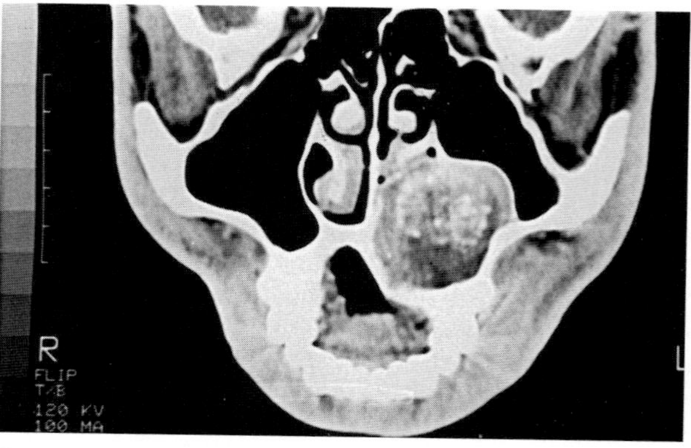

C

FIGURE 12–13.

Adenomatoid odontogenic tumor: Case in an 18-year-old man. A, Panoramic radiograph reveals only a few calcified flecks. B and C, Axial and coronal CT images show a distinct capsular space peripheral to the central area containing calcified flecks. The lesion tends to grow preferentially toward the antrum and nasal cavity. (Courtesy of Dr. C. S. Park, Yonsei University College of Dentistry, Seoul, Korea.)

slight buccal expansion of the cortex is evident in maxillary lesions, but significant expansion may be present in mandibular lesions. The expanded cortex may appear thick and firm or thin and yielding. In the maxilla, this lesion seems to grow preferentially in a medial direction, into the antrum and nasal fossa, because these lesions are large as a rule, without causing appreciable facial swelling at the time of diagnosis. Giansanti and colleagues (1970) pointed out that this lesion may encroach upon the antrum, completely obliterate it, and expand the orbital floor.

Radiopaque Flecks. Evidence of calcification within the lesion suggests the diagnosis. In their series, Giansanti and associates (1970) found that, in 52 cases, the presence or absence of calcifications in the lesion could be determined definitely. Among these cases, 65% had detectable radiopaque foci, with descriptions varying from faint to quite dense and radiopaque. Additionally, the radiopaque foci may be observed in just one area of the lesion, or the calcific material may predominate. The small calcifications may be arranged in many tiny patterns, including those resembling a snowflake, animal prints, hand or footprints, a doughnut shape, semicircles, and groups of dots. This undoubtedly results from the tendency to form glandule-like structures and rosettes, and the arrangement is reflected in the patterns in the calcifications. Although clumping of the radiopaque flecks has been shown, the predominant arrangement is an even distribution of the flecks throughout all of the lesion or a part of it, without much variation in size, shape, or distance from each other. One unique and previously unreported feature of the AOT is a well-defined radiolucent band, free of radiopaque flecks, that partly or, most often, com-

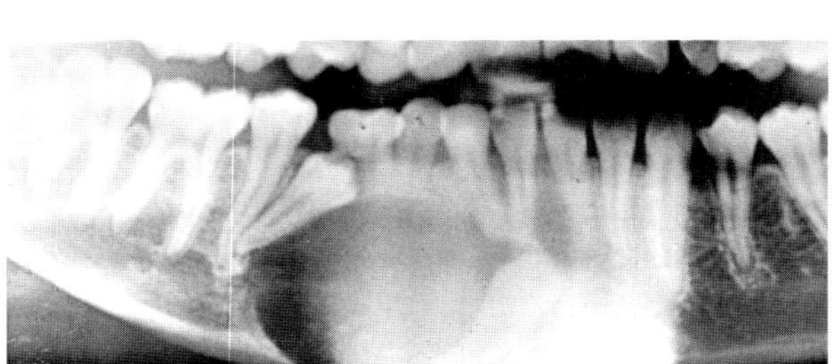

A

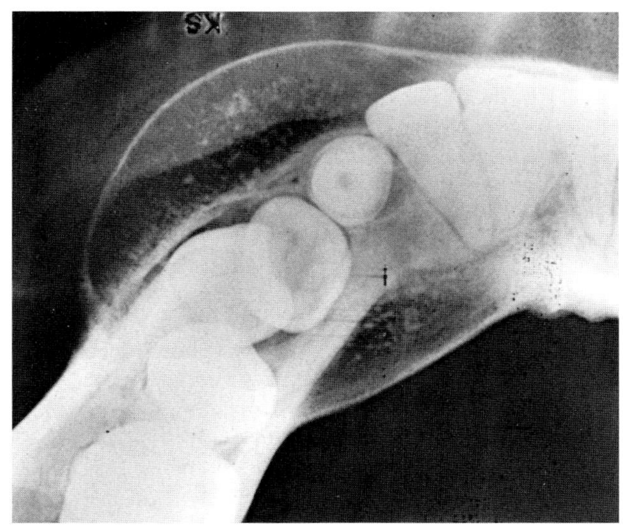

B

FIGURE 12–14.

Adenomatoid odontogenic tumor: Mandibular lesion in a 14-year-old girl. A, Unerupted canine is associated with radiolucent lesion. B, Tumorlike features of expanded cortex include unequal angles at the mandible, a slightly concave appearance anteriorly, and a cortex with varying thicknesses. The calcified flecks form tiny shapes, such as circles, semicircles, and groups of dots. (Courtesy of Dr. M. Van Dis, Indiana University, Indianapolis, IN.)

pletely surrounds the periphery of the lesion. This band is demarcated internally by a distinct margin formed by the outermost calcified flecks, and the peripheral extent of this band is defined by the outer margin of the lesion with the host bone. This band is referred to as the capsular space and may be approximately 0.3 to 0.8 cm wide. We also found that, although radiopaque flecks indicate a mature lesion, there is no relationship to the size of the lesion. We observed a small lesion approximately 1.5 cm in diameter with distinct radiopaque flecks in the central area; we also have seen very large lesions, approximately 3 cm or more in diameter, with no radiopaque flecks. If radiopaque flecks represent a sign of maturity, however, their presence may signal that the lesion has a significantly reduced potential to grow.

Relationship to Teeth

According to Giansanti and colleagues (1970), unerupted permanent teeth were associated with 74% of the cases, and the most common tooth was the canine (68%) among the 53 cases in which the specific unerupted tooth was mentioned. A few patients may have several unerupted teeth. To our knowledge, the AOT never has been reported in association with an unerupted primary tooth or with unerupted permanent first or second molars. Although the unerupted tooth usually is entirely within the central or upper part of the lesion, occasionally it is displaced to one side by the lesion.

Giansanti and colleagues (1970) found that there was separation of roots or displacement of adjacent erupted teeth in 26 cases; however, root resorption occurred in only 2 cases. They also observed that the most common radiologic presentation resembles that of a dentigerous cyst, but with one important difference: A dentigerous cyst usually does not extend apically beyond the cementoenamel junction (the cyst wall remains attached to the cementoenamel junction), whereas this lesion has a tendency to extend apically and eventually may surround or appear to surround the whole tooth.

AMELOBLASTIC FIBRO-ODONTOMA

(Odontoameloblastic fibroma)

In 1967, with a series of 26 cases, Hooker (1967) coined the term ameloblastic fibro-odontoma, distinguishing it as a separate entity. Before that time, no distinction was made between this lesion and the ameloblastic odontoma. Hooker (1967) stated that the histologic features consisted of all of the elements of ameloblastic fibroma, as well as the presence of a compound or complex odontoma. In a review of 706 odontogenic tumors, Regezi and colleagues (1978) found that 2% were ameloblastic fibro-odontomas, showing roughly the same incidence as for the ameloblastic fibroma.

Pathologic Characteristics

According to Gardner (1984), the ameloblastic fibro-odontoma does not appear in most classifications of odontogenic tumors, including that of the World Health Organization (WHO); thus, there is some controversy among pathologists concerning this lesion. Slootweg (1981) concluded that the ameloblastic fibroma is a separate entity, whereas the ameloblastic fibro-odontoma represents an immature odontoma. Anneroth and colleagues (1982) did not believe this lesion is a true neoplasm and recommended that it be regarded as a hamartoma, at least in children.

Clinical Features

Several series of cases have been reported, including 26 cases discussed by Hooker (1967), 50 cases by Slootweg (1981), and 7 cases by Miller and colleagues (1976). In the series of Slootweg (1981), the mean patient age was 8 years; Miller and colleagues (1976) reported that the average age was 10 years; and Hooker (1967) stated a mean age of 12 years. In a review of the literature by Reich and colleagues (1984), most cases occurred in patients younger than 20 years; in Hooker's series (1967), 73% of patients were younger than 15 years and all but two patients were younger than 20 years. One also should remember that odontomas usually develop during the tooth-forming years and these lesions also occur during the same period. Most studies indicate that more cases occur in male patients. Minderjahn (1979) reported a male-to-female ratio of 1.7:1, whereas in Hooker's (1967) series this ratio was 3.3:1. Trodahl (1972) pointed out that Hooker's (1967) material came from the Armed Forces Institute of Pathology, where the male-to-female ratio of the sample population is 2.5:1; thus, Hooker's (1967) 3.3:1 male-to-female ratio probably represents an actual ratio of 1.2:1. This is very similar to that found by Slootweg (1981) in his review of 50 cases in the literature, in which the ratio was 1.3:1, favoring male patients.

Because the lesions expand slowly, they expand without causing symptoms. Consistently, in most of these cases the lesion is associated with an impacted or unerupted tooth; thus, the missing tooth leads to additional investigation. In a recent series of seven cases reported by Miller and associates (1976), the chief presenting complaints were noneruption of one or several permanent teeth, facial swelling, and facial asymmetry.

Treatment/Prognosis

This lesion is not considered aggressive and may be treated by simple enucleation or curettage. The seven cases of Miller and associates (1976) were observed for an average of 4.7 years, with follow-up ranging from 3 months to 12 years; no recurrence was reported. In other studies, one or two recurrences have been reported, including that of Tsaganis (1972). Hooker (1967) emphasized the importance of recognizing the ameloblastic fibro-odontoma as a separate lesion from the ameloblastic odontoma because the former rarely recurs; however, the latter usually shows aggressive, locally destructive behavior and tends to recur, and its biologic behavior is similar to that of an ameloblastoma.

Howell and Burkes (1977) reported malignant transformation of an ameloblastic fibro-odontoma to an ameloblastic fibrosarcoma. This outcome is exceedingly rare.

◆ *RADIOLOGY (Figs. 12–15 to 12–17)*

The ameloblastic fibro-odontoma has few specific features, although these are suggestive of this lesion: (1) it occurs in the posterior jaws; (2) the odontoma component is observed but has a more radiolucent component than most odontomas; and (3) it is associated with an impacted tooth.

Location

In the series reported by Hooker (1967), most cases were in the posterior jaws, with an equal distribution between the upper and lower jaws, as with the odontoma component. In the study of Miller and colleagues (1976), six of seven cases developed in the posterior mandible and the remaining case was in the maxilla. In Hooker's (1967) series, approximately 25% occurred in the anterior regions, with the anterior lesions divided roughly equally between the maxilla and mandible. In Slootweg's (1981) review of 50 cases, 54% developed in the posterior mandible and 8% in the anterior mandible; maxillary cases were divided almost evenly, with 20% in the anterior and 18% in the posterior. Of all these cases, 72% occurred in the posterior jaws.

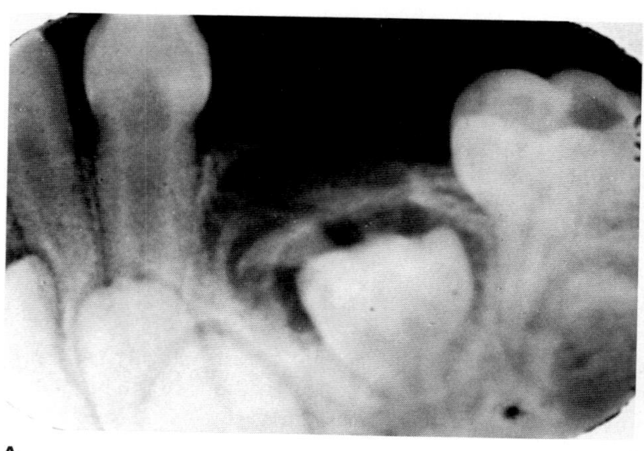

A

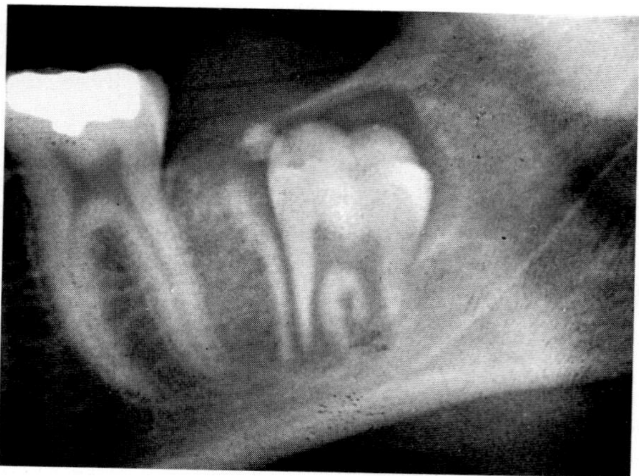

B

FIGURE 12–15.

Ameloblastic fibro-odontoma: Small lesions. A, Case is associated with noneruption of the primary first molar. In view of the small-sized lesion, notice the severe displacement of the erupted second primary molar. B, Lesion interfering with eruption of second molar. Notice the degree of distal displacement for such a small lesion.

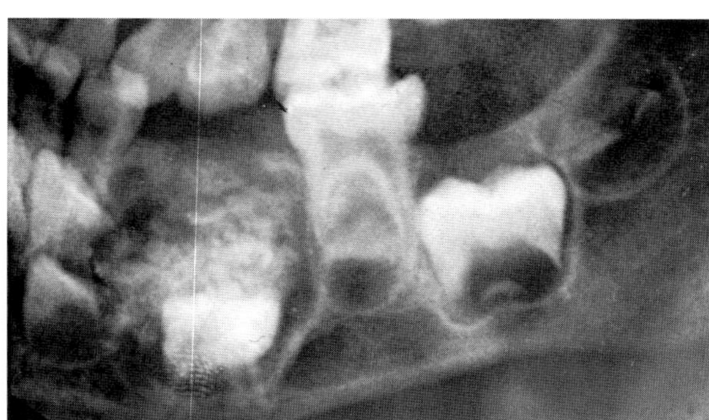

A

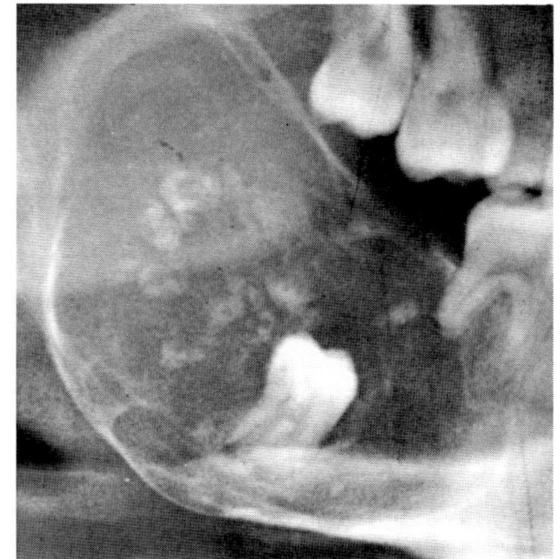

B

FIGURE 12–16.

Ameloblastic fibro-odontoma: A, Washer-like structures predominate, making it impossible to distinguish this from an odontoma. (Courtesy of Dr. E. Romero, Monterrey, Mexico.) B, Predominance of the ameloblastic fibroma component suggests the diagnosis. Notice the resorption of one of the first molar roots. (Courtesy of Drs. L. Archila, F. Erales, and R. Carlos, Guatemala City, Guatemala.)

Radiologic Features

The pericoronal radiolucency may vary from very small to large, sometimes expanding into the ramus, but maintains a smooth, well-defined cortical outline. When several large, mature ameloblastic fibro-odontomas are examined, it appears that they usually maintain a variable radiolucent zone (several millimeters to 1 cm in thickness) between the central odontomatous mass and expanded cortical plate.

Radiopaque Flecks. The central radiopaque area may resemble a composite or complex odontoma, or it may consist of nonspecific radiopaque flecks distributed throughout the lesion. The radiopaque component may be minimal, composed of one or several calcified areas, or it may predominate, depending on the degree of lesion development. In some instances, individual radiopaque structures appear very distinct and noncoalescent, with very round outlines; these may range from 1 or 2 mm to 1 cm in diameter. When identifiable tooth-like structures are seen, the odontoma component is recognized more easily. On cross-section, the tooth-like structures sometimes have a washer-like appearance, consisting of a thick radiopaque rim, representing enamel and dentin, and a radiolucent center, indicating pulp-like material.

Relationship to Teeth

The most striking feature of the 26 cases reported by Hooker (1967) and those reported by Miller and associates (1976) is that all cases were associated with an impacted or unerupted tooth. In a case reported by Daley and Lovas (1982), the maxillary lesion that was predominantly radiolucent occupied the entire maxillary sinus, and the involved second molar was displaced upward to a position just beneath the floor of the orbit. Although almost any of the odontogenic tumors and cysts can displace erupted and unerupted teeth, the degree of displacement often is proportional to the lesion

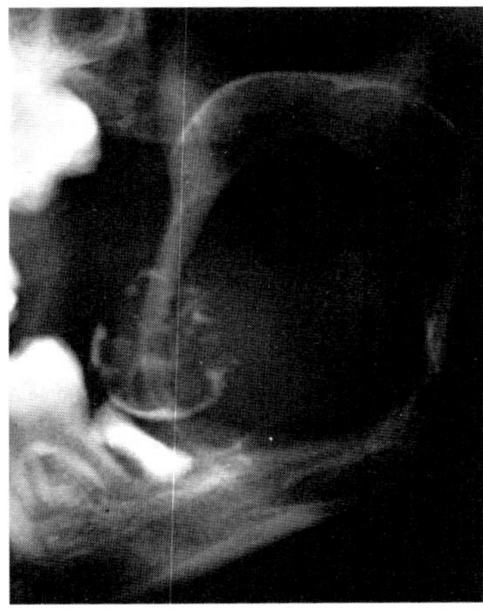

A

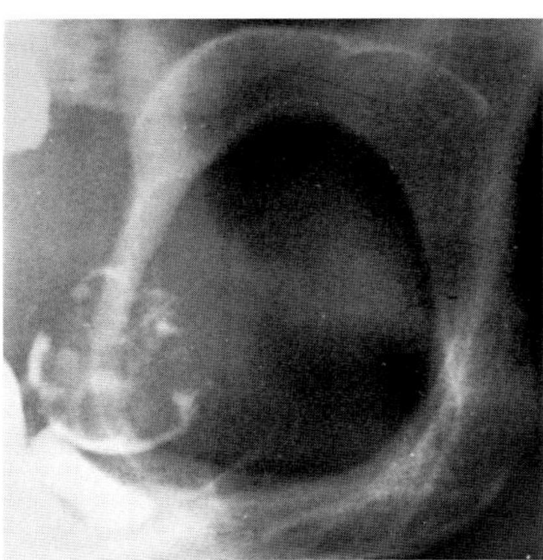

B

FIGURE 12–17.

Ameloblastic fibro-odontoma: A, In the early stage of development, the odontoma is large. There is overexposure of the lesion resulting from extensive destruction. B, Magnified bright light view shows bony details.

size. Curiously, even very tiny ameloblastic fibro-odontomas cause relatively more tooth displacement than other odontogenic lesions the same size. This may be one of the most diagnostic features of this lesion, particularly early small lesions.

ODONTOMA (Odontome, compound composite odontome, complex composite odontome, compound odontoma, complex odontoma, solid odontogenic tumor)

The term odontome first was coined by Broca in 1866 to designate all tumors of odontogenic origin. In 1946, Thoma and Goldman developed a classification limiting the use of the term odontome to lesions composed of tooth-like structures. They included the terms compound composite odontome and complex composite odontome, as well as several other subclassifications. In 1961, Gorlin and associates eliminated the term composite, considering it redundant, and classified odontomas as compound or complex. During this period, the English term odontoma, as derived from the original French term odontome, became popular. In 1971, the WHO (Pindborg and colleagues) defined two types of odontomas: (1) the compound odontoma is a malformation in which all of the dental tissues are represented and arranged in an orderly pattern such that the lesion resembles several or many tooth-like structures; and (2) the complex odontoma is a malformation in which all of the dental tissues are represented, and the individual tissues are well formed but arranged in a disorderly pattern such that the lesion does not resemble a tooth-like structure. In 1989, Kaugars and colleagues found no reason to differentiate between compound and complex and suggested they all be termed odontoma because "no appreciable clinical difference separates them." In light of the current practice, we will continue to refer to the two subtypes of odontoma because they appear different radiographically but concede that such a distinction may be academic.

According to Regezi and colleagues (1978), who reviewed 706 odontogenic tumors sent for biopsy, 37% were compound odontomas and 30% were complex odontomas. Together, odontomas represented 67% of their sample. Devildos (1972) studied 511 odontogenic tumors, with odontomas representing 54% of the sample. The odontoma is one of the most common abnormalities in the jaws.

Pathologic Characteristics

Although the odontoma once was considered a benign tumor of mixed origin, most investigators now believe it is a hamartoma. Several large studies have been published, including 149 cases reviewed by Budnick (1976), 167 cases reported by Toretti and colleagues (1984), and, most recently, 351 previously unpublished odontomas reviewed by Kaugars and colleagues (1989). Microscopically, the sine qua non for the diagnosis of odontoma is the identification of enamel matrix, the uncalcified precursor to enamel. Enamel usually is lost in the decalcification process; in addition, dentin, cementum, and pulp are seen. These are arranged as tooth-like structures or in a haphazard arrangement corresponding to the compound and complex subtypes.

Clinical Features

Kaugars and colleagues (1989) reported a median age of 16 years at diagnosis; 54% of cases were found in the second decade of life and only 15% in patients older than 30 years. Morning (1980) found an average age of 11 years at diagnosis and asserted that this was because a routine radiographic examination is provided for fourth graders in Denmark by the Public Service. Slootweg (1981) and Kaugars and colleagues (1989) determined that the average age was 17 years for compound odontoma and 22 years for complex odontoma. Morning (1980) found that 65% of compound odontomas (11 of 17 cases) associated with impacted teeth were diagnosed in children between 6 and 10 years of age, whereas 72% of complex odontomas associated with impacted teeth (10 of 14 cases) were diagnosed in patients between 11 and 20 years of age.

In the series of Kaugars and colleagues (1989), 68% of cases occurred in white patients, 31% in black patients, and 2% in patients of other races. Because only 15% of their biopsy specimens were from black patients, the incidence of odontoma in this group was double that expected. Budnick (1976) and Slootweg (1981) found a slight preponderance in male patients, 59% and 65%, respectively, whereas Toretti and colleagues (1984) and Kaugars and co-workers (1989) found an equal sex distribution. According to Morning (1980), dentists usually discover cases because of noneruption of a permanent tooth and sometimes because of persistence of the primary tooth. Other clinical findings include asymptomatic mild swelling, observed by Kaugars and colleagues (1989) in 8%, and displacement of erupted teeth, pain, or pressure. Morning (1980) stated that many are serendipitous radiologic findings. Shafer and colleagues (1983) believed that most odontomas are discovered by routine radiologic examinations.

Treatment/Prognosis

Kaugars and colleagues (1989) recommended surgical excision of odontomas and their surrounding soft tissue. Among their 351 odontomas, no recurrence was reported. At surgical enucleation, it is important to remember that the following lesions may share some of the radiographic features of odontoma: cystic odontoma, ameloblastic odontoma, ameloblastic fibro-odontoma, and keratinizing and calcifying odontogenic cyst type 1B; thus, it is equally important to remove surrounding soft tissue and submit it for pathologic study.

Morning (1980) discussed the post-treatment outcome of 42 cases of impacted teeth sometimes associated with odontomas. In 45% of the cases, these teeth erupted after simple enucleation of the odontoma. Reoperation was performed on the remainder, with exposure of the crown and removal of fibrous tissue; this produced eruption in 71% of these teeth. An additional eight teeth were treated by reoperation and orthodontic traction, and seven of eight eventually were

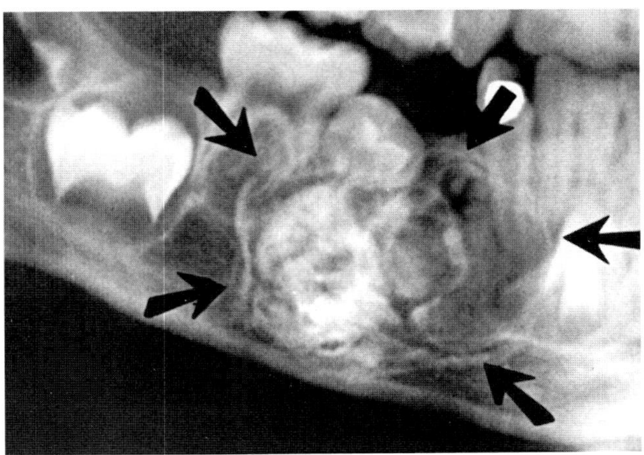

FIGURE 12–18.

Developing complex odontoma: Distal third is most developed; the middle third is partially opacified; and the anterior third is still radiolucent (arrows).

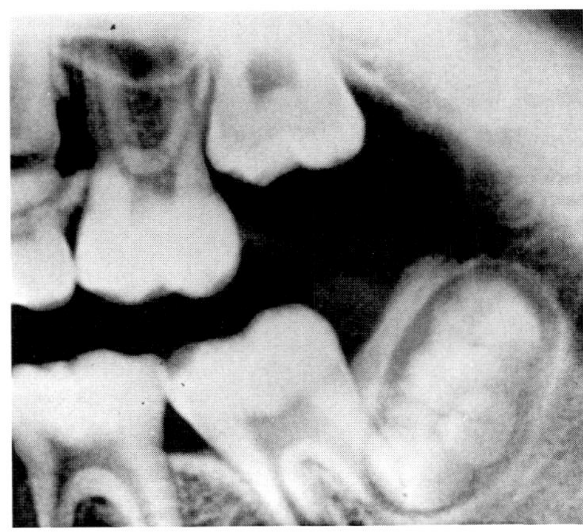

FIGURE 12–20.

Compound odontoma: Rare posterior case has morphologic characteristics of molars and developed in lieu of third molar. (Courtesy of Dr. M. E. Parker, University of the Western Cape, Tygerberg, South Africa.)

brought into occlusion. Overall, 32 of the 42 impacted teeth erupted fully with the varying forms of treatment mentioned. According to Morning (1980), the impacted tooth may be removed with the odontoma if it is displaced to an extreme degree or if the root morphologic characteristics are altered excessively, principally by dilaceration. An impacted or unerupted tooth with completely formed roots has very little potential of erupting on its own.

Complex odontomas may be attached to an adjacent erupted tooth, which has been reported by Worth (1963) and Al-Sahhar and Putrus (1985). When this occurs, they are difficult to remove and attempts to excoriate the mass result in movement of the attached tooth. In such cases, the odontoma must be separated surgically from the adjacent erupted tooth.

◆ RADIOLOGY (Figs. 12–18 to 12–22)

Odontomas usually are not difficult to diagnose. Kaugars and co-workers (1989) found that the clinical diagnosis correlated with the histologic diagnosis in most instances.

Location

Many studies have mentioned location, including those of Budnick (1976), Morning (1980), Toretti and colleagues (1984), Kaugars and co-authors (1989), and Minderjahn (1979). Their findings are summarized and interpreted as follows: Odontomas may occur anywhere in the jaws. The most common location is the anterior maxilla, and approximately two thirds of all odontomas occur in the anterior jaws. Roughly 60 to 70% of compound odontomas are seen anteriorly, with a maxilla-mandible ratio of 2:1; approximately 60% of complex odontomas are found in the posterior regions, with a slight predilection for the mandible. With each successive decade of life, there is a gradual increase in the percentage of odontomas posterior to the mesial surface of the first molar. Slightly more odontomas are located on the right side.

Radiologic Features

In the early stages, odontomas are radiolucent; and radiopaque flecks develop as the teeth begin to calcify. All odontomas are surrounded by a thin radiolucent zone consisting

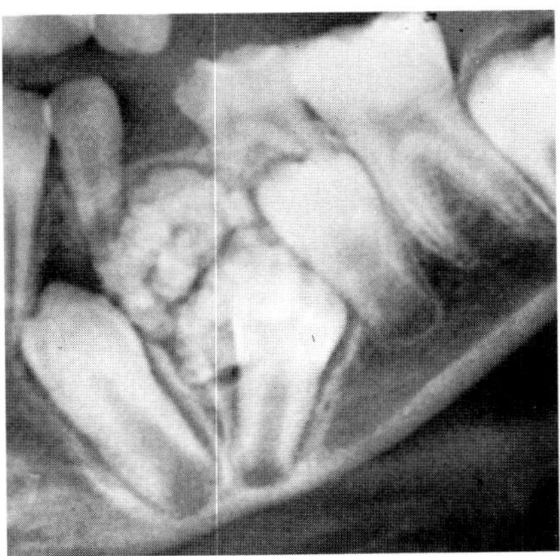

A

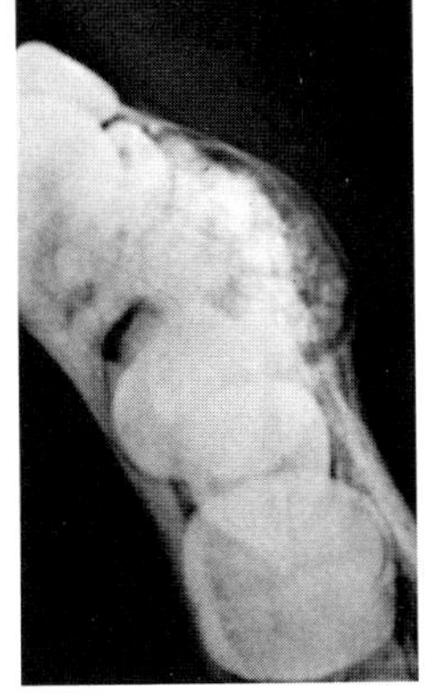

B

FIGURE 12–19.

Compound odontoma: Case in a 10-year-old boy. A, Lesion resembling tiny premolar crowns and a few washer-like shapes. The density is the same as that of teeth. B, Buccal expansion. (Courtesy of Drs. M. Araki, K. Hashimoto, and K. Honda, Nihon University School of Dentistry, Tokyo, Japan.)

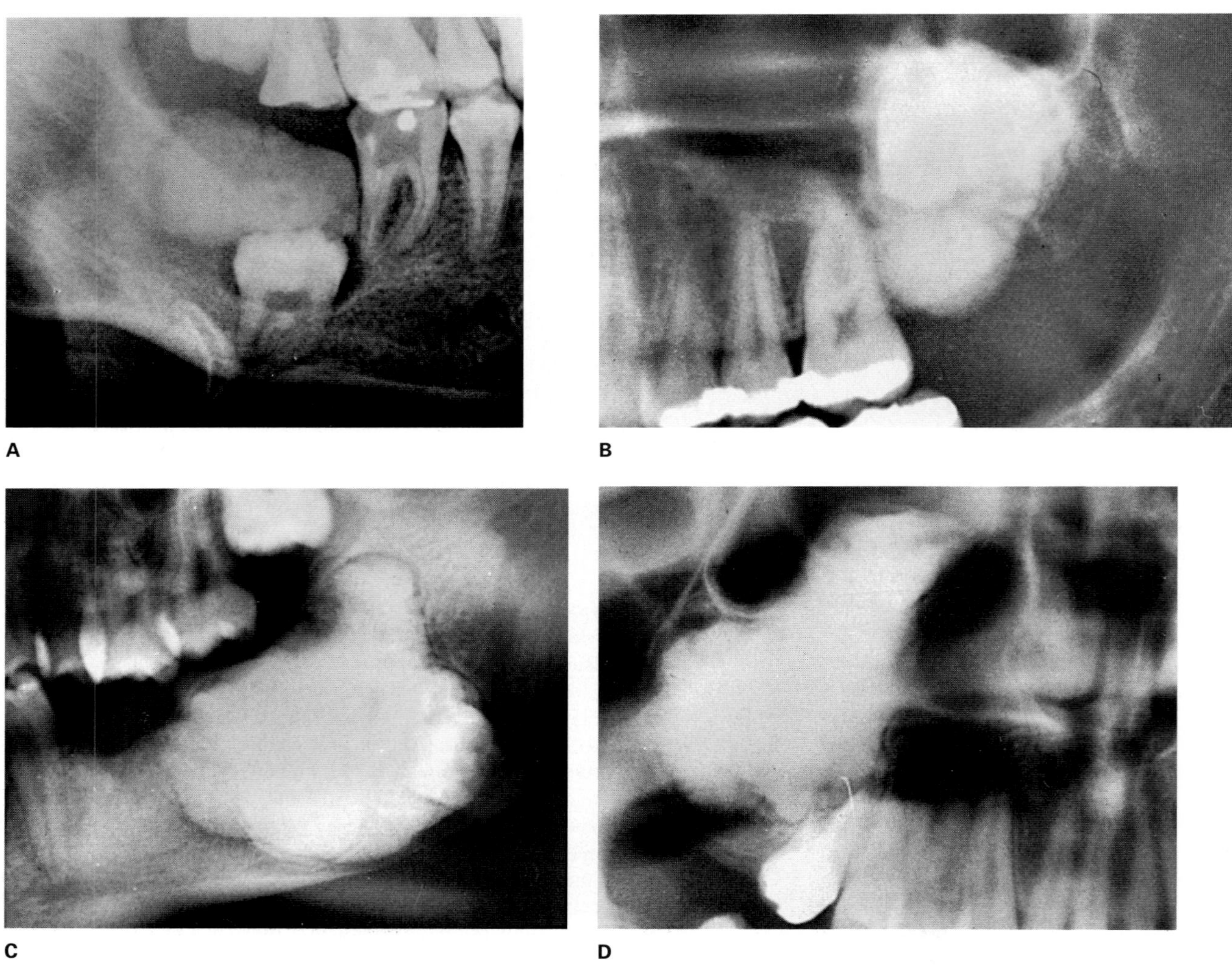

FIGURE 12–21.

Complex odontoma: A and B, Moderately sized lesions. (A, Courtesy of Drs. M. Araki and K. Hashimoto, Nihon University School of Dentistry, Tokyo, Japan.) C and D, Large lesions; impacted tooth may be difficult to see because of adjacent odontoma, which is of a similar density. (C, Courtesy of Professor T. Noikura, Kagoshima University, Ito Dental Clinic, Kagoshima, Japan.)

of a connective tissue capsule corresponding in all respects to the follicle of a normal tooth. Beyond this area, the lesion is surrounded by a thin sclerotic line corresponding in every way to the cortical outline of a normal tooth crypt. An important feature of odontomas is their tendency to cause only the mild expansion needed to accommodate the odontoma in the involved bone. Kaugars and colleagues (1989) observed that only 8% of patients had swelling clinically. Significant expansion in association with an odontoma leads one to consider another associated diagnosis such as cystic odontoma or ameloblastic odontoma.

The compound odontoma consists of several to literally dozens of tooth-like structures. This hamartoma usually does not exceed the diameter of a tooth; however, it occasionally may enlarge significantly. The tooth-like structures resemble small rudimentary teeth, their morphologic characteristics varying with the location in the jaws. For example, in the anterior area, the rudimentary teeth may resemble tiny incisors or they may be conical. On cross-section, they may have a washer-like appearance with a radiolucent center representing pulp. The rudimentary teeth have the same radiologic density as teeth.

The complex odontoma is a single radiopaque mass with a density somewhat greater than that of bone. It usually does not exceed the diameter of the teeth in the region; however, Worth (1963) stated that the largest complex odontoma is in a museum at Guy's Hospital in London and weighs 11 ounces. The radiopaque mass invariably is round or ovoid and usually has smooth margins. The margins sometimes appear lobulated or spikelike. The internal elements occasionally have a mottled appearance because of the varying densities of the mineralized components, consisting of enamel, dentin, and cementum versus dental papilla-like material, pulp and uncalcified enamel matrix, dentinoid, and cementum. At other times, the calcified mass takes on a sunburst appearance, with radiating lines of alternating den-

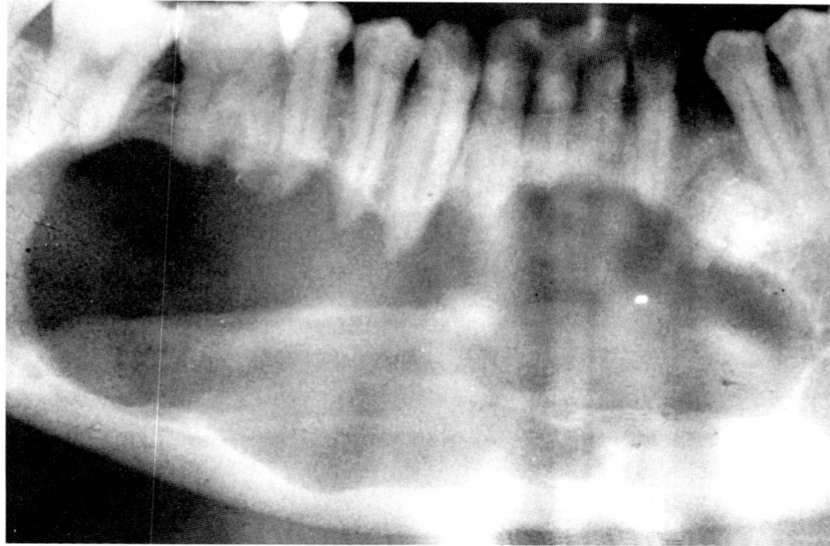

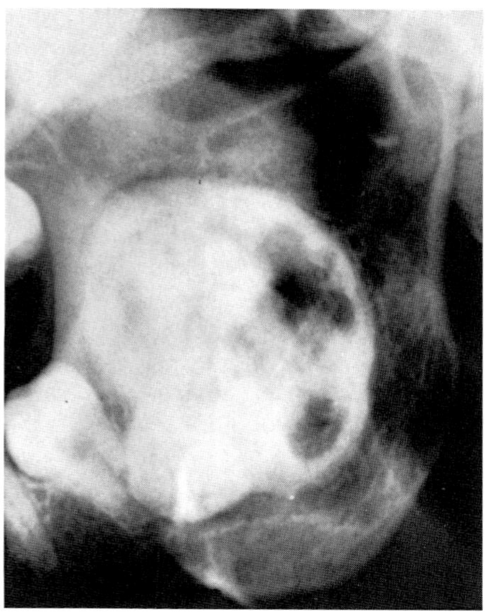

A B

FIGURE 12–22.

Cystic odontoma: A, Compound odontoma is in the left canine area. Dentigerous cyst may have arisen from impacted left canine at lower border of mandible or the compound odontoma. (Courtesy of L. Archila, F. Erales, and R. Carlos, Guatemala City, Guatemala.) B, Dentigerous cyst extends to angle and condyle areas in association with complex odontoma in ramus.

sities presumably resulting from a more orderly arrangement of calcified versus uncalcified elements.

In their series of 351 odontomas, Kaugars and co-workers (1989) found multiple odontomas in two patients. In one patient the lesions were in the right and left anterior maxilla, whereas the other pair was in the mandibular right premolar area and anterior mandible. We have seen several cases in which the odontomas were symmetrically bilateral.

Relationship to Teeth

Kaugars and colleagues (1989) found that 48% of all odontomas are associated with an unerupted tooth. In the maxilla, cases associated with an impacted tooth were divided almost equally between the anterior and molar regions, with the fewest in the premolar area. Among cases in the mandible, those in the molar area were most likely to be associated with an impacted tooth, followed by cases in the anterior region and then the premolar area. Odontomas generally are found between the roots of erupted teeth or they may cause impaction of an unerupted member of the normal complement of teeth.

Morning (1980) analyzed the relationship of odontomas to the impacted tooth and found that they could be above, next to, or around the tooth. Of complex odontomas, 50% of cases were above, 31% next to, and 19% around the tooth. Among compound odontomas, 60% of cases were next to, 30% above, and 10% around the tooth. Morning (1980) also studied the impacted tooth. It was normal in 55% of cases associated with compound odontomas and 63% of cases with complex odontomas; 50% of these impacted teeth erupted after removal of the odontoma. The root of the impacted tooth was abnormal in 53% of compound odontomas and 25% of complex odontomas, and only 36% of these teeth erupted after removal of the odontoma. Most of the normal and abnormal teeth erupted after retreatment. The crown of an impacted tooth was abnormal in only one case, a compound odontoma. At times, a complex odontoma may be attached to an adjacent erupted tooth, especially when in an inter-radicular location. Complex odontomas may completely surround an associated unerupted tooth, obliterating it entirely. A bright light may be helpful in finding such teeth; tomograms also are useful. Extra radiographs may be necessary to assess this possibility.

Cystic Odontoma

Odontomas may be associated with the development of a dentigerous cyst. Kaugars and colleagues (1989) reported a 28% incidence of cystic odontoma in their series. In complex odontomas, Worth (1963) stated that the radiolucent area surrounding the mass is increased when cystic transformation has occurred. The cyst may be slightly or much larger than the odontoma. The complex odontoma may be in the center of the cystic cavity or to one side. At other times, a bony sheath may partially surround part of the complex odontoma, with the thin capsule lying between the odontoma and bone; the cystic lesion can be seen on the other side. Thus, the odontoma may lie relatively free within the cystic cavity, or it may be surrounded partially by a bony sheath and not be free within the cystic cavity. This distinction will be important to the surgeon because the latter lesion may be more difficult to remove. Compound odontomas also may become cystic. In the several cases observed, we found that the little tooth-like structures become much more separated when cystic transformation has occurred. Normally they tend to be bunched up with very little space intervening. This separation of the tooth-like structures is an important sign of cystic degeneration. At other times, the tooth-like structures remain bunched-up, and cystic changes much like those we described for the complex odontoma are seen. Worth (1963) also commented on the presence of infection, which he says is a rare complication of cystic odontoma; however, in such instances, the thin rim of sclerotic bone that surrounds the cystic wall is lost. This finding may correlate with occasional symptoms of swelling, pain, and suppuration. Goldberg and colleagues (1981) reported two cases of cystic odontoma. Both cases were complex odontomas associated with impacted mandibular second molars. One patient was a 14-year-old girl and the other was a 30-year-old man.

AMELOBLASTIC ODONTOMA

(Odontoameloblastoma, adamanto-odontoma, soft and calcified odontoma, adamantine epithelioma)

The ameloblastic odontoma is rare. The first definitive report may have been by Kemper and Root in 1944. In 1967, Olech and Alvares reviewed the literature and found only nine cases, including their own. Since then, we discovered six more reported cases. We reviewed all 15 cases while compiling the information in this section.

Pathologic Characteristics

Shafer and colleagues (1983) stated that the ameloblastic odontoma is an odontogenic neoplasm of mixed tissue origin. It is composed essentially of tissues consistent with ameloblastoma and odontoma. The ameloblastoma component is identical to other ameloblastomas histologically. The odontoma element may consist of either the compound or complex variants. Shafer and colleagues (1983) emphasized that this tumor does not represent two separate conditions growing in unison, but consists of one neoplastic process with relatively undifferentiated and highly differentiated tissues in the same tumor.

Clinical Features

The patients' ages ranged from 5 to 35 years. Except in the 35-year-old patient, all cases occurred in patients 20 years of age or younger. Among these, 43% were in the first decade of life and 57% in the second decade. The male-to-female ratio was equal. Invariably, patients had painless swelling of several months' duration, with the time period ranging from several weeks to 18 months. Clinically, the swelling usually occurred in the buccal cortex, with diminution of the depth of the mucobuccal fold. Palpation of the swollen area usually does not elicit pain, and the overlying soft tissue appears normal. In a number of instances, the dental visit was scheduled because a primary or permanent tooth had not erupted.

Treatment/Prognosis

Most of the reported cases were treated conservatively by local excision, curettage, or enucleation. Among the 15 cases we found, recurrence was not mentioned in 7. The others were treated conservatively, and the follow-up ranged from 9 months to 10 years. As reported by Frissell and Shafer (1953), only one case recurred, and did so twice. Shafer and colleagues (1983) stated that the lesion must be considered to behave like the ameloblastoma component, and the treatment philosophy should be based on this predicate. In our review, some cases were managed adequately by conservative measures. In recurrent cases, more extensive excisions may be necessary. Because recurrence is possible, long-term radiologic follow-up is recommended.

◆ *RADIOLOGY (Fig. 12–23)*

In the differential diagnosis, ameloblastic fibro-odontoma, compound and complex odontomas, cystic odontoma, ameloblastic fibro-odontoma, and odontoma-associated Gorlin cyst, type IB, should be considered. The most challenging aspect of the radiologic interpretation is identification of the ameloblastoma component.

Location

Ameloblastic odontomas may locate preferentially, according to the odontoma component. Although the 15 cases we reviewed were distributed equally between the maxilla and mandible, 33% were in the maxillary incisor-canine regions, and 60% were in the anterior regions of the maxilla and mandible. The remaining cases occurred in the molar regions, with 27% in the mandible and 13% in the maxilla. In no instance was the premolar region solely involved, but one mandibular lesion occurred between the canine and premolar and one maxillary lesion was between the second bicuspid and first molar. Although we observed a slight tendency of anterior lesions to consist of the compound type and posterior lesions the complex type, there is too little information to indicate a trend.

Radiologic Features

We observed that lesions usually were either small or very large. Smaller lesions are between teeth and confined to the alveolar bone between the crest of the ridge and the apices of the teeth. Although small lesions tended to be well defined, a sclerotic margin usually was absent. Expansion of the cortex, often toward the buccal, was present consistently, even for smaller lesions. The odontoma component could be seen in various stages of development, with early lesions having a predominantly radiolucent appearance with some radiopaque flecks and more mature lesions having a better developed odontoma component, either resembling teeth or as a nonspecific mass representing a complex odontoma. Among these more mature lesions, there was often very little suggesting that they consisted of anything other than an odontoma, whereas others had a significant radiolucent component, suggesting a coexistent abnormality.

Although large lesions extend beyond the apical region, they appear to enlarge more in an anteroposterior direction, with rare involvement of the inferior cortex of the mandible. Large lesions may occupy an entire quadrant or extend into the ramus. In the maxilla, encroachment upon the sinus may occur. Expansion of the cortex invariably is present, al-

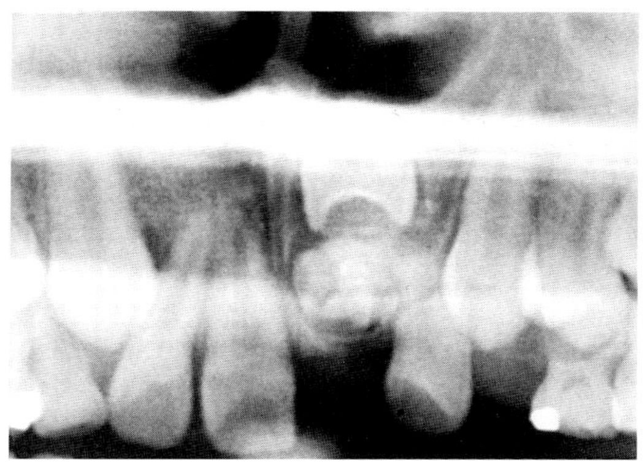
A

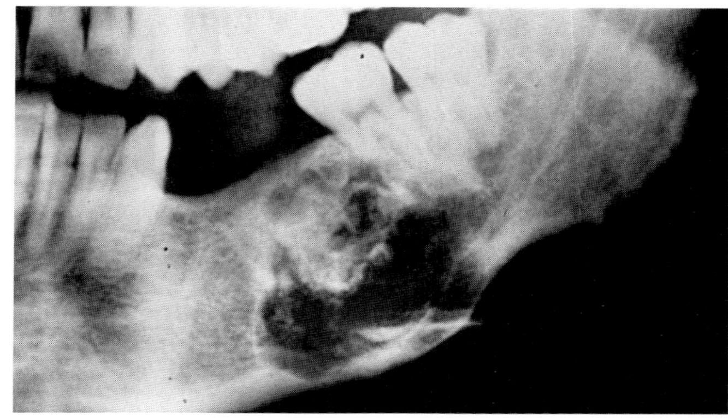
B

FIGURE 12–23.

Ameloblastic odontoma: A, Small lesion in the anterior maxilla interferes with permanent incisor. (Courtesy of Drs. A. and G. Castro Delgado, Universidad Javeriana, Santa Fé de Bogotá, Columbia.) B, Figure shows small washer-like structures throughout and bowing of the inferior border of the mandible. Although the lesion resembles an ossifying fibroma, the washer-like structures rule out that diagnosis. (Courtesy of Dr. N. Fuentes, Santiago, Chile.)

though it tends to be more in a buccolingual direction. Expansion of the inferior cortex is rare. Any suggestion of multilocularity with mild scalloping at the margins or one or more curved internal septa help differentiate this lesion from a cystic odontoma. In larger lesions, the margins usually are well defined and sometimes may be sclerotic, although focal areas of perforation may be present.

Relationship to Teeth

Regardless of size, most ameloblastic odontomas appear to be associated with one or more impacted or unerupted teeth, which may be severely displaced. In some instances, the roots of the adjacent erupted teeth were displaced to accommodate the lesion. Resorption of associated roots was not a feature, especially among permanent teeth. Thus, the several cases with resorption of primary teeth may have been physiologic.

AMELOBLASTIC FIBRODENTINOMA

(Immature dentinoma, fibroameloblastic dentinoma, calcifying fibroadamantoblastoma)

The ameloblastic fibrodentinoma is an extremely rare tumor of odontogenic origin. It first was reported by Field and Ackerman in 1942. Some believe the lesion is an immature dentinoma. In their review of the literature, Azaz and colleagues (1967) found nine cases reported between 1942 and 1967. Pindborg also reviewed the literature in 1955.

Pathologic Characteristics

According to Shafer and colleagues (1983), the epithelial component proliferates in a neoplastic fashion, along with the connective tissue portion of the lesion, with dysplastic dentin being formed. McKelvy and Cherrick (1976) stated that a peripheral variant of the ameloblastic fibrodentinoma exists; however, the distinction between this lesion and the peripheral odontogenic fibroma (WHO type) is not clear, and there may be a relationship between the ameloblastic fibrodentinoma and central odontogenic fibroma (WHO type). Gardner (1984) believed there is no histologic resemblance to the odontogenic fibroma (WHO type); thus, he suggested that the two terms should not be used synonymously. Because there are so few cases, no consensus has been reached by most pathologists.

Clinical Features

Azaz and colleagues (1967) reported the gender for eight of the nine patients; five were male and three female. The average age was 16 years (range, 4.5 to 63 years). If the 63-year-old patient is eliminated, the average age is 11 years. The age and slight male predilection are very similar to those for ameloblastic fibro-odontoma, and the age is somewhat younger than the average patient age for dentinoma. A number of lesions were associated with an unerupted primary incisor or a permanent molar, in a pattern much like the dentinoma. Three of the cases were associated with a primary incisor, two maxillary and one mandibular, with all occurring in 4-year-old children. Three were associated with mandibular first molars, in patients 8, 9, and 13 years of age, and with mandibular second molars, in patients 20 and 22 years of age. There is a pattern of increasing age with posterior location. In many instances, the patient is brought to the dental office because a primary incisor or permanent first or second molar has not erupted. Facial swelling may be observed in some patients. The lesions are painless.

Treatment/Prognosis

In most instances the lesions can be enucleated, and recurrence is not expected. If the involved tooth is not displaced severely, it may remain, so that it can erupt. The lesional tissue has been described as "mushroom-like" and whitish at surgery.

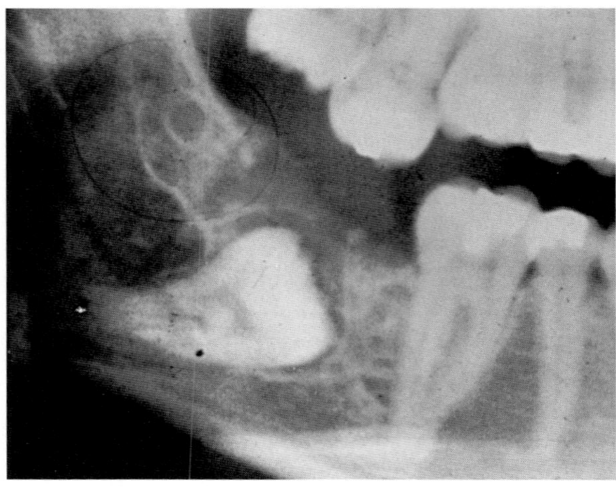

A

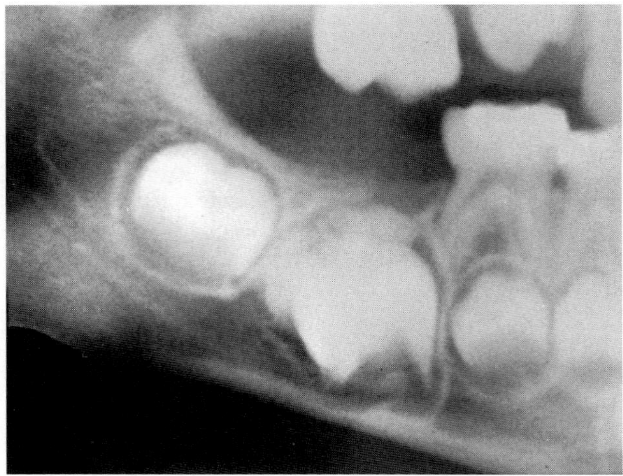

B

FIGURE 12–24.

Ameloblastic fibrodentinoma: A, Lesion is associated with impacted molar and extends into ramus. (Courtesy of Dr. G. Kaugars, Medical College of Virginia School of Dentistry, Richmond, VA.) B, Lesion resembles odontoma or small ameloblastic fibro-odontoma. (Courtesy of Dr. L. Roy Eversole, University of California at Los Angeles, Los Angeles, CA.)

◆ *RADIOLOGY (Fig 12–24)*

During the first decade of life, these lesions most often occur in the maxillary and mandibular anterior regions; in the second decade, the mandibular molar region is the most common location. According to Eversole (1985), many cases are associated with an unerupted tooth. The lesion is predominantly radiolucent; however, radiopaque flecks consisting of calcified dentinoid may be seen within the lesion. Eversole (1985) stated that radiopaque flecks may assume a target configuration, with zones of lucency interspersed between circular zones of radiopaque material. The lesion usually is well demarcated by a thin rim of sclerotic bone, and, according to Eversole (1985), multilocular lesions are possible. The follicular sac of the unerupted tooth may be enlarged. In the case of Azaz and colleagues (1967), the mandibular primary central incisor had not erupted, and the lesion was entirely radiolucent and diagnosed clinically as a dentigerous cyst. The case illustrated by Eversole (1985) consisted of an impacted first molar in a 7-year-old child. The follicular sac appeared slightly enlarged and contained several aggregations of mineralized material in close proximity to the crown. Several radiating spicules could be identified within the radiopaque material, resembling the radiating striae in some complex odontomas. In a 9-year-old patient reported by Field and Ackerman (1942), the lesion appeared to develop in place of the second permanent molar.

DENTINOMA (Mature dentinoma)

The dentinoma is an extremely rare tumor of odontogenic mesenchymal origin. It was reported initially by Straith in 1936. Since then, 2 variants of dentinoma have been described: dentinoma and ameloblastic fibrodentinoma, which was discussed previously. This section is limited to the dentinoma. Azaz and colleagues reviewed the literature in 1967 and found only 18 cases. Strangely, most cases seem to have been reported between 1936 and 1955. Perhaps this is because many pathologists no longer distinguish between dentinoma and ameloblastic fibrodentinoma. This discussion may serve only a historic purpose, although it would seem more orderly to consider the dentinoma as a mature ameloblastic fibrodentinoma.

Pathologic Characteristics

According to Shafer and colleagues (1983), the dentinoma is composed of odontogenic epithelium, irregular or dysplastic dentin, and immature connective tissue, resembling dental papilla. Strictly speaking, there should be dentinal tubules in the dentin for a diagnosis of dentinoma. In addition, a fibrous connective tissue capsule is present.

Clinical Features

In the review of Azaz and colleagues (1967), there were five male and three female patients. Although the average age was 20 years, there were two cases each in the first, second, third, and fourth decades of life. The youngest patient was 4 years old and the oldest was 36 years. Facial swelling has not been a feature of dentinoma; however, intraoral swelling of the alveolar ridge is observed invariably, along with noneruption of the corresponding tooth. The patient may visit the dental office because of mild discomfort in the region of an unerupted tooth or alveolar ridge swelling.

Treatment/Prognosis

Treatment usually consists of surgical enucleation, along with curettage of the capsule. In some instances, the associated unerupted tooth has been removed; however, this is not necessary if the tooth is essential to the patient's dentition. If root formation is incomplete at surgery, the tooth can be expected to erupt, especially if all fibrous connective tissue is curetted away from the coronal area of the unerupted tooth. Otherwise, the tooth can be brought into occlusion by orthodontic traction. Recurrence has not been a feature.

◆ RADIOLOGY (Fig. 12–25)

Although Worth (1963) stated that no particular radiologic features distinguish dentinoma from the complex odontoma, the dentinoma is sufficiently characteristic to be added to the differential diagnosis when these features are present: (1) a mandibular molar location (six cases), (2) an association with an unerupted molar (five cases), (3) a location directly over the occlusal surface of the impacted tooth (five cases); and (4) a size rarely exceeding 1.5 cm in diameter. Obviously, these features may be seen in the more common odontoma.

Location

As Kaugars and colleagues (1989) observed in their study of odontomas, dentinoma cases follow the pattern of increasing patient age with posterior location. For cases associated with the first molar, the patients' ages were 16 and 19 years; the second molar, 23 years; and the third molar, 25 and 30 years. The only case involving an unerupted primary tooth was the mandibular left primary lateral incisor in a 4-year-old boy; it was impacted and directly above the incisal edge, and it was approximately the same diameter as the tooth. In two cases reviewed by Azaz and associates (1967), the lesion was in the maxillary sinus area.

Radiologic Features

The dentinoma consists of a homogeneous or mottled radiopaque mass with a density similar to that of dentin. The mass is circular or ovoid, and rarely several masses may be grouped closely together. The margins of the mass may be smooth, lobulated, spiked, or a combination of these. The remainder of the lesion is surrounded by a thin radiolucent line corresponding to the capsule and, beyond this, a thin rim of condensed bone, very similar to the crypt of a developing tooth. If infection were present, the latter feature might be absent. To our knowledge, cystic degeneration has not been reported. According to Shafer and colleagues (1983), some dentinomas may be entirely radiolucent. It is possible that some of these more radiolucent lesions could have been ameloblastic fibrodentinomas because some authors group these with dentinomas.

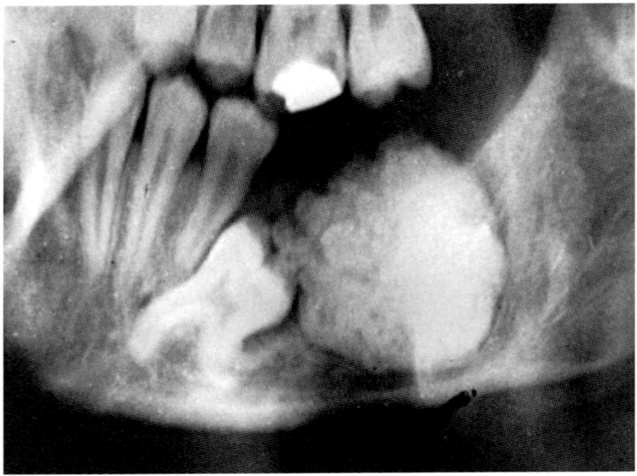

FIGURE 12–25.

Dentinoma: Sixteen-year-old patient with large, round, radiopaque structure situated in mandible surrounded by a definite radiolucent zone indicating encapsulation. The tumor was diagnosed as a dentinoma first by Dr. K.H. Thoma. (From Thoma KH: Oral Pathology: A Historical, Roentgenological and Clinical Study of the Diseases of the Teeth, Jaws and Mouth. St. Louis:CV Mosby, 1941, p. 951.)

Relationship to Teeth

There is a strong tendency for the dentinoma to occur directly above the coronal portion of an impacted tooth, usually a mandibular molar. This association appears to be rather intimate because the dentinoma points the same way as the impacted tooth.

References

Calcifying Odontogenic Cyst

Altini M, Farman AG: The calcifying odontogenic cyst. Oral Surg Oral Med Oral Pathol 40:651, 1975.

Friedman PD, Lumerman H, Gee JK: Calcifying odontogenic cyst. Oral Surg Oral Med Oral Pathol 40:93, 1975.

Gorlin RJ, Pindborg JJ, Clausen FP, Vickers RA: The calcifying odontogenic cyst: a possible analogue of the cutaneous calcifying epithelioma of Malherbe. Oral Surg Oral Med Oral Pathol 15:1235, 1962.

Ikemura K, Horie A, Tashiro H, Nandate M: Simultaneous occurrence of a calcifying odontogenic cyst and its malignant transformation. Cancer 56:2861, 1985.

Kaugars GE, Miller ME, Abbey LM: Odontomas. Oral Surg Oral Med Oral Pathol 67:172, 1989.

Nagao T, Nakajima T, Fukushima M, Ishiki T: Calcifying odontogenic cyst: a survey of 23 cases in the Japanese literature. J Maxillofac Surg 11:174, 1983.

Praetorius F, Hjorting-Hansen E, Gorlin RJ, Vickers RA: Calcifying odontogenic cyst: range, variation and neoplastic potential. Acta Odontol Scand 39:227, 1981.

Regezi JA, Kerr DA, Courtney RM: Odontogenic tumors: analysis of 706 cases. J Oral Surg 36:771, 1978.

Rykwind AW: Beitrag zur Pathologie der Cholesteatome. Virchows Arch Pathol 283:13, 1932.

Seeliger JE, Reyneke JP: The calcifying odontogenic cyst: report of a case. J Oral Surg 36:469, 1978.

Shear M: Cysts of the jaws, recent advances. J Oral Pathol 14:43, 1985.

Shear M: Cysts of the Oral Regions. 2nd Ed. Bristol:Wright PSG, 1983, p. 79.

Wright BA, Bhandwaj AK, Murphy D: Recurrent calcifying odontogenic cyst. Oral Surg Oral Med Oral Pathol 58:579, 1984.

Calcifying Epithelial Odontogenic Tumor

Basu MK, Matthews JB, Sear AJ, Browne RM: Calcifying epithelial odontogenic tumor: a case showing features of malignancy. J Oral Pathol 13:310, 1984.

Damm DD, et al: Combined epithelial odontogenic tumor: adenomatoid odontogenic tumor and calcifying epithelial odontogenic tumor. Oral Surg Oral Med Oral Pathol 55:487 1983.

Ficarra G, Hansen LS, Stiesmeyer EH: Intramural calcifying epithelial odontogenic tumor. Int J Oral Maxillofac Surg 16:217, 1987.

Franklin CD, Pindborg JJ: The calcifying epithelial odontogenic tumor: a review and analysis of 113 cases. Oral Surg Oral Med Oral Pathol 42: 753, 1976.

Goaz PW, White SC: Oral Radiology Principles and Interpretation. St. Louis:CV Mosby, 1987, p. 534.

Ismail IM, Al-Talabani NG: Calcifying epithelial odontogenic tumor associated with dentigerous cyst. Int J Oral Maxillofac Surg 15:108, 1986.

Jones HH, McGowan DA, Gorman JM: Calcifying epithelial odontogenic and keratinizing odontogenic tumors. Oral Surg Oral Med Oral Pathol 25:465, 1968.

Pindborg JJ: A calcifying epithelial odontogenic tumor. Cancer 2:838, 1958.

Pindborg JJ: Calcifying epithelial odontogenic tumors [abstract]. Acta Pathol Microbiol Scand [Suppl] 111:71, 1955.

Shafer WG, Hine MK, Levy BM: A Textbook of Oral Pathology. 4th Ed. Philadelphia:WB Saunders, 1983, p. 286.

Siar GH, Ng KH: Combined calcifying epithelial odontogenic tumor and adenomatoid odontogenic tumor. Int J Oral Maxillofac Surg 16:214, 1987.

Smith RA, et al: The calcifying epithelial odontogenic tumor. J Oral Surg 35:160, 1977.

Takeda Y, Kudo K: Adenomatoid odontogenic tumor associated with calcifying epithelial odontogenic tumor. Int J Oral Maxillofac Surg 15:469, 1986.

Adenomatoid Odontogenic Tumor

Ajagbe HA, Daramola JO, Junaid TA, Ajagbe AO: Adenomatoid odontogenic tumor in a black African population: report of 13 cases. J Oral Maxillofac Surg 43:683, 1985.

Courtney RM, Kerr DA: The odontogenic adenomatoid tumor. Oral Surg Oral Med Oral Pathol 39:424, 1975.

Giansanti JS, Someren A, Waldron CA: Odontogenic adenomatoid tumor (adenoameloblastoma): survey of 11 cases. Oral Surg Oral Med Oral Pathol 30:69, 1970.

Miles DA, Van Dis M, Kaugars GE, Lovas JGL: Oral and Maxillofacial Radiology: Radiologic/Pathologic Correlations. Philadelphia:WB Saunders, 1991, p. 64.

Regezi JA, Kerr DA, Courtney RM: Odontogenic tumors: analysis of 706 cases. J Oral Surg 36:771, 1978.

Stafne EC: Epithelial tumors associated with developmental cysts of the maxilla: report of 3 cases. Oral Surg Oral Med Oral Pathol 1:887, 1948.

Stroncek GG, Aeevodo A, Higa LH: Atypical odontogenic adenomatoid tumor and review of the literature. J Oral Med 36:102, 1981.

Ameloblastic Fibro-odontoma

Anneroth G, Modeer T, Twetman S: Ameloblastic fibro-odontoma in the maxillae: a case report. Int J Oral Surg 11:130, 1982.

Daley TD, Lovas GL: Ameloblastic fibro-odontoma: report of a case. J Can Dent Assoc 48:467, 1982.

Gardner DG: The mixed odontogenic tumors. Oral Surg Oral Med Oral Pathol 57:395, 1984.

Hooker SP: Ameloblastic odontoma: an analysis of twenty-six cases [abstract]. Oral Surg Oral Med Oral Pathol 24:375, 1967.

Howell RM, Burkes EJ: Malignant transformation of ameloblastic fibro-odontoma to ameloblastic fibrosarcoma. Oral Surg Oral Med Oral Pathol 43:391, 1977.

Miller AS, Lopez CF, Pullon PA, Elzay RP: Ameloblastic fibro-odontoma: report of seven cases. Oral Surg Oral Med Oral Pathol 41:354, 1976.

Minderjahn A: Incidence and clinical differentiation of odontogenic tumors. J Maxillofac Surg 7:142, 1979.

Regezi JA, Keer DA, Courtney RM: Odontogenic tumors: analysis of 706 cases. J Oral Surg 36:771, 1978.

Reich RH, Reichart PA, Ostertag H: Ameloblastic fibro-odontoma: report of a case with ultrastructural study. J Maxillofac Surg 12:230, 1984.

Slootweg PJ: An analysis of the interrelationship of the mixed odontogenic tumors: ameloblastic fibroma, ameloblastic fibro-odontoma and the odontomas. Oral Surg Oral Med Oral Pathol 51:266, 1981.

Trodahl JH: Ameloblastic fibroma: a survey of cases from the Armed Forces Institute of Pathology. Oral Surg Oral Med Oral Pathol 33:547, 1972.

Tsaganis GT: A review of the ameloblastic fibro-odontoma. Master's Thesis, George Washington University, Washington, D.C., 1972, p. 12.

Odontoma

Al-Sahhar WF, Putrus ST: Erupted odontoma. Oral Surg Oral Med Oral Pathol 58:225, 1985.

Broca P: Traite des tumeurs. Asselin. Paris 1:350, 1866.

Budnick SD: Compound and complex odontomas. Oral Surg Oral Med Oral Pathol 42:501, 1976.

Devildos LR: The calcifying odontogenic cyst: a clinical pathologic study. Thesis, Indiana University School of Dentistry, Indianapolis, Indiana, 1972, p. 36.

Goldberg H, Schofield IDF, Popwich LD, Wakeham D: Cystic complex-composite odontoma: report of two cases. Oral Surg Oral Med Oral Pathol 51:16, 1981.

Gorlin RJ, et al: Odontogenic tumors. Cancer 14:73, 1961.

Kaugars GE, Miller ME, Abbey LM: Odontomas. Oral Surg Oral Med Oral Pathol 67:172, 1989.

Minderjahn A: Incidence and clinical differentiation of odontogenic tumors. J Maxillofac Surg 7:142, 1979.

Morning P: Impacted teeth in relation to odontomas. Int J Oral Surg 9:81, 1980.

Regezi JA, Kerr DA, Courtney RM: Odontogenic tumors: analysis of 706 cases. J Oral Surg 36:771, 1978.

Shafer WG, Hine MK, Levy BM: A Textbook of Oral Pathology. 3rd Ed. Philadelphia:WB Saunders, 1983, p. 308.

Slootweg PG: Analysis of the interrelationship of the mixed odontogenic tumors: ameloblastic fibroma, ameloblastic fibro-odontoma and the odontomas. Oral Surg Oral Med Oral Pathol 51:266, 1981.

Thoma KH, Goldman HM: Odontogenic tumors: a classification based on observation of the epithelial, mesenchymal and mixed varieties. Am J Pathol 4:433, 1946.

Toretti E, Miller AS, Peezick B: Odontomas: an analysis of 167 cases. J Pedod 8:282, 1984.

Pindborg JJ, Kramer IRH, Torconi H: Histologic Typing of Odontogenic Tumors. Jaw Cysts and Allied Lesions. International Classification of Tumors. No. 5. Geneva:World Health Organization, 1971, p. 30.

Worth HM: Principles and Practice of Oral Radiologic Interpretation. Chicago:Year Book Medical Publishers, 1963, p. 420.

Ameloblastic Odontoma

Frissell C, Shafer W: Ameloblastic odontoma: report of a case. Oral Surg Oral Med Oral Pathol 6:1129, 1953.

Kemper J, Root R: Adamanto-odontoma: report of a case. Am J Orthod Oral Surg 30:709, 1944.

Olech E, Alvares O: Ameloblastic odontoma: report of a case. Oral Surg Oral Med Oral Pathol 23:487, 1967.

Shafer WG, Hine MK, Levy BM: A Textbook of Oral Pathology. 4th Ed. Philadelphia:WB Saunders, 1983, p. 311.

Ameloblastic Fibrodentinoma

Azaz B, Ulmansky M, Lewin-Epstein J: Dentinoma: report of a case. Oral Surg Oral Med Oral Pathol 24:659, 1967.

Eversole LR: Clinical Outline of Oral Pathology. 2nd Ed. Philadelphia: Lea & Febiger, 1985, p. 272.

Field HJ, Ackerman AA: Calcifying fibroadamantoblastoma. Am J Orthod Oral Surg 38:543, 1942.

Gardner OG: The mixed odontogenic tumors. Oral Surg Oral Med Oral Pathol 57:395, 1984.

McKelvy BD, Cherrick HM: Peripheral ameloblastic fibrodentinoma. J Oral Surg 34:826, 1976.

Pindborg JJ: On dentinomas: with report of a case. Acta Pathol Microbiol Scand [Suppl] 105:135, 1955.

Shafer WG, Hine MK, Levy BM: A Textbook of Oral Pathology. 4th Ed. Philadelphia:WB Saunders, 1983, p. 303.

Dentinoma

Azaz B, Ulmansky M, Lewin-Epstein J: Dentinoma: report of a case. Oral Surg Oral Med Oral Pathol 24:659, 1967.

Kaugars GE, Miller ME, Abbey LM: Odontomas. Oral Surg Oral Med Oral Pathol 67:172, 1989.

Shafer WG, Hine MK, Levy BM: A Textbook of Oral Pathology. 4th Ed. Philadelphia:WB Saunders, 1983, p. 303.

Straith EF: Odontoma: a rare type. Report of a case. Dent Digest 42:196, 1936.

Worth HM: Principles and Practice of Oral Radiologic Interpretation. Chicago:Year Book Medical Publishers, 1963, p. 426.

Chapter 13

Multilocular Radiolucencies

ODONTOGENIC KERATOCYST (Primordial cyst)

The term odontogenic keratocyst (OKC) first was suggested by Philipsen in 1956. Shear (1960) and Pindborg and colleagues (1962) established the histologic criteria for these cysts with parakeratotic and orthokeratotic variants. In 1960, Gorlin and Goltz described the syndrome bearing their name. A separate discussion of this syndrome follows in this chapter. In 1981, Wright suggested that the orthokeratinized variant be considered a distinct clinicopathologic entity. This cyst is discussed in Chapter 11. According to Hjorting-Hansen and colleagues (1969) and Toller (1972), the percentage of OKCs versus other cysts of the jaws was 11%; Brannon (1976) and Payne (1972) reported that it was 9%, and Pindborg and Hansen (1963) stated that it was 7%.

Pathologic Characteristics

As described by Brannon (1977), the epithelial lining is very thin and uniform in thickness, with little evidence of rete ridges. The basal layer is prominent and often palisaded, and the spinous layer is thin and may exhibit intracellular edema. Keratinization is predominantly parakeratotic (with nuclei) but may be orthokeratotic. The keratin layer often is corrugated. In addition, the fibrous connective tissue wall is generally thin and inflammation is absent. Other authors, such as Browne (1977) and Magnusson (1978), observed a tendency for the epithelium to separate from the connective tissue lining. In some instances, "abtropfung" or dropping down phenomenon of epithelial elements in the connective tissue wall has been observed. Payne (1972) found that this budding-like hyperplastic proliferation of the basal layer was suggestive of a dental lamina structure and that it was present in 85% of patients with the jaw cyst-basal cell nevus-bifid rib syndrome, 45% of patients with recurrent OKCs, and 8% of patients with nonrecurring OKCs. Payne (1972) also observed that so-called microcysts, daughter cysts, or satellite cysts were in the connective tissue wall in 78% of the patients with the jaw cyst-basal cell nevus-bifid rib syndrome, 18% of patients with recurrent OKCs, and 4% of patients with nonrecurring OKCs.

Clinical Features

The OKC may occur in people of any age. In Browne's (1970) series of 90 OKCs, the peak frequency occurred in the second and third decades of life. Shear (1983) found 40% of cases in this age range. In a review of 32 cases, Park and Kim (1985) found 56% of cases in patients younger than 30 years of age. Brannon (1976) and Browne (1970) reported that this cyst is rare in children younger than 10 years of age. In the series of Park and Kim (1985), no patient was younger than 10 years. More male patients tend to be affected than female patients; however, Pindborg and Hansen (1963), Soskolne and Shear (1967), and Park and Kim (1985) reported a 1:1 ratio. In contrast, Panders and Hadders (1969) reported a male-to-female ratio of 3:1; Magnusson (1978), 2.6:1; Shear (1983), 1.9:1; and Brannon (1976), 1.4:1. Our overall estimate of the male-to-female ratio is 1.7:1. The most frequent initial complaint is a painless swelling or intraoral drainage; other symptoms include pain or paresthesia.

Treatment/Prognosis

Most cases are treated by enucleation; however, marsupialization of larger cysts has been effective. Resection has been necessary in a few patients with multiple recurrences. At surgery, the cystic contents consist of a cheesy, curdy, caseous semisolid material. When enucleation occurs easily, the bony walls tend to be smooth; when enucleation is difficult, the bony walls usually are ragged, with internal spiculation and loculations. It may be difficult to remove the lesion in one piece because the epithelium tends to separate from the connective tissue wall. OKCs recur much more frequently than do other jaw cysts, which have an overall recurrence rate of approximately 5%. Table 13–1 lists the recurrence rates for OKCs that we found in our review of the literature.

Recurrences developed within 10 months to 25 years; they usually occur within 2 to 5 years after removal. Multiple recurrences also are possible, and the reported range was two to five recurrences within the same patient. Emerson and colleagues (1972) mentioned two recurrences in soft tissue, whereas Attenborough (1974) reported a recurrence in a bone graft from the iliac crest, well away from the junction with the mandible.

The following criteria may be helpful in predicting recurrence of OKCs:

1. "Abtropfung" is present histologically, as reported by the pathologist.
2. Daughter cysts are seen histologically, as reported by the pathologist.
3. The epithelium is separated from the connective tissue histologically.
4. Cysts are a component of the jaw cyst-basal cell nevus-bifid rib syndrome.
5. Radiologically, the cyst is large and multilocular, and especially if there is evidence of perforation and/or internal spiculation of the bony wall.
6. Enucleation tends to be difficult at surgery.

TABLE 13–1
Recurrence Rates for Odontogenic Keratocysts

Authors	Recurrence Rate (%)
Brannon (1977)	12
Panders and Hadders (1969)	14
Browne (1970)	25
Park and Kim (1985)	27
Rud and Pindborg (1969)	33
Eversole and colleagues (1975)	20 (2 years); 35 (5 years)
Vedtofte and Praetorius (1979)	51
Toller (1972)	58
Pindborg and Hansen (1963)	63

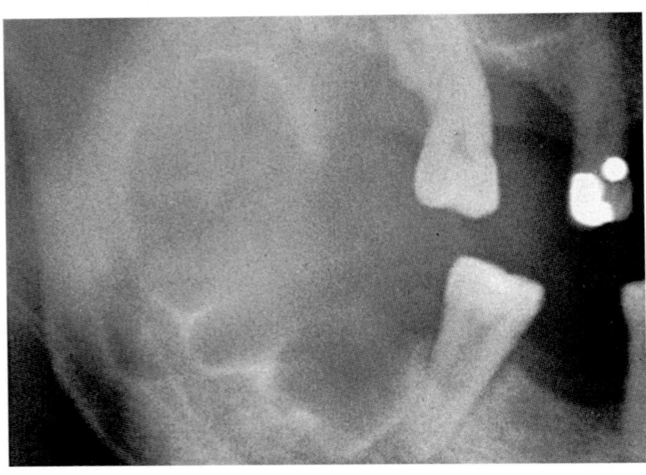

FIGURE 13–1.

Odontogenic keratocyst: seen as a primordial cyst: Case in a 47-year-old man shows scalloped margins, a cloudy lumen, perforation at the anterior border of the ramus, and soft tissue herniation. There is no expansion.

The following factors may indicate a diminished potential for recurrence of an OKC:

1. The previously outlined histologic criteria are absent.
2. The OKC is the orthokeratinized (without nuclei) variant.
3. The cyst is small and unilocular, especially in the maxilla.
4. Enucleation occurs with ease.

Most authors suggest frequent radiographic follow-up for at least 5 to 10 years. There is some debate as to whether OKCs can give rise to central squamous cell carcinoma in the jaws.

◆ RADIOLOGY (Figs. 13–1 to 13–8)

The typical features of OKCs are as follows:

1. There is enlargement at the expense of medullary space, often with only minimal expansion as a late feature, which is especially notable on computed tomography (CT) scans.
2. Mandibular OKCs tend to enlarge and fill the whole ramus.
3. The margins tend to be densely sclerotic, with a scalloped outline, especially in larger, older lesions.
4. Focal areas of perforation may be seen in plain radiographic and CT images.
5. The lumen may be cloudy because of keratin; the CT number of the luminal contents would be higher than for the cystic fluid of other cysts.
6. Maxillary lesions tend to be smaller and unilocular, with a smooth margin; large maxillary lesions are de-

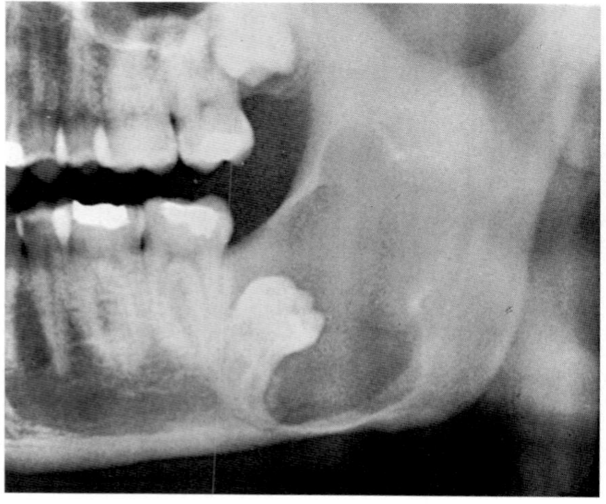

A

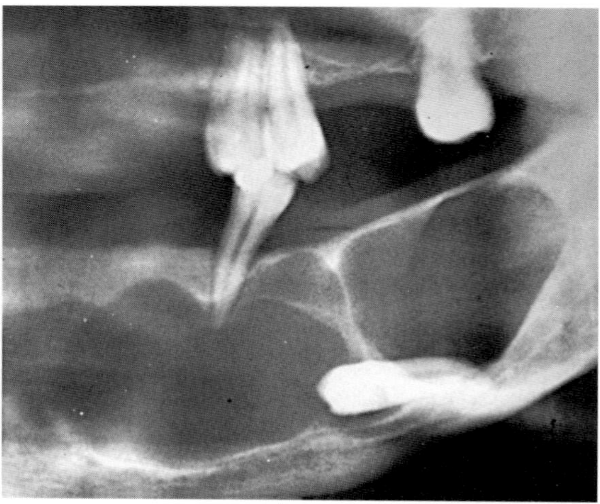

B

FIGURE 13–2.

Odontogenic keratocyst: mimicking a dentigerous cyst: A, Scalloping at margins and cloudy lumen. B, Bilocular appearance.

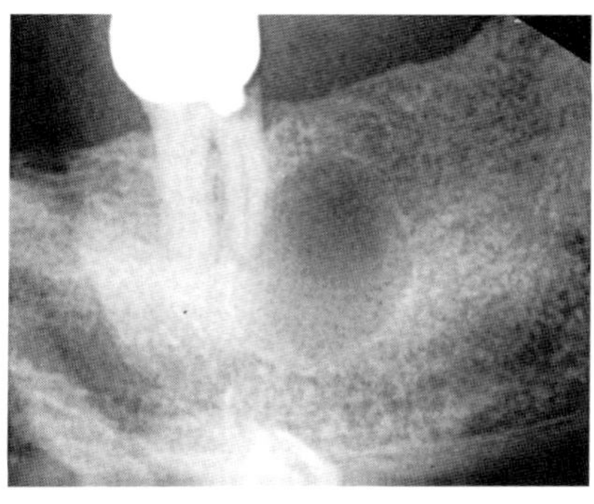

A

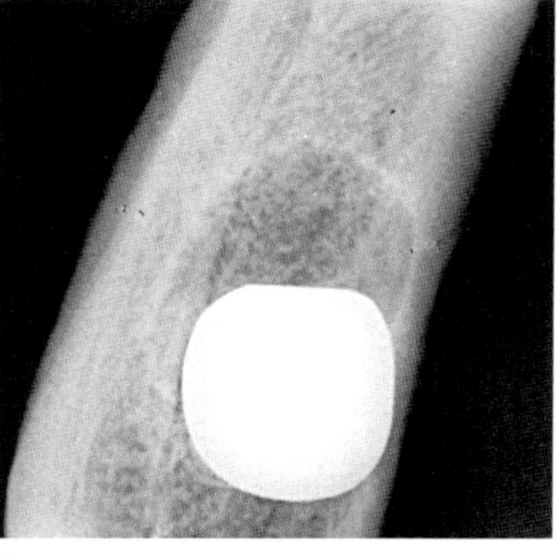

B

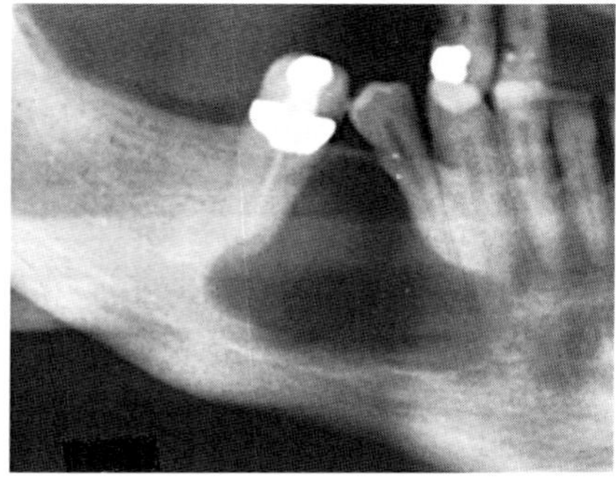

C

FIGURE 13–3.

Odontogenic keratocyst: mimicking lateral periodontal cyst: A and B, Figures show a cloudy lumen and lack of expansion. C, Case resembles botryoid lateral periodontal cyst and shows displacement of adjacent roots.

structive, may be expansile, and usually involve the sinus.

7. Although developing teeth may be displaced, the OKC usually does not resorb teeth.
8. The OKC may be seen bilaterally or in both jaws in patients younger than 10 years of age, in which case the Gorlin-Goltz syndrome should be suspected.

Location

Haring and Van Dis (1988) reviewed 60 cases of OKC and correlated the radiographic, clinical, and histopathologic findings. The most common location is the mandible. Brannon (1976) found 65% in the mandible; Haring and Van Dis (1988), 68%; McIvor (1972), 79%; and Browne (1970), 83%. Within the mandible, the most common site is the molar-ramus region. In a series of 14 OKCs studied by Isberg-Holm (1977), 42% were in the third molar-ramus area. McIvor (1972) stated that a radiolucency in the ramus not contacting any teeth is most likely an odontogenic keratocyst.

Radiologic Features

The radiographic patterns are listed in Table 13–2.

From these data, it seems that the OKC often may appear

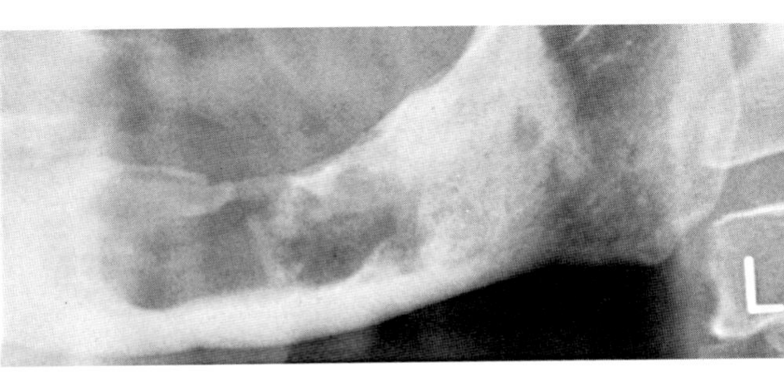

A

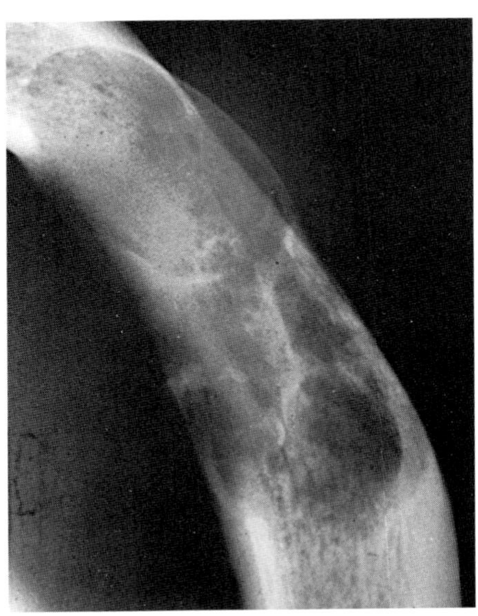

B

FIGURE 13–4.

Odontogenic keratocyst: mimicking residual cyst with infection: A, Irregular margins and relative lack of sclerosis indicating secondary infection. B, Large size with minimal expansion. Tiny radiolucent areas at anterior and posterior margins resemble permeative change; however, these are surrounded by a distinct sclerotic margin, are characteristic of inflammation in alveolar bone, and seem to precede lysis.

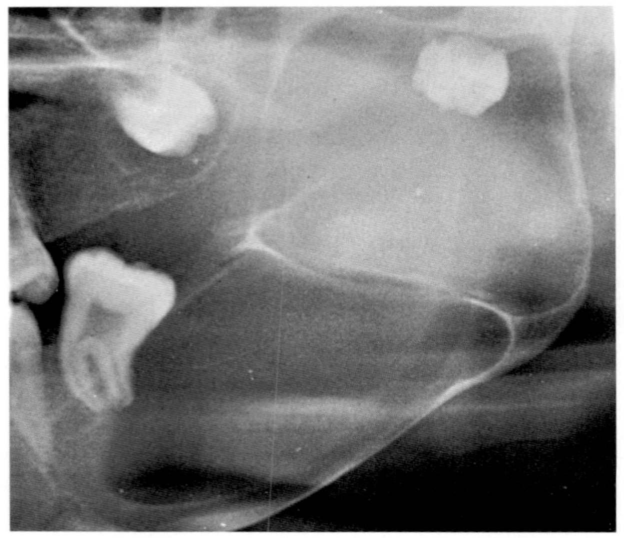

FIGURE 13–5.

Odontogenic keratocyst: mimicking mural ameloblastoma: There is displacement of the developing third molar and deformity of the root of the second molar. The keratocyst is bilocular and large, with minimal expansion. There is downward displacement of the inferior alveolar canal.

as a unilocular radiolucency, although lesions with scalloped margins and bilocular and multilocular patterns occur. Most OKCs are well developed at diagnosis; in a series of 14 cases reported by Isberg-Holm (1977), the average diameter was 3 cm. A thick sclerotic margin usually is present. In Browne's (1970) radiographic series of 90 OKCs, this feature was seen in 76%; Haring and Van Dis (1988) observed this in 45%. Three of Brannon's (1976) 52 cases with radiographs had a poorly defined periphery. Although minimal expansion often is present, even for huge cysts, this feature is not readily visible if only a single plain radiograph is taken. On CT scans, minimal expansion or a lack of expansion is a diagnostic feature in large lesions. In the series of Park and Kim (1985), 9 of 22 mandibular cysts exhibited expansion, whereas Haring and Van Dis (1988) found expansion in 27% of their cases.

Perforation may be seen commonly, but not always, especially on plain radiographic studies. When the perforation occurs at right angles to the plane of the film (i.e., at the margins of the cyst), perforation may be evidenced by focal discontinuity or the absence of sclerosis at the peripheral margin. In such instances, herniation of the cystic contents may occur. When the perforation is on the same plane as the film (i.e., within the luminal portion of the cyst), focal, more radiolucent or punched-out areas may be seen within the lumen. These usually are circular or ovoid and are approximately 1 cm or more in diameter.

In some instances, the luminal area of OKCs is notable because of the radiologic appearance of desquamated keratin accumulation. It may have a uniform consistency or appear in whorls and does not necessarily fill the entire lumen. We have termed this a cloudy or ''milky-way'' lumen; however, Park and Kim (1985) coined the phrase ''luminal haze'' to describe this feature and observed it in 5 of their 32 cases.

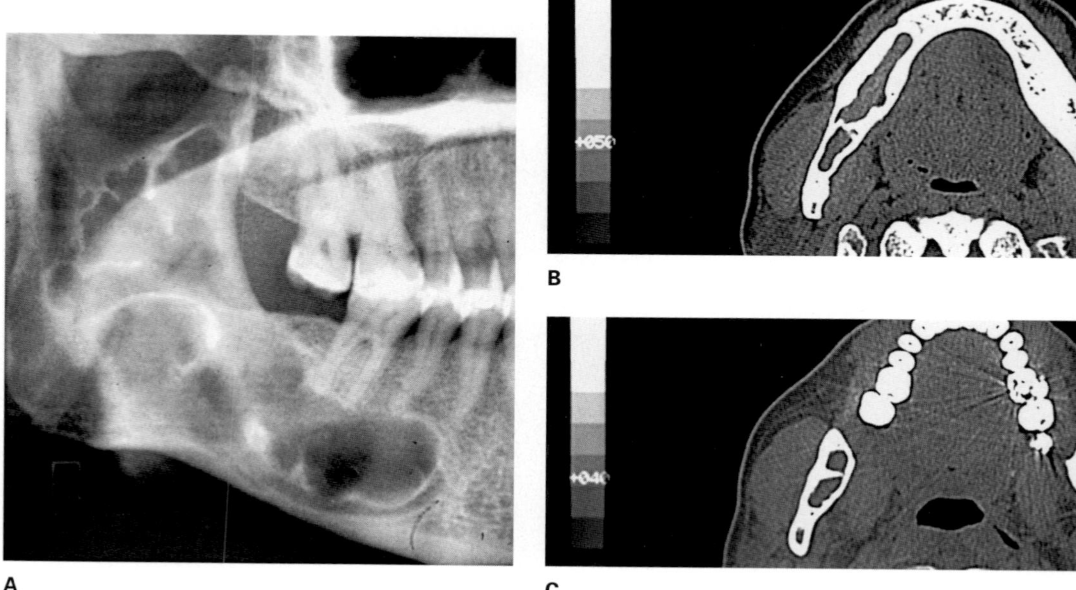

FIGURE 13–6.

Odontogenic keratocyst: CT workup of a large mandibular cyst: A, Figure shows a thick, densely sclerotic, scalloped margin and cloudy lumen. B and C, There is enlargement at the expense of the medullary space, with minimal expansion of the cortex. The pointed spikes at the endosteal margin directed toward the lumen may predict recurrence. (Courtesy of Drs. M. Araki, K. Hashimoto, and K. Honda, Nihon University School of Dentistry, Tokyo, Japan.)

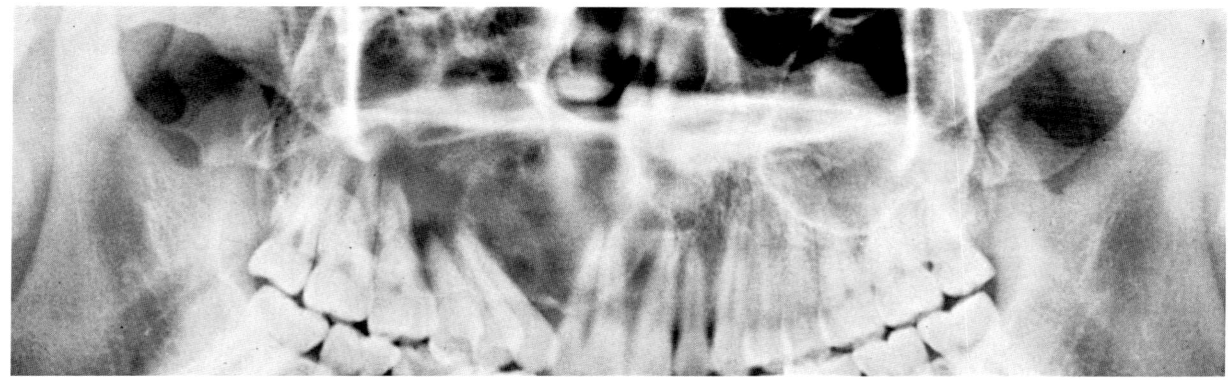

A

B

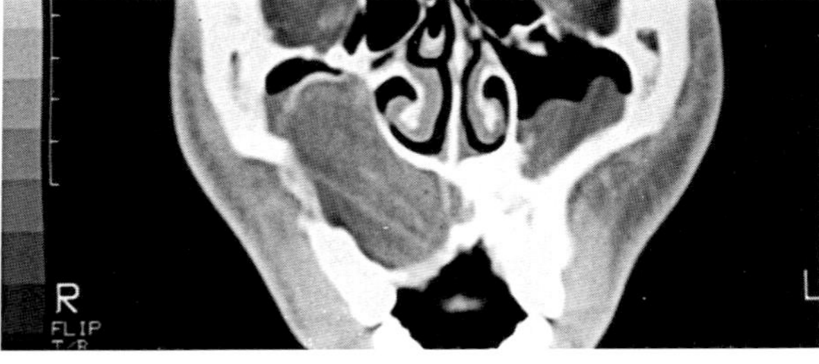

C

FIGURE 13–7.

Odontogenic keratocyst: CT workup of a large maxillary cyst. A, Large, poorly defined radiolucency in the right maxilla extending into sinus. B, Cortical expansion with spiking at internal margins, and slight density variations in the lumen caused by desquamated keratin within. C, Coronal image showing extension into most of the right sinus. The left sinus shows a soft tissue density with a polypoid configuration overlying a greatly thickened sinus wall, consistent with chronic osteomyelitis and inflammatory polyp formation. (Courtesy of Dr. Chang S. Park, Department of Dental Radiology, Yonsei University College of Dentistry, Seoul, Korea.)

Association with Teeth

Brannon (1976) reported tooth involvement in 14% of his cases. The most common of these findings was displacement of an unerupted or impacted tooth, occurring in 26% of the cases involving teeth. Other less common findings include displacement of erupted teeth, extrusion of erupted teeth, divergence of roots of erupted teeth, and, rarely, root resorption of adjacent teeth. Haring and Van Dis (1988) observed root resorption in 5% of their cases.

Maxillary Odontogenic Keratocysts

Maxillary OKCs appear to be somewhat different from mandibular lesions. McIvor (1972) discovered that maxillary lesions occurred in older age groups, were smaller, and usually did not recur. Browne (1970) reported that 93% of his maxillary lesions were unilocular, with a smooth periphery. In the series of Park and Kim (1985), 70% of the 10 maxillary cysts had a smooth, rounded margin; however, 90% of cases involved the antrum. Woo and colleagues (1987) reported

TABLE 13–2
Reported Radiologic Patterns of Odontogenic Keratocysts

	Unilocular			Multilocular		
	Poorly Defined	**Unilocular**	**With Scalloped Border**	**Bilocular**	**Multilocular**	**Total (cases)**
Brannon (1977)	(3%)	(62%)	—	(10%)	(23%)	52
Browne (1970)	—	(57%)	(21%)	—	(23%)	90
Isberg-Holm (1977)	—	(57%)	(33%)	—	(10%)	—
Park and Kim (1985)	—	(73%)	(27%)	—	—	22

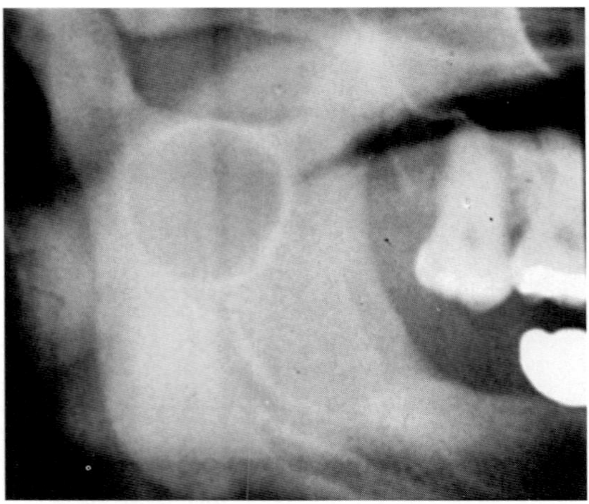

FIGURE 13–8.

Odontogenic keratocyst: Recurrent OKC 20 years after surgery. (Courtesy of Dr. H. Schwartz, Kaiser Permanente Medical Group, Los Angeles, CA.)

two cases of OKC in the maxillary anterior region, one of which simulated an incisive canal cyst.

Mimicry of OKCs

Despite the previously discussed features, only half or less of all OKCs are identified or suspected radiologically. In a series of 21 cases analyzed by Rud and Pindborg (1969), 48% were correctly diagnosed clinically, and in the series of Isberg-Holm (1977), 50% were diagnosed correctly from the radiographs. Haring and Van Dis (1988) had correct diagnoses in 26% of the cases sent for biopsy; the most frequent incorrect diagnosis was dentigerous cyst. The OKC may mimic many other cysts of the jaws: (1) a primordial cyst of the non-OKC type by the American definition; (2) a dentigerous cyst; from our review of various reports, such as that of Altini and Cohen (1982), the OKC may resemble a dentigerous cyst in 7 to 32% of cases; (3) a lateral periodontal cyst; in Brannon's series (1976), this was observed in 24% of cases; (4) idiopathically, an OKC in any location beyond the apices of the teeth; some have occurred in the mandibular molar region; (5) a radicular cyst; Wright and colleagues (1983) discussed four such cases; (6) a residual cyst; 12% of Brannon's (1976) cases had this appearance; and (7) a ''globulomaxillary'' cyst or ''median mandibular'' cyst.

Computed Tomography

On CT scans, the presentation is unique. The entire medullary space may be destroyed. Sometimes rough, irregular internal margins are seen, especially in the ramus on axial CT scans. The cortex may appear thickened and slightly bowed because of mild expansion. Severe expansion is present only rarely. Spiculation at the internal margins and the lack of significant expansion in a large lesion separates the OKC from all others on CT scans. In maxillary lesions, a CT scan is mandatory if the sinus is involved. The value of CT scans in assessment of these cysts has been emphasized by MacKenzie and colleagues (1985) and Lund (1985). In the antrum, the cystic margins tend to be smoother and more regular; however, perforations into the buccal space and nasal fossa often are seen.

JAW CYST-BASAL CELL NEVUS-BIFID RIB SYNDROME (Nevoid basal cell carcinoma syndrome, basal cell nevus syndrome, multiple basal cell nevi syndrome, Gorlin-Goltz syndrome)

This syndrome first was described by Gorlin and Goltz in 1960. In 1987, Gorlin presented the findings from an additional 53 patients and reviewed the literature extensively. Another case series was published by Woolgar and colleagues (1987).

Pathologic Characteristics

The pathogenesis of the syndrome is unknown; however, it is transmitted by a single autosomal dominant gene with complete penetrance and variable expressivity. Thus, male and female patients are affected equally, and everyone manifests some of the traits; however, some patients have more than others. Gorlin (1987) stated that approximately 60% of patients do not have an affected parent; thus, many cases represent new mutations. Cotten and colleagues (1982) reported squamous odontogenic tumor-like proliferation in the wall of the OKCs. Gorlin (1987) reported that ameloblastoma and squamous cell carcinoma have arisen in the wall of these cysts.

Clinical Features

In their review of the literature on the incidence of the most common features, Breytenbach and colleagues (1975), Van Dijk and Sanderink (1967), and Kamiya and colleagues (1985) reported their findings. Less common abnormalities were reviewed in 1987 by Gorlin. Other reports have been published by Cotten and colleagues (1982) and Donatsky and co-authors (1976).

Nevoid Basal Cell Carcinomas

Features of the basal cell nevus syndrome as reviewed by several authors are shown in Table 13–3. Gorlin (1987) reported that the nevoid basal cell carcinomas appear in patients between puberty and 35 years of age, although they have been observed at birth. The lesions are papular; may be pink, pale brown, or dark brown; and vary from 1 to 10 mm in diameter. There may be a few lesions or thousands. Although they may occur anywhere, there is a predilection for the the neck, upper trunk, and skin of the face, especially around the eyes, nose, mouth, and ears. The lesions may be isolated or grouped. Some lesions regress spontaneously, but this is rare. Metastasis is extremely uncommon, and management is surgical or by topical chemotherapy with agents such as 5-fluorouracil and oral administration of 13-cis-retinoic acid to prevent new lesions and arrest the growth of existing basal cell carcinomas.

Jaw Cysts

The jaw cysts are odontogenic keratocysts (OKCs), which develop during the first decade and peak during the second

TABLE 13–3
Characteristics of Basal Cell Nevus Syndrome

	Kamiya (1985) (%)	Van Dijk (1967) (%)	Breytenbach (1975) (%)
Basal cell carcinoma	15	—	81
Jaw cysts	100	81	90
Rib abnormalities	55	48	44
Hypertelorism	60	37	24
Palmar or plantar pits	65	24	23
Ectopic calcification	80	21	35
Scoliosis and kyphosis	40	20	25
Vertebral abnormalities	—	20	10
Hand abnormalities	—	12	10
Prognathism	55	9	49

and third decades of life. This behavior is somewhat different from that of the isolated OKC, which usually does not appear until the second decade of life. They are bilateral and may involve both jaws. In their review of the Japanese literature, Kamiya and colleagues (1985) found 20 reported cases and added 3 new cases. In their series, the most common feature of the syndrome was jaw cysts. According to Gorlin (1987), only 15% of these patients do not have radiologically demonstrable cysts by 40 years of age.

Rib Abnormalities

Gorlin (1987) stated that approximately 60% of patients have rib abnormalities, including anterior splaying, fusion, partially missing ribs, hypoplastic ribs, or bifid ribs. Cervical ribs are seen frequently. Almost all authors report rib involvement in approximately 50% of cases.

The most frequent initial complaint, as outlined by Kamiya and colleagues (1985), was swelling in the cheek region. Three patients had a "pus" discharge, three cases were detected on routine examination, and one patient had pain in the molar region of the mandible.

Treatment/Prognosis

Jaw cysts are treated by enucleation, and, as previously stated, there is a greater chance of recurrence than for isolated OKCs. The recurrence rate ranges from 30 to 60% within 3 to 5 years after enucleation.

◆ *RADIOLOGY (Figs. 13–9 to 13–11)*

Radiologic Features of the Jaws

The radiologic jaw changes in this syndrome are a result of the OKCs present. These syndrome OKCs have the same features as the isolated OKCs previously described. OKCs of the syndrome often are bilateral and may involve all four quadrants. They occur three times more commonly in the mandible. Woolgar and colleagues (1987) found that the mandibular molar region was the most common site, followed by the maxillary molar area. In a child younger than 10 years of age, detection of OKCs in the jaws should lead to an additional workup to determine whether the patient has the syndrome. In children, the cysts often cause displacement of developing teeth.

Radiologic Features of the Skull

Gorlin (1987) summarized these findings as follows: The calvaria usually is enlarged, with frontal and biparietal bossing, a low occiput, and a mildly increased interorbital distance. Lamellar calcification of the falx cerebri appears early in life and is seen in approximately 85% of these patients

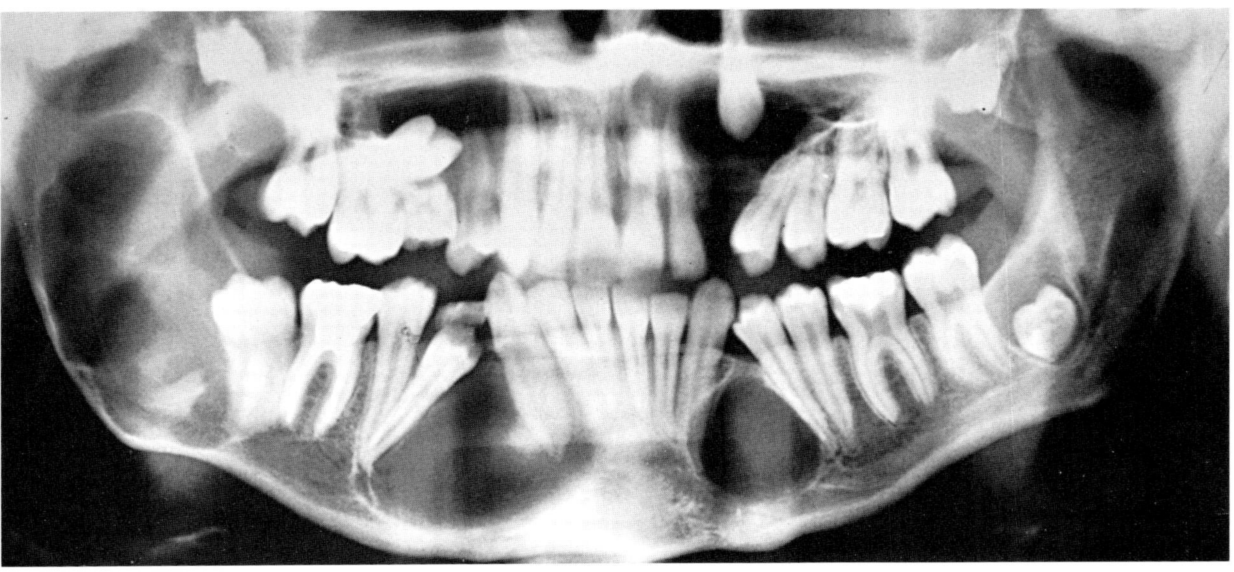

FIGURE 13–9.

Jaw cyst-basal cell nevus-bifid rib syndrome: Classic presentation with OKCs in all four quadrants. (Courtesy of Dr. M. Lamberg, Department of Oral Surgery, University of KUOPIO, Kuopio, Finland.)

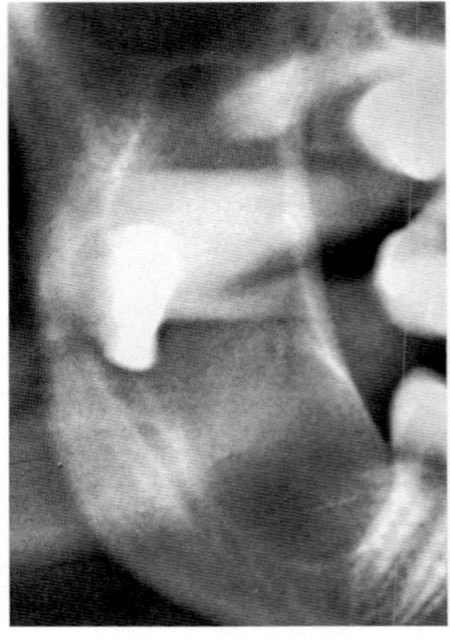

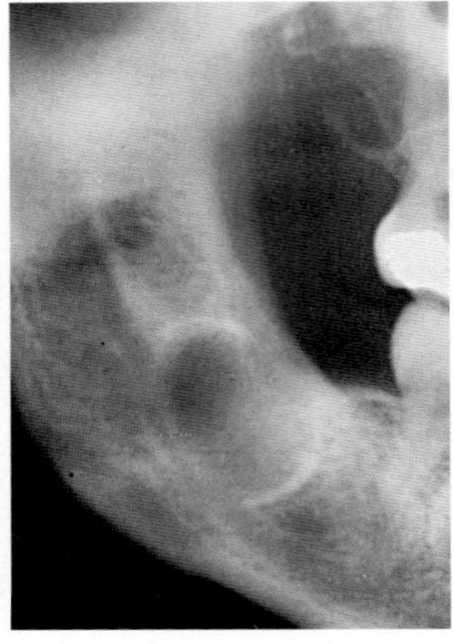

A B

FIGURE 13–10.

Jaw cyst-basal cell nevus-bifid rib syndrome: Recurrent OKC. A, Patient at 12 years of age. B, Six years after surgery. (Courtesy of Drs. F. Sammis and C. Portales, San Antonio, TX.)

compared with 5% in the normal population. Other ectopic calcifications may be seen in the tentorium cerebelli (40%), petroclinoid ligament (20%), and the dura, pia, and choroid plexus. There is hyperpneumatization of the sinuses in 60% because septa are absent. Bridging of the sella turcica by calcification of the diaphragma sellae is seen in 60 to 80% of cases as compared with 4% in the normal population. The sella is small and often asymmetric because of hyperpneumatization of the sphenoid sinus.

Other Radiologic Findings

In the vertebral spine, kyphoscoliosis is observed in 30 to 40% of patients, and spina bifida occulta is seen in the thoracic and cervical vertebrae in 60%. There are malformations at the occipitovertebral junction, including a short atlas, agenesis of the odontoid process, a third occipital condyle, or basilar agenesis. Fusion of cervical or upper thoracic vertebrae is seen in 40%, and lumbarization of the sacrum occurs in 40%. Other bony abnormalities include polydactyly of the hands and feet, hallux valgus, and syndactyly of the second and third fingers. Scapular and clavicular abnormalities also have been reported. Small pseudocystic lytic bone

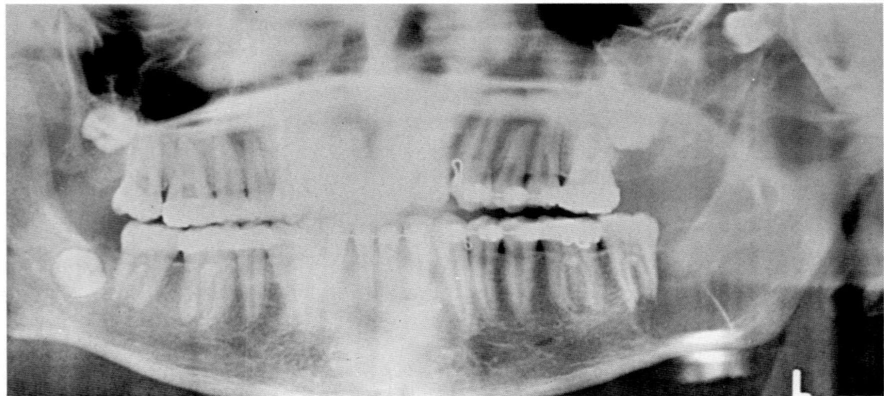

A

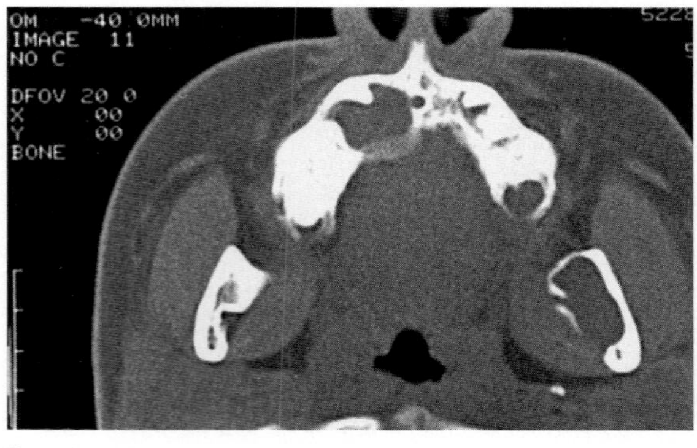

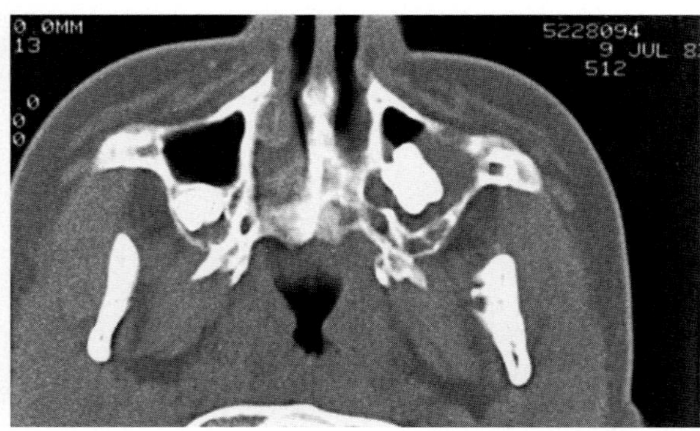

B C

FIGURE 13–11.

Jaw cyst-basal cell nevus-bifid rib syndrome: A, OKCs in jaws. B and C, CT images showing additional OKC in anterior maxilla and perforation in left ramus. Both sinuses contain OKCs and displaced teeth.

(*continued*)

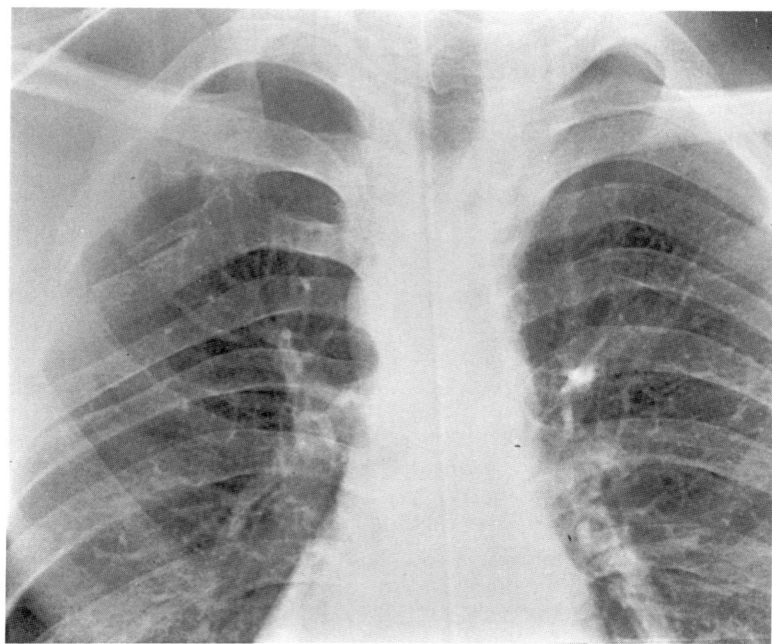

D

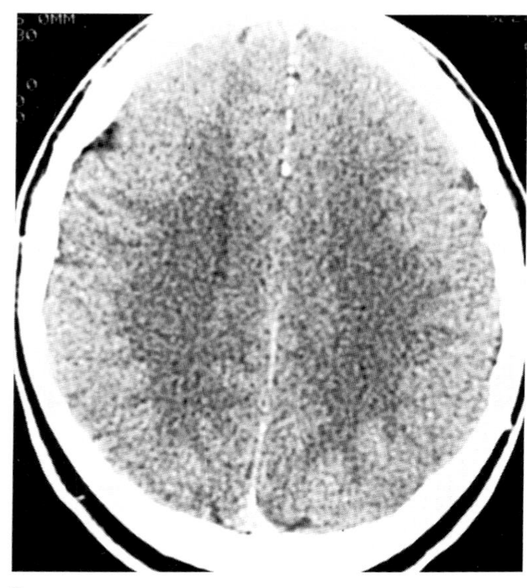

E

FIGURE 13–11. *(continued)*

D, Bifid ribs, upper right chest. E, Intracranial calcifications. (A, C, and D, Courtesy of Dr. H. Schwartz, Kaiser Permanente Medical Group, Los Angeles, CA; B, Courtesy of Professor P. Dhiravarangkura, Chulalonghorn University School of Dentistry, Bangkok, Thailand.)

lesions have been found in 35 to 40%, especially in the pelvis, calvaria, phalanges, and metacarpal, carpal, tarsal, and long bones. Subcutaneous calcification of the fingers and scalp has been reported, as well as calcified ovarian fibromas. The fourth metacarpals (type-E brachydactyly) are short in 15 to 45%; this is seen in approximately 20% of the normal population.

BOTRYOID ODONTOGENIC CYST (Botryoid lateral developmental periodontal cyst)

The botryoid (grapelike) odontogenic cyst first was reported by Weathers and Waldron in 1973. The earliest report may have been by Standish and Shafer in 1958, in which one of a series of five lateral periodontal cysts resembled a botryoid odontogenic cyst (BOC). It is the multicystic variant of the lateral (developmental) periodontal cyst. We estimate that approximately 15 to 20 cases of BOC have been reported. The most compelling reason for this separate discussion is that some BOCs recur approximately 8 to 10 years after surgery.

Pathologic Characteristics

In 1980, Wysocki and colleagues further clarified the histogenesis of the BOC. They proposed that the BOCs arise from clear cell rests of the dental lamina and represent a polycystic variant of the lateral developmental periodontal cyst. Although the BOC has been described as polycystic grossly, histologically, and radiologically, Greer and Johnson (1988) observed that 8 of their 10 cases were unilocular radiologically. They summarized the histologic findings as follows: There is a relatively thin nonkeratinized squamous epithelial lining with plaquelike thickenings that bulge into the cystic cavity. Zones of clear cells usually are dispersed throughout the epithelium and sometimes within the connective tissue wall. The connective tissue wall is invariably free of inflammatory infiltrate. Kaugars (1986) emphasized that, for a diagnosis of BOC, the lesion must be multicystic histologically.

Clinical Features

Kaugars (1986) summarized the clinical findings of five cases reported in the literature. Additionally, Greer and Johnson reported 10 new cases in 1988. The patients' ages ranged from 26 to 81 years. In Kaugars' (1986) series, the mean age was 61 years, whereas Greer and Johnson (1988) reported a mean age of 51 years; there was an average patient age of 46 years among these 15 reported cases we reviewed. The cases occurred in nine men and six women. All 10 patients reported by Greer and Johnson (1988) were white. The most common findings were swelling or expansion, which may be tender or associated with drainage. Among the 15 cases, approximately 6 seemed to be asymptomatic.

Treatment/Prognosis

Most BOCs are treated by simple enucleation; however, the BOC may recur approximately 8 to 10 years after surgery.

We have identified five reported recurrences, for a recurrence rate of 30 to 50% among reported cases. The first recurrence was reported by Phelan and colleagues (1988) and occurred roughly 9 years after removal by enucleation. A second patient was a 20-year-old woman; the original lesion was unilocular radiologically and resembled a lateral (developmental) periodontal cyst between the mandibular canine and lateral incisor; the recurrent BOC was detected 3 years after surgery and contained two locules radiologically. Approximately 1.5 years after the recurrent cyst was removed, it recurred a second time as a unilocular lesion. Roughly 6 months after this third operation, there was no evidence of healing and a fourth operation was performed. The surgical site appeared to be healing on follow-up. In the series of Greer and Johnson (1988), three lesions represented recurrences 8, 10, and 10 years after previous surgical removal. One patient was a 53-year-old man, a second was a 54-year-old man, and the third was a 28-year-old woman. Because the BOC tends to recur, often 8 to 10 years after surgery, long-term radiologic follow-up is recommended for these patients.

◆ RADIOLOGY (Figs. 13–12 to 13–14)

Kaugars (1986) emphasized that characterization of this lesion as multilocular is appropriate only with respect to the histologic findings of some lesions. Even lesions that are unilocular radiologically are multicystic or multilocular histologically.

Location

In our analysis of 15 lesions as reviewed by Kaugars (1986) and Greer and Johnson (1988), 14 of the 15 occurred in the mandible and 1 (which recurred) was in the maxilla. Six cases were associated with the canines on the anterior side. Four involved the premolars, four were in the incisor or midline region of the mandible, and one was associated with a mandibular third molar. The maxillary lesion was between the premolars. One lesion arose in an edentulous area. Among these 10 cases, 6 were associated with a mandibular canine, with 4 occurring on the left side and 2 on the right. Six of 10 cases reported by Greer and Johnson (1988) were on the left side, two were in the midline, one was in the midline and extended to the second premolar area, and one was between the right canine and first premolar.

Radiologic Features

Among the lesions reported by Greer and Johnson (1988), the average size was 1.6 cm and the median approximately 1.3 cm. The recurrent lesions were largest, being 1.8 cm and unilocular, 3.0 cm and multilocular, and 4.5 × 1.2 cm and unilocular. Thus, size eventually might correlate with propensity for recurrence. Of the five cases summarized by Kaugars (1986), one was unilocular, one was bilocular, and three were multilocular radiologically. Among the 10 new cases reported by Greer and Johnson (1988), 8 were unilocular and 2 multilocular.

We analyzed all of the reported multilocular lesions carefully. Although it is said that the radiologic features of this lesion are similar to those of other multilocular lesions, we are impressed with the following features gleaned from the five cases discussed by Kaugars (1986):

1. One of the locules occupies the same location as the lateral periodontal cyst (four cases).
2. When teeth are present, the lesion appears to cause resorption of the lamina dura in areas where it extends onto the roots of adjacent teeth (two cases).
3. The lesion appears high on the alveolar crest (four cases).
4. When the lesion extends beyond the apical region, this extension appears to be limited to approximately 1 cm (two cases).

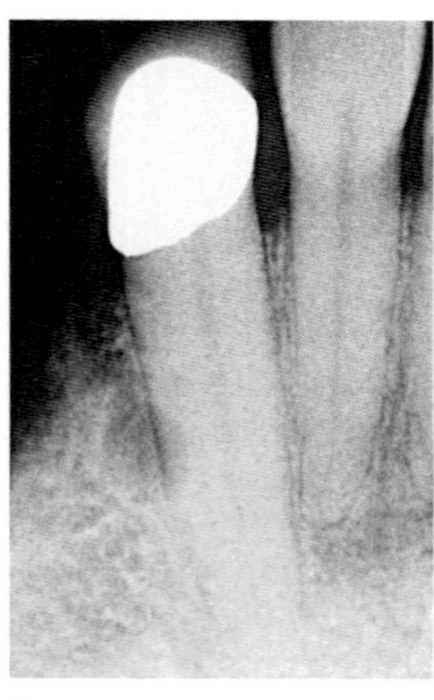
A

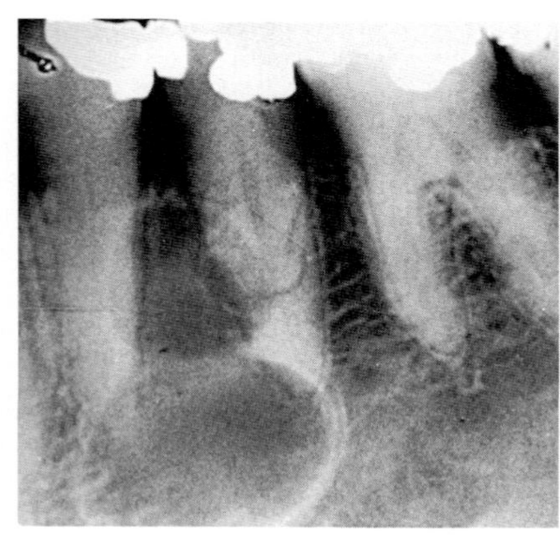
B

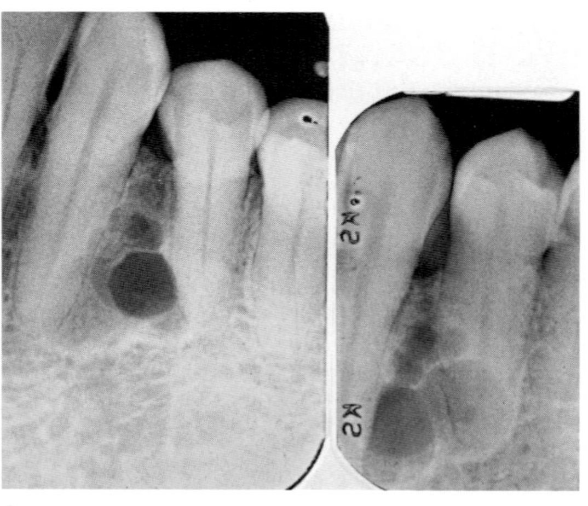
C

FIGURE 13–12.

Botryoid odontogenic cyst: A, Unilocular. (From Greer RO Jr, Johnson M: Botryoid odontogenic cyst: clinicopathologic analysis of ten cases with three recurrences. J Oral Maxillofac Surg 46:574, 1988.) B, Bilocular. (Courtesy of Drs. G. Kaugars and J. Whitney, Richmond, VA.) C, Multilocular. (Courtesy of Dr. S. Bricker, University of Indiana School of Dentistry, Indianapolis, IN.)

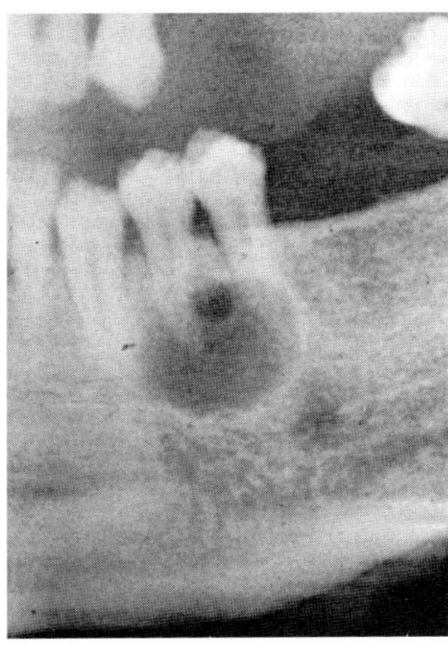
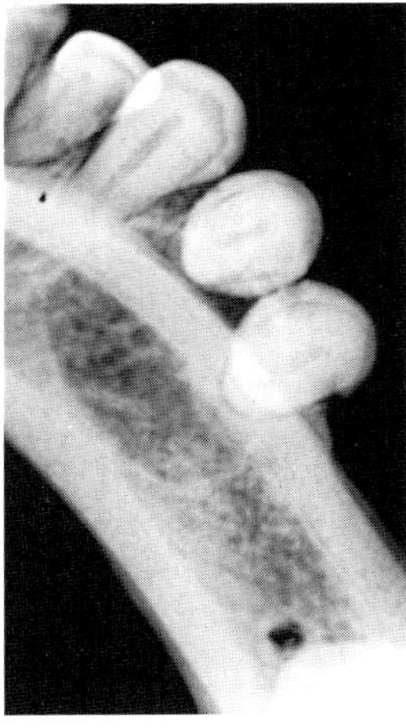

A B

FIGURE 13–13.

Botryoid odontogenic cyst: Bilocular lesion. A, Panoramic view. B, Occlusal view. (Courtesy of Dr. G. Kaugars, Medical College of Virginia School of Dentistry, Richmond, VA.)

5. The periphery of the locules shows continuous cortication with well-defined, intact borders (five cases).
6. Internal loculations were mostly absent, with more of a scalloped outline (four cases).
7. When present, internal loculations were circular and well corticated, with a relative lack of linear striations and septa (one case).

In the case with multiple recurrences reported by Phelan and colleagues (1988), all these features were observed in the bilocular recurrent lesion. Both unilocular lesions (the original and second recurrence) appeared in a slightly more apical position than most lateral developmental periodontal cysts. The original lesion appeared to be approximately 0.8 cm in diameter, resembled a lateral (developmental) periodontal cyst in all respects, and was anterior to the left mandibular canine. Kaugars (1986) showed an excellent series of radiographs taken from the same case in 1976, 1977, and 1982. The initial lesion appeared to involve the apices of the mandibular incisors; the lesion was approximately 3 cm in diameter, and either did not heal after enucleation or recurred; the second lesion finally was excised in 1985, after paresthesia developed in the anterior mandible.

ODONTOGENIC SIALOCYST (Sialo-odontogenic cyst, glandular odontogenic cyst)

The first sialo-odontogenic cyst was reported by Gardner in 1984 in a paper presented at a meeting in the Netherlands. The first cases in the literature were reported by Padayachee and Van Wyk in 1987. Some features of this condition are similar to those of the BOC and central mucoepidermoid tumor. Ten cases have been reported. The histologic features have been described in detail by Gardner and associates (1988). The 10 reported cases occurred in six female and four male patients, with ages ranging from 19 to 85 years (average age, 52 years). Four patients had clinical swelling. The remainder of the lesions were discovered on routine radiographs. Pain is not a feature. Cases most often have been in the mandibular midline or premolar areas. Most cases were treated by enucleation. Four cases recurred (40%), all within 2 to 4 years.

◆ *RADIOLOGY (Fig. 13–15)*

Most lesions (60%) were in the midline of the mandible, usually extending posteriorly to the premolars bilaterally.

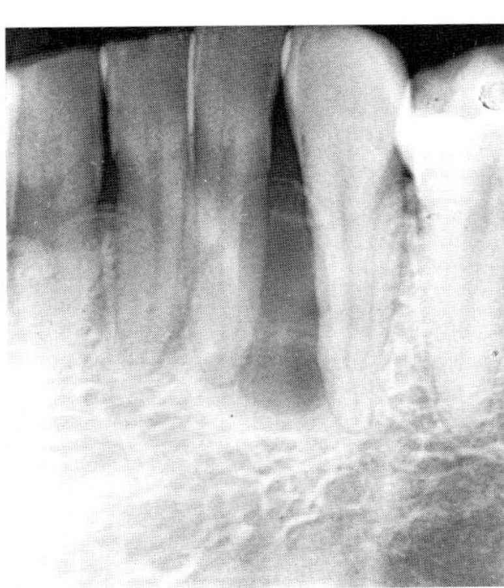
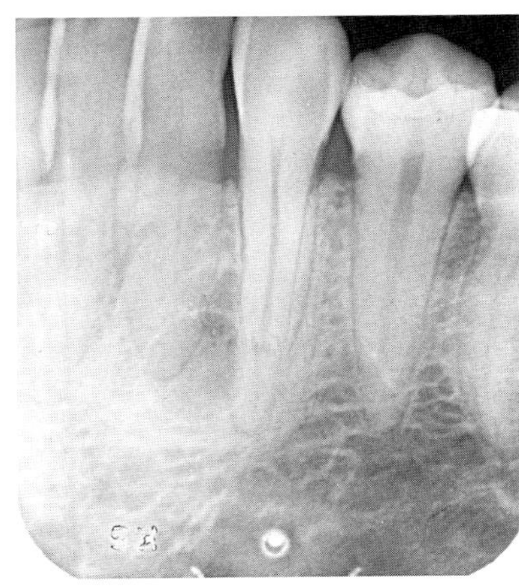

A B

FIGURE 13–14.

Recurrent botryoid odontogenic cyst: Original lesion was unilocular and approximately 0.5 cm on the panoramic view. A, First recurrence 17 months after surgery. B, Second recurrence 6 months after second excision. (From Phelan JA, et al: Recurrent botryoid odontogenic cyst [lateral periodontal cyst]. Oral Surg Oral Med Oral Pathol 66:345, 1988.)

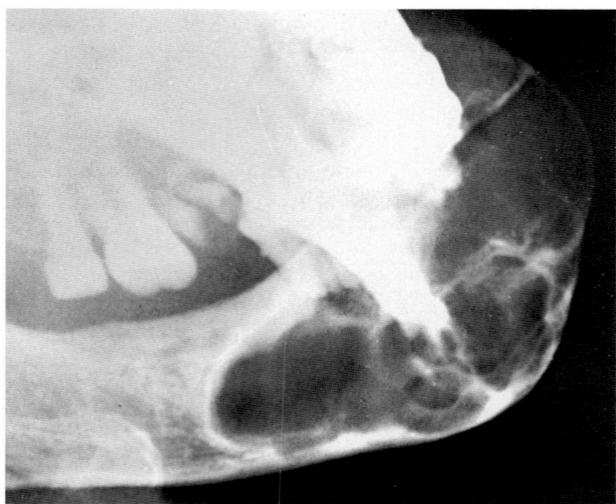

FIGURE 13–15.

Odontogenic sialocyst: Expansile multilocular radiolucency in the anterior mandible.

One lesion occupied the entire body of the mandible. Two lesions were confined to the mandibular premolar area; one resembled a lateral developmental periodontal cyst and was approximately 1.5 cm in diameter, whereas the other looked like a small central giant cell granuloma that was approximately 2 cm in diameter. The two maxillary cases were between the lateral and canine teeth, resembling the so-called "globulomaxillary" cyst.

The reported size of the lesions varies, ranging from 1 or 2 cm to 5 or 6 cm in diameter. They probably grow very slowly. The cortex was probably expanded in four cases, and at least three were multilocular. The remainder were unilocular radiolucencies. Smaller lesions seem to extend approximately half or two thirds of the way up between the roots of adjacent teeth and roughly 1 cm beyond the apex. Only the largest lesions were multilocular. Although the lesions were well demarcated, with a narrow transition zone, the thin sclerotic rim associated with most cysts sometimes was absent or inapparent; however, there was evidence of a wider, more diffuse band of reactive bone at the margins in many published radiographs. Root resorption is not a feature, but it did appear to be present in one case.

AMELOBLASTOMA (Adamantinoma, adamantoblastoma, multilocular cyst)

This tumor probably was recognized first by Cusack in 1827 and described in detail by Falksson in 1879. In 1885 Malassez introduced the term adamantinoma, and in 1930 Ivey and Churchill used the name ameloblastoma. The histologically **benign** ameloblastoma can be divided into three clinicopathologically distinct types: (1) classic ameloblastoma, (2) "malignant" ameloblastoma, and (3) mural ameloblastoma. There is a histologically **malignant** ameloblastoma referred to as ameloblastic carcinoma. In 1978, Shteyer and colleagues estimated that approximately 3000 cases had been reported. While reviewing 706 odontogenic tumors, Regezi and colleagues (1978) found that ameloblastoma accounted for 11% of the sample.

Pathologic Characteristics

The ameloblastoma is a benign, locally aggressive, infiltrative, odontogenic lesion. It is a true neoplasm of enamel organlike tissue but does not differentiate sufficiently to form enamel. The tissue of origin is not known, but most believe it arises from some source of odontogenic epithelium. A variety of histologic variants of ameloblastoma have been described: The follicular or simple type consists of a peripheral layer of cuboidal or columnar cells that resemble ameloblasts containing well-polarized nuclei, with a central mass of cells resembling stellate reticulum. The stellate reticulum sometimes breaks down, leaving only the peripheral cells. Thus, the simple type may be termed histologically as solid or cystic. Other well-described histologic types include plexiform, acanthomatous, granular cell, basal cell, and desmoplastic. Waldron and El-Mofty (1987) reviewed the desmoplastic type, which is characterized by an extensive collagenized stroma containing small islands of tumor epithelium, with a scant tendency to form cystic structures. It is said that there is no difference in clinical behavior between the histologic subtypes; however, Wood and Goaz (1991) pointed out that the subtypes that tend to be more cellular may behave more aggressively, whereas those containing more fibrous connective tissue or large cystic spaces tend to be less aggressive. The ameloblastoma may be a central lesion in bone and, rarely, a peripheral, epulis-like lesion. The peripheral type has been reviewed by Woo and colleagues (1987).

Clinical Features

The ameloblastoma may develop in patients of any age, including children. In a review by Small and Waldron (1955), the average patient age was 33 years. Sirichitra and Dhiravarangkura (1984) analyzed 147 Thai patients, and Ajagbe and Daramola (1987) studied 199 Nigerian people; both series had an average patient age of 32 years. In his series of 109 Nigerian patients, Adekeye (1980) discovered that 68% were in the third and fourth decades of life, and 80% were younger than 40 years. There is a slight preponderance in men. Fifty-two percent of the cases reported by Small and Waldron (1955) occurred in male patients and 48% in female patients. Sirichitra and Dhiravarangkura (1984) reported a male-to-female ratio of 1.1:1; Ajagbe and Daramola (1987), 4:3; and Adekeye (1980), 1.7:1.

The ameloblastoma is characterized by slow growth and painless swelling. Because most lesions are in the posterior mandible, the facial swelling is in this area. In their study of 102 ameloblastomas, Ueno and colleagues (1986) reported that 26% of patients had pain and discomfort; in 29%, ulceration or fistula formation occurred in the gingiva overlying the tumor. Other signs and symptoms include tooth mobility, paresthesia, purulent discharge, trismus, and ill-fitting dentures; only 4 of 102 cases were discovered on routine radiographic examination.

Treatment/Prognosis

Irrespective of treatment modality, Robinson and Martinez (1977) found an overall 67% recurrence rate; Gardner and colleagues (1987) reported a 71% recurrence rate. Among 24 cases in the maxilla, Tsaknis and Nelson (1980) found that 75% of recurrences involved the maxillary sinus. In an analysis of various treatment modalities in 72 patients with ameloblastoma of the mandible and 20 with maxillary lesions, Sehdev and colleagues (1974) found that curettage resulted in a 90% recurrence rate for mandibular lesions and 100% for maxillary lesions. Recurrent lesions were managed by marginal resection, in which a portion of the inferior cortex was left intact; segmental resections, in which the inferior cortex was removed; or hemisections, in which a portion of the body and entire ramus were removed. Such retreatments were successful in treating 80% of recurrent mandibular lesions. Maxillary lesions were more difficult to manage, especially when the antrum was involved. Sehdev and colleagues (1974) recommended more aggressive treatment for all maxillary lesions. Since the 1974 discussion of Sehdev and colleagues, a guardedly more conservative approach has evolved for some ameloblastomas, especially unilocular mandibular lesions and those that are diagnosed as mural ameloblastomas. At least enucleation should be performed, followed by thorough curettage or marginal osteotomy, because the lesion will recur if all of the lesional tissue infiltrating bone trabeculae beyond the visible margins is not removed. For large ameloblastomas, various forms of resection may be considered. Dolan and colleagues (1981) reported a recurrence in an autogenous rib graft. Radiation therapy alone or in conjunction with surgery has not been useful and is not recommended.

Malignant Ameloblastoma (Metastatic ameloblastoma)

The malignant ameloblastoma is the most aggressive form of histologically benign ameloblastoma, and metastasis often is associated with prior multiple recurrences and retreatments. In a review of 20 cases, Slootweg and Müller (1984) reported an average patient age of 31 years. Any histologic type may be involved. According to Buff and associates (1980), who reviewed 22 cases, the tendency for malignant ameloblastoma to metastasize cannot be predicted from the histologic appearance of the primary lesion. Most authors agree that metastasis occurs in association with multiple recurrences and surgical treatments. Three methods of metastasis have been suggested by Buff and colleagues (1980):

1. Aspiration of cells during surgery or when there is spread into the nasal passages.
2. Lymphatic spread to regional and distant nodes.
3. Hematogenous spread to distant organs.

They believe that all three modes have been responsible. According to Buff and colleagues (1980), most metastatic lesions were in the lung or pleura; however, there were metastases in the regional nodes, thoracic nodes, liver, brain, neck, diaphragm, cervical spine, spleen, kidney, ribs, and thoracic and lumbar spine. In one case of ameloblastoma in the ileum, it was suspected that prior transplantation of tumor cells occurred when a bone graft was taken during surgery. This case emphasizes the importance of using separate instruments for harvesting bone graft donor sites when bone grafts are placed at the same time resection is performed. In most cases, death occurred within a few months to several years after the initial treatment. Shafer and co-authors (1983) estimated that less than 2% of all ameloblastomas may behave in this way. Because most benign ameloblastomas probably are not reported any longer, and whereas most malignant ameloblastomas continue to be reported, we estimate that only 0.1 to 0.2% of all histologically benign ameloblastomas metastasize to become malignant ameloblastomas.

◆ RADIOLOGY (Figs. 13–16 to 13–30)

The ameloblastoma classically is described as a multilocular, expansile radiolucency that occurs most frequently in the mandibular molar/ramus area. In fact, some consider it the archtypical multilocular lesion to which all others are compared.

Location

Approximately 85% of the lesions occur in the mandible. In their series of 102 cases, Ueno and colleagues (1986) found 93% in the mandible and 97% of these involved the molar region. Extension into the ramus occurred in 62%, whereas 29% included the symphyseal region and only two of these cases were restricted to the mandibular anterior region. According to Waldron and El-Mofty (1987), the desmoplastic variant occurs more frequently in the anterior mandible.

Radiologic Features

Miles and co-authors (1991), stated that the notion that ameloblastomas begin as unilocular lesions and evolve into mul-

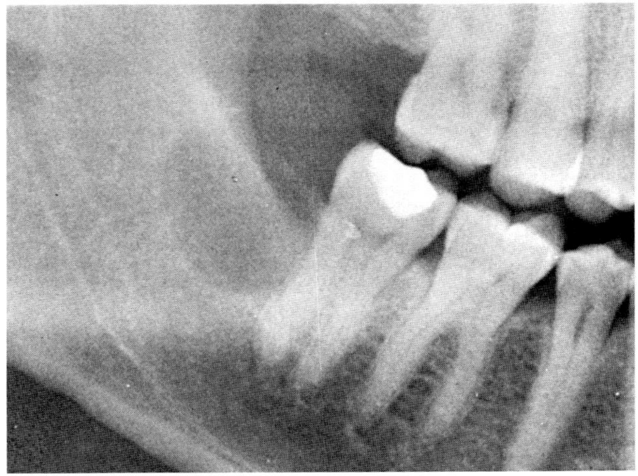

FIGURE 13–16.

Ameloblastoma: unilocular pattern: A 37-year-old man had his third molars removed 5 years previously. There is perforation at the crest of the ridge and soft tissue swelling. (Courtesy of Dr. C. Mader, Washington, D.C.)

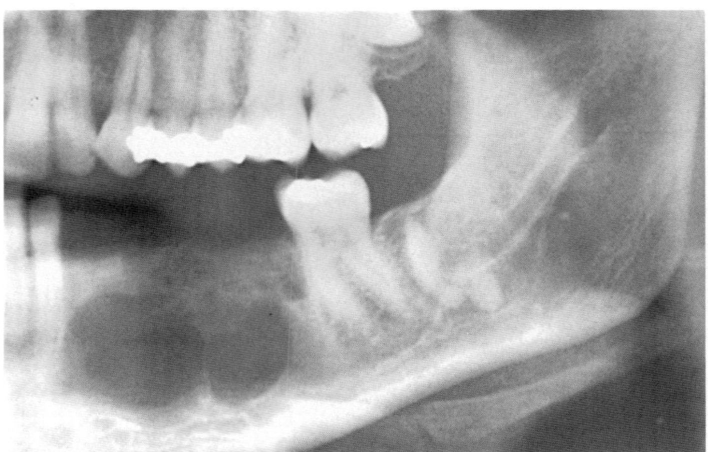

A

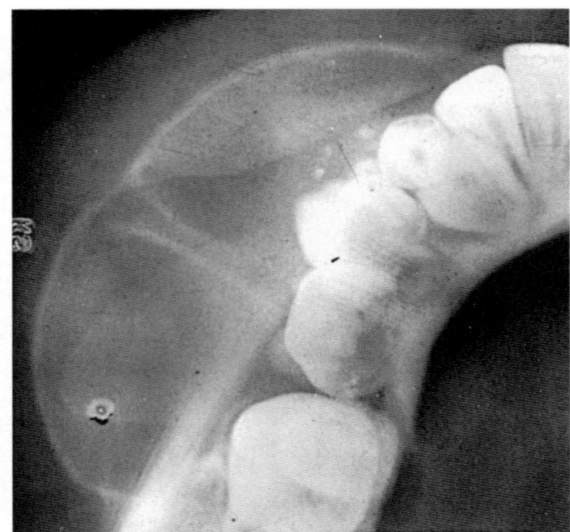

B

FIGURE 13–17.

Ameloblastoma: Bilocular pattern. A, Panoramic view. (Courtesy of D. Barnet, University of Oregon Health Science Center, Portland, OR.) B, Occlusal view, showing a tumorlike pattern of cortex expansion. (Courtesy of Professor P. Dhiravarangkura, Chulalonghorn University, Bangkok, Thailand.)

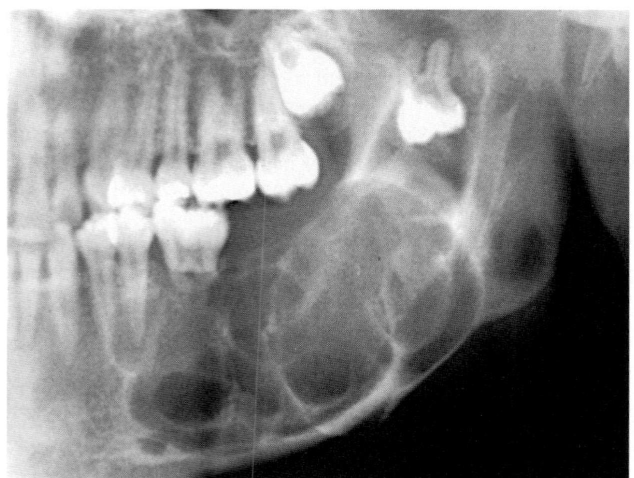

A

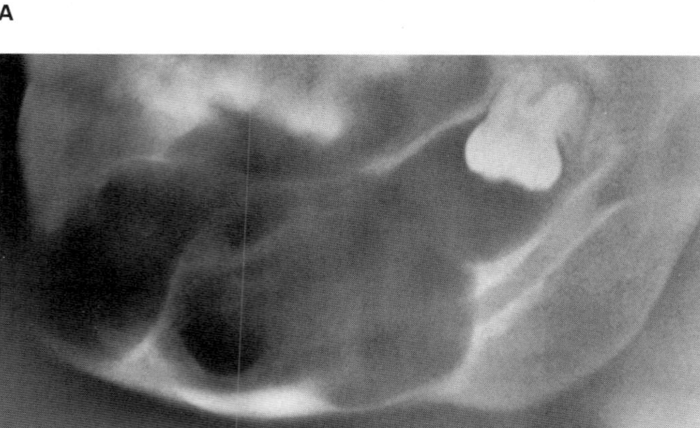

B

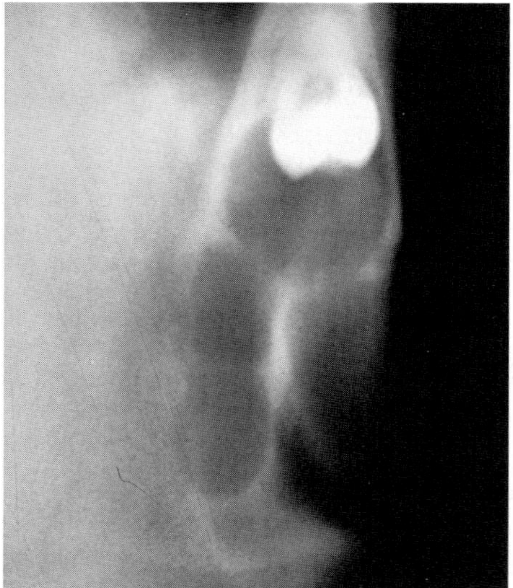

C

FIGURE 13–18.

Ameloblastoma: Multilocular soap-bubble pattern. A, B, and C, Root resorption and tooth displacement. Panel A shows a soap-bubble pattern. Panel C shows a spiderlike pattern. (Courtesy of Drs. M. Araki and K. Hashimoto, Nihon University School of Dentistry, Tokyo, Japan.)

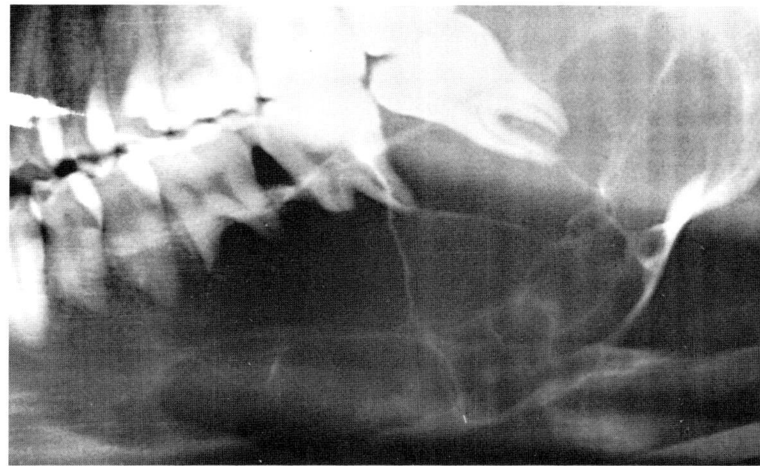

A

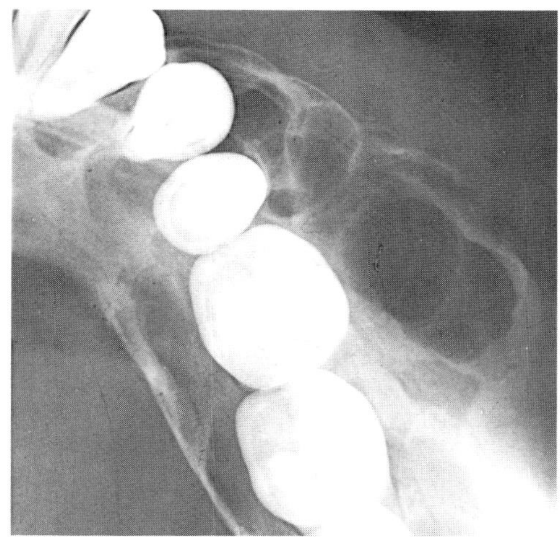

B

FIGURE 13–19.

Ameloblastoma: Multilocular spiderlike pattern. A, Long, straight septa emanate from the central area. (Courtesy of Dr. M. E. Parker, University of the Western Cape, Tygerberg, Republic of South Africa.) B, Another case shows buccal and lingual expansion. (Courtesy of Professor P. Dhiravarangkura, Chulalonghorn University School of Dentistry, Bangkok, Thailand.)

tilocular lesions is supported by the fact that the mean age of patients with unilocular lesions is 26 years, whereas it is approximately 38 years for those with multilocular ameloblastomas; they also stated that roughly 75% of ameloblastomas in people younger than 20 years of age are unilocular. The term unicystic should not be used to describe unilocular ameloblastomas because this is reserved for the mural ameloblastoma, which we discuss as a separate entity. The locules may be less than 1 cm in diameter, and in this instance they tend to be numerous, resembling a honeycomb. Larger locules tend to be fewer in number, and because expansion is invariably present, these are described as having a "soap bubble" appearance. Adekeye (1980) found that 10% were unilocular and 90% had a honeycomb or soap-bubble appearance. Ueno and colleagues (1986) analyzed 97 cases of ameloblastoma of the mandible and found that 47% were unilocular, 37% were multilocular, and 16% had a soap-bubble appearance.

Buccal and lingual expansion of the cortex invariably accompanies ameloblastomas. This is especially notable on

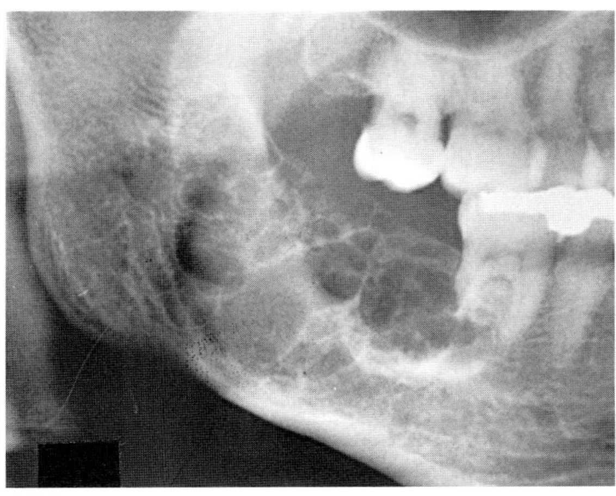

A

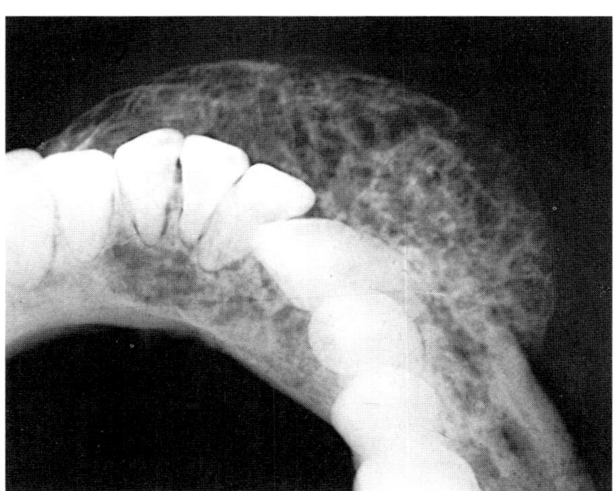

B

FIGURE 13–20.

Ameloblastoma: Multilocular honeycomb pattern. A, Figure shows root resorption and several larger locules. (Courtesy of Professor T. Noikura, First Oral Surgery Department, Kagoshima University, Kagoshima, Japan.) B, Figure shows the tumorlike manner in which the expanded margin meets the buccal plate. (Courtesy of Professor P. Dhiravarangkura, Chulalonghorn University, Bangkok, Thailand.)

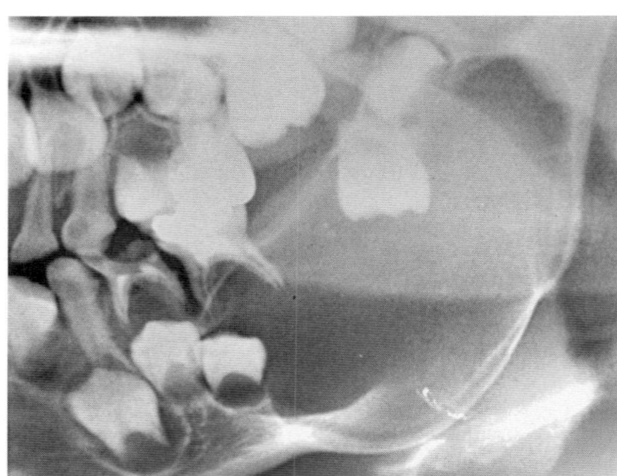
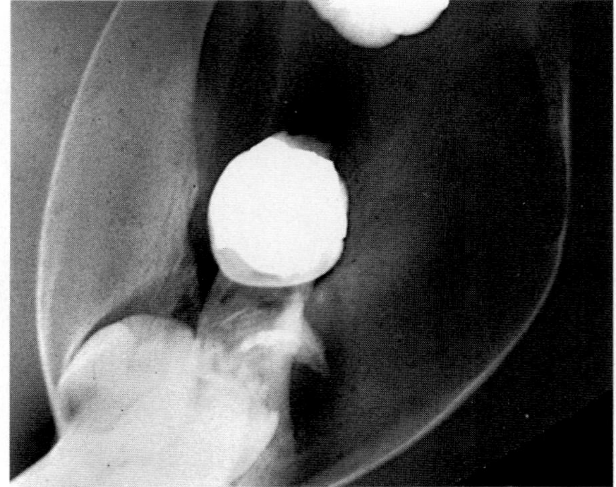

A B

FIGURE 13–21.

Ameloblastoma: Case with a dentigerous cyst-like appearance in a 7-year-old boy. A, First molar rarely gives rise to dentigerous cyst. B, Figure shows eggshell-thin expansion of buccal and lingual cortex. The buccal and lingual expansion and slight variations in the thickness of the expanded buccal cortex suggest tumor rather than a cyst. (Courtesy of Drs. M. Araki, K. Hashimoto, and K. Honda, Nihon University School of Dentistry, Tokyo, Japan.)

axial CT images and helps to distinguish ameloblastoma from the dentigerous cyst, which usually expands in only one direction, most often to the buccal. The expanded cortex of the ameloblastoma may be significantly thinned and intact, with an eggshell-like appearance, or in some instances perforations may be seen. The expanded cortex may show a tumor effect, with the greatest degree of expansion occurring along the vector of tumor growth.

Relationship to Teeth

Ueno and colleagues (1986) observed that an impacted tooth was involved in 38%; of these, 82% were third molars. Five cases affected a lower second molar, and in two cases the tooth was a premolar. Sirichitra and Dhiravarangkura (1984) found root resorption in 39% of the cases. With ameloblastoma, the root resorption has a knife edge pattern because all of the adjacent roots are cut off along a single linear

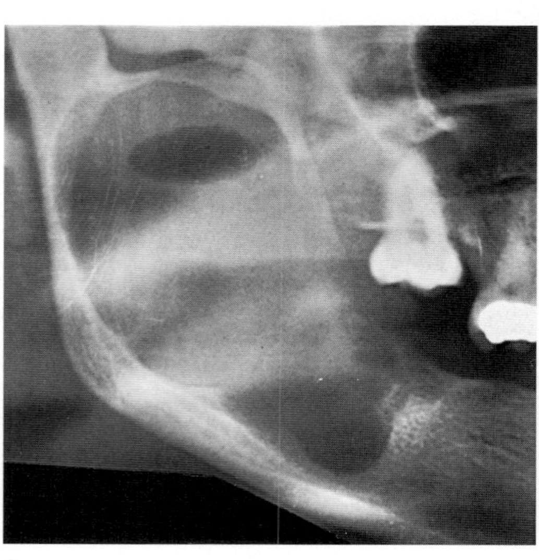
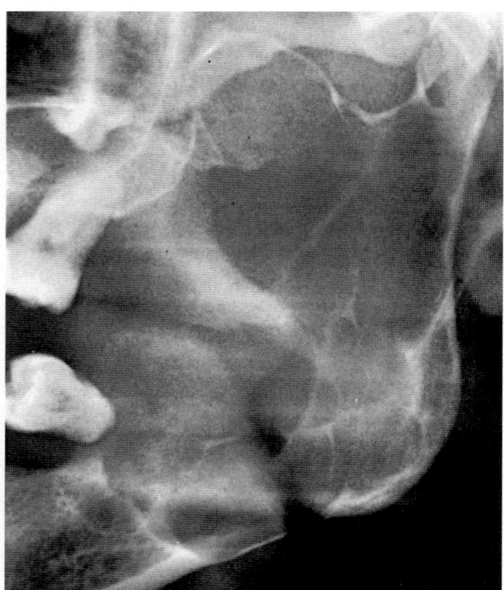

A B

FIGURE 13–22.

Ameloblastoma: A and B, Pattern characterized by invasion into the ramus, with destruction of the anterior ramus wall and crest of ridge, while the angle remains unaffected.

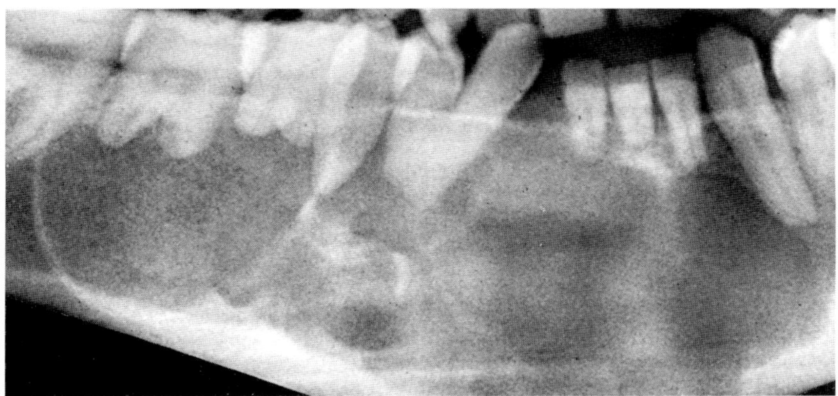

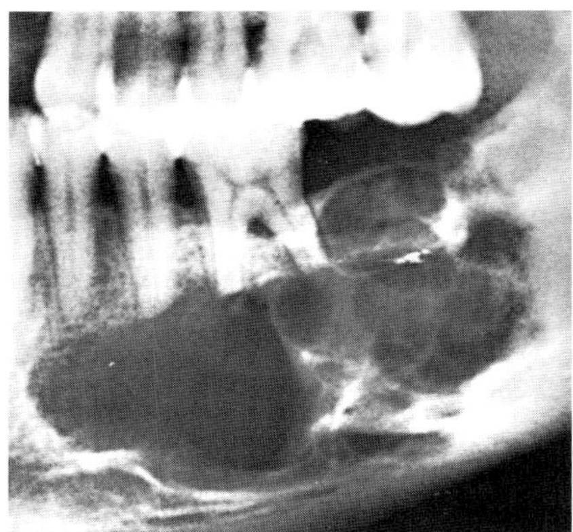

FIGURE 13–23.

Ameloblastoma: patterns of root resorption: A, Multiplanar pattern. B, Knife edge pattern, characteristic of ameloblastoma. (Courtesy of Dr. M. E. Parker, University of the Western Cape, Tygerberg, Republic of South Africa.)

plane, corresponding to the margin of the lesion. When roots are not resorbed, they tend to extend into the lesion rather than straddle it.

Worth's Classic Descriptions of Ameloblastoma

Worth's (1963) descriptions are especially applicable to mandibular lesions. He divided the ameloblastoma into four possible radiologic manifestations: The first resembles a dentigerous cyst without septa within the lesion, which is seen most frequently in the ramus, and suspicion of ameloblastoma increases when the patient is older than 30 years. Another sign of ameloblastoma is extension of a lesion in the body of the mandible into the ramus. The presence of some septa, even if they are slight, also increases the possibility of ameloblastoma greatly, especially if partial loculation can be seen. If a portion of the ramus wall is lost, especially the anterior wall or, less frequently, the superior wall, it is very possible that the lesion is an ameloblastoma. When, according to Worth (1963), there is a cystlike cavity with some deficiency of the wall, and faint septa are observed within the lesion, then the diagnosis is almost certainly an ameloblastoma.

Worth's (1963) second category, which he believed is the most common, consists of a cystic-appearing cavity with distinctive septa. The trabeculae vary widely in their shapes and arrangements, but one frequently sees strands radiating from a common center. Worth (1963) said that a gross caricature of a spider may be seen in some cases, and he believed this finding is almost pathognomonic of ameloblastoma. The trabecular arrangement usually is disordered. Some of the trabeculae are curved, suggesting that they may be embrac-

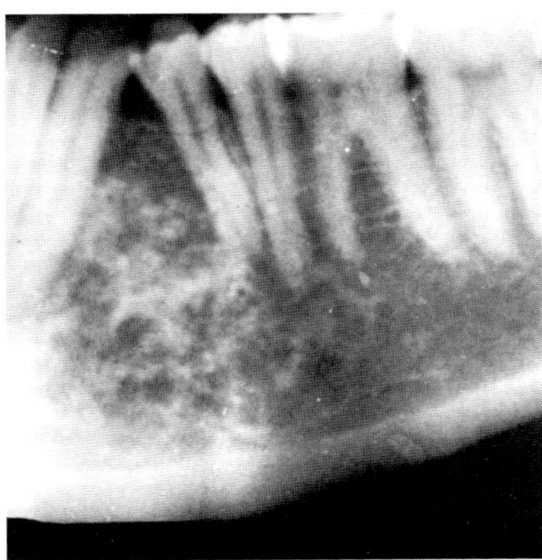

FIGURE 13–24.

Ameloblastoma: Typical desmoplastic histologic type. (Courtesy of Dr. E. Romero, Monterrey, Mexico.)

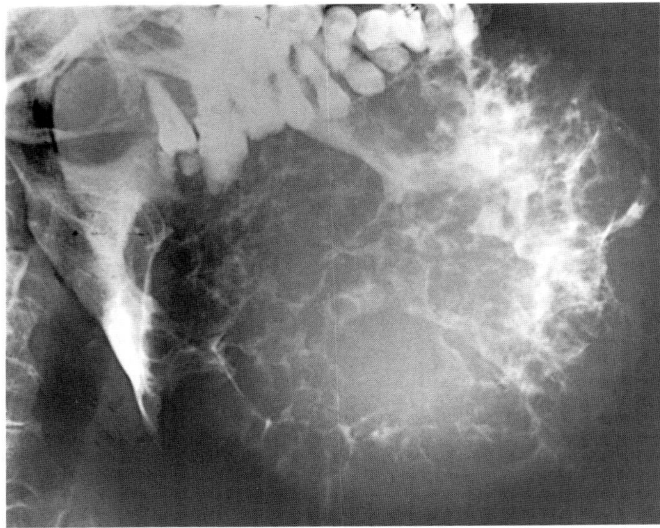

FIGURE 13–25.

Ameloblastoma: Case with tremendous growth potential. There are limitations of the plain views in determining the extent of the large lesions. (Courtesy of M. E. Parker, University of the Western Cape, Tygerberg, Republic of South Africa.)

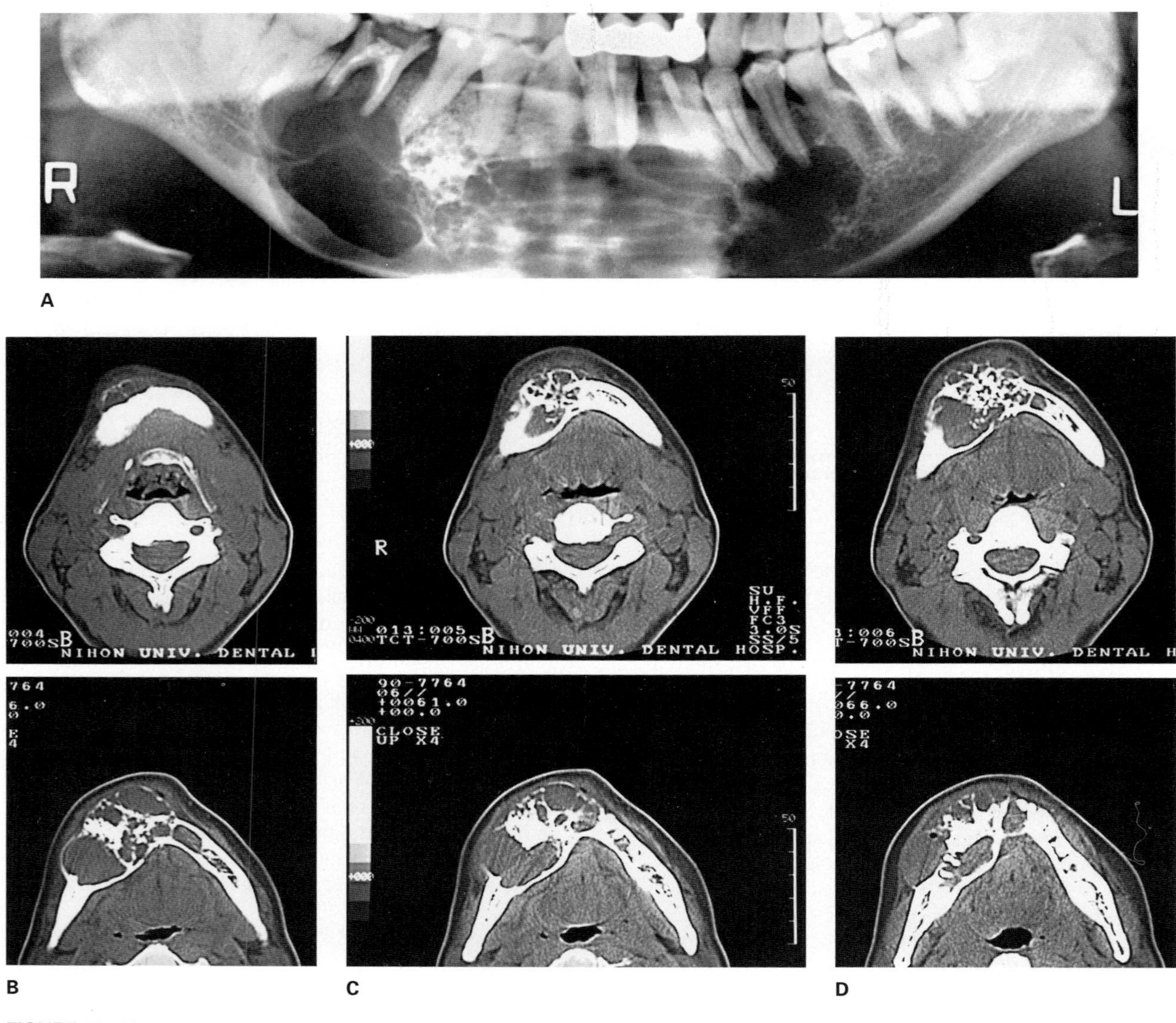

FIGURE 13–26.

Ameloblastoma: CT workup of large mandibular lesion. A, Panoramic view. B to D, CT images showing buccal and lingual expansion and eggshell-thin expanded cortices with perforations. (Courtesy of Drs. M. Araki, K. Hashimoto, and K. Honda, Nihon University School of Dentistry, Tokyo, Japan.)

ing cystic areas. They also may be thin or coarse, with some more than 2 mm wide. When there is also a defect in the wall of the cystlike lesion, it is almost certainly an ameloblastoma. The defect in the wall is usually at the anterior surface of the ramus or the superior border of the body of the mandible. Characteristically, the angle of the mandible invariably is preserved. The inferior aspect may be ballooned out, with a significant smooth downward convexity that may be eggshell thin and intact.

The third pattern specified by Worth (1963) is less common than the second but more common than the first. According to him, this one has a multilocular cystic appearance. It is seen most frequently in the posterior portion of the mandible and ramus. Two, three, or more cavities may appear in continuity, with thin septa separating them. The patient's age, especially if he or she is older than 30 years, and the loss of continuity of one of the free walls are suggestive of ameloblastoma. In this instance, there also may be a significant downward enlargement of the inferior border of the jaw, which maintains a convex lower border. In the maxilla, this multilocular pattern is highly suggestive of ameloblastoma.

Worth's (1963) fourth category is associated with what he terms the solid variety of the tumor. In this instance, normal bone is replaced with a honeycomb appearance in which cavities are relatively small and fairly uniform in size, although there are some variations between compartments. The honeycomb may consist of a few to hundreds of little cavities. The cavity walls are coarse, and the margins of the lesion are lobulated in conformity with the adjacent cavities.

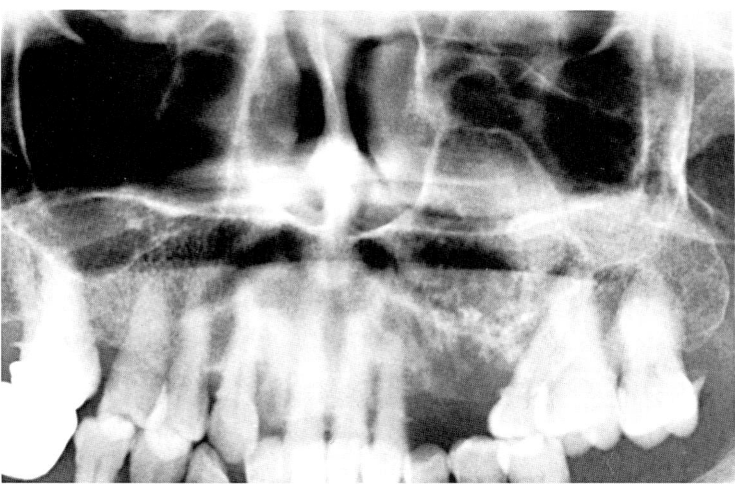

A

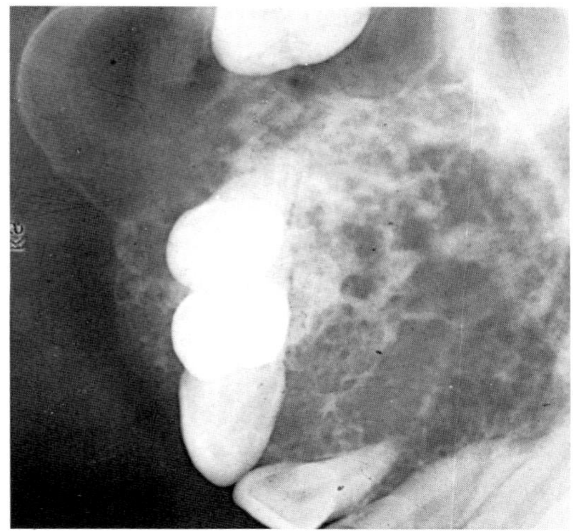

B

FIGURE 13–27.

Ameloblastoma: Maxillary lesions: plain views. A, Panoramic view of lesion extending into the left antrum. (Courtesy of Professor T. Noikura, Department of Dental Radiology, Kagoshima University, Kagoshima, Japan.) B, Occlusal view. (Courtesy of Professor P. Dhiravarangkura, Chulalonghorn University School of Dentistry, Bangkok, Thailand.)

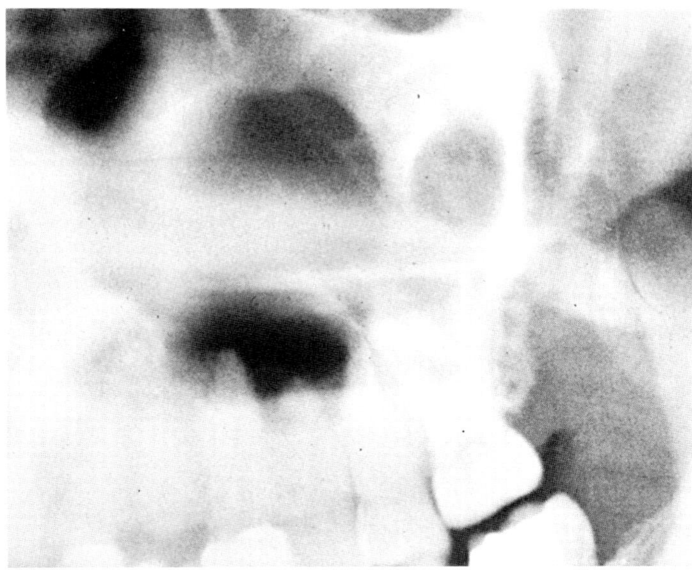

A

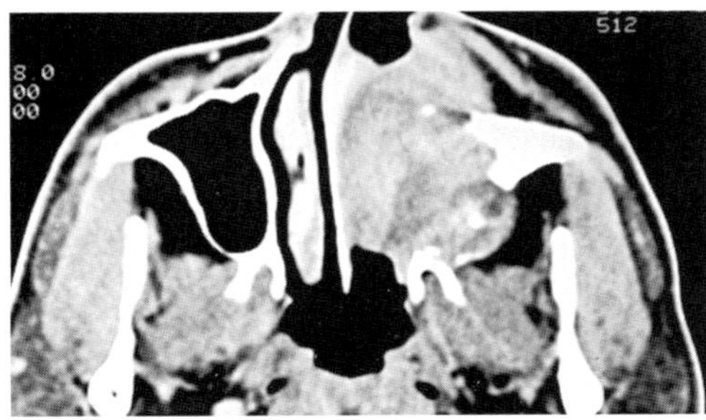

B

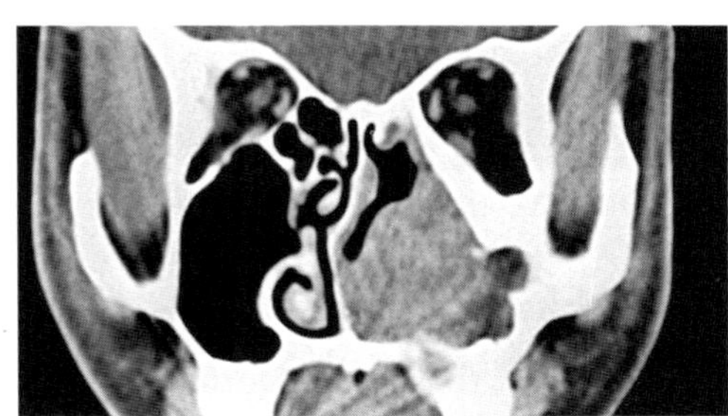

C

FIGURE 13–28.

Ameloblastoma: Maxillary lesion as seen on plain radiograph and CT scan. A, Panoramic view provides limited information. B and C, Lesion actually occupies most of antrum; destruction extends to nose and the root of the zygoma. (Courtesy of Dr. C. S. Park, Department of Radiology, Yonsei University College of Dentistry, Seoul, Korea.)

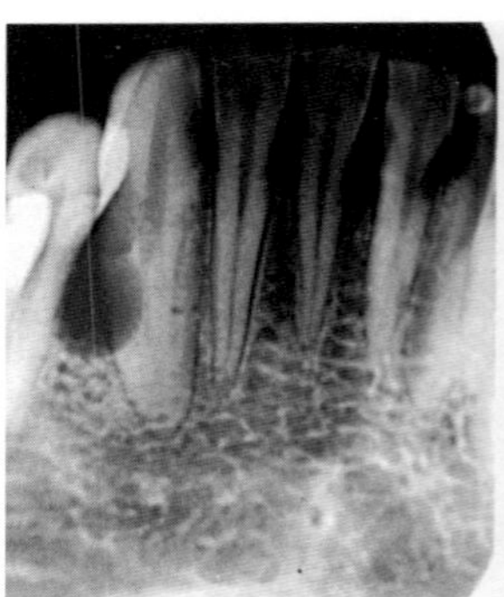
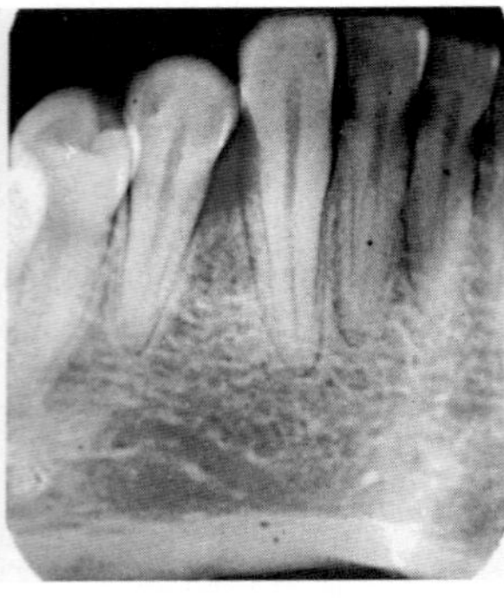
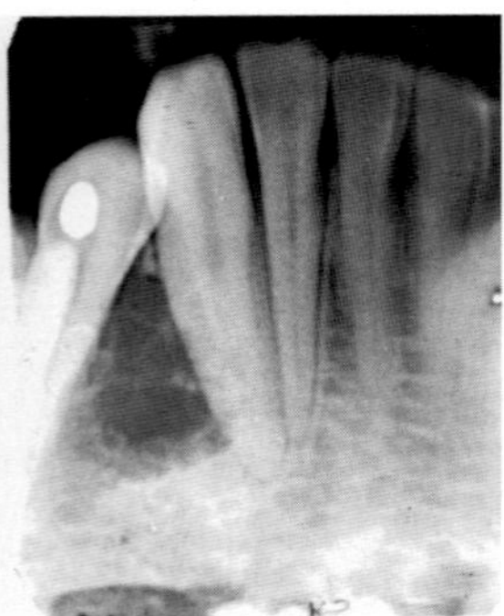

FIGURE 13–29.

Ameloblastoma arising in a cyst: The original lesion (left) was diagnosed as an OKC. One year later, the area appeared to be filling in (middle); 4 years later, the lesion recurred as an ameloblastoma (right).

The margins separating normal bone from tumor are denser than normal bone, and although this may be interpreted as a cortex, it is wider and less etched than most cortices of cysts or benign tumors. According to Worth (1963), it is unusual for any unerupted tooth to be associated with this presentation of the tumor. A combination of cystic and solid types often is found. Some patterns described by Worth (1963) actually may have consisted of mural ameloblastomas as we know them today.

Radiologic Features of Maxillary Ameloblastomas

Maxillary ameloblastomas are important because they often extend into adjacent facial structures, have an increased potential for recurrence, and may result in significant disfigurement after treatment. There are several reports of ameloblastomas in the maxilla, including those by Imai and colleagues (1980), who reviewed 77 maxillary ameloblastomas and added five new cases, and Tsaknis and Nelson (1980), who reported an analysis of 24 cases from the Armed Forces Institute of Pathology. A great deal of the data in this discussion is from these two reports. In their review of the Japanese literature, Imai and colleagues (1980) found that only 6% of ameloblastomas occurred in the maxilla. Male-to-female ratios of 1.5:1 (Imai and colleagues, 1980) and 2.4:1 (Tsaknis and Nelson, 1980) were reported. The average patient age is 46 years. Imai and colleagues (1980) stated that 75 to 90% occurred in the premolar-molar region. Tsaknis and Nelson (1980) observed that the maxillary antrum was involved in 12 of 24 cases and six of the eight recurrences showed sinus involvement. Radiologically, when the antrum was involved there was destruction of the antral walls, antral cloudiness, and thickening of the lining membrane. The same general radiomorphologic patterns reported for the mandible are seen in the maxilla, but three of the five cases of Imai and colleagues (1980) were unilocular; however, these authors and Worth (1963) reported that a scalloped band of bone resorption could be seen at the margin in most cases on careful observation, even though the lesion appeared unilocular. They also observed a knife edge appearance when the maxillary teeth are resorbed.

Radiologic Features of Malignant Ameloblastoma

In a discussion of malignant ameloblastoma by Buff and colleagues (1980), the primary lesion was in the mandible in 80% of cases, and 70% of all primary lesions occurred in the third-molar region. Of 20 malignant ameloblastomas

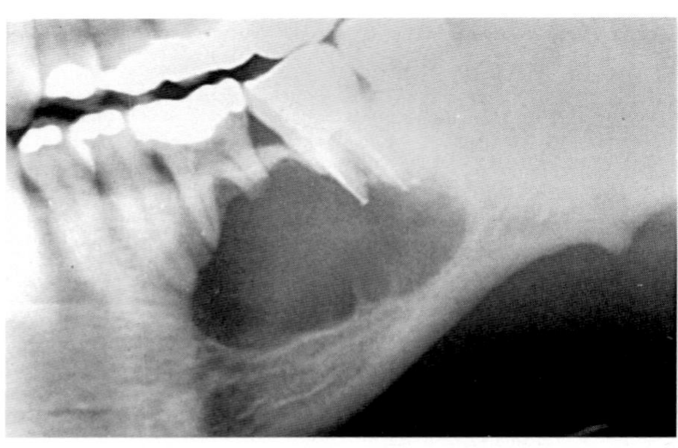

A

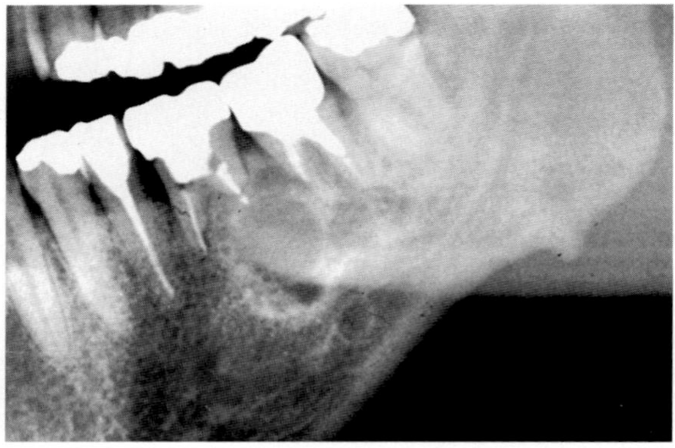

B

FIGURE 13–30.

Ameloblastoma arising in a cyst: The original lesion was interpreted as a radicular cyst of the second molar; endodontic therapy was performed. A, Three years later, healing had not occurred. The first molar and second premolar were treated endodontically. The lesion was excised and proved to be a radicular cyst histologically. B, Seven years after removal of the radicular cyst, this lesion proved to be an ameloblastoma. (Courtesy of Professor G. Tronje, Karolinska Institutet, Stockholm. Sweden.)

reviewed by Slootweg and Müller (1984), 90% were in the mandible. None of the radiologic characteristics of malignant ameloblastoma suggests its nature or is different from the features of ordinary ameloblastomas. Buff and colleagues (1980) expected the CT numbers in the pulmonary metastatic lesions to be equal to or less than those of the adjacent soft tissues. The observation of higher CT numbers usually indicates calcification and, thus, a benign pulmonary lesion. In this case, the CT numbers in the metastatic lesion were higher than those of the adjacent soft tissue, suggesting a benign pulmonary lesion with calcification. These authors attributed the higher CT number to a dense fibrous stoma in some ameloblastomas.

Advanced Imaging of Ameloblastomas

Cohen and colleagues (1985) discussed the utility of CT in evaluating four extensive cases involving the mandible and one in the maxilla. In the maxillary case, extension into the infratemporal fossa was seen clearly on the CT scan but was not observed on the conventional plain radiographs or tomography. They found that CT was superior to conventional radiography in showing the soft tissue extent of ameloblastomas, which may be seen only if hard and soft tissue windows are ordered. On axial CT scans, buccal and lingual expansion and a CT number similar to that of gingival epithelium help distinguish the ameloblastoma from similar-appearing cystic lesions on plain radiographs.

Heffez and colleagues (1988) discussed the role of magnetic resonance imaging (MRI) in the evaluation of ameloblastomas. They quoted Schaefer and colleagues (1985), stating that decreased CT attenuation resulting from fibrosis and edema may make it difficult to delineate the interface of tumor and normal tissue, especially after radiation therapy or previous surgery. Heffez and co-authors (1988) explained that MRI distinguishes variation in the time-dependent behavior of hydrogen nuclei, known as the relaxation phenomenon, and not the variation in electron density as with CT. T2-weighted images allow the clinician to differentiate more easily between solid structures and fluid. Heffez and colleagues (1988) explained that the ameloblastoma shows a significant increase in signal intensity on T2-weighted images. Thus, the tumor-scar tissue interface was identified readily. In one of their recurrent ameloblastomas, edge definition was assessed from CT images, and histopathologic examination later showed that the margin obtained was larger than necessary. In another case, MRI was used to plan the surgical margins, and a more conservative procedure resulted, with clear margins.

ODONTOGENIC MYXOMA (Odontogenic fibromyxoma, odontogenic myxofibroma)

According to Farman and colleagues (1977 to 1978), Virchow (1863) probably was the first to describe the histologic features of odontogenic myxoma, which did not appear in the dental literature until the 1947 report of Thoma and Goldman. In reports by Regezi and colleagues (1978) and Minderjahn (1979), the odontogenic myxoma accounted for 3 to 6% of all odontogenic tumors. It occurs two to four times less frequently than the ameloblastoma.

Pathologic Characteristics

The odontogenic myxoma is a locally aggressive benign neoplasm. It is believed to arise from odontogenic mesenchymal elements of the dental papilla, which it closely resembles histologically, or the dental follicle or periodontal ligament. The histologic appearance of the odontogenic myxoma typically consists of loosely arranged rounded or angular cells lying in an abundant mucoid stroma. The tissue does not appear highly cellular. Remnants of odontogenic epithelium have been observed occasionally. There are usually a few capillaries and occasionally strands of collagen.

Clinical Features

Several large reviews have been reported, including 95 cases by Barros and colleagues (1969), 99 cases by White and associates (1975), and 213 cases by Farman and colleagues (1977 to 1978). Adekeye and co-authors (1984) recently reported 18 new cases. The lesion is rare in children younger than 10 years and in people older than 50 years. Only 14 of 213 cases reported by Farman and colleagues (1977 to 1978) occurred in the first decade of life. According to these authors, the mean patient age varies slightly according to sex and location. Although the mean age ranged from 25 to 35 years, mandibular lesions occurred 5 years earlier than maxillary lesions, and lesions were seen approximately 5 years earlier in male patients compared with female patients. Minderjahn (1979) and Barros and co-workers (1969) reported an equal male-to-female ratio; in an analysis of 176 reported cases for which sex was specified, Farman and colleagues (1977 to 1978) found that 99 occurred in female and 77 in male patients, for a ratio of 3:2. Most lesions grow slowly and painlessly, and the teeth usually are not affected clinically. In the mandible, buccal and lingual swelling occurs, but in the maxilla, swelling is seen mainly when the sinus is not involved. When there was sinus involvement, less swelling was observed. In such instances, exophthalmos and nasal obstruction may occur.

Treatment/Prognosis

Smaller lesions usually are treated by curettage, with or without cautery. Larger lesions sometimes are treated by resection. At surgery the tissue consists of a pale brownish, gelatinous substance. Most surgeons consider this pathognomonic. In other instances, when the lesion is more fibrous, the tumor consists of a glistening bosselated mass, with a color varying from gray-white to amber. When a flat instrument is placed on the cut surface, clear slimy filaments are seen as the instrument is drawn away.

Farman and colleagues (1977 to 1978) found that wide resection resulted in fewer recurrences, whereas treatment by curettage or enucleation, with or without electrocautery, resulted in recurrence in 6 of 19 (32%) cases. Barros and colleagues (1969) studied 50 cases for which follow-up data were available. Of these, 13 (26%) recurred. Among the recurrences, 10 were treated by curettage and 1 by resection; treatment for the remaining 2 was not specified.

◆ RADIOLOGY (Figs. 13–31 to 13–35)

Allen (1980) emphasized the importance of taking a panoramic radiograph versus the full-mouth survey. He reported a case occurring in a 27-year-old black woman. The patient had yearly dental examinations with a full intraoral series of radiographs, with the last being taken 10 months before the lesion was detected. The lesion was not noticed on these views, however, because it was confined to the angle-ramus region and it occupied almost all of the ramus-angle area at diagnosis. The patient required mandibular resection from the first premolar up to and including the condyle.

Location

In most series, the mandible is favored over the maxilla. Farman and associates (1977 to 1978) found 132 reported cases in the mandible and 91 in the maxilla. In 18 cases studied by Adekeye and associates (1984), 11 were mandibular and 7 maxillary. Like most odontogenic tumors, it develops most often in tooth-bearing areas—in this case the molar region, followed by the premolar area. Farman and associates (1977 to 1978) found that this lesion may cross the midline, especially in the mandible; maxillary midline lesions usually did not involve the sinus. Maxillary lesions often affect the antrum, with 40 (44%) of the 91 lesions in this study involving the ipsilateral sinus. Occasionally mandibular lesions have been reported in non-tooth-bearing areas such as the upper ramus and condyle, without extension into the body of the mandible. Farman and associates (1977 to 1978) found reports of three such cases.

Radiologic Features

Barros and colleagues (1969) proposed that the radiologic appearance of the odontogenic myxoma consists of one of two patterns, depending on the evolution of the tumor: The first stage begins with an osteoporotic appearance, with more prominent medullary spaces separated by thin septa of bone. These septa become thinner and more elongated as the tumor infiltrates locally, forming larger areas of osteolysis. During this stage, the lesion acquires its classic radiographic appearance, which consists of a multilocular radiolucency with well-developed locules, composed of trabeculae tending to intersect at right angles. The bony septa forming the locules usually are straight, thin, elongated, and lacy. Eversole (personal communication, 1980) once said that the internal configuration of the bony septa resembled ''lichen planus of the jaw bone.'' Although some authors have described these as having a soap-bubble or honeycomb appearance, many lesions tend to form more angular locules, resembling the strings of a tennis racket. Other shapes include small or large triangles, diamonds, squares, rectangles, and X, Y, and V figures. The margin frequently is poorly defined, even in the first stage.

As defined by Barros and colleagues (1969), the second stage consists of the breakout or destructive phase characterized by a loss of internal locules, significant expansion, and

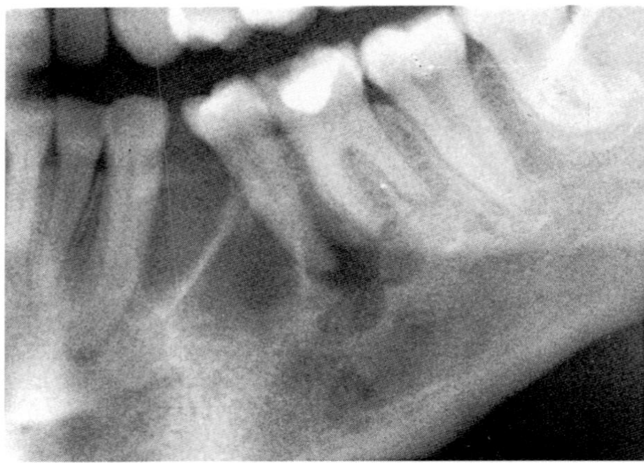

A

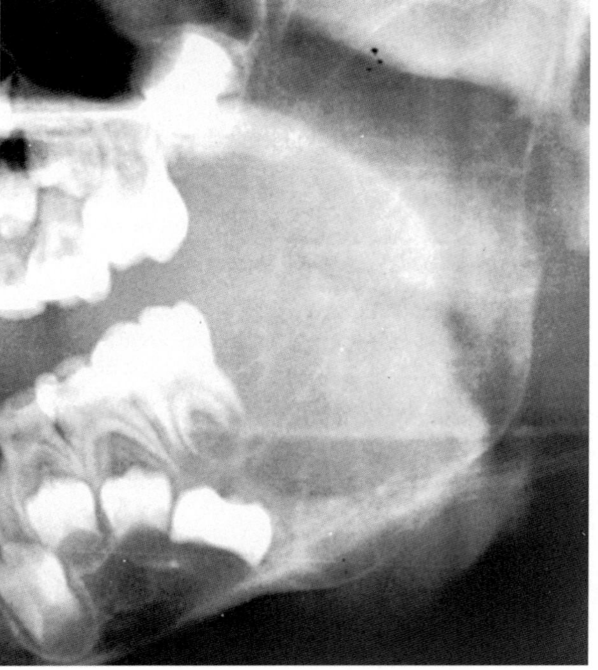

B

FIGURE 13–31.

Odontogenic myxoma: Case in the early stage. A, The single septum is straight and very thick. The distinct sclerotic margin is focally absent. B, Thin, elongated, interlacing septa are seen, and there is involvement of the angle. (Courtesy of Drs. L. Archila, F. Erales, and R. Carlos, Guatemala City, Guatemala.)

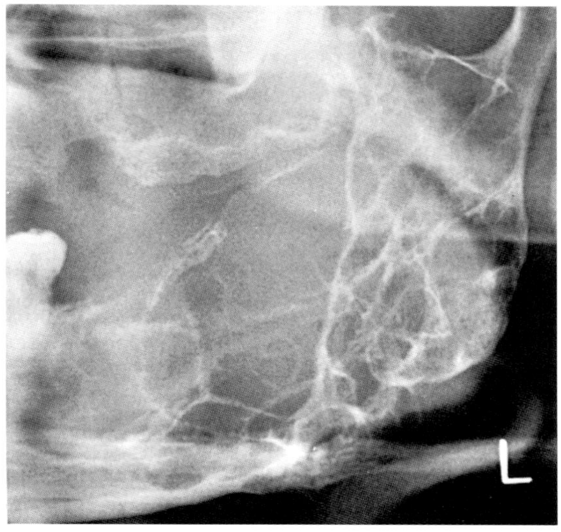

A

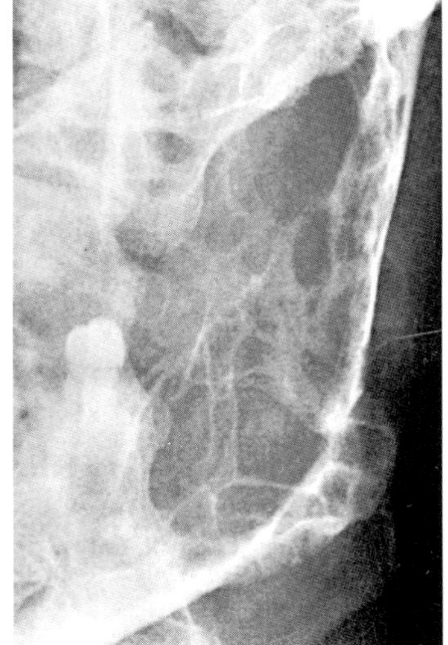

B

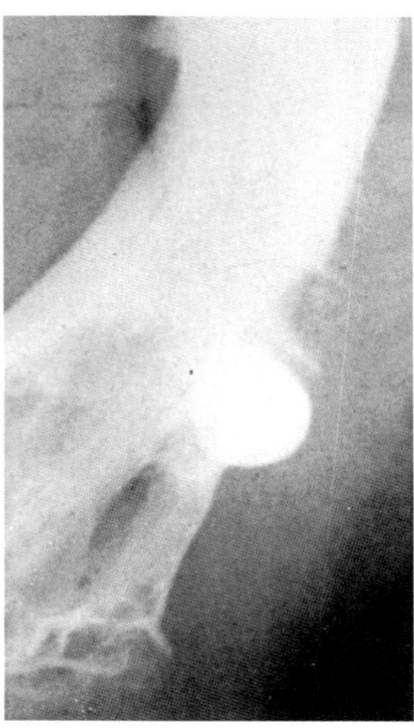

C

FIGURE 13–32.

Odontogenic myxoma: Case in the breakout phase. A, Locules form typical diamond, triangular, and rectangular shapes. Figure shows angle involvement. B, Almost imperceptible septa extend peripherally for a short, equal distance at right angles to the lateral margin of the ramus. C, Figure shows several peripheral extensions of septa on the buccal side. (Courtesy of Professor T. Noikura, Second Oral Surgery Department, Kagoshima University, Kagoshima, Japan.)

perforation of the cortex with invasion into the surrounding soft tissues; in the maxilla, there is extension into the antrum. We believe that an early feature of this stage is the appearance of septa beyond the peripheral margin of the lesion, extending at right angles to the margin, thus imparting a hairbrush or sunburst appearance. This feature has been described by Chuchurru and colleagues (1985), Farman and associates (1977 to 1978), and Cohen and Hertzanu (1986) and represents bony septa being carried into the soft tissues with the tumor mass. On axial CT scans, internal septa usually were absent in the large lesions reported by Cohen and Hertzanu (1986). In the maxilla, the CT scans also showed complete filling of the maxillary sinus, with extension into the nasal fossa and zygoma and thinning of the orbital floor and hard palate.

In 14 of 18 cases described by Adekeye and associates (1984), the internal configuration was described as soap-bubble (8 cases), showing "trabeculation" (6 cases), and multilocular (1 case), and 4 cases had no internal elements. The margins were poorly defined in 14 of the 18 cases. All

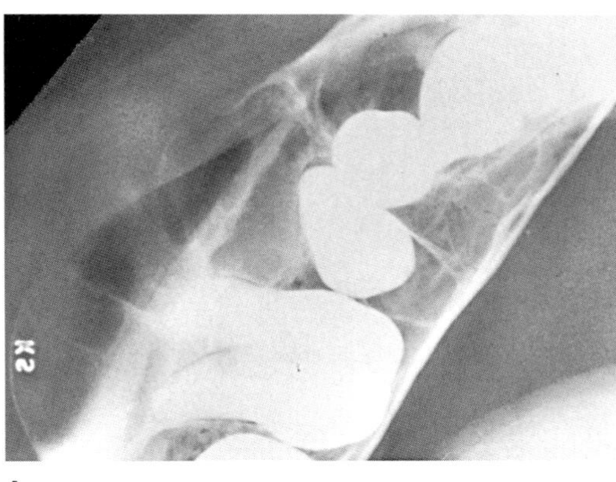

A

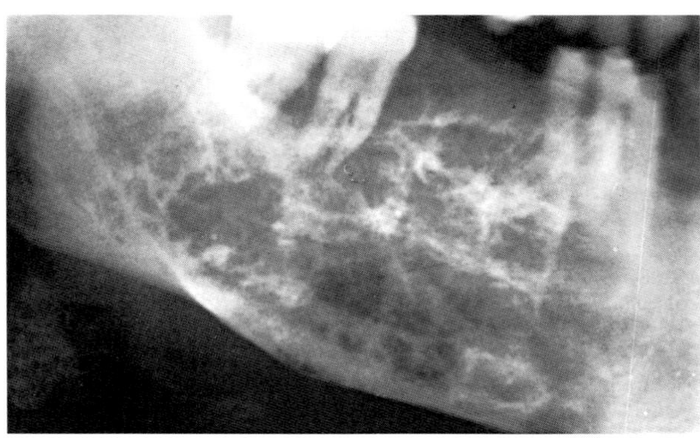

B

FIGURE 13–33.

Odontogenic myxoma: Peripheral septal extensions indicate the breakout stage. A, Septa are at right angles to the long axis of the mandible but remain within the inner confines of the lesion. (Courtesy of Professor L. Alfaro, University of Chile School of Dentistry, Pathology Referral Center, Santiago, Chile.) B, Septa extend beyond the superior margin of the lesion. (From Farman AG, Nortjé CJ, Wood RE: Oral and Maxillofacial Diagnostic Imaging. Philadelphia:Mosby, 1993, p. 12.)

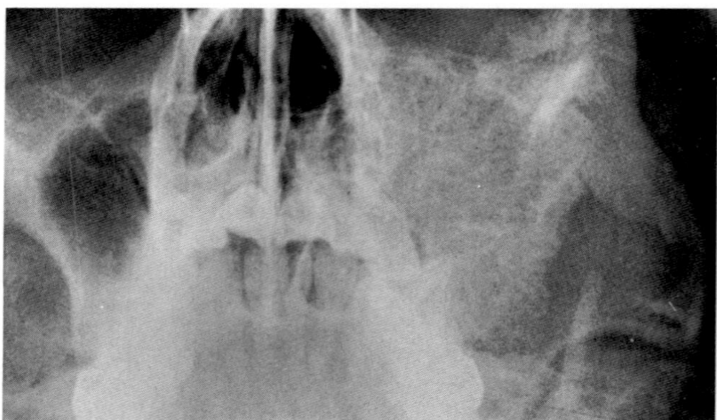

A

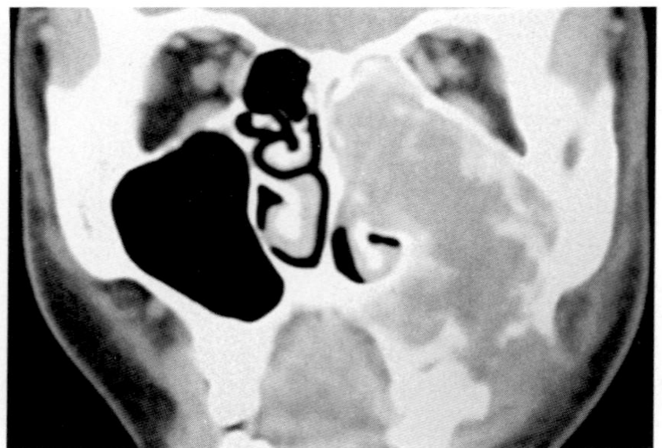

B

FIGURE 13–34.

Odontogenic myxoma: Two cases simulating a typical large maxillary lesion. A, Case 1: Plain view showing involvement of the maxilla, with peripheral extension of septa, and spread to the maxillary sinus. (Courtesy of Professor T. Noikura, First Oral Surgery Department, Kagoshima University, Kagoshima, Japan.) B, Case 2: Extensive destruction of the left maxilla with breakout into soft tissues, involvement of the maxillary sinus and nasal fossa, extension into the anterior ethmoids, and deformity of the medial orbital margin.

four cases described as well defined contained internal septa, and all four cases without internal elements were poorly defined. The odontogenic myxoma may destroy the angle of the mandible; the ameloblastoma almost never does this.

Farman and colleagues (1977 to 1978) pointed out that areas of opacity may be present in some myxomas and cited four such cases in the literature. Rennie and associates (1985) reported such a case in a 5-year-old boy. The lesion was in the mandibular molar-ramus area, with severe displacement of the developing second permanent molar. Just distal to the partially erupted first molar, a 1 × 1 cm calcified mass was observed. The lesion resembled a cystic odontoma. Histologically, the calcified tissue looked like the hard tissues seen in ossifying or cementifying fibromas.

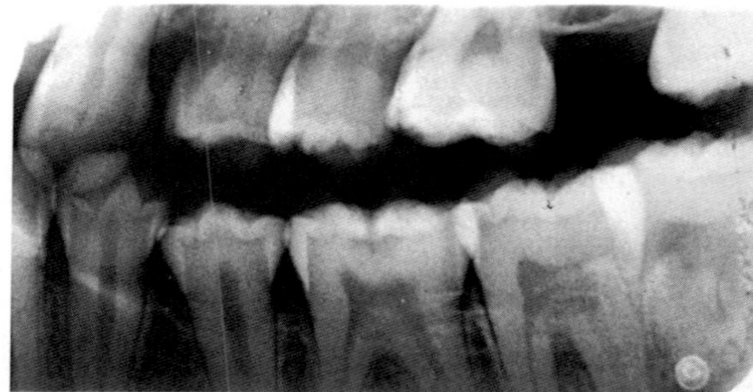

A

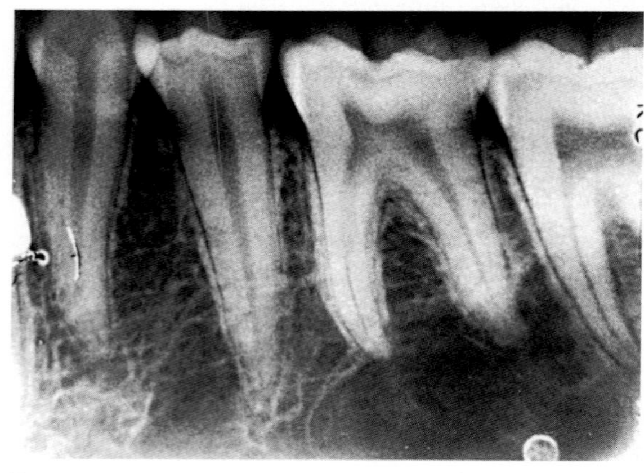

B

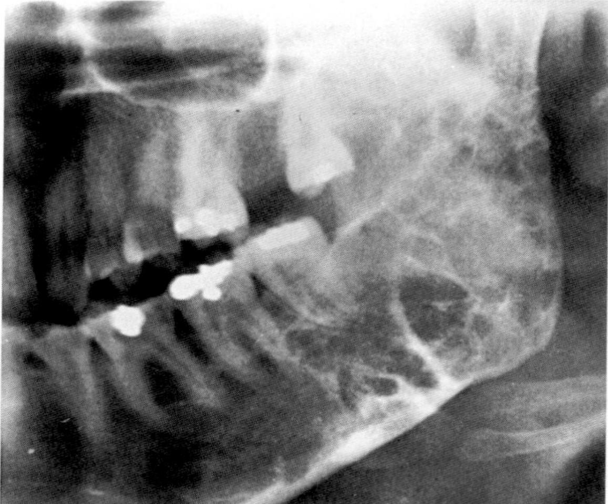

C

FIGURE 13–35.

Odontogenic myxoma: A and B, Intraoral radiographs from patient with no symptoms who was examined regularly this way. C, Ten months after radiographs A and B were taken, the lesion was detected on this radiograph. (From Allen PS: Fibromyxoma of the mandible: case report and radiographic considerations. J Am Dent Assoc 101:930, 1980.)

Relationship to Teeth

During the breakout phase, root resorption and tooth displacement may occur. Farman and associates (1977 to 1978) found that involvement of adjacent teeth was rare. In 5 of 18 large odontogenic myxomas reported by Adekeye and associates (1984), the teeth were displaced and only 1 case had root resorption. We observed a case in which the adjacent teeth were "cut off," with a knife edge effect high up on the roots and only approximately one third of the root length remaining.

Extragnathic Odontogenic Myxoma

Although it is said that the odontogenic myxoma occurs exclusively in the jaws, Farman and associates (1977 to 1978) found several reports, including one by Stout (1948) and one by Marcove (1964), in which this lesion was detected in tissues outside the jaws. Farman and associates (1977 to 1978) pointed out that soft tissue myxomas seem to be at least as common as the jaw lesions. Although most occur in the somatic tissues, isolated cases have developed in the parotid region, lower lip, cheek, and soft palate.

CENTRAL GIANT CELL GRANULOMA

(Central giant cell reparative granuloma, osteoclastoma, giant cell tumor of bone)

The original term central giant cell granuloma (CGCG) was coined by Jaffe in 1953, when he suggested this lesion should be distinguished from the giant cell tumor (GCT) of bone. Jaffe believed that the CGCG is a reactive lesion, whereas the GCT is a neoplasm. In 1988, Auclair and colleagues found no reliable histologic data supporting the separation of these two entities. In their report of 37 cases, Eisenbud and colleagues (1988) observed that CGCG was the most common jaw lesion, after odontogenic and nonodontogenic cysts.

Pathologic Characteristics

According to Miles and colleagues (1991), the CGCG may consist of one of several related reactive lesions resulting from trauma or vascular insult producing intramedullary hemorrhage. If the blood supply is cut off completely, no giant cell reaction occurs and the traumatic bone cyst results. Conversely, if the blood supply is maintained fully, an arteriovenous malformation (AVM) develops; however, if the blood supply is maintained only partially, the aneurysmal bone cyst or CGCG could result. We believe the CGCG begins as a single resorption lacuna that enlarges in conjunction with the formation of adjacent resorption lacunae. V-shaped bony ridges separate the resorption lacunae and create a multilocular appearance. With additional growth, most of these ridges are lost as new resorption lacunae form at the crests of the ridges. Ultimately, the trabeculae disappear, causing the mature lesion to have no internal structure. One or a few V-shaped ridges of bone may remain at the periphery, which have been described as crenations.

Some lesions have reactive bone appearing as a sclerotic margin; these changes may occur slowly and asymptomatically, and such lesions are classed as nonaggressive. This process also may occur more rapidly and symptomatically; these CGCGs are considered aggressive. In either case, the classic histologic appearance of the tissue consists of a loose connective tissue stroma with many fibroblasts and capillaries. Multinucleated giant cells, with a few to 20 or more nuclei, are interspersed within the connective tissue stroma. There are foci of old extravasated blood and hemosiderin pigment, with some phagocytosed by macrophages. New trabeculae of osteoid or bone often are present, especially at the periphery. A histologically identical lesion occurs with the brown tumors of hyperparathyroidism, a completely separate condition, discussed elsewhere in this text. Many believe the GCT occurs only in the bones of the skeleton and not in the jaws, and it is said that the CGCG does not occur outside the jaws; however, there are a few reports of GCT in the jaws and CGCG outside the jaws. Some were published by Sturrock and colleagues (1984), Caskey and coauthors (1985), and Bertheussen and co-workers (1983). In the jaws, CGCG arises in association with Paget's disease, whereas GCTs arise in the skeleton in patients with this disease. Although GCTs occur more in men older than 20 years of age, approximately 15% develop in patients between 10 and 20 years of age. Auclair and colleagues (1988) concluded that, although the two lesions sometimes may be distinguished on the basis of histologic features, the overlap in their study indicates that the CGCG and GCT represent a continuum of a single disease process modified by the patient's age, the location of the lesion, and possibly other factors. We believe the nonaggressive lesions may represent CGCGs, whereas the aggressive type may consist of GCTs in the jaws.

Clinical Features

According to Waldron (1953), 60% of CGCGs in the jaws occur in patients younger than 20 years. In their review of 37 cases, Eisenbud and colleagues (1988) found that 43% occurred in patients between 10 and 19 years of age, 68% in those younger than 30 years, and only four cases in patients older than 50 years. Waldron and Shafer (1966) reported that the lesion is more common in female patients, with a female-to-male ratio of 2:1. Eisenbud and associates (1988) found that 62% of cases occurred in female patients. In 1986, Chuong and colleagues suggested differentiation of CGCGs into aggressive and nonaggressive behavior patterns. The basis for this division consisted of histologic, clinical, and radiologic factors. The following histologic features indicate the behavior pattern: the relative size of the giant cells, stromal characteristics, mitotic index, presence of inflammation, and amount of hemosiderin. The clinical features of a more aggressive pattern include pain, rapid growth, swelling, and recurrence; the nonaggressive lesion tends to be asymptomatic, exhibits slow growth, and seldom recurs. The radiologic features of the aggressive type include resorption of the adjacent root apices, perforation of the expanded cortex, and a diameter exceeding 2 cm; nonaggressive lesions are characterized by an absence of root resorption, intact cortices, and possibly a diameter smaller than 2 cm. A peripheral variant of this lesion occurs on the gingiva and produces an epulis-like soft tissue mass in the gingival area. In edentulous areas, it may result in a nodule or swelling on the alveolar ridge.

Treatment/Prognosis

CGCGs are known to recur, and recurrence is a feature of the aggressive type. In a study of 57 cases, Piekarczyk and Kozlowski (1984) reported a 10% recurrence rate; Andersen and colleagues (1973), 13% among 129 cases; and Eisenbud and co-workers (1988), 16% among 37 cases. In 1983, Cherrick studied 292 CGCGs and observed that recurrence was related to size. Twelve percent of lesions smaller than 2 cm in diameter recurred, whereas 37% of lesions larger than 2 cm in diameter recurred. In 49 CGCGs, Auclair and colleagues (1988) found no correlation between lesion size and recurrence; however, they did find that a young age may be a predictor of recurrence. Among the five patients with recurrences, the average age was 11 years, and all of these patients were younger than 17 years. The average age of patients without recurrence was 29 years. Lesions with an aggressive pattern as described by Chuong and associates (1986) recur; the nonaggressive type does not recur.

According to Miles and co-authors (1991), simple curettage should produce excellent results in nonaggressive lesions; however, more aggressive lesions may require curettage plus peripheral ostectomy, with large burs used to remove the superficial bone layer lining the surgical cavity down to a hard burnished surface. According to Chuong and colleagues (1986), surgery in combination with radiation therapy has been successful in some aggressive maxillary lesions; however, Miles and colleagues (1991) warned that radiation therapy may induce malignant transformation. In cases with multiple recurrences of "central giant cell granuloma," the brown tumor of hyperparathyroidism should be suspected strongly.

Although malignant CGCGs are rare, Bondi and co-authors (1974) stated that approximately 10% of GCTs may undergo sarcomatous transformation. Mintz and colleagues (1981) reported a malignant GCT in the mandible.

◆ RADIOLOGY (Figs. 13–36 to 13–42)

The following is a summary of the radiologic features of CGCG as we understand it:

1. In the mandible, lesions are located in the tooth-bearing areas previously occupied by the primary dentition and may cross the midline. A peripheral variant also may be seen, in a similar location.
2. The central lesion develops through three stages. First, it begins as a simple cystlike radiolucent resorption lacuna, often smaller than 2 cm. Then enlargement occurs, producing several interadjacent resorption lacunae, with a multilocular pattern within the bone and expansion at the periphery. In the mature lesion, there are few internal septa; however, crenations produce scalloping of the margins.
3. The margins of the CGCG may be sclerotic. Internally, the lesion may be radiolucent or granular, or contain thin, wispy septa. These latter may be attached to the marginal crenations.
4. There are aggressive and nonaggressive subtypes. The primary radiologic features of the aggressive type include perforation of an expanded cortex and resorption of adjacent teeth. An additional characteristic may be a diameter greater than 2 cm in a patient younger than 17 years and clinical features of rapid growth and pain.

Location

Miles and co-authors (1991) observed that the CGCG occurs primarily in the mandible, anterior to the first molars. The lesion may cross the midline. Approximately one third of the cases reported by Eisenbud and colleagues (1988) occurred in the maxilla. In addition, some cases may extend into the third molar area but rarely into the ramus. Several

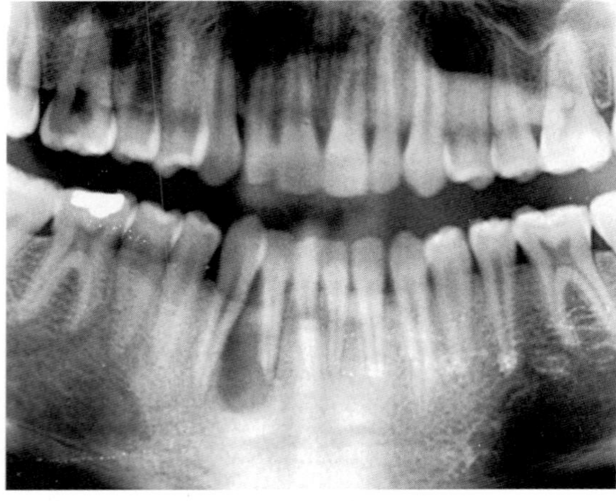

A

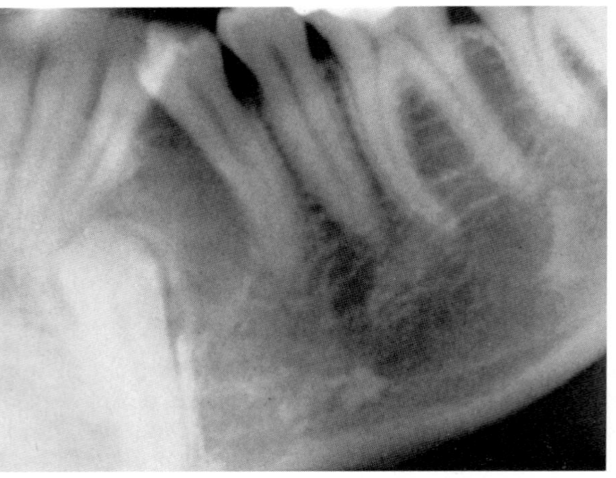

B

FIGURE 13–36.

Central giant cell granuloma: Early first-stage (unilocular) lesion. A, In a 14-year-old boy, there is diffuse sclerosis at the margin. B, Case resembles a dentigerous cyst, but follicle is not enlarged.

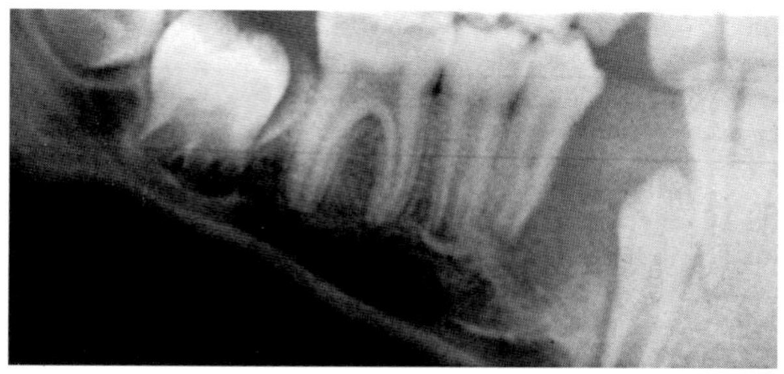

FIGURE 13–37.

Central giant cell granuloma: Small second-stage (multilocular) lesion, with wispy septa within.

CGCG cases have been reported in the upper ramus at the base of the condylar neck.

Radiologic Features of Central Jaw Lesions

In this section, we suggest a chronology of events through which the various radiologic appearances of CGCG evolve, and we attempt to ascribe some meaning to these findings with respect to the diagnostic features and clinical behavior of the lesion. Radiologically, all CGCGs enlarge in a sequence of three phases:

1. Early, smaller lesions begin as a cystlike radiolucency.
2. As the lesion enlarges, adjacent areas of bone are replaced, and septa may separate adjacent lacunae of resorbed bone, thus forming a multilocular appearance. At the same time, there is expansion and thinning of the peripheral cortex. According to Poyton (1982), sometimes a double margin can be seen when expansion is present.
3. Ultimately, the septa are resorbed from the most central part of the lesion toward the periphery, leaving only crenations at the margins.

Within the three phases of development, the following radiologic features are specifically suggestive of CGCG: (1) the margins may be sclerotic, and marginal sclerosis is poorly opacified when present; (2) on close inspection, the margin may appear to be a thin, slightly irregular area of reactive bone; (3) the buccal or lingual cortex may be expanded and perforated in some cases; (4) the internal septa are thin and wispy; and (5) triangular crenations are observed at the margins. Cohen and Hertzanu (1988) reviewed the radiologic features of 16 cases and found that 50% were multilocular and the remainder were unilocular. Fifty percent of these had a smooth margin, and 50% had a scalloped margin. Also, 9 of 16 cases had a well-defined margin and 7 cases had a poorly defined margin.

In the nonaggressive type, radiologic evidence of an intact, slightly more radiodense margin can be seen. We have encountered CGCG cases, however, in which the sclerotic bone at the periphery is discontinuous and wispy; in some

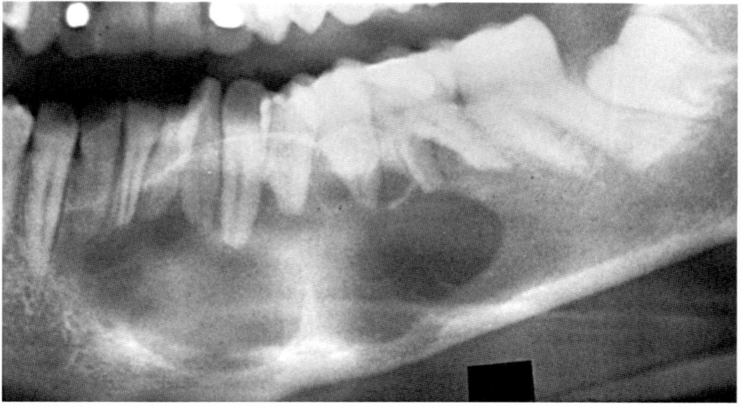

A

B

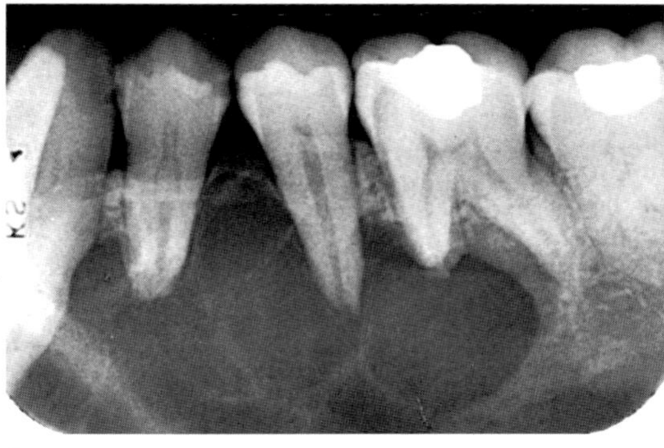

C

FIGURE 13–38.

Central giant cell granuloma: Late second-stage (multilocular) lesion in a 16-year-old girl. A to C, Figures show wispy septa, large marginal crenation, and multiplanar root resorption. An age less than 17 years, large size, expansion, and root resorption indicate that the lesion is the aggressive type and recurrence may develop.

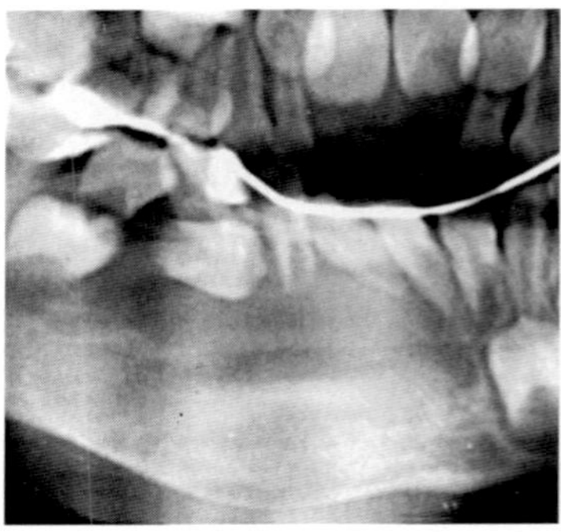

A

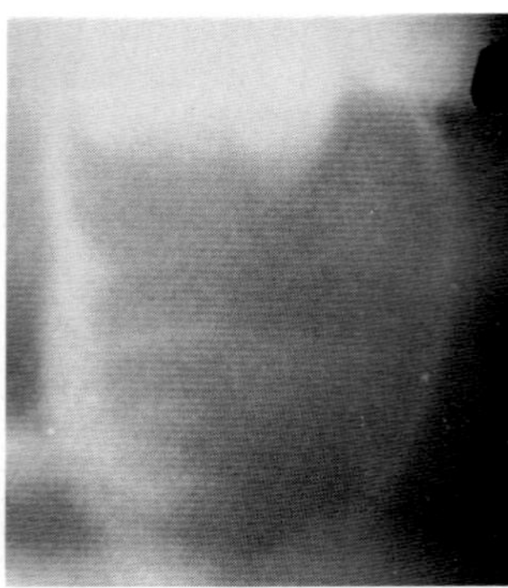

B

FIGURE 13–39.

Central giant cell granuloma: Large third-stage lesion (unilocular with marginal crenations) in a 6.5-year-old girl. A, A midline lesion displaces erupted and unerupted teeth. B, A cross-sectional tomogram shows wispy crenations at the lingual margin. The expanded cortex is intact. (Courtesy of Drs. Alvaro Castro Delgado and Gabriel Castro Delgado, Universidad Javeriana, Santa Fé de Bogotá, Colombia).

instances, no sclerotic margin can be detected. When present, this wispy discontinuous marginal bone may represent trabecular and cortical remnants carried outward with the growing lesion, as in the GCT, which behaves more aggressively than the CGCG and recurs more frequently when treated by simple curettage.

Relationship to Teeth

An important feature of CGCG is its relationship to teeth. Any CGCG may envelop the roots of adjacent teeth completely, causing the roots to protrude into the lesion. It also may cause divergence of the roots of adjacent erupted teeth and displacement of unerupted teeth. Cohen and Hertzanu (1988) described divergence of the roots of adjacent teeth in 10 cases (71%) and root resorption in 3 (21%). Resorption of adjacent root apices is a sign of an aggressive, usually benign lesion. According to Miles and co-authors (1991), the CGCG tends to resorb the root apex in a slightly concave-cervical direction, creating a curved appearance. In other instances, root resorption may have occurred in two different planes on the same root and at two or more locations on an adjacent root.

Advanced Imaging of Central Giant Cell Granuloma

Cohen and Hertzanu (1988) emphasized the value of CT when larger lesions have perforated and expanded into the floor of the mouth, maxillary antrum, or nasal fossa. The CT images indicated perforation at the margins, and expansion was present when perforation occurred. On CT scans, the internal septa were much less radiodense than the surrounding bone, and in one case internal septa were absent. These authors stressed the advantage of both coronal and axial CT views to delineate the full soft tissue extent of larger lesions. They found that CT was superior to conventional radiography because it clearly showed the soft tissue mass of a lesion, extension into adjacent structures, and bony destruction.

Radiologic Features of Peripheral Lesions

When associated with teeth, the peripheral giant cell granuloma may cause resorption of the underlying interseptal bone, more so than the pyogenic granuloma or the peripheral odontogenic fibroma with calcifications. Often, no radiologic changes are seen. Edentulous areas show two patterns of bone change: First, a characteristic ''peripheral cuff'' of bone, representing buttress formation, may be seen at the crestal periphery of the lesion. This cuff or buttress tends to be more triangular and thicker at its base and thins out progressively as it surrounds the superficial part of the lesion; it rarely extends along the full peripheral margin. Beneath this area, there is destruction of alveolar bone, sometimes with a wispy multilocular pattern, with smaller locules than in the central lesion. The margin at the base of the lesion may be crenated, with perhaps one or two longer trabeculae of bone extending from the tips of the crenations into the lesion. In rare instances, the internal morphologic features of the lesion may be granular. The second manifestation in edentulous areas, as described by Gibilisco (1985), is saucerization of the edentulous ridge, without tumefaction of the underlying alveolar bone; however, there is a diffuse zone of reactive sclerotic bone beneath the peripheral lesion. Our case occurred in a 59-year-old man taking aspirin daily as an anticoagulant. He wore a removable partial denture that was loose, unstable, and in poor occlusion with an upper removable partial denture. Clinically, the lesion was completely flat and reddish and resembled a vascular lesion or hematoma.

Giant Cell Tumor of Bone

The essential radiologic features of GCT as it occurs in the skeleton are as follows: The lesion begins as a radiolucency in the metaphyseal end of a long bone, in an eccentric position. The distal femur, proximal tibia, and distal radius are favored sites. It grows slowly and ultimately may occupy the entire diameter of the bone. The most important diagnostic factor is that it produces no new bone formation, periosteally or endosteally. Expansion may appear to be present, but this is cortex displaced by the tumor mass. The lesion may perforate the cortex, carrying with it wispy remnants of the original cortex, causing the bone outline to appear enlarged. The fine lines that crisscross the lesion are remnants of destroyed bone and are not new bone trabeculae. Although the lesion usually is fairly well defined, the margins are not sharp. The peripheral portion of the lesion occasionally does not have a bony outline, and the internal elements are almost entirely radiolucent, with no evidence of remaining bone. The lesion may perforate through and cross a joint space. Multifocal cases involving several bones have been reported.

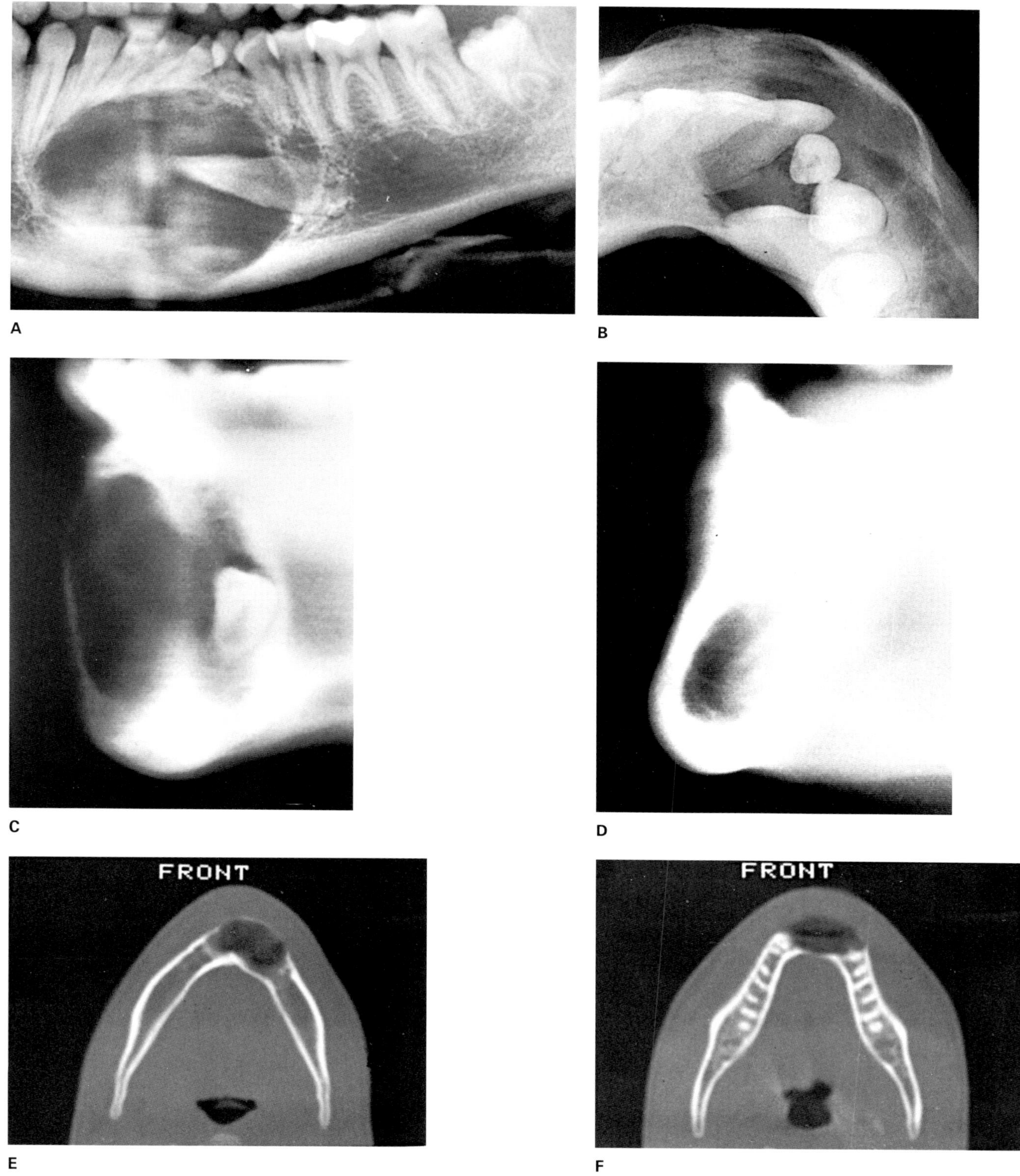

FIGURE 13–40.

Central giant cell granuloma: Third-stage (unilocular) lesion in a 14-year-old boy with no symptoms. A, Lesion resembles dentigerous cyst. There is tipping and resorption of the roots of the teeth. B, Buccal expansion is unlike that in cysts. The canine has a lingual position. C, The cross-sectional tomogram shows buttress formation at the expanded buccal cortex and perforation superiorly. D, Figure shows wispy septa. E and F, The bone window on axial CT images shows a wavy expanded buccal cortex of uneven thickness with reduced density inferiorly and perforation at the level of the root apices. (Courtesy of Dr. B. Potter, Medical and Dental College of Georgia, Augusta, GA.)

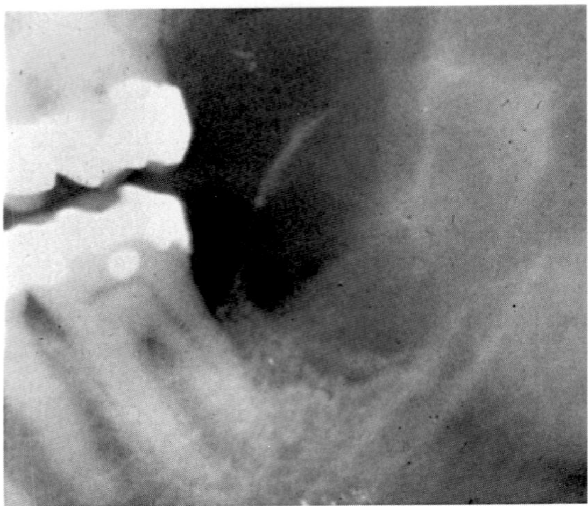

FIGURE 13–41.

Peripheral giant cell granuloma: Case shows the characteristic peripheral cuff of bone and a single crenation at the mesial crestal margin.

ANEURYSMAL BONE CYST

The aneurysmal bone cyst (ABC) first was reported in the bony skeleton by Jaffe and Lichtenstein in 1942 and received this name because of its ballooned-out radiologic appearance. This lesion first was reported in the jaws by Bernier and Bhaskar in 1958.

Pathologic Characteristics

The lesion is characterized by a fibrous connective tissue stroma containing many cavernous or sinusoidal blood-filled spaces. There are many fibroblasts, as well as numerous multinucleated giant cells with a similar appearance and distribution to those in the CGCG. Hemosiderin is present, and osteoid and new bone formation often are seen. Currently, many believe the histogenesis is related to another primary bone lesion that initiates the development of a secondary reactive lesion, namely the ABC. In 66 cases, Biesecker and associates (1970) found that 32% of ABCs had an accompanying benign primary bone lesion. In their study of 57 cases of secondary ABC, Levy and colleagues (1975) found that the most common associated lesions were the traumatic bone cyst and CGCG; others included osteosarcoma, nonossifying fibroma, osteoblastoma, hemangioendothelioma, and hemangioma. Five cases occurred in association with a fracture or other bone trauma. Other reported associated lesions summarized by Struthers and Shear (1984b) included ossifying fibroma, cementifying fibroma, GCT of bone, fibrous dysplasia, chondroblastoma, chondromyxoid fibroma, myxofibroma, and sarcoma. Veth and colleagues (1985) reported an ABC associated with Van Buchem's disease. Nadimi and colleagues (1987) discovered an ABC occurring along with a dentigerous cyst.

Clinical Features

In an extensive literature review, Struthers and Shear (1984a) found 42 well-documented cases of ABC in the jaws and reported 4 new cases. Ninety-three percent occurred in the first three decades of life, with most developing in the second decade. Sixty-four percent of cases occurred in patients younger than 20 years of age. In their series, there was a slight predilection for female patients (62%). Studies by Ruiter and co-workers (1972), Biesecker and associates (1970), and Tillman and colleagues (1968) analyzed a total of 263 extragnathic cases. Seventy-eight percent occurred in patients younger than 20 years, and 58% occurred in female patients. In jaw lesions, most patients had swelling; in 16 cases it was possible to document that the swelling was rapid, whereas in only 4 cases it was gradual. Pain was reported in 13 cases; however, it is not considered a significant feature of ABCs.

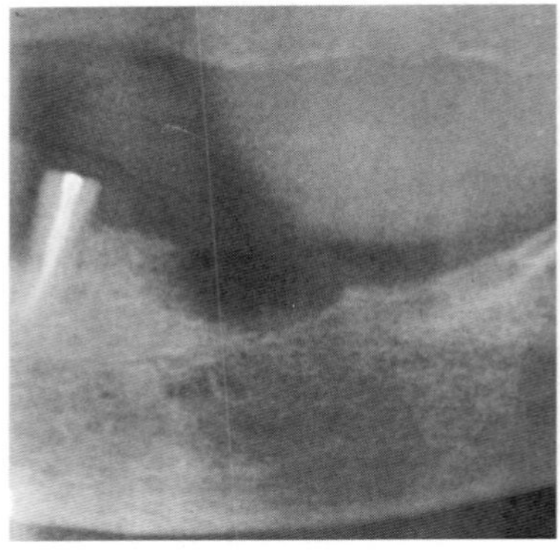

A

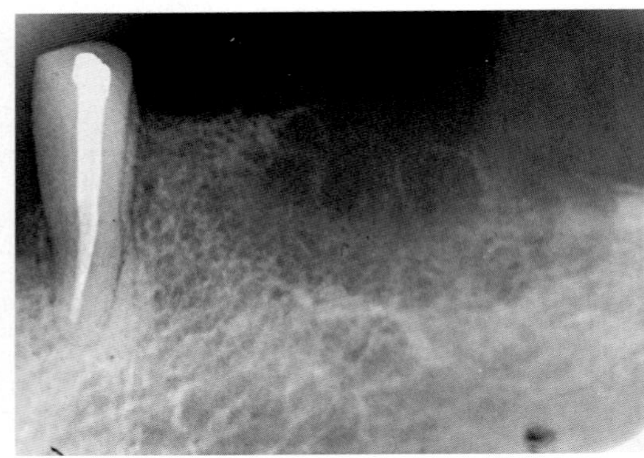

B

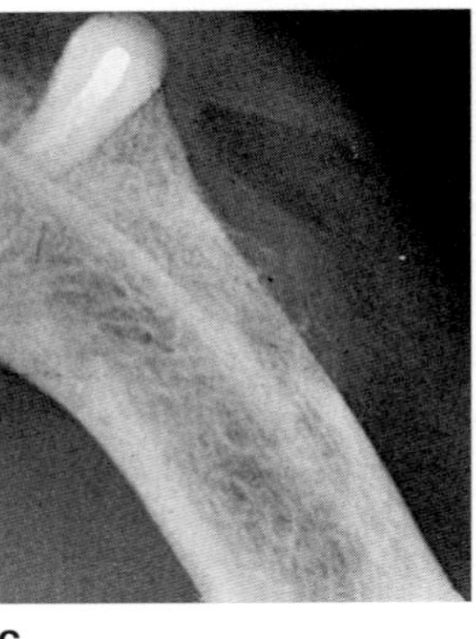

C

FIGURE 13–42.

Peripheral giant cell granuloma: A, Few diagnostic features are seen. B, Multiple crenations are observed along the internal margins. There is a wide transition zone between the lesion and healthy bone. C, Case shows slight buccal expansion but with perforation and a few wispy septa; the remainder of the lesion appears as a central osteoporotic area with marrow spaces of diminished density and more prominent trabeculae. (Courtesy of Dr. S. Prapanpoch, Bangkok, Thailand.)

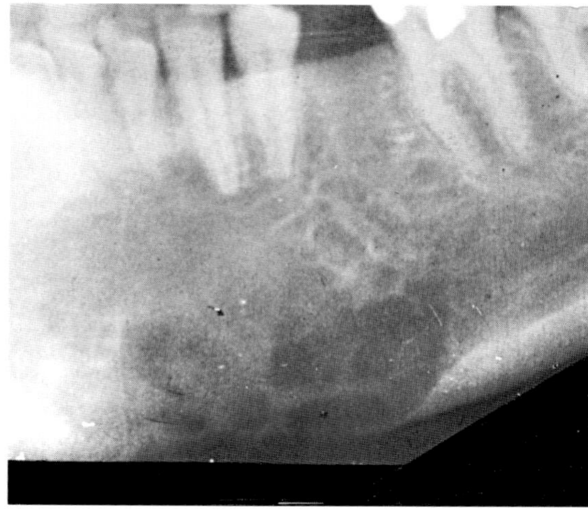

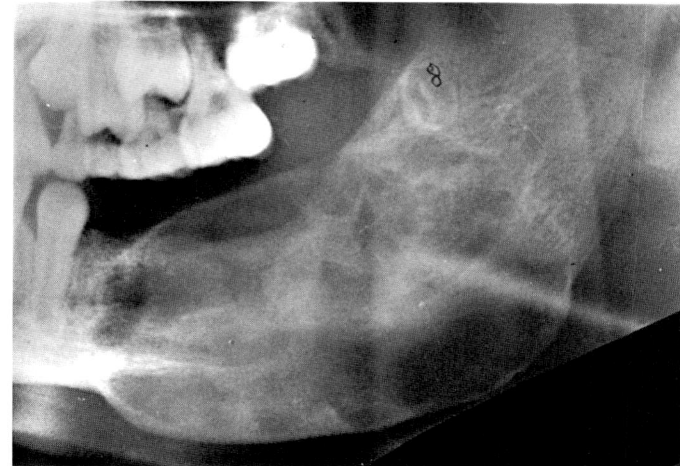

A B

FIGURE 13–43.

Aneurysmal bone cyst: A, Growth phase shows erosion of the inferior cortex, internal septa forming loculations, and a wide zone of transition between lesional bone and normal bone. (Courtesy of Dr. G. Pappas, Columbus, OH.) B, Figure shows ballooned-out appearance of the third or stable phase. (Courtesy of Drs. L. Archila, F. Erales, and R. Carlos, Guatemala City, Guatemala.)

Treatment/Prognosis

When the lesion is opened surgically, blood wells up. As reported by Struthers and Shear (1984a), the ABC has a higher recurrence rate than the CGCG. Among 46 jaw lesions reported by Struthers and Shear (1984a), recurrence developed in 53% after curettage, and this is similar in the skeleton. The treatment of choice is thorough curettage with careful follow-up. Supplemental procedures, such as cautery, cryotherapy, and radiation therapy, generally have been unsuccessful or, after radiation therapy, Tillman and colleagues (1968) reported sarcomatous changes.

◆ *RADIOLOGY (Figs. 13–43 to 13–47)*

Radiologic Features of the Jaws

This lesion classically is described as an eccentrically located, ballooned-out, multilocular radiolucency with a honeycomb or soap-bubble appearance. On close examination, the multilocular pattern may consist of very dense filamentous septa converging toward the center of the lesion. There may be thinning or destruction of the cortex, and a periosteal reaction may be observed, though it is rare in the jaws.

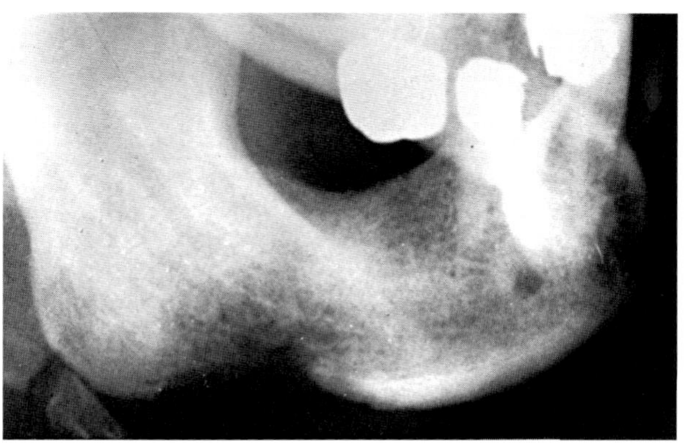

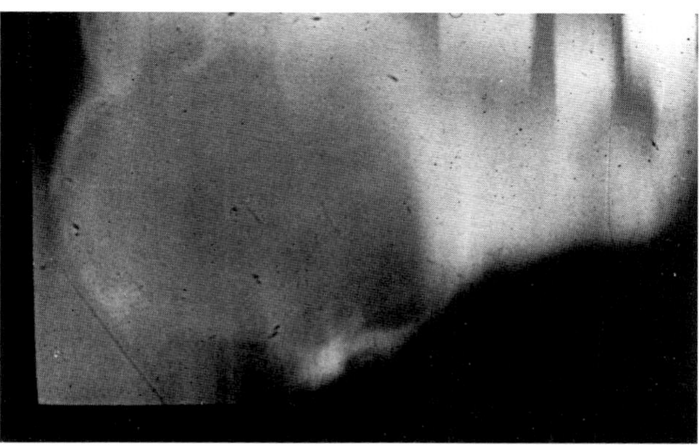

A B

FIGURE 13–44.

Aneurysmal bone cyst: A, Initial presenting lesion in growth phase, with irregular erosion of inferior cortex. Remainder of lesion appears geographic, with a wide zone of transition at the margin. B, Same lesion 9 months later, with ballooned-out appearance of stable phase and a few faint internal septa. (From Eisenbud L, Attie J, Garlick J, Platt N: Aneurysmal bone cyst of the mandible. Oral Surg Oral Med Oral Pathol 64:202, 1987.)

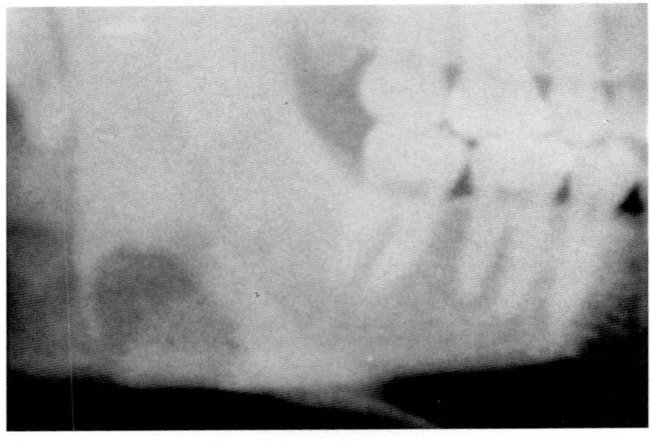

A

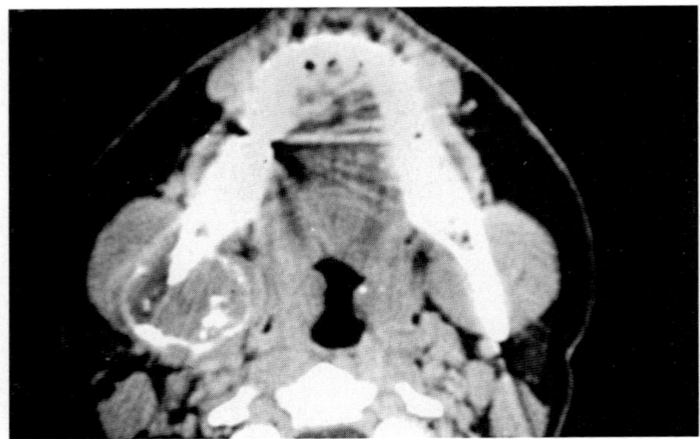

B

FIGURE 13–45.

Aneurysmal bone cyst: A 28-year-old white man with swelling at angle of mandible. A, Panoramic radiograph shows lesion. B, Axial CT scan shows ballooned-out appearance of the third or stable phase. (Courtesy of Dr. H. Schwartz, Kaiser Permanente Medical Group, Los Angeles, CA.)

Location

Of 46 cases reported by Struthers and Shear (1984a), 28 occurred in the mandible and 18 in the maxilla. The molar region was the most common site, and the anterior region of the mandible rarely was involved. Some mandibular lesions extended into the angle and ramus.

Radiologic Features

Buraczewski and Dabska (1971) defined three radiologic stages in ABC development. The initial stage is characterized by an **osteolytic phase,** with a nonspecific radiologic appearance. The second phase, or the **growth phase,** shows significant bone destruction, indistinct margins, the appearance of internal septa, and the first signs of a bony shell. In the third phase, or the **stabilization phase,** the fully developed radiologic picture is seen, with a balloonlike expansion of the cortex, a sclerotic lining that may be interrupted, and a soap-bubble or honeycomb pattern of the internal elements. Supporting this idea of development in phases, Eisenbud and colleagues (1987) reported a case in which a 48-year-old man had an irregular, lytic, destructive, poorly demarcated radiolucency involving the inferior border of the mandible

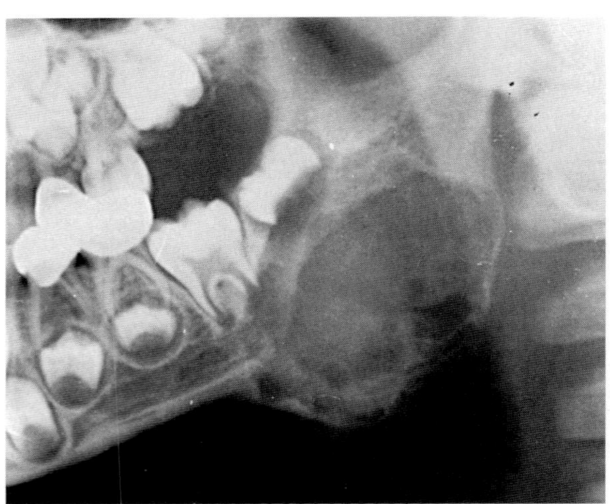

A

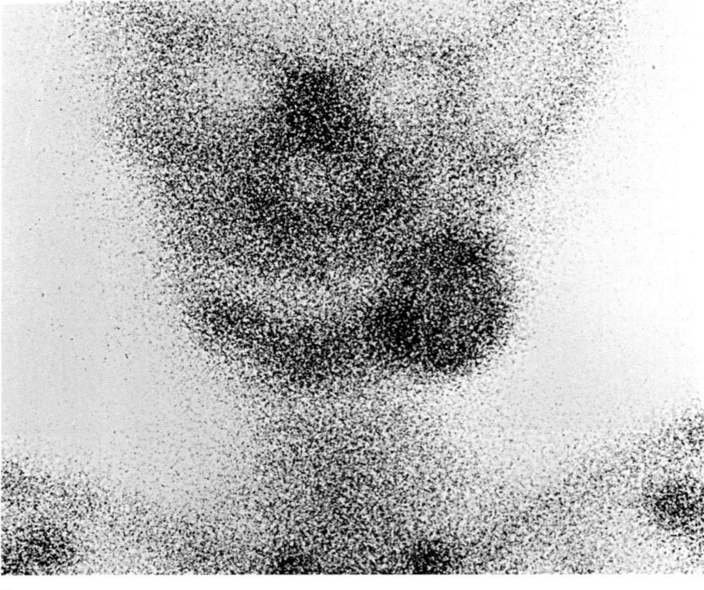

B

FIGURE 13–46.

Aneurysmal bone cyst: Radionuclide and vascular workup in a 6-year-old boy. A, Panoramic radiograph shows classic ballooned-out appearance. B, Bone scan with 10 mCi of ^{99m}technetium MDP shows intense accumulation around bony wall of lesion.

(*continued*)

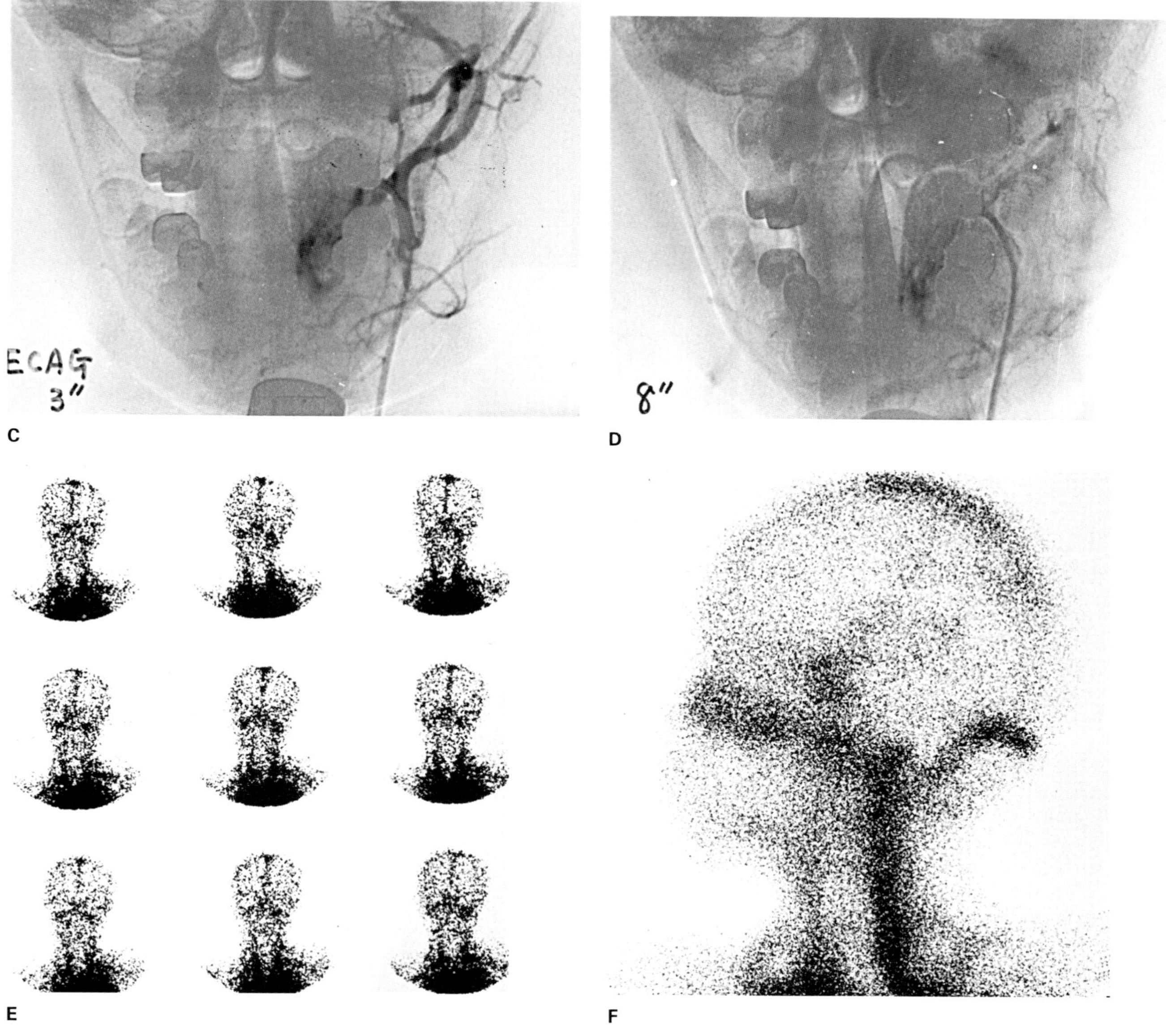

FIGURE 13–46. *(continued)*

C and D, Left external carotid angiograms 3 and 8 seconds after injection, showing hypovascular or avascular nature of lesion. E, Radionuclide angiography consisting of dynamic serial images taken at 2-second intervals and showing no hypervascularization of the lesion. F, Pool scan 1 hour after radionuclide angiography showing no concentration of radioactive material in bone. (From Okuyama T, et al: Diagnosis of aneurysmal bone cyst of the mandible: a report of two cases with emphasis on scintigraphic approaches. Clin Nucl Med 10:786, 1985.)

in the third molar region. A biopsy of the lesion was performed, and radiation therapy resulted in a 30% reduction. Nine months later, the lesion had enlarged and was seen as a clearly defined, expansile, multilocular radiolucency that had expanded to the first molar and angle regions. Although there was some extension in a superior direction, the lesion appeared to have expanded eccentrically in a more inferior direction. On the first occasion the lesion was in the first stage, but the second time the findings were consistent with the third stage. In our review of numerous case reports, we found that most radiologic descriptions fell within one of these stages.

Relationship to Teeth

El Deeb and colleagues (1980) reported occasional root resorption of adjacent teeth, whereas Bhaskar and colleagues (1959) illustrated several cases with root displacement in erupted teeth.

Angiography

Using external carotid arteriography, Okuyama and colleagues (1985) showed that an ABC in the angle-ramus region appeared hypovascular or even avascular throughout the arterial and venous phases. This supports the idea that the blood-filled sinusoidal spaces consist of essentially non-

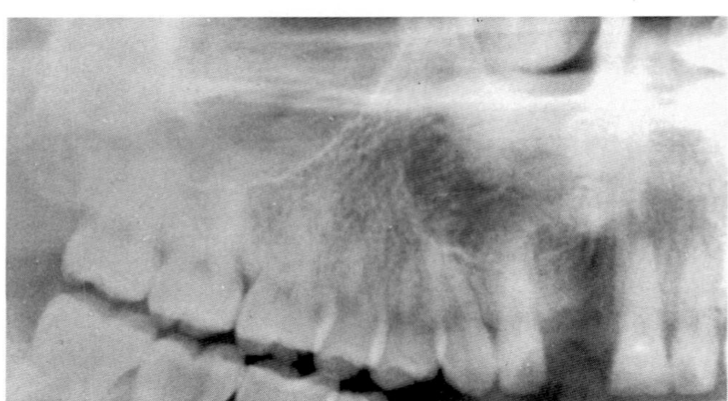

A

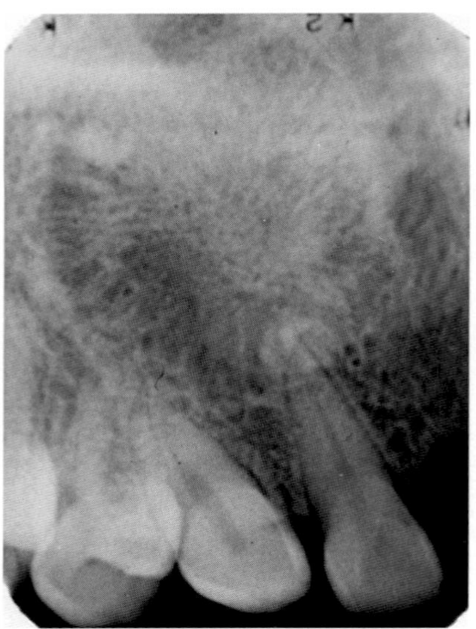

B

FIGURE 13–47.

Aneurysmal bone cyst: Maxillary lesion. A, Panoramic radiograph shows lesion apical to canine. B, Small foramen-like radiolucencies and septa radiate toward the central part of the lesion. (Courtesy of Dr. G. Terezhalmy, Case Western Reserve School of Dentistry, Cleveland, OH.)

circulating blood. Using 10 millicuries of ^{99m}technetium MDP in the same patient, they showed an intensive, thick, doughnutlike accumulation of technetium around the bony wall of the lesion, with little accumulation of radionuclide in the central portion. In a similar study of a mandibular lesion, Ueno and colleagues (1982) showed normal findings with angiograms of the right common carotid artery. When they injected water-soluble radiopaque contrast medium directly into the lesion, an oval radiopacity was observed on contrast radiographs; 7 days later, there was no residual contrast medium.

Radiologic Features of the Bony Skeleton

According to Edeiken (1981), the ABC received its name from its dramatic blown-out radiologic appearance; it is one of the few lesions named after its radiologic features. Generally speaking, skeletal ABCs seem to follow the three stages outlined by Buraczewski and Dabska (1971), namely osteolysis, growth, and stable phases. In addition, Edeiken and Hodes (1963) stated that they may arise intraosseously or extraosseously. The intraosseous lesions seem to balloon the cortex as they enlarge, whereas the extraosseous lesions appear in soft tissue and erode the underlying bone. The lesion is osteolytic, develops eccentrically, and is nonspecific in its early stages. In its mature stage, it is characterized by a ballooned-out cortex that may be thin enough to seem absent radiologically. Lesions often develop at the end of a long bone, and a periosteal reaction may be observed at the advancing edge of the lesion. The internal elements are characterized by bony septa, which are curved, forming a honeycomb or soap-bubble appearance. In a review of 26 skeletal cases of ABC, Morton (1986) showed that 16 cases occurred in the long bones, 5 in the vertebrae, 1 in the clavicle, 1 in the pelvis, and 3 in the tarsus.

CENTRAL HEMANGIOMA (Vascular nevus, juvenile hemangioendothelioma)

The literature is inconsistent regarding the various types of vascular lesions. In some instances, the terms hemangioma and arteriovenous malformation (AVM) are used synonymously. We believe there are two groups of lesions: hemangiomas and AVMs. Therefore, we offer separate discussions for these lesions, although there are points of overlap in the text.

Pathologic Characteristics

Although quite common in soft tissue, the hemangioma occurs much less frequently as a central bone lesion. Histologically, Shafer and co-authors (1983) described the capillary hemangioma as the most common form, consisting of many small capillaries lined by a single layer of endothelial cells supported by a connective tissue stroma. A variant has been termed juvenile hemangioendothelioma because it occurs in children and has a more cellular pattern. Singh and colleagues (1977) reported a case in an 8-year-old girl. The cavernous form of hemangioma consists of much larger blood-filled sinusoidal spaces, each lined by endothelial cells and supported by a connective tissue stroma. It is disputed whether the hemangioma is a true neoplasm or whether it is a hamartomatous malformation because many are present at birth.

Clinical Features

Watson and McCarthy (1940) reviewed 1563 vascular tumors and found that 85% were evident in the first year of life and 73% were present at birth. In a review of 35 cases of hemangioma in the jaws, Lund and Dahlin (1964) discovered that most developed in the first two decades of life. They also observed that female patients were affected more often than male patients, with a ratio of 2:1.

According to reviews by Sadowsky and colleagues (1981) and Anderson and associates (1981) and other reports we studied, the following clinical signs and symptoms may be associated with vascular lesions. Hemangiomas may have been present since the first year of life, whereas AVMs may develop in a teenager, possibly after trauma. Facial asymmetry, especially over the mandible, may result from swelling or hypertrophy. The overlying skin may be as much as 2° F warmer, and it may be moist. The skin or mucosa may be bluish, purplish, or reddish. The patient may complain of pain or paresthesia. Other symptoms include pulsatile or swishing noises, tinnitus or impaired hearing, blurred vision, and epistaxis. A highly characteristic sign is blood oozing spontaneously from the gingival sulcus of one or more teeth that may be loose. The tooth may exhibit a pumping movement when pressure is applied to it and released. There also may be premature exfoliation of the primary teeth and delayed eruption of the permanent teeth, as well as congenitally missing teeth, in the region of the lesion. Expansion of the alveolar process may be observed, with a diminished depth of the mucobuccal fold. Central hemangiomas may yield blood readily on aspiration, whereas the AVM may cause the syringe to fill without aspiration of the plunger.

Treatment/Prognosis

Although spontaneous regression of some central hemangiomas has been discussed by Shira and Guernsey (1965), most must be treated. Treatment modalities usually involve surgical removal; however, other techniques, using radiation therapy, sclerosing agents, and embolization, have been used. Thorn and colleagues (1986) discussed a refinement of embolization techniques and used them successfully to manage two maxillary lesions. In many instances, the workup involves bone scans, angiograms, and magnetic resonance flow studies. A vascular surgeon often is involved in the surgery and ligates the carotid artery before entering the jaw lesion. Even with this precaution, hemostasis problems may occur.

Lamberg and colleagues (1979) discovered that 10 deaths occurred during treatment for central hemangiomas and reported a new case. Nine of the cases were in the mandible and two in the maxilla. The patients' ages ranged from 11 to 26 years. According to Lamberg and colleagues (1979), extraction of teeth extending into a hemangiomatous region seems to be the most common cause of fatal bleeding, and the tooth was a molar in all cases. They also found that, in 8 of the 11 instances in which the patient died, the operator was aware of or suspected a hemangioma. These authors stressed the importance of suspecting this lesion in young patients with suspect gingival bleeding and mobile teeth and recommended delay of treatment until all contingencies can be planned for and managed in a hospital setting.

◆ RADIOLOGY (Figs. 13–48 to 13–53)

Radiology of Jaw Lesions

The radiology of central hemangioma should be understood clearly by all dentists who interpret radiographs. This knowledge can be lifesaving to the patient.

Location. Lund and Dahlin (1964) found that central hemangiomas are twice as common in the mandible versus the maxilla. In their review of 61 mandibular cases, Maurizi and colleagues (1982) reported that the body of the mandible may be involved slightly more frequently than the ramus or symphyseal areas.

Radiologic Features. Classically, central vascular lesions usually consist of a multilocular, expansile lesion, which may be associated with displacement and resorption of unerupted and erupted teeth. The cortex usually remains intact. Nevertheless, many variations and combinations of changes may lead the clinician to suspect a vascular lesion; thus, careful attention to all of the figures in this section is important. In forming the basic multilocular pattern, the delicate radiopaque striations may constitute a few or many locules

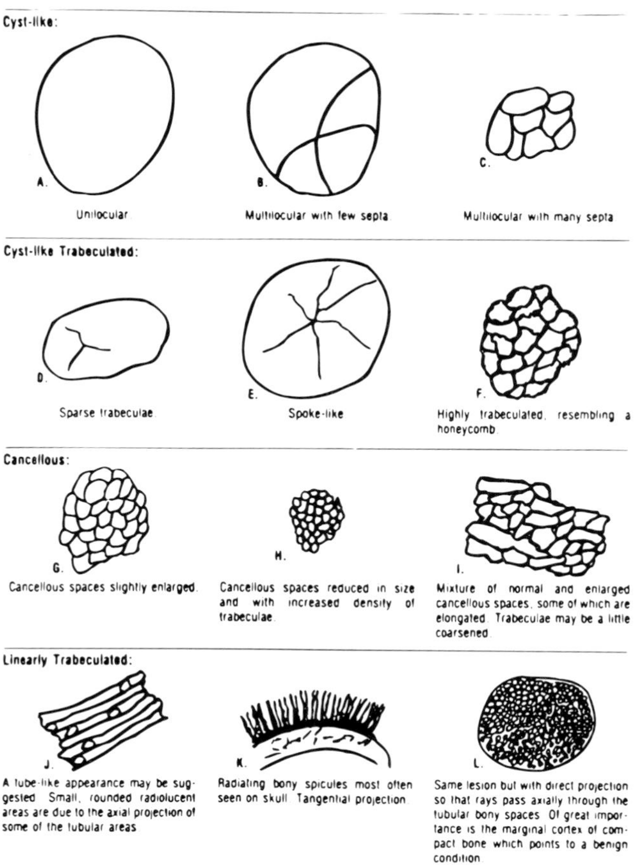

FIGURE 13–48.

Central hemangioma: Various appearances of central hemangioma. (Courtesy of Drs. H. M. Worth, and D. Stoneman, Toronto, Canada, and Eastman Kodak Company, Rochester, NY.)

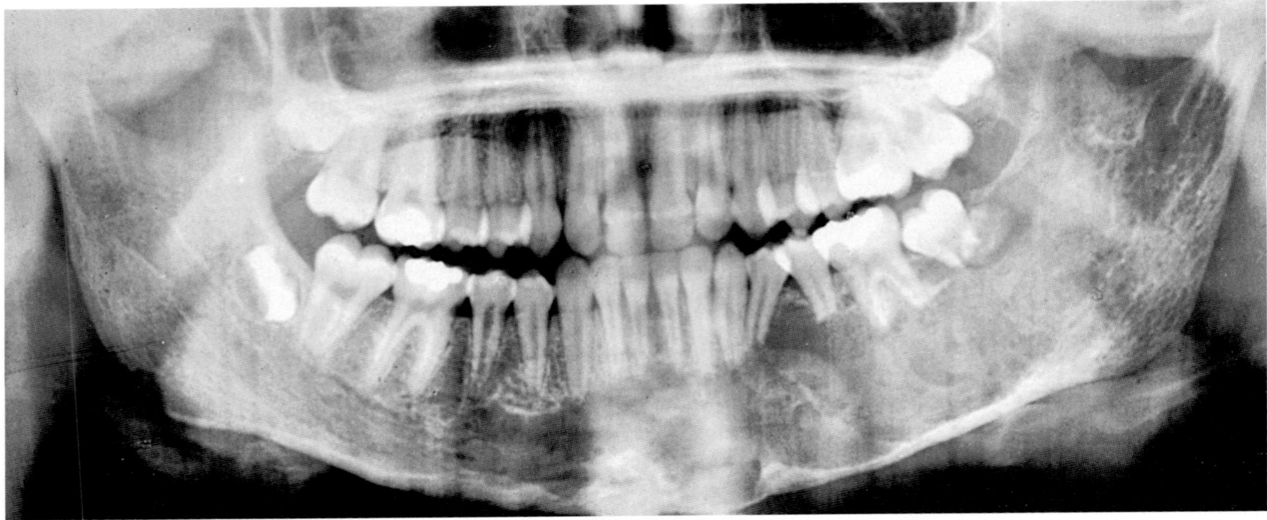

A

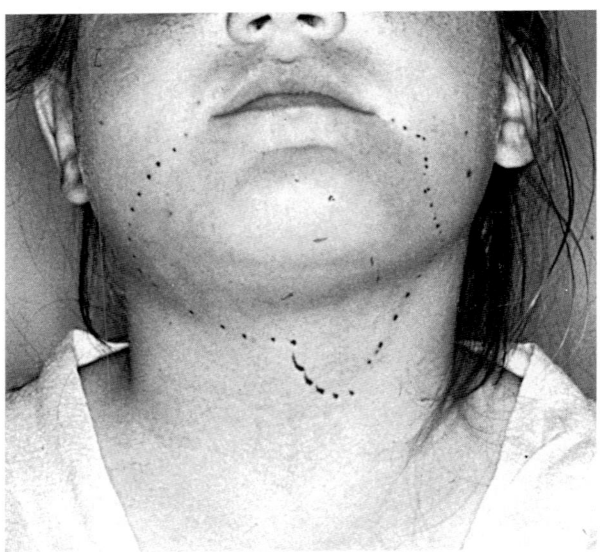

B

FIGURE 13–49.

Central hemangioma: This case is illustrated because the patient died of the treatment, although all possible precautions were taken before and during the procedure. A, Numerous clusters of noncorticated foramina and resorption of many root tips. In the posterior ramus, fine trabeculae are arranged in a parallel fashion, with noncorticated foramina interspersed. B, Clinical appearance. (From Lamberg MA, Tasanen A, Jääskkeläinen J: Fatality from central hemangioma of the mandible. J Oral Surg 37:578, 1979.)

and be arranged in a hub, spokelike, or honeycomb pattern. According to Worth (1963) and Worth and Stoneman (1979), the slightest hint of a hub is strongly suspect. These findings may be accompanied by several noncorticated foramina, which may be distributed singly throughout the lesion or occur in groups of two or three. Additionally, these foramina may be associated with a parallel or tubelike arrangement of radiopaque striae. No other lesion shows this latter pattern. In another variation, the striae are arranged in a sunburst or sunray pattern, resembling an osteogenic sarcoma, chondrosarcoma, or complex odontoma. The radiographic findings may be limited to a central, unilocular, well-corticated, cystlike radiolucency; in other cases, no bony lesion may be apparent, and only the trabecular pattern and size of the marrow spaces in the affected area may be altered. The presence of phleboliths or a wavy doughnut-shaped radiopacity representing a large calcified blood vessel wall is helpful. A difference in the vertical height of the mandible on the affected side compared with the other is suggestive, but may be seen in lymphangioma, neurofibroma, and fibrous dysplasia. The lesions often are well delineated, but a sclerotic margin is a variable feature. We have seen it in approximately half of the cases. Its absence may indicate that the lesion is inactive, whereas its presence may indicate active growth.

Radiologic Features of the Skull

According to Edeiken (1981), hemangiomas are located most often in the vertebral column and calvarium of the skull. They are rare in the axial skeleton. Edeiken (1981) stated that hemangiomas may appear anywhere in the calvaria. They may be small, only a few millimeters in diameter, or they may exceed 3 cm. Most calvarial lesions are osteolytic and round, with or without a sclerotic margin. Calvarial hemangiomas often have a sunburst pattern of radiating bone septa. One may differentiate the septa from those of osteosarcoma by studying the margins in radiographs perpendicular to the lesions. The margins in this case will be well defined

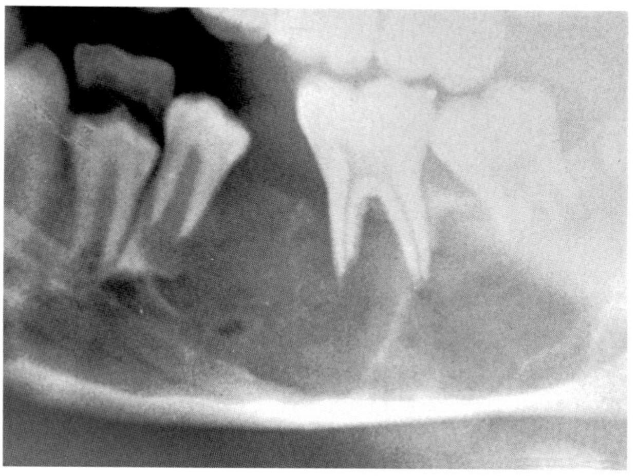

A

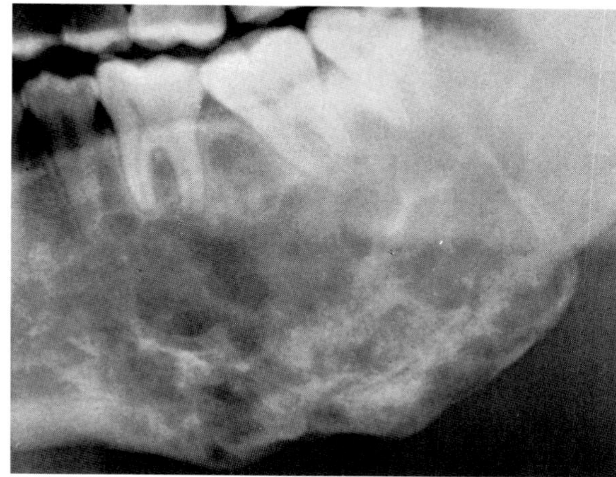

B

FIGURE 13–50.

Central hemangioma: A, Root resorption of first molar and widening of the periodontal membrane space around the mesial root. Tooth was compressible in socket. Separation of teeth and multiple foramen-like structures are seen. (Courtesy of Dr. G. Pappas, Columbus, OH.) B, Multilocular pattern. Inferior alveolar canal ends in several smaller vascular channels, with many noncorticated foramina. There is also expansion of the inferior cortex. (Courtesy of Drs. Alvaro Castro Delgado and Gabriel Castro Delgado, Universidad Javeriana, Santa Fé de Bogotá, Colombia.)

and sometimes corticated. A palpable bump and history of painless slow growth indicate the diagnosis. This sunburst appearance is seen much more frequently in the skull than in jaw lesions.

When discussing skull manifestations of hemangioma, it is important to recognize the intracranial calcifications in Sturge-Weber syndrome, also known as encephalotrigeminal angiomatosis, characterized by unilateral soft tissue hemangiomas on the face along the first, second, or third branches of the trigeminal nerve. Superficial cervical branches also may be involved. Vascular lesions sometimes develop intracranially, especially involving the leptomeninges. These lesions are responsible for the neurologic symptoms in most patients. There is convolutional calcification of masses of vessels on the surface of the brain, described as "tram-line" calcifications because of the parallel calcified vessel walls. They are seen most often in the occipital region. The pattern consists of a convoluted, curving series of anastomosing lines with a more densely calcified central area and fading and narrowing of the calcified channels toward the periphery. Typically, the calcified channels seem to occur on the same plane as the film in lateral views rather than in cross-section, as is observed often in soft tissue hemangiomas.

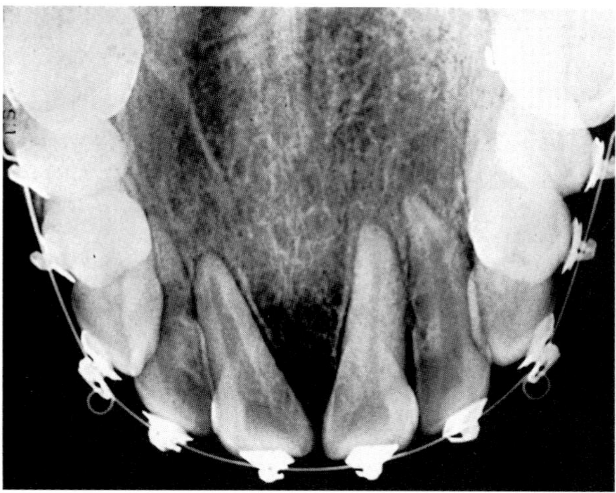

FIGURE 13–51.

Central hemangioma: Maxillary lesion. The trabeculae have a fine honeycomb pattern. (Courtesy of Professor H. Fuchihata, Dean, Osaka University School of Dentistry, Osaka, Japan.)

Radiologic Features of the Zygomatic Bone

Har-El and colleagues (1987) reported two new cases and found six others in the literature. Histologically, 75% were the cavernous type. Five of eight patients were female, and, unlike other central hemangiomas, seven of the eight occurred in patients in the fourth, fifth, or sixth decades of life. The usual complaint was an infraorbital bony hard mass, sometimes with cosmetic deformity. One patient had exophthalmia. The external carotid artery was clamped in only one patient, and an external approach with an infraorbital incision was used in seven patients. Operative blood loss was not notable in any patient. Har-El and colleagues (1987) believed that the radiologic appearance of zygomatic hemangiomas is pathognomonic, although various patterns were presented. Most showed an irregular bony tumor, with a reticulated or honeycomb internal pattern. One showed a typical sunray appearance, and two were simply irregular without an internal architecture. On arteriography, one case showed a prominent blood supply to the lesion.

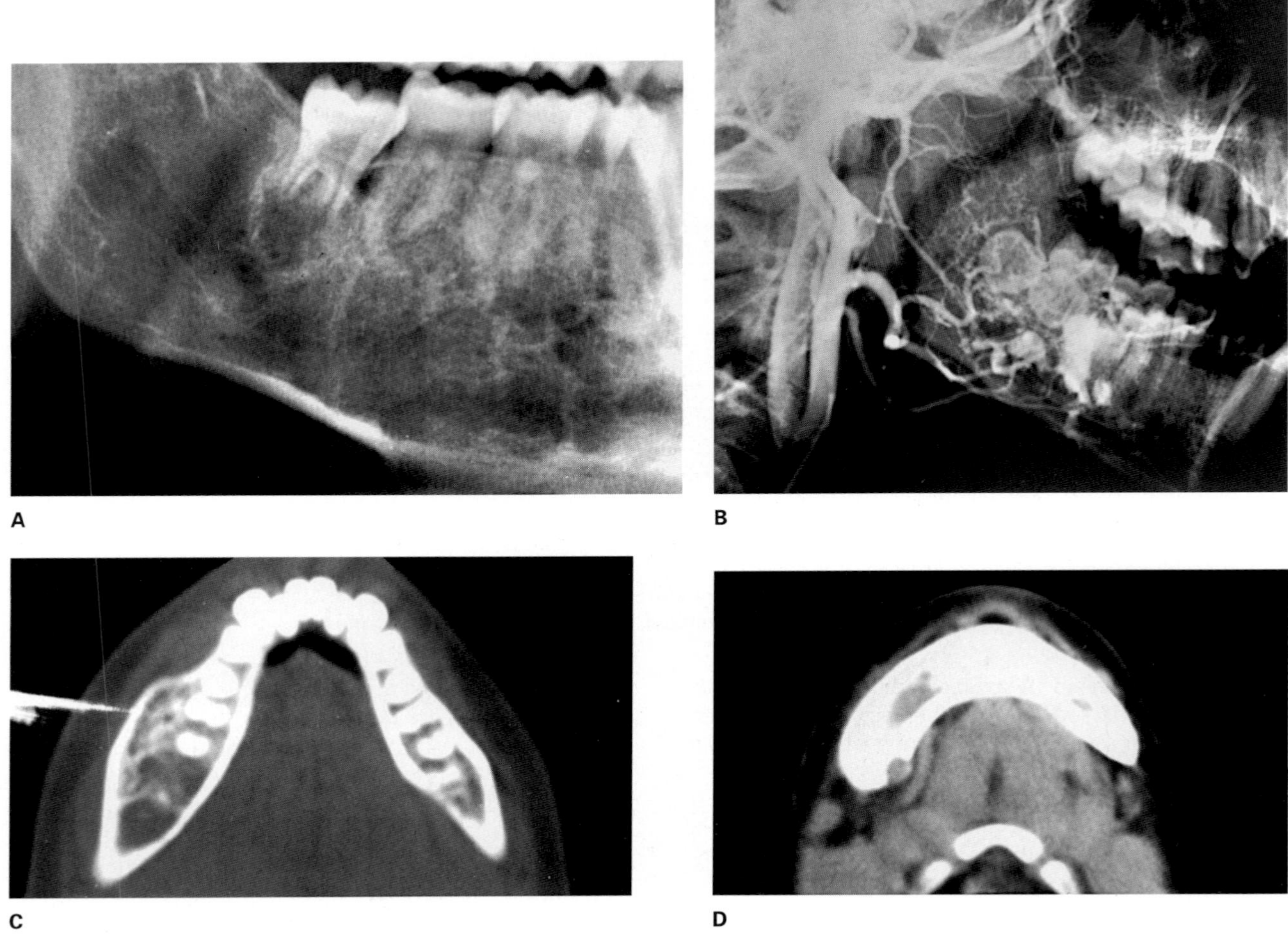

FIGURE 13–52.

Central hemangioma: A, Widening of inferior alveolar canal and multiple tiny foramen-like structures. Approximately 1 cm apical to the first molar, there are fine, parallel trabeculae with tiny radiolucent areas interspersed. Erosion of the cortex also is seen. B, External carotid angiogram showing filling of the lesion immediately after injection. C, Expansion of buccal cortex, and a foramen-like structure. D, Vascular impression on lingual cortex made by major feeder vessel. (Courtesy of Dr. H. Schwartz, Kaiser Permanente Medical Group, Los Angeles, CA.)

ARTERIOVENOUS MALFORMATION

(Arteriovenous malformation, arteriovenous shunt, arteriovenous aneurysm [arteriovenous fistula or plexiform hemangioma])

The diagnosis of a vascular lesion can be the most important clinical diagnosis a practitioner can make; even with careful planning, the lesions are difficult to treat. If a vascular lesion is not recognized, the patient ultimately may die during treatment.

Pathologic Characteristics

Shafer and co-authors (1983) divided arteriovenous (AV) aneurysms into three basic types: (1) a cirsoid aneurysm, consisting of a tortuous mass of small arteries and veins linking a larger artery and vein; (2) a varicose aneurysm, consisting of an endothelial-lined sac linking an artery and vein; and (3) an aneurysmal varix, which is a direct connection between an artery and dilated vein. All AVMs are characterized by some form of direct connection between an artery and vein without intervening capillary circulation.

Clinical Features

Gomez (1970) reviewed 151 AVMs seen at the Mayo Clinic and found that 92% were congenital. Anderson and colleagues analyzed the literature in 1981 and found 60 reported AVMs affecting the mandible. Maurizi and colleagues (1982), in their review of 61 AVMs in the jaws, cited many reports supporting the idea that maxillary AVMs occur much less frequently than mandibular lesions. These authors found

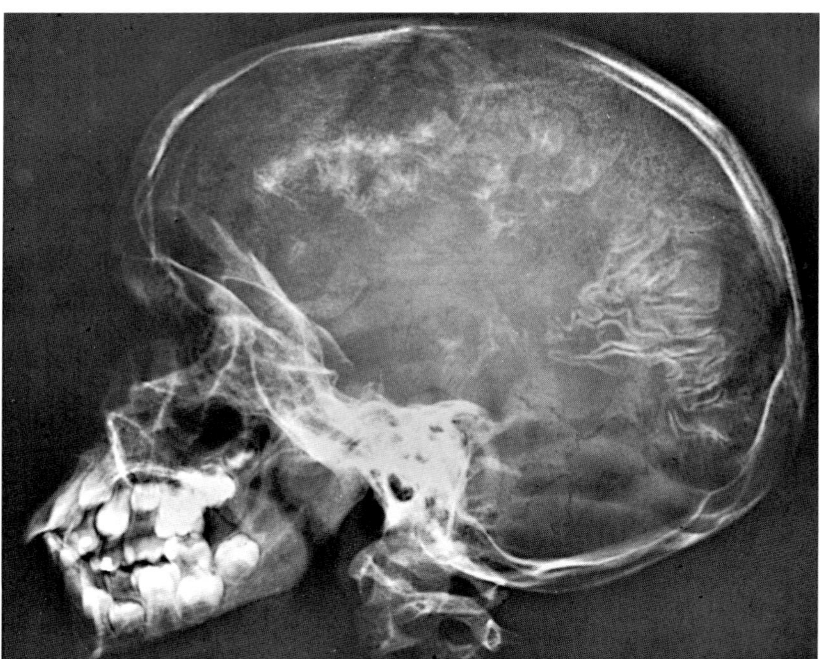

FIGURE 13–53.

Sturge-Weber syndrome: Characteristic pattern of "tram-line" calcifications of intracranial vascular lesions. In some cases, phleboliths are superimposed on the maxillofacial region from the facial hemangioma. (From Farman AG, Nortjé CJ, Wood RE: Oral and Maxillofacial Diagnostic Imaging. Philadelphia:Mosby, 1993, p. 151.)

only a slight female predilection; 34 cases were in female patients and 27 in male patients. The peak incidence was in the second decade of life, with 26 cases occurring at this time; only 3 developed in children younger than 10 years.

According to reviews by Sadowsky and colleagues (1981) and Anderson and associates (1981), as well as other reports that we studied, the following clinical signs and symptoms may be associated with vascular lesions. Hemangiomas may have been present since the first year of life, whereas AVMs may develop in a teenager, possibly after trauma. There may be asymmetry of the face, especially over the mandible, resulting from swelling or hypertrophy (from the increased blood supply). The overlying skin may be as much as 2° F warmer, and it may be moist. The skin or mucosa may be bluish, purplish, or reddish. The patient may complain of pain or paresthesia. Other symptoms include pulsatile or swishing noises, tinnitus, or impaired hearing. Blurred vision or epistaxis also may be reported. A highly characteristic finding is blood oozing spontaneously from the gingival sulcus of one or more teeth that may be loose. The tooth also may exhibit a pumping movement when pressure is applied to it and released. In addition, there may be premature exfoliation of the primary teeth and delayed eruption of the permanent teeth, as well as congenitally missing teeth, in the region of the lesion. Expansion of the alveolar process may be observed, with a diminished depth of the mucobuccal fold. With AVMs, an easily audible bruit and palpable thrill (vibration) may be felt. Secondary to AVMs, heart size and blood pressure frequently are increased. Holman (1962) further reported an increase in blood volume, heart rate, total cardiac output, stroke volume, left atrial pressure, and pulmonary arterial pressure. Central hemangiomas may yield blood readily on aspiration; however, the pressure of the central AVM may drive the plunger out of the syringe!

Treatment/Prognosis

Treatment modalities have been reviewed by Halazonitis and co-workers (1982) and Sadowsky and colleagues (1981). Some of these include radiation therapy, which has questionable value; cryosurgery; and injection of sclerosing agents such as sodium morrhuate or sodium tetradactyl sulfate, with unpredictable results. Embolization (occlusion) of feeder arteries has been useful; however, Orbach (1976) warned of complications, including thrombus formation, spasm of the artery, rupture of dilated vessels, passage of the embolus into a normal artery or through the lesion, and proximal arrest of the embolus. Schultz and colleagues (1988) treated a central AVM with cyanoacrylate injection directly into the feeder vessel, using a microballoon catheter, as the only mode of therapy; after 4 years, there was no evidence of the lesion and a complete regeneration of bone. Surgical approaches, including curettage, resection, or subperiosteal resection of the involved segment, have been the most common. Svane and colleagues (1989) reported excellent results with a graft of porous hydroxyapatite block.

Ligation of the feeder vessels has been tried in an attempt to control bleeding or minimize blood loss during surgery, but with inconsistent results. To illustrate this point, Kelly and colleagues (1977) confirmed an AVM in the right posterior mandible by arteriography. The main feeder vessels appeared to be the right lingual and facial arteries. The right inferior alveolar artery could not be shown to communicate with the AVM. Blood filled the AVM from the anterior to the posterior, exiting from the mandible through the mandibular foramen through the inferior alveolar veins. Also, an arteriogram of the left common carotid artery, with a basilar view, showed no contributions to the AVM from the left side. The right external carotid artery was ligated above the superior thyroid artery. When the area was entered carefully, copious hemorrhage occurred with every attempt to proceed with the surgery. To achieve hemostasis, the area was packed and surgery was continued subsequently. Once surgery was complete, the surgical defect was packed with two 2 × 8 cm sheets of Gelfoam (Upjohn, Kalamazoo, MI), and the flaps were closed with continuous sutures. The procedure required 6 hours. The patient, a 25-year-old white man, lost 2200 ml of blood. He received 1500 ml of Plasma-Lyte (Travenol, Deerfield, IL) and three units of blood. Kelly and colleagues (1977) pointed out that even though the right external carotid artery was ligated and the left carotid did not contribute to the lesion, a copious blood flow occurred throughout the surgical procedure. They illustrated the important contribution of venous back flow after forward pressure has been removed by ligation of the external carotid artery. These venous connections cannot be seen on arteriography because the dye-filled lesion would mask them. Batson's plexus is a system of paravertebral vessels with no valves. Blood can flow up or down, and vessels to the mandible connect with this plexus. The paravertebral plexus flows independently of the heart-lung circulation.

◆ RADIOLOGY (Figs. 13–54 and 13–55)

Radiologic Features of the Jaws

Miles and co-authors (1991) stated that AVMs have very few specific radiologic features, summarizing them as follows:

1. They are multilocular lesions with expansion and thinning of the cortex but without perforation.
2. They show a sunray appearance.
3. They appear as ill-defined or well-defined radiolucencies.
4. There is variable tooth displacement and root resorption.

Many of the features of central hemangiomas may be present in AVMs. In addition, AVMs may present as enlargements of the inferior alveolar canal.

Angiography of Hemangiomas and AVMs

Zou and colleagues (1983) analyzed 70 cases for the use of angiography for maxillofacial vascular lesions in the hard and soft tissues. They found that plain radiographs can show signs such as phleboliths, peripheral compressive destruction of the jaws, and widening of the canal within the jaws. Worth (1963) also pointed out the importance of calcified blood vessel walls in some soft tissue hemangiomas, but, unfortunately, phlebolithiasis and calcified blood vessel walls are not seen in central bony lesions. Angiography is useful in determining the extent, location, and type of vascular tumor and in assessing the blood supply and drainage. Zou and associates (1983) stressed that, in some AV fistulas, small shunts are not shown on angiograms. These may be responsible for unexpected bleeding at surgery, as well as tumor recurrence. They also stated that some cavernous hemangiomas with demonstrable venous drainage have many small arteries at the periphery, which is why such hemangiomas cannot be shown by arterial angiography. Spatz and colleagues (1985) stated that angiography is the best diagnostic tool for diagnosing vascular malformations definitively; however, they believed that the arteriogram cannot be relied on to show the full extent of the lesion. Often vascular channels that have been dormant and are not visible on angiograms become active when the main afferent vessels are ligated at surgery, sometimes resulting in massive hemorrhage. Gelfand and colleagues (1975) stated that arteriography has no use in hemangiomas. Orbach (1976) asserted that AVMs almost invariably are larger and more extensive than

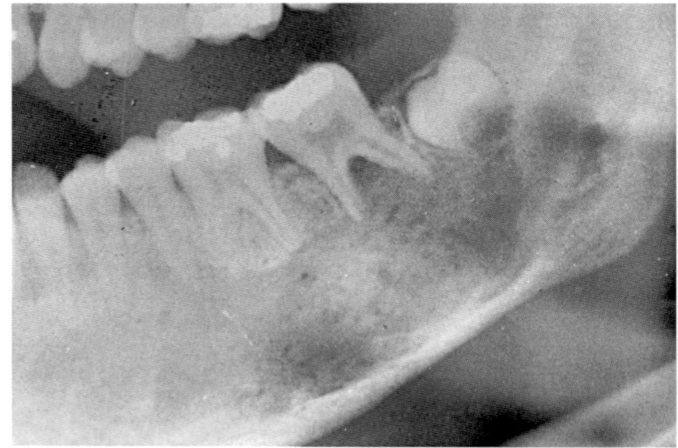

A

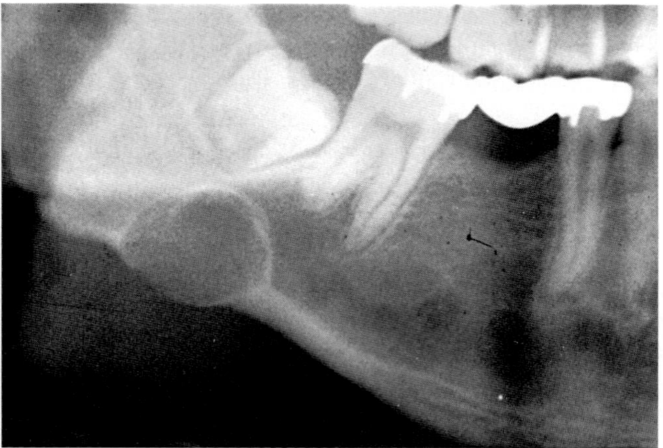

B

FIGURE 13–54.

Arteriovenous malformation: A, Figure shows numerous foramen-like structures; a small, very round, prominent radiolucent foramen-like area in the angle region, most likely caused by a feeder vessel; endosteal thinning of the inferior cortex; and disappearance of the inferior alveolar canal. (Courtesy of Dr. C. Parks, San Francisco, CA.) B. Figure shows a large vascular impression in the region of the facial artery and enlargement and deformity of the inferior alveolar canal anterior to the depression, whereas the canal appears normal posteriorly. (Courtesy of Dr. D. Stoneman, Toronto, Canada.)

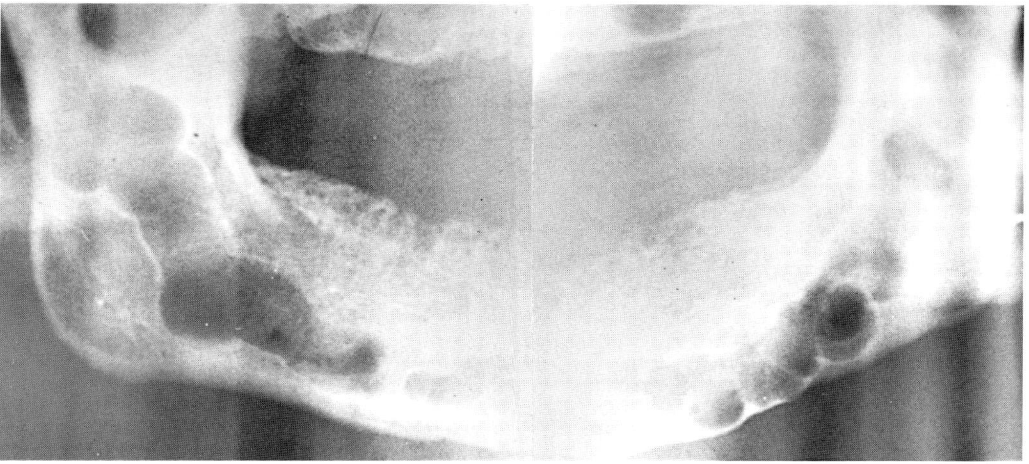

FIGURE 13–55.

Arteriovenous malformation: Bilateral AVMs associated with gross enlargement of the inferior alveolar canals, creating the illusion of a bilateral multilocular lesion. (Courtesy of Dr. B. Collett, Gainesville, FL.)

the arteriograms indicate. According to Orbach (1976), the arteriographic features of AVM are as follows:

1. Dilatation and lengthening of afferent arteries.
2. Early and preferential filling of shunts.
3. Decreased and delayed filling of associated normal arteries.
4. Early opacification of draining veins.
5. Rapid flow to collateral vessels.

Orbach (1976) stated that the main feeder vessels can be seen only during competent, extensive procedures, often requiring selective study of the vertebral artery, thyrocervical trunk, and external and internal carotid arteries.

CHERUBISM (Familial fibrous dysplasia of the jaws, familial multilocular cystic disease of the jaws, disseminated juvenile fibrous dysplasia, familial fibrous swelling of the jaws, hereditary fibrous dysplasia of the jaws)

Cherubism first was described by Jones in 1933 as a ''familial multilocular cystic disease of the jaws.'' Although he later introduced the term cherubism because of the similarity to the cherubic facial appearance of children depicted in renaissance art, it appears that Jones' original term was derived from the radiologic appearance. Anderson and McClenden (1962) reviewed 65 cases from 21 families and suggested that the pattern of inheritance was autosomal dominant, with 100% penetrance in male family members and 50 to 70% penetrance in female members. Although cherubism is diagnosed from the radiographs, the tissue sometimes is examined microscopically. Histologically, there is a highly vascular fibrous stroma, sometimes arranged in a whorled pattern containing large numbers of plump fibroblasts. Numerous multinucleated giant cells are present, with prominent nuclei and nucleoli. There are often hemorrhagic foci, and hemosiderin may be seen. A characteristic feature, when present, is the perivascular eosinophilic cuffing of the small capillaries in the lesion. In more mature lesions, collagenous and fibrous tissues predominate, whereas the number of giant cells is diminished. Remnants of odontogenic epithelium from developing teeth may be scattered throughout the lesion. These lesions have been detected in children as young as 2 years of age, and clinical evidence of the condition usually appears by the time a child is 5 years old. Bilaterally swollen cheeks develop, and, when the maxillary sinus is involved, exophthalmia may be seen. Some patients exhibit café au lait pigmentations. Spontaneous regression usually occurs before a patient is 20 years of age, but in rare instances lesions may remain until a person is 30 years old. Cosmetic recontouring sometimes is performed during adolescence. Unerupted and ectopically erupted permanent teeth may be treated orthodontically. Radiation therapy is contraindicated. An association with other disorders and malignant transformation have not been reported.

◆ *RADIOLOGY (Figs. 13-56 to 13-59)*

Cherubism classically is described as a bilateral, multilocular, multicystic-appearing expansile lesion usually affecting the mandible and sometimes the maxilla of children. The condyles usually are spared. In its classic presentation, cherubism is radiologically pathognomonic.

Location

It usually is located bilaterally in the mandibular angle. Davis and colleagues (1983) reported that the next two most common locations are the mandibular molar region and coronoid process. The changes begin at the angle and spread anteriorly and posteriorly. In a review of 20 cases from one family, Peters (1979) found that the condyle always was spared. The lesions tend to be symmetrically bilateral, although Reade and colleagues (1984) reported a case of uni-

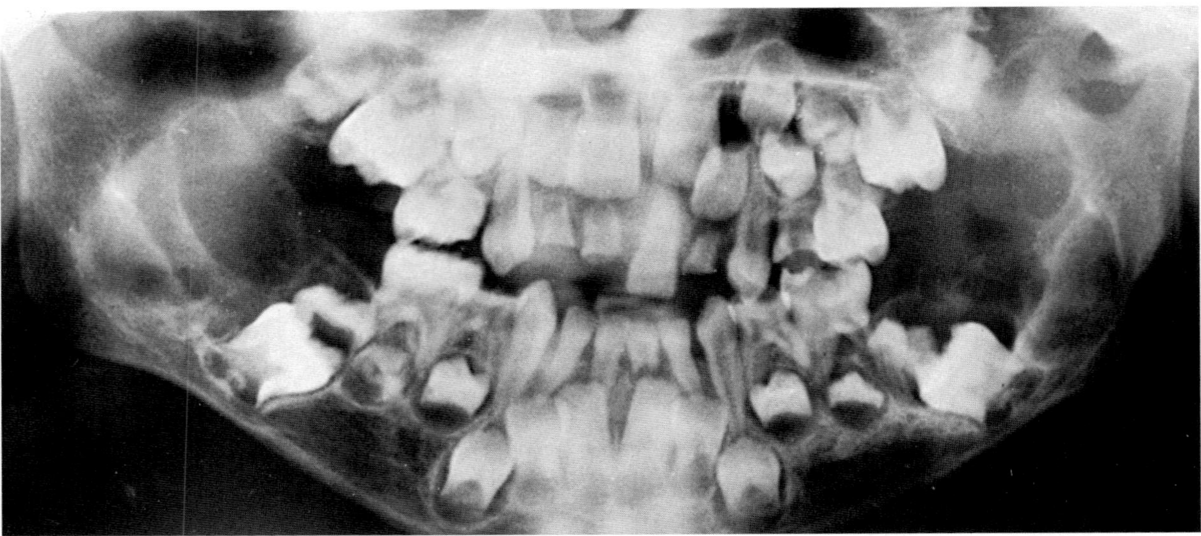

FIGURE 13–56.

Cherubism: Mild presentation in a 5-year-old boy, with expansion in the ramus angle area and multiple locules beginning to form. (From Bianchi SD, Boecardi A, Mela F, Romagnoli R: The computed tomographic appearances of cherubism. Skeletal Radiol 16:60, 1987.)

lateral involvement of the mandibular angle in a 16-year-old boy.

Radiologic Features

Invariably, consistent features include expansion, thinning of cortices, and little or no reactive subperiosteal new bone formation. Although perforation of the cortex is seen sometimes, pathologic fracture is not a feature. Cherubism may affect the central and buccal aspects of the jaws preferentially, with less effect on the lingual cortex. The locules of cherubism are almost always multiple, with excellent opacification of the septa defining them. In well-developed cases, multiple locules may be seen within large lucunae of bone destruction. The sizes usually are mixed, and large, medium, and small cystlike spaces occur in the same patient. Although the locules often are round or ovoid, they also assume larger, less regular shapes, but the contours tend to be rounded. In some instances, the internal loculations become indistinct, leaving only a scalloped peripheral outline similar to that of the OKC. The disappearance of internal loculations is a sign of resolution. When the maxilla is involved, the tuberosity is the most common location. Maxillary lesions often expand at the expense of the maxillary sinus. Many of these children have a poorly developed antrum. The antral lesions may cause bowing of the floor of the orbit and exophthalmia clinically.

Bianchi and colleagues (1987) studied six cases of cherubism with CT scans. None of their cases showed involve-

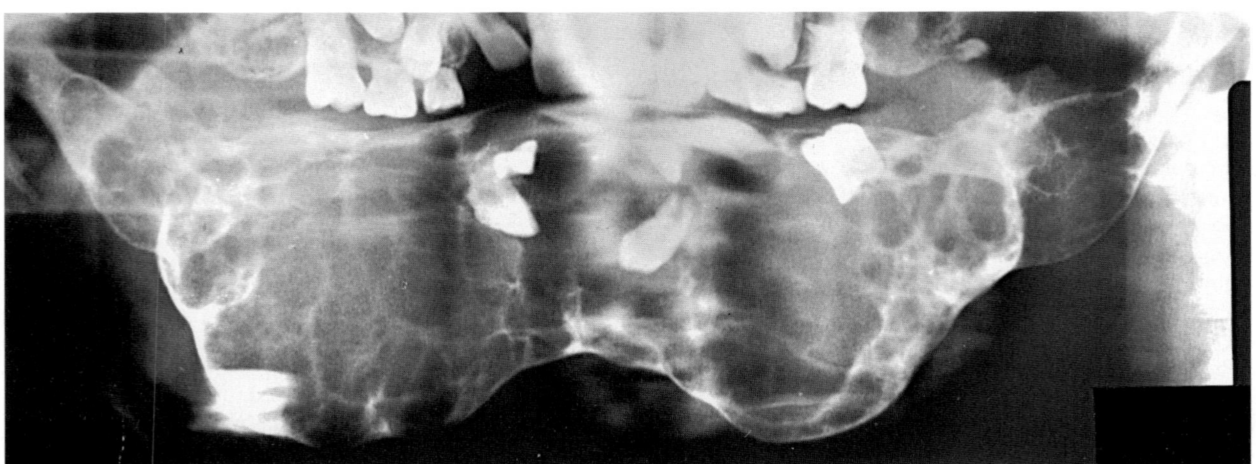

FIGURE 13–57.

Cherubism: Case in a 9-year-old boy. The condyles remain unaffected. (Courtesy of Dr. H. Schwartz, Kaiser Permanente Medical Group, Los Angeles, CA.)

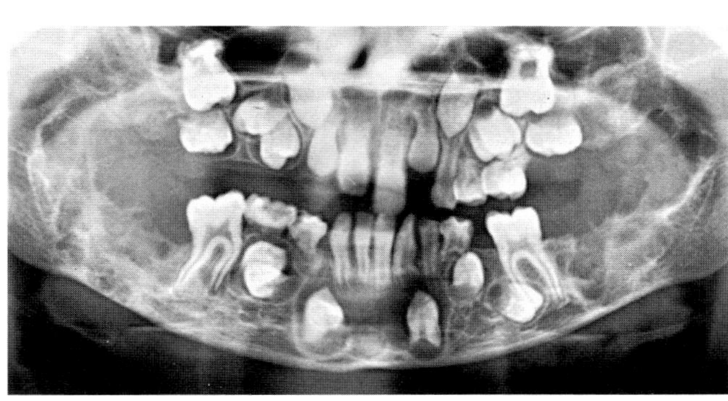

A

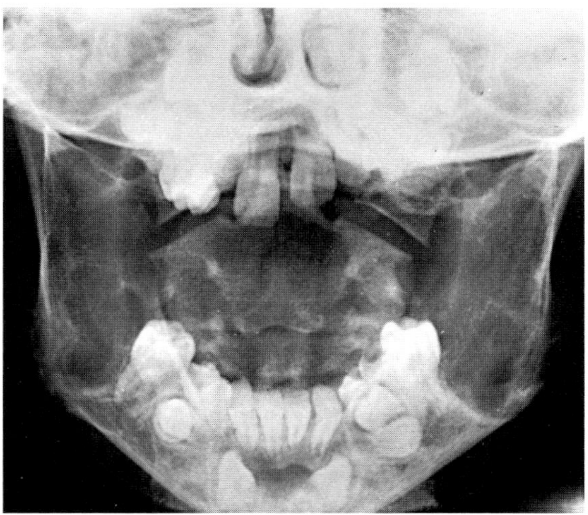

B

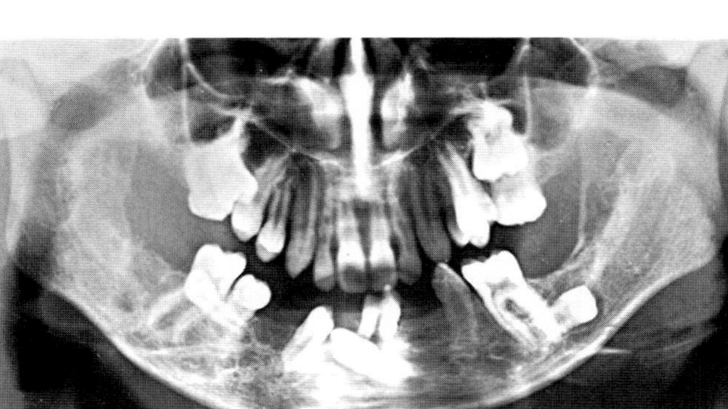

C

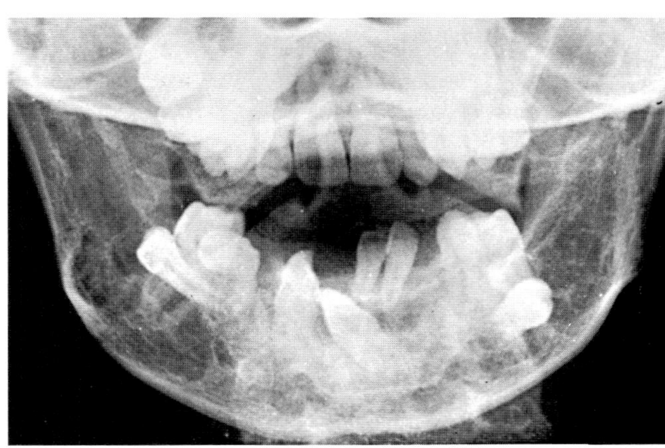

D

FIGURE 13–58.

Cherubism: A and B, Patient at 6 years of age. C and D, Patient at 12 years of age. Resolution is evident in posterior mandible, and there is more distinctive pneumatization of the maxillary sinus.

ment of the other facial bones. These authors also demonstrated that mandibular lesions seemed closer to the buccal cortex, which was expanded, thinned, and discontinuous. There was much less involvement of the lingual cortex. In two early cases in a 5-year-old boy and a 9-year-old girl, the authors detected maxillary lesions that could not be seen on conventional radiographs. They also showed extensive multilocular involvement of the hard palate and rare involvement of the right condyle in a 17-year-old boy.

Radiologic Signs of Regression

In cherubism, evidence of regression consists of a loss of the internal loculations, diminished expansion of the buccal cortical plate, gradual replacement of internal elements with a granular appearance, and, finally, the return of a normal-appearing trabecular pattern. In some instances, a few radiolucent areas with patches of irregular sclerosis or a dense granular appearance may persist after a patient is 30 years of age. In many cases, the last area to resolve is the mandibular angle-ramus area. The clues are the bilateral location, evidence of resolution, and family history of cherubism. It is possible that cherubism begins in the angle area and spreads to the mandibular body and ramus bilaterally, with regression occurring in the reverse order.

Relationship to Teeth

Although one often sees developing teeth floating within the cystic-appearing spaces, many permanent teeth may have erupted. Physiologic resorption of the primary roots sometimes is accelerated, resulting in early exfoliation. Root deformities and displacement of developing permanent teeth may be seen. There may be ectopic eruption of some permanent teeth and impaction of others.

Extragnathic Cherubism

It is said that cherubism affects only the jaws and indirectly the antrum and orbital floor. The remainder of the face and skull are not affected. Although the rest of the skeleton usu-

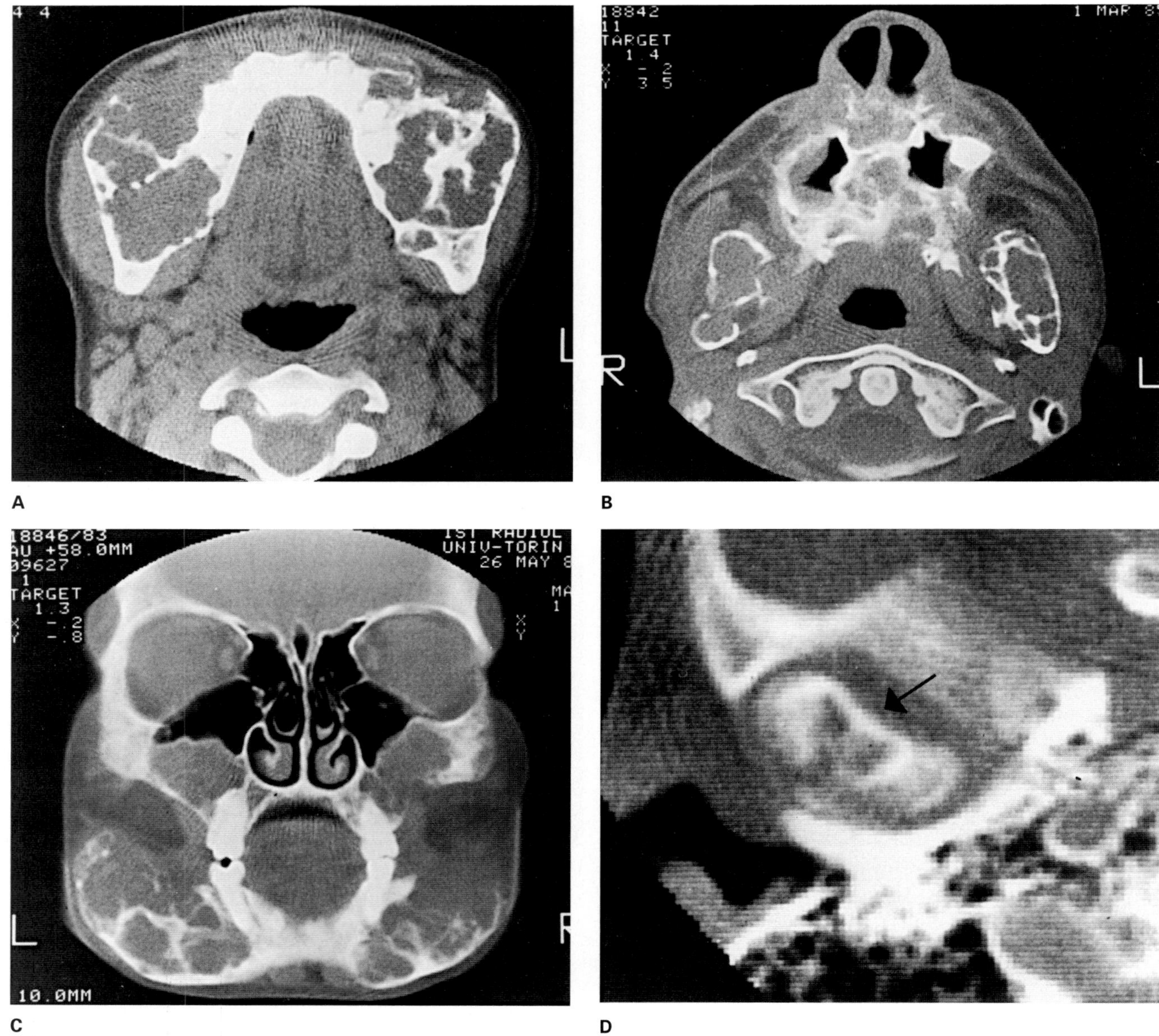

FIGURE 13–59.

Cherubism: A to D, CT study showing severe expansion of the mandible, involvement of the ramus, and rare involvement of the condyle in a 17-year-old patient. (From Bianchi SD, Boecardi A, Mela F, Romagnoli R: The computed tomographic appearances of cherubism. Skeletal Radiol 16:60, 1987.)

ally is not involved, Davis and colleagues (1983) cited reports of rare occurrences in the ribs, humerus, and femur. Cherubism is histologically similar to several other fibro-osseous lesions with giant cells.

CENTRAL ODONTOGENIC FIBROMA

(Simple variant, World Health Organization [WHO] variant, and granular cell variant)

Shafer and colleagues (1983) stated that, of all the odontogenic tumors, this lesion has the most poorly defined parameters. One must be careful when assessing the literature because some authors have lumped the central and peripheral variants into one group. Sepheriadou-Mavropoulou and colleagues (1985) reviewed cases of central odontogenic fibroma and found only 13 cases, including their own.

Pathologic Characteristics

Central odontogenic fibromas classically have been divided into two histologically distinct variants, and a third type was suggested recently. The first, which has been called the simple type, resembles the dental follicle and consists of a very bland connective tissue mass that is described in this way because the many plump fibroblasts appear to be equidistant from each other. There are a few small islands of odontogenic epithelium scattered throughout the lesion. The second type, designated the WHO type, contains mineralized material that has been interpreted as osteoid, cementumlike, or dysplastic dentin. Dysplastic dentin usually is found in close to the odontogenic epithelium. The WHO type has more islands of odontogenic epithelium. Gardner (1980) discussed the histologic characteristics of these two types in detail. Most believe the WHO type occurs much less commonly. Wesley and colleagues (1975) showed that only 1 of 8 lesions had calcifications. Among the 13 cases of Sepheriadou-Mavropoulou and colleagues (1985), 5 specimens contained calcifications; however, several cases in their series did not contain odontogenic epithelium.

The third type, suggested by Vincent and colleagues (1987), should be referred to as the granular cell variant of central odontogenic fibroma. This lesion has been known as granular cell ameloblastic fibroma, central granular cell tumor of the jaws, granular cell odontogenic fibroma, and spongiocytic adamantinoma. In their literature review, Vincent and colleagues (1987) found 10 cases, beginning with the first definitive report by Couch and colleagues in 1962, and added 2 new cases. These authors believed that this mixed lesion is derived primarily from odontogenic mesenchyme and secondarily contains odontogenic epithelium. Histologically, the lesion is characterized by large, round to polygonal stromal cells with a finely granular, eosinophilic cytoplasm and often eccentrically located ovoid to round nuclei. The granular cells are arranged in lobules and separated by a thin connective tissue septum containing small, thin-walled vessels. The granular cells sometimes were associated with cementumlike material. Within the lobules of granular cells there were abundant, small, ovoid or sometimes elongated islands of cuboidal to low columnar epithelial cells. Amorphous eosinophilic material often was found in the center of these epithelial cell clusters, and some centers had a stellate reticulumlike appearance. Vincent and colleagues (1987) stated that because of the abundant and relatively uniform distribution of the odontogenic epithelium, this lesion is a specific variant of the WHO type.

Clinical Features

In the review by Dahl and associates (1981), the mean patient age was 34 years, with a range of 11 to 80 years. Among the cases analyzed by Sepheriadou-Mavropoulou and coauthors (1985), 9 of 13 occurred in patients in the second and third decades of life; however, the average patient age was 31 years. There does not appear to be a sex predilection. Most lesions are seen as a painless swelling. In the granular cell variant, 10 of 12 cases reviewed by Vincent and colleagues (1987) occurred in female patients; the average age was 51 years. Among the female patients, 9 of the 10 cases occurred in 50- to 60-year-old women, and 1 case developed in a 65-year-old woman. In men, the lesions occurred when the patients were 27 and 39 years old.

Treatment/Prognosis

Curettage is the treatment of choice. The only known recurrence was reported by Heimdal and colleagues (1980), which was treated by enucleation and appears to have been the simple type histologically; it recurred after 9 years. This case emphasizes the importance of long-term radiologic follow-up. Most cases of the granular cell variant were treated by surgical excision or curettage; in 10 of 12 cases in the series, the patients were observed for 6 months to 12 years, with no recurrences reported.

◆ *RADIOLOGY (Figs. 13–60 to 13–63)*

The radiologic features of central odontogenic fibroma have not been well described because the lesion is rare. The only feature that we have identified that would help separate this lesion from all others is its propensity to occur in the mandible.

Location

The overwhelming majority of these cases occur in the mandible. Among 13 cases reported by Sepheriadou-Mavropoulou and colleagues (1985), only 2 occurred in the maxilla. One appeared to be the simple type and the other a WHO type. The molar region is the most common area affected, with lesions being fairly large at diagnosis, involving large

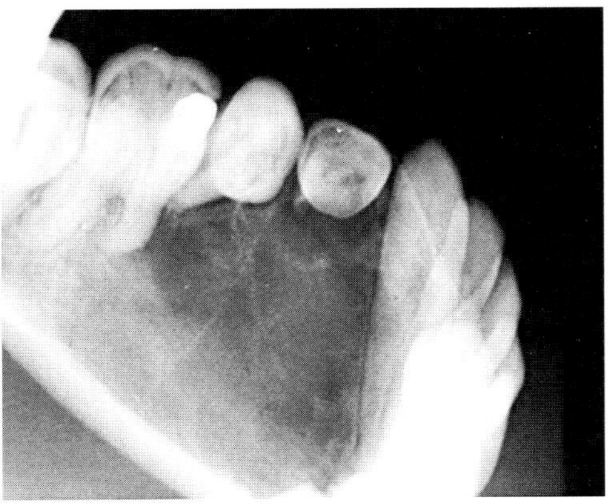

A

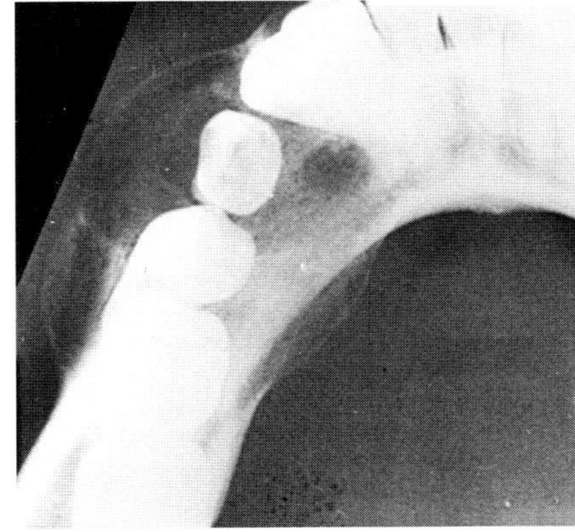

B

FIGURE 13–60.

Odontogenic fibroma: The histologic subtype is not known. A, Oblique occlusal view showing a multilocular pattern and lack of sclerosis at the margin. B, Occlusal view of the same case shows expansion of the buccal and lingual cortices, which are thinned but remain intact.

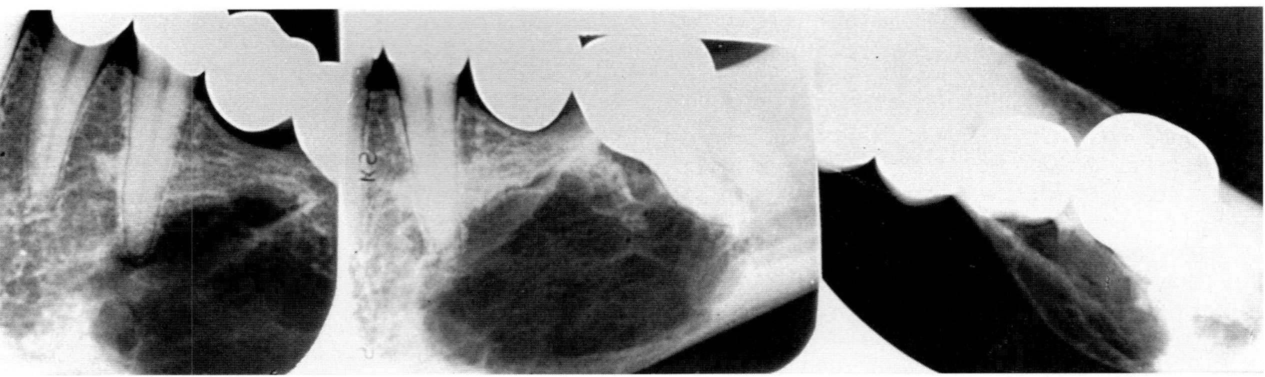

FIGURE 13–61.

Odontogenic fibroma: The histologic subtype is not known, but this Swedish case may represent a WHO type. This 31-year-old woman had a history of previous tumor, and teeth were removed when she was 21 years of age. The figure shows multiple faint locules and a thin, but intact, expanded margin. (Courtesy of Professor G. Tronje, Karolinska Institutet, Stockholm, Sweden.)

portions of the body of the mandible. Several lesions extended into the ramus. The anterior mandible was affected in four cases; however, there was usually extension posteriorly to the premolar or molar regions.

Among cases of the granular cell variant, a huge majority were in the mandible, with 10 of 11 cases with a reported location occurring in the mandible. Of these, seven (58%) were in the molar region, with one case extending to the angle and none involving the ramus. Several cases in the molar region extended to the premolar area. Two cases were in the canine area, and one was in the premolar region. The maxillary lesion was in the premolar region.

Radiologic Features

Most lesions appear moderately destructive. A multilocular pattern was observed in at least half of the cases, whereas the others were described as unilocular, irregularly osteolytic, or radiolucent. Expansion of the cortex occurs in large lesions, and perforation of the cortex probably is not a feature. The margins are well defined in most cases, but there is usually no sclerotic margin. The septa of bone forming the locules may not appear as radiopaque as those in ameloblastoma but slightly more so than those in the central giant cell granuloma. It is possible that some lesions contain radiopaque flecks. In rare instances, the lesion may appear as a homogeneous radiopaque mass. Several cases were associated with an impacted or unerupted tooth. Teeth may be displaced, and root resorption was observed in one case.

The details of the radiologic features of the granular cell variant are scant; however, a less aggressive appearance is seen. All lesions were described as radiolucencies. The lesion is said to be well demarcated, circumscribed, or well defined; however, a sclerotic margin may be present. Most lesions appear to be unilocular, and internal features such as loculations rarely are mentioned. In one instance, focal radiodensities were observed in the central part of the lesion. Other features include slight downward displacement of the inferior alveolar canal and expansion of the inferior cortex

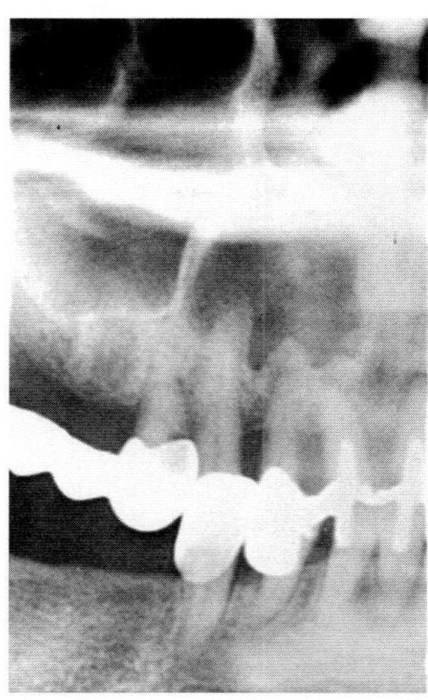

A

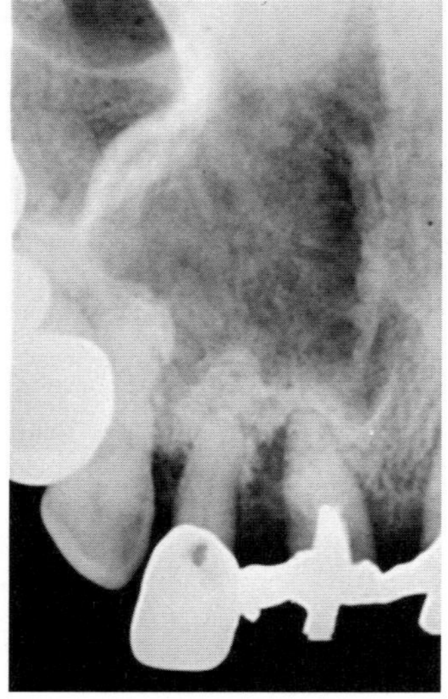

B

FIGURE 13–62.

Odontogenic fibroma: A and B, The histologic subtype is not known, but this Japanese case may represent the WHO type. The case has a rare maxillary location. There is no tendency to infiltrate into the sinus, although the wall is deformed and thickened. Internal elements consist of septa and calcified flecks. (Courtesy of Professor T. Noikura, First Oral Surgery Department, Kagoshima University, Kagoshima, Japan.)

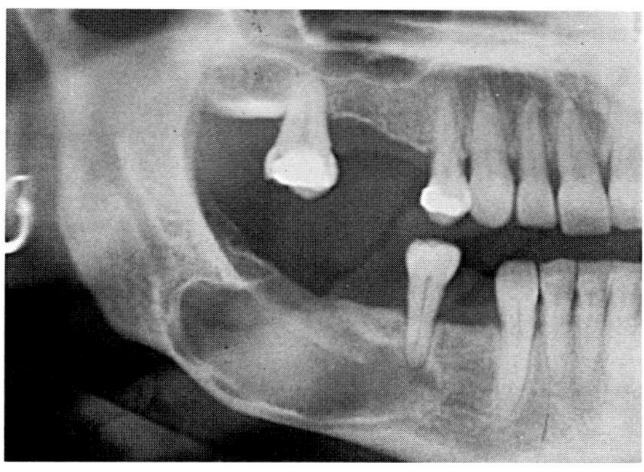

FIGURE 13–63.

Odontogenic fibroma: granular cell variant: This is typical of the few reported lesions. (From Vincent SD, Hammond HL, Ellis GL, Juhlin JP: Central granular cell odontogenic fibroma. Oral Surg Oral Med Oral Pathol 63:715, 1987.)

of the mandible. Although these lesions may be medium to large, they do not seem to grow to huge, disfiguring proportions.

DESMOPLASTIC FIBROMA (Intraosseous desmoid tumor, osseous fibromatosis)

Desmoplastic fibroma (DF) of bone first was described by Jaffe in 1958. In 1965, Griffith and Irby reported the first case in the jaws. It is a rare lesion; however, in the skeleton, it occurs most often in the mandible. Hashimoto and colleagues (1991) presented an excellent review. According to Ackermann and Rosai (1974), DF of bone represents the osseous counterpart of soft tissue fibromatosis or desmoid tumors, which are more common and tend to occur in the abdominal wall. In a review of 8542 bone tumors, Dahlin and Unni (1986) found that 315 cases (3.7%) were fibrous tumors and only 9 (0.1%) were DFs. In the bone tumor registry in Japan (1985), 14,977 primary bone tumors were registered between 1972 and 1985, and only 54 (0.4%) were DFs. In 1989, Crim and colleagues found only 114 cases in the world literature. The most common location was the mandible, accounting for 26% of the cases. In their review, Hashimoto and colleagues (1991) found 50 cases in the jaws.

Pathologic Characteristics

The DF is a locally aggressive lytic benign tumor of bone. According to Hashimoto and colleagues (1991), the benign nonossifying tumors of the jaws are classified as follows: (1) odontogenic fibroma, (2) desmoplastic fibroma, and (3) nonossifying fibroma. The odontogenic fibroma may contain mineralized material, but it is not osseous. The cause of desmoplastic fibroma is unknown, but trauma may play a role in its development. On gross examination, the tumor is white to tan and firm and rubbery. Histologically, Jaffe (1958) said that the tumor was composed of small spindle-shaped fibroblasts in a setting of abundant intercellular material that usually is rich in mature collagen fibers. Microscopic evidence of muscular infiltration by tumor was present in 42% of the cases reviewed by Freedman and colleagues (1978). Histologically, it may be very difficult to distinguish this lesion from grade 1 fibrosarcoma and grade 1 fibroblast predominant osteosarcoma.

Clinical Features

In a review of 114 DFs in all skeletal locations, Crim and colleagues (1989) reported a mean patient age of 21 years at diagnosis (age range, 15 months to 75 years). Reviewing 26 cases in the jaws, Freedman and co-authors (1978) found a mean age of 16 years (age range, birth to 36 years). In the series of 50 jaw lesions reviewed by Hashimoto and colleagues (1991), 80% were diagnosed in patients younger than 30 years of age, with 36% of cases occurring in the first decade, 18% in the second decade, and 26% in the third decade of life. All studies showed an equal distribution among male and female patients. According to Hashimoto and colleagues (1991), the most common presenting complaint is painless swelling, intraorally or extraorally, in approximately 90% of the cases; a history of trauma was found in 20% of the cases. Pain is a variable feature and seems to occur more frequently in extragnathic sites, although it may be present rarely in the jaws. Although pathologic fracture is seen in 9% of all skeletal lesions, it has not been reported with jaw lesions. Other signs and symptoms include deviation of the mandible on opening, malocclusion, and trismus, especially when the swelling is at the angle of the mandible. Strangely, hypoplasia of the mandible was reported in these cases. Freedman and colleagues (1978) stated that the time lapse between when the patient became aware of the swelling and then sought treatment ranged from 2 days to 8 years. The mean elapsed time was 17 months; however, 61% of the patients sought treatment within 6 months.

Treatment/Prognosis

In their review of 26 cases in the jaws, Freedman and colleagues (1978) studied biologic behavior and treatment. Their findings did not fully corroborate the original recommendation of Jaffe (1958), who advised segmental resection as the treatment of choice. In addition, Freedman and co-authors (1978) could not correlate recurrence consistently with cortical perforation or histologic evidence of muscle infiltration by tumor. They observed cortical perforation in 77% and muscular infiltration by tumor in 42% of the cases. Among the 26 cases reviewed, 16 were treated by simple excision (presumably with thorough curettage), 7 by resection, and 1 each by biopsy only (extent unspecified), segmental resection, and radiation therapy. With a follow-up of 3 months to 8 years, 19 (73%) of these cases did not recur. Among the nonrecurrent cases, 12 were treated by excision, 6 by resection, and 1 by radiation therapy. No follow-up data were available for 4 cases (15%). Thus, the recurrence rate is between 10% and 30%. The case treated by biopsy alone was congenital and totally regressed by the time the patient was 7 years old. The one treated by segmental resection was reported by Van Blarcom and colleagues (1971) and recurred as a grade 2 fibrosarcoma with metastases.

◆ RADIOLOGY (Figs. 13–64 and 13–65)

In a review of the radiologic features of 114 cases of DF in gnathic and extragnathic locations, Crim and colleagues (1989) observed the following radiologic features among 83 patients with available radiographs:

1. The most common skeletal location was the mandible (26%).
2. There was a geographic pattern of bone destruction with a narrow transition zone and nonsclerotic margins (96%).
3. Internal pseudotrabeculation was seen (91%).
4. Expansion was observed (89%), although distinct periosteal new bone was seen in only two cases (2%).
5. Perforation of the cortex was present (28%).
6. Three cases arose in the periosteum and were differentiated radiologically from desmoid (fibrous) tumors of intraosseous or soft tissue origin.

Location

In a review of 114 DFs in all skeletal sites, Crim and coauthors (1989) reported the following locations: mandible (26%), maxilla (2%), femur (14%), innominate bone of the pelvis (14%), humerus (11%), radius (9%), tibia (7%), and, in descending order of frequency, the scapula, metatarsal, rib, skull, fibula, vertebra, calcaneus, clavicle, ulna, metacarpal, and sacrum (1 to 3% each). Thus, 28% of the lesions occurred in the jaws, and tumors may develop in almost any bone. In the series of 50 jaw lesions reviewed by Hashimoto and colleagues (1991), 84% occurred in the mandible and 16% in the maxilla. Most of the mandibular lesions were posterior to the molar region in the angle-ramus area, 12% were anterior to the premolar region, and one crossed the midline. In the maxilla, tumor extension into the maxillary sinus occurred in 7 of 8 cases. The remaining maxillary lesion was limited to the alveolar bone in the molar area, although there seemed to be a suggestion of extension in the antrum on the plain radiographs.

Radiologic Features

The radiologic features of DF have been well described by Crim and colleagues (1989). The DF is a locally aggressive lesion. It is purely lytic and does not contain mineralized matrix. The pattern is predominantly geographic; this means that the lesions appear as single or, more often, multiple relatively large radiolucent areas, without a well-defined margin, although the margins can be located on close inspection. There is a narrow transition zone representing areas of partial infiltration by tumor between distinct foci of lysis and normal bone. Marginal sclerosis is seen rarely and is limited to small regions of the tumor margin. A multilocular pattern is produced by the pseudotrabeculae, which result from uneven bone destruction, leaving ridges of intact bone near the periphery of the tumor. These pseudotrabeculae may vary in appearance from coarse linear strands to a thinner, more delicate, lacelike pattern. Rarely, a motheaten pattern is seen. Expansion often is present; in such cases, cortical perforation may be observed and the herniated soft tissue mass may displace adjacent muscles. The DF is characteristically hypovascular on angiograms. When a DF arises from the periosteum, cortical destruction originates at the periosteal surface.

Hashimoto and colleagues (1991) analyzed the radiologic findings in 47 cases with available radiographs. Forty cases were in the mandible and 7 in the maxilla. Among the mandibular cases, 28 (70%) were well defined, and these were categorized as multilocular (64%) or unilocular (36%). The remaining 12 mandibular cases (30%) were described as poorly circumscribed radiolucencies. Expansion of cortical bone and thinning or perforation were observed in 58% of

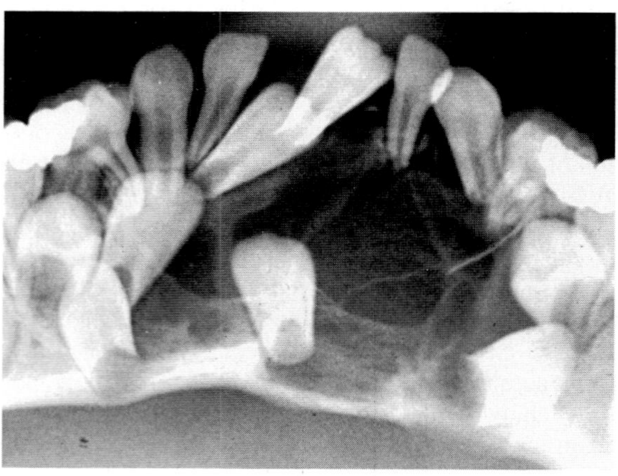

A

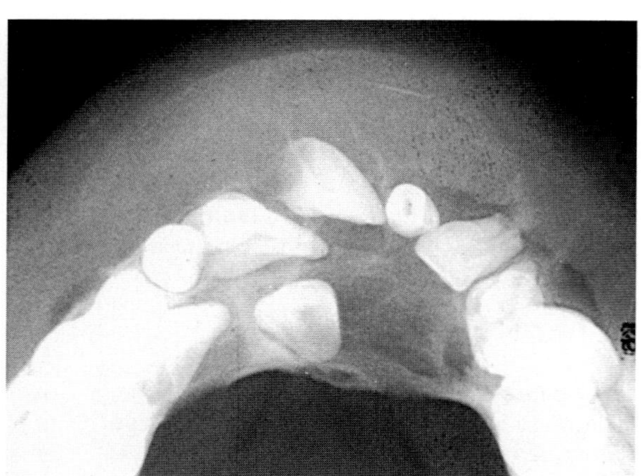

B

FIGURE 13–64.

Desmoplastic fibroma: A, Panoramic view, using an intraoral source, shows a similarity to the odontogenic fibroma. B, In the occlusal view, the similarity to odontogenic fibroma ends. The case shows an expanded, perforated cortex, and bony remnants form pseudotrabeculae. (From Araki M, Hashimoto K, Honda K: Desmoplastic fibroma of the mandible. Oral Radiol 3:71, 1987.)

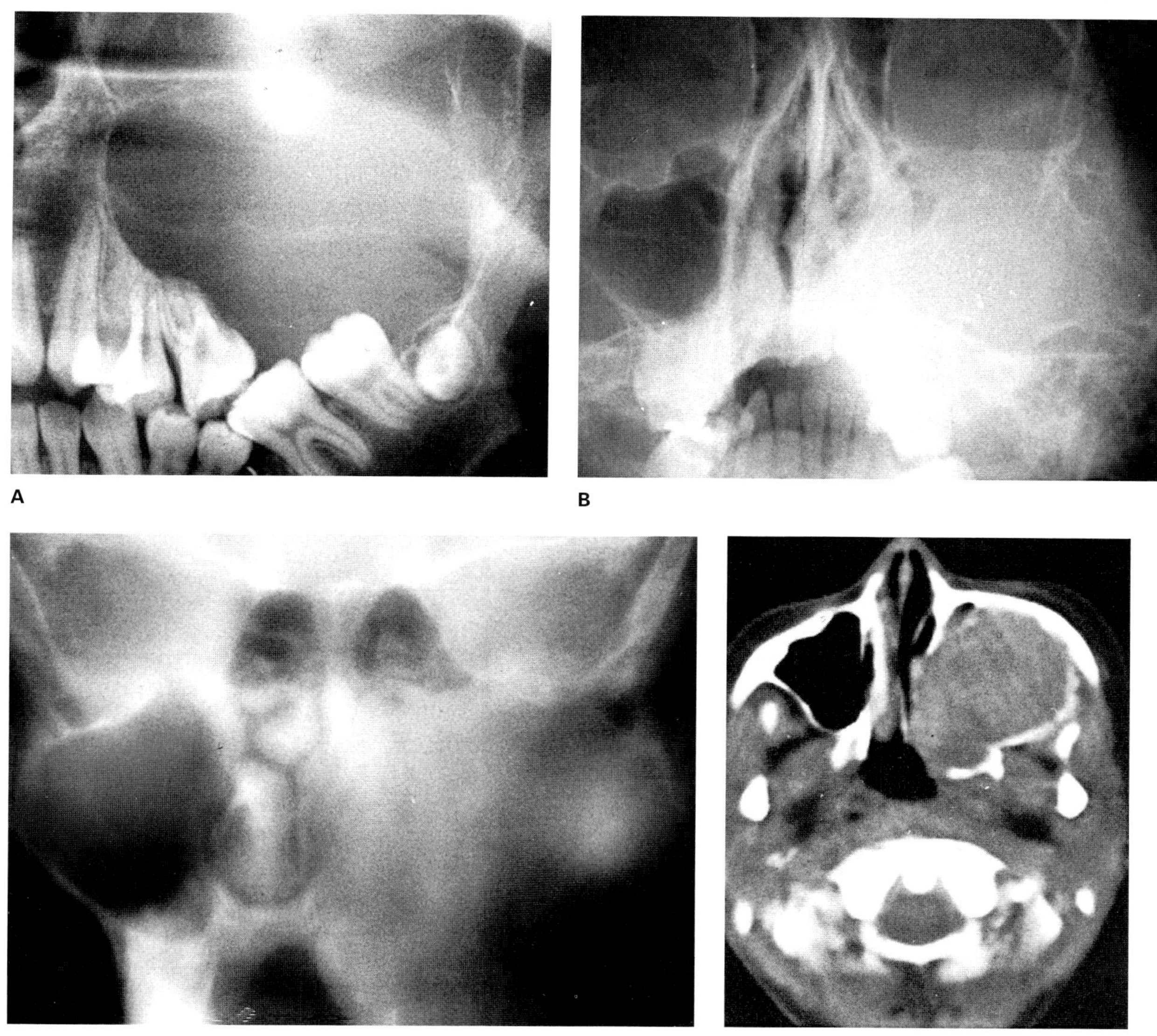

FIGURE 13–65.

Desmoplastic fibroma: A, In a panoramic view, it is impossible to determine the extent of the lesion. B, Waters view shows infiltration into the left maxillary sinus and erosion of the lateral wall and orbital roof. C, Posterior-anterior tomogram shows extensive destruction of the maxilla, sinus, and nasal fossa contents and superior expansion of the orbital floor. D, Axial CT scan shows the extent of involvement of the upper sinus and nasal fossa. (From Hashimoto K, et al: Desmoplastic fibroma of the maxillary sinus: report of a case and review of the literature. Oral Surg Oral Med Oral Pathol 72:126, 1991.)

the cases; however, a distinct periosteal reaction was found in only 2 cases (5%).

Hashimoto and colleagues (1991) analyzed six previously reported cases involving the maxillary sinus and reported a new case. Features included increased opacification of the sinus space and thinning or perforation of the sinus wall. There may be extension into the nasal cavity, with obliteration of structural detail by tumor infiltration. Bowing and possibly perforation of the nasal septum may occur in extensive cases. On CT scans, the tumor appears as a homogeneous mass with a CT number similar to that of muscle. In their case, the tumor in the maxillary sinus caused posterior displacement of the posterior sinus wall and the coronoid process. In the other maxillary case, a soap-bubble pattern was observed within the alveolar bone in the molar region, and plain radiographs appeared to show a faintly more radiopaque area within the sinus.

Many authors have discussed the difficulty of histologically distinguishing DF from grade 1 fibrosarcoma and fibroblastic osteosarcoma. Crim and colleagues (1989) pointed out that the radiologic changes in fibrosarcoma are permeative, meaning that the lytic areas are very tiny and numerous and they tend to infiltrate the cortex without expansion; additionally, the transition zone is wider, producing an ill-defined tumor-host bone interface. In DF, the pattern is almost always geographic, with a narrow transition zone providing well-defined margins. In osteosarcoma, mineralized tumor matrix and periosteal reactions are present, producing various patterns discussed in Chapter 16 (''Focal Radiopacities''), which covers osteosarcoma.

Relationship to Teeth

In their analysis of 23 cases with available radiographs of the teeth, Freedman and colleagues (1978) found no tumors associated with an embedded tooth. This lack of involvement with an impacted tooth is paradoxic because the ages during which this tumor is diagnosed involve active tooth formation and eruption. Resorption of adjacent root apices has been observed. Freedman and co-authors (1978) reported a 34% incidence among 23 cases; however, Hashimoto and co-authors (1991) found a 6% incidence among 48 patients with teeth.

NONOSSIFYING FIBROMA (Fibrous defect of bone, nonosteogenic fibroma, metaphyseal fibrous defect, fibrous xanthoma, central fibroma of bone)

The nonossifying fibroma is a common lesion in the long bones of children. Cale and colleagues (1989) suggested that this is one of a group of lesions that they classified as the fibrohistiocytic lesions of bone. We are including a brief review to provide a better understanding of this confusing group of rare lesions. Sources of additional information include Edeiken (1981), Sutton (1975), Liaw and colleagues (1979), Cale and colleagues (1989), and Anavi and co-authors (1989). The Cale (1989) classification is shown in Table 13–4.

The nonossifying fibroma first was recognized by Jaffe and Lichtenstein in 1942. The first definitive report of a jaw lesion probably was written by Rudy and Scheingold in 1964 and identified it as a xanthogranuloma, although a previous report was published by Agazzi in 1951. Recently, Elzay and colleagues (1984) presented a review of jaw lesions and reported two new cases. They identified five true cases of nonossifying fibroma, all occurring in the mandible. The other cases were reported by Rudy and Scheingold (1964), Liaw and colleagues (1979), and Makek (1980). According to Cale and co-authors (1989), the case of Liaw and co-workers (1979) was a benign fibrous histiocytoma.

TABLE 13–4
Fibrohistiocytic Lesions of Bone: A Classification

Benign
1. Metaphyseal fibrous defect
    a. Fibrous cortical defect
    b. Nonossifying fibroma
2. Benign fibrous histiocytoma

Malignant
1. Malignant fibrous histiocytoma

(From Cale AE, Freedman PD, Kerpel SM, Lumerman H: Benign fibrous histocytoma of the maxilla. Oral Surg Oral Med Oral Pathol 68:444, 1989.)

Fibrohistiocytic Lesions of Bone: A Brief Review

Fibrous Cortical Defect

The fibrous cortical defect is seen primarily in the metaphyses of long bones. It is thought to be a reactive lesion arising when fibrous tissue from the periosteum invades the underlying cortex. There may be a history of trauma in some cases. Outside the jaws, this condition is very common, and as many as 30 to 40% of all children are affected. The age range of patients is 2 to 14 years, and the male-to-female ratio is 2:1. This lesion may regress spontaneously within 2 weeks to 2 years or may persist and evolve into a nonossifying fibroma.

Nonossifying Fibroma

Jaffe and Lichtenstein (1942) believed that the nonossifying fibroma arises de novo or is part of a continuum, with the lesion beginning as a fibrous cortical defect, becoming a nonossifying fibroma, and ultimately ending up as a sclerotic bone island. This sequel is the exception rather than the rule. The lesion occurs in older children and adolescents between 8 and 20 years of age, and the male-to-female ratio is 2:1. This lesion is characterized by pain and possible pathologic fracture and may regress spontaneously. Sclerotic bone islands may develop idiopathically or as a sequel to other conditions such as a fibrous cortical defect, a nonossifying fibroma, and other unrelated conditions. The lesion consists of compact bone and sometimes cartilage. It can develop in patients of any age but grows more rapidly in children. The male-to-female ratio is equal. This condition may be analogous or similar to the jaw lesion we describe as osteosclerosis.

Benign Fibrous Histiocytoma

The benign fibrous histiocytoma first was described by Stout and Lattes in 1967. It is seen most often as a soft tissue neoplasm. Occasional bone lesions have been reported, including four cases in the jaws. Dahlin and Unni (1986) examined 8542 bone lesions and found 10 benign fibrous histiocytomas. All patients were adults, and eight had pain in the lesion area. As opposed to the lesions in children and adolescents, which occur in the metaphyses of the long bones, the benign fibrous histiocytoma tends to develop in the diaphysis, epiphysis, or bones with no metaphysis such as the sacrum, ilium, or vertebrae. All of the skeletal lesions produced well-defined radiolucencies; two recurred and necessitated amputation of the involved limbs.

The jaw lesions were reported by Remagen and associates (1986), White and Makar (1986), Liaw and co-authors (1979), and Cale and co-workers (1989). The three mandibular lesions were in the angle-ramus area and were well-defined radiolucencies associated with clinical swelling; extension into the adjacent soft tissues probably occurred in all three cases. The case of Cale and co-authors occurred in the maxillary premolar region of a 13-year-old boy with asymptomatic swelling in the area. The lesion appeared poorly defined, with resorption of the root of the erupted first premolar. Cale and co-authors (1989) pointed out that the fibrous cortical defect in children and nonossifying fibroma in adolescents have been reported as variants of the fibrous histiocytoma in bone. They showed evidence that some bone lesions have a benign fibrohistiocytic appearance histologically, resembling the fibrous cortical defect and nonossifying fibroma, but with different clinical and radiographic features. In summary, they said that benign fibrous histiocytoma can be diagnosed in the jaws under two circumstances: (1) when the tissue exactly resembles one of the two metaphyseal fibrous defects microscopically, but clinically the patient is an adult and has pain or swelling with radiologic evidence of a locally destructive radiolucent lesion, most often in the mandibular angle-ramus area; or (2) when the jaw lesion more exactly resembles the features of the soft tissue benign fibrous histiocytoma on microscopic examination; in this instance, the microscopic features take prevalence over the clinical features in the diagnosis. Their patient was 13 years old and had a painless swelling in the maxillary premolar region, a profile suggestive of the metaphyseal fibrous defects. A case of benign fibrous hystiocytoma may be seen in Figure 13–66.

Malignant Fibrous Histiocytoma

Malignant fibrous histiocytoma (MFH) is the most common malignant mesenchymal tumor in adults, but the incidence of MFH in bones is rather low compared with that in soft tissues. Two reports involving jaw lesions were published by Anavi and colleagues (1989), who reviewed the literature and found 14 cases, and Abdul-Karim and co-workers (1985), who reported 11 new cases from the M. D. Anderson Cancer Center in Houston, Texas. Approximately 25 cases of MFH in the jaws have been reported. At least 5 occurred in teenagers, 2 in newborns or very young children (1.5 years), and 18 in adults. Most patients had swelling or pain and a poorly defined radiolucent lesion in the mandibular ramus. Treatment consists of varying combinations of radiation therapy, chemotherapy, and surgery. The recurrence rate is at least 50%, and metastasis occurs in a minimum of 50%. The 5-year survival rate is almost 50%.

Pathologic Characteristics of Nonossifying Fibroma in the Jaws

According to Liaw and colleagues (1979), the nonossifying fibroma completely lacks osteogenic activity and epithelial elements. The general pattern consists of whorled bundles of spindle-shaped fibroblasts in a connective tissue matrix. Interspersed in this tissue, there are varying numbers of giant cells and xanthic or foam cells. A connective tissue capsule is present. Elzay and colleagues (1984) believed the nonossifying fibroma in the jaws is a reactive fibrous lesion.

Clinical Features

The patients' ages ranged from 11 to 49 years (average, 22 years). Four of the five patients were younger than 21 years of age. All of the lesions occurred in the mandible and were sufficiently posterior to the tooth-bearing areas to eliminate any suspicion of an odontogenic origin. They were all asymptomatic.

Treatment/Prognosis

The lesions were treated by excision or curettage, and no recurrences were reported for follow-up periods ranging from 10 to 36 months.

◆ *RADIOLOGY (Figs. 13–66 and 13–67)*

General Radiologic Features

The nonossifying fibroma has been reviewed by Edeiken (1981) and Makek (1980). It is found most often in the long bones, especially the femur and tibia, and usually is an incidental finding on radiographs. The lesion occurs in the metaphysis toward one end of the bone. It usually extends toward the diaphysis and sometimes the epiphysis. In the beginning, the lesion tends to be eccentric but ultimately may occupy the entire bone diameter. The lesions are multilocular, with a V or U shape at one end. The cortical margin tends to be thin, with slight expansion, and the medullary margin usually is thin and sclerotic. A periosteal reaction is seen only with pathologic fracture; otherwise it is absent. There may be minimal to mild radionuclide uptake. Most radiologists consider this lesion pathognomonic radiologically.

Radiologic Characteristics of Nonossifying Fibroma in the Jaws

All five jaw lesions occurred in the mandible. As explained by Elzay and colleagues (1984), the mandible grows by apposition along the posterior border and concomitant resorption along the anterior border. All five mandibular lesions occurred within this mandibular growth zone.

The first lesion of Elzay and colleagues (1984) was oval and paralleled the long axis of the ramus. The margins were smooth, with slight expansion of the posterior border of the ramus, and a sclerotic margin was present. There were two locules, with the smaller locule at the inferior end having a definite U shape. A second lesion was in the lower central aspect of the ramus. It was multilocular, with an outer periphery consisting of a prominent sclerotic rim ranging from 1 to 3 mm. A distinct and marked V shape was observed at the superior margin of the lesion. The septa forming the locules appeared to be 1 to 3 mm thick, with a density slightly less than that of cortical bone. The case reported by Liaw and colleagues (1979) consisted of an ovoid, unilocular, well-defined radiolucent lesion, occupying much of the angle and lower ramus. No internal bony septa were observed. The cortex was excessively thin and appeared to be absent at the buccal, lingual, and inferior aspects. The periosteum was elevated; however, no periosteal reaction was apparent. Makek's (1980) case was a multilocular eccentric radiolucency at the posterior margin of the condylar neck. The posterior margin did not appear expanded; how-

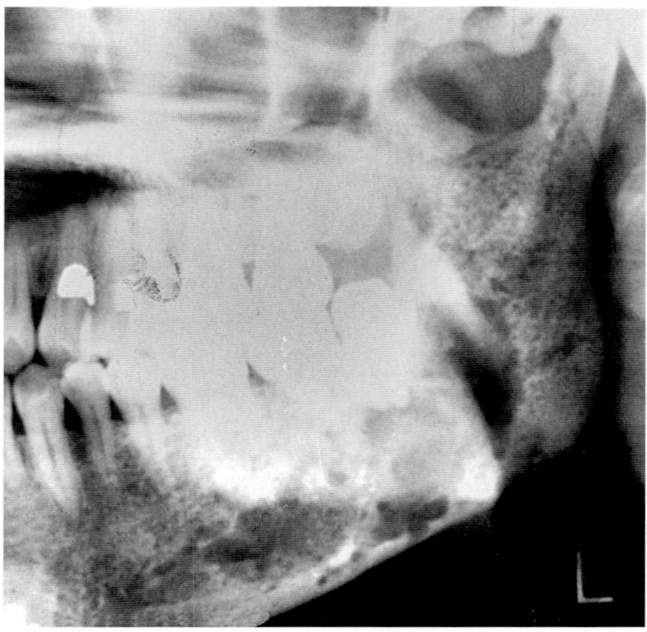

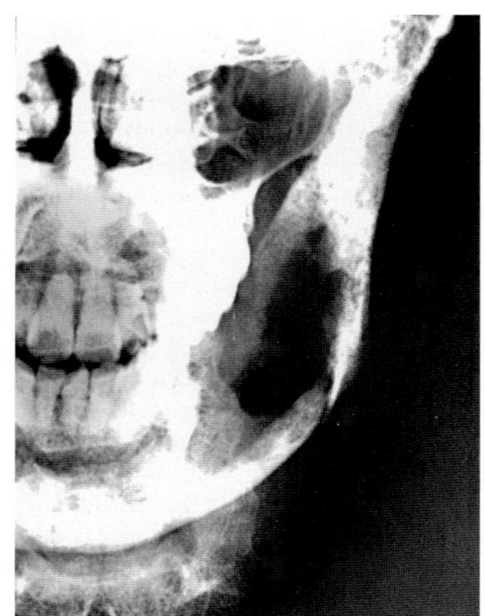

A B

FIGURE 13–66.

Benign fibrous hystiocytoma: Case in a 40-year-old woman, treated by hemimandibulectomy. A, Large area of geographic bone destruction with multiple permeative areas throughout the body and ramus of the mandible. Reactive bone is absent at the margins. B, Posterior-anterior view showing pathologic fracture with no apparent periosteal reaction. (Courtesy of M. Araki and K. Hashimoto, Nihon School of Dentistry, Tokyo, Japan.)

ever, the cortex was thin at its endosteal surface. The margin appeared moderately thick and sclerotic. The trabeculae forming the five locules appeared to have the same density as normal bone in the area. The lesion was 3.5 × 2 × 1 cm and ovoid, with its long axis parallel to the condylar neck. A rounded U shape was seen easily at the inferior leading margin.

CHONDROMYXOID FIBROMA

The chondromyxoid fibroma in the jaws was reported initially by Jaffe and Lichtenstein in 1948. Dahlin (1967) stated that this lesion accounts for 2% of all benign bone tumors in the skeleton. In 1970, Feldman and associates found 199 skeletal lesions. Damm and colleagues (1985) and Lustman

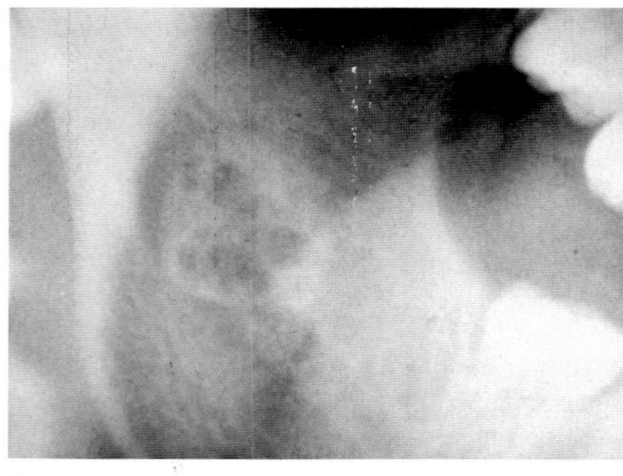

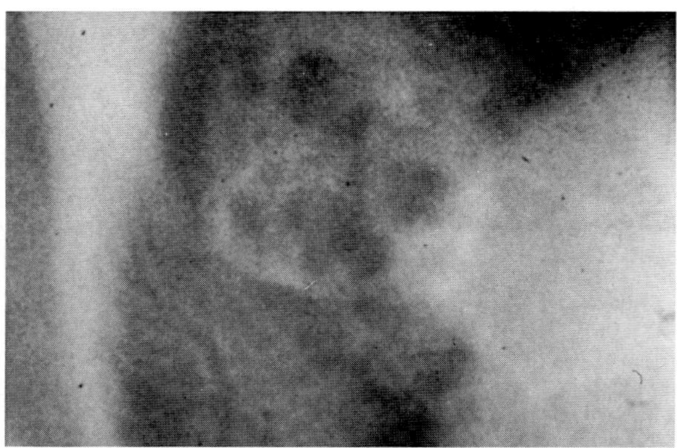

A B

FIGURE 13–67.

Nonossifying fibroma: Case in a 16-year-old girl. A, Multiple locules and thick sclerotic margins. B, Magnified view of the same case showing another lesion developing immediately inferior to the multilocular area. The second lesion has a broad, V-shaped inferior margin, pointing toward the bottom of the illustration. (Courtesy of Dr. G. Taybos, Indianapolis, IN.)

and associates (1986) reviewed the literature; of these cases, approximately 14 occurred in the jaws. For the pathologist, one of the major difficulties with this lesion is differentiating it from chondrosarcoma, which it greatly resembles histologically. Paul's (1951) case in a 67-year-old man was reported as a well-differentiated chondrosarcoma; however, after close scrutiny, this lesion was accepted as a chondromyxoid fibroma. The lesion Grotepass and colleagues (1976) reported as a chondromyxoid fibroma in a 16-year-old white girl ultimately recurred as a chondrosarcoma. Chondromyxoid fibroma is rare in patients younger than 10 years and in those older than 60 years. Most cases occurred in the second and third decades of life. There is a slight preponderance of male patients. The lesion usually grows slowly and does not appear to be aggressive, but pain is a symptom. Jaw lesions have been treated with curettage, enucleation, block excision, and resection. Although the reported recurrence rate of skeletal chondromyxofibromas is 13 to 25%, there is only one documented jaw recurrence, treated by curettage. Because histologic diagnosis is difficult, close scrutiny of the radiographs and radiologic follow-up are suggested for these cases.

◆ *RADIOLOGY (Figs. 13–68 to 13–70)*

Location

All but 2 of the 14 reported jaw lesions occurred in the mandible. Four of the mandibular lesions were in the anterior region, with two in the symphysis. Most of the remaining lesions occurred in the molar-premolar region. One case was in the angle, and the case of Grotepass and colleagues (1976) extended posteriorly from the angle, involving the entire ramus and sparing only the condyle and coronoid process. Both maxillary cases occurred in the lateral incisor region. Toremalm and associates (1976) also reported a case on the posterior wall of the maxillary sinus and involving the pterygopalatine space.

Radiologic Features

All jaw lesions were radiolucent. Reported diameters ranged from 1 to 4.5 cm, with most in the 1- to 2-cm range. Three lesions were multilocular. The case of Grotepass and colleagues (1976) may be seen in Figure 13–68. One case was described as a mottled radiolucency; perhaps flecks of calcific material were evident. Others were described as vague and ill defined, with no mention of internal architecture. Perhaps smaller earlier lesions are predominantly osteolytic, with a sclerotic margin and internal loculations or calcific deposits developing as the lesion matures.

INTRAOSSEOUS ANGIOLIPOMA

This is an extremely rare lesion, with only two cases reported in the jaws. The first was described by Polte (1976) and colleagues and the second by Lewis and associates (1980). As proposed by Lewis and associates (1980), this lesion may represent fatty infiltration of a postsurgical defect, with subsequent or concurrent vascularization. Both cases occurred in middle-aged patients—a 39-year-old man and a 56-year-old woman. In both patients, teeth were extracted from the area. The two patients complained of hyperesthesia of the lower lip.

◆ *RADIOLOGY*

General Radiologic Features

Jaffe (1968) stated that angiolipomatous lesions of the vertebral bodies are common at autopsy. Lichtenstein (1977)

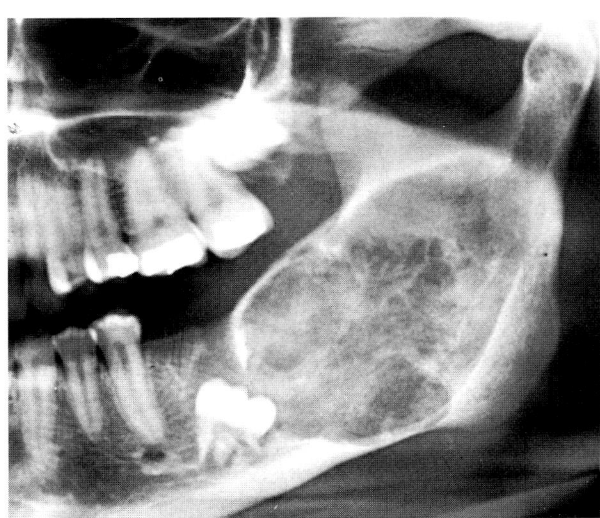

A

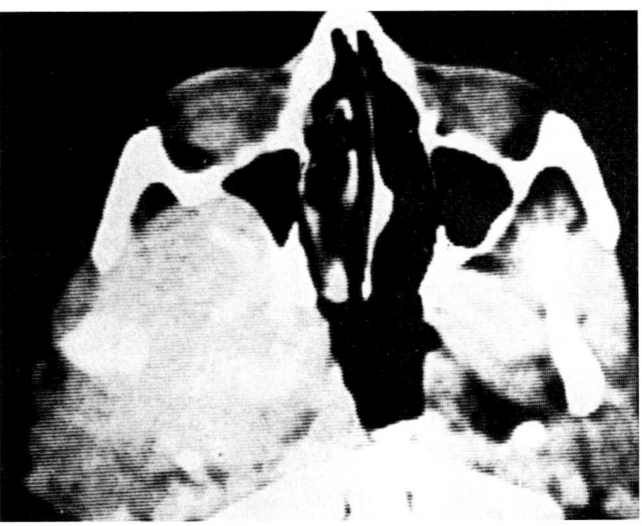

B

FIGURE 13–68.

Chondromyxoid fibroma: A, Presenting lesion with typical features of chondromyxoid fibroma. B, CT image of recurrent lesion in left mandible at level of condyle and infiltrating into maxilla. The recurrent tumor was a chondrosarcoma. (Courtesy of Franz Grotepass, Universiteit von Stellenbosch, Tygerberg, Republic of South Africa.)

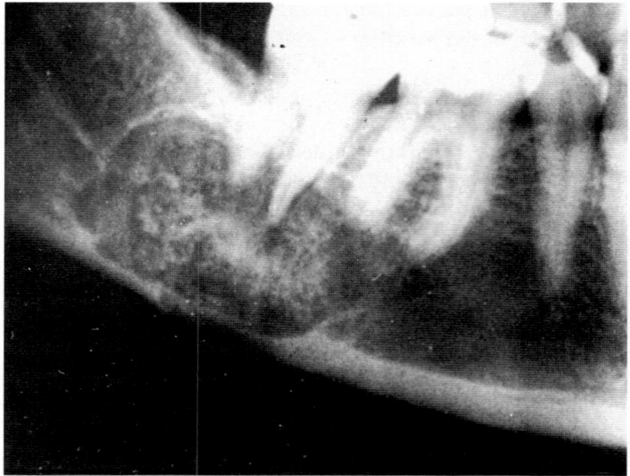

A

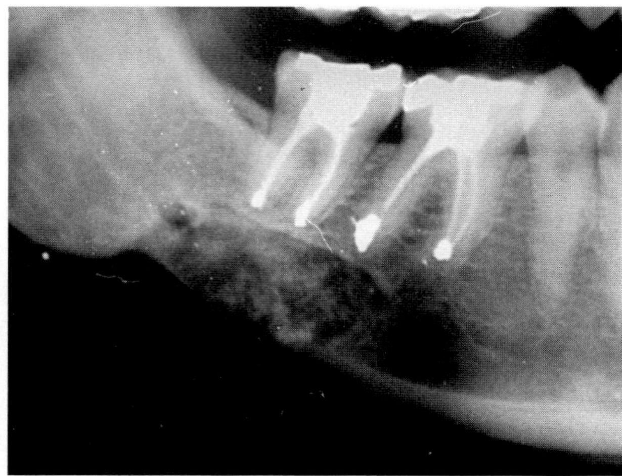

B

FIGURE 13–69.

Chondromyxoid fibroma: A, Presenting lesion. The dotlike appearance of the mineralized flecks greatly resembles the typical calcific foci seen in cartilaginous lesions. The calcific foci group into snowflakelike shapes and have a density somewhat less than or similar to that of bone. B, Recurrent lesion. (From Danielsen B, Ritzau M, Wenzel A: Recurrence of chondromyxoid fibroma: a case report. Dentomaxillofac Radiol 20:65–67, 1991.)

stated that they cause no symptoms and are not seen on radiographs. As Lewis and associates (1980) indicated, they are of interest because of their histologic similarity to the intraosseous angiolipoma and the vertebral body is a common location for hemangioma.

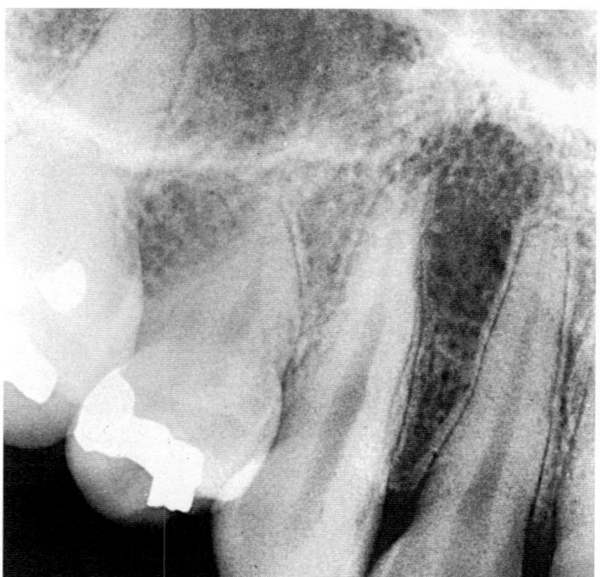

FIGURE 13–70.

Chondromyxoid fibroma: Early lesion in anterior maxilla, between the canine and lateral incisor. The lesional area appears more osteoporotic, with permeative changes within. (From Damm D, et al: Chondromyxoid fibroma of the maxilla. Oral Surg Oral Med Oral Pathol 59:176, 1985.)

Radiologic Features of the Jaws

Both jaw lesions were extensive multilocular radiolucencies in the left mandibular molar area. The case of Lewis and colleagues (1980) extended anteriorly to the canine area. Root resorption was seen in one tooth in the region. Expansion was not reported. The multilocular appearance resembled hyperplastic marrow spaces, but red or fatty marrow was not seen. Some trabeculae at the periphery appeared thin, wispy, and somewhat discontinuous. In the central portion of the lesion, three or four well-opacified striae appeared to radiate from a central point. Although the lesion could be separated clearly from the adjacent normal bone, the margins were not distinct and did not appear corticated.

References

Odontogenic Keratocyst

Altini M, Cohen M: The follicular primordial cyst: odontogenic keratocyst. Int J Oral Surg 11:175, 1982.

Attenborough NR: Recurrence of an odontogenic keratocyst in a bone graft: report of a case. Br J Oral Surg 12:33, 1974.

Brannon RB: The odontogenic keratocyst: a clinicopathologic study of 312 cases. Part I: Clinical features. Oral Surg Oral Med Oral Pathol 42:54, 1976.

Brannon RB: The odontogenic keratocyst: a clinicopathologic study of 312 cases. Part II: Histologic features. Oral Surg Oral Med Oral Pathol 43: 233, 1977.

Browne RM: The odontogenic keratocyst: clinical aspects. Br Dent J 128: 225, 1970.

Browne RM: The odontogenic keratocyst: histological features and their correlation with clinical behavior. Br Dent J 131:249, 1977.

Emerson TG, Whitlock RIH, Jones JH: Involvement of soft tissue vs odontogenic keratocysts (primordial cysts). Br J Oral Surg 9:181, 1972.

Eversole LR, Sabes WR, Rovin S: Aggressive growth and neoplastic potential of odontogenic cysts. Cancer 35:270, 1975.

Gorlin RJ, Goltz RW: Multiple nevoid basal cell epithelioma, jaw cysts and bifid rib syndrome. N Engl J Med 262:908, 1960.
Haring JI, Van Dis ML: Odontogenic keratocysts: a clinical, radiographic, and histopathologic study. Oral Surg Oral Med Oral Pathol 66:145, 1988.
Hjorting-Hansen E, Andreason JO, Robinson LH: A study of odontogenic cysts with special reference to location of keratocysts. Br J Oral Surg 7:15, 1969.
Isberg-Holm A: Odontogenic keratocysts: roentgenological aspects. Dentomaxillofac Radiol 6:17, 1977.
Lund VJ: Odontogenic keratocyst in the maxilla: a case report. Br J Oral Maxillofac Surg 23:210, 1985.
Magnusson BC: Odontogenic keratocysts: a clinical and histological study with special reference to enzyme histochemistry. J Oral Pathol 7:8, 1978.
McIvor J: The radiological features of odontogenic keratocysts. Br J Oral Surg 10:116, 1972.
MacKenzie GD, Oatis GW Jr, Mullen MP, Grisius RJ: Computed tomographs in the diagnosis of an odontogenic keratocyst. Oral Surg Oral Med Oral Pathol 59:302, 1985.
Panders AK, Hadders HN: Solitary keratocysts of the jaws. J Oral Surg 27:931, 1969.
Park TW, Kim SR: Clinical and radiographic study of odontogenic keratocyst. Oral Radiol 1:45, 1985.
Payne TF: An analysis of the clinical and histopathological parameters of the odontogenic keratocyst. Oral Surg Oral Med Oral Pathol 33:538, 1972.
Philipsen HP: Om keratocyster (kolesteatomer) I Kaeberne. Tandlaegebladet 60:963, 1956.
Pindborg JJ, Hansen J: Studies on odontogenic cyst epithelium. Part II: Clinical and roentgenographic aspects of odontogenic keratocysts. Acta Pathol Microbiol Scand 58:283, 1963.
Pindborg JJ, Philipsen HP, Henniksen J: Studies on odontogenic cyst epithelium. Fundamentals of Keratinization, publication no. 70. Washington, DC:American Association for the Advancement of Science, 1962, p. 151.
Rud J, Pindborg JJ: Odontogenic keratocysts: a follow-up study of 21 cases. J Oral Surg 27:323, 1969.
Shear M: Cysts of the Oral Regions. 2nd Ed. Bristol:Wright and Sons, 1983, p. 4.
Shear M: Primordial cysts. J Dent Assoc S Afr 15:211, 1960.
Soskolne WA, Shear M: Observations on the pathogenesis of primordial cysts. Br Dent J 123:321, 1967.
Toller PA: Newer concepts of odontogenic cysts. Int J Oral Surg 1:3, 1972.
Vedtofte P, Praetorius F: Recurrence of the odontogenic keratocyst in relation to the clinical and histological features. Int J Oral Surg 8:412, 1979.
Woo S-K, Eisenbud L, Kleiman M, Assael N: Odontogenic keratocysts in the anterior maxilla: report of two cases, one simulating a nasopalatine cyst. Oral Surg Oral Med Oral Pathol 64:463, 1987.
Wright BA, Wysocki GP, Larder TC: Odontogenic keratocysts presenting as periapical disease. Oral Surg Oral Med Oral Pathol 56:425, 1983.
Wright JM: The odontogenic keratocyst: orthokeratinized variant. Oral Surg Oral Med Oral Pathol 51:609, 1981.

Jaw Cyst-Basal Cell Nevus-Bifid Rib Syndrome

Breytenbach HS, et al: Die klimiese eienskappe en genetiese identiteit von die basaalsel nevus sindrom. S Afr Med J 49:544, 1975.
Cotten S Jr, Super S, Sunder-Ray M, Chaudhry A: Multiple nevoid basal cell carcinoma syndrome. J Oral Med 37:69, Jul-Sept 1982.
Donatsky O, Hjörting-Hansen E, Philipsen HP, Fejerskov O: Clinical, radiologic and histopathologic aspects of 13 cases of nevoid basal cell carcinoma syndrome. Int J Oral Surg 5:19, 1976.
Gorlin RJ, Goltz RW: Multiple nevoid basal-cell epithelioma, jaw cysts and bifid rib. A syndrome. N Engl J Med 262:908, 1960.
Gorlin RJ: Nevoid basal cell carcinoma syndrome. Medicine 66:98, March 1987.
Kamiya Y, et al: Familial odontogenic keratocysts: report of three cases and review of Japanese dental literature. Int J Oral Surg 14:73, 1985.
Van Dijk E, Sanderink JFH: Basal cell carcinoma syndrome. Dermatologica 134:101, 1967.
Woolgar JA, Rippin JW, Browne RM: The odontogenic keratocyst and its occurrence in the nevoid basal cell carcinoma syndrome. Oral Surg Oral Med Oral Pathol 64:727, 1987.

Botryoid Odontogenic Cyst

Greer RO Jr, Johnson M: Botryoid odontogenic cyst: clinicopathologic analysis of ten cases with three recurrences. J Oral Maxillofac Surg 46: 574, 1988.
Kaugars GE: Botryoid odontogenic cyst. Oral Surg Oral Med Oral Pathol 62:555, 1986.
Phelan JA, et al: Recurrent botryoid odontogenic cyst (lateral periodontal cyst). Oral Surg Oral Med Oral Pathol 66:345, 1988.
Standish SM, Shafer WG: The lateral periodontal cyst. J Periodontol 29: 27, 1958.
Weathers DR, Waldron CA: Unusual multilocular cysts of the jaws (botryoid odontogenic cysts). Oral Surg Oral Med Oral Pathol 36:235, 1973.
Wysocki GP, Brannon RB, Gardner DG, Sapp P: Histogenesis of the lateral periodontal cyst and the gingival cyst of the adult. Oral Surg Oral Med Oral Pathol 50:327, 1980.

Odontogenic Sialocyst

Gardner DG, Kessler HP, Morency R, Schaffner DL: The glandular odontogenic cyst: an apparent entity. J Oral Pathol 17:359, 1988.
Gardner DG: Unusual odontogenic cyst (mucous producing odontogenic cyst; sialo-odontogenic cyst). Case from Dr. Renald Morency, Quebec City, Canada. Presented at the IAOP Meeting, The Netherlands, 1984.
Padaychee A, Van Wyk CW: Two cystic lesions with features of both the botryoid odontogenic cyst and the central mucoepidermoid tumor: sialo-odontogenic cyst? J Oral Pathol 16:499, 1987.

Ameloblastoma

Adekeye EO: Ameloblastoma of the jaws: a survey of 109 Nigerian patients. J Oral Surg 38:36, 1980.
Ajagbe HA, Daramola JO: Ameloblastoma: a survey of 199 cases in the University College Hospital, Ibadan, Nigeria. Natl Med Assoc 79:324, 1987.
Buff SJ, Chen JT, Ranin CC, Moore JO: Pulmonary metastasis from ameloblastoma of the mandible: report of a case and review of the literature. J Oral Surg 38:374, 1980.
Cohen MA, Hertzanu Y, Mendelsohn DB: Computed tomography in the diagnosis and treatment of mandibular ameloblastoma: report of cases. J Oral Maxillofac Surg 43:796, 1985.
Cusack JW: Report of amputations of portions of the lower jaw. Dublin Hosp Rec 4:1, 1827.
Dolan EA, Angelillo JC, Georgiade NG: Recurrent ameloblastoma in autogenous rib graft: report of a case. Oral Surg Oral Med Oral Pathol 51: 357, 1981.
Daramola JO, Abioye AA, Ajagbe HA, Aghadiumo PU: Maxillary malignant ameloblastoma with intraorbital extension: report of a case. J Oral Surg 38:203, 1980.
Falksson R: Zur kenntnis der kieferzysten. Virchows Arch [A] 76:504, 1879.
Gardner DG, Marton TH, Warsham JC: Plexiform unicystic ameloblastoma of the maxilla. Oral Surg Oral Med Oral Pathol 63:221, 1987.
Heffez L, Mafee MF, Vaiana J: The role of magnetic resonance imaging in the diagnosis and management of ameloblastoma. Oral Surg Oral Med Oral Pathol 65:2, 1988.
Imai K, et al: Ameloblastoma of the maxilla: report of five cases. Dentomaxillofac Radiol 9:41, 1980.
Ivey RH, Churchill HR: The need of a standardized surgical and pathological classification of tumors and anomalies of dental origin. Am Assoc Dent Sch Trans 7:240, 1930.
Malassez L: Sur le rôle des débris épithéliaux paradentoires. Arch Physiol Norm Pathol 5:309; 6:379, 1885.
Miles DA, Van Dis M, Kaugars GE, Lovas JG: Oral and Maxillofacial Radiology. Philadelphia:WB Saunders, 1991, p. 52.
Regezi JA, Kerr DA, Courtney RM: Odontogenic tumors: analysis of 706 cases. J Oral Surg 36:771, 1978.
Robinson L, Martinez MG: Unicystic ameloblastoma: a prognostically distinct entity. Cancer 40:2278, 1977.
Schaefer SD, et al: Magnetic resonance imaging versus computed tomography: comparison in imaging oral cavity and pharyngeal carcinomas. Arch Otolaryngol 11:730, 1985.
Sehdev MK, et al: Ameloblastoma of the maxilla and mandible. Cancer 33:324, 1974.

Shafer WG, Hine MK, Levy BM: A Textbook of Oral Pathology. 4th Ed. Philadelphia:WB Saunders, 1983, p. 276.

Shteyer A, Lustmann J, Lwin-Epstein J: The mural ameloblastoma: a review of the literature. J Oral Surg 36:866, 1978.

Sirichitra V, Dhiravarangkura P: Intrabony ameloblastoma of the jaws: an analysis of 147 Thai patients. Int J Oral Surg 13:187, 1984.

Slootweg PJ, Müller H: Malignant ameloblastoma or ameloblastic carcinoma. Oral Surg Oral Med Oral Pathol 57:168, 1984.

Small IA, Waldron CA: Ameloblastomas of the jaws. Oral Surg Oral Med Oral Pathol 8:281, 1955.

Tsaknis PJ, Nelson JF: The maxillary ameloblastoma: an analysis of 24 cases. J Oral Surg 38:336, 1980.

Ueno S, Nakamura S, Mushimoto K, Shirasu R: A clinicopathologic study of ameloblastoma. J Oral Maxillofac Surg 44:361, 1986.

Waldron C, El-Mofty S: A histopathologic study of 116 ameloblastomas with special reference to the desmoplastic variant. Oral Surg Oral Med Oral Pathol 63:441, 1987.

Wood NK, Goaz PW: Differential Diagnosis of Oral Lesions. 4th Ed. St. Louis:Mosby-Yearbook, 1991, p. 391.

Woo S-B, Smith-Williams JE, Sciubba JJ, Lipper S: Peripheral ameloblastoma of the buccal mucosa: case report and review of the English literature. Oral Surg Oral Med Oral Pathol 63:78, 1987.

Worth HM: Principles and Practice of Oral Radiologic Interpretation. Chicago:Year Book Medical Publishers, 1983, p. 476.

Odontogenic Myxoma

Adekeye ED, Avery BS, Edwards MB, Williams HK: Advanced central myxoma of the jaws in Nigeria. Int J Oral Surg 13:177, 1984.

Allen PS: Fibro myxoma of the mandible: case report and radiographic considerations. J Am Dent Assoc 101:930, 1980.

Barros RE, Dominquez FV, Cabrini RL: Myxoma of the jaws. Oral Surg Oral Med Oral Pathol 27:225, 1969.

Chuchurru JA, Luberti R, Cormcelli JC, Dominquez FV: Myxoma of the mandible with unusual radiographic appearance. J Oral Maxillofac Surg 43:987, 1985.

Cohen MA, Hertzanu Y: Myxofibroma of the maxilla: a case report with computed tomogram findings. Oral Surg Oral Med Oral Pathol 61:142, 1986.

Farman AG, et al: Myxofibroma of the jaws. Br J Oral Surg 15:3, 1977–1978.

Marcove RC, Kambolis C, Bullogh PG, Jaffe HL: Fibromyxoma of bone. Cancer 17:1209, 1964.

Minderjahn A: Incidence and clinical differentiation of odontogenic tumors. J Maxillofac Surg 7:142, 1979.

Regezi JA, Kerr DA, Courtney RM: Odontogenic tumors: analysis of 706 cases. J Oral Surg 36:771, 1978.

Rennie JS, MacDonald DG, Critchlow HA: Unusual myxomatous odontogenic tumor with calcification. Int J Oral Surg 14:307, 1985.

Stout AP: Myxoma: the tumor of primitive mesenchyme. Ann Surg 127: 706, 1948.

Thoma KH, Goldman HM: Central myxoma of the jaw. Am J Orthod 33: 532, 1947.

Virchow R: Die Krankhaften Geshwulste. Bd. I. Berlin:Verlag August Hirschwald, 1863, p. 369.

White DK, Chen SY, Mohnac AM, Miller AS: Odontogenic myxoma: a clinical and ultrastructural study. Oral Surg Oral Med Oral Pathol 39: 901, 1975.

Central Giant Cell Granuloma

Andersen L, Fejerskov O, Philipsen HP: Oral giant cell granulomas: a clinical and histologic study of 129 new cases. Acta Pathol Microbiol Immunol Scand [A] 81:606, 1973.

Auclair PL, et al: A clinical and histomorphologic comparison of the central giant cell granuloma and giant cell tumor. Oral Surg Oral Med Oral Pathol 66:197, 1988.

Bertheussen KJ, Holck S, Schiodt T: Giant cell lesion of bone in the hand with particular emphasis on giant cell reparative granuloma. J Hand Surg 8:46, 1983.

Bondi R, Urso C, Santucci B, Santucci M: Giant cell lesion of the jaw: case report. Tumori 74:479, 1974.

Caskey P, Wolf MD, Fechner RE: Multicentric giant cell reparative granuloma in the small bones of the hand: a case report and review of the literature. Clin Orthop 193:199, 1985.

Cherrick HM: Presentation to the American Association of Oral and Maxillofacial Surgeons, Las Vegas, Sept 1983.

Chuong R, Raban CB, Kozakewich H, Perez-Atayde A: Central giant cell lesions of the jaws: a clinical pathologic study. J Oral Maxillofac Surg 44:708, 1986.

Cohen MA, Hertzanu Y: Radiologic features including those seen with computed tomography of central giant cell granuloma of the jaws. Oral Surg Oral Med Oral Pathol 65:255, 1988.

Eisenbud L, Stern M, Rothberg M, Sachs SA: Central giant cell granuloma of the jaws: experience in the management of 37 cases. J Oral Maxillofac Surg 46:376, 1988.

Gibilisco JA: Stafne's Oral Radiographic Diagnosis. 5th Ed. Philadelphia: WB Saunders, 1985, p. 221.

Jaffe HL: Giant cell reparative granuloma, traumatic bone cyst and fibrous (fibro-osseous) dysplasia of the jaw bones. Oral Surg Oral Med Oral Pathol 6:159, 1953.

Miles DA, Van Dis M, Kaugars GE, Lovas JG: Oral and Maxillofacial Radiology: Radiologic/Pathologic Correlations. Philadelphia:WB Saunders, 1991, p. 159.

Mintz GA, et al: Primary malignant giant cell tumor of the mandible: report of a case and review of the literature. Oral Surg Oral Med Oral Pathol 51:164, 1981.

Piekarczyk J, Kozlowski K: Central giant cell granuloma in the mandible of children: report of 4 cases. Australas Radiol 28:149, 1984.

Poyton HG: Oral Radiology. Baltimore:Williams & Wilkins, 1982, p. 281.

Sturrock BD, Marks RB, Gross BD, Carr RF: Giant cell tumor of the mandible. J Oral Maxillofac Surg 42:262, 1984.

Waldron CA, Shafer WG: The central giant cell reparative granuloma of the jaws. Am J Clin Pathol 45:437, 1966.

Waldron CA: Giant cell tumors of the jaw bones. Oral Surg Oral Med Oral Pathol 6:1055, 1953.

Aneurysmal Bone Cyst

Bernier JL, Bhaskar SN: Aneurysmal bone cysts of the mandible. Oral Surg Oral Med Oral Pathol 11:1018, 1958.

Bhaskar SN, Bernier JL, Godby F: Aneurysmal bone cyst and other giant cell lesions of the jaws: report of 104 cases. J Oral Surg Anesth Hosp D Serv 17:30, 1959.

Biesecker JL, Marcone RC, Huvos A, Mike V: Aneurysmal bone cysts: a clinicopathologic study of 66 cases. Cancer 26:615, 1970.

Buraczewski J, Dabska P: Pathogenesis of aneurysmal bone cyst: relationship between the aneurysmal bone cyst and fibrous dysplasia of bone. Cancer 28:597, 1971.

Edeiken J, Hodes PJ: Giant cell tumors versus tumors with giant cells. Radiol Clin North Am 1:75, 1963.

Edeiken J: Roentgen Diagnosis of Diseases of Bone. 3rd Ed. Baltimore: Williams & Wilkins, 1981, p. 149.

Eisenbud L, Attie J, Tarlick J, Platt N: Aneurysmal bone cyst of the mandible. Oral Surg Oral Med Oral Pathol 64:202, 1987.

El Deeb M, Sedano HO, White DE: Aneurysmal bone cysts of the jaws. Int J Oral Surg 9:301, 1980.

Jaffe HL, Lichtenstein L: Solitary unicameral bone cyst with emphasis on the roentgenographic picture, pathologic appearance and pathogenesis. Arch Surg 44:1004, 1942.

Levy W, Miller AS, Bonakdarpour A, Aegerter E: Aneurysmal bone cyst secondary to other osseous lesions: report of 57 cases. Am J Clin Pathol 63:1, 1975.

Morton KS: Aneurysmal bone cyst: a review of 26 cases. Can J Surg 29: 110, 1986.

Nadimi H, et al: Aneurysmal bone cyst associated with a dentigerous cyst: report of a case. J Am Dent Assoc 115:859, 1987.

Okuyama T, et al: Diagnosis of aneurysmal bone cyst of the mandible: a report of two cases with emphasis on scintigraphic approaches. Clin Nucl Med 10:786, 1985.

Ruiter DJ, van Rijssel TG, van der Velde EA: Aneurysmal bone cysts: a clinicopathological study of 105 cases. Cancer 39:2231, 1972.

Struthers PJ, Shear M: Aneurysmal bone cyst of the jaws. Part I: Clinicopathological features. Int J Oral Surg 13:85, 1984a.

Struthers PJ, Shear M: Aneurysmal bone cyst of the jaws. Part II: Pathogenesis. Int J Oral Surg 13:92, 1984b.

Tillman BP, Dohlin DC, Liscomb P, Stewart JR: Aneurysmal bone cyst: an analysis of 95 cases. Mayo Clin Proc 43:478, 1968.

Ueno S, et al: Aneurysmal bone cyst of the mandible. J Oral Maxillofac Surg 40:680, 1982.

Veth RPH, et al: Van Buchem's disease and aneurysmal bone cyst: a case history. Arch Orthop Trauma Surg 104:65, 1985.

Central Hemangioma

Anderson JH, Grisius RJ, McKean TW: Arteriovenous malformation of the mandible. Oral Surg Oral Med Oral Pathol 52:118, 1981.

Edeiken S: Roentgen Diagnosis of Diseases of Bone. 3rd Ed. Baltimore: Williams & Wilkins, 1981, p. 127.

Har-El G, Hadar T, Zinkin HY, Sidi J: Hemangioma of the zygoma. Ann Plast Surg 18:533, 1987.

Lamberg MA, Tasanen A, Jääskkeläinen J: Fatality from central hemangioma of the mandible. J Oral Surg 37:578, 1979.

Lund BA, Dahlin DC: Hemangiomas of the mandible and maxilla. J Oral Surg 22:234, 1964.

Maurizi M, Fiumicelli A, Paludetti G, Simoncelli C: Arteriovenous fistula of the mandible: a review of the literature and report of a case. Int J Pediatr Otorhinolaryngol 4:177, 1982.

Sadowsky D, et al: Central hemangioma of the mandible: literature review, case report and discussion. Oral Surg Oral Med Oral Pathol 52:471, 1981.

Shafer WG, Hine MK, Levy BM: A Textbook of Oral Pathology. 4th Ed. Philadelphia:WB Saunders, 1983, p. 156.

Shira RB, Guernsey LH: Central cavernous hemangioma of the mandible: report of a case. J Oral Surg 23:636, 1965.

Singh J, Sidhu BS, Kareta S: Hemangioendothelioma of the mandible: report of a case. J Oral Surg 35:673, 1977.

Thorn JJ, Worsage N, Gyldensted C: Arterial embolization in the treatment of central hemangiomas of the maxilla: report of two cases. Br J Oral Maxillofac Surg 24:114, 1986.

Watson SL, McCarthy WD: Blood and lymph vessel tumors. Surg Gynecol Obstet 71:569, 1940.

Worth HM: Principles and Practice of Oral Radiologic Interpretation. Chicago:Year Book Medical Publishers, 1963, p. 522.

Worth HM, Stoneman DW: Radiology of vascular abnormalities in and about the jaws. Dent Radiogr Photogr 52:1, 1979.

Arteriovenous Malformation

Anderson JH, Grisius RJ, McKean TW: Arteriovenous malformation of the mandible. Oral Surg Oral Med Oral Pathol 52:118, Aug 1981.

Gelfand G, Dixon RA, Gans BJ: Central cavernous hemangioma of the mandible. J Oral Surg 33:448, 1975.

Gomez MMR: Arteriovenous fistula: review of 10 year experience at the Mayo Clinic. Mayo Clinic Proc 45:81, 1970.

Halazonitis JA, Kountouris J, Halazonitis NA: Arteriovenous aneurysm of the mandible: report of a case. Oral Surg Oral Med Oral Pathol 53:454, 1982.

Holman E: Contributions to cardiovascular physiology gleaned from clinical and experimental observations of abnormal arteriovenous communications. J Cardiovasc Surg 3:48, 1962.

Kelly DE, Terry BC, Small EW: Arteriovenous malformation of the mandible: report of a case. J Oral Surg 35:387, 1977.

Maurizi M, Fiumicelli A, Paludetti G, Simoncelli C: Arteriovenous fistula of the mandible: a review of the literature and report of a case. Int J Pediatr Otorhinolaryngol 4:171, 1982.

Miles DA, Van Dis M, Kaugars G, Lovas JG: Oral and Maxillofacial Radiology: Radiologic/Pathologic Correlations. Philadelphia:WB Saunders, 1991, p. 173.

Orbach S: Congenital arteriovenous malformations of the face: report of a case. Oral Surg Oral Med Oral Pathol 42:2, July 1976.

Sadowsky D, et al: Central hemangioma of the mandible: literature review, case report and discussion. Oral Surg Oral Med Oral Pathol 52:471, 1981.

Schultz RE, Kempf KK, George ED: Treatment of a central arteriovenous malformation of the mandible with cyanoacrylate: a 4-year follow-up. Oral Surg Oral Med Oral Pathol 65:267, 1988.

Shafer WG, Hine MK, Levy BM: A Textbook of Oral Pathology. Philadelphia:WB Saunders, 1983, p. 154.

Spatz S, Kaltman S, Farber S: Vascular malformation: report of a case with eight-year follow-up. J Oral Maxillofac Surg 43:281, 1985.

Svane TJ, Smith BR, Wolford LM, Pace LL: Arteriovenous malformation of the mandible and its treatment: a case report. Oral Surg Oral Med Oral Pathol 67:379, 1989.

Worth HM: Principles and Practice of Oral Radiologic Interpretation. Chicago:Year Book Medical Publishers, 1963, p. 522.

Zou Z, et al: Clinical application of angiography of oral and maxillofacial hemangiomas: clinical analysis of seventy cases. Oral Surg Oral Med Oral Pathol 55:437, 1983.

Cherubism

Anderson BE, McClenden JC: Cherubism: hereditary fibrous dysplasia of the jaws. Part I: Genetic considerations. Oral Surg Oral Med Oral Pathol 15:5, 1962.

Bianchi SD, Boecardi A, Mela F, Romagnoli R: The computed tomographic appearances of cherubism. Skeletal Radiol 16:60, 1987.

Davis GB, Sinn DP, Watson SW: Cherubism: clinicopathologic conferences. J Oral Maxillofac Surg 41:119, 1983.

Jones WA: Familial multilocular cystic disease of the jaws. Am J Cancer 17:946, 1933.

Peters WJN: Cherubism: a study of twenty cases from one family. Oral Surg Oral Med Oral Pathol 47:307, 1979.

Reade PC, McKellar GM, Radden BG: Unilateral mandibular cherubism: brief review and case report. Br J Oral Maxillofac Surg 22:189, 1984.

Central Odontogenic Fibroma

Couch RD, Morris EE, Vellios F: Granular cell ameloblastic fibroma: report of 2 cases in adults with observations on its similarity to the congenital epulis. Am J Clin Pathol 37:398, 1962.

Dahl EC, Walfson SH, Haugen JC: Central odontogenic fibroma: review of literature and report of cases. J Oral Surg 39:120, 1981.

Gardner DG: The central odontogenic fibroma: an attempt at clarification. Oral Surg Oral Med Oral Pathol 50:425, 1980.

Heimdal A, Isacsson G, Nilsson L: Recurrent central odontogenic fibroma. Oral Surg Oral Med Oral Pathol 50:140, 1980.

Sepheriadou-Mavropoulou TH, Patrikiou A, Sotiriadou S: Central odontogenic fibroma. Int J Oral Surg 14:550, 1985.

Shafer WG, Hine MK, Levy BM: A Textbook of Oral Pathology. 4th Ed. Philadelphia:WB Saunders, 1983, p. 294.

Vincent SD, Hammond HL, Ellis GL, Juhlin JP: Central granular cell odontogenic fibroma. Oral Surg Oral Med Oral Pathol 63:715, 1987.

Wesley RK, Wysocki GP, Mintz SH: The central odontogenic fibroma. Oral Surg Oral Med Oral Pathol 40:235, 1975.

Desmoplastic Fibroma

Ackermann LV, Rosai J: Surgical Pathology. 5th Ed. St. Louis:CV Mosby, 1974, p. 1065.

Crim J, et al: Desmoplastic fibroma of bone: radiographic analysis. Radiology 172:827, 1989.

Dahlin DC, Unni KK: Bone Tumors: General Aspects and Data on 8542 Cases. 4th Ed. Springfield, IL:Charles C Thomas, 1986, p. 375.

Freedman PD, Cardo VA, Kerpel SM, Lummerman H: Desmoplastic fibroma (fibromatosis) of the jawbones: report of a case and review of the literature. Oral Surg Oral Med Oral Pathol 46:386, 1978.

Griffith JG, Irby WB: Desmoplastic fibroma: report of a rare tumor of the oral structures. Oral Surg Oral Med Oral Pathol 20:269, 1965.

Hashimoto K, et al: Desmoplastic fibroma of the maxillary sinus: report of a case and review of the literature. Oral Surg Oral Med Oral Pathol 72:126, 1991.

Jaffe HL: Tumors and Tumorous Conditions of the Bones and Joints. Philadelphia:Lea & Febiger, 1958, p. 298.

Van Blarcom CW, Masson JK, Dahlin DC: Fibrosarcoma of the mandible. Oral Surg Oral Med Oral Pathol 32:4289, 1971.

Bone Tumor Registry in Japan: The Incidence of Bone Tumors in Japan: 1985. Tokyo:Tokyo National Cancer Center, 1985, p. 134.

Non-ossifying Fibroma

Abdul-Karim FW, et al: Malignant fibrous histiocytoma of the jaws: a clinicopathologic study of 11 cases. Cancer 56:1590, 1985.

Agazzi C: Nonosteogenic fibroma of the jaw. Ann Otol Rhinol Laryngol 60:365, 1951.

Anavi Y, Herman GE, Graybill S, MacIntosh RB: Malignant fibrous histiocytoma of the mandible. Oral Surg Oral Med Oral Pathol 68:436, 1989.

Cale AE, Freedman PD, Kerpel SM, Lumerman H: Benign fibrous histiocytoma of the maxilla. Oral Surg Oral Med Oral Pathol 68:444, 1989.

Dahlin DC, Unni KK: Bone Tumors: General Aspects and Data on 8542 Cases. 4th Ed. Springfield, IL:Charles C Thomas, 1986, p. 141.

Edeiken J: Roentgen Diagnosis of Diseases of Bone. 3rd Ed. Baltimore: Williams & Wilkins, 1981, p. 113.
Elzay RP, Mills S, Kay S: Fibrous defect (non ossifying fibroma) of the mandible. Oral Surg Oral Med Oral Pathol 58:402, 1984.
Jaffe HL, Lichtenstein L: Non-osteogenic fibroma of bone. Am J Pathol 18:205, 1942.
Liaw WJ, So TK, Yao YT: Non-ossifying fibroma of the mandible. J Formosan Med Assoc 78:795, 1979.
Makek M: Non-ossifying fibroma of the mandible. Arch Orthop Trauma Surg 96:225, 1980.
Remagen W, Nidecker A, Prein J: Case report 359. Skeletal Radiol 15: 251, 1986.
Rudy NR, Scheingold SS: Solitary xanthogranuloma of the mandible. Oral Surg Oral Med Oral Pathol 18:262, 1964.
Stout AP, Lattes R: Tumors of soft tissue. Atlas of Tumor Pathology. Section II, Fascicle I. Washington, DC: Armed Forces Institute of Pathology, 1967, p. 38.
Sutton D: A Textbook of Radiology. 2nd Ed. Edinburgh:Churchill Livingstone, 1975, p. 138.
White RD, Makar J: Xanthofibroma of the mandible. J Oral Maxillofac Surg 44:1010, 1986.

Chondromyxoid Fibroma

Dahlin DC: Chondromyxoid Fibroma: Bone Tumors. 2nd Ed. Springfield, IL:Charles C. Thomas, 1967, p. 48.
Damm D, et al: Chondromyxoid fibroma of the maxilla. Oral Surg Oral Med Oral Pathol 59:176, 1985.
Feldman F, Hecht HL, Johnston MD: Chondromyxoid fibroma of bone. Radiology 94:249, 1970.
Grotepass FW, Farman AG, Nortjé CJ: Chondromyxoid fibroma of the mandible. J Oral Surg 34:988, 1976.
Jaffe HL, Lichtenstein L: Chondromyxoid fibroma of bone: distinctive benign tumor likely to be mistaken for chondrosarcoma. Arch Pathol 45: 541, 1948.
Lustmann J, Gazit D, Ulmansky M, Lewin-Epstein J: Chondromyxoid fibroma of the jaws: a clinicopathologic study. J Oral Pathol 15:343, 1986.
Paul JK: Chondromyxosarcoma of the mandible. J Oral Surg 9:319, 1951.
Toremalm NG, Lindstrom C, Malm L: Clinical records: chondromyxoid fibroma of the pterygopalatine space. J Laryngol Otol 90:971, 1976.

Intraosseous Angiolipoma

Jaffe HL: Tumors and Tumorous Conditions of Bones and Joints. Philadelphia:Lea & Febiger, 1968, p. 224.
Lewis DM, Brannon RB, Isaksson B, Larsson A: Intraosseous angiolipoma of the mandible. Oral Surg Oral Med Oral Pathol 50:156, Aug 1980.
Lichtenstein L: Bone Tumors. 5th Ed. St. Louis:CV Mosby, 1977, p. 160.
Polte HW, Kolodny SC, Hooker SP: Intraosseous angiolipoma of the mandible. Oral Surg Oral Med Oral Pathol 41:637, 1976.

Chapter 14

Poorly Defined Radiolucencies

CHRONIC RAREFYING OSTEOMYELITIS

Osteomyelitis is an inflammatory reaction of bone and bone marrow that clinically produces pus. It is an inflammation of the soft parts of the medullary and haversian systems and extends to involve the periosteum. The calcified portion takes no active part in the process, but it is affected secondarily by the loss of blood supply; as a consequence, a greater or lesser portion of the bone dies. In less advanced societies, it usually is caused by gram-positive microorganisms; the most common are Staphylococcus aureus and Staphylococcus epidermidis, which are estimated to be responsible for 80 to 90% of cases of osteomyelitis of the jaws; mixed bacterial cultures, hemolytic streptococcus, pneumococcus, typhoid and acid-fast bacilli, Escherichia coli, and actinomyces account for the remaining infections. In modern societies there has been a decline in the predominance of staphylococcal osteomyelitis. It is thought to be attributed to the use of antibiotics and improved diagnostic methods. For instance, only half of the cases of osteomyelitis of the jaws are believed to be caused by Staphylococcus aureus, and the remainder are attributed to anaerobes, particularly Bacteroides fragilis and melaninogenicus, fusobacteria, anaerobic cocci, and gram-negative organisms such as klebsiella, pseudomonas, and proteus. Therefore, samples of bone and pus must be obtained for both aerobic and anaerobic culture. In a series reported by Silberman and associates (1974), 40% of the patients were infected with gram-negative bacilli; 35% had streptococcus as the predominant organism, and only 20% had staphylococcus as the major or only pathogen. They suggested that some gram-negative infections, especially in the mandible, originate from the patient's own microbiota but most result from nosocomial infections (originating in the hospital).

Osteomyelitis may be acute or chronic, suppurative or nonsuppurative and may involve various reactions of bone. In the acute stage there are little or no visible effects on the bone radiologically; in the chronic stage a variety of bone responses are possible. It can produce radiopaque lesions such as those seen in focal sclerosing osteomyelitis, chronic diffuse sclerosing osteomyelitis, or Garrè's osteomyelitis. The brief discussion in this chapter will be limited to a reaction that involves lysis of bone and is termed chronic rarefying osteomyelitis. Osteomyelitis may be hematogenous or blood borne in origin or nonhematogenous with an associated contiguous focus of infection. In children and adolescents, osteomyelitis usually results from hematogenous infection, the common causative organism being Staphylococcus aureus. The bones most often affected in hematogenous osteomyelitis are the femur and tibia because of their exposure to trauma and strain, followed by the humerus. In adults hematogenous infection is rare, and when it does occur the disease is much less severe. Osteomyelitis of the jaws is usually nonhematogenous in origin and often follows periapical and periodontal infections and trauma, especially compound fractures.

Pathologic Characteristics

Osteomyelitis is a rare disease in normal healthy people living in modern society. Systemic diseases with accompanying changes in host defenses may influence the onset and course of the disease. Osteomyelitis is associated with diabetes, agranulocytosis, neutropenias, leukemia, uremias, sickle cell anemia, severe anemia, febrile diseases such as typhoid, malnutrition, traumas, complications of fractures, and previous ionizing radiation to the bone. Silberman and colleagues (1974) reported an increased frequency of osteomyelitis in chronic alcoholics and drug abusers. Furthermore, certain diseases that alter the vascularity of bone may predispose someone to osteomyelitis (e.g., osteoporosis, Paget's disease, fibrous dysplasia, bone malignancy, and bone necrosis resulting from mercury, bismuth, and arsenic exposure). Steroids and immunosuppressive drugs also increase the susceptibility to osteomyelitis by decreasing the ability of the host to limit the infection.

The microorganisms cause an intense inflammatory reaction within the bone marrow, which will produce hyperemia, increased capillary permeability, and infiltration of chiefly neutrophilic polymorphonuclear leukocytes and occasional lymphocytes and plasma cells. Proteolytic enzymes are liberated, causing the destruction of bacteria and vascular thrombosis, which in turn results in tissue necrosis. Pus is produced and will travel through the haversian and nutrient canals and accumulate beneath the periosteum; it lifts the periosteum from the bone and, at the same time, makes its way along the outside of the bone. From there the pus may penetrate the Volkmann's canals, which are small vascular channels that run at right angles to the surface of the bone, and infect bone marrow in an adjacent area. Because of the inflammatory swelling, there is a great increase in tension within the rigid walls of the cancellous spaces and the haversian canals so vessels are compressed and their lumina obliterated. This results in vascular collapse, venous stasis, and thrombosis. Several factors—(1) the raising of the periosteum from the bone that it supplies with blood, (2) the increased tension and vascular compression within the bony canals, and (3) the resultant thrombosis—have one effect in common: They cut off the blood supply from the calcified portion of the bone, resulting in bone death.

After variable periods of time, when the disease has become chronic, portions of dead bone become partially or completely separated from the host bone. These fragments are covered with granulation tissue, which occupies the site of destruction. The separated or partially separated dead bone, called sequestrum, can be lifted out freely when exposed at surgery.

Meanwhile, the periosteum is not inactive. Although it has been separated from the bone, some of the cells of the osteogenic layer usually survive, and, when the acuteness of the infection is past, osteoblasts lay down new bone over the sequestrum to form a sheath or case of new bone called the involucrum. Surgical removal of too much of the involucrum may lead to fracture of the jaw, and if displacement of fragments occurs, it may be difficult to replace and maintain the bone fragments in position.

If the infection is very severe, all the osteoblasts may be destroyed so that no new bone is formed. The involucrum becomes perforated, and these small holes form tracts or cloacae through which pus passes from the sequestrum to the epithelial surface, which may be red because of inflammation.

Clinical Features

There is a history of a debilitating systemic disease or fractures in chronic rarefying osteomyelitis. According to Wood and Goaz (1978), the male-to-female incidence of osteomyelitis is 5:1, and the usual age is between 30 and 80 years. Osteomyelitis is found more frequently in men because they are involved in traumatic episodes more often and their bones are usually denser. The mandible is affected three times more frequently than the maxilla, and the prominent regions are the mandibular premolar-molar region and symphysis. The mandible is involved more often than the maxilla for the following reasons: mandibular bone is much less vascular than the maxilla; spontaneous drainage is initiated more readily in the maxilla because the cortical plates are thinner; and the body of the mandible is the most common site of compound fractures.

The chief complaint is tenderness or pain and swelling over the affected area. The patient may experience trismus if there is spread to a muscle of mastication. Regional lymphadenopathy is a constant finding. The patient's temperature will be elevated, and he or she may be dehydrated. A sinus from an abscess within the bone frequently will open on the face or mucosal surface. There may be pain and tenderness on palpation, and the bone may appear swollen. This swelling results from the formation of pus or edema under considerable pressure beneath the periosteum. The overlying soft tissues often have a reddish surface. Pressure on the swelling may cause the expression of pus from a sinus opening. The patient may complain of fetid breath, and the teeth may be mobile and sensitive to percussion. Paresthesia and anesthesia of the lip are common developments in cases of mandibular involvement, probably because of compression of the neurovascular bundle.

Treatment/Prognosis

First, it must be determined whether an underlying debilitating systemic disease is present; if so, the disease must be controlled with the cooperation of the patient's physician as soon as possible. Laboratory tests are helpful in establishing a diagnosis of chronic osteomyelitis of the jaws or underlying predisposing systemic disease. The leukocyte count will be moderately elevated and the erythrocyte sedimentation rate may be slightly elevated.

Therapy for chronic osteomyelitis of the jaws should include a combined therapeutic and surgical approach consisting of 6 weeks of parenteral antibiotics and removal of devitalized bone. Surgery should include the removal of persistently loose teeth or sequestra. If an open wound is present, it must be irrigated frequently with a solution of 3% hydrogen peroxide and normal saline (1:1). Oral hygiene must be excellent. In addition, oral antibiotic therapy is given for another 2 to 6 months. Topazian (1981) suggested that specimens must be obtained for Gram's staining, and aerobic and anaerobic cultures for sensitivity testing. As soon as these results are available, specific antibiotic therapy should be initiated in adequate doses for a suitable period of time. If the stain shows a predominance of gram-positive cocci in clumps suggestive of staphylococcus, penicillinase-resistant penicillin alone is recommended. Continued drainage from fistulas and failure to form sequestra may indicate a need to change antibiotics. A gram-stained slide consisting predominantly of gram-negative rods establishes a working diagnosis of an anaerobic bacteroides infection; initially, aqueous penicillin is given intravenously, followed by oral penicillin V after systemic signs have subsided. If both gram-positive cocci in clumps and gram-negative rods are seen, both penicillin and penicillinase-resistant penicillin should be given. If the patient is allergic to penicillin, clindamycin is recommended as a first alternate because it is effective against penicillinase-producing staphylococci, streptococci, and anaerobic bacteria, including bacteroides; if colitis develops it is usually transient and resolves on withdrawal of the medication. Cephalosporins are not recommended as the primary substitute for penicillin allergy because they are only moderately effective against oral anaerobes and their broad-spectrum coverage increases antibiotic complications.

Nakajima and associates (1977) suggested that surgical saucerization may be necessary if drainage continues through the sinus despite appropriate antibiotic coverage. If too much bone is lost, a bone graft may be required. Hart and Mainous (1976), Goupil and colleagues (1978), and Young and Bump (1978) have reported that the use of hyperbaric oxygen in conjunction with antibiotics has proved to be extremely beneficial in treating chronic osteomyelitis.

◆ *RADIOLOGY (Figs. 14–1 to 14–6)*

General Features

In the acute and subacute phases, a variable-sized region will begin to show lysis at approximately 7 days. The affected part is generally warm, red, and tender. Pus builds up until vessels are occluded, leading to focal bone infarction and sequestra of dead bone form. The pus permeates from the haversian system, lifting up the periosteum in the process. By 2 weeks after inception, the periosteum begins to lay down reactive bone, referred to as the involucrum. If the pressure within the periosteum is high enough, the cortical vessels will close, causing cortical bone sequestration. The edema from the infection imparts a grayish foggy appearance

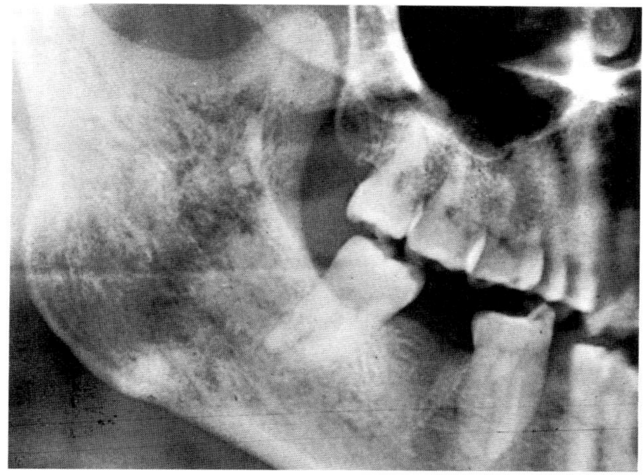

FIGURE 14–1.

Chronic Rarefying Osteomyelitis: The early changes are permeative and tractlike areas in ramus.

that obscures normal bone and fat shadows in the radiograph. This is a valuable radiologic sign because malignant tumors rarely cause this degree of soft tissue edema. Chronic rarefying osteomyelitis appears as a thickened, irregular region of sclerotic bone containing several radiolucent areas and an elevated periosteum. Uncommonly, a lytic area may develop rapidly at the site of a chronic draining sinus.

Positive findings may be seen on the bone scan 24 hours after onset, whereas conventional radiographic changes may not be seen until 7 to 14 days. The role of the bone scan includes early detection, differentiation of osteomyelitis from cellulitis, and identification of renewed activity in cases of chronic osteomyelitis. The standard technique is the use of technetium phosphate. Localized increased radioisotope uptake in the involved area is seen as a positive finding. If the technetium phosphate bone scan shows normal findings in patients with suspected osteomyelitis, a ^{67}Ga scan is indicated. Gallium is less dependent than technetium on blood flow; thus, it may localize the site of infection before the technetium phosphate scan.

The angiographic features of acute osteomyelitis are similar to those of other infections. There are dilated arteries, veins, and capillaries. Gradually, with progression of the disease and the development of necrosis, the angiographic picture will change.

Computed tomography (CT) scans can show more cortical sequestra, cloacae, and soft tissue abscesses than conventional radiographs. Ram and colleagues (1981) stated that, with CT scans, the detection of gas within the medullary spaces is an infrequent but reliable diagnostic sign of osteomyelitis that may not be evident on plain film radiographs; it is analogous to the presence of gas within soft tissue abscesses.

The sensitivity of magnetic resonance imaging (MRI) to the detection of acute osteomyelitis is greater than that of plain film radiography and CT, although the specificity of the technique is not clear. According to Runge (1992), MRI has been found to be very sensitive for detecting osteomyelitis. Unfortunately, the MRI findings are unspecific, and it can be difficult to differentiate osteomyelitis from trauma or a neoplasm.

Radiologic Features of the Jaws

Bone changes consistent with chronic osteomyelitis may not be seen for at least 7 days or longer after the onset of acute symptoms and may be delayed for as long as 1 month. It generally is considered that there must be a loss of 30 to 60% of the mineral content of bone for the radiographs to show any change. The earliest radiographic change is seen in the trabeculae in the involved area; they become thin, of poor density, and slightly unsharp or blurred. It appears as though the film has been wiped when wet, making the trabeculae appear fuzzy. The trabeculae soon lose their continuity and opacity, and frank destruction of bone becomes apparent. Periosteal elevation usually occurs at the same time the osteolytic lesions become evident. The radiolucent lytic areas are usually irregular in character, with ragged and poorly defined borders separated by islands of normal-appearing bone. Such islands of normal or nearly normal bone, separated by irregular areas of bone destruction, present a radiographic picture that is highly suggestive of osteomyelitis. The bone often takes on a ''motheaten'' appearance because of the enlargement of the medullary spaces and widening of the Volkmann's canals subsequent to bone destruction and its replacement with granulation tissue. With the passage of time, there is a tendency for the radiolucent areas to become confluent and enlarge at the expense of the islands.

Osteomyelitis of the mandible sometimes overwhelms the greater part of the bone, and large portions may die quickly. The result is the formation of large sequestra and sometimes a few smaller ones. Dark lines appear at the sites of separation of the dead fragments or sequestra from living bone. Later, after removal of the dead bone, a structureless gray space remains in which it is not yet possible to see any evidence of new bone, although there is probably some involucrum present.

Periosteal new bone formation is not sufficiently marked in most adults to produce more than a slight suggestion of a gray shadow parallel to the inferior margin of the mandible. In some adults there is a well-formed sheath of new bone (involucrum), and one or more cloacae (holes for drainage) may be seen in occlusal radiographs as dark linear shadows passing from the surface of the bone to the depths, where a sequestrum is usually visible. Bone sclerosis and new bone formation usually suggest that the disease has been present for longer than 1 month.

It is sometimes important to determine whether a bone fragment is vital, and in some cases help may be obtained from radiographic examinations. Bone that is inflamed tends to lose calcium, a condition known as hyperemic decalcification. This can occur only if there are blood vessels present that permit the removal of the calcium. If the fragments of bone become increasingly radiolucent during a 3-week period, it is reasonable to assume that there is still a blood supply to the fragment. If the fragment retains its density, this suggests that the fragment has lost its blood supply and has become a sequestrum.

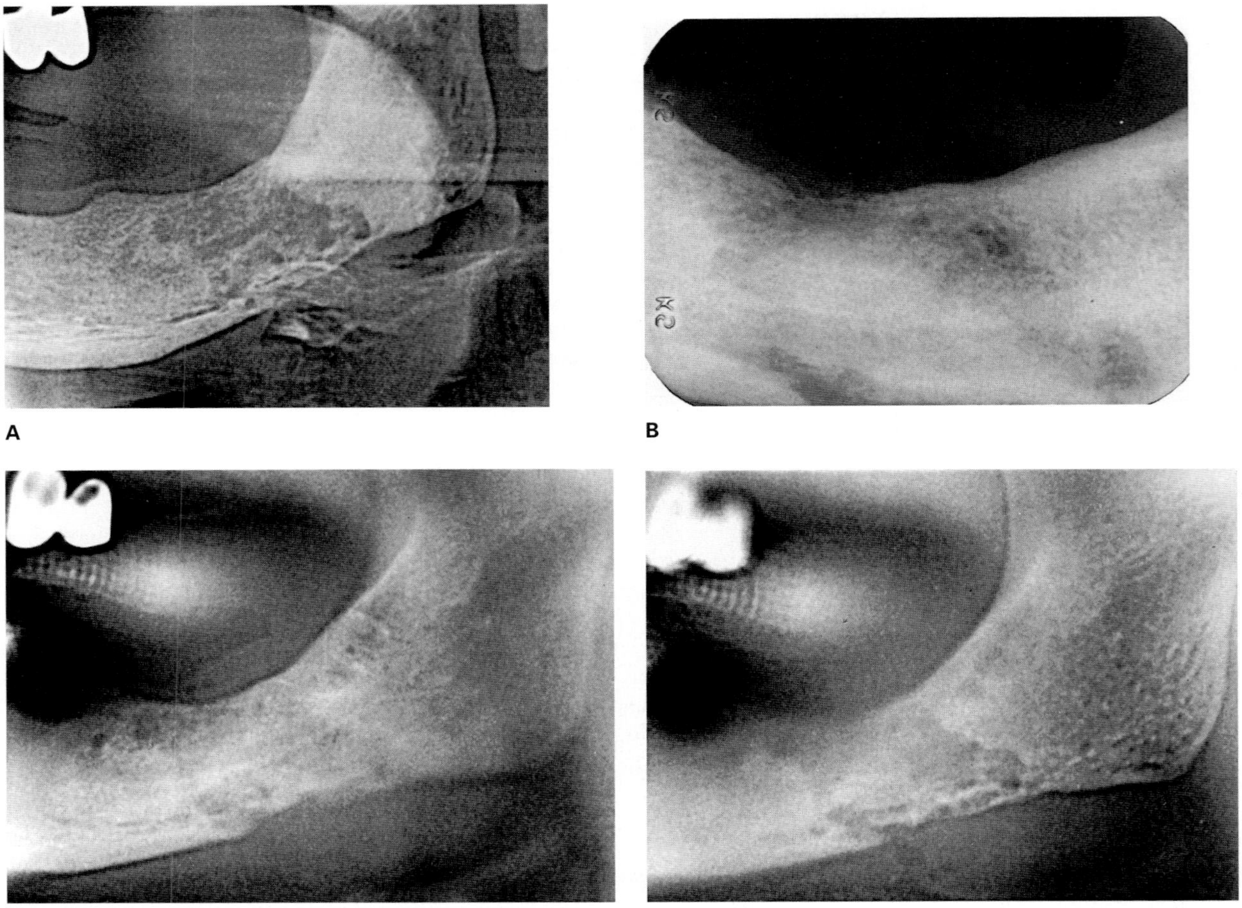

A

B

C

D

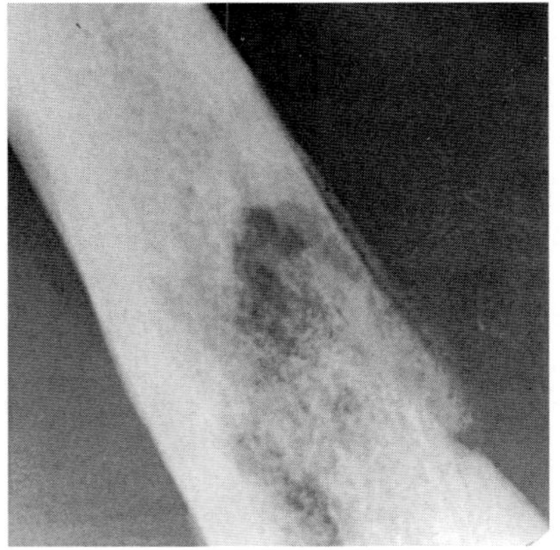

E

FIGURE 14–2.

Chronic Rarefying Osteomyelitis in a 63-year-old Man: A, Panoramic radiograph shows geographic area of bone demineralization with several motheaten areas within and erosion of cortex. Image is sharp because of digital reprocessing. B, Periapical radiograph shows haziness of structures resulting from edema. Rarefied areas appear more confluent, forming a central island of bone susceptible to infarction. C, The lingual tomogram is similar to the panoramic radiograph (A). D, Buccal tomogram shows possible infarction because sequestrum is of same density as surrounding bone. E, Occlusal radiograph shows permeative and motheaten changes, fistula for drainage, and periosteal reaction. (Courtesy of Professor T. Noikura, Kagoshima University First Oral Surgery Department, Kagoshima, Japan.)

OSTEORADIONECROSIS OF JAWS

Osteoradionecrosis (ORN) is a pathologic process that sometimes follows heavy irradiation of bone and is characterized by a chronic, painful necrosis accompanied by late sequestration and sometimes permanent deformity. ORN first was reported by Regaud in 1922. The pathology of ORN first was described by Ewing in 1926 under the name radiation osteitis. McLenna (1955) reported that ORN of the jaws became a frequent finding in the 1950s as irradiation of oral malignant neoplasms became a well-established practice. Orthovoltage radiation ranging from 150 to 250 keV was used before the 1960s. The absorbed dose at this energy level has a greater damaging effect on bone than soft tissue; consequently, orthovoltage is used infrequently today. More recently, megavoltage with an energy level of 1.2 meV, commonly obtained from cobalt 60 teletherapy, and the linear accelerator with a photon energy of 6.7 meV have supplanted

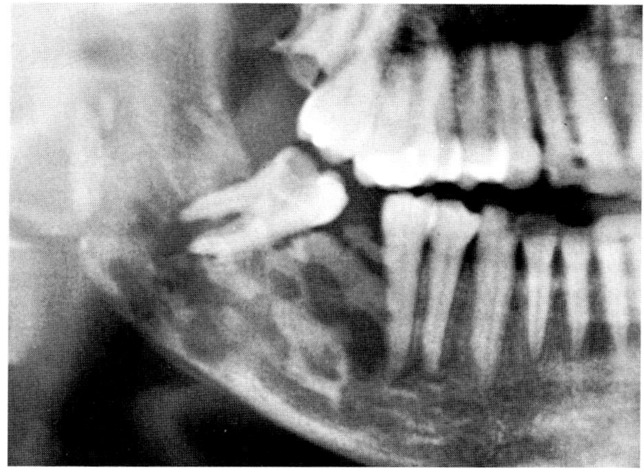

A

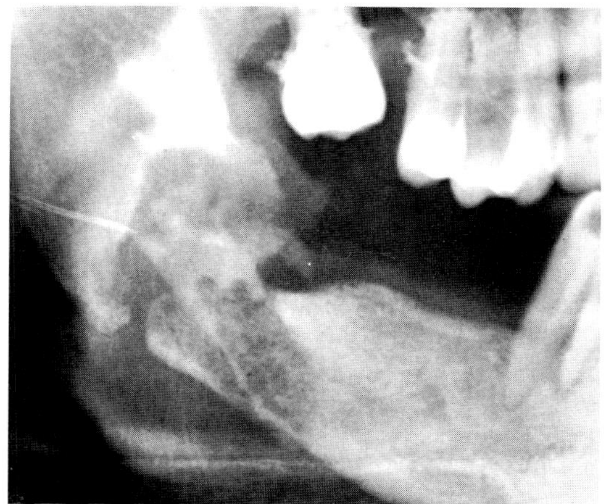

B

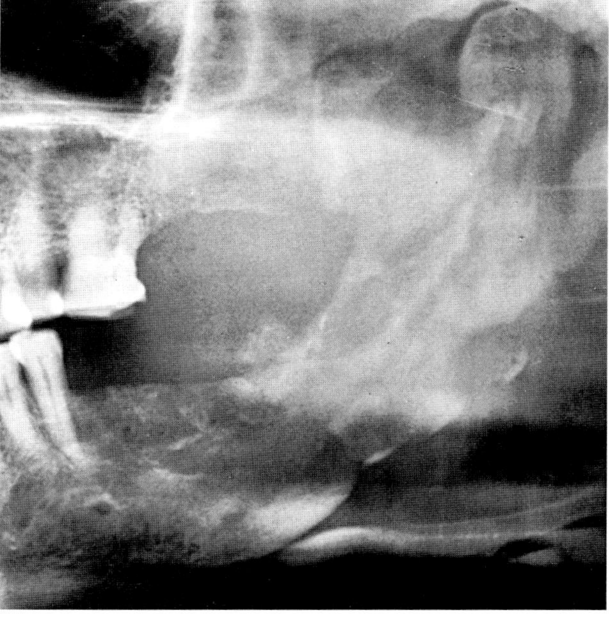

C

FIGURE 14–3.

Chronic Rarefying Osteomyelitis: A, Typical motheaten pattern. Radiopaque areas represent sequestra, and lucent areas represent lysis and replacement with granulation tissue. There is a faint periosteal reaction at angle. (Courtesy of Drs. Lilian and Israel Chilvarquer, Sao Paulo, Brazil.) B, Large sequestrum and pathologic fracture. C, Large areas of rarefaction, sequestrum formation, and pathologic fractures at the angle and condylar neck.

orthovoltage. At this high energy level, bone and soft tissues tend to absorb approximately the same energy; this has been termed the "bone sparing" effect of cobalt 60 and is the major factor in its widespread use today.

In 1970, Meyer defined the classic triad of ORN as radiation, trauma, and infection. He described the role of trauma, usually consisting of tooth removal, to be the portal of entry for oral bacterial flora into the underlying bone. In a study of Marx in 1983(a), no microorganisms could be cultured or observed in deep, so-called "infected bone" of ORN. The results of this investigation indicate that microorganisms play a minor role in the pathophysiology of ORN of the jaws; they appear to act more as surface contaminants than infective agents. Similarly, the direct role of trauma is questioned. Of the 26 cases of ORN reviewed by Marx (1983a), 35% could not be correlated with an episode of trauma; of the 17 cases related to trauma, 15 were associated with postirradiation tooth removal (88%). Daly and Drane (1973) reported a 39% incidence of ORN unassociated with any specific trauma. The mechanism of ORN seems to be an inability of both the soft and hard tissues to keep up with cellular turnover and collagen synthesis after high radiation doses. Marx (1983a) offered a new tetrad in ORN consisting of (1) radiation; (2) hypoxic-hypovascular-hypocellular tissue, referred to as the "three H" principle; (3) tissue breakdown consisting of cellular death and collagen lysis exceeding synthesis and cellular replication; and (4) a nonhealing wound in which energy, oxygen, and metabolic demands exceed the supply. The overall conclusion is that ORN is a problem of wound healing rather than infection.

In a study of 100 patients receiving radiation therapy for head and neck carcinoma, Morrish and colleagues (1981) stated that the most important risk factor in the development of osteonecrosis was the total radiation delivered to the bone, particularly the less vascular mandible. ORN developed in 85% of the dentate patients and 50% of the edentulous patients who received more than 75 Gy (7500 rads) to the bone;

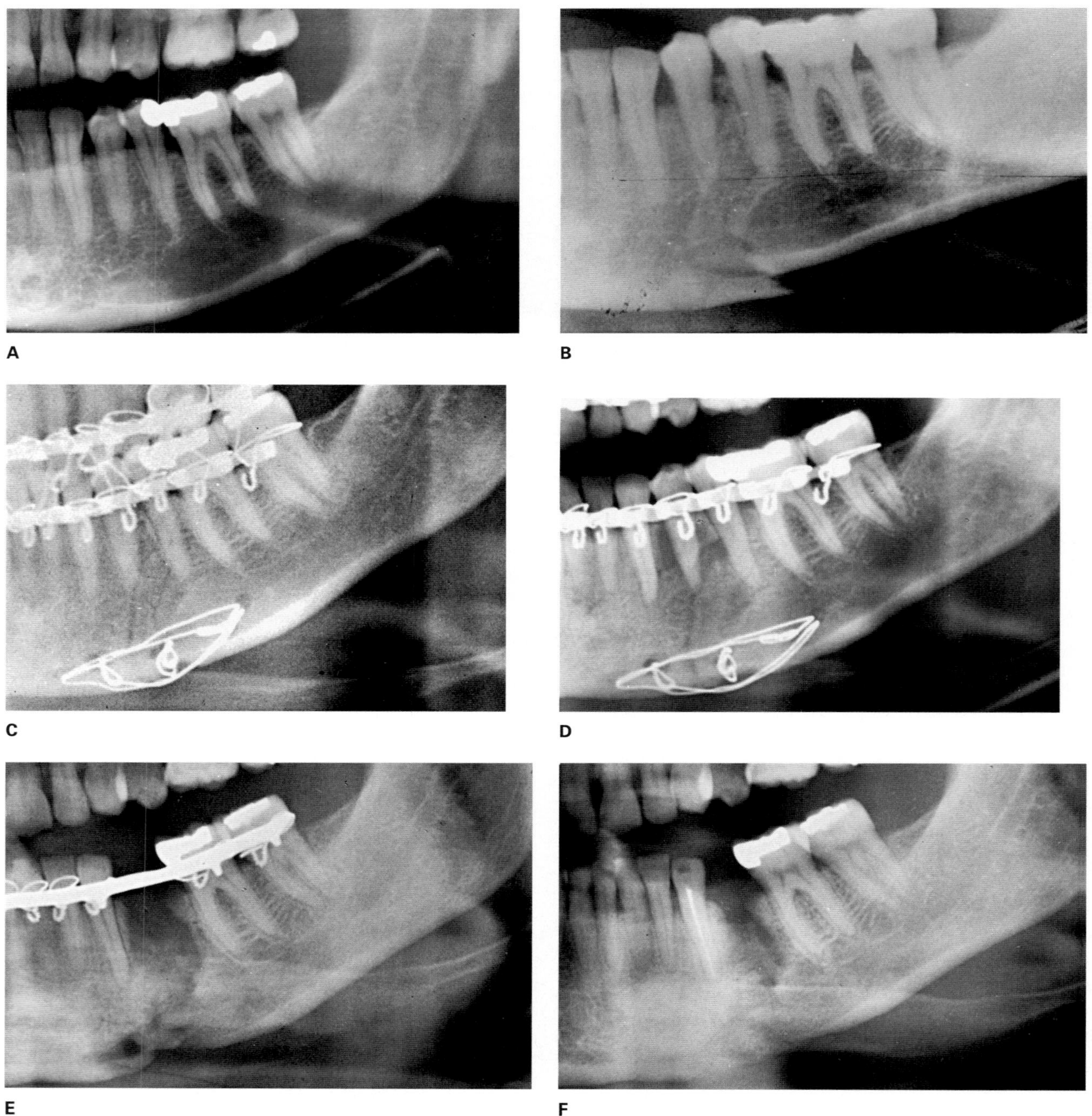

FIGURE 14–4.

Chronic Rarefying Osteomyelitis: A, Before fracture. B, Fracture before reduction. C, Fracture reduced with excellent alignment of fracture segments. The image is sharp in the area of fracture lines, and two premolars straddle fracture lines. D, Two months after reduction. Haziness in area results from edema. There are broader, more ragged fracture lines, and rarefaction of bone is seen around the first and second premolars. E, Premolars extracted. There is chronic osteomyelitis in the region. F, Nine months after fracture, with healing in progress. (Courtesy of Dr. D. Miles, Indiana University, Indianapolis, IN.)

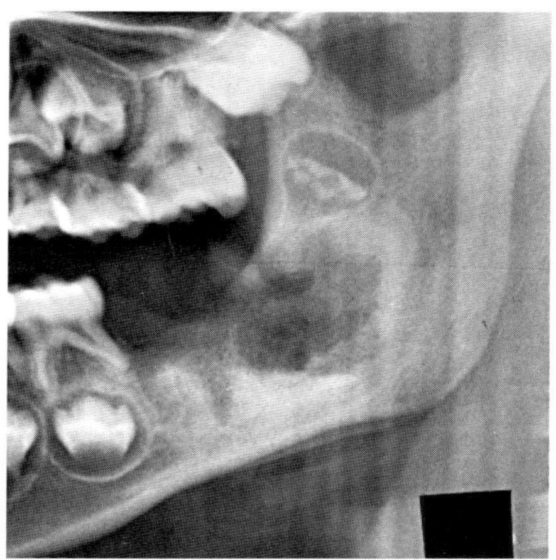

A

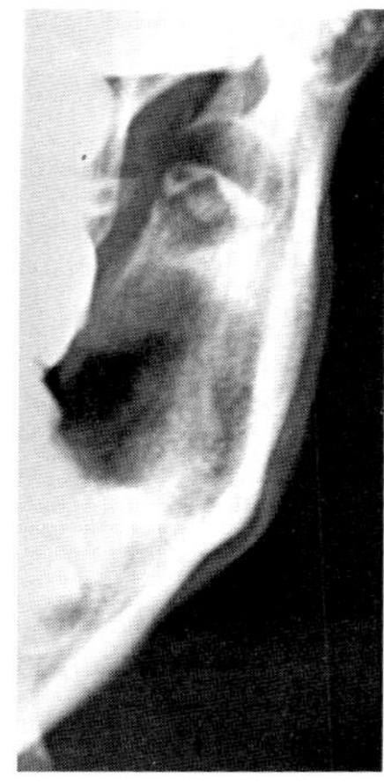

B

FIGURE 14–5.

Chronic Tuberculous Osteomyelitis: A, Lesion in ramus and displacement of permanent third molar tooth bud. B, Periosteal reaction.

none of the patients who received less than 65 Gy had ORN develop.

Pathologic Characteristics

Ionizing radiation has a profound effect on hard and soft tissues. The radiation effects are endothelial cell death, hyalinization resulting from amyloid degeneration, and thrombosis of vessels. The periosteum undergoes fibrosis, and bone osteocytes and osteoblasts become necrotic, with fibrosis of the marrow spaces. Bone trabeculae are reduced in width and number so that there is an increase in the size of the marrow spaces, which contain necrotic debris. These changes are progressive and lead to necrosis of bone and sequestration, although there is no clear line of demarcation between vital and nonvital bone. The mucosa and skin become fibrotic, with significantly diminished cellularity and vascularity of the underlying connective tissue.

Clinical Features

Epstein and associates (1981) suggested that the incidence of ORN ranges from 5 to 22%, with a mean incidence of 10 to 18%. The incidence depends on the reporting institution, aggressiveness of the radiation therapy, and follow-up time. ORN is a disease of the elderly with a male predilection. It is more common in the mandible. In a series reviewed by Mizuno and co-authors (1978), 95% of cases occurred in the

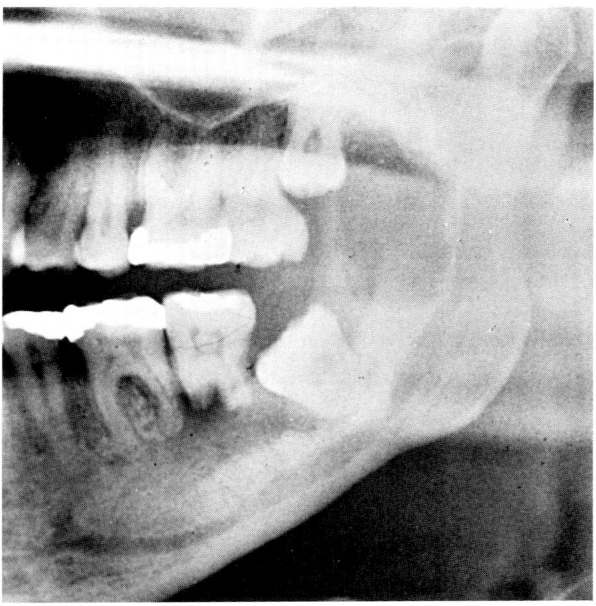

A

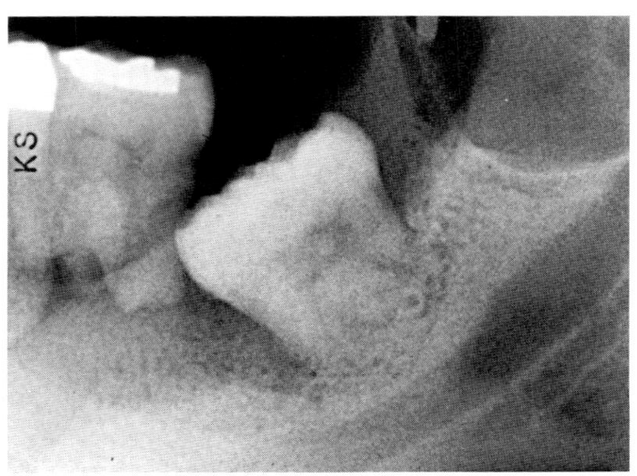

B

FIGURE 14–6.

Chronic Actinomycotic Osteomyelitis: A, Radiolucent area in ramus is odontogenic keratocyst. There is resorption of apices of second molar and rarefaction in area. B, Periapical view of area. (Courtesy of Dr. D. Barnett, University of Oregon Health Sciences Center, Portland, OR.)

mandible and 5% in the maxilla. Komisar and co-workers (1985) reported that the incidence is less than 2% for the maxilla even though the maxilla may be included in the radiation portal. Pain and evidence of exposed bone of more than 3 months' duration without healing are the chief features of ORN of the jaws. The exposed bone is gray to yellow in color and has a rough surface texture that may cause additional irritation to adjacent soft tissue. Suppuration is not evident in most cases. Associated symptoms of xerostomia, fetid breath, perversion of taste, and food impaction in the area of the lesion may be present. Trismus and difficulty in mastication, swallowing, and speech also may accompany ORN. Progression of the condition may lead to pathologic fracture and intraoral and extraoral fistulas.

Treatment/Prognosis

The degree of radiation-related tissue injury varies greatly between patients even with identical doses and fractionations. Some patients have a greater residual and peripheral cellular pool that can respond better to the radiation injury. An accurate assessment of oral health before radiation therapy, followed by appropriate treatment and aggressive oral hygiene maintenance, offers the most promising means of reducing the incidence and severity of ORN. Morrish and co-authors (1981) stated that removal of diseased teeth within the radiation portals, particularly in the mandible, will prevent ORN; extensive alveoloplasty should be performed to permit primary mucoperiosteal closure. Radiation therapy should be delayed for 10 to 14 days to allow initial healing; all remaining teeth should be restored and periodontal therapy completed within this 2-week period. A customized tray should be provided to apply fluoride to the teeth after flossing.

After radiation therapy, dental extraction is an inadvisable method of handling diseased teeth within the portals of irradiation. A safer alternative is to treat infected teeth with root canal therapy; after such therapy these teeth can be amputated at the gingival margins, exposing areas of difficult access for cleaning. A saliva substitute should be used by the patient if radiation-induced xerostomia is present. The solution is intended to facilitate rehardening of tooth surfaces and minimize xerostomia-induced soft tissue disorders. When the radiation dose is relatively low (less than 60 Gy) and most of the bone exposures remain within the zone of the attached gingiva, ORN can be treated conservatively by the following measures:

1. The patient must abstain from alcohol or tobacco.
2. The patient must practice good oral hygiene.
3. The exposed bone should be irrigated with saline water or diluted hydrogen peroxide, and purulent wounds should be covered with a packing containing zinc peroxide and neomycin.
4. Antimicrobial treatment of ORN is of questionable value; however, when a reliable culture identifies pathogens, the appropriate antibiotic should be used.
5. Analgesics are prescribed for pain.
6. Supportive treatment with fluids and a liquid or semiliquid diet high in protein and vitamins is desirable.
7. Rough, irregular, exposed bone is smoothed and sequestra are removed gently when accessible.

Bone necrosis occurring after administration of a dose greater than 65 Gy does not respond favorably to conservative treatment measures. In advanced cases of ORN in which there is a large portion of exposed bone extending beyond the mucogingival junction and involving the buccal and lingual plates of bone, hyperbaric oxygen is a useful adjunct to therapy, particularly when combined with surgical sequestrectomy or mandibular resection.

Marx (1983b) used hyperbaric oxygen and aggressive surgery in a progressively staged manner to achieve complete resolution of ORN of the mandible in 58 patients. This success may be explained by the alteration of the existing hypoxia, hypocellularity, and hypovascularity of the tissues; the intermittent elevations of tissue oxygen tension stimulate collagen synthesis and fibroblastic proliferation.

◆ *RADIOLOGY (Figs. 14–7 to 14–10)*

The radiographic picture begins with an irregular radiolucency, usually in the mandible, with very indistinct borders. The progression of the bone change is so slow and slight that extension of the disease is recognized only in comparisons with previous radiographs. If not controlled, areas of rarefaction eventually spread to large portions of the mandible. A typical motheaten pattern of bone is seen, with poorly defined, ragged borders; enlarged and irregular trabecular spaces; and, often, evidence of bone sequestration.

Sometimes a dark line is seen to enclose portions of bone of variable size, some of which may be quite large. The dark line is the site of separation of a nonviable portion of the bone (sequestrum) that eventually will be thrown off if not removed surgically. Pathologic fracture also may be seen. In advanced cases, the condition is difficult to distinguish

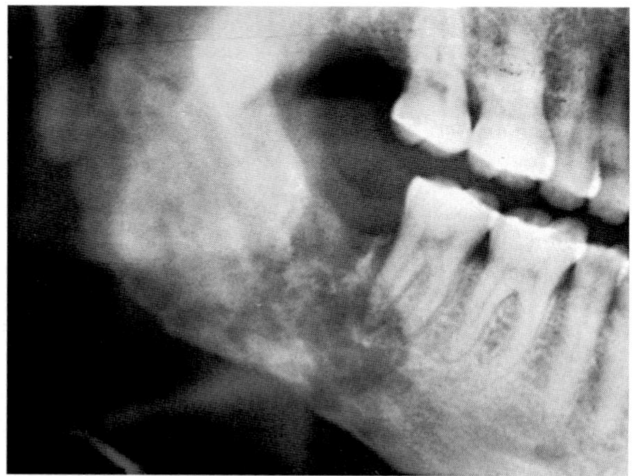

FIGURE 14–7.

Osteoradionecrosis in 60-year-old Man: There was a history of carcinoma in tonsillar fossa and metastatic neck nodes, treated by radiation therapy 7 years previously. Radiograph was taken several months after third molar extraction. (Courtesy of Dr. D. Miles, Indiana University, Indianapolis, IN.)

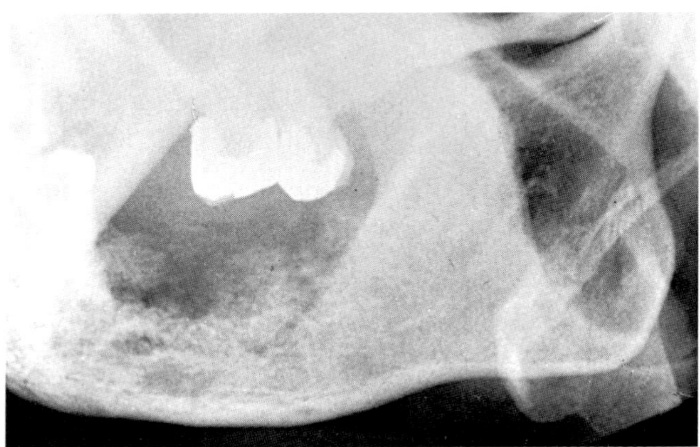

FIGURE 14–8.

Osteoradionecrosis in a 45-year-old Man: A benign condition was treated by radiation therapy in lieu of appropriate dental treatment. Ultimately, the hemimandible was lost.

from chronic rarefying osteomyelitis of a pure microbial origin. One distinguishing feature of ORN is the absence of any form of periosteal reaction, which often may be present in chronic rarefying osteomyelitis. Epstein and associates (1981) and Bergstedt (1975) reported that bone scintigraphy may be of some assistance in determining the degree of bone involvement by showing a lack of labeling in the area of the lesion.

NEURALGIA-INDUCING CAVITATIONAL OSTEONECROSIS (NICO, Idiopathic jawbone cavities of Ratner)

Since John Locke first described the symptoms of trigeminal neuralgia in 1677, very few investigators have seriously considered the possibility of a dental cause. According to Wepsic (1973), it has been estimated that trigeminal neuralgia afflicts 15,000 new patients in the United States each year. Trigeminal neuralgia, or tic douloureux, is a disorder of the sensory nucleus of the trigeminal nerve, producing bouts of severe, seconds-long, lancinating pain in the distribution of one or more divisions of the trigeminal nerve, most often the mandibular or maxillary divisions. The disease is unilateral in nearly all cases, and the pain seldom, if ever, crosses the midline. Janetta (1967) has discounted a dental cause on the basis that many patients are totally, or at least partially, edentulous in the area of the pain, and extraction of the remaining teeth did not alter the pain. Neurologists such as Harris (1926), and Kinnier Wilson and Bruce (1955) believed dental and oral pathosis might be an important contributing factor in the onset of trigeminal neuralgia. In 1979, Ratner and associates, in a series of 38 patients with idiopathic trigeminal neuralgia and 23 patients with atypical neuralgia, found that, in nearly all instances, the painful phenomena associated with both disorders were related to the presence of maxillary and mandibular bone cavities at previous tooth extraction sites. Later, fenestrations and periodontal defects were implicated in dentate areas.

Pathologic Characteristics

When radiographically localized areas were exposed by standard oral surgical procedures, the areas were found to consist of bone cavities at the sites of previous tooth extractions, with dimensions up to 2 cm or more in a given axis. Often, narrow tracts lead from the cavity in an irregular fashion through adjacent bone for distances up to 2 cm. In the mandible, these tracts always opened at the site of the mandibular canal. In the maxilla, the tracts ended in a second bone cavity, which might be larger than the first, and at times would continue to a third cavity; occasionally it was found that these tracts communicated with the nasal cavity or antrum. Nerve fibers often were exposed in the walls of the cavities as a result of the bone destruction.

The material removed from the cavities was characterized histopathologically by Ratner and associates (1979) as showing a highly vascular abnormal healing response of bone; some lesions had a mild lymphocytic infiltration and fibrous tissue, and others ranged from void spaces to abnormal-appearing osteoid tissue. Preliminary microbiologic studies of material from the walls of the cavities showed the existence within them of a complex polymicrobial mix of aerobic and anaerobic flora.

Clinical Features

Older patients usually are affected by facial neuralgias; the disease seldom occurs in people younger than 35 years of age. It is a well-established fact, but a completely unexplained one, that the right side of the face is affected in more patients than the left by a ratio of approximately 1.7 to 1. In a controlled study of 526 patients with trigeminal neuralgia, Rothman and Monson (1973) found that the female-to-male sex distribution was 1.17:1. The history usually is typical and diagnostic. The pain of trigeminal neuralgia is of a searing or

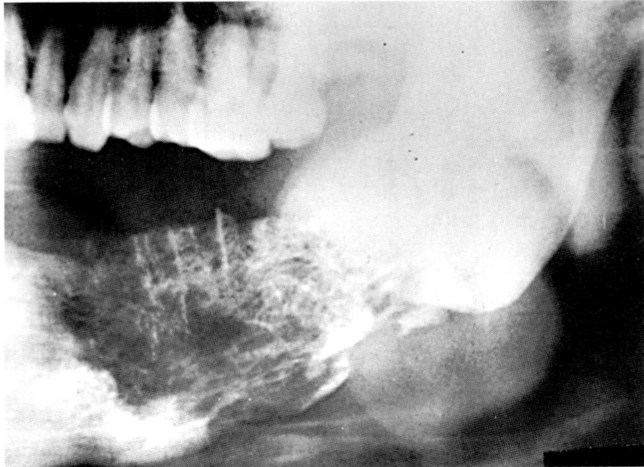

FIGURE 14–9.

Osteoradionecrosis in a 63-year-old Man: There was a history of irradiation to the neck area 5 years previously. Extractions were performed in area within portal of radiation; sockets have not healed 5 months after extraction. A periosteal reaction is absent, and there is pathologic fracture.

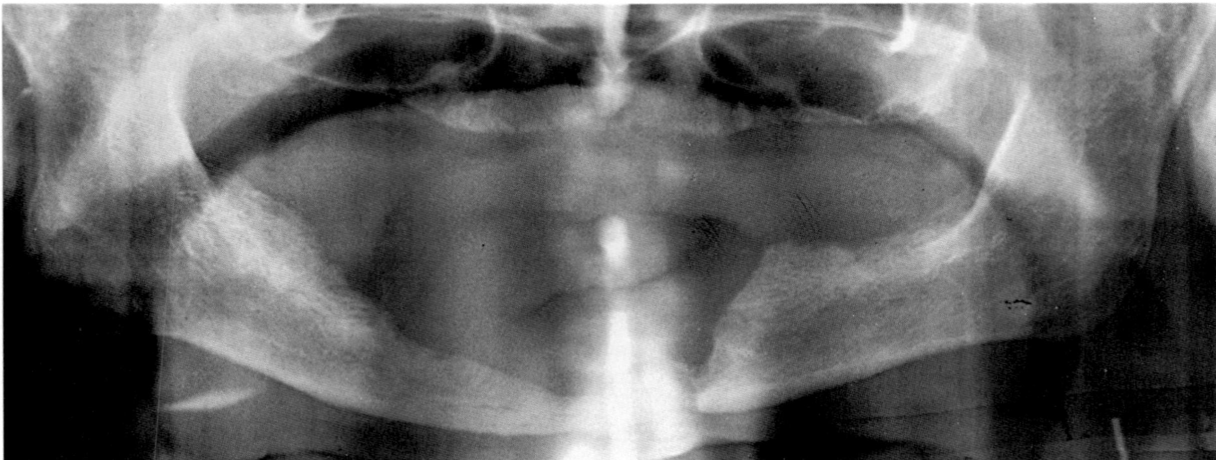

A

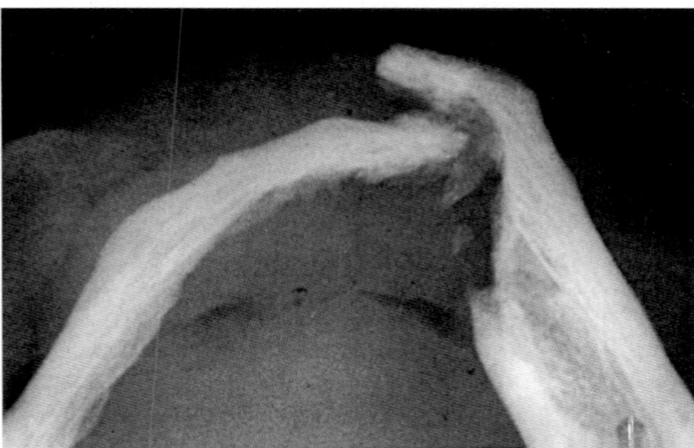

B

FIGURE 14–10.

Osteoradionecrosis in a 37-year-old Man: There was a history of radiation therapy to the neck for Hodgkin's disease 15 years previously, and teeth were extracted before radiation therapy. The lesion began as a simple denture ulcer. Radiographs were taken 1 year later. A major portion of the mandible required resection. A, Panoramic view. B, Occlusal view. (Courtesy of Dr. D. Miles, Indiana University, Indianapolis, IN.)

lancinating type and is often set off by touching a trigger point or by an activity such as chewing or brushing the teeth. In the early stages of the disease, the pain is relatively mild, sometimes described as dull, burning, or resembling a sharp toothache. Later, the pain becomes intense, and although each bout is brief, successive bouts may incapacitate the patient. Roberts and Person (1979) and Shaber and Krol (1980) separately found that the interval between extraction and onset of pain ranged from months to many years later.

As outlined by Roberts and Person (1979), carefully mapping out the distribution of the pain indicates patterns that suggest the location of the cavity in the jaws. Further localization is provided by injecting a drop or two of local anesthetic in the mucobuccal fold adjacent to the suspected area. Immediate cessation of the pain, which must be present during this test, further points to the location and is highly suggestive of the diagnosis. After this, the radiographs are studied for the presence of the subtle changes suggestive of a cavity.

Treatment/Prognosis

Carbamazepine (200 to 1600 mg/day) is generally effective, and the benefit often is sustained; liver and hematopoietic functions should be monitored. Phenytoin (300 to 600 mg/day) or baclofen (15 to 40 mg/day) is effective in some cases. Surgical approaches have been used, such as the separation of arteries pressing against the trigeminal root in the posterior fossa, direct surgical treatments of the Gasserian ganglion, and surgical sectioning of the fifth nerve fibers proximal to the Gasserian ganglion at the brain stem level.

Treatment of the neuralgia-inducing cavitational osteonecrosis consisted of vigorous curettage of the bone cavities, which was repeated if necessary, plus administration of antibiotics to induce healing and filling of the cavities with new bone. Responses of patients to this treatment consisted of significant to complete pain remission, the longest of which lasting 9 years. Mathis and co-workers (1981) found that after similar treatment their results were in agreement with those of Ratner and co-workers (1979), Roberts and Person (1979), and Shaber and Krol (1980) in that healing of the bony defects resulted in some measure of pain relief for all the patients who received surgery.

◆ *RADIOLOGY (Figs. 14–11 and 14–12)*

Because the cavities are within the medullary bone of the jaws and do not tend to affect the endosteal surface of the cortex, the cavities generally have not been observed clearly in radiographs. This is especially so in periapical radiographs. With the use of panoramic radiographs, it may be possible to detect cavities more readily, possibly because of

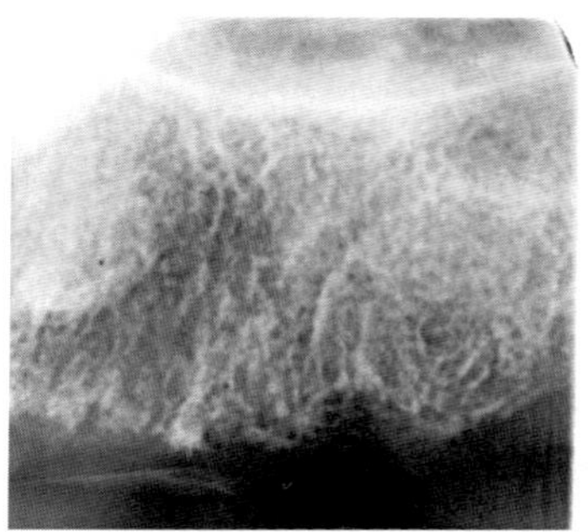
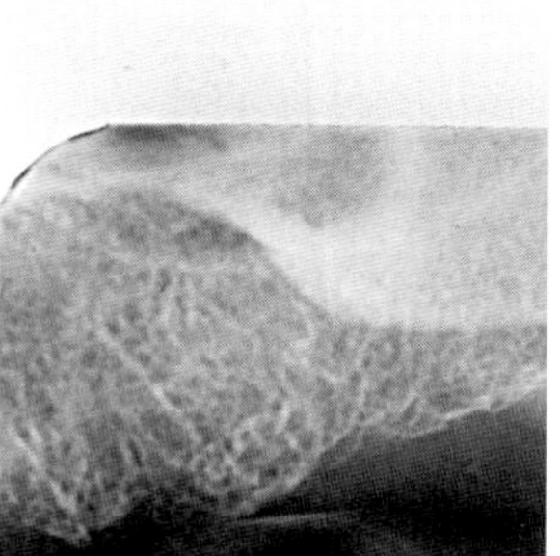

FIGURE 14–11.

Idiopathic Jawbone Cavity of Ratner in a 49-year-old Woman: She was edentulous for 20 years and had atypical facial neuralgia on left. The area of the left canine and first premolar is focally more osteoporotic. There are a few elongated, coarser trabeculae and some lamina dura residues. There was significant pain relief after curettage of the area. The removed tissue consisted of normal bone and bone marrow, some fibrous connective tissue, and a few lymphocytes.

the increased latitude of some panoramic radiographic film, the greatly diminished amount of radiation used, and the tomographic effect in all panoramic radiographs.

Although Ratner and co-workers (1979) initially found that bone cavities could not be detected on radiographs, Roberts and Person (1979) observed that they could detect radiographic changes in the jawbones that ordinarily would be considered as normal variations but which, in these patients with facial pain, reflect the existence of pain-related bone cavities. In their series of cases, the radiographic appearance of the bone-related cavities varied considerably, and none of the radiographic changes was pathognomonic for trigeminal or atypical facial neuralgias but all were considered suspect and worthy of additional exploration. They described four distinct radiographic variations as follows: (1) discrete, clearly demarcated ovoid or triangular radiolucent areas; (2) irregular radiolucencies with sparse, thickened, and disorganized trabeculae; (3) osteoporotic regions consisting of demineralized-appearing bone; and (4) vestiges of lamina dura or distorted bone trabeculae outlining the site of an abnormally healed tooth socket, often of many years' duration. Other less well-described appearances include moth-eaten radiolucencies, poorly demarcated nonexpansile radiolucencies, soap bubble radiolucencies, radiopaque flecks and "peau d'orange" or stippled radiopacities, radiopacities resembling cotton-wool, ground-glass radiopacities, remnants of horizontal inter-radicular trabeculae in edentulous areas, unremodeled sockets at extraction sites, and focal areas of resorption of the inferior alveolar canal or maxillary sinus walls. These changes are extremely subtle, and in many other patients without symptoms these have been considered variations of asymptomatic lesions or normal changes.

GIANT CELL HYALIN ANGIOPATHY

(Calcifying odontogenic hyalin ring granuloma, pulse granuloma, granulation tissue with giant cells and hyalin change)

Giant cell hyalin angiopathy is a rare pathologic entity that first was recognized in 1977 by Dunlap and Barker, although the first report probably was made by Adkins in 1972. The true nature of this lesion still remains uncertain, but it is of little apparent clinical significance. This condition is considered very rare.

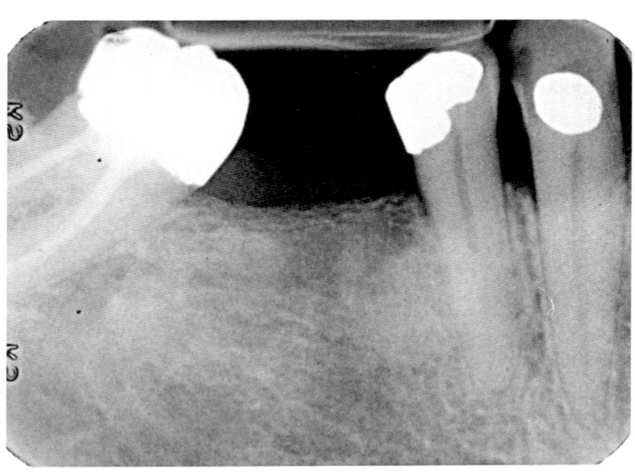

A

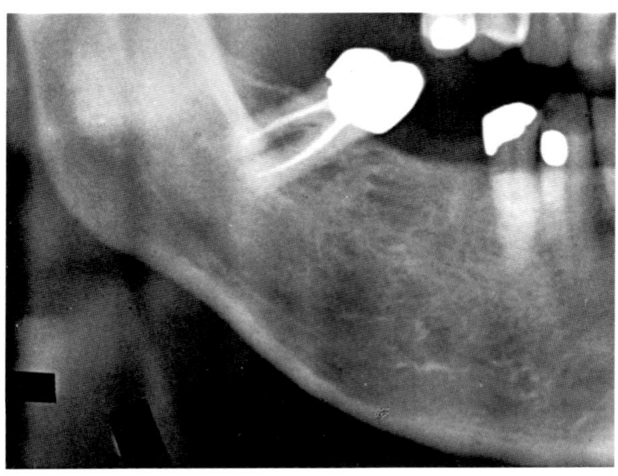

B

FIGURE 14–12.

Idiopathic Jawbone Cavity of Ratner in a 56-year-old Man: There was a history of severe tic douloureux on the right side. A and B, Both radiographs were taken on the same day. The panoramic radiograph shows focal osteoporotic area in first molar region not apparent in periapical view and elongated trabeculae in region. A slight condensation of bone surrounds the area. After two curettages, a small block resection, and removal of molar, the patient was pain free for 6 years. Biopsy specimens consisted of collagenous tissue, normal bone, marrow, and a few lymphocytes.

Pathologic Characteristics

In 1972, Adkins described 15 histologic specimens as granulomas obtained from edentulous portions of maxilla (2 cases) and the mandible (13 cases). All of these lesions contained areas of fibrous tissue with coarse collagen bundles and mature fibroblasts, highly cellular areas with vacuolated macrophages, foamy histiocytes, and lymphocytic predominance. In addition, lobulated, circularly arranged, deeply stained areas of calcification with numerous multinucleated foreign body giant cells around and within pale eosinophilic rings were apparent. Dunlap and Barker (1977) concluded that the lesion is a form of acute vasculitis with subsequent thickening and hyalinization of vessel walls. Other theories have been postulated by Mincer and associates in 1979, El-Labban and Kramer in 1981, and McMillan and co-workers in 1981.

Ciola and associates (1983) described a 67-year-old man with a history of peptic ulcer who had a well-defined, linear ulceration in the mucobuccal fold of the left mandibular region. A 3.0- by 3.0-cm hard exophytic mass, apparently fixed to the periosteum, was palpable along the left lateral border of the mandible. No paresthesia was observed, and the mass was not tender to palpation. The patient only complained of a sensation ''like ants are eating my jawbone'' (formication). Aspiration of the mass produced a small amount of bloody aspirant. Multiple biopsy specimens and cytologic smears were taken, and treatment with 250 mg ampicillin four times a day was started at the request of the gastroenterologist.

Treatment/Prognosis

In the case of Ciola and co-workers (1983), the radiographic findings were consistent with an inflammatory process. The manner in which the lesion responded to antibiotic therapy and then readily recurred after cessation of antibiotic therapy was consistent with a bacterial infection. The regrowth of the lesion in the period after initial cessation of antibiotic therapy and its resolution after 16 weeks of penicillin administration suggested an infectious process akin to actinomycosis; however, no organism or foreign body could be identified. The patient's immediate postoperative course was uneventful, with a progressive decrease in the size of the lesion.

◆ *RADIOLOGY (Fig. 14–13)*

In the case of Ciola and co-workers (1983), bone scans of the head and neck showed abnormal uptake in the left mandible. In the panoramic radiograph, a considerable amount of bone destruction was apparent, extending from the alveolar ridge to the mandibular canal, with varying degrees of resorption. The margins of the lesion were irregular, and, in general, the lesion could be described as motheaten. Two distinct circumscribed lytic areas were superimposed on the mandibular canal. The radiographic findings were consistent with an inflammatory process. In the development of a radiographic differential diagnosis, the following lesions were considered: osteomyelitis, actinomycosis, multiple myeloma, neurilemoma, squamous cell carcinoma, and metastatic malignant neoplasms. This lesion is illustrated in Figure 14–13.

PRIMARY INTRAOSSEOUS CARCINOMA OF THE JAWS (Primary intra-alveolar epidermoid carcinoma of jaws, central epidermoid carcinoma)

According to Morrison and Deeley (1962), Loos first described primary intraosseous carcinoma (PIOC) of the jaws in 1913. In a recent review by Elzay in 1982, only 12 reported cases were accepted as sufficiently documented for acceptance as true cases. It is classified by the World Health Organization as an odontogenic carcinoma consisting of a squamous cell carcinoma arising within the jaws, having

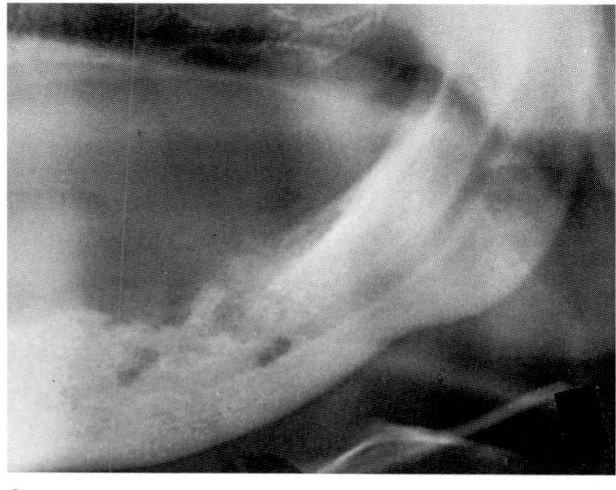

A

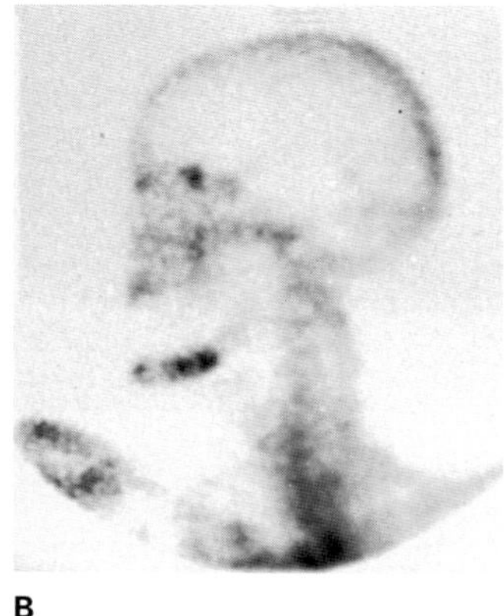

B

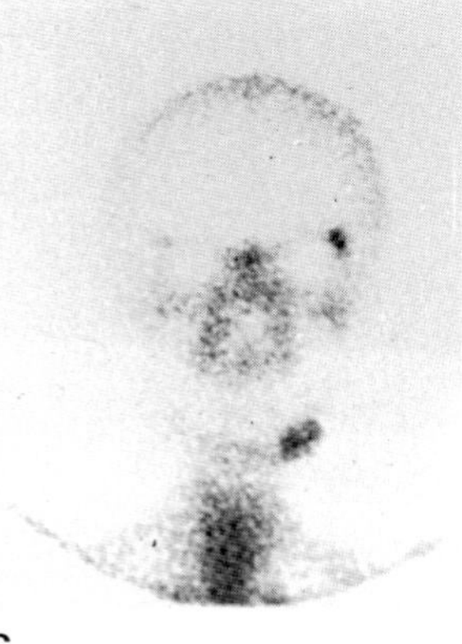

C

FIGURE 14–13.

Giant Cell Hyalin Angiopathy in a 67-year-old Man: Lesion appears motheaten. A, Panoramic view. B and C, Increased uptake in bone scan. (Courtesy of Dr. B. Ciola, Westhaven, CT.)

no initial connection with the oral mucosa, and presumably developing from residues of odontogenic epithelium. Stoll and co-workers (1957) stated that intraosseous carcinomas are rare in bones other than the jaws, which supports the concept that PIOCs are odontogenic in origin. In the case of Van Wyk and colleagues (1987), the growth pattern of the tumor that developed around the teeth points to a possible origin from the cell rests of Mallasez.

Pathologic Characteristics

Among the 12 cases reported by Elzay (1982), 7 were characterized as being nonkeratinizing, whereas 5 exhibited varying degrees of keratinization. Alveolar and plexiform patterns were observed. Of the 12 cases, 7 showed palisading or regimentation of the epithelial cells, but no palisading was reported in 5 cases. Elzay (1982) has proposed a classification of PIOCs into three types, according to the odontogenic tissue from which they originate:

1. Those arising from odontogenic cysts.
2. Those arising from an ameloblastoma, either well differentiated (malignant ameloblastoma) or poorly differentiated (ameloblastic carcinoma).
3. Those arising de novo from odontogenic epithelial residues and varying in their ability to form keratin.

Clinical Features

Shear (1969), McGowan (1980), and Elzay (1982) reported data regarding the patients' ages and sex and the location of the lesion that indicated that the tumors occur mainly in adults in the sixth to seventh decades, the male-to-female incidence ratio is 3:1, and the tumor usually is situated in the posterior mandible. The condition may be asymptomatic or painful and may mimic localized periodontal disease. Of practical dental importance is that mobility of the teeth is one of the first clinical signs. Paresthesia or a burning sensation is another symptom. The regional lymph nodes may be enlarged and nontender. An extraction tooth socket may be present at the time of diagnosis, and there may be an extension of the tumor mass protruding into the oral cavity through the tooth socket. Within the fungating, friable soft tissue tumor mass, floating teeth may be evident, and some teeth may have exfoliated spontaneously.

Treatment/Prognosis

The initial treatment of PIOC is surgical excision or resection and ipsilateral neck node dissection if there is clinical evidence of nodal spread. Shear (1969) reported a 5-year survival rate of 30 to 40%. In Elzay's (1982) review of 12 cases, 4 of 10 patients (40%) were reported to have survived more than 2 years after therapy.

◆ *RADIOLOGY (Fig. 14–14)*

With the proliferation of more malignant cells, bone destruction becomes more rapid and random. One of the earliest and most characteristic signs of malignancy is the lack of a well-defined border with, or most frequently without, marginal sclerosis. The cortex often is resorbed in an irregular motheaten or permeative fashion without appreciable expansion. Cortical perforations may be observed. Generally, there are two reasons why resorption and displacement of teeth are not features of this tumor: (1) PIOC tends to grow too rapidly and is too destructive to produce these features; and (2) it tends to grow around obstructions such as teeth rather than displace them because invasion probably occurs along the path of least resistance. Also, the margin of the lesion may consist of large eroded areas within which smaller areas

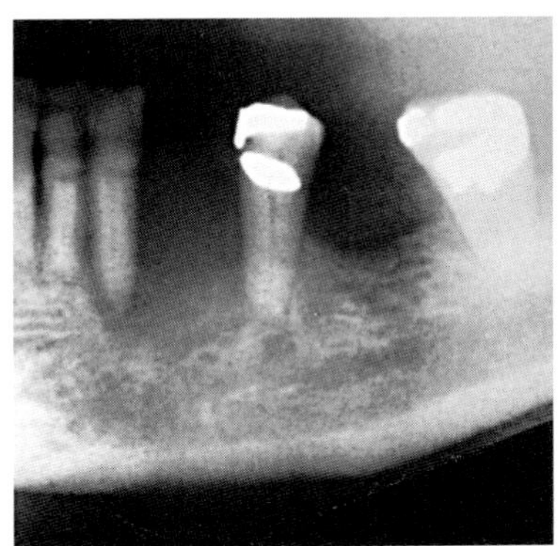

A

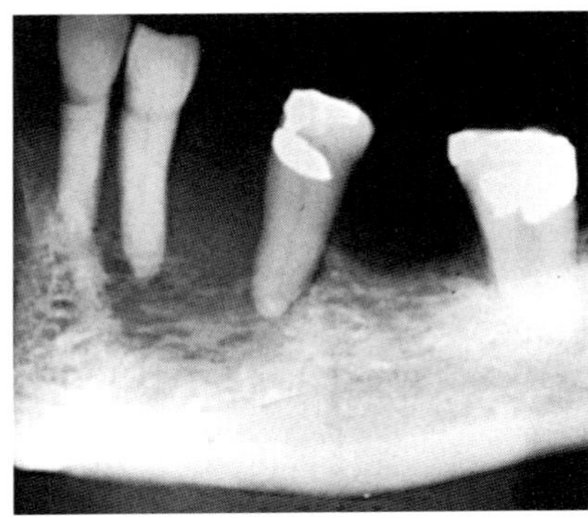

B

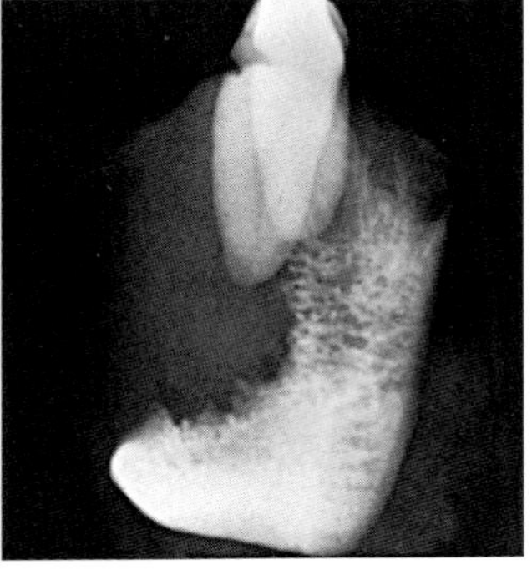

C

FIGURE 14–14.

Primary Intraosseous Carcinoma: A, Panoramic radiograph shows nonspecific area of rarefaction in canine-premolar region without evidence of sclerosis at margins. B and C, Radiographs of resected specimen show changes more clearly. Geographic area results from total destruction of buccal half of mandible. Permeative areas represent tumor infiltration into remaining bone. Permeative changes, lack of marginal sclerosis, and absence of periosteal reaction indicate a malignant process but do not indicate the specific disease. (From Van Wyk CW, Padayachee A, Nortjé CJ, von der Heyden U: Primary intraosseous carcinoma involving the anterior mandible. Br J Oral Maxillofac Surg 25:427, 1987.)

of bone destruction are present. This pattern has been described as "bays within bays." Larger geographic areas of alveolar bone destruction may be present, with only the inferior cortex intact. Pathologic fracture may occur, and osteomyelitis may be present.

GINGIVAL CARCINOMA

According to Shafer and co-authors (1983), gingival carcinoma accounts for approximately 10 to 12% of all oral carcinomas. Almost all of the tumors occurred in people older than 40 years of age and 82% occurred in men. Etiologic factors associated with gingival carcinoma include poor oral hygiene, excessive alcohol intake, use of tobacco, and advancing age. The specific cause remains unknown. It appears to occur more frequently in the mandible, although many cases of maxillary gingival carcinoma have been reported. Gingival carcinoma may be seen clinically as a white leukoplakic or reddened erythroplakic area. Hard, unmovable, nontender neck nodes are often palpable in the anterior triangles of the neck and in the submandibular region. The skin overlying these nodes often contains many fine telangiectatic vessels, causing the skin in the area to appear reddened. Ultimately, a soft tissue mass is visible, and invasion of the alveolar bone occurs. This causes loosening of the associated teeth; thus, the condition may resemble periodontal disease. Approximately 50% of the cases will have metastasized at diagnosis, and the 5-year survival rate is only approximately 25%.

◆ *RADIOLOGY (Figs. 14–15 to 14–20)*

Location

Gingival carcinoma may be found slightly more frequently in the mandible.

"Floating Tooth"

Initially there are no radiologic changes. With progression, the condition may mimic periodontal disease, with varying amounts of bone loss and ultimately the floating tooth appearance. There are five subtle radiologic differences between the floating tooth as seen in periodontal disease and that seen in gingival carcinoma:

1. In periodontal disease, the radiolucent area surrounding the floating tooth does not contain any trabecular remnants, whereas in gingival carcinoma, trabecular remnants may be present.
2. In periodontal disease, the free margin of alveolar bone surrounding the defect is smooth, whereas in gingival carcinoma it is ragged.
3. In periodontal disease, the free margin of alveolar bone is distinct, with a punched-out appearance, whereas in gingival carcinoma there may be a wide zone of transition between the free margin and normal bone.
4. In periodontal disease, reactive sclerotic bone may be seen at the margin, whereas in gingival carcinoma marginal sclerosis often may be absent.
5. In periodontal disease, the condition often affects adjacent teeth, and local factors such as calculus can be seen. In gingival carcinoma, the bone loss often is

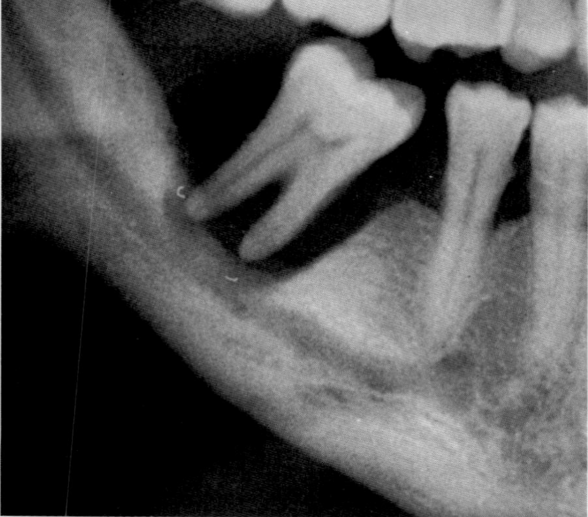

A

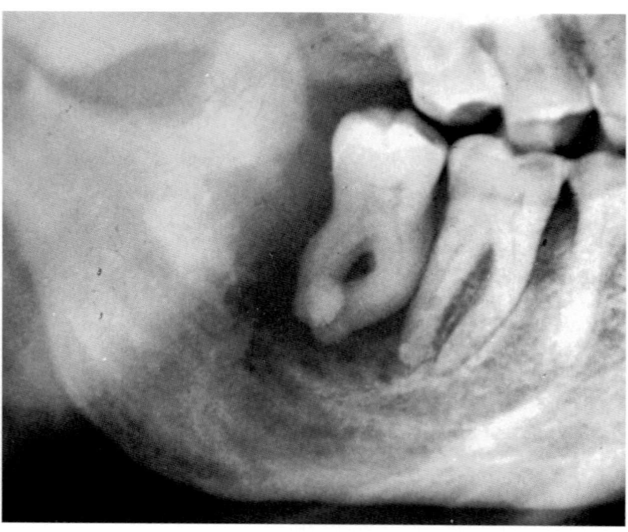

B

FIGURE 14–15.

Floating Tooth: A, Periodontal disease, with sharp, punched-out free margin of alveolar bone around periodontal defect. There are no trabecular remnants within the periodontal defect. There is reactive sclerosis at some parts of the margin. Periodontal disease and calculus are seen in adjacent areas. B, Gingival carcinoma, with a poorly defined, ragged free margin of alveolar bone around rarefied area. There are trabecular remnants within the radiolucent area, and no reactive sclerosis is seen at the margin. A permeative pattern of bone destruction is seen, and there is a milder degree of periodontal disease in adjacent teeth.

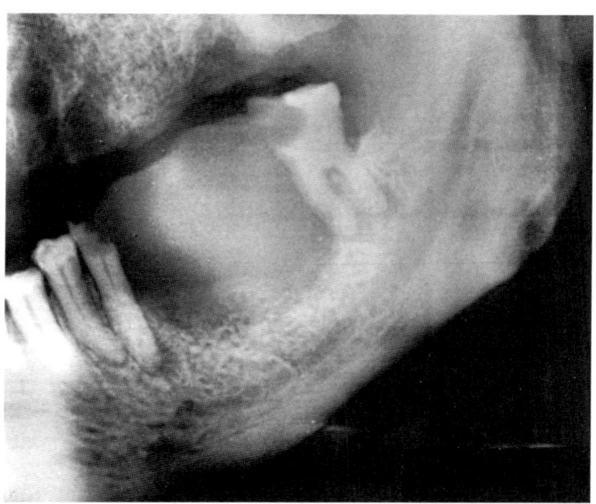

A

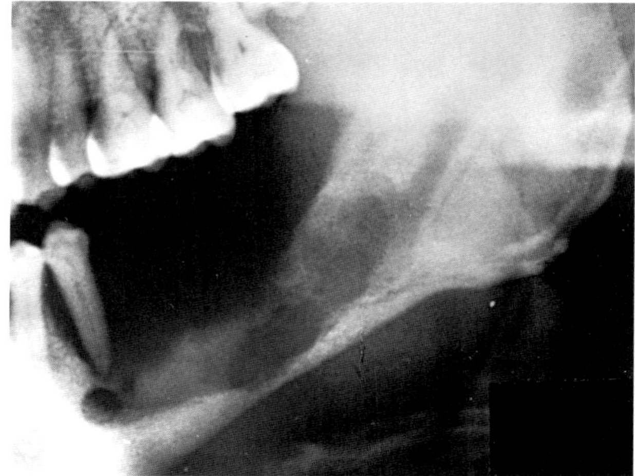

B

FIGURE 14–16.

Gingival Carcinoma: There is saucerization of the alveolar ridge. A, Wide transition zone containing trabecular remnants, reactive sclerosis indicating a slower process, and a large soft tissue mass. B, Geographic area of bone destruction and smaller areas of lysis within, described as "bays within bays," a sign highly suggestive of malignancy. There is a wide transitional zone distally, little reactive sclerosis, and endosteal lysis of the cortex without any periosteal reaction.

limited to a single tooth, and a similar degree of periodontal bone loss is absent in other parts of the dentition.

Saucerization

Another appearance of gingival carcinoma occurs when the area is edentulous. There is saucerization of the crestal portion of the alveolar ridge, and beneath this area there may be a wide transition zone and a relative lack of sclerosis at the margin. Remnants of alveolar bone within the area of tumor invasion are seen relatively infrequently in primary disease in comparison with metastatic disease, where this finding is more frequent. At times, large areas of geographic bone destruction are seen, and in other instances the changes

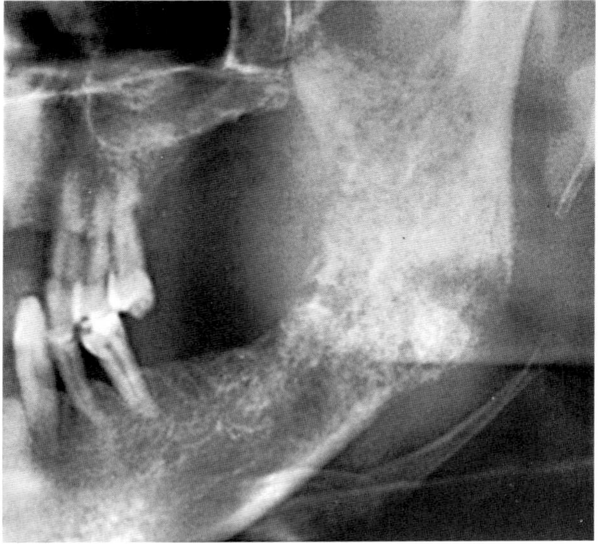

A

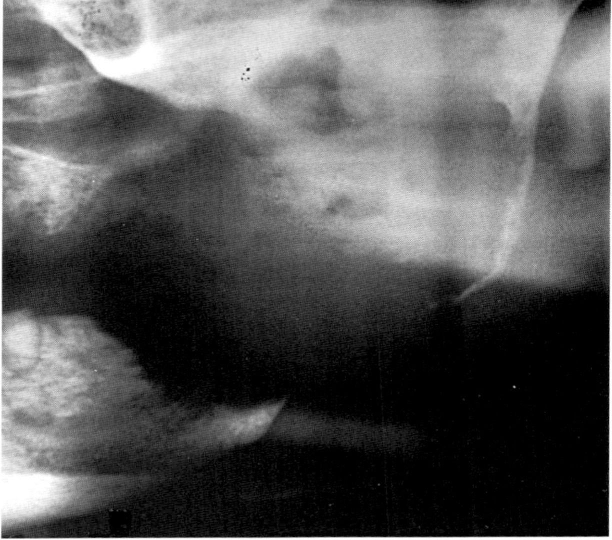

B

FIGURE 14–17.

Gingival Carcinoma: A, Permeative pattern of bone destruction in ramus. The permeative changes in the cortex are strongly suggestive of a malignant neoplasm. (Courtesy of Professor T. Noikura, First Department of Oral Surgery, Kagoshima University, Kagoshima, Japan.) B, Geographic pattern of bone destruction in ramus and pathologic fracture.

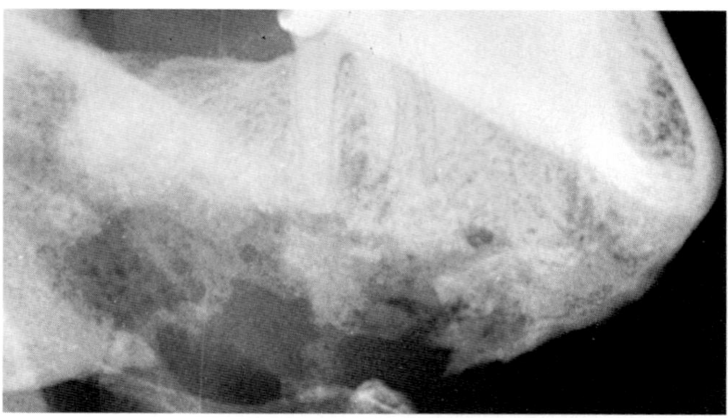

FIGURE 14–18.

Carcinoma of the Floor of the Mouth: Carcinoma spread to the gingiva, then mandible. There is destruction of the inferior cortex, a wide zone of transition with permeative changes within, and lack of sclerosis at the margin. (Courtesy of Professor T. Noikura, First Oral Surgery Department, Kagoshima University School of Dentistry, Kagoshima, Japan.)

have a motheaten appearance or are permeative. A soft tissue mass also may be evident overlying the cupped-out area of the ridge.

Other Features

Gingival carcinoma has another appearance when there is superficial spread to the floor of the mouth before invasion into the underlying bone. In this instance, the destruction begins at the inferior border of the mandible and spreads superiorly. There may be motheaten and permeative patterns of bone destruction within the inferior cortex and bone. Large geographic areas of bone destruction also may be present.

In the maxilla, similar changes are seen, though we have observed fewer cases. In the maxilla, invasion into the antrum, nasal fossa, and orbit may occur rapidly and probably diminishes the prognosis.

CENTRAL MUCOEPIDERMOID CARCINOMA

Although Linell (1948) and Hertz (1952), in separate accounts, credited Lepp with the original documentation of central mucoepidermoid carcinoma in 1939, in 1963 Bhaskar was the first to describe two cases definitively. Mucoepidermoid carcinoma is an unusual type of salivary gland tumor composed of mucous-secreting cells and epidermoid-type cells in varying proportions. Foote and Frazell (1954) and Chaudry and colleagues (1961) stated that mucoepidermoid carcinoma accounts for 11% of major and 8% of minor salivary gland malignant neoplasms; as a central lesion within the jaws, it is quite uncommon, accounting for only 2 to 3% of all mucoepidermoid carcinomas. A complete search of the English language literature by Gingell and co-workers in 1984 showed that the total number of documented cases of central mucoepidermoid carcinoma was approaching 60.

Pathologic Characteristics

The histologic appearance is similar to that seen in mucoepidermoid tumors arising in salivary glands. Three basic cell

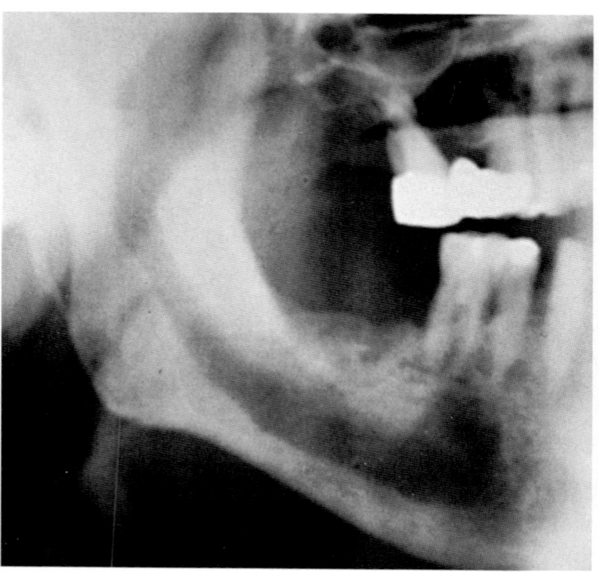

A

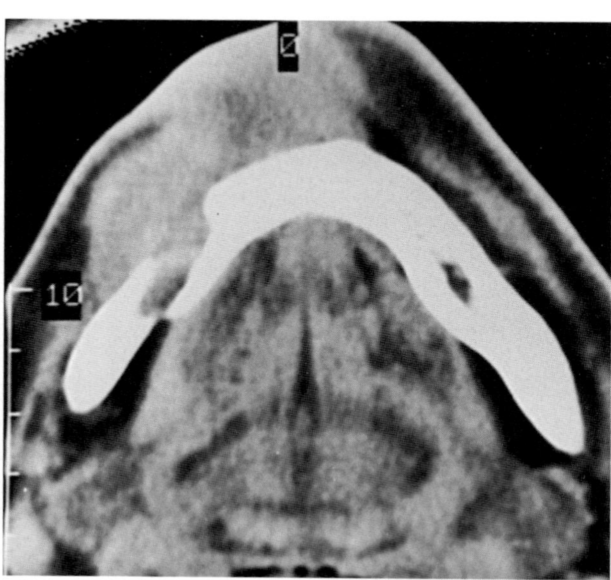

B

FIGURE 14–19.

Carcinoma of the Lip: The carcinoma spread to the gingiva and inferior alveolar canal through the mental foramen. A, Widened inferior alveolar canal. B, CT scan shows soft tissue mass and invasion through the mental foramen (compare with the left side). There is a pathologic fracture of the mandible. (Courtesy of Dr. H. Schwartz, Kaiser Permanente Medical Group, Los Angeles, CA.)

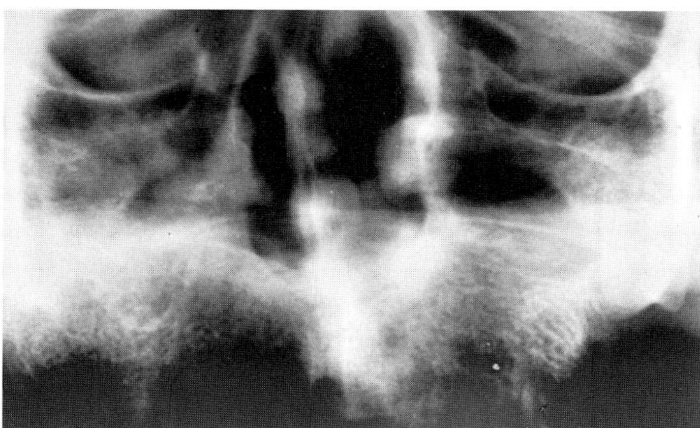

A

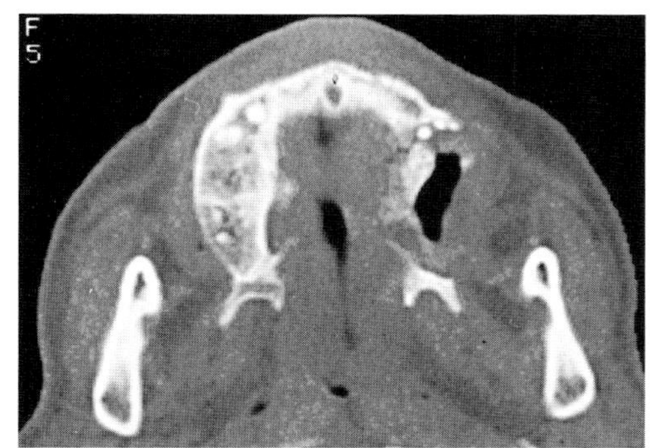

B

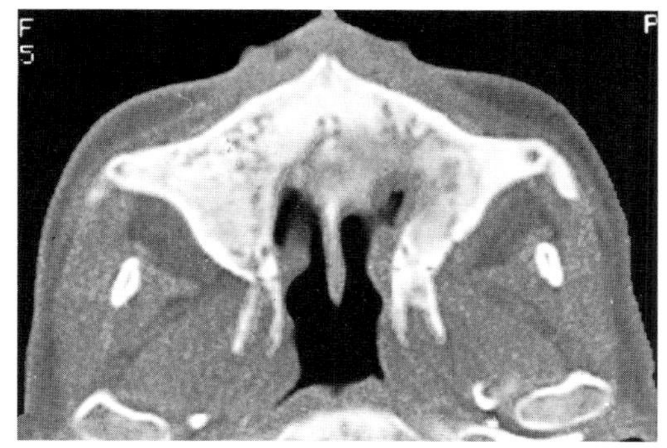

C

FIGURE 14–20.

Carcinoma of the Maxillary Gingiva: A, Rarefaction in canine premolar area of left maxilla. B, Destruction of left maxilla from the canine area to pterygoid plates. C, Geographic destruction in left side and permeative changes in right maxilla. (Courtesy of Professor T. Ohba, Kyushu Dental College, Kitakyushu, Japan.)

types are present in varying proportions, shown mostly by mucus and epidermoid cells with lesser numbers of intermediate cells. Most reported cases would fall into the well-differentiated category. Mucus secretion is a constant and typical feature. A dense proliferation of epidermoid or intermediate elements with a limited amount of mucus indicates more anaplastic and aggressive behavior. Lesions displaying mucous cell predominance or multiple cell types in a more diverse arrangement of cystic, papillary, and cleftlike formations appear to be less inclined to metastasize. Bhaskar and Bernier (1962) and Melrose and associates (1973) have classified these latter lesions as benign. Sonesson (1950), Dhawan and associates (1970), and Chaudry and colleagues (1961) have stated that, because of the recognized potential for recurrence of mucoepidermoid carcinoma and an irregular clinical course, all such lesions should be considered malignant.

With the demonstration of mucous cells within the lining of odontogenic cysts, Marano and Hartman (1974), Brown and colleagues (1966), Smith and associates (1954), and Browand and Waldron (1975) speculated considerably on the relationship of the pluripotential capabilities of odontogenic epithelium and the development of central salivary gland tumors. In addition to metaplastic tendencies, a neoplastic transformation of the cyst wall into benign odontogenic and malignant nonodontogenic tumors has been reported. It also has been observed that ordinary or nonkeratinizing odontogenic cysts, such as apical periodontal cysts, may give rise to central mucoepidermoid carcinoma on rare occasions.

Clinical Features

In a review of 50 cases by Stoch and Smith (1980), the youngest patient was a 1-year-old girl and the oldest was an 85-year-old woman. Most patients were between 40 and 60 years of age. Eversole and colleagues (1975) reported 27 acceptable cases of central mucoepidermoid carcinoma and showed that 65% of cases occur in people in the fifth through eighth decades of life. Smith and associates (1968) reported 9 cases at the Mayo Clinic and found the average age at diagnosis to be 46 years. Marano and Hartman (1974), Smith and associates (1968), and Browand and Waldron (1975) reported that females are affected twice as frequently as males; however, Eversole and colleagues (1975) reported the sex distribution as equal. According to Silverglade and associates (1978), the tumor's usual clinical manifestation is a swelling caused by bony expansion, which may cause facial asymmetry. Eversole and colleagues (1975) found that swelling was a finding in 81% of the cases, pain in 40%, paresthesia in 11%, and palpable nodes in 26%. Smith and associates (1968) determined that there was an average of 5 years' duration from the onset of symptoms before patients sought any treatment; Silverglade and colleagues (1978) found that period to vary between 3 weeks and 20 years. Rarely, firm, nontender lymph nodes may be palpated; Stoch and Smith (1980) stated that metastases, though limited to the regional lymph nodes, occurred in only 4 of their 50 documented cases. It is only in the later stages, when the tumor reaches significant proportions, that definitive signs appear or sensory changes occur. Toothache or neurologic pain may be the only symptom. If the tumor becomes infected, infection-related symptoms may occur. Infection and infiltration of muscle lead to trismus.

The following criteria for diagnosis were established by Silverglade and associates (1978), Alexander and associates (1974), and Schultz and Whitten (1969): (1) the presence of intact cortical plates, (2) radiographic evidence of bone destruction, and (3) histopathologic confirmation, positive mucin staining, absence of primary lesions in salivary glands or other tissues, and exclusion of an odontogenic tumor.

Treatment/Prognosis

The preferred therapy for the well-differentiated, largely cystic, and clinically slow-growing central lesion remains a matter of controversy. Alexander and associates (1974) and Dhawan and co-authors (1970) recommended wide surgical excision as a minimum procedure. Browand and Waldron (1975), Silverglade and others (1978), and Schultz and Whitten (1969) reported good results after simple enucleation. Eversole and associates (1975) recommended en bloc resection with preservation of the inferior border of the mandible, if possible, as the treatment of choice for lesions that have not produced extensive osseous destruction. The more anaplastic and poorly differentiated cases dictate a more radical surgical treatment, with removal of any regional metastases.

Among the 50 documented cases of Stoch and Smith (1980), 13 cases recurred and 4 deaths were attributed to the tumor. Of the 27 cases reviewed by Eversole and co-authors, 8 patients (30%) had recurrence 6 months to 10 years after surgery. The survival rate of 15 patients at 2 years and 9 patients at 5 years was 100%; an additional patient died of the disease 14 years after diagnosis, one patient was alive with the disease at 10 years, and one patient had uncontrollable disease at 4 months.

◆ *RADIOLOGY (Figs. 14–21 to 14–25)*

Location

In the study of Browand and Waldron (1975), most of the lesions occurred in the mandible, although a few developed in the maxilla. Smith and associates (1968) and Browand and Waldron (1975) reported that, in the mandibular premolar-molar region, most lesions appeared to occur above the mandibular canal; although these did not extend anteriorly beyond the premolar region, some lesions may be located in the mandibular midline.

Radiologic Features

Most reported cases have been described as radiolucent and often multilocular; others have been described as solitary cystic and multicystic with well-defined margins. In other instances, margins have been described as diffusely destructive and poorly defined. The most frequent clinical and radiographic diagnosis was ameloblastoma or dentigerous cyst. Marano and Hartman (1974) reported a case in which the periapical radiographs showed a well-circumscribed radiolucent lesion resembling a cyst, distal to the maxillary third molar; a Waters' view disclosed a domelike extension of the cystic lesion into the maxillary antrum, and the posteroanterior radiograph showed pronounced bony destruction of the floor and walls of the maxillary antrum.

Relationship to Teeth

This lesion often appears as a diffuse radiolucency at the apices of posterior teeth, mimicking periapical abnormalities associated with nonvital teeth; however, the radiolucency persists after root canal therapy. At other times, the lesion is associated with an impacted tooth, usually a third molar.

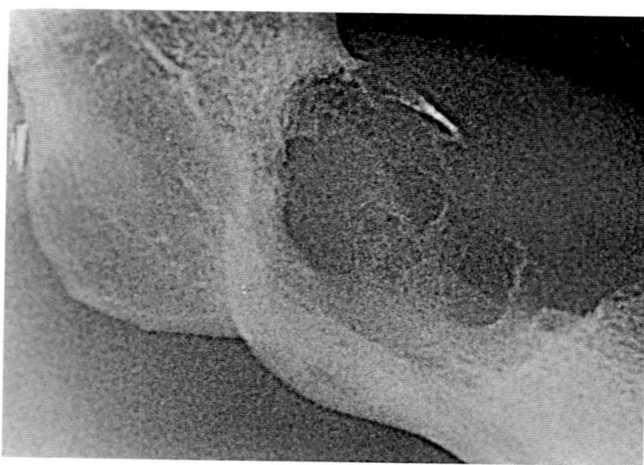

A

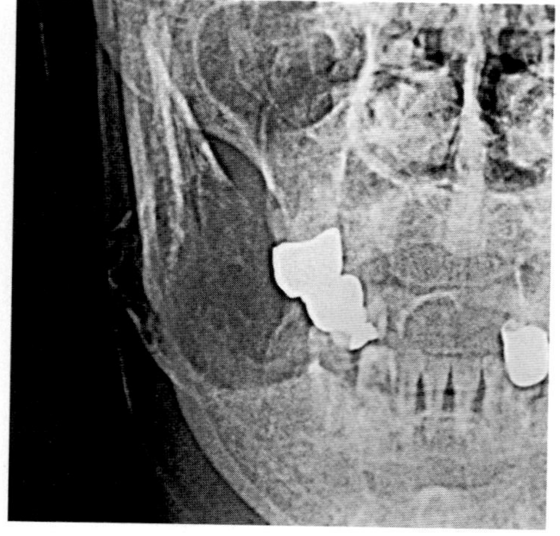

B

FIGURE 14–21.

Central Mucoepidermoid Carcinoma: Digitally reprocessed images. A, Multilocular lesion in retromolar area, expansion of cortex, and perforation at crest of ridge. B, Expanded margin is wavy and perforated. (Courtesy of Professor T. Noikura, Second Oral Surgery Department, Kagoshima University School of Dentistry, Kagoshima, Japan.)

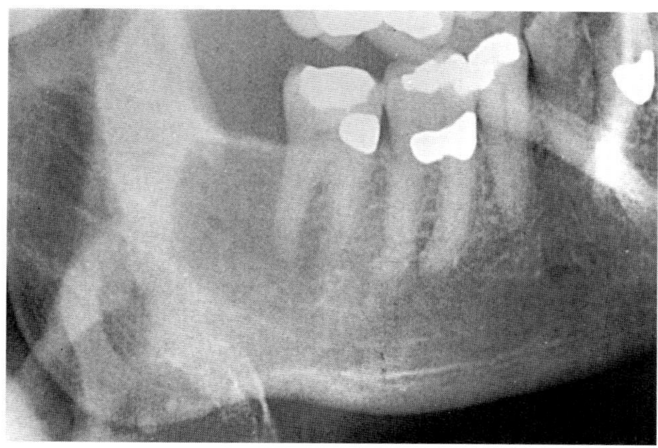

A

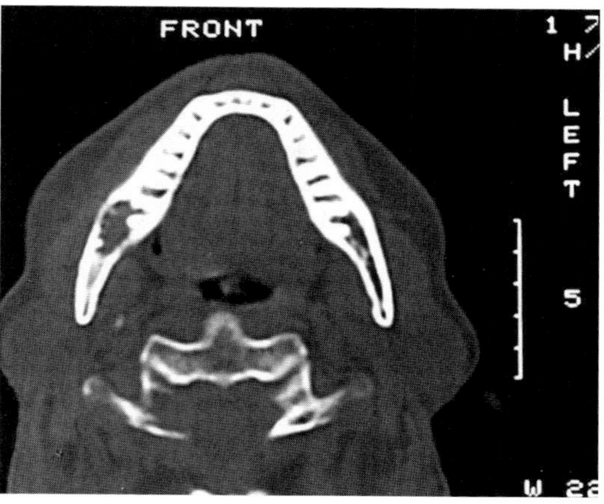

B

FIGURE 14–22.

Central Mucoepidermoid Carcinoma: A, Well-defined punched-out geographic area, with permeative changes within the radiolucency. B, Demineralization of the buccal cortex.

Grubka and associates (1983) reported that most lesions were associated with third molars or arose in the area of a previously extracted third molar. Fredrickson and Cherrick (1978) reported a case of a mixed radiolucent/opaque lesion that extended from the maxillary first premolar to the maxillary third molar and exhibited root resorption of the premolars and molar. Because central mucoepidermoid carcinoma occasionally may appear as a pericoronal radiolucency, this entity should be included in the differential diagnosis of pericoronal radiolucencies.

CENTRAL CLEAR CELL CARCINOMA

The clear cell carcinoma first was recognized in 1956 and is a tumor of salivary gland origin. It is seen primarily in the parotid gland, although it may be seen in the accessory salivary glands in the oral cavity. It is considered a rare lesion when central in bone. Clear cell carcinoma has been reviewed by Corio and colleagues (1982) and Shafer and co-authors (1983). These lesions are classified as low-grade malignant neoplasms. Histologically, the lesion consists of

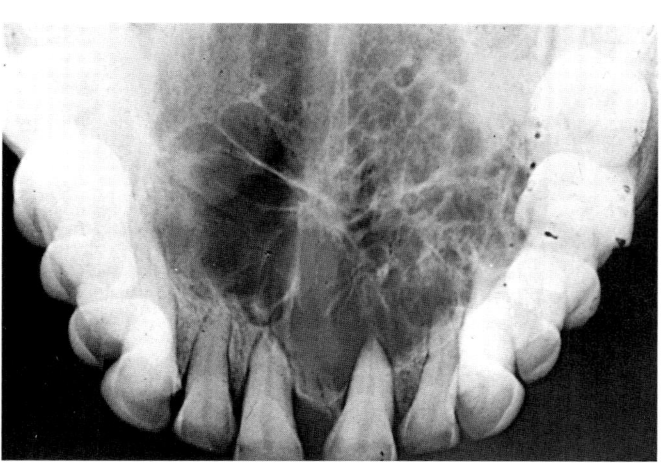

A

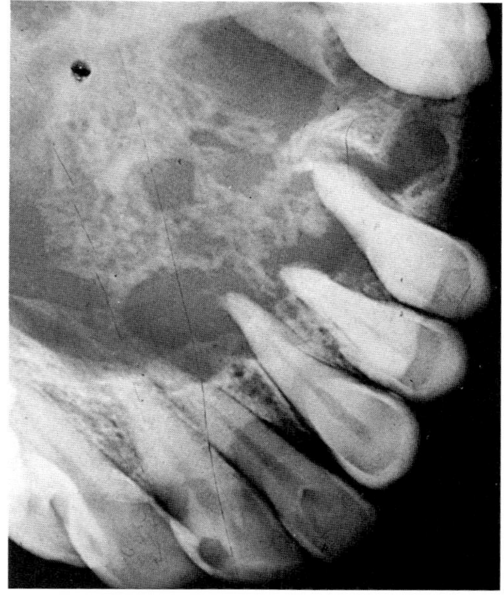

B

FIGURE 14–23.

Central Mucoepidermoid Carcinoma: A, Benign locally aggressive appearance, with soap bubble and honeycomb patterns. B, Malignant appearance, with admixture of permeative and motheaten changes without reactive sclerosis. (Courtesy of Dr. P. Dhiravarangkura, Chulalonghorn University, Bangkok, Thailand.)

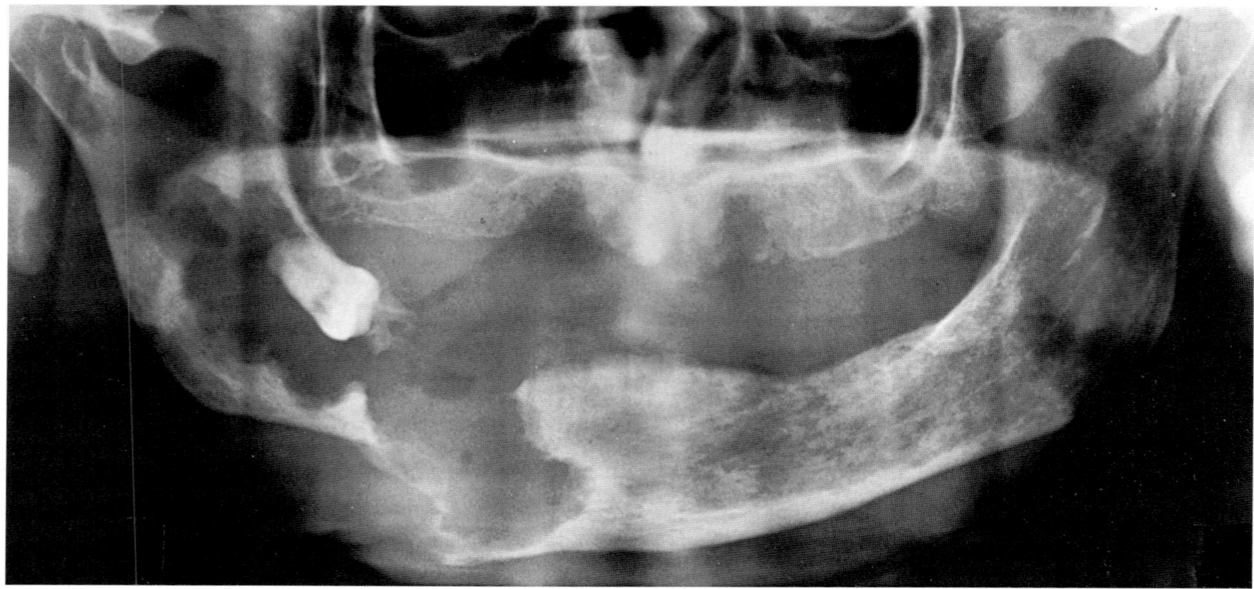

FIGURE 14–24.

Central Mucoepidermoid Carcinoma: Pathologic fracture in 80-year-old man with pain. He had a slim build, did not smoke or consume alcohol, and never wore a denture although he was edentulous for 50 years. The histologic diagnosis was central mucoepidermoid carcinoma arising in the wall of a dentigerous cyst.

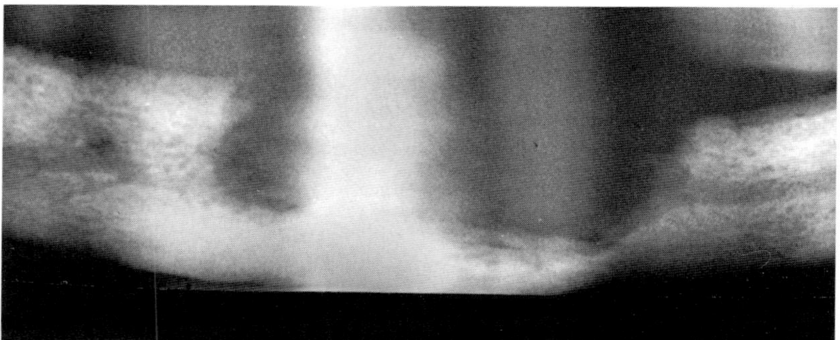

A

FIGURE 14–25.

Central Mucoepidermoid Carcinoma: Metastasis. A, Primary lesion in anterior mandible. B, Metastatic lesion in right fourth rib, with pathologic fracture; it can be seen just to left (patient's right) of inferior tip of tracheostomy device. (Courtesy of Dr. H. C. Shwartz, Kaiser Permanente Medical Group, Los Angeles, CA.)

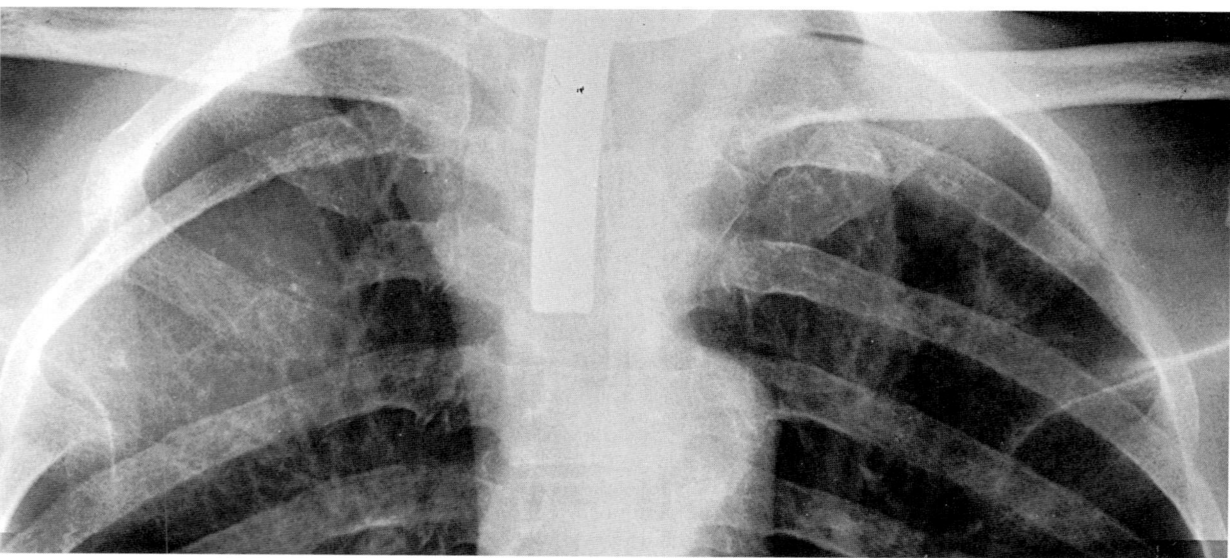

B

clusters of clear cells surrounded by a thin layer of connective tissue, thus giving the lesion an organoid appearance. A variant has been termed epithelial-myoepithelial carcinoma of intercalated duct origin. These lesions are seen more frequently in elderly women. The lesion is treated by surgery, and the prognosis is considered relatively good. According to Shafer and co-authors (1983), fewer than one third recur and fewer still metastasize.

◆ *RADIOLOGY (Fig. 14–26)*

Very little is known about the radiologic features of the central lesion. It is a low-grade malignant neoplasm, so features similar to those of benign locally aggressive lesions might be expected. Because the lesion bears considerable histologic similarity to clear cell carcinoma of the kidney (hypernephroma), the possibility of metastatic hypernephroma should be explored when a central bony lesion is diagnosed as clear cell carcinoma.

ODONTOGENIC GHOST CELL CARCINOMA

The odontogenic ghost cell carcinoma is a malignant counterpart of the keratinizing and calcifying odontogenic cyst originally described in 1962 by Gorlin and co-workers and in 1963 by Gold, and redefined in 1981 by Praetorius and associates. In 1983, Pindborg and Rick agreed that a keratinizing and calcifying odontogenic cyst that was cytologically malignant and that recurred and metastasized should be designated as an odontogenic ghost cell carcinoma. In 1985, Ikemura and co-workers reported the simultaneous occurrence of a calcifying odontogenic cyst and its malignant transformation. In 1986, Ellis and Shmookler reported three cases of ghost cell tumor with malignant clinical and histologic features. Grodjesk and colleagues (1987) reported a patient with an unusual malignant odontogenic tumor containing large numbers of ghost cells. Surgical excision is the treatment of choice. In the case reported by Grodjesk and colleagues (1987) in the right maxilla, treatment consisted of a right hemimaxillectomy; later, a course of cobalt 60 radiation therapy was administered to the neck and right maxilla regions. Approximately 6 months later, a chest radiograph showed multiple well-circumscribed nodular densities in both lungs, suggestive of metastatic disease. Shortly after, the patient died.

◆ *RADIOLOGY*

Odontogenic ghost cell carcinoma may be located in any of the sites in the jaws in which its benign counterpart, the Gorlin cyst, is reported to occur. Very little is known about the radiologic features of this lesion. A panoramic radio-

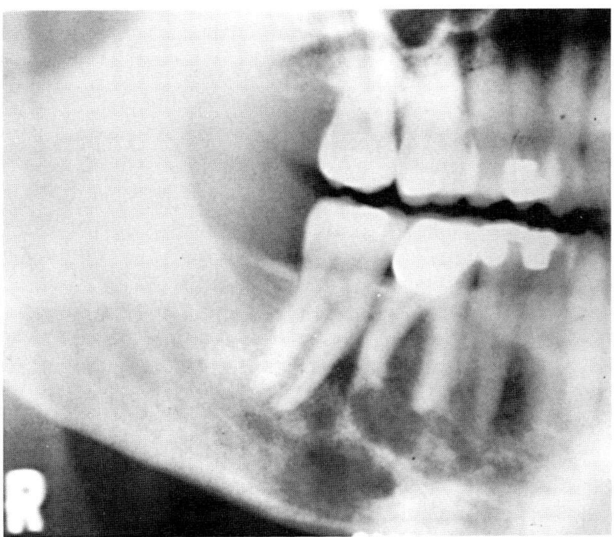

A

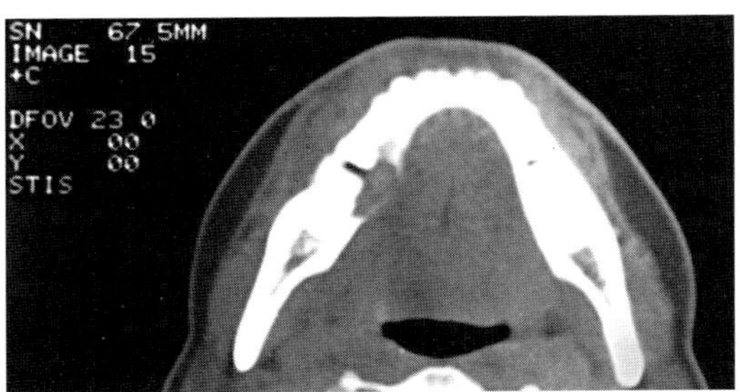

B

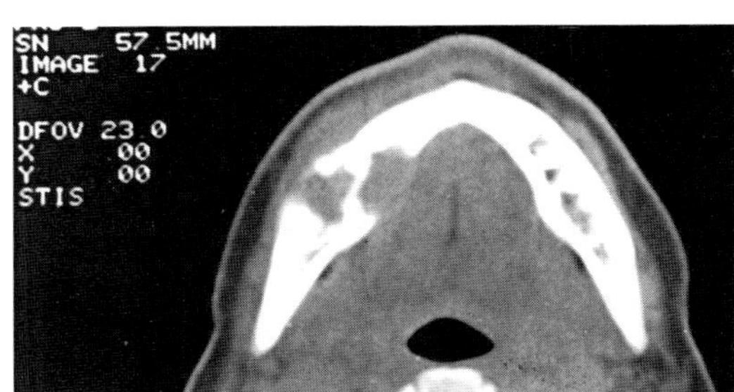

C

FIGURE 14–26.

Central Clear Cell Carcinoma in Elderly White Woman: A, Motheaten and permeative changes and lack of reactive sclerosis at margins. These findings are suggestive of a malignant neoplasm. B and C, Expansion of buccal and lingual cortices and very thin, almost imperceptible layer of subperiosteal new bone at expanded margin. These findings are suggestive of a locally aggressive benign lesion. (Courtesy of Dr. H. Schwartz, Kaiser Permanente Medical Group, Los Angeles, CA.)

graph of Grodjesk and colleagues (1979) showed destruction of the right maxilla with obliteration of the maxillary sinus. Occlusal and periapical radiographs showed an ill-defined area of moderate density in which partially resorbed tooth fragments were embedded. Facial bone radiographs, including tomographs, showed opacification of the right maxillary antrum extending into the nasal cavity with erosion of the medial wall. The inferolateral wall of the antrum appeared to be eroded, with extension of the mass into the oral cavity. In the basal or axial view, apparent extension into the ethmoid sinuses could be seen; the orbital wall was intact. A ^{99m}technetium scan showed focal satellite accumulation of tracer material in the right maxilla; the remaining skeleton appeared normal.

AMELOBLASTIC CARCINOMA

Slootweg and Muller (1984) and Corio and associates (1987) defined ameloblastic carcinoma as any ameloblastoma in which there is histologic evidence of malignant disease in the primary or recurrent tumor, regardless of whether it has metastasized. There is obvious histologic transformation of the epithelial component indicating carcinoma, usually epidermoid carcinoma.

The term malignant ameloblastoma should be confined to ameloblastomas that metastasize yet show an apparent ''benign'' appearance in primary and metastatic lesions. In other words, the metastatic tumor still resembles the primary ameloblastoma, which is benign in appearance, with no histologic evidence of malignant transformation. This lesion was discussed under ''ameloblastoma''.

Pathologic Characteristics

In the eight cases of ameloblastic carcinoma reported by Corio and associates (1987), the individual epithelial cells often displayed dysplastic changes, including an increased nuclear/cytoplasmic ratio, nuclear hyperchromatism, and mitosis in increased numbers with abnormal forms. Necrosis and dystrophic calcification in the centers of some islands were also significant histologic features not usually observed in the typical ameloblastoma. In four cases of Corio and colleagues (1987), the neoplasia may have arisen from a cystic lining; in two cases, typical ameloblastoma was observed in some areas, whereas other fields exhibited histologic evidence of malignancy.

Clinical Features

In 1987, Corio and associates reported eight cases of ameloblastic carcinoma from the Armed Forces Institute of Pathology. The mean patient age was 30 years (range, 15 to 84 years). The incidence of male and female patients was equal. Two patients were white, three were black, and the races of three were unspecified. The duration was stated in four instances and ranged from 2 months to 1 year. Signs and symptoms varied; the most common symptom was swelling (six cases), followed by pain or rapid growth (three cases each), trismus (one case), and dysphonia (one case). Clinically, the ameloblastic carcinoma is more aggressive than most typical ameloblastomas, with perforation of cortical bone, extension into surrounding soft tissue, numerous recurrent lesions, and metastasis to cervical lymph nodes.

Treatment/Prognosis

The treatment of choice for ameloblastic carcinoma is surgery, and the 5-year survival rate is 30 to 40% according to Shear (1969); metastasis to regional lymph nodes is common. In the eight cases of ameloblastic carcinoma reported by Corio and associates (1987), four cases were treated with resection, one with enucleation, and three with unspecified surgery.

◆ *RADIOLOGY*

In the cases of ameloblastic carcinoma reported by Corio and colleagues (1987), seven cases involved the mandible and only one occurred in the maxilla. Four of these involved the posterior mandibular region, and two affected much of the mandibular body and ramus and extended into the contiguous soft tissues. The size of the tumor was stated in five cases and ranged from 1.5 to 7 cm. The radiographic findings were suggestive of ameloblastoma, except that some radiographs also exhibited focal radiopacities, apparently reflecting dystrophic mineralization. In one case there was obliteration of the sinus. In other cases root resorption was observed. These lesions were uniformly aggressive in appearance: three tumors perforated cortical bone, and two extended into the floor of the mouth and adjacent soft tissues.

METASTATIC DISEASE OF THE JAWS

A metastasis can be defined as a spontaneous neoplastic lesion that arises from another cancer with which it is no longer in continuity. In 1891, von Recklinghausen hypothesized that osseous metastases probably originated in bloodborne tumor emboli rather than from lymphatic spread. Bones with red marrow, such as the trunk bones, ribs, skull, proximal femur, and humerus, are the preferential sites of metastasis. Metastases to bones distal to the knees or elbows are rare.

A skeletal focus of metastatic cancer is often the presenting lesion and may be the only demonstrable tumor; in other cases, the skeleton may be riddled with metastases while the lungs and viscera are clear. These apparent dilemmas can be explained by the studies of Batson (1957). He showed an extensive communicating plexus of veins surrounding the vertebral column; these veins communicate directly with the proximal half of the lower extremities through the inferior vena cava and with the proximal half of the upper extremities, head, and neck through the superior vena cava. This venous plexus is unique in that there are no valves to control blood flow. As a result, when pressure in the lungs or abdomen increases, as in expiration, blood may either bypass or flow from the caval systems into the vertebral plexus of veins, which in turn, connect with the venous and sinusoidal system of the bones of the spine, shoulder girdle, skull, mandible, or even up to the region of the elbows or knees without having to flow through the heart, lungs, or liver. It is through this route that the principal metastases from carcinoma of the breast, prostate, and kidney are believed to occur, without necessarily involving the lungs, liver, or parenchymal organs.

Pathologic Characteristics

The microscopic picture of metastatic bone disease is one of nests, islands, and cords of neoplastic epithelium supported by a fibrous stroma. The individual tumor cells show keratinizing, adenoid, or anaplastic morphologic characteristics, depending on the site of origin of the primary tumor. Of the tumors known to metastasize to bone, the most common primary sites are the breast, prostate, and lung. Catalona and co-workers (1991) measured the blood levels of prostate-specific antigen in 1600 men who were 50 years of age and older. These authors reported that the prostate-specific antigen test correctly identified 36% more prostate cancer cases than did rectal examinations and detected 40% more cases than did an ultrasound scope, a device used by some urologists to examine the gland visually.

Clinical Features

Worth (1963) and Lichtenstein (1952) stated that metastatic carcinoma is the most common malignant tumor of bone. In a large autopsy series by Mirra (1989), the ratio of skeletal metastases to primary bone tumors was approximately 125 to 1. Of patients with metastatic disease, 15 to 20% have clinically evident skeletal metastases; at autopsy, after bone sampling, this number increases to 70%. More than 80% of bone metastases are from carcinoma of the breast, prostate, lung, kidney, and thyroid. Stypulkowska and associates (1979) and Bhaskar (1973) reported that metastatic malignant neoplasms in the oral cavity are rare and account for only 1% of all oral neoplasms. The average age of patients with bone metastasis is 55 years. Galasko (1975) reported that pain is the most frequent symptom of bone metastases and occurs in approximately two thirds of patients with lesions detectable by standard radiography. Clausen and Poulsen (1963) observed that the most common symptoms are swelling and pain. They emphasized that paresthesia and anesthesia are especially ominous features, when present. Other symptoms are loosening of teeth, trismus, periodontal abscess, facial paralysis, and, rarely, pathologic fracture. Metastatic disease of the jaws may be asymptomatic. With respect to cancer of the skeletal system, hypercalcemia and hypertrophic pulmonary osteoarthropathy are important systemic manifestations. Massive rapid bone destruction—particularly in association with high-grade lytic breast, lung, or kidney metastases and myeloma—may lead to severe hypercalcemia, causing symptoms such as lethargy, anorexia, nausea, dehydration, confusion, and coma. Hypertrophic pulmonary osteoarthropathy is characterized by periosteal thickening and pain, predominantly of the long and short tubular bones; swollen joints in 30 to 40% of patients; and, often but not invariably, clubbing of the digits. Most cases are associated with benign and malignant pulmonary disease such as bronchogenic carcinoma, mesothelioma, and Hodgkin's disease. Pathologic fracture may be seen in jaw metastases.

Clausen and Poulsen (1963) reported 97 cases of metastatic carcinoma of the jaws and found that the most common primary tumors were as follows: breast (31%); lung (18%); kidney (15%); thyroid, prostate, and colon (6% each); and stomach carcinoma (5%) and melanocarcinoma (5%); 82% of cases were found in the mandible. Meyer and Shklar (1965) reported that 70% of their 20 cases of metastasis to the oral cavity were adenocarcinomas and 85% occurred in the mandible.

In men older than 50 years of age, prostate carcinoma is the most common cancer that metastasizes to bone. Approximately 35% of patients with prostate cancer show radiographic evidence of bone metastases. Roughly 30,000 men die of this disease in the United States each year, in part because 70% of all cases go undetected until the carcinoma has spread beyond the prostate gland.

Approximately 15% of lung cancers metastasize to bones, including those of the hands and feet. In the past, lung cancer has been chiefly a tumor of male cigarette smokers, but Ciola and Yesner (1977) reported that the incidence among women has been increasing and the male-to-female ratio at Memorial Hospital in New York was 2:1. With the increase in lung cancer in women, it can be expected that the number of oral carcinomas in women resulting from metastatic sources also will increase.

In 83 cases of neuroblastoma of the adrenal glands reported by Stern and associates (1974), 25% of the cases were metastatic to the jaws. Approximately 85% of patients with neuroblastoma are younger than 10 years of age. In any patient younger than 20 years with a malignant-appearing bone tumor, metastatic neuroblastoma and lymphoma/leukemia are the prime considerations. Only 16% of patients with Ewing's sarcoma and 8% with primary osteosarcoma are younger than 10 years of age.

Clausen and Poulsen (1963) provided the following criteria for identifying metastatic diseases of the jaws:

1. The lesion must be a true metastasis localized to the bone tissue, as distinguished from direct invasion by a primary tumor of contiguous structure.
2. The lesion must be verified microscopically as carcinoma.
3. The primary site of the lesion must be known.

Treatment/Prognosis

The occurrence of metastatic growth in the jaws usually carries a grave prognosis. Clausen and Poulsen (1963) reported that 70% of patients reviewed died within 1 year. In jaw metastases from thyroid and renal cell carcinoma, particularly to the mandible and showing an isolated nodule, Gorlin and Goldman (1970) reported that the prognosis is more favorable. A variety of measures have been used to provide considerable symptom relief and prolonged pain palliation, including, singly or in combination, radiation therapy, administration of sex hormones, adrenalectomy, chemotherapy, and even hypophysectomy. Invariably, however, the disease is fatal.

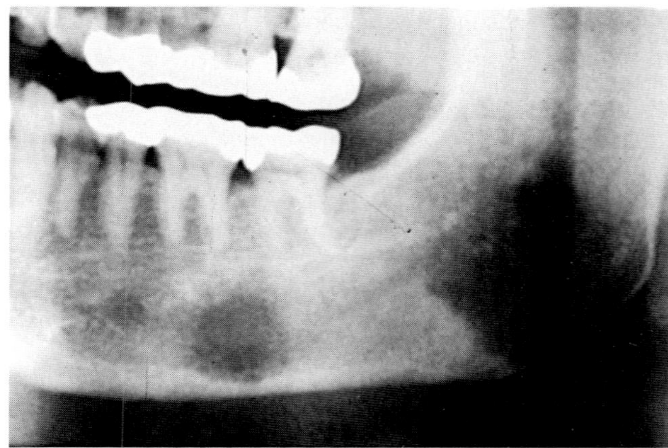

FIGURE 14–27.

Metastatic Disease: Adenocarcinoma of the Lung: A 51-year-old white man had paresthesia in the left lower lip and shortness of breath. A geographic pattern is seen with trabecular remnants within. There is endosteal erosion of the inferior cortex with permeative changes at the lytic margin. (Courtesy of Dr. H. Schwartz, Kaiser Permanente Medical Group, Los Angeles, CA.)

◆ RADIOLOGY (Figs. 14–27 to 14–35)

General Radiologic Features

Most bone metastases are purely lytic. Solitary lesions are less common than multiple lesions. Mirra (1989) specified the ''when you see..., think...'' rule of bone metastases: In a patient with multiple bone lesions that appear malignant, one should consider metastases first, lymphoma/leukemia second, osteosarcoma third, and other possibilities last. Multiple lytic defects in the skull are particularly common in multiple myeloma, metastatic carcinoma, neuroblastoma, and Hand-Schüller-Christian (HSC) disease. Carcinomatous skull metastases are typically from primary tumors of the breast or lung. The preferential sites of the metastatic deposits from breast cancer are the spine, pelvis, ribs, skull, femur, humerus, and scapula. Pathologic fractures most commonly occur in the spine, neck of femur, and ribs. Approximately 65% of breast metastases are lytic, roughly 25% are mixed lytic and blastic, and the remaining 10% are blastic. Occasionally, the lesions are entirely blastic in one bone and purely lytic in another.

Cawson (1959) showed that bone resorption was most active where metastatic tumor cells were plentiful; however, in areas where tumor cells were sparse, there was an abundance of new bone formation. Metastasis from prostate carcinoma characteristically produces an osteosclerotic appearance on radiographs, but occasionally thyroid or breast carcinoma metastases have an identical appearance. Prostatic metastases are blastic in approximately 75% of cases, lytic in 10%, and mixed in 15%. Occasional cases are associated with a focal, periosteal ''sunburst'' appearance. Approximately 80% of lung carcinoma metastases are lytic, 15% mixed lytic-blastic, and 5% blastic.

Renal cell and thyroid carcinomas are the two metastatic cancers most likely to be associated with a solitary metastasis because they are associated most frequently with pure lysis. The edge of the lesion may appear ''sharp'' to ''nibbled,'' whereas the shape can vary from round to oval to loculated; many cases show fusiform to an eccentric ''blowout'' type of expansion, frequently with total loss of cortical borders.

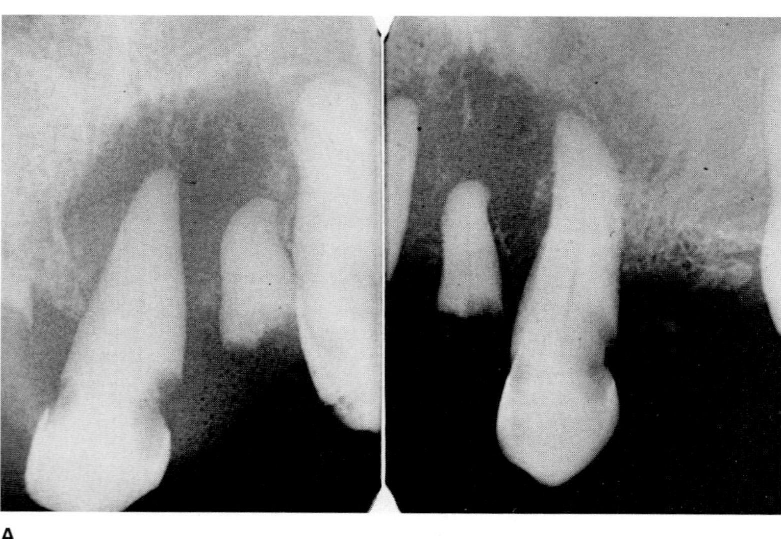

A

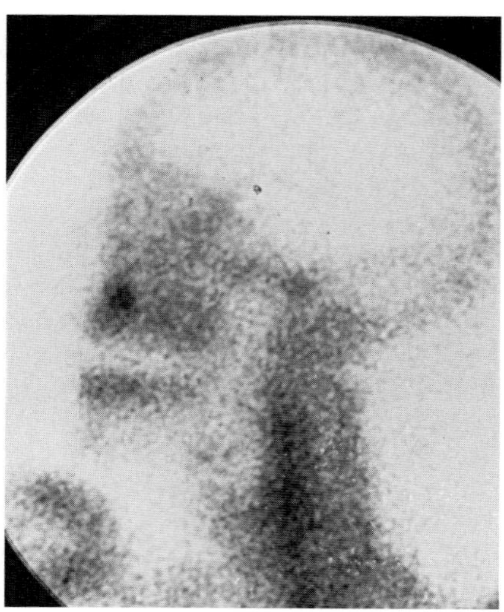

B

FIGURE 14–28.

Metastatic Disease: Adenocarcinoma of the Lung: A, Central and lateral incisor roots show floating tooth appearance, with one important difference from gingival carcinoma: in metastatic disease there are often multiple trabecular remnants (From Ciola B, Yesner R: Radiographic manifestations of a lung carcinoma with metastases to the anterior maxilla. Oral Surg 44:811, 1977.) B, Technetium scan shows a single hot spot in region of lesion. (Courtesy of Drs. B. Ciola and R. Yesner, West Haven Veterans Administration, West Haven, CT.)

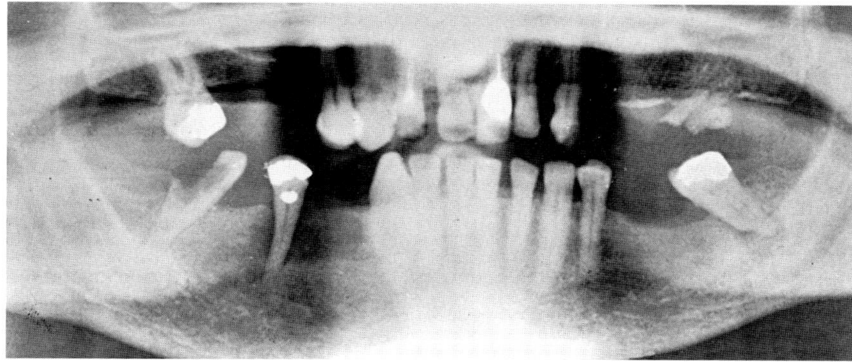

A

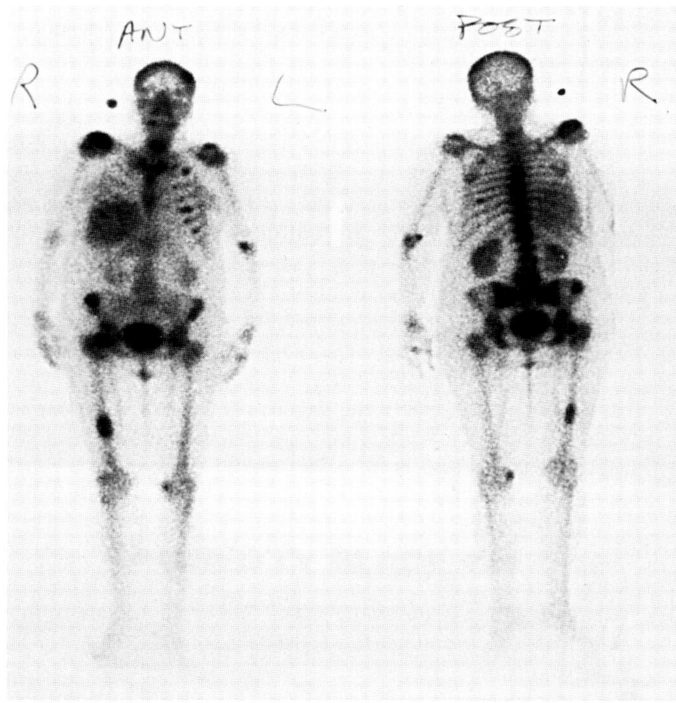

B

FIGURE 14–29.

Metastatic Disease: Adenocarcinoma of the Lung: A, Bilateral metastases to mandibular premolar areas. B, Technetium scan shows bilateral metastases to mandible. Other metastases include clavicles, ribs, pelvis, and right femur, with the primary tumor in the right lung. Hot spots in the joints represent arthritic disease. The central hot spot in the pelvis is accumulated radionuclide in the bladder, and the kidneys are seen in posterior view for the same reason. (Courtesy of Dr. G. Naylor, National Naval Dental Center, Bethesda MD.)

Pathologic fracture occurs in approximately 33% of cases. Mirra (1989) stated that in patients older than 30 years with solitary or multiple purely lytic malignant tumors with fusiform bone expansion, one should consider renal cell metastasis first, thyroid metastasis second, and then other possibilities.

Radiologic Features of the Jaws

Location. The most frequent sites of metastasis to bone are areas occupied by red bone marrow. Most carcinomas that occur in the jaws from metastasis often arise in the central portion of the jaws, an area richest in red marrow. When bone is involved in metastatic disease, the jaws rarely are affected. According to Worth (1963), metastases may occur anywhere in either jaw, but there seems to be a preference for the third molar region of the mandible.

Radiologic Features. Metastases in bone show two main radiographic appearances: frank destruction of an area of bone without new bone formation within the lesion or adjacent bone, and an appearance mimicking osteomyelitis.

In the first radiographic appearance, the lytic area is termed geographic if a single large focus of bone has been destroyed. In this instance, the lesion is considered to be relatively slow growing and less aggressive than other malignant presentations, such as motheaten and infiltrative patterns. The margin shows the same suggestion of infiltration as in primary malignant tumors; when there is only one such lesion, it may not be possible to distinguish whether it is primary or metastatic. The combination of a geographic area of osteolysis with very irregular margins and islands of bone within the radiolucent area is an appearance highly suggestive of metastasis. These islands of bone may differ in size, but they all tend to have irregular margins and represent

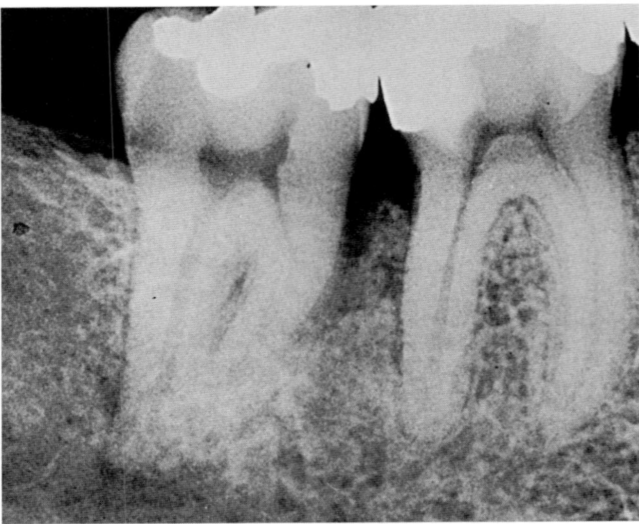

FIGURE 14–30.

Metastatic Disease: Metastatic Adenocarcinoma of the Breast: Very subtle permeative changes at apex of second molar mimic pulpal infection; however, additional permeative change is present in area. (Courtesy of C. Thompson, M. Bartley, and L. Woolley, Department of Oral Pathology, University of Oregon Health Sciences Center, Portland, OR.)

bone fragments that have been separated by an infiltrating malignant process; these are not masses of new bone, as in some osteogenic sarcomas. If there is more than one such area, the diagnosis of metastatic carcinoma is almost certain. A primary malignant tumor tends to cause lysis of all of the host bone as it advances, without leaving islands of bone behind. The absence of clinical or radiographic evidence of swelling may suggest that the lesion is metastatic.

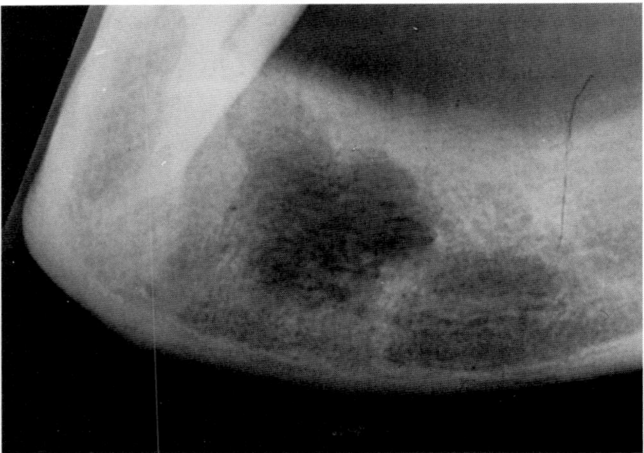

FIGURE 14–31.

Metastatic Disease: Breast Adenocarcinoma: A 43-year-old woman complained of left temporomandibular joint pain of several months' duration. There is a geographic area of lysis within which multiple permeative changes are seen. Slight sclerosis is seen in some areas of margin, and there is a wide transition zone in the upper mesial part of the lesion.

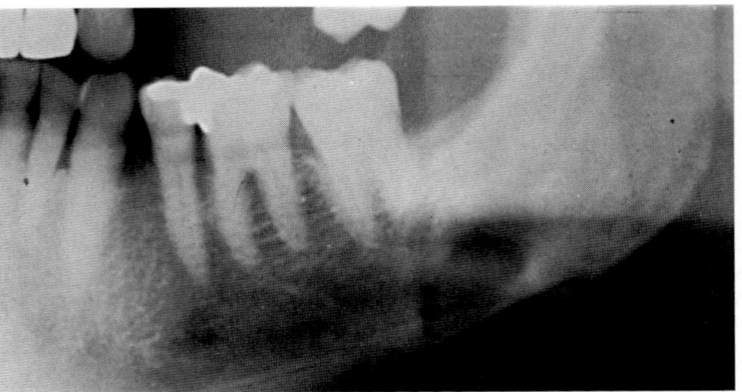

FIGURE 14–32.

Metastatic Disease: Prostate Carcinoma: Resembles salivary gland depression. A diffusely rarefied area is seen anterior to the lesion. (Courtesy of Dr. T. Underhill, Winston-Salem, NC.)

The second radiographic appearance of the lytic or radiolucent type of metastasis in the jaw has considerable resemblance to some manifestations of osteomyelitis characterized by the presence of many areas of bone destruction, some of which may not be more than 2 mm in diameter. Generally, osteomyelitis consists of a motheaten pattern only, and on careful inspection with low-kilovoltage occlusal and lateral views, a periosteal reaction can be seen. In metastatic disease, although motheaten patterns may be seen, a permeative pattern of bone destruction is invariably present in lytic metastatic disease. There may be destruction of the cortex, and a periosteal reaction is notably absent. Pathologic fracture may be seen in the area of rarefaction.

Although most of the lesions that metastasize to the jaws are osteolytic, certain tumors may produce osteoblastic lesions characterized by the production of bone. Such lesions are manifested as radiopaque areas and are associated most often with carcinoma of the prostate and, occasionally, the breast and lung.

Metastatic carcinoma of the jaws also may mimic periodontal and periapical disease. Metastatic disease often is diagnosed only when the socket of a previously extracted tooth does not heal. As emphasized by Clausen and Poulsen (1963), loss of bony support or thickening of the periodontal ligament space involving one or several adjacent teeth in the absence of generalized periodontitis is an important sign of metastatic disease.

It should be understood that, although radiographic examination is valuable in the study of metastatic tumors in bone, conventional radiography alone does not exclude their presence. It is very common for widespread bone involvement to be present without any radiographic evidence of abnormality. In such instances, bone scintigraphy with technetium usually shows the lesions.

In a study of 25 cases of malignant tumors metastatic to the jaws, Meyer and Shklar (1965) observed that 5 led to the discovery of the primary lesion. In a study of 97 cases, Clausen and Poulsen (1963) found that the oral metastasis was discovered before the primary lesion in 33 cases.

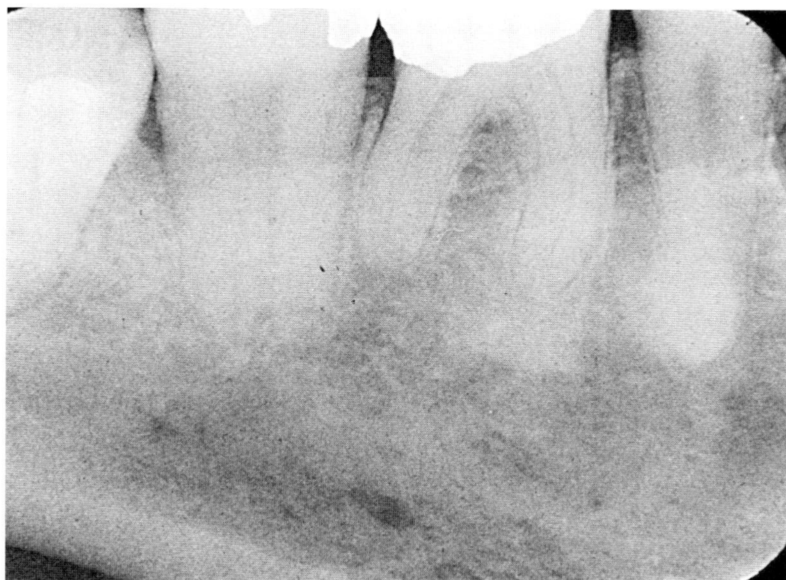

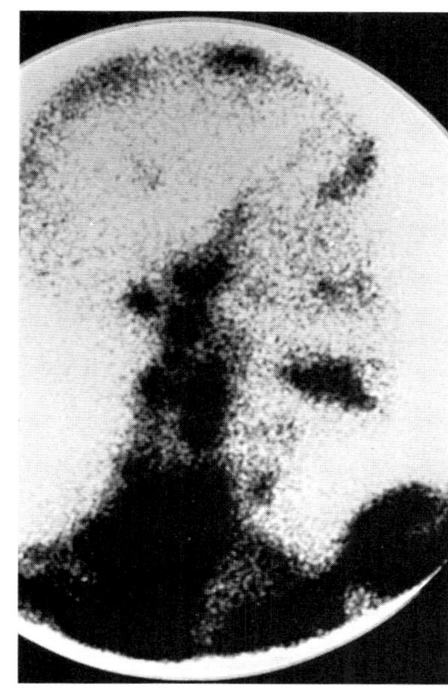

A B

FIGURE 14–33.

Metastatic Disease: Prostate Carcinoma: A, Permeative changes within rarefied area and indistinct trabecular pattern. B, Technetium scan shows multiple metastases in the mandible, cervical spine, auditory portion of the temporal bone, and calvarium of the skull. The lesser hot spots in the maxillary and frontal regions probably represent sinus infection. (From Ciola B: Oral radiographic manifestations of a metastatic prostatic carcinoma. Oral Surg 52:105, July 1981.)

FIBROSARCOMA OF BONE

Fibrosarcoma is a rare malignant primary tumor of bone characterized histologically by poorly differentiated to well-differentiated fibrous tissue proliferation that is not associated with the production of cartilage, osteoid, or bone. As early as 1943, Budd and MacDonald advocated the distinction of fibrosarcoma from osteogenic sarcoma. Phemister (1948) suggested that this occurs more frequently in the medullary region than in the periosteum. Dahlin (1978) and

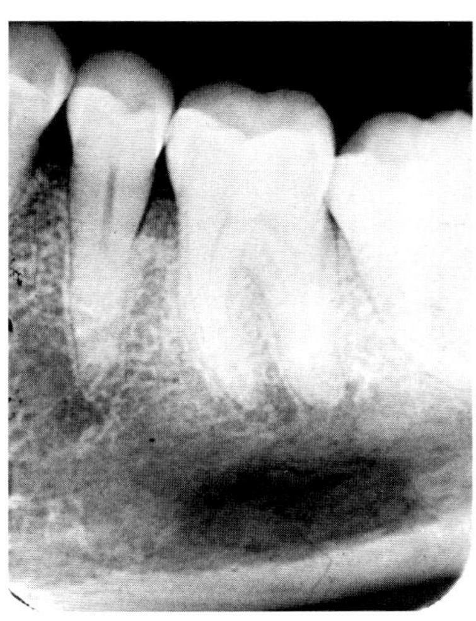

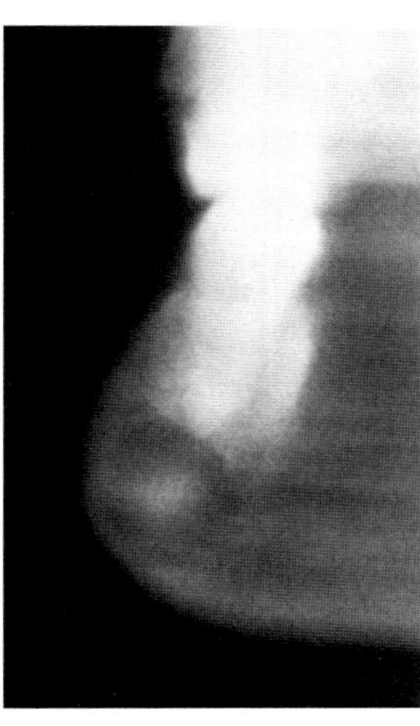

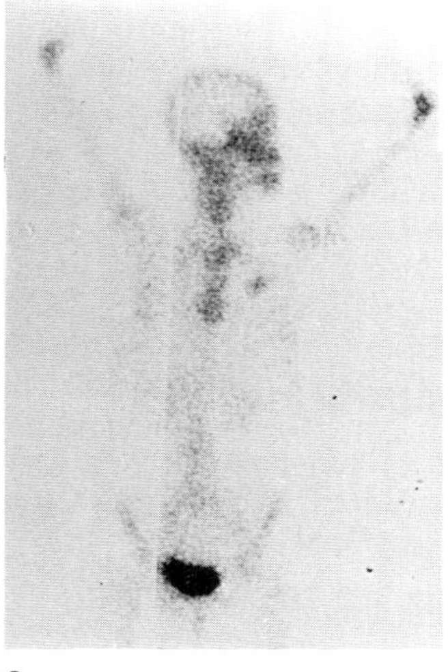

A B C

FIGURE 14–34.

Metastatic Disease: Melanoma: A 46-year-old woman had a history of melanoma on the neck, which was removed 3 months previously. The current complaint was paresthesia in the left lower lip. A, Geographic rarefaction and permeative changes within. B, Tomogram of same area shows large residue of bone within rarefied area. C, Area of increased uptake in mandible. (Courtesy of Dr. T. Underhill, Winston-Salem, NC.)

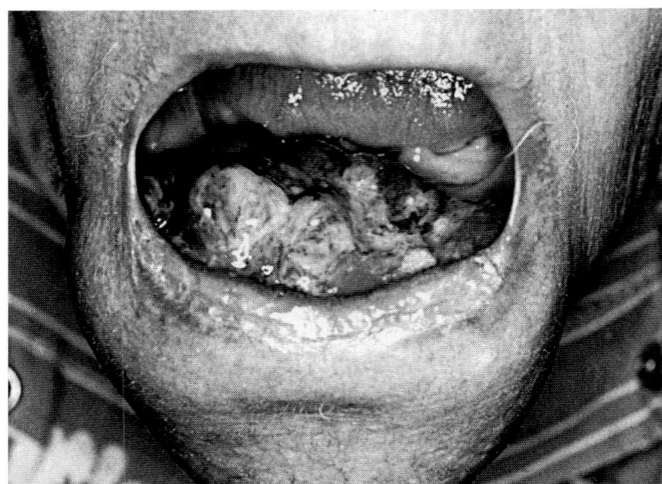

A

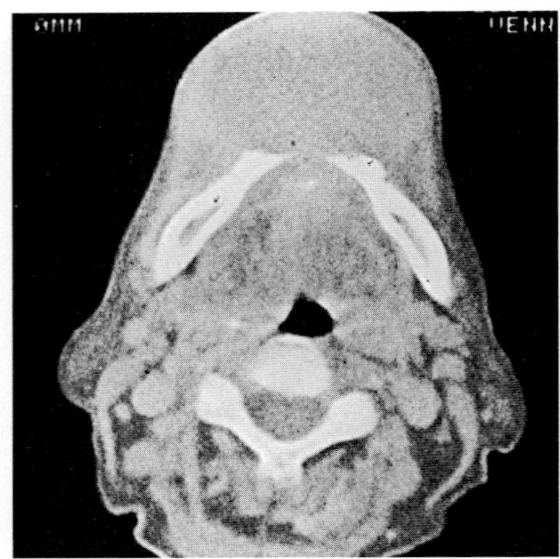

B

FIGURE 14–35.

Metastatic Disease: Colon Adenocarcinoma: An 85-year-old woman had a history of lower bowel resection for cancer. She was well for 18 months until she discovered several loose anterior teeth; after these were removed, large swelling developed rapidly and a biopsy was performed subsequently. A, Clinical presentation of mass. B, CT image of lesion. (From Mast HL, Nissenblatt MJ: Metastatic colon carcinoma and review of literature. J Surg Oncol 34:202, 1987.)

Schajowicz (1981) stated that most fibrosarcomas occur de novo but may arise secondarily from Paget's disease, bone damaged by radiation, ameloblastic fibroma, chronic osteomyelitis, and, rarely, fibrous dysplasia.

Pathologic Characteristics

Microscopically, the tumor tissue may be well differentiated, poorly differentiated, or anaplastic. Patient survival rates are lower among those with the poorly differentiated type. Well-differentiated fibrosarcomas are composed of elongated and spindle-shaped tumor cells with small and uniform nuclei. Dahlin and Ivins (1969) stated that intercellular collagen formation may be so abundant that the tumor may be misinterpreted as a desmoplastic fibroma. The tumor cells of well-differentiated fibrosarcomas characteristically are arranged in interesting fascicles, producing a herringbone pattern. In less well-differentiated fibrosarcomas, there is increased cellularity, with cells arranged more closely and a corresponding decrease in the amount of collagen. The nuclei are larger, ovoid or round, and more irregular. The chromatin is coarse, clumped, and distributed more irregularly. Mitotic activity is increased. The herringbone pattern is less evident and may be absent.

Clinical Features

Fibrosarcoma of bone occurs distinctly less frequently than osteogenic sarcoma or chondrosarcoma. The relative incidence of fibrosarcoma of bone ranges from approximately 3.5% of all primary malignant bone tumors, as reported by Larsson and colleagues (1976), to 12%, as reported by McKenna and co-authors (1966). Fibrosarcoma of the bone is observed in men and women with approximately equal frequency. The age distribution of patients varies widely, from 8 to 88 years; of the 200 cases reported by Stout (1948), 45% of the cases occurred in patients between the ages of 20 and 40 years. In a series of 117 patients with fibrosarcoma reported by Taconis and Van Rijssel (1986), 14 patients (10%) had fibrosarcoma of the jaws. Of these, 10 (72%) were male and 4 (28%) were female. The patients' ages ranged from 8 to 59 years (mean, 30 years). From the files at the Mayo Clinic, Van Blarcom and associates (1971) reported the cases of 13 patients with fibrosarcoma of the mandible. Seven patients were male and six were female. At diagnosis, their ages ranged from 12 to 49 years; six patients were in the fourth decade of life. Paresthesia was a presenting complaint of four patients, and two patients had trismus. Other clinical findings include local pain, swelling, and limited motion, which usually are of less than 6 months' duration. Pathologic fracture is present at the time of the initial evaluation in approximately 33% of patients.

Treatment/Prognosis

Generally, fibrosarcoma is resistant to radiation therapy, and chemotherapy does not control the disease. Therefore, the usual therapy has been surgical removal. Osseous fibrosarcomas are aggressive and have a tendency for one or more recurrences. The recurrence rate and likelihood of patient survival correlate with the histologic grade of the neoplasm. The lesion tends to metastasize to the lungs and bones, even when wide surgical excision has been performed. Differentiation between fibrosarcoma of bone and soft tissue fibrosarcoma has prognostic significance. Pritchard and associates (1977) reported that the 5-year survival rate for patients with soft tissue fibrosarcoma was approximately 60%, as opposed to a 4.2% 5-year survival rate as reported by Larsson and associates (1976) and 32% rate as reported by McKenna and co-workers (1966) for patients with central fibrosarcoma of the bone. Toconis and Van Rijssel (1986) stated that the 5-year survival rate of 71% for fibrosarcoma of the jaws is more favorable than the rate for fibrosarcoma in the remainder of the skeleton. Dahlin (1978), Mirra (1981), Pritchard and associates (1977), and Schajowicz (1981) reported a 5-year survival rate of 25 to 34% for fibrosarcoma in the skeleton. In the Mayo Clinic series of bone sarcomas (Dahlin and Ivins [1969], Van Blarcom and colleagues [1971]), mandibular fibrosarcoma exhibited a 5-year survival rate of 40%, which is a more favorable outcome than the 29% rate found in the whole series. Huvos and Higinbotham (1975) studied the Memorial Sloan-Kettering Cancer Center series and observed that the better prognosis for jaw fibrosarcoma became apparent only in the long term. The 5-year survival rate was 27% for both long bone and jaw cases, whereas this figure decreased to 17% in 20 years for long bone fibrosarcomas but remained constant at 27% for jaw fibrosarcomas throughout the 20-year observation period.

◆ RADIOLOGY (Fig. 14–36)

General Radiologic Features

Dahlin (1978), Pritchard and associates (1977), and Bertoni and associates (1984) reported that the skeletal distribution of fibrosarcoma of the bone is similar to that of osteosarcoma and malignant fibrous histiocytoma. The tubular bones are affected more often in younger patients, but older patients have a tendency toward flat bone involvement. The femur is involved in 40% of cases, tibia in 16%, and humerus in 10%. The bones around the knee account for 33 to 80% of all fibrosarcomas.

The tumor usually occurs eccentrically in the metaphysis of a long bone but may extend into the epiphysis. The chief radiographic feature is a destructive osteolytic lesion with a geographic, motheaten, or permeative pattern of bone destruction and, generally, a wide zone of transition between normal and abnormal bone. There is rarely a reactive sclerosis at the margin, and periosteal reactions are infrequent. When present, periosteal bone formation is variable in appearance, showing lamellar or spiculated patterns or a Codman's triangle. Cortical destruction and soft tissue masses are seen. There is no neoplastic new bone formation, and flocculent calcifications cannot be seen within the radiolucent areas as seen in osteosarcomas and chondrosarcomas. A common finding is a bone sequestrum, varying in size, which may be present in the tumor; these sometimes are related to pathologic fracture. Fibrosarcoma is the only malignant bone tumor in which sequestration is found frequently; sequestration also has been described in the intracortical Ewing's sarcoma. Massive expansion may be present, simulating an aneurysmal bone cyst.

Radiologic Features of the Jaws

Location. In a series of 117 patients with fibrosarcoma described by Taconis and Van Rijssel (1986), the incidence of fibrosarcoma in the jaws was 1% (14 patients); primary soft tissue fibrosarcoma with secondary involvement of the bone was excluded. Van Blarcom and co-workers (1971) and Slootweg and Muller (1984) reported that the mandible (5% of cases) and maxilla (2% of cases) are uncommon sites of fibrosarcomas. In the 14 cases of fibrosarcoma of the jaw described by Taconis and van Rijssel (1986), 10 cases were located in the mandible and 4 in the maxilla. Of the tumors located in the mandible, three were located in the body, three in the angle, and four in the ramus.

Radiologic Features. In the 13 cases of fibrosarcoma of the mandible reviewed by Van Barcom and associates (1971), the essential destructive nature of this tumor was

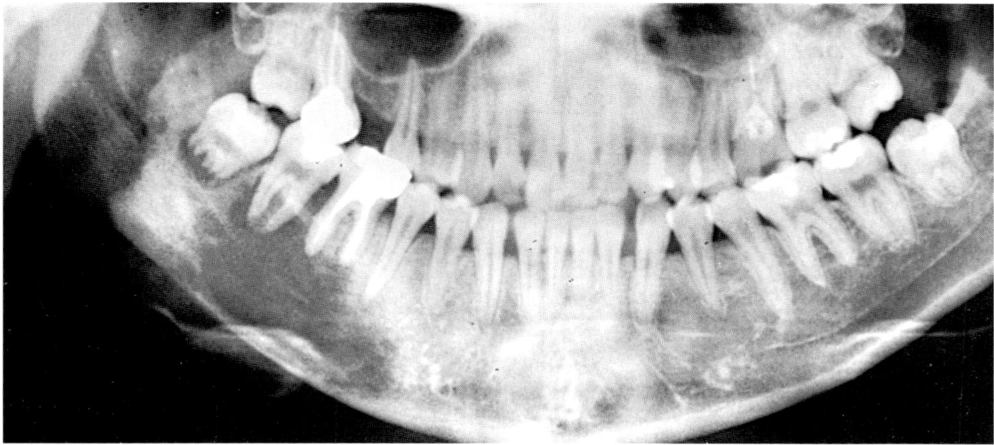

FIGURE 14–36.

Fibrosarcoma in a 17-year-old Girl: Geographic area of rarefaction with trabecular remnants within lesion. There is a permeative change in ramus; irregular, ragged margins; erosion of the endosteal surface of the cortex without periosteal reaction; enlarged, increased lucency of dental papilla; and retarded development of third molar. (Courtesy of Drs. M. Araki, K. Hashimoto, and K. Honda, Nihon University School of Dentistry, Tokyo, Japan.)

recognized readily, although there were no features that distinguished fibrosarcomas from other malignant osteolytic tumors. Every patient had a radiolucent defect of variable size, without evidence of nodular or diffuse calcifications within. There was a characteristic ill-defined zone of radiolucency that was usually smaller than the actual tumor, and the peripheral invading portions of which may not have destroyed sufficient bone to be radiographically visible. A wide zone of transition may be seen at the margin. When teeth were in contact with the tumor, the root surface frequently was resorbed. Cortical perforation, occasionally associated with subperiosteal reactive new bone, was usually a late finding and always provided additional evidence of tumor aggressiveness. Two of the cases appeared as cystlike lesions, both having originated in ameloblastic fibromas. One case was diagnosed originally as desmoplastic fibroma and was well circumscribed at the outset. Permeation of bone with invasion of the cortex was common and helped differentiate these tumors from benign fibrous lesions.

In a study of seven cases of fibrosarcoma of the jaws by Slootweg and Muller (1984), the tumors were seen as radiolucent lesions, and all but one case exhibited poorly defined margins. When there was extensive destruction of alveolar bone, the involved teeth in two cases appeared to be hanging in the air or floating. Motheaten bone destruction as evidenced by multiple small and irregular radiolucencies was seen in one case in which there was also a pathologic fracture. In another case, a rather circumscribed radiolucency surrounded the crown and coronal half of the root of an impacted premolar; the presumptive diagnosis in this case was a follicular cyst or benign odontogenic tumor.

In 14 cases of fibrosarcoma of the jaws reported by Taconis and van Rijssel (1986), all but one of the lesions measured 2 to 2.5 cm in width. All were lytic. Three cases had a motheaten pattern, three showed unilocular geographic areas of destruction, one was a multilocular lesion with sclerotic margins, and two showed total destruction of the mandible in the region with a soft tissue mass and floating teeth. No periosteal bone reaction was seen, and soft tissue extension could not be found, except in two cases with total bone destruction.

All four cases in the maxilla were located in the central region, with destruction of the bone of the lateral wall of the sinus and the orbital floor, with soft tissue extension. CT is the best diagnostic procedure for delineating the extension of the tumor, especially in the maxillary region. In one case, there was a geographic-type lesion with ill-defined margins.

EWING'S SARCOMA (Ewing's tumor)

Ewing's sarcoma is a highly malignant primary bone sarcoma, usually affecting children and young adults. It is a distinctive, small round cell neoplasia that is the sixth most common malignant tumor of bone. The origin of the round cells has been questioned since the original description of the tumor in 1921 by James Ewing, who believed the round cells were derived from marrow endothelium. Because the nature of the parent cell is still in dispute, use of the eponym "Ewing's sarcoma" is still appropriate to distinguish this entity. Ewing's sarcoma constituted 9% of the malignant bone tumors in Schajowicz' (1981) files and 6% of the malignant bone tumors in Dahlin's series (1978). Mirra (1989) reported that 5% of all bone tumors are Ewing's sarcoma; it is the sixth most common biopsy-proven malignant bone tumor, ranking behind myeloma, osteosarcoma, chondrosarcoma, malignant lymphoma, and giant cell tumor. Wood and associates (1990) reviewed 105 cases of Ewing's sarcoma of the jaws and found that there were 98 primary lesions compared with 7 metastatic lesions (ratio, 14:1).

Pathologic Characteristics

The origin of Ewing's sarcoma is controversial. Most authors no longer believe it is derived from endothelium, the hematopoietic system, or neuroblasts. Currently, it is generally believed that the basic tumor cells are derived from reticuloendothelial cells or undifferentiated mesenchymal cells of bone marrow, as postulated by Navas-Palacios and co-workers (1984), Dickman and associates (1982), and Miettinen and colleagues (1982). Histologically, the lesion is characterized by sheets of small, blastlike round cells that typically contain intracytoplasmic glycogen, lack well-demarcated cell borders, and have a modest reticulin production. Tumor bone or cartilage formation is absent. The tumor is divided into strands or lobuli by conspicuous septa of fibrous tissue. Mitoses are present but infrequent. Hemorrhagic areas of extensive necrosis are common, sometimes producing an apparent perithelial arrangement of the viable cells as the necrosis of the tumor tissue occurs at some distance from the blood vessels. This appearance prompted the term "perithelioma" in older literature.

Clinical Features

Neff (1986), Kissane and associates (1983), and Arafat and colleagues (1983) reported that people affected by this tumor are, on the average, younger than those affected by any other primary malignant bone tumor. Approximately 75% of patients with this neoplasm are between the ages of 10 and 25 years at the time of clinical presentation. Fewer than 1% of the patients are 1 year of age or younger. In patients younger than 5 years, the diagnosis of metastatic neuroblastoma is more probable. deSantos and Jing (1978) reviewed 48 cases of Ewing's sarcoma of the jaws and reported that the average age of onset was 15 years for cases in the mandible and 16 years for those in the maxilla. In a series of 105 patients with Ewing's sarcoma of the jaws reported by Wood and associates (1990), reliable age figures were available for 77 patients; the average age at diagnosis was 16 years (range, 2 to 44 years). Ewing's sarcoma was reported to be approximately twice as common in male compared with female subjects in series of cases reported by Geschickter and Copeland (1949), Dahlin (1978), and Pomeroy and Johnson (1975). Greenfield (1986) reported that the sex distribution was equal or indicated a slight prevalence in male subjects. In a series of 105 jaw lesions reported by Wood and co-workers (1990), the gender was specified in 78 cases; 45 occurred in male patients, resulting in a male-to-female ratio of 1.5:1. Fraumeni and Glass (1970) found a slight male predilection

(60%) and an overwhelming predominance of white patients (95%); Resnick and Niwayama (1988) stated that the rarity of Ewing's sarcoma in black people (1 or 2%) deserves emphasis.

The chief complaint is often local pain, usually of several months' duration, which increases persistently in severity. The duration of pain is diagnostically important because a patient with osteomyelitis may have a similar clinical and radiologic picture, but a history of pain of only a few weeks' duration. Swelling from extension of the tumor into the soft tissues is the second most common symptom or sign; a tender soft tissue mass is usually present but is not warm. Regional dilated veins may be present. Wood and associates found that swelling was the most frequent complaint of their patients, occurring in 39%; pain was also a prominent complaint, as reported by Hardy and Gibbs (1984), Brownson and Cook (1969), and Salman and Darlington (1944), although some cases were painless. The tumor tends to become necrotic, which contributes to systemic findings consisting of malaise, fever sometimes as high as 105° F, leukocytosis, anemia, and an elevated erythrocyte sedimentation rate. These findings are confused easily with those of osteomyelitis and are ominous when seen with Ewing's sarcoma, usually signifying a fulminating course.

Treatment/Prognosis

As recently as 10 years ago, approximately 90% of patients with Ewing's sarcoma died within 2 years of the initial diagnosis. Bone metastases are found at autopsy in roughly 60% of patients. Fordham and associates (1982) reported that bone metastases were present in 12% of children at clinical presentation and 33% had metastases on subsequent examinations. Weir and co-workers (1979) reported that Ewing's sarcoma metastatic to the jaws is a rare occurrence. There are no known reports in the literature of metastasis to the jaws without evidence of other primary osseous involvement. In a study before the advent of modern chemotherapy, Telles and associates (1978) studied 26 patients with Ewing's sarcoma and reported that the frequency of metastases to various organs was as follows: lungs, 85%; bones, 69%; pleura, 46%; lymph nodes, 46%; dura or meninges, 27%; and central nervous system, 12%. Rosen and co-workers (1981), Bacci and colleagues (1982), and Wilkins and associates (1986) stated that, with modern therapeutic practices of local ablative surgery in combination with chemotherapy and radiation therapy in selected cases, long-term survival rates have improved dramatically to an average 79% 2-year disease-free survival rate. In a series of 105 jaw lesions reported by Wood and associates (1990), the survival length ranged from 12 days to 17 years; there were no follow-up data for 52 patients; of the remaining patients, 30 died of the disease, 19 had no evidence of disease at their last checkup, and 4 were alive with the disease.

◆ *RADIOLOGY (Figs. 14–37 to 14–41)*

General Radiologic Features

Although Ewing's sarcoma may develop in virtually any bone in the human body, it principally affects the lower segment of the skeleton, with the sacrum, innominate bone, and bones of the lower extremity accounting for approximately two thirds of all cases. This figure is supported by the reviews of Kissane and co-workers (1983), Wang and Schulz (1953), Falk and Alpert (1965), and Campanacci and colleagues (1979). According to Resnick and Niwayama (1988), the most frequent sites of involvement are the femur (22%), ilium (12%), tibia (11%), humerus (10%), fibula (9%), and ribs (8%). Ewing's sarcoma is relatively uncommon in the vertebrae above the sacrum (6%) and the mandible and maxilla (2%); it is rare in the skull (1%) and facial bones (0.5%). According to Greenfield (1986), the tubular bones are most likely to be involved in a younger patient, but in patients older than 20 years of age, the flat bones are the most frequent sites.

The fundamental radiographic findings in Ewing's sarcoma reflect the aggressive nature of this lesion, including osteolysis, cortical erosion, periostitis, and a soft tissue mass. Permeative destruction is a major feature of Ewing's sarcoma and is seen in approximately 90% of cases. The zone of transition between the area of destruction and healthy host bone is broad, vague, and imperceptible. The appearance of bone destruction can range from permeative pinhead-sized holes; to motheaten, "rotten wood"; to geographic or nearly purely lytic patterns. Wilner (1982) reported that approximately 33% of cases show a characteristic "cracked ice"

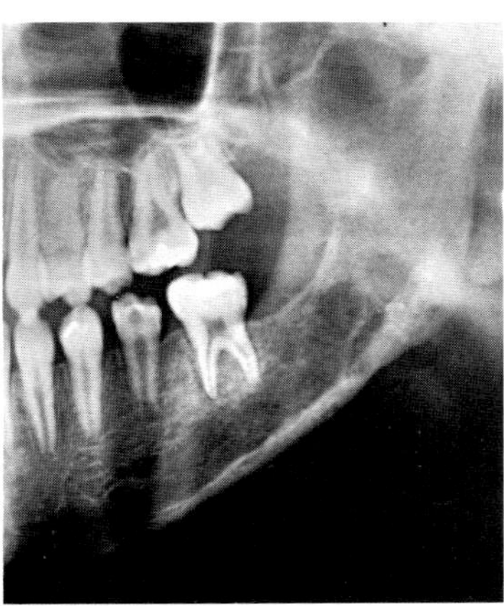

A

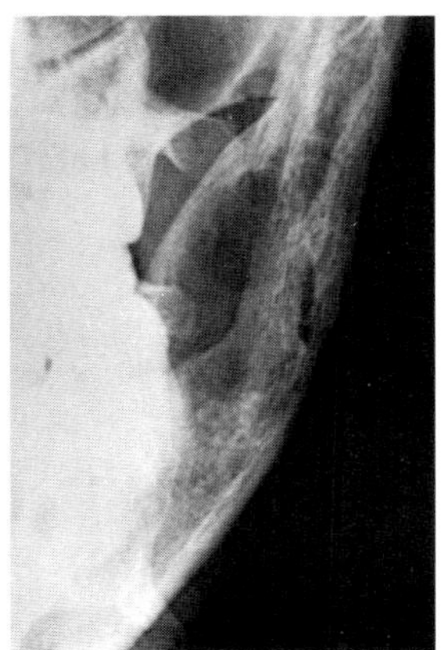

B

FIGURE 14–37.

Ewing's Sarcoma in a 12-year-old Girl: A, Panoramic changes are subtle. There is erosion of the endosteal surface of the cortex in the lesional area. B, Geographic pattern of bone destruction in angle ramus area. (Courtesy of Professor H. Fuchihata, Dean, Osaka University School of Dentistry, Osaka, Japan.)

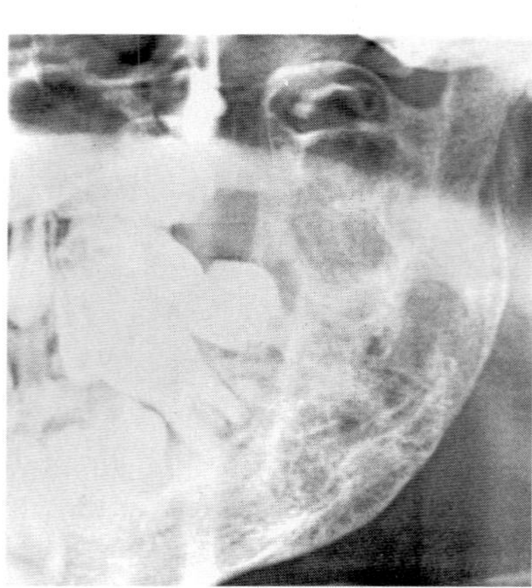

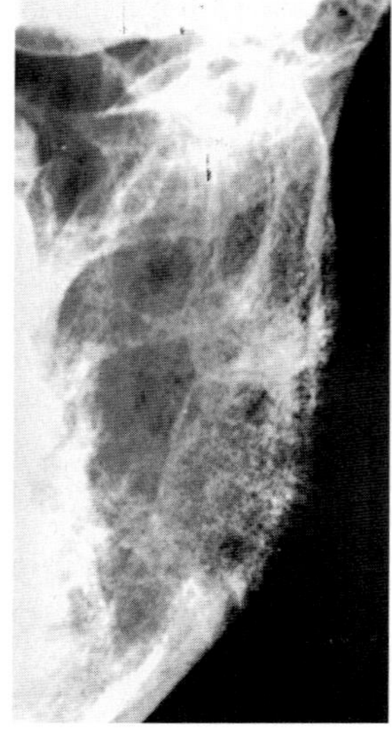

A B

FIGURE 14–38.

Ewing's Sarcoma in a 10-year-old Girl: A, Expansion, locules, and fine striations. B, Hair-on-end periosteal reaction. (Courtesy of Professor H. Fuchihata, Dean, Osaka University School of Dentistry, Osaka, Japan.)

pattern. Other patterns can be described as fine, reticulated, honeycombed, punched out, or circumscribed. Because of these variable patterns, Ewing's sarcoma can mimic most malignant and a few benign entities of bone, such as osteomyelitis, eosinophilic granuloma (EG), giant cell tumor, simple bone cyst, and aneurysmal bone cyst, and generally there are no great problems in distinguishing these disorders histopathologically. In almost all cases, the cortex is affected, and partial to complete erosion or a permeative, "lacelike" to "ratty" loss of the normally sharp and dense cortical density is evident; these cortical changes are often subtle. A soft tissue mass is a common finding; close to 90% of Ewing's sarcomas show a soft tissue mass or swelling resulting from one or more "ominous" periosteal reactions, such as an onion skin pattern. The soft tissue mass may be difficult to see with standard radiographs; CT scanning or MRI more effectively shows soft tissue masses emanating from bone. Pathologic fracture occurs in 5 to 10% of patients with Ewing's sarcoma because of the significant destructive capabilities of the tumor.

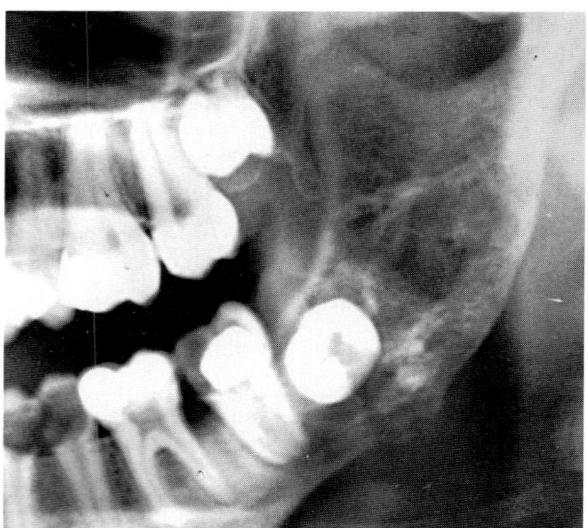

FIGURE 14–39.

Ewing's Sarcoma in a 13-year-old Girl: Area of rarefaction contains fine reticulated pattern, and there is erosion of the cortex. (Courtesy of Dr. José Ribamar De Azevedo, Instituto Odonto-Radiologico de Brasilia, Brasilia, Brazil.)

Periosteal reactions are seen in approximately 50% of cases and usually indicate late or advanced disease. The periosteal response is exuberant and may consist of multiple layers of new bone with a variety of appearances: onion skin or orange-peel patterns, single or multiple horizontal lines, perpendicular striations or a "hair-on-end" pattern, and "Codman's triangles." McCormack and associates (1952) referred to Ewing's sarcoma as the "great imitator of bone pathology" because of its variability.

As in most aggressive osseous neoplasms, scintigraphy with a bone-seeking radiopharmaceutical agent generally shows increased uptake of the radionuclide in foci of Ewing's sarcoma; however, Bushnell and colleagues (1983) reported exceptions in which a photon-deficient region or "cold" lesion is evident. The major usefulness of radionuclide bone scanning in Ewing's sarcoma is evaluation of metastases, both initially and on follow-up; it is also useful for monitoring responses to therapy.

Ginaldi and de Santos (1980), Vanel and associates (1982), and Turoff and Becker (1978) reported that CT scanning is used best in defining the extraosseous extent of a Ewing's sarcoma, especially in the skull, spine, ribs, and pelvis. This technique is also helpful in evaluating the tumor's response to radiation therapy or chemotherapy and in delineating the precise portals to be used during radiation therapy. MRI provides similar information that can be obtained with CT, but the accuracy of some margins may be assessed more readily with MRI.

Angiography in Ewing's sarcoma is most useful when the lesion involves the flat bones or vertebrae. In the flat bones and small bones, the radiographic appearance of Ewing's sarcoma and osteomyelitis is quite similar. Angiogra-

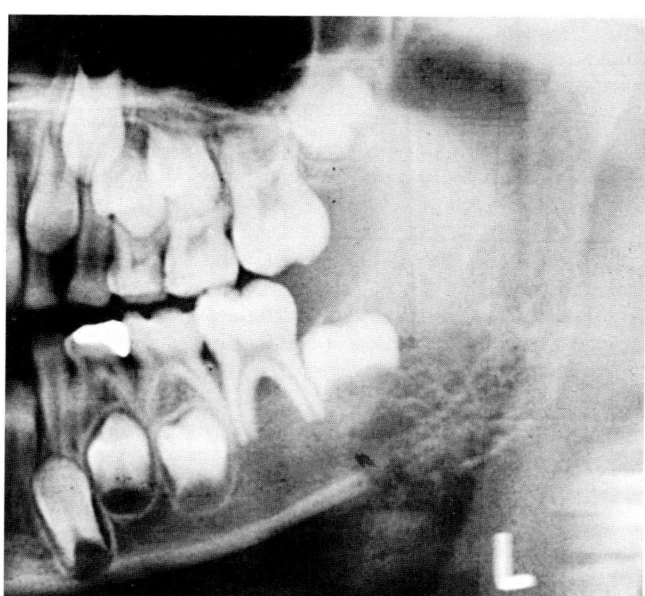

A

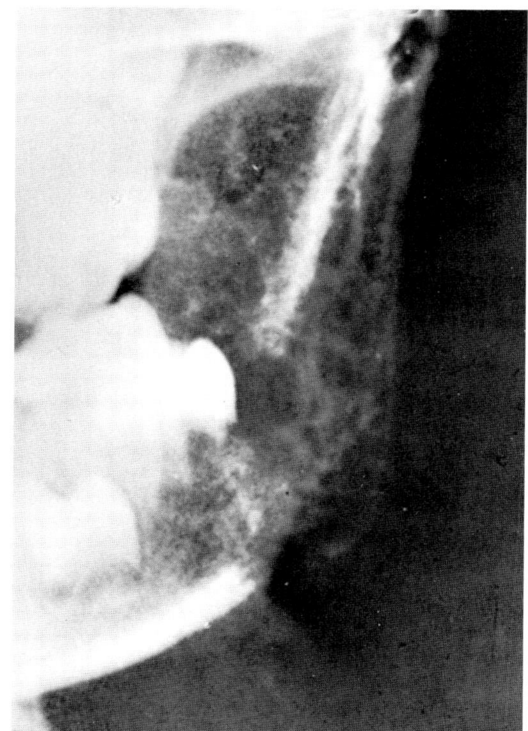

B

FIGURE 14–40.

Ewing's Sarcoma in an 8-year-old Girl: A, Panoramic radiograph. B, Anteroposterior radiograph. There is a cracked-ice pattern of fine reticulations; cortical expansion, erosion, and perforation; and a faintly seen hair-on-end periosteal reaction in molar area. (From Farman AG, Nortjé CJ, Wood RE: Malignancies affecting the jaws. In: Oral and Maxillofacial Diagnostic Imaging. St. Louis:CV Mosby, 1993, p. 296.)

phy can be valuable in their differentiation. Ewing's sarcoma is a vascular tumor and has angiographic features typical of malignant hypervascular bone lesions.

Radiologic Features of the Jaws

Location. With regard to the jawbones, de Santos and Jing (1978), Arafat and colleagues (1983), and Bacchini and co-workers (1986) reported that mandibular lesions are more frequent than those of the maxilla (ratio, approximately 3: 1). Roca and co-workers (1968) reported that the mandibular ramus is the most common location in the mandible. Wood and associates (1990) found 66 cases in the mandible and 31 in the maxilla (2.1:1); posterior parts of the jaws were favored over anterior parts of the jaws by a 4:1 ratio when the site was specified accurately.

Radiologic Features. According to de Santos and Jing (1978), the most frequent radiologic findings in jaw lesions were permeative bone destruction, periosteal reactions, and an adjacent soft tissue mass. Ewing's sarcoma of the jaws has radiographic features similar to those seen in the remainder of the skeleton. These include a permeative destructive pattern characteristic of small round cell tumors such as non-Hodgkin's lymphoma (NHL), neuroblastoma, and rhabdomyosarcoma and periosteal reactions that were seen in more than half of the cases in the peripheral skeleton. The laminated onion skin periosteal reaction is not pathognomonic of Ewing's sarcoma and need not be present for a diagnosis. In a series of 105 cases reported by Wood and associates (1990), the laminar periosteal response was not a common feature of Ewing's sarcoma of the jawbones; they reported that a poorly defined osteolytic lesion that may have associated sunray spicules of periosteal bone is a more common radiologic manifestation.

Other common radiologic signs of the jaws as cited by Wood and associates (1990) include a soft tissue mass adjacent to the destructive site, with destruction of the cortices of unerupted tooth follicles. The incidence and characteristics of the soft tissue mass in the mandible were similar to those seen in the peripheral skeleton. In a series of Ewing's sarcoma of the jaws reported by de Santos and Jing (1978), teeth were involved in 75% of the cases by displacing developing tooth follicles or erupted permanent teeth.

HISTIOCYTOSIS X

Histiocytosis X is a group of nonlipid histiocytoses characterized by proliferation of histiocytes in which no heritable disorder of lipid metabolism is demonstrable; the cause is

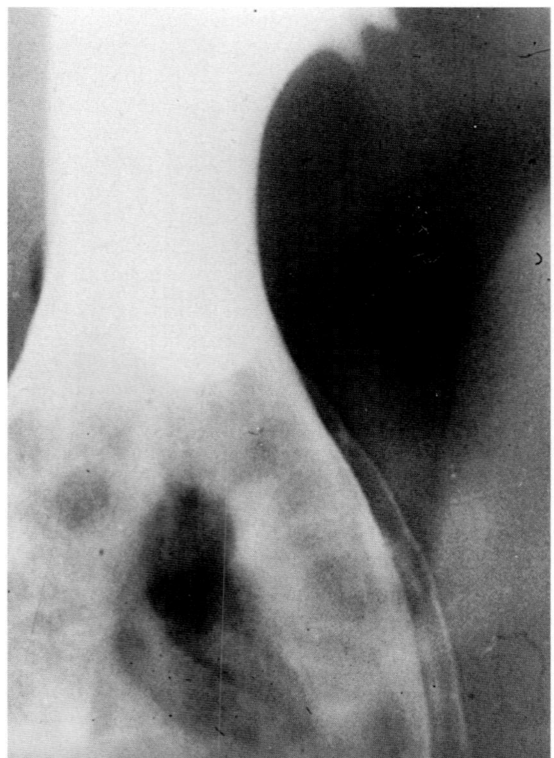

FIGURE 14–41.

Ewing's Sarcoma: Occlusal view shows onion skin periosteal reaction on lingual cortex. The tumor is relatively advanced. (Courtesy of Dr. Jaime San Pedro, University of Chile School of Dentistry, Chilean Referral Center for Pathology, Santiago, Chile.)

unknown. Historically, the nonlipid histiocytoses are categorized into three disorders:

1. Letterer-Siwe disease, the acute form, occurs in children younger than 3 years and is usually fatal; there is rapid dissemination of disease to skin, lymph nodes, bone, liver, and spleen. Letterer (1924), and later Siwe (1933), delineated the features of this disease occurring in infants.
2. HSC disease, the most varied chronic form, usually begins in early childhood, but can appear in late middle age, with chronic dissemination mainly to the bones and lungs and sometimes other organs; a triad of bone defects, exophthalmos, and diabetes insipidus occurs rarely. HSC disease and eosinophilic granuloma first were described by Hand in 1893, Schuller in 1915, and later Christian in 1920.
3. Eosinophilic granuloma, the mildest form, occurs most commonly in people between 20 and 40 years of age and characteristically involves bone; however, approximately 20% of patients have lung infiltration, and sometimes the lungs are involved exclusively.

Farber (1941) and Green and Farber (1942) were the first to group the three conditions HSC disease, Letterer-Siwe disease, and EG as different forms of a unique pathologic entity. Lichtenstein, in his classic review article in 1953, proposed the term histiocytosis X for the disease as a whole. The name histiocytosis was proposed because it denoted an inflammatory, proliferative reaction of histiocytes, and the letter X denoted the unknown origin of the condition. The histiocytosis X classification proposed by Lichtenstein in 1953 included the following: (1) acute disseminated histiocytosis X (Letterer-Siwe disease), with multiple systemic involvement; (2) chronic disseminated histiocytosis X (HSC disease), with osseous lesions, which are frequently multiple, and extraskeletal lesions, especially in the lungs; and (3) chronic, localized histiocytosis X (EG), with solitary or multiple skeletal lesions and occasional extraskeletal involvement, especially in the lungs. Schajowicz and Polak (1947) and Mirra (1989) agreed that the entities of histiocytosis X are not diseases, but rather syndromes; that is, the entities are different but often are not well delimited and are clinical manifestations of the same basic disorder.

Pathologic Characteristics

Clear separation among the three forms of histiocytosis is difficult on the basis of histologic manifestations. Proliferation of histiocytes, eosinophilic granulocytes, and other inflammatory cells is characteristic of each of these disorders. The aggressive phagocytic activity of the histiocytes is evidenced by the intracellular accumulation of hemosiderin and lipid, leading to their designation as foam or xanthomatous cells. The histiocytes in the histiocytosis X disorders may accumulate intracytoplasmic lipids, but unlike the inherited metabolic disorders such as Gaucher's, Niemann-Pick, and Tay-Sachs diseases, these lipids accumulate from the ingestion of necrotic debris from the lesions rather than as an inborn error of metabolism. The Langerhans' cells are believed to be of histiocytic origin and virtually diagnostic of histiocytosis X. Letterer-Siwe disease is characterized by a massive histiocytic proliferation, but few if any eosinophilic or any other chronic inflammatory cells; the development of foam cells is possible if the infant survives for 10 to 12 months or more. HSC disease is characterized by sheets of histiocytes with scattered accumulations of eosinophils around areas of necrosis. In EG, eosinophils are seen singly, in sheets, and in focal clusters around small vessels. Within a few weeks to months, the macrophage system of histiocytes begins to convert the ingested debris into lipids, their cytoplasm becomes pale to foamy, and the histiocytes are referred to as foam cells. In the late phase of EG, masses of foaming histiocytes mixed with scar tissue are found.

Clinical Features

The manifestations of histiocytosis X vary, and the diagnosis must be confirmed by biopsy and immunologic studies to ascertain the nature of the cells involved in this lesion. From 1982 to 1984, Nakajima and co-workers (1928), Rowden and associates (1983), and Ide and co-authors (1984) demonstrated a particular protein, the S-100 protein, in lesions of histiocytosis X, now considered to be the most reliable diagnostic indicator for histiocytosis X. The function of the S-100 protein is unknown, but it is normally present in glial cells, myoepithelial cells, Langerhans' cells, melanocytes, and reticulum cells of lymph nodes. The term Langerhans' cell dates back to 1868 and refers to neural dendritic cells of the epidermis described by Langerhans. It's now believed that Langerhans' cells are a specialized form of histiocyte. The term Langerhans' cells and the entire system of dendritic cells are virtually synonymous.

Acute disseminated histiocytosis X is seen most frequently in children younger than 3 years of age, although occasionally there are cases in patients in late childhood or young adulthood. This form is very rare, accounting for only 0.1% of all primary bone tumors on which biopsies have been performed; Mickelson and Bonfiglio (1977) reported that the frequency of this form of histiocytosis is lower than that of EG and HSC disease, accounting for approximately 10% of all of the histiocytoses. It is characterized by sudden onset and a rapidly progressive malignant course, with fever, hemorrhagic tendency, progressive anemia, hepatosplenomegaly, lymphadenopathy, and hyperplasia of the gingiva. Characteristic maculopapular skin lesions and petechiae are seen. Patients are prone to infections.

Chronic disseminated histiocytosis X most commonly occurs in children younger than 5 years of age. Mirra (1989) stated that most patients are seen initially before the age of 15 years and 66% are younger than 5 years. The male-to-female ratio is 1.3:1. The incidence is rare, approximately 0.3% of primary bone tumors on which biopsies have been performed. Otitis media is the most frequent complaint. The classic triad of bone lesions (usually calvarial defects in the skull), diabetes insipidus, and exophthalmos occurs in approximately 10 to 15% of patients. Roughly 50% have diabetes insipidus, and exophthalmos is present in approximately 25% of the patients. Mobility of teeth and bleeding gingivae are common with jaw involvement. Neurologic complaints are seen with involvement of the spinal bones, leading to wedge fractures and vertebra plana. Vertebra plana is spondylitis or inflammation of vertebrae in which the vertebral body is reduced to a sclerotic disk. Lymphadenopathy and hepatosplenomegaly result from disseminated granulomatous lesions of the reticuloendothelial system. With extensive bone involvement, anemia is possible; when present, it is a grave prognostic sign. A low-grade fever occurs in some patients.

EG can affect any organ system, but most cases involve tissues of the reticuloendothelial system such as bones, lymph nodes, liver, and spleen. The incidence of EG is rare; it represents 1% of primary bone tumors on which biopsies have been performed. The solitary type of EG is approximately twice as common as the multiple variants of osseous EG, including those with extraosseous spread. Resnick and Niwayama (1988) reported that EG represents approximately 70% of the total number of cases of histiocytosis X. Mirra (1989) stated that most patients are 1 to 15 years of age when seen initially; approximately 90% are 5 to 15 years of age (average age, 10 to 12 years). The male-to-female ratio is 2:1. It is more common in white than black people. Clinical signs and symptoms of EG include local pain, tenderness, and swelling related to adjacent skeletal lesions. A palpable soft tissue mass is common. Low-grade fever and redness are possible. Jaw involvement can cause tooth mobility because of localized bone loss. If there is early spinal involvement, collapse of the vertebral body may occur, causing neurologic complaints resulting from nerve impingement or spinal cord compression. Pathologic fracture of the long bones or significant limitation of motion of an affected limb is rare. Leukocytosis may be apparent, and eosinophilia is observed occasionally when the blood is examined. Moderate elevation of the erythrocyte sedimentation rate and normochromic anemia are found occasionally.

There are conflicting reports as to the incidence of oral involvement in histiocytosis X. Blevins and colleagues (1959) suggested that oral manifestations occur more often than previously suspected. In Sleeper's (1951) patients, 62% had oral involvement, and 77% of the patients studied by Sedano and associates (1969) had dental symptoms. In Hartman's (1980) review of 114 patients with oral involvement, 67% of the lesions occurred as intraosseous defects within the jaws, whereas 33% of the lesions occurred in oral soft tissues. Seventy-six percent of the intraosseous lesions occurred in the mandible, and the posterior portion of the jaws was the predominant site of occurrence in two thirds of the cases. Many patients simultaneously exhibited oral soft tissue involvement and intraosseous involvement. The presence of jaw swelling or a palpable epulislike mass was the most common presenting oral symptom in Hartman's review; pain, gingivitis, and mobility of teeth were frequent complaints. The incidence of extraoral lesions was 70%, with the most common sites of involvement being the skull and lower extremities. In the study of Jones and colleagues (1970), many children with histiocytosis X had precocious exfoliation of primary teeth, followed by the eruption and mobility of the permanent teeth caused by intraosseous lesions. The appearance of advanced periodontal disease in young children is suggestive of histiocytosis X, as is the failure of a socket to heal after extraction of a loose tooth that caused tenderness. Frequently, diabetes insipidus and regional lymphadenopathy are seen with oral involvement.

Treatment/Prognosis

The acute form causes a rapid downhill course; more than 95% of infants who acquire this disease before 1 year of age die within 6 months to 1 year. Some of the survivors have a prolonged clinical course, showing features of the chronic form of the disease. There have been no consistent effective therapeutic measures for the acute form. Chemotherapy may enable the child to survive the reticuloendothelial histiocytic onslaught and enter the chronic stage of the disease. The course of chronic disseminated disease cannot be defined adequately by histologic criteria alone. Greenfield (1986) reported that the course of the disease is chronic, with remissions and exacerbations. Prognostic indicators are related to the numbers of organ symptoms involved, coupled with progression of the disease. According to Lahey (1962), the prognosis of HSC disease worsens with involvement of multiple organ systems; the disease is fatal in 10 to 30% of such cases. Overall, the mortality rate is 13%. Death usually results from respiratory or cardiac failure.

Cohen and colleagues (1980) and Capanna and associates (1985) reported that the course of EG is usually benign, with healing occurring after simple curettage or local injection of steroids. Those with very large tumors that may lead to pathologic fracture and lesions of vertebral bodies have been treated successfully with low-dose radiation therapy (ranging from 6 to 10 Gy [600 to 1000 rads]), low doses of methotrexate or vinblastine, and local steroid injections. Patients with EG with bone and skin lesions tend to fare better than those with EG in multiple organ sites. Individual skeletal lesions usually heal within a few years, although shorter periods are possible. In general, the disease runs a protracted course, sometimes extending over 10 to 20 years. In patients with femur involvement, the skull probably should be radiographed; the opposite should be done if the skull is involved. A radionuclide bone scan also may be warranted to confirm other bone sites. Greenfield (1986) stated that 35% of bone scans were normal in patients with extensive radiographic evidence of skeletal disease. Bone scans are more reliable in follow-up examinations and for detection of recurrences. If no other lesions are discovered or become manifest after 1 year, additional lesions rarely will develop.

In general, the prognosis of any of the types of histiocytosis X is relative to the location and extent of organ involvement, so that clinical, radiologic, and laboratory evaluation of the patient must include an examination of all potential target areas of the disease. The greater the number of tissues or systems that are affected, the poorer the prognosis, especially if abnormalities of the liver, lung, or hematopoietic system are identified. The prognosis of histiocytosis X also is related to the age of the patient at the time of the onset of clinical abnormalities; generally, the younger the person, the poorer the prognosis.

Complicating any analysis of prognosis is the documentation that osseous and extraosseous lesions may resolve spontaneously at a rate unaffected by the mode of therapy. Therefore, reports on the effectiveness of treatment, such as partial or complete surgical removal, radiation therapy or chemotherapy, or corticosteroid administration, alone or in combination, must be interpreted cautiously.

◆ RADIOLOGY (Figs. 14–42 to 14–45)

General Radiologic Features

Radiologically, bone lesions may or may not be seen in acute or chronic disease. When present, they result from bone destruction by granulation tissue and are similar in all three forms of histiocytosis X. The basic lesion is an area of osteolysis that may involve any portion of any bone.

Radiologic Features of Acute Disseminated Disease (Letterer-Siwe Disease)

Generally, the disease may affect all bones during its clinical course. Because of the rapid progression of the disease, many cases of Letterer-Siwe disease show no radiologic findings or the findings are subtle. When lesions are visible, they usually consist of a generalized osteopenia or reduced bone mass, followed by permeative changes appearing as a myriad

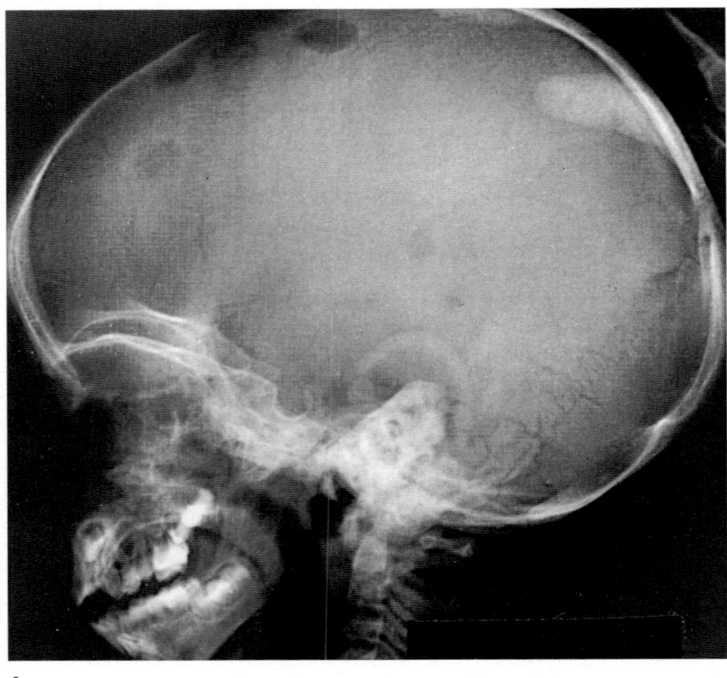

A

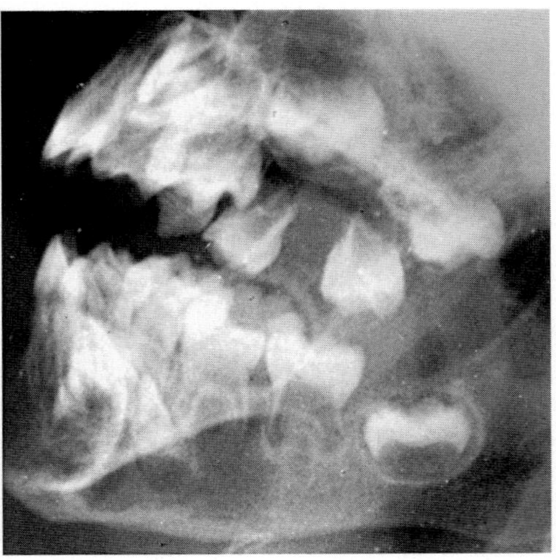

B

FIGURE 14–42.

Hand-Schüller-Christian Disease: A 3-year-old boy, believed to be in remission, had an epulis-like lesion in the maxillary left molar region. A, Multiple punched-out lesions in skull. B, Separation between maxillary primary molars, and alveolar bone destruction in association with soft tissue mass.

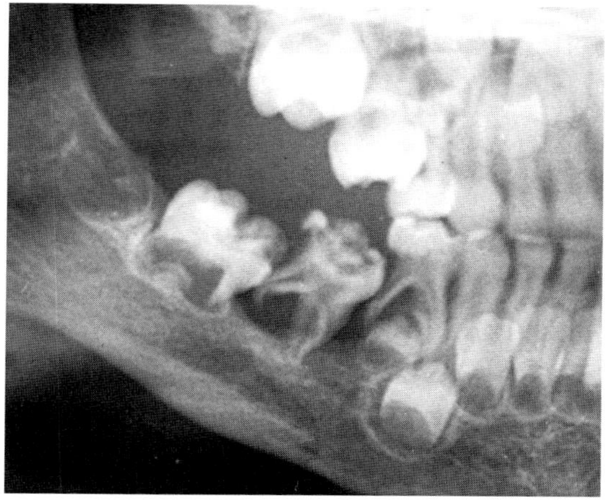

A

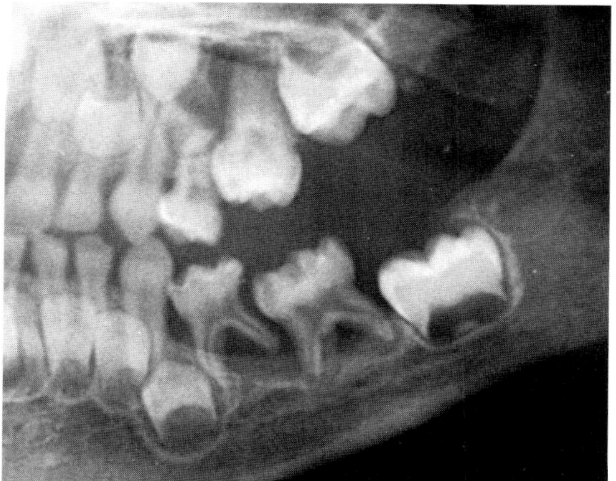

B

FIGURE 14–43.

Hand-Schüller-Christian Disease in a 4-year-old Girl: A and B, The pattern of alveolar bone destruction resembles that of juvenile periodontitis.

of small fine holes in the bone. Later, larger lytic defects or holes may appear. Most bone lesions are disseminated and minute, from 1 mm to several millimeters in size. Single or multiple areas of bone destruction are observed, particularly in the calvarium, base of the skull, and mandible. Longitudinally oriented periosteal lamellae may be seen at any time during the course of the disease. Even so, the radiographic findings of Letterer-Siwe disease are not specific.

Radiologic Features of Chronic Disseminated Disease (Hand-Schüller-Christian Disease)

This disease may involve any bone; however, more than 90% of patients have cranial involvement. Approximately 7% of the patients may have one or more lesions in the hands and feet. The lesions may range from 1 to 25 cm; the huge lesions probably represent confluence of many smaller lesions. Special features include bone expansion, geographic

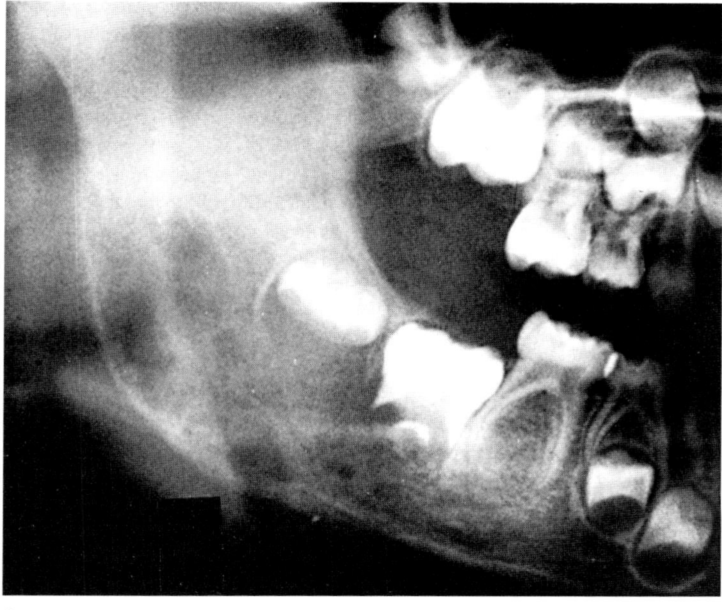

A

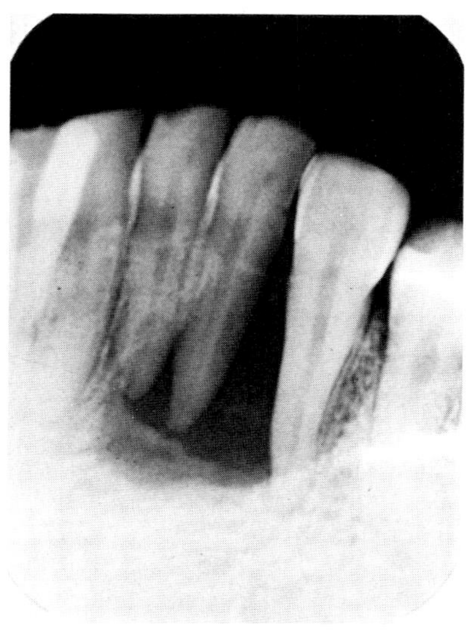

B

FIGURE 14–44.

Eosinophilic Granuloma: A, In a 5-year-old boy, there is a motheaten appearance, expansion and thinning of the cortex, and involvement of developing dental follicle. B, In a 28-year-old man, the lesion resembles a local periodontal defect, gingival carcinoma, or squamous odontogenic tumor. (Courtesy of Drs. M. Araki and K. Hashimoto, Nihon University School of Dentistry, Tokyo, Japan.)

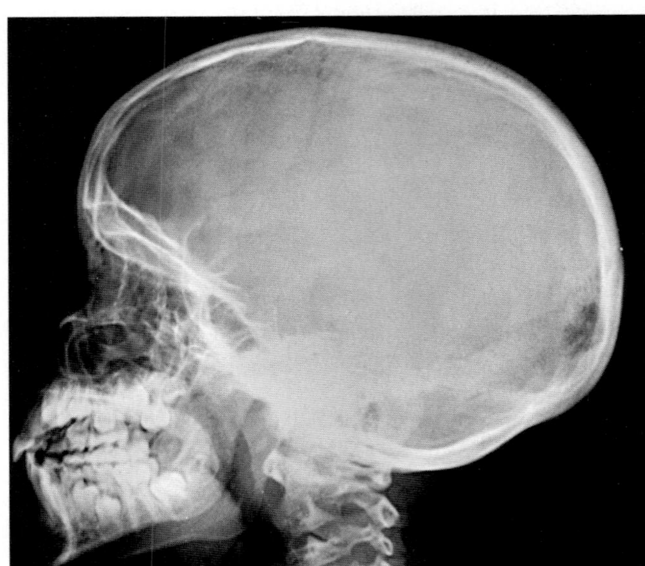

A

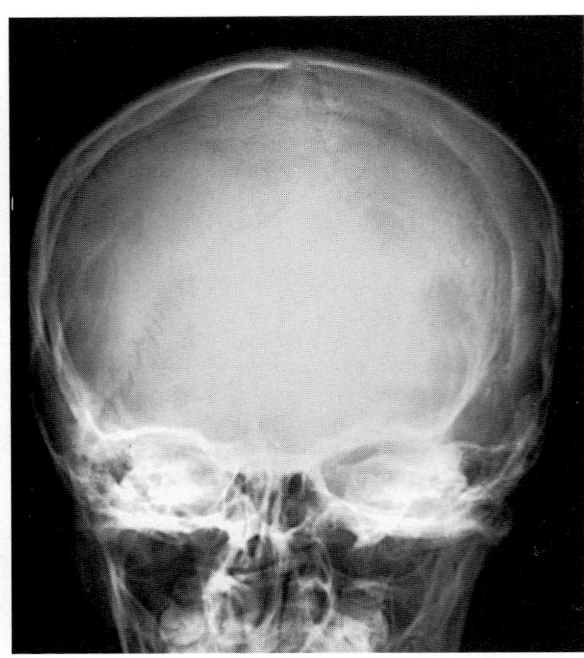

B

FIGURE 14–45.

Eosinophilic Granuloma in a 9-year-old Boy: A and B, The geographic area of bone destruction in the skull is in the occipital area, on the left side.

skull, hole-within-a-hole effect, and soft tissue mass. Because of the numbers and sizes of lesions, bones frequently become expanded and multilocular in the midphase to late phase of the disease. The epiphyseal regions almost always are spared. The skull lesions typically begin as small "punched-out" areas originating in the diploe, then expand and perforate the inner and outer tables unevenly, leading to an appearance of a double contour or hole-within-a-hole overlap, giving a three-dimensional effect to the lesion in some cases. There is a peculiar beveling with multiple undulating contours of the margin, also characteristic of EG.

Extensive confluence of cranial lesions may develop later, giving a maplike or geographic skull appearance in the disseminated forms of the disease. Occasionally the cortex may be destroyed with the penetration and outgrowth of a soft tissue mass.

Radiologic Features of Eosinophilic Granuloma

EG has a peculiar distribution. Mirra (1989) reported that nearly 70% of lesions involve the flat bones such as the skull (25%), jawbones (4%), spine (9%), pelvis (12%), and ribs (9%); approximately 30% of the lesions occur in the long bones. Involvement is rare in the sacrum and bones of the hands and feet. Jennings and associates (1982) stated that fewer than 1% of the cases of solitary EG involve the bones of the hand. In the long bones, most lesions involve either the metaphysis (28%), diaphysis (58%), or metadiaphysis (12%). The vertebral body is affected more often than the arch. Involvement of the disk space is rare, unlike in osteomyelitis. The lesion size ranges from 1 to 15 cm (average, 4 to 6 cm). In the incipient stage of EG, the lesion usually begins as a small, centrally placed, lytic process with shaggy, poorly delineated margins. There is a permeative to moth-eaten pattern of destruction. The cortices often are focally eroded, and the periosteum may be stimulated to produce one or more parallel lamellae of variable thickness. In the midphase, the lesion still may enlarge, but its borders become more sharply delineated; the outer contours vary from round to oval to irregularly lobulated. During the midphase, the lesion may reach its maximum size, after which a continuous peripheral rind of reactive benign host bone sclerosis may form, which is thin at first and thickens with time. Periosteal reactions still may be prominent or begin to abate. In the late phase, the tumor's appearance is very similar to that during the midphase except for resolution of periosteal lamellae, sharper circumscription of the lesion, and, occasionally, a thick rind of sclerosis. Sometimes lesions that are many years old may resolve completely without surgery.

There are four unusual radiologic variants of EG: (1) the beveled-edge lesion of the skull, (2) the button sequestrum of the skull, (3) the vertebra plana, and (4) the soft tissue mass. The beveled-edge lesion of the skull is an uneven destruction of the outer as compared with the inner table of the skull, which gives rise to the so-called beveled-edge appearance. The button sequestrum or "bull's-eye" appearance of the skull is rare and consists of a radiolucent area with a dense central nidus of intact bone. Compere and coworkers (1954) reported that vertebral involvement by EG leads to insidious collapse of the vertebral body without loss of disk space. Eventually the vertebral body may be compressed into a thin wafer. This extreme flattening is known as vertebra plana or Calve's (1925) syndrome. Schlesinger and colleagues (1986) reported that a soft tissue mass may form in 5 to 10% of patients with EG, ranging in size from a few millimeters to several centimeters, which is highly suggestive of a malignant tumor.

Radiologic Features of Histiocytosis X of the Jaws

Location. In the acute form, jaw changes are seen rarely. If bony changes are seen, it is of prognostic significance because they may signal the beginning of the chronic stage, which has a better prognosis. In Mirra's (1989) study of 240 cases of solitary EG, 4% of the cases had mandibular involvement. The lesions usually appeared in the molar and premolar regions.

Radiologic Features. If the jaws are affected in HSC disease, the change usually consists of localized alveolar bone loss resembling focal periodontal disease, with or without an associated epulislike gingival mass. Conversely, the patient may have a generalized loss of alveolar bone, with multiple mobile primary or permanent teeth. In chronic cases, patients may lose all of their teeth by the time they are 14 to 16 years of age.

In a review of EG by Jones and associates (1970), the radiographic examination generally showed a nonspecific radiolucent appearance, common to any destructive process. Margins of individual lesions may be well defined or indistinct, and osseous expansion usually is not observed, although this feature might be observed more frequently with more consistent use of the occlusal view. Perforation of the cortical plate is a common finding, particularly with large lesions. In many instances, the EG lesions may resemble localized periodontal disease; however, the bony defect resembling vertical bone loss may have a double density along its vertical height, producing a beveled effect as is seen in the skull. Hartman (1980) and Keusch and colleagues (1966) found that the amount of bone loss varied but frequently the destruction of the supporting alveolar bone was severe enough to allow displacement of teeth and, in some cases, was so severe that the teeth appeared to be floating in air. The margins of the jaw lesions, within the alveolar bone or in association with teeth, may or may not be lined by reactive host bone. An absence of reactive marginal sclerosis indicates active disease with additional growth of tumor possible; the initial appearance of a thin rind of reactive marginal sclerosis indicates a diminished growth rate of the lesion, and a thick rind indicates a more exuberant host bone response to an active lesion. Pathologic fractures of the jaws may occur but were not reported in Hartman's study.

MULTIPLE MYELOMA (Plasmacytic myeloma, plasma cell myeloma, myelomatosis, Kahler's disease, plasmacytoma)

Myeloma is a neoplastic proliferation of plasma cells that may occur in several forms. Plasma cells are found in various areas of the human body, particularly in the lymph nodes, bone marrow, and submucosa of the gastrointestinal tract. They are the functional unit of the B-cell line of the immune system and are responsible for the production of immunoglobulin (Ig), proteins of high molecular weight that function as antibodies as they circulate throughout the tissues. When infectious disease and other disorders are present, the number of plasma cells increases within the bone marrow, resulting in a similar increase in the production of immunoglobulins. This response is termed plasmacytosis and is a normal consequence of infection. When plasma cell proliferation appears as an inappropriate or uncontrolled event, a disease state exists. Several diseases can be manifested in this fashion, and Isobe and Osserman (1971) and Osserman (1979) grouped these diseases together as plasma cell dyscrasias. The clinical manifestations of these diseases result from the effects of expanding collections of cells or abnormal accumulations of substances produced by these cells. Plasma cell dyscrasias include the following: (1) multiple myeloma, characterized by an increase in abnormal plasma cells; (2) Waldenström's macroglobulinemia, in which there is an increase in plasmacytoid lymphocytes; and (3) amyloidosis, in which there is deposition of a specific Ig in tissue.

According to Clamp (1967), the first patient known to have multiple myeloma was Thomas Alexander Bean in 1845; during the 17 months of his illness, he had several recurrences of pain and his urine contained unusual "animal matter" that became soluble when boiled and formed again when cooled. Several years later, a young physician and chemist, Henry Bence Jones, described the protein in detail. Kyle (1975) reported that the term multiple myeloma was introduced by Rustizky in 1873; Kahler described a striking case in 1889; and, in 1900, Wright recognized that myeloma tumors consisted of plasma cells. In 1939, Longsworth and associates applied electrophoretic techniques to the study of multiple myeloma, and immunoelectrophoresis was described by Grabar and Williams in 1953; these two procedures have facilitated diagnosis of the disease.

Most patients with plasma cell disorders have increased concentrations of homogeneous proteins termed "M" or monoclonal components of the serum, which are Igs. There are five major classes of Igs: IgG, IgM, IgA, IgD, and IgE. These have identical heavy or "H" chains and identical light kappa or lambda chains. The type of Ig that is being elaborated abnormally can be identified by its electrophoretic pattern and varies among plasma cell dyscrasias. Patients with plasma cell myeloma are grouped according to the type of Ig produced by the tumor; approximately 55 to 60% have IgG myeloma, 20% have IgA myeloma, and 1 to 2% have IgD myeloma. Furthermore, in multiple myeloma large quantities of Bence Jones proteins representing free light kappa or lambda chains are common and may be identified in the urine in approximately 50% of cases.

Multiple myeloma is a progressive and ultimately fatal neoplastic disease characterized by plasma cell tumors in the bone marrow and overproduction of an intact monoclonal Ig (IgG, IgA, and IgD) or Bence Jones protein (free monoclonal kappa or lambda light chains). The studies of Mundy and colleagues (1974) and Durie and associates (1981) showed that plasma cells can produce an osteoclastic stimulating factor possibly responsible for the osteolytic lesions characteristic of myeloma; this factor also leads to inhibition of osteoblasts. Often, back pain, anemia, renal damage, numerous osteolytic lesions, hypercalcemia, and increased susceptibility to bacterial infection may be associated. The cause of plasma cell proliferation in plasma cell myeloma is unknown.

Dahlin (1978) stated that myeloma is the most common biopsy-analyzed primary bone tumor and accounts for approximately 35% of all bone tumors and 45% of all malignant bone tumors. Multiple myeloma, a multifocal type of myeloma associated with back pain and anemia, is the most common form of myeloma, accounting for more than 50% of cases. This type of myeloma accounts for 10% of all malignant disease and more than 10% of hematologic cancers.

Pathologic Characteristics

Myeloma is composed of nodular or diffuse aggregates of plasma cells. The infiltrate of plasma cells is pure to almost totally pure, with an absence of fibrosis and marrow fat cells. A total absence of bone spicules also is observed in the lesional infiltrates, which explains the radiologic evidence of lysis. Diffuse infiltrates of plasma cells result in the generalized form of myeloma, the nodular foci result in multiple myeloma, and a single nodular mass results in the solitary form. When distinguishing benign plasma cell infiltrates from myeloma, it should be realized that myelomatous regions are composed purely of plasma cells that obliterate the marrow. Normal marrow aspirates contain few plasma cells, approximately 3% or less. Conditions such as infections, rheumatoid arthritis, and cirrhosis may contain many plasma cells (as many as 30%), but the plasma cells are admixed with other cell types and the marrow fat is not totally obliterated.

Clinical Features

Multiple myeloma is the most common form of myeloma, accounting for more than 50% of cases. Generalized myeloma is the diffuse skeletal form of the disease, can be mistaken easily for osteoporosis, and accounts for approximately 15% of all myelomas. Solitary myeloma represents 25% of all myelomas. Kyle (1975) based his diagnosis of multiple myeloma on the following criteria: increased numbers of abnormal, atypical, or immature plasma cells in the bone marrow or histologic proof of plasmacytoma, as well as the presence of a monoclonal protein in the serum or urine, or bone lesions consistent with those of myeloma. In multiple myeloma, there are many abnormalities in the laboratory test results: (1) anemia is seen in most patients; (2) plasma Ig levels are increased; (3) there is a monoclonal spike in the globulin fraction of serum electrophoresis; (4) Bence Jones proteins are found in the urine; (5) hypercalcemia is seen in 25% of patients; (6) serum alkaline phosphatase levels are increased in 25% of patients; and (7) results of renal function studies are abnormal.

Kyle (1975), in a review of 869 cases, and Carson and colleagues (1955), in a review of 90 cases, reported that the disease usually occurs in patients between the ages of 25 and 80 years (average age, 62 years). Hewell and Alexanian (1976) stated that myeloma is rare in childhood and unusual in people younger than 40 years of age. Mirra (1989) reported that approximately 67% of patients with multiple myeloma are men, for a male-to-female ratio of 2:1. Goodman (1986) reported that myeloma is particularly common in black people. In Kyle's (1975) study, bone pain occurred in 68% of patients with myeloma; this is to be expected because myeloma is predominantly a disease of the bone marrow. The pain often is characterized as an aching, ''rheumatism-like'' pain that is intermittent at the onset, is aggravated or precipitated by movement, and does not occur at night except with a change of position. This is in contrast to the pain of metastatic carcinoma, which frequently is worse at night. The pain of myeloma increases in severity, becomes more prolonged, and may necessitate the use of narcotics for relief. The pain is localized most often in the lower back but also is encountered in the upper spine, pelvis, ribs, and sternum; it is associated frequently with bone tenderness. Low back or chest pain associated with osteopenia of the spine in middle-aged men should be investigated promptly to rule out multiple myeloma. Pathologic fracture is observed frequently, especially in the spinal bones; persistent localized pain or tenderness of sudden onset usually indicates a pathologic fracture, which often occurs with only minimal trauma.

The patient's height may be shortened by several inches because of vertebral collapse and kyphosis. Other symptoms include weakness, easily induced fatigue, anorexia, weight loss, and vomiting, most of which are related to the ensuing anemia and ''toxins'' released by the masses of neoplastic cells. Anemia was present initially in two thirds of Kyle's (1975) patients; pallor is a common finding and reflects anemia. Weight loss and night sweats usually are not prominent until the disease is advanced. In Kyle's (1975) patients, spontaneous bleeding occurred in 7%, which most often took the form of epistaxis, but gastrointestinal bleeding also was observed. These bleeding occurrences relate to the neoplastic replacement of normal hematopoietic marrow, resulting in decreased platelet and leukocyte production. Splenomegaly and lymphadenopathy are uncommon, with lymphadenopathy detected in only 4% of Kyle's (1975) patients. In a number of patients, submandibular swelling occurred from macroglossia, which resulted from amyloidosis. The relationship of altered proteins in multiple myeloma and the formation of amyloid is well established. In some patients the occurrence of congestive heart neuropathy may be associated with amyloidosis.

Oral manifestations may be the first signs or symptoms of multiple myeloma. Bhaskar (1975) estimated that 12 to 15% of patients and Bruce and Royer (1953) indicated that 12% of 59 patients in their series had oral signs and symptoms. Epstein and co-workers (1984) reviewed 783 cases from the literature and found oral manifestations in 14%; this estimate is probably low because many studies involved material from medical records, without oral or dental examinations and dental radiographs. In a study of 44 patients, Cataldo and Meyer (1966) found that 31% had oral signs or symptoms; however, 70% of patients with adequate jaw radiographs had signs of disease. In 33 patients with oral signs and symptoms, Smith (1957) showed that swelling was reported most commonly (76%), pain was less common (39%), and ulceration, loosening of teeth, and miscellaneous symptoms occurred in 18% of patients.

Treatment/Prognosis

Multiple myeloma is a highly malignant disease of hematopoiesis. It is progressive, but optimal management improves the quality and duration of life. The prognosis is related to the extent of the disease at diagnosis, adequacy of supportive measures, and response to chemotherapy. Approximately 60% of treated patients show objective improvement; the median survival time for responding patients is 2 to 3 years. High levels of M-protein in serum or urine, diffuse bone lesions, hypercalcemia, pancytopenia, and renal failure are unfavorable signs.

Maintenance of ambulation is vital. Analgesics and palliative doses of radiation therapy (10 to 20 Gy) to localized areas of symptomatic bone involvement relieve pain significantly. Adequate hydration is also essential because of renal functional impairment. In the later stages of the disease, renal insufficiency accounts for death in 50% of patients.

Prednisone (60 to 80 mg/day) is useful for hypercalcemia, and allopurinol (100 mg tid) controls hyperuricemia. Antibiotics are indicated for active bacterial infection, although prophylactic antibiotics are not recommended; monthly doses of gamma globulin may be helpful if bacterial infections recur. Transfusions of packed erythrocytes are indicated for severe anemia. Objective improvement, as documented by a 50% or greater reduction in serum or urine M-protein, usually follows chemotherapy with oral alkylating agents such as melphalan and cyclophosphamide. The median survival length may be extended threefold to sevenfold. The major causes of death of patients with multiple myeloma are infection and renal failure.

◆ *RADIOLOGY (Figs. 14–46 to 14–49)*

General Radiologic Features

Multiple myeloma can localize to any red marrow-containing bone in an adult. Therefore, the axial skeleton, ribs, skull, pelvis, and long bones often are affected; the bones of the hands and feet rarely show radiologic involvement. Mirra (1989) studied 720 cases of multiple myeloma, and 31% involved the skull and jaws.

Myeloma is characterized by sharply punched-out lytic areas, ranging in size from a few millimeters to several centimeters. Mirra (1989) reported that, in contrast to other lymphomas, particularly Hodgkin's disease, myelomatous infiltration usually causes cortical and medullary lysis without sclerosis in 98% of cases. In multiple myeloma, a subcortical circular or elliptical radiolucent shadow is particularly distinctive and is observed most often in the long, tubular bones. An associated mild periosteal proliferation may act as a buttress, preventing or resisting fracture. The subcortical defects cause erosion of the inner margins of the cortex and, when extensive, create a scalloped or wavy look throughout the endosteal surface. Other radiologic findings include a trabeculated appearance, consisting of normal-sized trabeculae; a reticulated appearance, consisting of a coarsening of trabeculae; a honeycombed appearance; and even bubbly patterns within a rarefied area. Lesions in the spine precipitate compression fractures.

Special Studies

Although radionuclide examination with technetium bone-seeking pharmaceutical agents is valuable in the early detection of most neoplastic processes involving the bony skeleton, the results of this examination are less predictable in patients with myeloma. Currently, it is believed that the radionuclide examination in patients with myeloma does not show all lesions and that conventional radiography is a more valuable technique in assessing the distribution of lesions, with the possible exception of rib abnormalities, which may be seen earlier with scintigraphy. Van Antwerp and colleagues (1975) stated that areas of increased uptake in some people may not indicate the presence of a tumor but would indicate amyloid deposition.

CT, with its considerable ability to detect changes in tissue density, is valuable in the delineation of lesions within the medullary spaces, whether these are sites of metastasis, infection, or primary disease. As opposed to plain film radiography, in which considerable osseous destruction is required before abnormalities become apparent, CT images may indicate minor alterations in radiodensity, reflecting the early presence of myelomatous foci. The technique is well suited for evaluating patients in whom myeloma is suspected on the basis of clinical findings of back pain and tenderness and laboratory changes in serum and electrophoresis parameters and in whom conventional radiographs are normal. Price and co-workers (1980) reported that CT scans can be used to detect the extent of osseous and soft tissue involvement in patients with well-documented myeloma, especially in areas of complicated anatomy, such as the spine, pelvis, and face.

Daffmer and colleagues (1986) showed that MRI can delineate the degree of marrow involvement in many disorders, including lymphoma, leukemia, Gaucher's disease, and multiple myeloma. The normally intense signal is derived from fatty marrow but is diminished by tumor or infiltration.

Radiologic Features of the Jaws

Location. In studies by Bruce and Royer (1953), Miller and colleagues (1969), Lewin and Cataldo (1967), Spitzer and Price (1948), and Ramon and co-workers (1978), mandibular abnormalities were observed in 20 to 33% of patients with myeloma and may be the first bony manifestation of the disease. Stafne (1958) reported that the mandibular premolar and molar regions and coronoid process are the more frequently reported sites; according to Worth (1969), lesions are more common in the posterior third and angle of the jaw.

In a study of 193 patients with multiple myeloma, Lambertenghi-Deliliers and associates (1988) found that none of their patients had osteolytic or osteoporotic lesions in the maxilla; mandibular lesions were never an isolated radiologic finding, but were observed only in patients in whom skeletal involvement included the skull as well as other bones. The authors suggested that radiologic involvement of the mandible indicated that the disease was in an advanced clinical stage and therefore had an unfavorable prognosis.

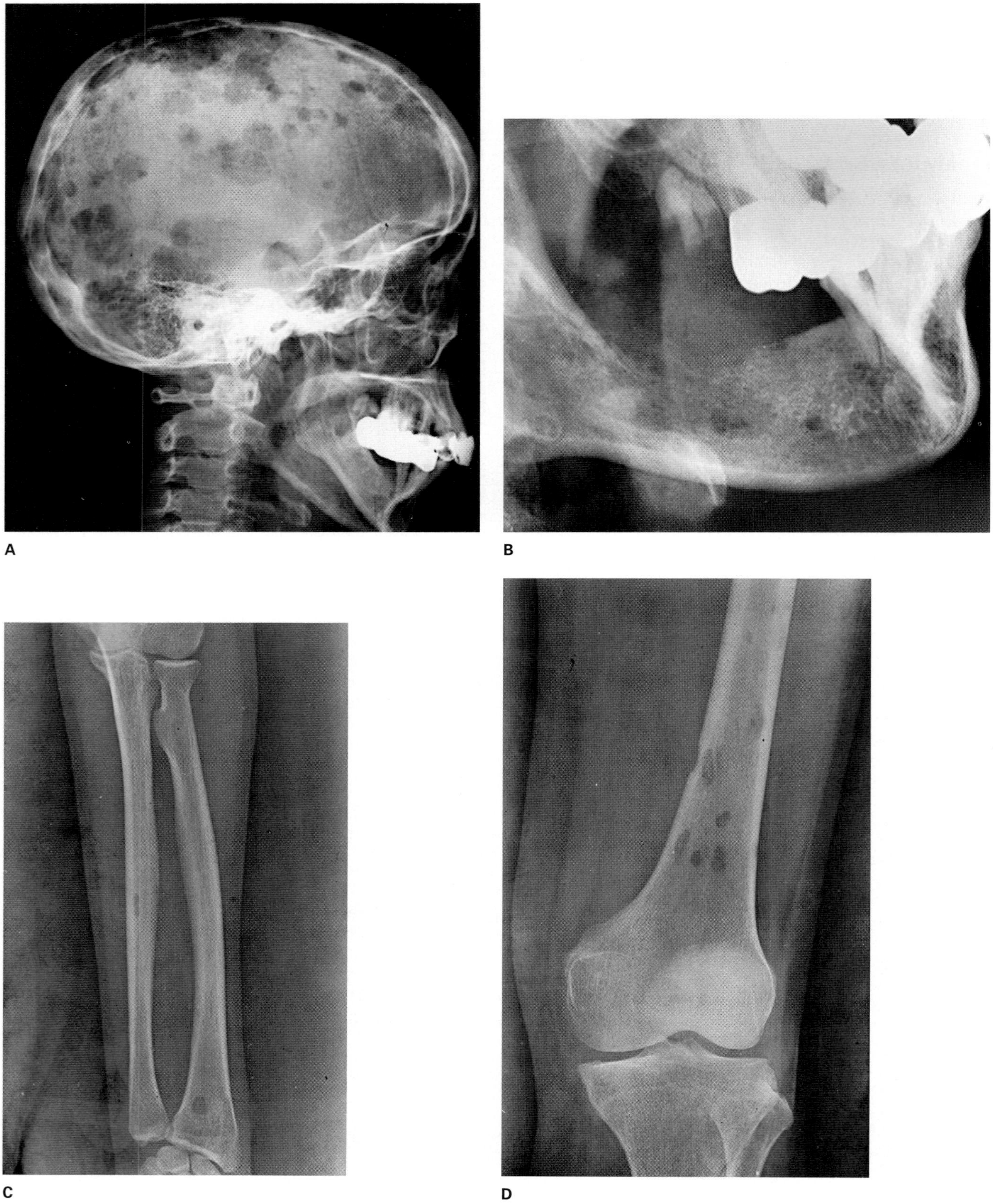

A

B

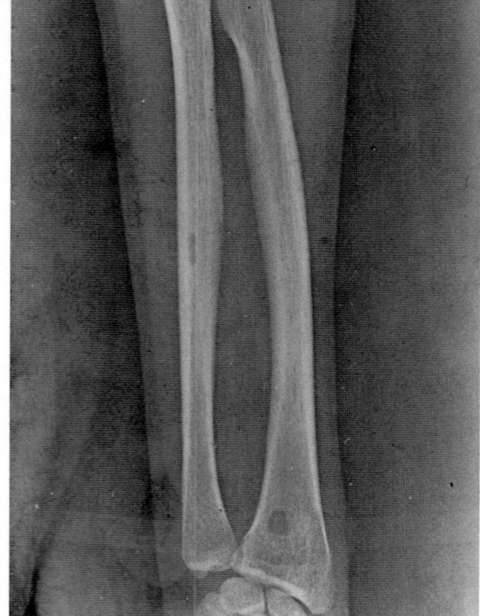

C

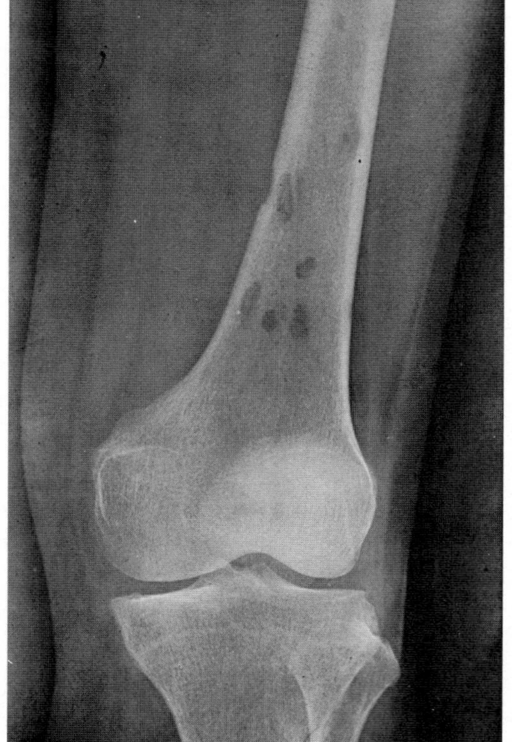

D

FIGURE 14–46.

Multiple Myeloma in a 50-year-old Woman: A, In the skull, there are multiple punched-out lesions. B, In the mandible, there are permeative changes within the larger osteoporotic area. C and D, In the long bones (mid ulna, distal radius, and femur), there are small punched-out lesions. (Courtesy of Professor T. Ohba, Kyushu Dental College, Kitakyushu, Japan.)

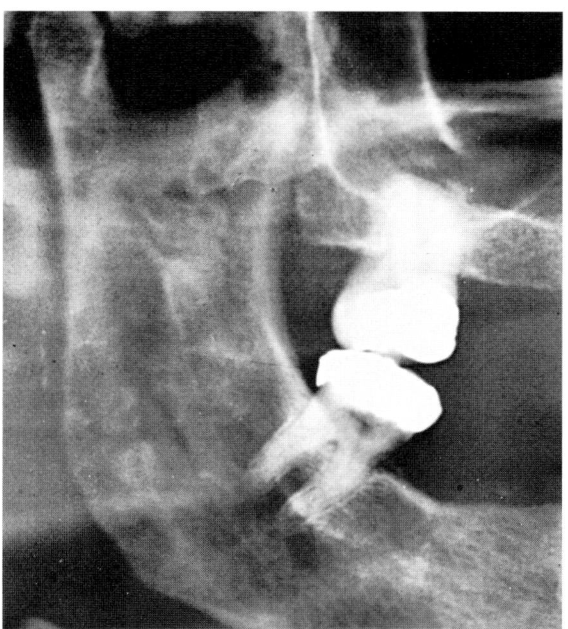

FIGURE 14–47.

Multiple Myeloma: Diffuse osteoporotic change, within which motheaten areas can be seen. There is endosteal erosion of the cortex at the angle.

Radiologic Features. Worth (1969) described the radiolucent lesions of multiple myeloma as rounded, with defined and noncorticated borders; no new bone formation occurs, even if destruction extends to the margin of the mandible. In the jaws the lesions may be geographic but irregular in outline. Diffuse involvement of the jaws may occur rarely, producing an appearance of osteoporosis with normal-sized or coarsened trabeculae. Rarely, honeycomb or multilocular patterns within a rarefied area are formed by the remaining trabeculae. Perforation of the cortex is more common than expansion in the mandible. The lamina dura may be destroyed in some cases. Radiolucent lesions may be associated with teeth and do not result characteristically in root resorption, although root resorption may occur rarely. A pathologic fracture of the condylar neck was observed in one of the cases of Bruce and Royer (1953). In a case reported by Ramon and associates (1978), the primary manifestation of their mandibular lesion was a very distinct sunray radiographic pattern. Jagger and co-workers (1978) described a case of multiple myeloma occurring in the mandibular condyle, affecting the function of the temporomandibular joint.

In a study of 17 patients with myeloma of the jaws reported by Bruce and Royer (1953), 15 underwent radiographic examination of the skull. The skull lesions were punched-out, rounded, and of various sizes, with little, if any, circumferential osteosclerotic bone reaction. The smaller lesions coalesce in some instances, thus forming larger radiolucent areas. The multiple punched-out vacuolated regions in the skull were observed occasionally, with larger regions of diffuse radiolucency with hazy, ill-defined margins.

NON-HODGKIN'S LYMPHOMA

(Lymphosarcoma, reticulum cell sarcoma)

NHL is a heterogenous group of diseases, consisting of neoplastic proliferation of lymphoid cells that usually dissemi-

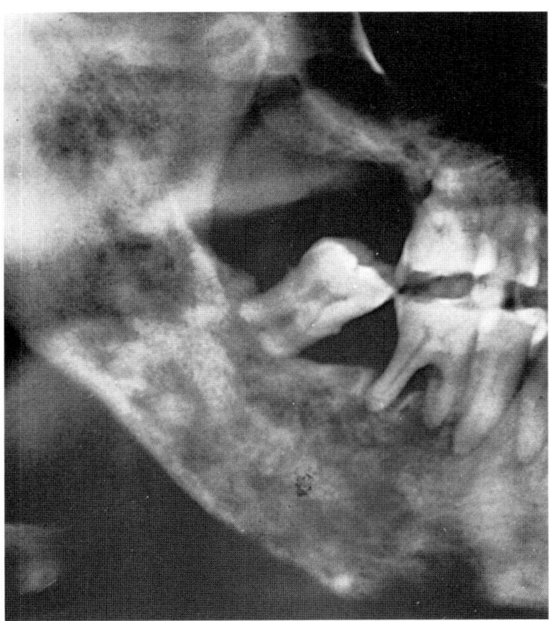

A

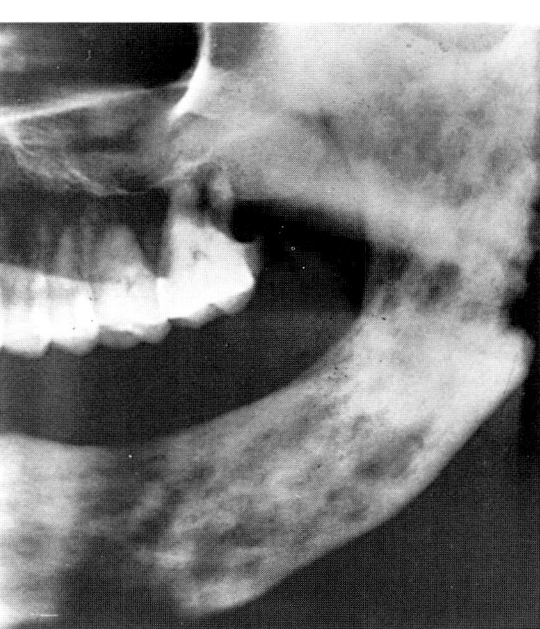

B

FIGURE 14–48.

Multiple Myeloma in a 60-year-old Man: A and B, Right and left sides of same patient, showing permeative and motheaten changes throughout. There are permeative changes within the cortex on the right side and endosteal erosion of the cortex.

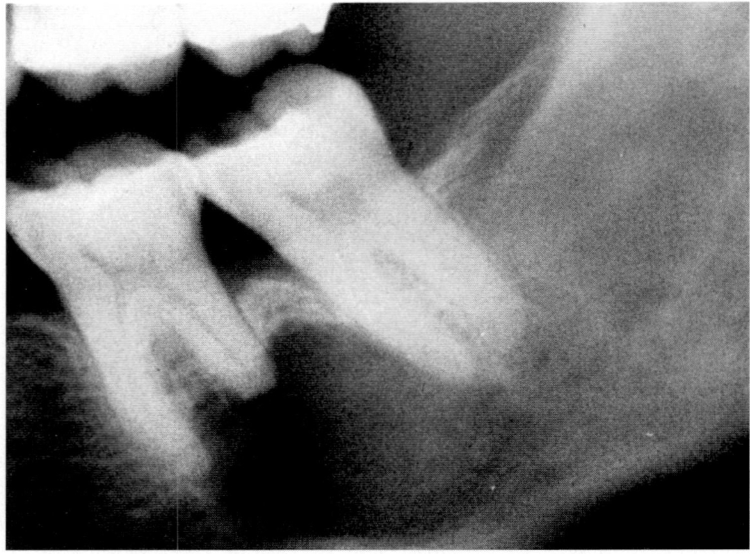

A

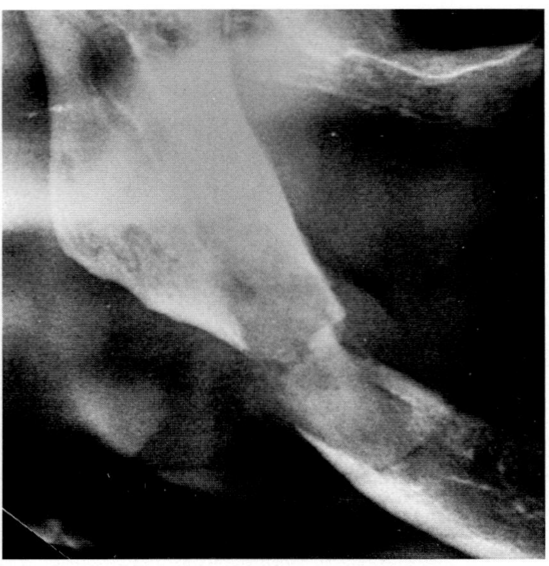

B

FIGURE 14–49.

Multiple Myeloma: Geographic pattern of destruction. A, Associated with resorption of root apices of adjacent teeth. (From Epstein JB, Voss NJS, Stevenson-Moore P: Maxillofacial manifestations of multiple myeloma. Oral Surg 57:267, March 1984.) B, Associated with pathologic fracture.

nate throughout the body. Their courses may range from rapidly fatal, to indolent and initially well tolerated. A leukemialike picture may develop in as many as 50% of children and 20% of adults with some type of NHL. In 1863 Virchow distinguished lymphosarcoma as a separate neoplastic entity arising in lymphoid tissue from leukemia originating in bone marrow. In 1893, Kundrat described gross and microscopic differences of lymphoid tumors and named the neoplasm lymphosarcoma. Greenfield (1878), Sternberg (1898), and Reed (1902) further clarified and separated Hodgkin's disease, with its characteristic giant cells, from other lymphoid tumors. A decade later, James Ewing (1913) recognized reticulum cell sarcoma as a variant of malignant lymphoma. NHL occurs more frequently than Hodgkin's disease, with 7000 to 8000 new cases diagnosed annually in the United States.

Pathologic Characteristics

The cause of NHL is unknown. Radiation and immune deficiencies have been implicated as possible etiologic factors. An increased incidence of NHL was observed in Hiroshima survivors, kidney transplant recipients undergoing immunosuppressive therapy, and patients with immune deficiency syndromes. A close association of human type C retrovirus with some adult leukemias and lymphomas composed of peripheral T cells has been shown recently.

The NHLs are currently in a state of change with respect to classification. Rappaport presented a new classification of malignant lymphomas including Hodgkin's disease in 1956 and revised this classification in 1966. Rappaport's classification of NHLs is used by many practicing diagnostic pathologists until final agreement on classification of malignant lymphoma is reached by hematopathologists. All classes of NHL are classified as nodular or diffuse except the lymphoblastic type and undifferentiated Burkitt's or non-Burkitt's (pleomorphic) types, which occur only in a diffuse pattern. The lymphocytic (nodular) and histiocytic (diffuse) types are the most common variants of NHL. NHL was classified by Rappaport according to the system shown in Table 14–1.

Clinical Features

In general, the lymphocytic (nodular) type (lymphosarcoma) of NHL occurs in older patients, whereas 35% of patients

TABLE 14–1
Malignant Lymphoma and Non-Hodgkin's Lymphoma as Classified by Rappaport

New System	Old System
1. Lymphocytic type (well or poorly differentiated)	Lymphosarcoma
2. Lymphoblastic type (diffuse pattern only)	
3. Histiocytic type	Reticulum cell sarcoma
4. Mixed lymphocytic–histiocytic type	Mixed lymphoma
5. Undifferentiated non-Burkitt's (pleomorphic) type	Stem cell lymphoma
6. Undifferentiated Burkitt's type	Stem cell lymphoma

with the histiocytic (diffuse) type (reticulum cell sarcoma) are younger than 40 years of age. The behavior of NHL generally can be predicted and correlated with the histologic classification. It occurs in all age groups, although the incidence increases with age.

Many patients have asymptomatic lymphadenopathy involving cervical or inguinal regions, or both. The enlarged lymph nodes are rubbery and discrete and later become matted. The tonsils are occasional sites of involvement. Mediastinal and retroperitoneal lymphadenopathy may cause pressure symptoms on various organs. Weight loss, fever, night sweats, and asthenia (weakness) indicate disseminated disease. Anemia is seen in approximately 33% of patients at diagnosis and ultimately develops in most. Hypogammaglobulinemia resulting from progressive disease in immunoglobulin production occurs in 15% of patients and may predispose the patient to serious bacterial infection. In 30% of cases of NHL, extranodal involvement may occur. Choukas (1948), Rollins and Thoma (1957), and Molander and Pack (1963) reported numerous cases of NHL involving the oral cavity. Gastric involvement may simulate gastrointestinal carcinoma or an intestinal lymphoma that may cause a malabsorption syndrome. Although any type of malignant lymphoma may originate occasionally in bone, most cases that do so result from histiocytic (diffuse) NHL; Coles and Schulz (1948) reported that in histiocytic NHL (reticulum cell sarcoma), bone involvement has been observed in 21% of cases, whereas in lymphocytic NHL (lymphosarcoma), the frequency of bone lesions is approximately 12%. Van Slyck (1972) reported that, in general, the more immature the cell composing the lesion, the greater the frequency of bone involvement either by hematogenous spread or direct invasion.

Resnick and Niwayama (1988) reported that in the disseminated forms of NHL, abnormalities of the axial skeleton predominate, with frequent involvement of the spine, pelvis, skull, and ribs. The presence of non-Hodgkin's lymphocytic lymphoma in the jaws is rare according to Gould and Main (1969); Sippel and Samartano (1971) reported that the maxilla seems to be affected more frequently than the mandible.

Treatment/Prognosis

Localized NHL does occur, but the disease is disseminated in approximately 90% of nodular types and 70% of diffuse cases when first recognized. Clinical staging procedures similar to those for Hodgkin's disease are indicated, except laparotomy and splenectomy rarely are necessary. Gould and Main (1969) and Carbone (1979) stated that, to accomplish staging and sequential comparison, the clinical and laboratory examinations should be supplemented with imaging and nonimaging techniques, including radioisotope studies, chest and abdomen radiographs, intravenous pyelograms, lymphography, and bone marrow biopsy. Herberg and associates (1984), Lee and associates (1984), and Holtas and coworkers (1986) reported that the precise role of CT and MRI in searching for sites of involvement (staging) is not clear, although both methods show promise in the detection of lymphadenopathy.

The final staging is based more often on clinical findings in non-Hodgkin's disease, whereas in Hodgkin's disease, pathologic staging is more critical for management decisions.

The prognosis and response to treatment are influenced significantly by histopathology, stage of disease, and, in some reports, results of surface marker studies. Favorable prognostic types include nodular histologic types and well-differentiated lymphocytic types that are usually B-cell (bone marrow-derived) lymphomas. The median survival times of these patients range from greater than 5 years to 7.5 years, but the patients eventually die of the disease. Unfavorable prognostic groups include patients with T-cell (thymus-derived) or lymphoblastic lymphomas or diffuse, poorly differentiated lymphocytic, histiocytic, and undifferentiated types (including Burkitt's lymphoma [BL]). These patients usually die within 1 year unless intensive treatment is given, in which case the prognosis may be good. Other factors that adversely affect prognosis are an age greater than 70 years, elevated lactic dehydrogenase levels, "bulky" masses greater than 10 cm in diameter, and more than two extranodal sites of disease.

Therapy of disseminated disease (Stage III or IV) of the favorable prognostic type is variable and includes radiation therapy and chemotherapy. Unfortunately, over a 2- to 6-year period, a slowly progressive disease that is resistant to most treatment programs develops in most patients. Advanced "unfavorable" prognostic types may respond dramatically to multiagent chemotherapy, and as many as 50% will have long-term remissions and may be cured. Patients with T-cell lymphoblastic lymphoma are treated similarly to those with acute childhood T-cell lymphocytic leukemia, with intensive chemotherapy regimens including prophylactic treatment of the central nervous system. There is an estimated 50% cure rate.

The overall survival rate of 30 to 40% is lower than that of Hodgkin's disease, but survival is higher in certain histologic subclassifications. Common causes of death in patients with NHL are infection, organ failure, hemorrhage, and disseminated tumor.

◆ *RADIOLOGY (Figs. 14–50 to 14–52)*

General Radiologic Features

Bone involvement in NHL is more commonly a manifestation of disseminated disease rather than a primary lesion. Greenfield (1978) estimated that the incidence of skeletal alterations in widespread NHL is 10 to 20% in adults and 20 to 30% in children. In the disseminated form, abnormalities of the axial skeleton predominate, with frequent involvement of the spine, pelvis, skull, ribs, and facial bones. In the series of Vieta and colleagues (1942), 85% of the bony lesions were osteolytic, with no new bone formation. Individual lesions are seen as areas of bone destruction, with irregular and infiltrating borders wiping out host bone architecture. Multiple osteolytic lesions with motheaten or permeative patterns of bone destruction predominate. Endosteal scalloping and cortical destruction are associated with spread to adjacent soft tissues. Periostitis occurs but is less frequent and severe than in Hodgkin's disease. On rare occasions,

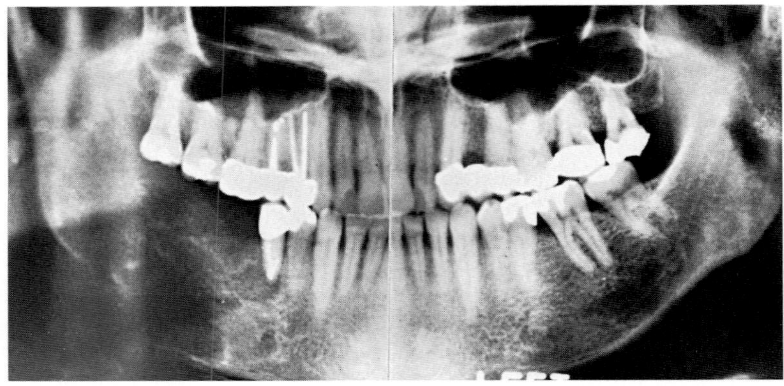

A

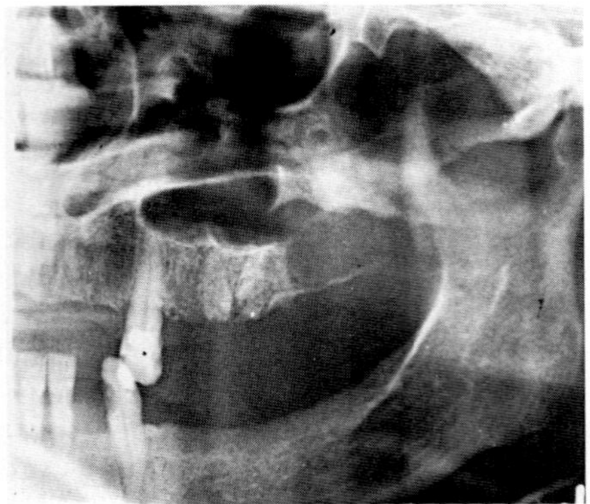

B

FIGURE 14–50.

Non-Hodgkin's Lymphoma: A, Bilateral lesions in mandible, geographic and motheaten changes, and perforation of the right cortex with no evidence of expansion. B, Geographic area of bone destruction in left posterior maxilla. (From Eisenbud L, Sciubba J, Mir R, Sachs SA: Oral presentations in non-Hodgkin's lymphoma: a review of thirty-one cases. Oral Surg 57:272, March 1984.)

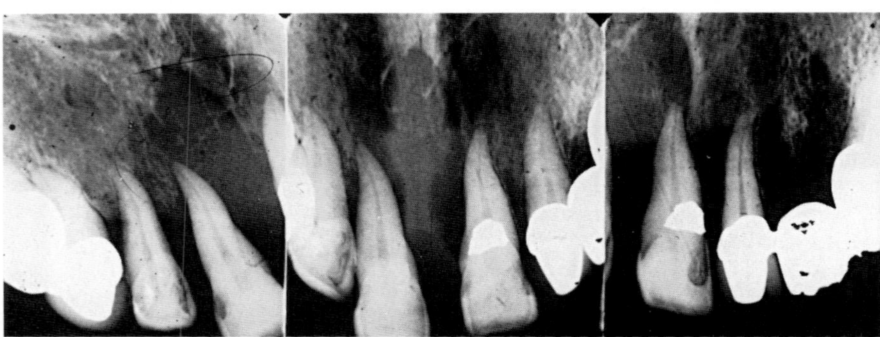

A

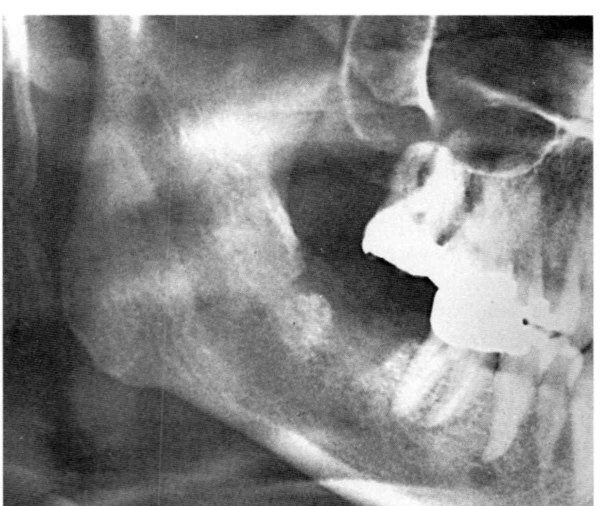

B

FIGURE 14–51.

Non-Hodgkin's Lymphoma: A, Seen as floating teeth in anterior maxilla. There are a few trabecular remnants, and motheaten and permeative changes in remaining alveolar bone. B, Seen as a diffuse widening of inferior alveolar canal with destruction of cortical walls of canal. (From Eisenbud L, Sciubba J, Mir R, Sachs SA: Oral presentations in non-Hodgkin's lymphoma: a review of thirty-one cases. Oral Surg 57:272, March 1984.)

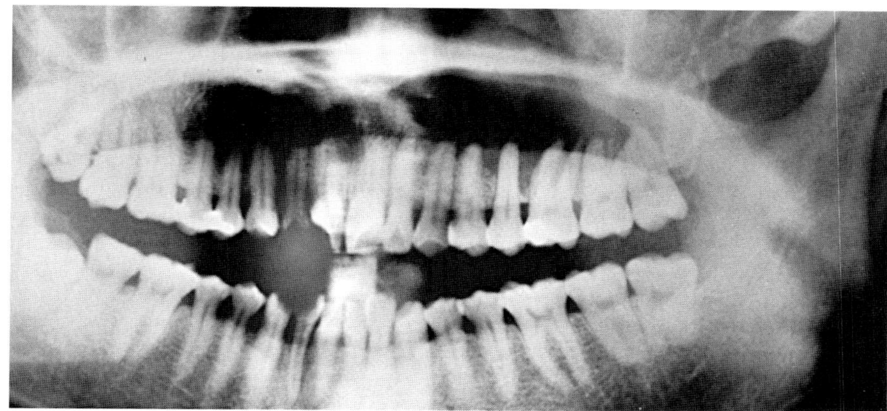

A

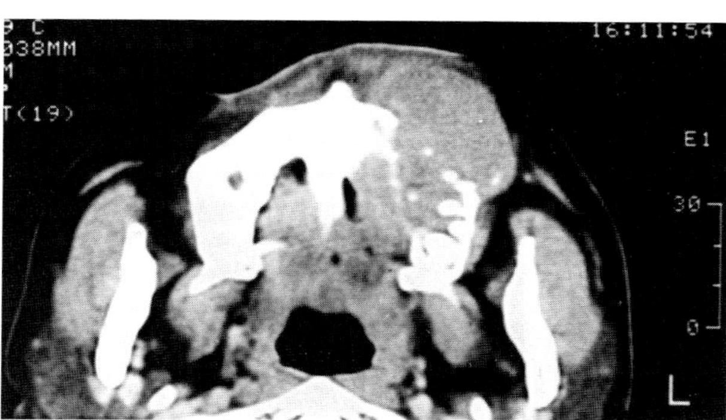

B

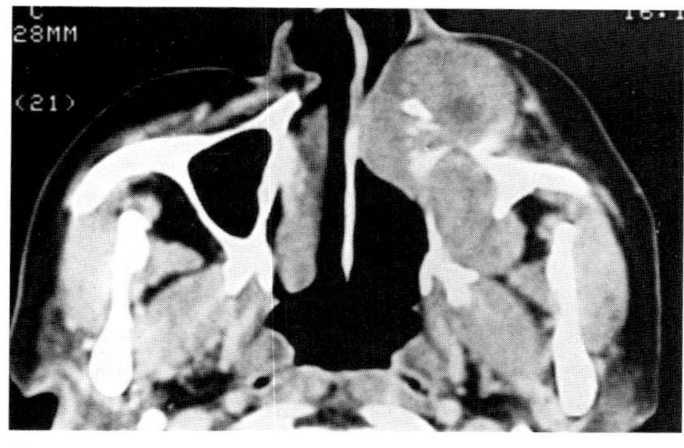

C

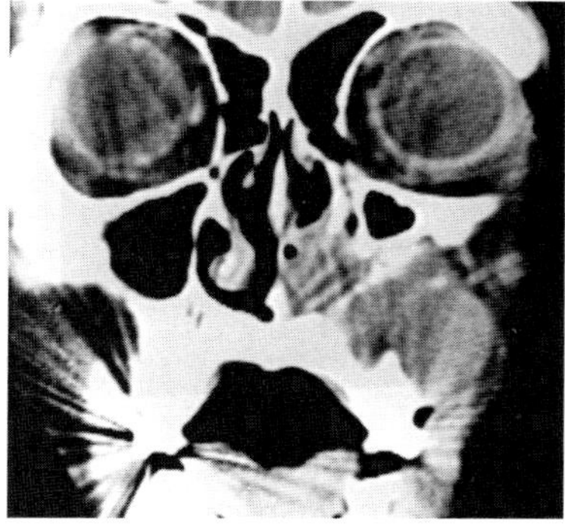

D

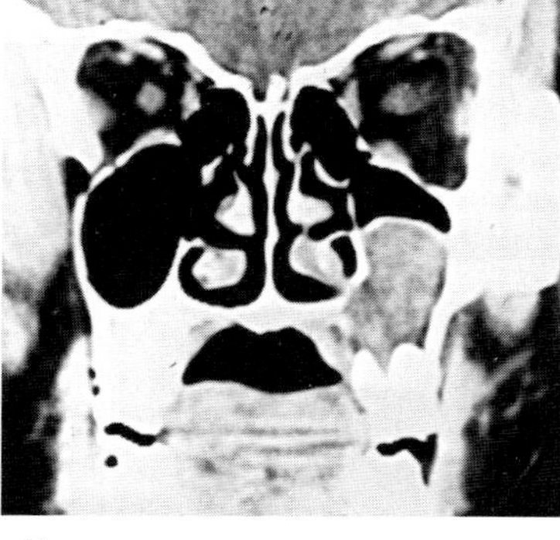

E

FIGURE 14–52.

Non-Hodgkin's Lymphoma: A, Lesion is in left maxilla and rendered invisible by glossopalatal air space, possibly because of soft tissue mass on palate preventing proper tongue placement against palate during exposure. B, C, D, and E, Destruction of left maxilla with tumor enlargement toward buccal and palatal sides. There is invasion into antrum, nasal fossa, and infratemporal space. (From Li TKL, MacDonald-Jankowski DS: An unusual presentation of a high-grade non-Hodgkin's lymphoma in the maxilla. Dentomaxillofac Radiol 19:224, Nov 1991.)

localized or diffuse osteosclerosis is evident, although this finding also is more common in Hodgkin's disease.

Radiologic Features of the Jaws

Jaw lesions may be purely destructive, or there may be some new bone formation in association with the osteolysis; the purely bone-forming changes do occur but are rare. When a lesion comes to the surface of the jaw, the bone is effaced and it is highly improbable that any new bone will be found beneath the periosteum; thus, expansion is absent. Multiple lesions occur, with several in many bones or the same bone. The margins of individual lesions are more irregular with non-Hodgkin's lymphocytic lymphoma (lymphosarcoma) than multiple myeloma. There may be destruction of the supporting bone of the teeth, resulting in mobility clinically. When the neoplasm involves the maxilla, there may be evidence of invasion of the lesion into the floor of the nasal cavity or maxillary sinus. Periosteal reactions are not seen.

PRIMARY NON-HODGKIN'S HISTIOCYTIC LYMPHOMA OF BONE

(Primary reticulum cell sarcoma of bone)

In 1939, Parker and Jackson (1939) first called attention to the lesion now known as ''primary non-Hodgkin's histiocytic lymphoma'' (primary reticulum cell sarcoma of the bone). The condition as reported by McCormack and associates (1952), Fripp and Sissons (1954), and Francis and coworkers (1954) is being established more and more definitely as a distinct clinicopathologic entity in a growing body of literature. The concept of this lesion grew out of the dilemma created by cases supposedly representing Ewing's sarcoma but not running the full clinical course typical of that disease. The cells of the primary non-Hodgkin's histiocytic lymphoma of bone apparently are derived from the primary mesenchyme in the marrow of the affected bone.

Pathologic Characteristics

The cytologic pattern of this osseous lesion is identical to that of non-Hodgkin's histiocytic lymphoma of the soft tissue (reticulum cell sarcoma); however, if one studies a biopsy specimen from a solitary destructive lesion, one must consider a number of diagnostic possibilities before calling a lesion a primary non-Hodgkin's histiocytic lymphoma (primary reticulum cell sarcoma of bone). For instance, under certain circumstances it may be difficult to distinguish cytologically between this disease and a form of cancer metastatic to bone, osteolytic osteosarcoma, plasma cell myeloma, and Ewing's sarcoma.

Clinical Features

According to Dahlin (1978), this condition has a male-to-female ratio of at least 3:2. Approximately half of the patients are younger than 40 years. The condition is rare in children younger than 10 years of age, although a fair proportion of the patients are between 11 and 20 years of age. Most of the remainder are between 40 and 60 years of age. With respect to age, primary non-Hodgkin's histiocytic lymphoma of bone contrasts with generalized non-Hodgkin's histiocytic lymphoma (reticulum cell sarcoma), with patients nearly all older than 40 years of age; it also contrasts with Ewing's sarcoma, with patients preponderantly younger than 25 years of age.

Clinical signs and symptoms are usually not striking except for the presence of localized swelling in the region of the involved bone, usually the mandible. In a 1955 review of all of the reported cases of primary reticulum cell sarcoma (primary non-Hodgkin's histiocytic lymphoma) of the mandible, Gerry and Williams reported that the principal presenting complaint is generally pain, often described as an aching in the area of the swelling. The patient usually has pain for several months to 1 year or more before seeking treatment. The oral mucosa seldom ulcerates over the involved bone site; however, the color of the tissue may change somewhat, appearing as a diffusely inflamed reddish area. The teeth are often mobile because of destruction of the alveolar bone. When the neoplasm involves the maxilla, there may be expansion of the lesion into the floor of the nasal cavity and sinus, but maxillary lesions are rare. Regional lymphadenopathy may be present, and, aside from local discomfort, the patient nearly always appears to be in reasonably good health without systemic signs or symptoms.

Treatment/Prognosis

After clinical and limited pathologic staging, early disease (Stage I or II) with "favorable" prognostic cell types may be cured by radiation therapy. Localized "unfavorable" prognostic types can be irradiated, and approximately half of Stage I types will be cured. Chemotherapy with or without radiation therapy is used with Stage II disease. The data of Coley and associates (1950) indicated a remarkably high 5-year survival rate of 73% when patients treated palliatively were excluded. In a series of primary non-Hodgkin's histiocytic lymphoma of bone reported by Boston and associates (1974), 98 patients with long-term follow-up had a 5-year survival rate of 44%.

◆ *RADIOLOGY (Figs. 14–53 to 14–56)*

General Radiologic Features

The leading radiographic feature is the presence of irregular patches of radiolucency representing osteolysis in the inferior portion of the affected bone part. There is a predilection for the long tubular bones, particularly the femur, tibia, and humerus. Localization to an innominate bone, scapula, rib, or some part of the vertebral column is not exceptional, but other localizations are definitely rare. In the long bone, the lesion may be located in the middle of the shaft or near one end of the bone. The foci of radiolucent osteolysis often are found intermingled with patchy areas of radiopacity that reflect reactive new bone formation at the site of the tumor. If the tumor has invaded the cortex it will be thinned; less frequently, part of the regional cortex may be thickened. In any event, the contour of the bone in the affected area does not seem to be distended very much. Sometimes periosteal new bone may be seen on the outer surface, but it usually is not striking. When the lesion has broken the bounds of the cortex and extended into the surrounding soft tissues, an extraosseous tumor mass of variable size will be apparent, but there is usually no evidence of ossification within this mass.

Radiologic Features of the Jaws

Primary non-Hodgkin's histiocytic lymphoma of bone is not a common disease of the jaws but appears to be somewhat more frequent in the mandible than the maxilla. Of the 150 primary cases of Dahlin (1978), 22 (15%) occurred in the mandible; there were no cases in the maxilla. In the jaws, the tumor usually gives rise to an irregular radiolucent area of bone destruction, with margins suggestive of infiltration; thus, the lesions are poorly defined, with a broad zone of transition between normal host bone and the central tumor mass within the mandible. Another frequent presentation in the jaws is that of a diffuse osteolytic lesion involving the alveolar bone that destroys the supporting bone of the teeth; the teeth become very mobile as this process progresses. Reactive new bone formation may be seen. This usually is seen at the margins of the lesion, although cortical thickening also may be seen. The reactive bone tends to be linear in character, although it may be more diffuse. According to Gerry and Williams (1955), radiating spicules of subperiosteal new bone that stand more or less perpendicular to the jaw also may be present rarely. After radiation therapy, new bone is laid down in tumors that resolve, but the trabecular pattern remains altered from that of normal bone.

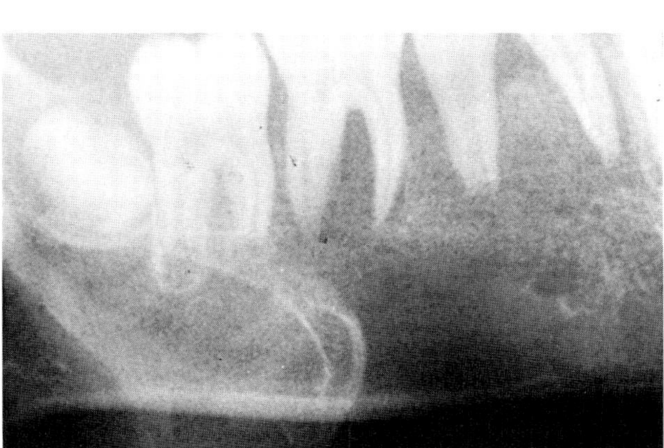

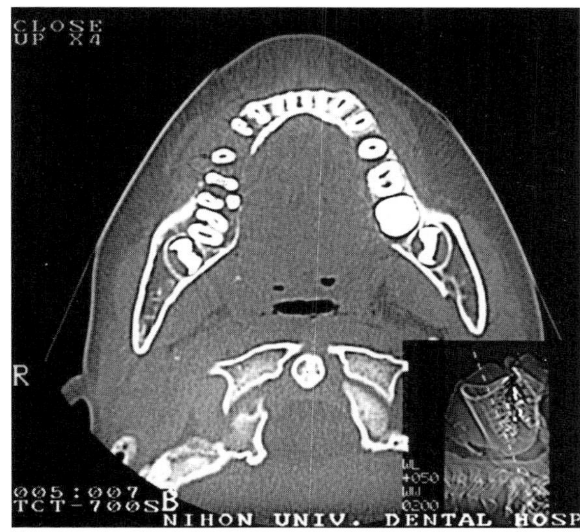

A B

FIGURE 14–53.

Primary Non-Hodgkin's Histiocytic Lymphoma of Bone in an 11-year-old Boy: A, Permeative changes throughout body of right mandible. B, Perforation of buccal and lingual cortices without expansion, and infiltration of tumor mass into adjacent soft tissues. (Courtesy of Drs. M. Araki, K. Hashimoto, and K. Honda, Nihon University School of Dentistry, Tokyo, Japan.)

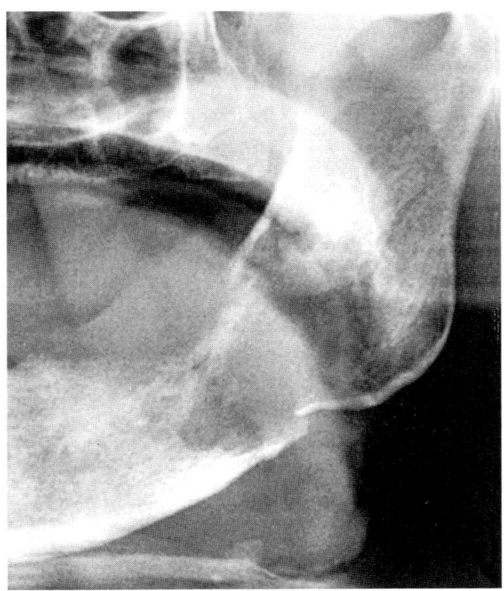

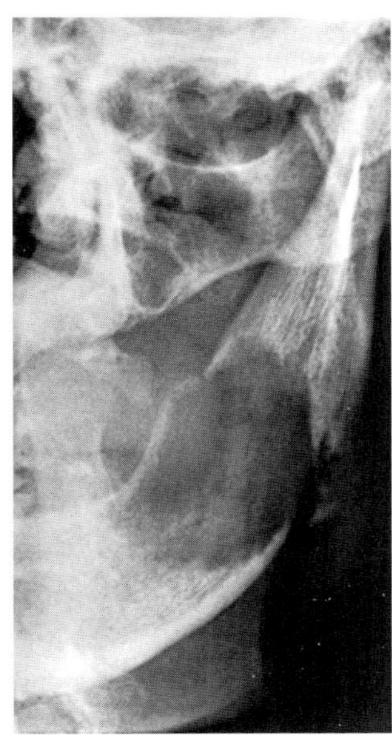

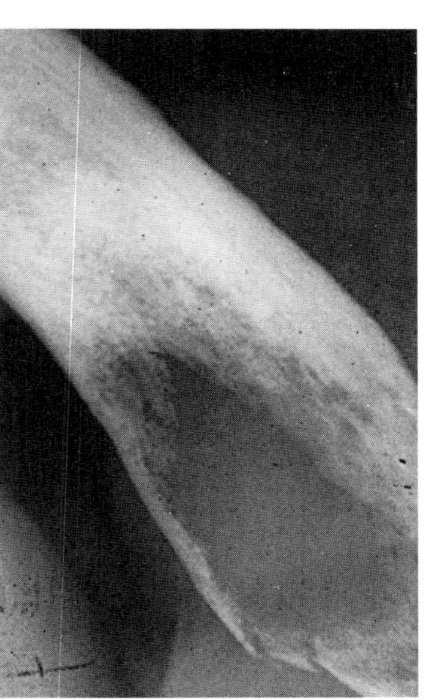

A B C

FIGURE 14–54.

Primary Non-Hodgkin's Histiocytic Lymphoma of Bone in a 65-year-old Man: A, Panoramic radiograph shows geographic bone destruction with poorly defined margins and discontinuity of inferior cortex. B, Posteroanterior radiograph of the mandible shows geographic bone destruction and pathologic fracture without periosteal reaction. C, Occlusal radiograph shows geographic destruction with permeative change at the margins representing tumor infiltration and pathologic fracture of the lingual cortex. (Courtesy of T. Noikura, First Oral Surgery Department, Kagoshima University, Kagoshima, Japan.)

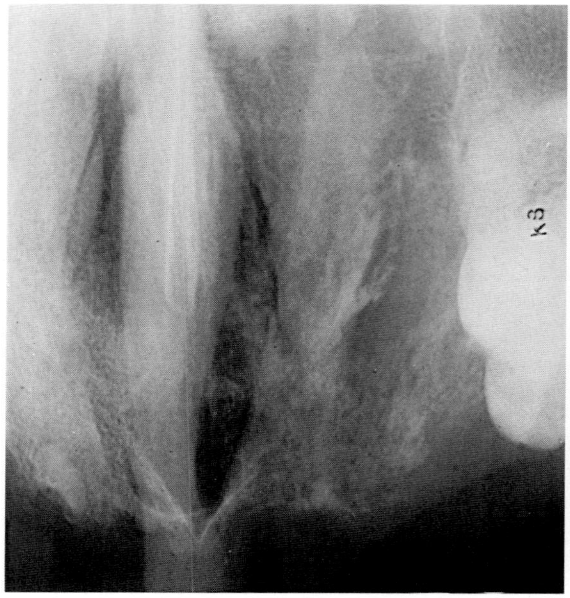

A

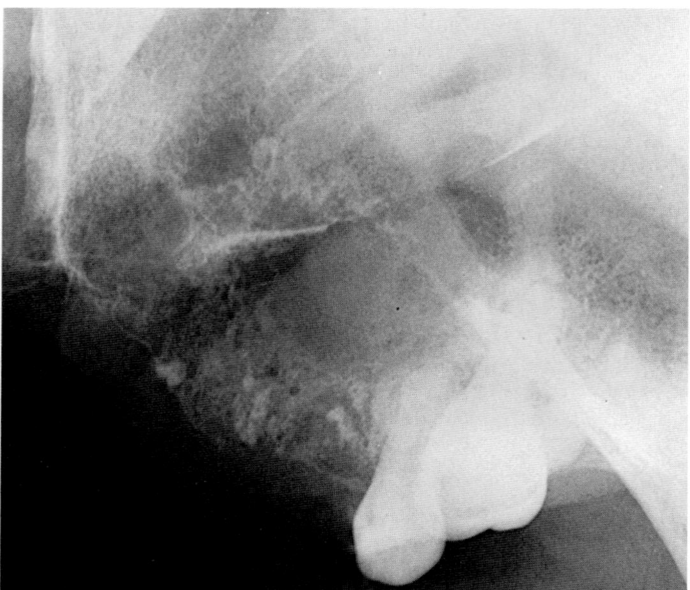

B

FIGURE 14–55.

Primary Non-Hodgkin's Histiocytic Lymphoma of Bone in a 66-year-old Man: A and B, Occlusal views show geographic and permeative changes in the left maxilla. (Courtesy of T. Noikura, First Oral Surgery Department, Kagoshima University, Kagoshima, Japan.)

BURKITT'S LYMPHOMA (African jaw lymphoma, American Burkitt's lymphoma)

BL is a stem cell lymphoma consisting of malignant proliferation of undifferentiated B-lymphocytes and is seen most often in children. It first was described in 1958 by Dr. Denis Burkitt, British missionary surgeon, in African children of the lowlands of Uganda, affecting the jaws and viscera. In 1962, Burkitt published the results of his African "tumor safari." This expedition showed that the lesion was found as far south as modern day Maputo (Mozambique) and extended north to Tanzania; the tumor never was seen at altitudes greater than 5000 feet (also true in the United States) or in areas where the temperature drops below 60° F. Additional

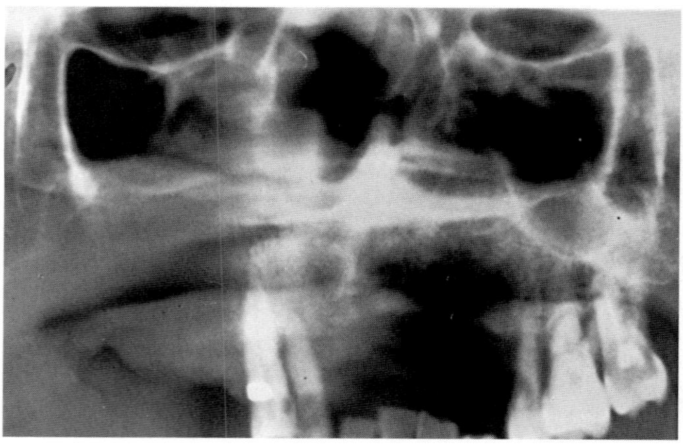

A

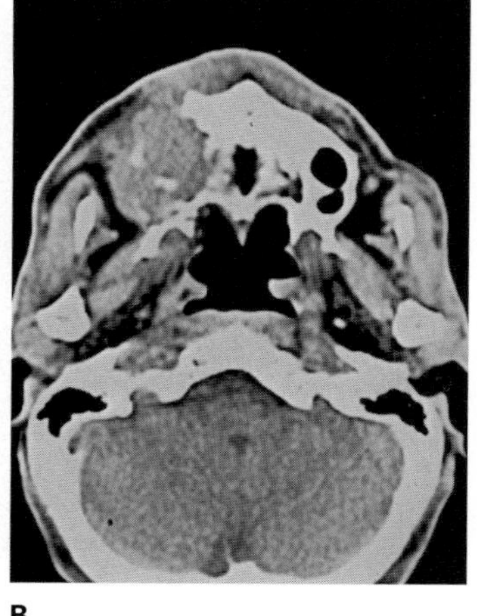

B

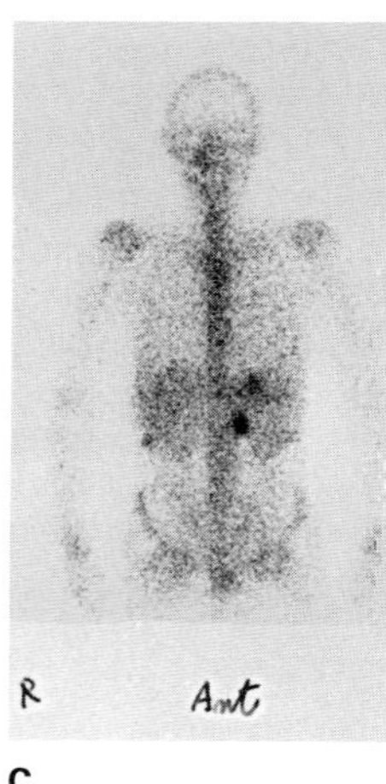

C

FIGURE 14–56.

Primary Non-Hodgkin's Histiocytic Lymphoma of Bone in a 55-year-old Man: A, Large area of destruction in right maxilla. B, CT image at level of sinus floor shows destruction of the right maxilla and sinus floor and a large tumor mass containing trabecular remnants. C, Technetium scan shows weak uptake in right maxilla, considering extent of lesion. Several hot spots in left liver indicate probable metastasis. (Courtesy of Professor T. Ohba, Kyushu Dental College, Kitakyushu, Japan.)

investigation prompted the designation of the "Burkitt's tumor belt," a geographic area in which Burkitt's tumors were recorded. This area correlated well with areas suitable for an insect-vectored disease, which prompted Burkitt and others to suggest such a transmission pattern. BL in Africa (endemic type) and outside Africa (nonendemic type) share similar histologic and cytochemical properties but differ in their clinical presentation. Involvement of facial bones is particularly characteristic in Africa, where it is seen in approximately 60% of all patients. Parker and associates (1980), Ziegler (1981), and Levine and Cho (1974) related that jaw involvement is less common in North America, where it is seen in 15 to 18% of patients; in this group the gastrointestinal tract alone is affected more frequently. Ziegler and associates (1977) reported that the two types of BL also showed differences in their relationship to the Epstein-Barr virus, which has been demonstrated in tumor cell cultures from African patients but not from patients outside Africa.

Levine and associates (1975) stated that 200 to 300 cases of BL are diagnosed annually in the United States. The National Cancer Institute reported that the annual rate for American BL was 0.05 cases per 100,000 persons from 1973 to 1977 in the United States.

Pathologic Characteristics

It is possible that Epstein-Barr virus is merely one of several co-factors required for induction of the disease, with malaria being another. Malaria or other chronic infections may alter the immune response of the host, thus promoting the oncogenic effect of the Epstein-Barr virus. The diagnosis of BL always is confirmed by microscopic examination of involved tissue taken from the oral cavity, lymph nodes, and bone marrow. Kramer (1965) related that the round or polyhedral medium-sized lymphocytes of BL have irregularly shaped nuclei and two or three prominent nucleoli per nucleus. Scattered throughout the masses of lymphocytes are large, pale-staining histiocytes (macrophages) in which remnants of phagocytized cells can be seen in the cytoplasm. O'Connor (1970) described the histiocytes as stars against a basophilic lymphocytic background, producing the characteristic starry sky histologic picture. This starry sky appearance is seen in other lymphomas, but it is more prominent in BL. Although clinical differences have been noticed between African endemic and American nonendemic cases, these tumors are identical histologically.

Clinical Features

In the endemic zones of Central Africa, BL is the most common childhood malignant neoplasm. The peak age of occurrence is stated to be 5 years by Burkitt (1962), 6 years by Kramer (1965), and 7 years by O'Connor (1970). In nonendemic areas, the mean peak age was 11 years, as reported by Areneau and associates in 1975. According to reports by Bhaskar (1973), Dean and associates, Levine and associates (1975), and Srivastava and associates (1976), there is a male predominance of 2:1 among those with African and nonendemic BL. Levine and associates (1975) found a male predominance of 3:1 in children younger than 15 years of age, whereas in patients older than 15 years, there is a female predominance, with a ratio of 3:2. The clinical signs of BL consist of abdominal masses, hepatomegaly, vomiting, ecchymosis, pallor, lymphadenopathy, and headache. The dentist may play an important role in the early diagnosis of BL by recognizing the clinical signs of unexplained multiple loose teeth, bilateral jaw tenderness, swollen gingiva, and cervical lymphadenopathy, coupled with the characteristic radiographic changes in the jaw.

Treatment/Prognosis

Successful treatment is related to an early diagnosis so that chemotherapy can be started before the disease becomes widespread. For instance, if an abdominal tumor already has reached the size at which it can be termed a mass, the chances of survival are greatly reduced. When present, manifestations in and around the jaws are among the earliest, if not the earliest, signs of the disease. Ziegler and associates (1979) stated that BL is the fastest growing of all tumors. In some instances, surgical debulking of up to 90% of the tumor mass is the first treatment performed, alone or in combination with radiation therapy, chemotherapy, or both. According to Abasa and associates (1981) and Beenson and McDermott (1975), the tumor responds dramatically to chemotherapy, which may result in the "tumor lysis" syndrome, however, characterized by gross and occasional lethal metabolic consequences from the release of intracellular products that lead to severe hyperuricemia, hypercalcemia, hyperphosphatemia, electrolyte disturbances, and renal malfunction. Tumor lysis can be offset by maintaining metabolic homeostasis with adequate hydration, allopurinol, alkalization of the urine, and concomitant monitoring of kidney function and blood chemistry.

The quicker the initial response to chemotherapy, the better the prognosis, which depends on the stage and extent at presentation and the absence or presence of visceral involvement. Stages A and B indicate single and multiple extra-abdominal sites; Stage C is defined by intra-abdominal disease involving the kidneys or gonads; and Stage D is similar to Stage C, but with involvement of extra-abdominal sites including the bone marrow or central nervous system. The prognosis can be improved when the bulk of abdominal tumors is resected. Intermittent intensive chemotherapy consisting of high doses of cyclophosphamide alone or lower doses combined with methotrexate and vincristine produces long-term disease-free survival in 70 to 80% of patients with Stage A or B disease and 30 to 40% of patients with Stage C and D disease.

In BL, virtually 100% of its cells are in active mitosis, so that the size of a tumor doubles every 24 hours. Without treatment, death may occur in 2 to 3 months. Because practically all cells in BL are in the mitotic cycle, it can be cured by a single dose of cyclophosphamide in a substantial percentage of patients. Most treatment failures result from central nervous system metastases, where highly active drugs cannot reach the tumor cells because of the blood-brain barrier.

◆ RADIOLOGY (Figs. 14–57 to 14–59)

General Radiographic Features

Fowles and associates (1983) and Wright (1964) have described lesions in the tubular bones and pelvis. The femur and tibia are especially vulnerable. There is an unusually high incidence of involvement of the proximal humerus, so Parker and associates (1980) suggested this bone should be radiographed early. Osteolytic foci develop in the medullary portion of the bone, coalesce, penetrate the cortex, produce periostitis, and lead to a soft tissue mass. The lesions are commonly multiple, bilateral, and even symmetrical in distribution. Accurate diagnosis on the basis of radiographic findings alone is difficult; however, the clinical features, including the absence of severe pain and toxemia and the presence of tenderness or local inflammation and a soft tissue mass, are helpful diagnostic clues.

Radiologic Features of the Jaws

Dental radiographs play an important part in the early diagnosis of BL. Adatia (1966a) reviewed the jaw radiographs of 63 patients with BL who were under the care of Dr. Denis Burkitt. Adatia (1966a) observed the greatest incidence of jaw tumors in 3-year-old children. The earliest radiologic evidence of disease is a loss of bone substance, which is subtle at first and consequently may be overlooked. The first loss of bone substance usually is found distal to the last developing mandibular molar in the arch, where the radiolucency is ill defined and may extend into the tooth crypt.

The radiographic changes enumerated by Cockshott (1965) and Adatia (1966a, 1966b) consisted of the following features: initial thinning and ultimate destruction of tooth crypts, widening of the follicular space, and displacement of developing and erupting teeth. There were also multiple areas of radiolucency that ultimately coalesced to form larger osteolytic lesions that rapidly destroy the lamina dura; in some instances, so much of the bone supporting the teeth was destroyed by the tumor that the teeth appeared to be floating in air. With perforation of the cortex, a soft tissue mass may extend into the buccal space, oral cavity, or maxillary antrum. When the tumor burst through the bone, sometimes it continued to grow subperiosteally, inducing

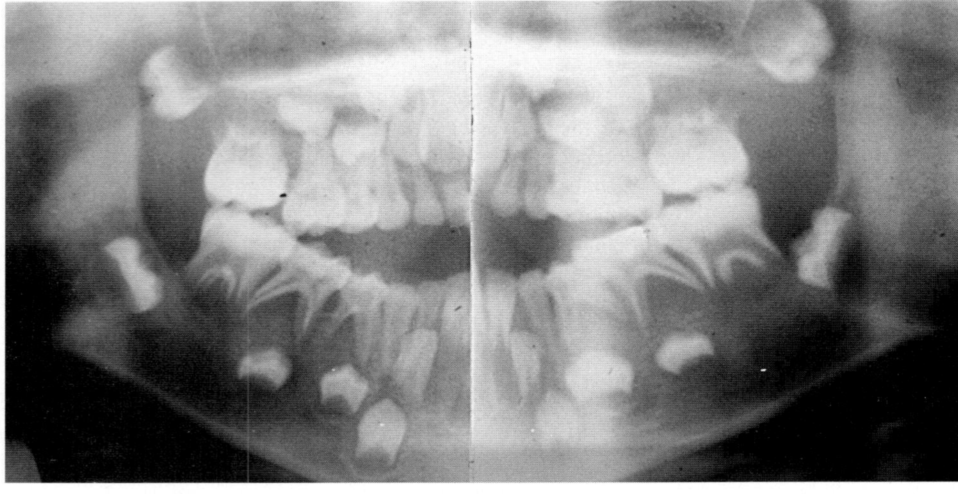

A

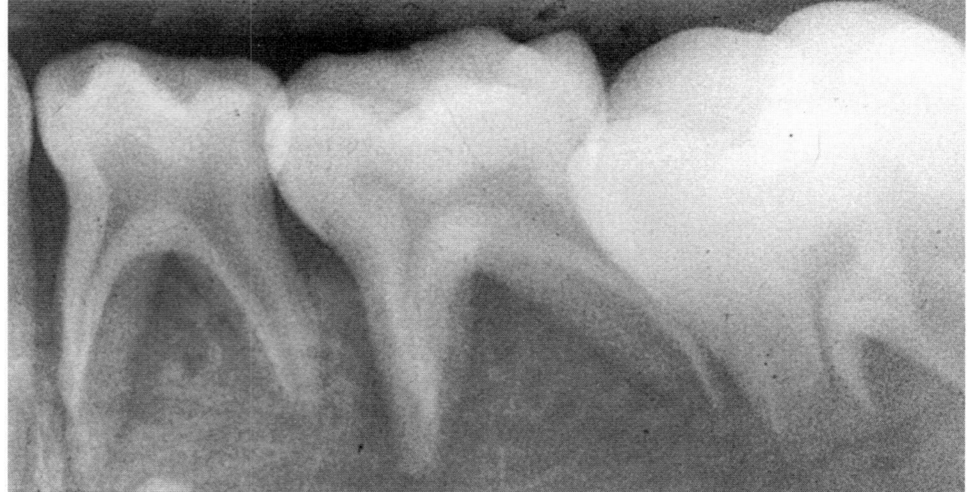

B

FIGURE 14–57.

Burkitt's Lymphoma in a 6-year-old Boy: A, Destruction of most radiopaque tooth crypt walls bilaterally in mandible and displacement of developing maxillary second molars, thus suggesting extent of disease. B, Generalized loss of lamina dura and concomitant widening of periodontal membrane space. (From Hupp JR, Collins FJV, Ross A, Myall RNT: A review of Burkitt's lymphoma. J Oral Maxillofac Surg 10:193, 1982.)

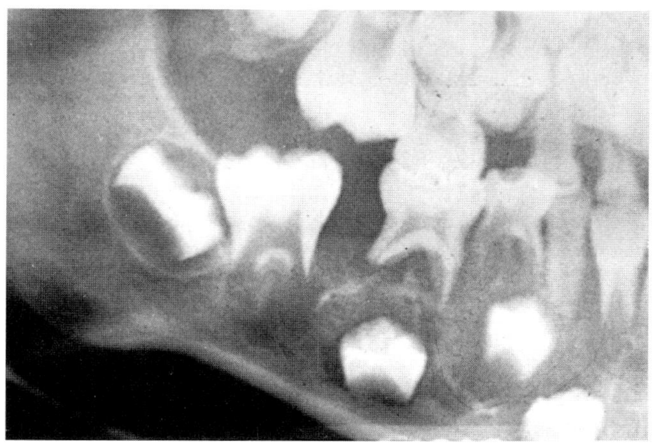

FIGURE 14–58.

Burkitt's Lymphoma: Displacement of erupting first molar and developing teeth in a 6-year-old American boy. There is partial erosion of tooth crypt walls, enlargement of follicular space of developing teeth, and loss of lamina dura with concomitant widening of the periodontal membrane space. (Courtesy of Drs. F. Sammis and C. Portales, San Antonio, TX.)

subperiosteal reactive bone formation and appearing radiographically as sunray spicules. Fourteen percent of Adatia's (1966b) radiographs showed that the sunray phenomenon is associated with mandibular lesions. These radiographic changes are not unique to BL. He observed no root resorption in association with any of the lesions studied. In endemic cases, Adatia (1966a, 1966b) reported that the radiologic changes in the jaws usually are detected before the appearance of any clinical signs of the disease.

Shortly after successful chemotherapy and clinical regression of the tumor, the crypts of developing teeth and the lamina dura are reformed, the teeth return to their normal position in the jaws, and the normal architecture of the bone is re-established. According to Adatia (1966a), odontogenesis of developing teeth will resume after successful treatment.

Alling and associates (1973) believed that the clinical and radiographic differential diagnosis should include histiocytosis X and pediatric solid tumors, such as Wilms' tumor, retinoblastoma, plasmacytoma, Ewing's sarcoma, metastatic neoplasms, and fibro-osseous lesions. If the lesion is unilateral, it may be suggestive of leukemia or lymphoma, but osteomyelitis also should be considered. When the radiolucency is bilateral, there is a strong likelihood that the patient has a lymphoma or possibly leukemia.

HODGKIN'S DISEASE (Hodgkin's lymphoma)

Hodgkin's disease is a chronic disorder of the reticuloendothelial system, with lymphoreticular proliferation of unknown cause that may be seen in localized or disseminated form. It accounts for 40% of all lymphomas. Kaplan (1980) reported that the disease first was described by Thomas Hodgkin in 1832, when he reported seven patients with a common lymph node and splenic enlargement, cachexia, and fatal termination. In 1856, Wilks concluded a detailed study of Hodgkin's cases, added 11 of his own, and named the condition Hodgkin's disease. This disease is primarily one of lymph nodes and lymphoid organs. The lymph nodes of the cervical chain are often the initial site of involvement. In the United States, 5000 to 6000 new cases of Hodgkin's disease are diagnosed annually.

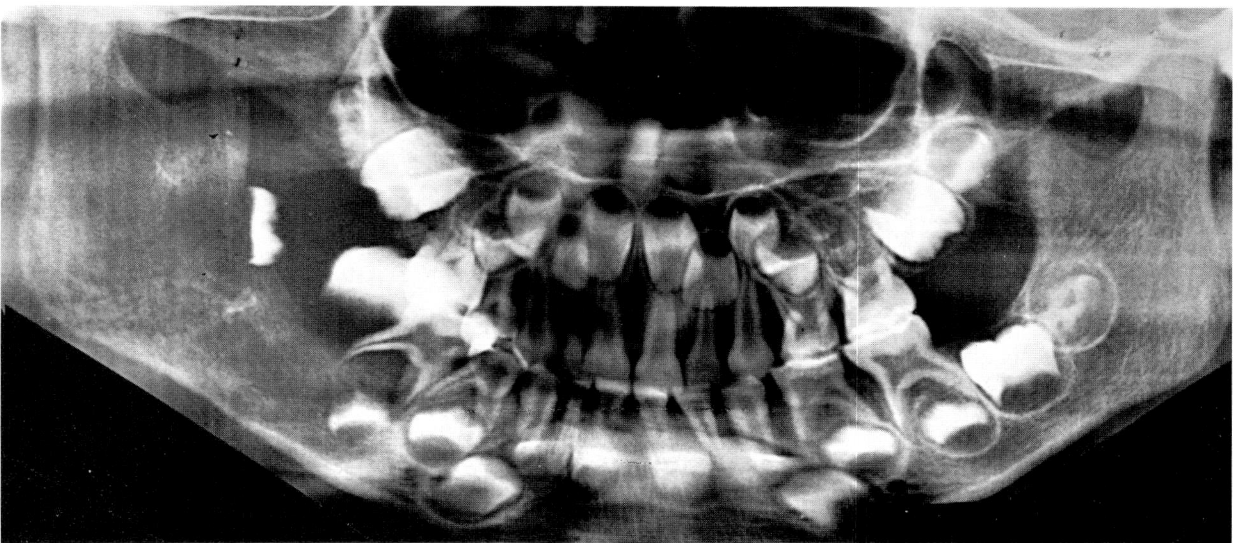

FIGURE 14–59.

Burkitt's Lymphoma: Osteoporotic change in right body and ramus of mandible in 5-year-old African boy. There is apparent early eruption of first and second molars resulting from their inclusion in the tumor mass, loss of crypt wall around the developing second premolar, and loss of alveolar bone around the second primary molar.

Pathologic Characteristics

From epidemiologic studies, there is no evidence of horizontal spread. Hodgkin's disease resembles a low-grade graft-versus-host reaction, and recent evidence of tumor-associated antigens in Hodgkin's tissue is consistent with this interpretation. A number of infectious agents, including viruses such as Epstein-Barr virus, are postulated as causes. Although the cause of Hodgkin's disease remains unknown, genetic and environmental factors appear to be involved.

Diagnosis depends on identification of large multinucleated reticulum cells (Sternberg-Reed [SR] cells) in lymph node lesions or other sites. Sternberg (1898) and Reed (1903) distinguished Hodgkin's disease, with its characteristic giant cells, from other lymphoid tumors. Hodgkin's infiltrates are heterogeneous and consist of abnormal reticulum cells, histiocytes, lymphocytes, monocytes, plasma cells, and eosinophils. The essential histologic feature of Hodgkin's disease consists of the multinucleated SR cell in an appropriate cellular background. The SR cell is a large, multinucleated reticulum cell measuring up to 400 μm in diameter; it has an abundant cytoplasm that is irregular in shape and varies in its staining reaction from acidophilic to basophilic. Some investigators consider the SR cells to be derived from B lymphocytes, and others advocate a monocyte-macrophage derivation. Generally the prognosis is worse when there are many SR cells.

The classification of Hodgkin's lymphoma was devised originally by Lukes and co-workers (1966a) and modified by a panel of experts who met in Rye, New York, in 1966. Lukes and associates (1966b) reported on the Rye classification, established in 1966, and it is used universally by pathologists today. There are four histopathologic classifications of Hodgkin's disease, and the microscopic distinction between the types of Hodgkin's disease has clinical and prognostic significance. For example, the lymphocyte predominant and nodular sclerosis types generally tend to be localized, and the prognosis is best in these types. The mixed cellularity and lymphocytic depletion types are more likely to be of widespread distribution, with a poorer prognosis.

Clinical Features

This disease is rare in children younger than 10 years of age; however, there is a bimodal age distribution, with one peak at ages 15 to 34 and another after the age of 54. The peak age range is 20 to 29 years. The overall male-to-female ratio is 1.4:1. Boys are affected predominantly in childhood (5:1), and men and women are affected approximately equally after age 70. Mayer and Smalley (1983) reported that 60 to 80% of patients with Hodgkin's disease have painless, asymmetric, "rubbery" lymphadenopathy in the cervical area. One fourth to one third of patients also have associated symptoms of unexplained weight loss in excess of 10% in 6 months, a temperature higher than 100.4° F, and night sweats. Malaise and pruritus may be present. Splenomegaly is observed in 50 to 70% of patients, but, despite enlargement, the spleen may not be involved histologically. Other constitutional symptoms include a dry cough and dysphagia, with mediastinal involvement and lower extremity edema or organ obstruction with abnormal involvement. A mild normocytic and normochromic anemia with or without eosinophila, neutrophilic leukocytosis, and autoimmune hemolytic anemia is present in 30 to 50% of patients. Bone abnormalities are more common in adults than children. The tumor may reach the osseous tissue by hematogenous dissemination or direct spread from contiguous diseased lymph nodes. Parker and associates (1980) observed that hematogenous spread is associated with a poorer prognosis. Appell and co-workers (1948) stated that direct spread from lymph nodes is especially common in the sternum, ribs, and spine. Pain, tenderness, swelling, and a palpable mass in the bone are the most common signs.

Treatment/Prognosis

In the United States, 1900 people die of Hodgkin's disease each year. The expected overall 5-year survival rate is 50 to 60%. Proper treatment of Hodgkin's disease can lead to long-term remission and even cure. Radiation therapy and combination chemotherapy clearly have been effective. The most important prognostic determinates are the histiologic type and clinical stage of the disease. The lymphocyte predominate type has the most favorable prognosis, followed by the nodular sclerosis type, mixed cellularity type, and lymphocyte depletion type, with the least favorable prognosis. Localized or Stage 1 disease is limited to one anatomic lymph node region and has a much better prognosis than disseminated or Stage IV disease, which indicates extranodal involvement of bone marrow, lung, or liver disease. Patchefsky and co-workers (1973) reported that male sex, older age, and systemic symptoms also are associated with a poorer prognosis.

Most patients with Hodgkin's disease have decreased or defective cellular immunity and demonstrable cutaneous anergy characterized by diminished reactivity to specific antigens. The decreased T-lymphocyte function may result from increased suppressor cell activity. The immunologic deficiency increases with advancing disease and increasing aggressive therapy, and there is a more pronounced effect in patients receiving both chemotherapy and radiation therapy. Because of their defective immune state, patients with Hodgkin's disease have a higher risk of infections caused by microorganisms and parasites that produce intracellular infection, including bacteria, such as Mycobacterium tuberculosis and listeria; fungi; and viruses including herpes zoster and protozoa, such as pneumocystis. Patients frequently die of sepsis.

◆ *RADIOLOGY*

General Radiologic Features

Primary Hodgkin's disease of bone is extremely rare, and its existence in a given patient is difficult to prove; the secondary form is common. Mirra (1989) found only 2 cases of primary Hodgkin's disease in bone among 3000 cases of Hodgkin's disease, for an incidence of 0.06%. The overwhelming majority of patients with Hodgkin's disease of bone have clinical evidence of lymph node involvement months to years before the process manifests in bone. Coles and Schulz (1948), O'Carroll and associates (1976), and Mussholf (1971) reported that 12 to 15% of patients with Hodgkin's disease have bone involvement shown either radiographically or by trephine biopsy. According to Steiner (1943), as many as 78% of patients with Hodgkin's disease have evidence of bone involvement at autopsy.

Most bone lesions in Hodgkin's disease are discovered in the vertebrae; other regions include the ribs, pelvis, and long bones, particularly the femur. Although any part of the bone may be involved, the metaphyses are most often affected in the long bones. The size of the lesion is extremely variable, from barely visible to involvement of an entire bone. Vieta and co-workers (1942) and Horan (1969) reported that bone lesions in Hodgkin's disease are usually polyostotic, as observed in 38 patients who collectively had involvement of 144 bones. Bone lesions are not distinctive. The lesions vary from poorly circumscribed and trabeculated, to loculated or showing a soap bubble appearance. Purely osteolytic lesions usually occur in the flat bones (i.e., ribs, sternum and pelvis). The osteolytic forms are those most often resulting in pathologic fracture. Parker and associates (1980) reported that the frequency of sclerotic lesions varies from 14 to 45%; these are excessively rare in the jaws but common in the vertebrae and pelvis. Purely osteoblastic lesions may affect a single vertebral body, causing an ''ivory vertebra'' appearance. Approximately 50% of all solitary ivory vertebrae are caused by Paget's disease, 30% by Hodgkin's disease, and 20% by other metastatic neoplasms. A sclerotic bone response may accompany direct invasion from an adjacent lymph node. For example, in the spine this appears as a scalloping of the anterior surface of the vertebral body. Widespread diffuse osteosclerosis may result from an osseous response to extensive bone marrow fibrosis rather than from frank involvement of the bone itself. Granger and Whitaker (1967) reported that one third of Hodgkin's disease cases are associated with longitudinal to perpendicular periosteal reactions, which mimic osteomyelitis or other highly malignant primary bone tumors.

The differential diagnosis between EG and chronic osteomyelitis is very important. Most patients with EG are children; most patients with Hodgkin's disease are young adults. Radiographically, lesions of solitary EG are purely lytic and relatively small, usually less than 5 cm in diameter; Hodgkin's disease entails multiple lesions that are purely lytic in only 15% of cases, and these are usually greater than 5 cm in diameter. Radiologically, chronic osteomyelitis usually is accompanied by a longitudinal periosteal reaction, which is found in less than 33% of patients with Hodgkin's disease.

The clinical staging of Hodgkin's disease is assessed by noninvasive procedures that include ultrasonography and CT scans of the abdomen and pelvis and, in selected cases, gallium body scans and bone scans. The role of MRI is being evaluated. Bipedal lymphangiograms generally are performed in patients with nodal disease because this is not seen readily on abdominal and pelvic CT scans.

Radiologic Features of the Jaws

Hodgkin's disease is rare in the jaws. Jackson and Parker (1947) and Vieta and associates (1942) did not find any cases in the jaws. Geschickter and Copeland (1949) did not mention the jaw in their account of the disease. Craver and Copeland (1934) found one case with mandibular involvement. The maxilla was affected in 1 of the 120 cases studied by Dresser and Spencer (1970). Foreman and Wesson (1970) reported a case secondarily involving the mandible and overlying alveolar mucosa.

LEUKEMIA

Leukemia is characterized by the progressive overproduction of leukocytes that usually appear in the circulating blood in an immature form. Because the proliferation of leukocytes or their precursors occurs in such an uncoordinated and independent fashion, leukemia generally is considered a true malignant neoplasm, particularly because the disease is often fatal.

Pathologic Characteristics

Although viruses cause several forms of animal leukemia, the cause of human leukemia is undefined. Only two viral associations have been identified: Epstein-Barr virus, a DNA virus, is associated with BL; and the human T-cell lymphotrophic virus, an RNA retrovirus, has been linked to some T-cell leukemias and lymphomas. Exposure to ionizing radiation and certain chemicals is associated with an increased risk of leukemia. Some genetic defects such as Down's syndrome and familial disorders such as Fanconi's anemia predispose people to leukemia. Whatever the etiologic agent, transformation to malignancy appears to occur in a single cell through two or more steps, with subsequent proliferation and clonal expansion.

Leukemias have been defined as acute or chronic. Although the original basis for this separation was life expectancy, these terms now are applied on the basis of cellular maturity. Thus, acute leukemias are predominantly undifferentiated cell populations and chronic leukemias more mature forms. Acute leukemias are divided into acute lymphoblastic leukemia (ALL) and acute nonlymphoblastic leukemia (ANLL). Chronic leukemias are separated into chronic myelocytic leukemia (CML) and chronic lymphocytic leukemia (CLL). CML is a clonal myeloproliferation caused by malignant transformation of a pluripotent stem cell and characterized clinically by a striking overproduction of granulocytes primarily in the bone marrow but also in extramedullary sites such as the spleen and liver. CLL is a clonal expansion of mature-appearing lymphocytes involving lymph nodes and other lymphoid tissues and progressive infiltration of bone marrow and circulation in blood. Thus, chronic leukemia is characterized by the appearance of mature lymphocytes in blood, bone marrow, and lymphoid organs. The acute leukemias usually progress rapidly and are characterized by replacement of normal marrow by blast cells of a clone arising from malignant transformation of a hematopoietic stem cell; the leukemia cells accumulate in the bone marrow, replace normal hematopoietic cells, and spread to the liver, spleen, lymph nodes, central nervous system, kidneys, and gonads.

Clinical Features

ALL is predominantly a childhood disease, with a peak incidence in children from 3 to 5 years of age. It is the most common childhood malignant condition, also occurring during adolescence and less commonly among adults. ANLL occurs in patients at all ages and is the most common acute leukemia among adults. It is the form usually associated with irradiation as a causative agent and occurring as a secondary malignant condition after cancer chemotherapy. CML may occur in people at any age; it is uncommon in those younger than 10 years of age and is seen most often in adults with a median age of 45 years. There is no significant sex preponderance. CLL is a disease of older people, with the average age at diagnosis being 60 years in 75% of cases. It is two to three times more common in males than females. The cause is unknown, but some cases are familial. The disease is rare in China and Japan.

According to Parker and associates (1980), among cases of acute leukemia among children, approximately 80% are lymphoblastic in origin, 10% are myeloblastic (nonlymphoblastic), and 10% are of another cellular origin. Acute leukemia can affect children and adults. The onset is sudden, characterized by weakness, fever, headache, generalized swelling of lymph nodes, evidence of anemia, and petechial or ecchymotic hemorrhages in the skin and mucous membranes, especially the soft palate. Cervical lymphadenopathy is often the first sign of the disease. Numerous organs such as the spleen, liver, and kidney become enlarged because of leukemic infiltration, especially in cases of long duration. Van Slyck (1972) reported that acute leukemia in adults is frequently nonlymphoblastic or myeloblastic (immature leukocyte) in cell origin. As a general rule, clinical and radiologic evidence of skeletal involvement in leukemia is less common in adults than children. Acute leukemia in adults may be associated with bone pain and tenderness. Thomas and co-workers (1961) reported that 5% of such patients had bone pain initially, and 50% had this symptom sometime during their illness.

Lynch and Ship (1967) studied 155 leukemic patients over a period of 10 years. Specific oral signs were present in 38% of patients with acute leukemia, and 4% had oral changes that were significant in the diagnosis of leukemia. The most common oral sign of leukemia occurring in the postdiagnostic period was spontaneous oral hemorrhage or petechiae. The second and third most common findings were mucosal ulcers and generalized gingival hyperplasia. In a review of 500 cases, Stafford and associates (1980) found that oral manifestations of leukemia were more common in patients with acute leukemia than those with chronic leukemia. The most frequent oral problems associated with ANLL were gingival oozing, petechiae, hematomas, or ecchymoses. Gingival enlargement, redness, and pain often were present. In this study, 65% of patients had some form of oral pathosis as their initial complaint.

Treatment/Prognosis

Before current treatments were available, the average patient with acute leukemia survived approximately 4 months after diagnosis. Now the treatment goal for all patients with ALL and ANLL should be cure. The first goal of treatment of acute leukemias is to achieve complete remission, which is associated with resolution of abnormal clinical features, return to normal blood counts, and hematopoiesis in the bone marrow with less than 5% blast cells.

Regardless of the risk factors, the likelihood of initial remission is greater than 90% in patients with ALL. Fifty percent of these children should have a continuous disease-free survival for 5 years. For patients with ANLL, reported remission induction rates range from 50 to 85%. A long-term disease-free survival is reported to occur in 20 to 40% of patients with acute leukemia. Bone marrow transplantation is reported to result in a 40 to 50% long-term disease-free survival rate. The most important prognostic clinical feature is age. Patients older than 50 years have less likelihood of an induced remission. Patients in whom ANLL develops after chemotherapy and radiation therapy have the poorest prognosis; however, the goal of treatment for all patients with acute leukemia is cure.

No significant improvement in survival has occurred in patients with chronic leukemia in recent years. In patients with CLL, the median survival length from diagnosis until death from all causes is approximately 6 years. Approximately 15 to 20% of these deaths are from causes unrelated to CLL. The median survival time of patients with CLL or its complications is approximately 10 years. The median survival length of patients with CML is 3 to 4 years after clinical onset. Approximately 10% of patients die of other causes; the rest die of ''blast crises'' or during an accelerated phase of the disease. The goal of treatment is palliation, not cure.

◆ *RADIOLOGY (Figs. 14–60 and 14–61)*

General Radiologic Features of Acute Leukemias

The osseous and articular manifestations of chronic leukemia are less common and less severe than those of acute leukemia. Greenfield (1986) reported that radiologically detectable skeletal involvement in leukemia occurs in 50 to 70% of cases of childhood leukemia and as many as 10% of cases in adults. These lesions do not represent metastases; they are primary lesions of bone from neoplastic proliferation of marrow elements.

The radiographic changes associated with acute leukemia were classified by Resnick and Niwayama (1988) as follows:

1. Diffuse osteopenia: This consists of a reduced bone mass and is a nonspecific finding simulating osteoporosis and other metabolic disorders. Benz and associates (1976), Simmons and co-workers (1968), and Thomas and associates (1961) believed that this diffuse decrease in radiodensity of the skeleton results from leukemic infiltration of the bone marrow. Epstein (1957) stated that medullary widening and cortical thinning in tubular bones and vertebral compression are encountered. The osteopenia in patients with leukemia who are being treated with steroids may be related to the therapy.

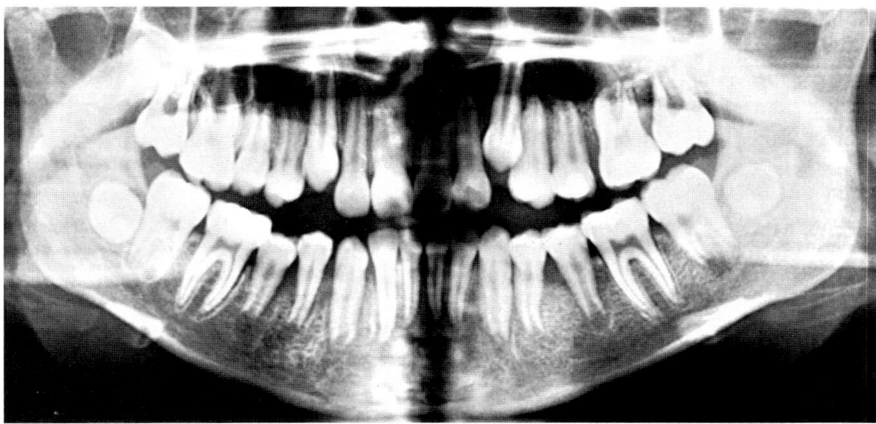

A

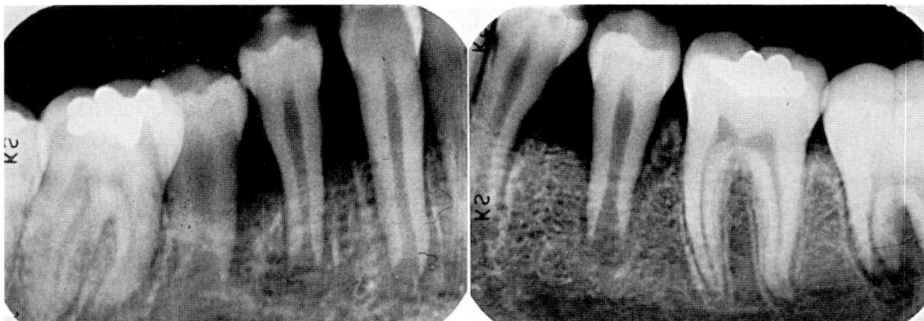

B

FIGURE 14–60.

Leukemia: Bilateral view of mandibular premolar area. A and B, Periodontal defect-like appearance, loss of lamina dura, and osteopenic appearance of alveolar bone with tiny more radiolucent marrow spaces, each appearing to have a zone of reactive sclerosis around it. (Courtesy of Drs. Alvaro and Gabriel Castro Delgado, Universidad Javeriana, Santa Fé de Bogotá, Columbia.)

2. Radiolucent and radiodense metaphyseal bands: Symmetric metaphyseal bandlike radiolucent areas are observed in acute leukemia and other chronic childhood illnesses. They are seen most commonly at sites of rapid bone growth, including the distal femur, proximal tibia, proximal humerus, and distal radius. Wilson (1959) stated that, after the age of 2 years, radiolucent metaphyseal bands are more characteristic of leukemia than other chronic childhood illnesses. Silverman (1948) mentioned that radiodense metaphyseal bands may be seen adjacent to the areas of increased radiolucency. In some cases the entire metaphysis is radiodense. Metaphyseal radiolucent bands occur less frequently in adults than in children with acute leukemia.
3. Osteolytic lesions: Becker and co-workers (1979) reported that multiple or solitary radiolucent lesions are encountered in tubular and flat bones, including the cranial vault, pelvis, ribs, and shoulder girdle. Melhem and Saber (1980) reported that the medial cortex of the proximal portion of the humerus is a characteristic site of involvement. The skull, which is involved rarely, may show areas of bone destruction. Nixon and Gwinn (1973) reported that sutural diastasis or separation in the skull is common in infants and children with leukemia. It is produced by increased intracranial pressure resulting from leukemic cell infiltration of the meninges or cerebrum or from intracerebral hemorrhage. Sullivan (1957) stated that, in older patients, sutural separation is rarely present, except after chronic chemotherapy.
4. Periostitis: Silverman (1948) reported that periosteal bone formation can be associated with lytic lesions. Proliferating leukemic cells in the marrow invade the cortex through haversian canals and extend to subperi-

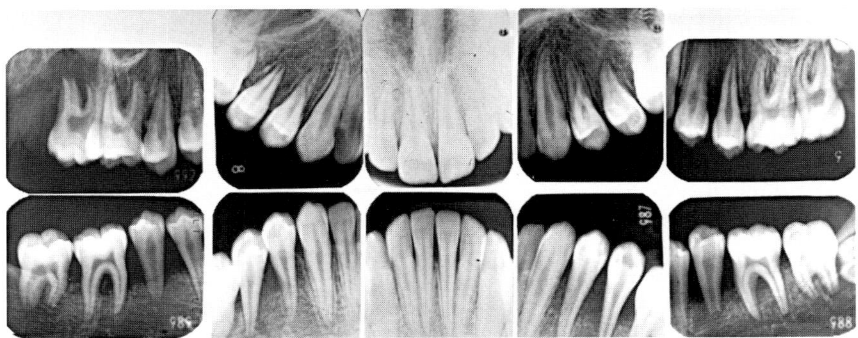

FIGURE 14–61.

Leukemia in a 12-year-old Girl: Changes resemble those of periodontal disease. (Courtesy of Professor H. Fuchihata, Dean, Osaka University, Osaka, Japan.)

osteal locations, causing elevation of the periosteal membrane; subperiosteal hemorrhage may be an associated finding. Nixon and Gwinn (1980) reported that periostitis is particularly prominent in the long bones, although it may occur elsewhere. Single or multiple areas may be found.

5. Osteosclerosis: Silverman (1948) reported that osteosclerosis is a relatively infrequent finding in leukemia. When present, it is particularly prominent in the metaphyses of long bones. Reactive bone formation in response to leukemic cell infiltration or infarction may be responsible for such sclerosis.

General Radiologic Features of Chronic Leukemias

Schabel and associates (1980) reported that marrow hyperplasia in some adults with chronic leukemia becomes evident as a nonspecific diffuse osteopenia, particularly in the axial skeleton. Redmond and co-workers (1983) observed discrete osteolytic lesions in fewer than 3% of their patients with chronic leukemia, occurring particularly in the femur and humerus. Rarely, widespread or multifocal bone sclerosis is evident; perhaps it is related to diffuse marrow fibrosis. Brownstein and associates (1980) stated that clinical and radiographic manifestations of skeletal involvement in chronic leukemia can become more prominent during a blast crisis, in which large numbers of myeloblasts appear in the marrow and peripheral blood and a downhill clinical course occurs, characterized by anemia, myelofibrosis, and, ultimately, death from infection or bleeding within 4 to 6 months.

Radiologic Features of the Jaws

Jaw involvement in leukemia first was described by Bender in 1944. According to Worth (1963), the jaws usually escape radiologic change, but when they are involved, there is a pattern consisting of a uniform osteoporosis leading to increased radiolucency and effacement of the lamina dura. The jaws of young people normally show less trabeculation than adult jaws, so osteoporosis may produce an appearance that could be mistaken for osteomyelitis.

The gingival tissues become enlarged from the leukemic infiltrate, and in some cases they undergo necrosis. This results in a proliferation of microorganisms that ultimately enter the periodontal tissues, destroying them. Alveolar bone is lost, and the radiologic appearance resembles that of periodontal disease. The periodontal changes most likely result from infection because of lowered resistance of the tissue, caused by the abnormal blood state. Just as the alveolar supporting bone is more prone to infection in leukemia, so are the deeper portions of the jaws, the body of the maxilla and mandible. The uncomplicated removal of a tooth may result in widespread osteomyelitis. If unerupted teeth are within their follicles, the walls of the follicles are lost; thus, the appearance may resemble that of hyperparathyroidism.

Williams and co-workers (1983) reported a case of ALL in a 7½-year-old girl. The radiographic examination of the posterior mandible showed an irregular radiolucent area in the region of the molars. There was loss of the lamina dura, and the roots of the first molar appeared pencil sharp as a result of resorption. Areas of radiolucency were visible around and between the roots, and the tooth appeared to be in danger of exfoliation. The mesial part of the crypt around the developing third molar had been destroyed, and the tooth was displaced in the direction of the ascending ramus. Peterson and co-workers (1983) reported an unusual instance of leukemic infiltrate at the apex of a mandibular second molar in an adult with relapsed ANLL. The oral symptoms resemble those of pulpal disease requiring root canal therapy.

Curtis (1971) studied 197 children with leukemia, and panoramic radiographs were taken during remission in 117 of these children with ALL; 76 (65%) were found to have abnormal radiologic findings. These abnormalities varied from obvious destruction of crypts and lamina dura or displacement of teeth, to more subtle changes in radiodensity of the alveolar bone. Crypt destruction was the most frequent finding. Curtis (1971) reported a high degree of correlation between radiographic evidence of destruction of alveolar bone and clinical evidence of active leukemia in children thought to be in remission. This author also stated that panoramic examinations are of diagnostic value, especially in instances of impending relapse. He described three patients in hematologic remission who exhibited radiologic changes and noticeable mandibular swelling. In two, relapse was confirmed by biopsy, and in the third patient the bone marrow relapse was swift. In most of the cases with radiologic abnormalities, regression to normal occurred after chemotherapy or, in symptomatic cases, local radiation therapy to the jaw.

References

Chronic Rarefying Osteomyelitis

Goupil MT, Steed DL, Kolodny SC: Hyperbaric oxygen in the adjunctive treatment of chronic osteomyelitis of the mandible: report of case. J Oral Surg 36:138, 1978.

Hart GB, Mainous EG: The treatment of radiation necrosis and hyperbaric oxygen. Cancer. 37:2580, 1976.

Nakajima T, Yagata H, Kato H, Tokiwa N: Surgical treatment of chronic osteomyelitis of the mandible resistant to intraarterial infusion of antibiotics: report of case. J Oral Surg 35:823, 1977.

Ram PC, et al: CT detection of intraosseous gas: a new sign of osteomyelitis. Am J Roentgenol 137:721, 1981.

Runge VM: Magnetic Resonance Imaging: Clinical Principles. Philadelphia:JB Lippincott, 1992, p. 341.

Silberman M, et al: Mandibular osteomyelitis in the patient with chronic alcoholism: etiology, management and statistical correlation. Oral Surg Oral Med Oral Pathol 38:530, 1974.

Topazian RG: Osteomyelitis of the jaws. In: Topazian RG, Goldberg MH, eds. Management of Infections of the Oral and Maxillofacial Regions. Philadelphia:WB Saunders, 1981, p. 240.

Wood NK, Goaz PW: Differential Diagnosis of Oral Lesions. 2nd Ed. St. Louis:CV Mosby, 1980, p. 448.

Young J, Bump R: Hyperbaric oxygenation: prosthodontics responsibilities. J Prosthet Dent 39:100, 1978.

Osteoradionecrosis

Bergstedt HS: Bone scintigraphy of facial skeleton with 99 Tcm-diphosphonate. Acta Radiol [Diagn] (Stockh) 16:337, 1975.

Daly TE, Drane JB: Management of teeth related to the treatment of oral cancer. National Cancer Conference Proceedings #7. New York:American Cancer Society, 1973, p. 147.

Epstein JB, Hatcher DC, Graham M: Bone scintigraphy of fibro-osseous lesions of the jaw. Oral Surg Oral Med Oral Pathol 51:346, 1981.
Ewing J: Radiation osteitis. Acta Radiol 6:399, 1926.
Komisar A, Silver C, Kalnicki S: Osteoradionecrosis of the maxilla and skull base. Laryngoscope 95:24, 1985.
Marx RE: A new concept in the treatment of osteoradionecrosis. J Oral Maxillofac Surg 41:351, 1983b.
Marx RE: Osteoradionecrosis: a new concept of its pathophysiology. J Oral Maxillofac Surg 41:283, 1983a.
McLenna W: Some aspects of the problems of radionecrosis of the jaws. Proc R Soc Med 48:1017, 1955.
Meyer I: Infectious diseases of the jaws. J Oral Surg 28:17, 1970.
Mizuno A, Sekiyama S, Seki S, Kojima M: Clinical observation on osteoradionecrosis of the mandible. Oral Surg Oral Med Oral Pathol 46:22, 1978.
Morrish RB et al: Osteonecrosis in patients irradiated for head and neck carcinoma. Cancer 47:1980, 1981.
Regaud C: Sur la necrose des os attients par un processus cancereux et traiters par les radiations. Comp Rend Soc Biol 87:417, 1922.

Neuralgia-Inducing Cavitational Osteonecrosis

Harris W: Neuritis and Neuralgia. London:Oxford University Press, 1926, p. 163.
Janetta PJ: Evidence for a peripheral etiology of trigeminal neuralgia. J Neurosurg 26:168, 1967.
Kinnier Wilson SA, Bruce AN: Neurology. Baltimore:Williams & Wilkins, 1955, p. 405.
Locke J: Letters to Dr. Mapletoft: Letter VII, Paris, August 9, 1677. European Magazine, Feb 1789, p. 89.
Locke J: Letters to Dr. Mapletoft: Letters IX, X, Paris, December 4, 1677. European Magazine, March 1789, p. 185.
Mathis BJ, Oatis GW, Grisius RJ: Jaw bone cavities associated facial pain syndromes: case reports. Milit Med 146:719, Oct 1981.
Ratner EJ, et al: Jawbone cavities and trigeminal and atypical facial neuralgias. Oral Surg Oral Med Oral Pathol 48:3, 1979.
Roberts AM, Person P: Etiology and treatment of idiopathic trigeminal and atypical facial neuralgias. Oral Surg Oral Med Oral Pathol 48:298, 1979.
Rothman KJ, Monson RR: Epidemiology of trigeminal neuralgia. J Chronic Dis 26:3, 1973.
Shaber EP, Krol AJ: Trigeminal neuralgia: a new treatment concept. Oral Surg Oral Med Oral Pathol 49:486, 1980.
Wepsic JC: Tic douloureux: etiology, refined treatment. N Engl J Med 288: 280, 1973.

Giant Cell Hyalin Angiopathy

Adkins KF: Granulomas in edentulous jaws. NZ Dent J 68:209, 1972.
Ciola B, Bahn SL, Yesner R: Radiographic changes associated with giant cell hyalin angiopathy. Oral Surg Oral Med Oral Pathol 55:108, 1983.
Dunlap CL, Barker BF: Giant cell hyalin angiopathy. Oral Surg Oral Med Oral Pathol 44:587, 1977.
El-Labban NC, Kramer RH: The nature of hyaline rings in chronic periostitis and other conditions: an ultra-structured study. Oral Surg Oral Med Oral Pathol 51:509, 1981.
McMillan MD, et al: Giant cell angiopathy or pulse granuloma. Oral Surg Oral Med Oral Pathol 52:178, 1981.
Mincer HH, McCoy JH, Turner JE: Pulse granuloma of the alveolar ridge. Oral Surg Oral Med Oral Pathol 48:126, 1979.

Primary Intraosseous Carcinoma of Jaws

Elzay RP: Primary intraosseous carcinoma of the jaws. Oral Surg Oral Med Oral Pathol 54:299, 1982.
McGowan RH: Primary intra-alveolar carcinoma: a difficult diagnosis. Br J Oral Surg 18:259, 1980.
Morrison R, Deeley TJ: Intra-alveolar carcinoma of the jaw: treatment by supervoltage radiotherapy. Br J Radiol 35:321, 1962.
Shear M: Primary intra-alveolar epidermoid carcinoma of the jaw. J Pathol 97:645, 1969.
Stoll HC, Marchetta FC, Schobinger R: Malignant epithelial tumors of the mandible and maxilla. Arch Pathol. 64:239, 1957.
Van Wyk CW, Padayachee A, Nortjé CJ, von der Heyden U: Primary intraosseous carcinoma involving the anterior mandible. Br J Oral Maxillofac Surg 25:427, 1987.

Gingival Carcinoma

Shafer WG, Hine MK, Levy BM: A Textbook of Oral Pathology. Philadelphia:WB Saunders, 1983, p. 124.

Central Mucoepidermoid Carcinoma

Alexander RW, Dupuis RH, Holton HH: Central mucoepidermoid of the mandible. J Oral Surg 33:541, 1974.
Bhaskar SN, Bernier JL: Mucoepidermoid tumors of major and minor salivary glands: clinical features, histology, variations, natural history and results of treatment for 144 cases. Cancer 15:801, 1962.
Bhaskar SN: Central mucoepidermoid tumors of the mandible. Cancer 12: 721, 1963.
Browand BC, Waldron CA: Central mucoepidermoid tumors of the jaws. Oral Surg Oral Med Oral Pathol 40:631, 1975.
Brown AM, Lucchesi FJ: Central mucoepidermoid tumor of the mandible: report of case. J Oral Surg 24:356, 1966.
Chaudry AF, Vickers RA, Gorlin RJ: Intraoral minor salivary gland tumors: an analysis of 1,414 cases. Oral Surg Oral Med Oral Pathol 14:1194, 1961.
Dhawan IK, Bhargava S, Nayah NC: Central salivary gland tumors of jaws. Cancer 26:211, 1970.
Eversole LR, Sabes WR, Robin S: Aggressive growth and neoplastic potential of odontogenic cysts. Cancer 35:270, 1975.
Foote FW, Frazell EL: Tumors of the major salivary glands. Cancer 6: 1065, 1953.
Fredrickson C, Cherrick HM: Central mucoepidermoid carcinoma of the jaws. J Oral Med 33:80, 1978.
Gingell JC, Beckerman T, Levy BA, Snider LA: Central mucoepidermoid carcinoma. Oral Surg Oral Med Oral Pathol 57:436, 1984.
Grubka JM, Wesley RK, Monaco F: Primary intraosseous mucoepidermoid carcinoma of the anterior part of the mandible. J Oral Maxillofac Surg 41:389, 1983.
Hertz J: Mucous secreting tumors of the jaws. Acta Chir Scand 103:276, 1952.
Linell F: Mucus-secreting and cystic epidermoid carcinomas of mucous and salivary glands. Acta Pathol Microbiol Scand 25:801, 1948.
Marano PD, Hartman KS: Central mucoepidermoid carcinoma arising in a maxillary odontogenic cyst. J Oral Surg 32:915, 1974.
Melrose RJ, Abram AA, Howell FV: Mucoepidermoid tumors of the intraoral minor salivary glands: a clinico-pathologic study of 54 cases. J Oral Pathol 2:314, 1973.
Schultz W, Whitten JB Jr: Mucoepidermoid carcinoma of the mandible. J Oral Surg 27:337, 1969.
Silverglade LB, Aluares OF, Oleche E: Central mucoepidermoid tumors of the jaws: review of the literature and case report. Cancer 22:650, 1968.
Smith AG, Broadbent TR, Zwaleta A: Tumors of oral mucous glands. Cancer 7:224, 1954.
Smith RL, Dahlin DC, Waite DC: Mucoepidermoid carcinoma of the jawbones. J Oral Surg 26:387, 1968.
Sonesson A: Intraosseous mucus-secreting and cystic epidermoid carcinoma of the jaw. Acta Radiol 34:25, 1950.
Stoch RB, Smith I: Mucoepidermoid carcinoma in the mandible: report of case. J Oral Surg 38:56, 1980.

Central Clear Cell Carcinoma

Corio RL, Sciubba JJ, Brannon RB, Batsakis JG: Epithelial-myoepithelial carcinoma of intercalated duct origin: a clinicopathologic and ultrastructural assessment of 16 cases. Oral Surg Oral Med Oral Pathol 53:280, 1982.
Shafer W, Hine MK, Levy B: A Textbook of Oral Pathology. 4th Ed. Philadelphia:WB Saunders, 1983, p. 251.

Odontogenic Ghost Cell Carcinoma

Ellis GL, Shmookler BM: Aggressive (malignant?) epithelial odontogenic ghost cell tumor. Oral Surg Oral Med Oral Pathol 61:471, 1986.
Gold L: The keratinizing and calcifying odontogenic cyst. Oral Surg Oral Med Oral Pathol 16:1414, 1963.
Gorlin RJ, Pindborg JJ, Clausen FP, Vickers RA: The calcifying odontogenic cyst: a possible analogue of the cutaneous calcifying epithelioma of Malherbe. Oral Surg Oral Med Oral Pathol 15:1235, 1962.

Grodjesk JE, et al: Odontogenic ghost cell carcinoma. Oral Surg Oral Med Oral Pathol 63:576, 1987.

Ikemura K, Horie A, Tashiro H, Nandate M: Simultaneous occurrence of a calcifying odontogenic cyst and its malignant transformation. Cancer 56:2861, 1985.

Pindborg JJ, Rick GM: Odontogenic tumors: classification and diagnostic problems: continuing education program. Am Acad Oral Pathol, 1983.

Praetorius F, Hjorting-Hansen E, Gorlin RJ, Vickers RA: Calcifying odontogenic cyst: range, variations, and neoplastic potential. Acta Odontol Scand 39:227, 1981.

Ameloblastic Carcinoma

Corio RL, Goldblatt LI, Edwards PA, Hartman KS: Ameloblastic carcinoma: a clinicopathologic study and assessment of eight cases. Oral Surg Oral Med Oral Pathol 64:570, 1987.

Shear M: Primary intra-alveolar epidermoid carcinoma of the jaw. J Pathol 97:645, 1969.

Slootweg PJ, Muller H: Malignant ameloblastoma or ameloblastic carcinoma. Oral Surg Oral Med Oral Pathol 57:168, 1984.

Metastatic Disease of the Jaws

Batson OV: The vertebral vein system. AJR 78:198, 1957.

Bhaskar SN: Synopsis of Oral Pathology. St. Louis:CV Mosby, 1973, p. 304.

Catalona WJ, et al: Measurement of prostate-specific antigen in serum as a screening test for prostate cancer. N Engl J Med 324(17):1156, 1991.

Cawson RA: Secondary carcinoma of the mandible. Dent Pract 9:240, 1959.

Ciola B, Yesner R: Radiographic manifestations of a lung carcinoma with metastases to the anterior maxilla. Oral Surg Oral Med Oral Pathol 44: 811, 1977.

Clausen F, Poulsen H: Metastatic carcinoma to the jaws. Acta Pathol Microbiol Scand 57:361 1963.

Galasko CSB: The pathological basis for skeletal scintigraphy. J Bone Joint Surg [Br] 57:353, 1975.

Gorlin RJ, Goldman HM: Thoma's Oral Pathology. Vol 1. St. Louis:CV Mosby, 1970, p. 573.

Lichtenstein L: Bone Tumors. St. Louis:CV Mosby, 1952, p. 281.

Meyer I, Shklar G: Malignant tumors metastatic to mouth and jaws. Oral Surg Oral Med Oral Pathol 20:350, 1965.

Mirra JM: Bone Tumors. Vol 2. Philadelphia:Lea & Febiger, 1989, pp. 1498, 1500.

Stern MH, Turner JE, Coburn TP: Oral involvement in neuroblastoma. J Am Dent Assoc 88:346, 1974.

Stypulkowska J, Bartkowski S, Panas M, Zalecka M: Metastatic tumors to the jaws and oral cavity. J Oral Surg 37:805:808, 1979.

von Recklinghausen RD: Fie Fibruse oder ceformirende Ostitis, die Osteomalacie und die osteoplastiche Carcinose in ihren gegenseitigen Beziehun. In: Festschrift Rudolf Virchow zu seinem, 71 Geburtstage gewidnet. Berlin, 1891, p. 1.

Worth HM: Principles and Practice of Oral Radiologic Interpretation. Chicago:Year Book Medical Publishers, 1963, p. 560.

Fibrosarcoma of Bone

Bertoni F, et al: Primary central (medullary) fibrosarcoma of bone. Semin Diagn Pathol 1:185, 1984.

Budd JW, MacDonald I: Osteogenic sarcoma: a modified nomenclature and review of 118 five-year cases. Surg Gynecol Obstet 77:413, 1943.

Dahlin CC: Bone Tumors: General Aspects and Data on 6,221 cases. 3rd Ed. Springfield, IL:Charles C Thomas, 1978, p. 315.

Dahlin DC, Ivins JC: Fibrosarcoma of bone: a study of 114 cases. Cancer 23:35, 1969.

Huvos AG, Higinbotham NL: Primary fibrosarcoma of bone: a clinicopathologic study of 130 patients. Cancer 35:837, 1975.

Larsson SE, Lorentzon R, Boquiest L: Fibrosarcoma of bone: a demographic, clinical and histopathological study of all cases recorded in the Swedish cancer registry from 1958 to 1968. J Bone Joint Surg [Br] 58-B:412, 1976.

McKenna RJ, Schwinn CP, Joong KY, Higinbotham NL: Sarcomata of the osteogenic series (osteosarcoma, fibrosarcoma, parosteal osteogenic sarcoma, and sarcomata arising from abnormal bone): an analysis of 552 cases. J Bone Joint Surg [Am] 48-A:1, 1966.

Mirra JM: Bone Tumors: Diagnosis and Treatment. Philadelphia:JB Lippincott, 1981, p. 276.

Phemister DB: Cancer of bone and joint. JAMA 136:545, 1948.

Pritchard DJ, et al: Fibrosarcoma of bone and soft tissues of the trunk and extremities. Orthop Clin North Am 8:869, 1977.

Schajowicz F: Tumors and tumor-like lesions of bones and joints. New York:Springer-Verlag, 1981, p. 342.

Slootweg PJ, Muller H: Fibrosarcoma of the jaws: a study of 7 cases. J Maxillofac Surg 12:157, 1984.

Stout AP: Fibrosarcoma: the malignant tumor of fibroblasts. Cancer 1:30, 1948.

Taconis WK, Van Rijssel TG: Fibrosarcoma of the jaws. Skeletal Radiol 15:10, 1986.

Van Blarcom CW, Masson JK, Dahlin DC: Fibrosarcoma of the mandible: a clinicopathologic study. Oral Surg Oral Med Oral Pathol 33:428, 1971.

Ewing's Sarcoma

Arafat A, Ellis GL, Adrian JC: Ewing's sarcoma of the jaws. Oral Surg Oral Med Oral Pathol 55:589, 1983.

Bacchini P, et al: Ewing's sarcoma of the mandible and maxilla. Oral Surg Oral Med Oral Pathol 6:278, 1986.

Bacci G, et al: The treatment of localized Ewing's sarcoma: the experience at the Instituto Orthopedico Rizzoli in 163 cases treated with and without adjuvant chemotherapy. Cancer 49:1561, 1982.

Brownson RJ, Cook RP: Ewing's sarcoma of the maxilla. Ann Otol Rhinol Laryngol 78:1299, 1969.

Bushnell D, Shiraz P, Khedkar N, Blank J: Ewing's sarcoma seen as a "cold" lesion on bone scans. Clin Nucl Med 8:173, 1983.

Campanacci M, Bacci G, Boriani S, Laus M: Ewing's sarcoma: a review of 195 cases. Ital J Orthop Traumatol 5:293, 1979.

Dahlin DC: Bone Tumors. 3rd Ed. Springfield, IL: Charles C Thomas, 1978, p. 227.

de Santos LA, Jing BS: Radiographic findings of Ewing's sarcoma of the jaws. Br J Radiol 51:609, 682, 1978.

Dickman PS, Liotta LA, Triche TJ: Ewing's sarcoma: characterization in established cultures and evidence of its histogenesis. Lab Invest 47: 375, 1982.

Ewing J: Diffuse endothelioma of bone. Proc NY Pathol Soc 21:17, 1921.

Falk S, Alpert M: The clinical and roentgen aspects of Ewing's sarcoma. Am J Med Sci 250:492, 1965.

Fordham EW, Ali A, Turner DA, Charters JR: Atlas of Total Body Radionuclide Imaging. Vol 1. Philadelphia:Harper and Row, 1982, p. 213.

Fraumeni JG, Glass AC: Rarity of Ewing's sarcoma among USA Negro children. Lancet 1:366, 1970.

Geschickter CF, Copeland M: Tumors of Bone. 3rd Ed. Philadelphia:JB Lippincott, 1949, p. 387.

Ginaldi S, de Santos LA: Computed tomography in the evaluation of small round tumors of bone. Radiology 134:441, 1980.

Greenfield GB: Radiology of Bone Diseases. 4th Ed. Philadelphia:JB Lippincott, 1986, p. 597.

Hardy P, Gibbs AR: Ewing's sarcoma of the mandible. Br J Oral Surg 22: 287, 1984.

Kissane JM, et al: Ewing's sarcoma of bone: clinicopathologic aspects of 303 cases from the intergroup Ewing's sarcoma study. Hum Pathol 14: 773, 1983.

McCormack LJ, Dockerty MB, Ghormley RK: Ewing's sarcoma. Cancer 5:85, 1952.

Miettinen Lehto UP, Virtanen I: Histogenesis of Ewing's sarcoma: an evaluation of intermediate filaments and endothelial cell markers. Virchows Arch [B] 41:277, 1982.

Mirra JM, Picci P, Gold RH: Bone Tumors: Clinical, Radiologic, and Pathologic Correlations. Vol. 2. Philadelphia:Lea & Febiger, 1989, p. 1089.

Navas-Palacios JJ, Aparicio-Duque R, Valdes MD: On the histogenesis of Ewing's sarcoma: an ultrastructural, immunohistochemical, and cytochemical study. Cancer 53:1882, 1984.

Neff JR: Nonmetastatic Ewing's sarcoma of bone: the role of surgical therapy. Clin Orthop 204:111, 1986.

Pomeroy TC, Johnson RE: Prognostic factors for survival in Ewing's sarcoma. AJR 123:598, 1975.

Resnick D, Niwayama G: Diagnosis of Bone and Joint Disorders. 2nd Ed. Vol 6. Philadelphia:WB Saunders, 1988, p. 3845.

Roca AN, Smith JL, McComb WS: Ewing's sarcoma of the maxilla and mandible. Oral Surg Oral Med Oral Pathol 25:194, 1968.

Roessner A, et al: Biologic characterization of human bone tumors: I. Ewing's sarcoma. A comparative electron and immunofluorescence microscopic study. J Cancer Res Clin Oncol 104:161, 1982.
Rosen G, et al: Ewing's sarcoma: ten year experience with adjuvant chemotherapy. Cancer 47:2204, 1981.
Salman I, Darlington G: Rare (unusual) malignant tumor of the jaws. Am J Orthod Oral Surg 30:725, 1944.
Schajowicz F: Tumors and Tumorlike Lesions of Bone and Joints. New York:Springer-Verlag, 1981, p. 244.
Som PM, Hermann G, Krespi Y, Shugar J: Ewing's sarcoma of the mandible. Am Otol Rhinol Laryngol 89:20, 1980.
Telles NC, Rabson AS, Pomeroy TC: Ewing's sarcoma: an autopsy study. Cancer 41:2321, 1978.
Turoff NB, Becker M, Lewis M: Ewing's sarcoma: unusual presentation delineated by computerized tomography. Report of a case. J Bone Joint Surg [Am] 60:1109, 1978.
Vanel D, et al: Computed tomography in the evaluation of 41 cases of Ewing's sarcoma. Skeletal Radiol 9:8, 1982.
Wang CC, Schulz MD: Ewing's sarcoma: a study of fifty cases treated at the Massachusetts General Hospital, 1930–1952 inclusive. N Engl J Med 248:571, 1953.
Weir JC, Amonett MR, Krolls SO: Tumorous conditions of the fibula, supraorbital area, and mandible. J Oral Pathol 8:313, 1979.
Wilkins R, Pritchard D, Burgert O, Unni K: Ewing's sarcoma of bone: experience with 140 patients. Cancer 58:2551, 1986.
Wilner D: Radiology of Bone Tumors and Allied Disorders. Vol. 3. Philadelphia:WB Saunders, 1982, p. 2467.
Wood RE, Nortje CJ, Hesseling P, Grotepac F: Ewing's tumor of the jaw. Oral Surg Oral Med Oral Pathol 69:120, 1990.

Histiocytosis X

Blevins C, et al: Oral and dental manifestations of histiocytosis X. Oral Surg Oral Med Oral Pathol 12:473, 1959.
Calve J: Localized affection of spine suggesting osteochondritis of vertebral body with clinical aspects of Pott's disease. J Bone Joint Surg [Am] 7: 41, 1925.
Capanna R, et al: Direct cortisone injection in eosinophilic granuloma of bone: a preliminary report on eleven patients. J Pediatr Orthop 5:339, 1985.
Christian HA: Defects in membranous bones, exophthalmos, and diabetes insipidus: an unusual feature of dyspituitarism. Med Clin North Am 3: 849, 1920.
Cohen M, et al: Direct injection of methylprednisolone sodium succinate in treatment of solitary eosinophilic granuloma of bone: a report of nine cases. Radiology 136:289, 1980.
Compere EL, Johnson WE, Conventry MD: Vertebra plana (Calve's disease) due to eosinophilic granuloma. J Bone Joint Surg [Am] 36A:969, 1954.
Farber SJ: The nature of "solitary or eosinophilic granuloma" of bone. Am J Pathol 17:625, 1941.
Green WT, Farber S: Eosinophilic or solitary granuloma of bone. J Bone Joint Surg [Am] 24:499, 1942.
Greenfield GB: Radiology of Bone Diseases. 4th Ed. Philadelphia:JB Lippincott, 1986, p. 501.
Hand A Jr: Polyuria and tuberculosis. Arch Pediatr 10:673, 1893.
Hartman KS: Histiocytosis X: a review of 114 cases with oral involvement. Oral Surg Oral Med Oral Pathol 49:38, 1980.
Ide F, et al: Immunohistochemical and ultrastructural analysis of the proliferating cells in histiocytosis X. Cancer 53:917, 1984.
Jennings CD, Stelling C, Powell D: Case report 199: eosinophilic granuloma of the right third metacarpal. Skeletal Radiol 8:229, 1982.
Jones John C, Lilly GE, Marlete RH: Histiocytosis X. J Oral Surg 28:461, 1970.
Keusch KD, Poole CA, King DR: The significance of "floating teeth" in children. Radiology 86:215, 1966.
Lahey M: Prognosis in reticulo-endotheliosis in children. J Pediatr 60:664, 1962.
Langerhans P: Veher die nerven der menschlichen Hant. Virchows Arch [A] 44:325, 1868.
Letterer E: Aleukamische retickulose (en Beitrag ze den proliferativen Erkvankungen des Retikuloendothellal-apparetes). Frank Zeit Pathol 30: 377, 1924.
Lichtenstein L: Histiocytosis X: integration of eosinophilic granuloma of bone: "Letterer-Siwe disease" and "Schüller-Christian disease" as related manifestations of a single nosologic entity. Arch Pathol Lab Med 56:84, 1953.
Mickelson MR, Bonfiglio M: Eosinophilic granuloma and its variations. Orthop Clin North Am 8:933, 1977.
Mirra JM: Bone Tumors. Vol 2. Philadelphia:Lea & Febiger, 1989, p. 1023.
Nakajima T, et al: An immunoperoxidase study of S-100 protein distribution in normal and neoplastic tissues. Am J Surg Pathol 6:715, 1928.
Resnick D, Niwayama AG: Diagnosis of Bone and Joint Disorders. 2nd Ed. Vol 4. Philadelphia:WB Saunders, 1988, p. 2431.
Rowden G, Connelly EM, Winklemann RK: Cutaneous histiocytosis X: the presence of S-100 protein and its use in diagnosis. Arch Dermatol 119:553, 1983.
Schajowicz F, Polak M: Contribucion al estudio del denominade "granuloma eosinofilico" y a sus reiaciones con la Xantomatosis osea. Rev Asoc Med Argent 61:218, 1947.
Schlesinger AE, Glass R, Young S, Fernbach S: Case report 342: eosinophilic granuloma of the right iliac wing. Skeletal Radiol 15:57, 1986.
Schüller A: Über eigenartige Schädeldefekte im Jugendalter. Fortschr Geb Rontgenstr 23:12, 1915.
Sedano HO, Cernea P, Hasxe G, Gorlin RJ: Histiocytosis X. Oral Surg Oral Med Oral Pathol 27:760, 1969.
Siwe S: Dieretikuloendotheliose-ein nues Krankheitsbild unter den Hepatosplenogeglien. Z Kinderheilkd 55:212, 1933.
Sleeper EI: Eosinophilic granuloma of bone: its relationship to Hand-Schüller-Christian and Letterer-Siwe's diseases with emphasis upon oral symptoms and findings. Oral Surg Oral Med Oral Pathol 4:896, 1951.
Thomas JS, et al: Combined immunological and histiochemical analysis of skin and lymph node lesions in histiocytosis X. J Clin Pathol 35:327, 1982.

Multiple Myeloma

Bhaskar SN: Synopsis of Oral Pathology. St. Louis:CV Mosby, 1975, p. 407.
Bruce KW, Royer RQ: Multiple myeloma occurring in the jaws: a study of 17 cases. Oral Surg Oral Med Oral Pathol 6:729, 1953.
Carson CP, Ackerman LV, Maltby JD: Plasma cell myeloma: a clinical, pathologic and roentgenologic review of 90 cases. Am J Clin Pathol 25:849, 1955.
Cataldo E, Meyer I: Solitary and multiple cell tumor of the jaws and oral cavity. Oral Surg Oral Med Oral Pathol 22:628, 1966.
Clamp JR: Some aspects of the first recorded case of multiple myeloma. Lancet 2:1354, 1967.
Daffmer RH, et al: MRI in the detection of malignant infiltration of bone marrow. AJR 146:353, 1986.
Dahlin DC: Myeloma in Bone Tumors. 3rd Ed. Springfield, IL: Charles C Thomas, 1978, p. 160.
Durie BGM, Salmon SE, Mundy GR: Relation of osteoclast activating factor production to extent of bone disease in multiple myeloma. Br J Haematol 47:21, 1981.
Epstein JB, Voss NJS, Stevenson-Moore P: Maxillofacial manifestations of multiple myeloma. Oral Surg 57:267, March 1984.
Goodman MA: Plasma cell tumors. Clin Orthop 204:86, 1986.
Grabar P, Williams CA: Méthode permettant l' étude contiguée des propriétés électrophorétiques et immunochimiques d'un mélange de protéınes: application au sérum sanguin. Biochim Biophys Acta 10:193, 1953.
Hewell GM, Alexanian R: Multiple myeloma in young person. Ann Intern Med 84:441, 1976.
Isobe T, Osserman EF: Pathologic conditions with plasma cell dyscrasias: a study of 806 cases. Ann NY Acad Sci 190:507, 1971.
Jagger RG, Helkimo M, Carlsson GE: Multiple myeloma involving the temporomandibular joint. J Oral Surg 35:557, 1978.
Kyle RA: Multiple myeloma: review of 869 cases. Mayo Clin Proc 50:29, 1975.
Lambertenghi-Deliliers G, et al: Incidence of jaw lesions in 193 patients with multiple myeloma. Oral Surg Oral Med Oral Pathol 65:533, 1988.
Lewin RW, Cataldo E: Multiple myeloma discovered from oral manifestations: report of a case. J Oral Surg 25:68, 1967.
Longsworth LG, Shedlovsky T, MacInnes DA: Electrophoretic patterns of normal and pathological human blood serum and plasma. J Exp Med 70:399, 1939.

Miller CD, Goltry RR, Shenaslky JH: Multiple myeloma involving the mandible. Oral Surg Oral Med Oral Pathol 28:603, 1969.
Mirra JM: Bone Tumors. Vol 2. Philadelphia:Lea & Febiger, 1989, p. 1123.
Mundy GR, et al: Evidence for the secretion of an osteoclast stimulating factor in myeloma. N Engl J Med 291:1041, 1974.
Osserman EF: Plasma Cell Dyscrasias. In: Beeson PB, McDermott W, Wyngaarden JB, eds. Cecils' Textbook of Medicine. 15th Ed. Philadelphia:WB Saunders, 1979, p. 1852.
Price HI, Danirger A, Wainwright HC, Batnitzky S: CT of orbital multiple myeloma. Am J Neuroradiol 1:573, 1980.
Ramon Y, et al: A large mandibular tumor with a distinct radiological ''sunray effect'' as the primary manifestation of multiple myeloma. J Oral Surg 36:52, 1978.
Smith DB: Multiple myeloma involving the jaws. Oral Surg 10:910, 1957.
Spitzer R, Price LW: Solitary myeloma of the mandible. Br Med J 1:1027, 1948.
Stafne EC: Oral Roentgenographic Diagnosis. Philadelphia:WB Saunders, 1958, p. 207.
Van Antwerp JD, O'Mara RE, Pitt MJ, Walsh S: Technetium-99m diphosphonate accumulation in amyloid. J Nucl Med 16:238, 1975.
Worth HM: Principles and Practice of Oral Radiologic Interpretation. Chicago:Year Book Medical Publishers, 1969, p. 582.

Non-Hodgkin's Lymphoma

Carbone PP: Introduction to lymphoreticular neoplasms. In Beeson PB, McDermott W, Wyngaarden JB, eds. Cecil Textbook of Medicine. 15th Ed. Philadelphia:WB Saunders, 1979, p. 1829.
Choukas NC: Lymphosarcoma of the maxilla. Oral Surg Oral Med Oral Pathol 23:567, 1967.
Coles WC, Schulz MD: Bone involvement in malignant lymphoma. Radiology 50:458, 1948.
Ewing J: Endothelioma of lymph nodes. J.M. Research 28, 1913.
Gould J, Main J: Primary lymphosarcoma of the maxillary alveolar processor. Oral Surg Oral Med Oral Pathol 28:106, 1969.
Greenfield WS: Specimens illustrating the pathology of lymphosarcoma and leukocythaemia. Tr Path Soc London 29:272, 1978.
Herberg E, Wolverson MK, Sundaran M, Shields JB: CT findings in leukemia. AJR 143:1317, 1984.
Holtas SL, Kido DK, Simon JH: MR imaging of spinal lymphoma. J Comput Assist Tomogr 10:111, 1986.
Kundrat H: Vebor Lymphosardo-matosic. Wien Klin Wochenschr 6:211, 1893.
Lee JKT, et al: Magnetic resonance imaging of abdominal and pelvic lymphadenopathy. Radiology 153:181, 1984.
Molander DW, Pack GT: Lymphosarcoma: choice of treatment and end-results in 567 patients. Rev Surg 20:3, Jan-Feb, 1963.
Rappaport H: Tumors of the hematopoietic system. In: Atlas of Tumor Pathology, section III, fascicle VIII. Washington, DC:Armed Forces Institute of Pathology, 1966.
Reed DM: On the pathologic changes in Hodgkin's disease with special reference to its relation to tuberculosis. Johns Hopkins Rep 10:133, 1902.
Resnick D, Niwayama G: Diagnosis of Bone and Joint Disorders. 2nd Ed. Vol 4. Philadelphia:WB Saunders, 1988, p. 2472.
Rollins FG, Thoma KH: Lymphosarcoma of the mandible. Oral Surg Oral Med Oral Pathol 19:350, 1957.
Sippel W, Samartano J: Leukemia manifested as lymphosarcoma of the mandible: report of case. J Oral Surg 29:363, 1971.
Sternberg C: Ueber eine Eigenärtige unter dem Bilde der Pseudoleukamie varlaufende Tuberculose des lymphatischen Apparates. Ztschr Heilk 19:21, 1898.
Van Slyck EJ: The bony changes in malignant hematologic disease. Orthop Clin North Am 3:733, 1972.
Vieta JO, Friedell HL, Craver LF: A survey of Hodgkin's disease and lymphosarcoma in bone. Radiology 39:1, 1942.
Virchow R: Die krankhoften Geschwulste. Vol 1. Berlin:A Hirschivald, 1863.

Primary Non-Hodgkin's Histiocytic Lymphoma of Bone

Boston HC, Dahlin DC, Ivins JC, Cupps RE: Cancer 34:1131, 1974.
Coley BL, Higinbotham NL, Groesbeck AP: Primary reticulum cell sarcoma of bone. Radiology 55:641, 1950.
Dahlin DC: Bone Tumors: General Aspects and Data on 6,221 Cases. 3rd Ed. Springfield, IL: Charles C Thomas, 1978, p. 174.
Francis KC, Higinbotham NL, Coley OL: Primary reticulum cell sarcoma of bone. Gynecol Obstet 99:142, 1954.
Fripp AT, Sissons HA: A case of reticulosarcoma (reticulum-cell sarcoma) of bone. Br J Surg 42:103, 1954.
Gerry RC, Williams SF: Primary reticulum cell sarcoma of the mandible. Oral Surg Oral Med Oral Pathol 8:568, 1955.
McCormack CJ, Ivins JC, Dahlin DC, Johnson EW Jr: Primary reticulum cell sarcoma of bone. Cancer 5:1182, 1952.
Parker F Jr, Jackson H Jr: Primary reticulum cell sarcoma of bone. Surg Gynecol Obstet 68:45, 1939.

Burkitt's Lymphoma

Abasa NA, Iczkovitz ML, Henefer EP: American Burkitt's lymphoma manifested in a solitary lymph node. Oral Surg Oral Med Oral Pathol 51: 121, 1981.
Adatia AK: Burkitt's tumor in the jaws. Br Dent J 120:315, 1966a.
Adatia AK: Radiology of Burkitt's tumor of the jaws. East Afr Med J 43: 290, 1966b.
Alling CC, Jackson RW, Martinez MC, Toman DE: Burkitt's lymphoma. J Oral Surg 31:463, 1973.
Areneau JC, et al: American Burkitt's lymphoma: a clinico-pathologic study of 30 cases. I. Clinical factors relating to prolonged survival. Am J Med 62:283, 1975.
Beenson PB, McDermott W: Textbook of Medicine. 14th Ed. Philadelphia: WB Saunders, 1975, p. 1507.
Bhaskar SN: Synopsis of Oral Pathology. 4th Ed. St. Louis:Mosby, 1973, p. 301.
Burkitt D: A sarcoma involving the jaws in African children. Br J Surg 46:218, 1958.
Burkitt D: A tumor safari in east and central Africa. Br J Cancer 16:379, 1962.
Cockshott WP: Radiological aspects of Burkitt's tumor. Br J Radiol 38: 172, 1965.
Dean AG, et al: Aetiology of Burkitt's lymphoma. Lancet 2:1225, 1973.
Fowles JV, et al: Burkitt's lymphoma in the appendicular skeleton. J Bone Joint Surg [Br] 65:464, 1983.
Kramer IRH: Malignant lymphoma of children in Africa. Int J Dent 15: 200, 1965.
Levine PH, Cho BR: Burkitt's lymphoma: clinical features of American cases. Cancer Res 34:1219, 1974.
Levine PH, et al: The American Burkitt Lymphoma Registry: a progress report. Ann Intern Med 83:31, 1975.
O'Connor GT: Persistent immunologic stimulation as a factor in oncogenesis with special reference to Burkitt's tumor. Am J Med 46:279, 1970.
Parker BR, Marglin S, Castellino RA: Skeletal manifestations of leukemia, Hodgkin's disease and non-Hodgkin's lymphoma. Semin Roentgenol 15:302, 1980.
Srivastava AB, Pant GC, Kaur KJ, Gupta S: Burkitt's lymphoma. J Ind Dent Assoc 48:77, 1976.
Surveillance Epidemiology and End Results incidence and mortality data, 1973–1977. NCI Monogr no. 57, NIH publ. no. 81–2330, 1981.
Wright DH: Burkitt's tumor: a post-mortem study of 50 cases. Br J Surg 51:245, 1964.
Ziegler JC: Burkitt's lymphoma. N Engl J Med 305:735, 1981.
Ziegler JL, Magrath IT, Gerber P, Levine PH: Epstein-Barr virus and human malignancy. Ann Intern Med 86:323, 1977.
Ziegler JL, Magrath IT, Olweny CLM: Cure of Burkitt's lymphoma. Lancet 2:2:936, 1979.

Hodgkin's Disease

Appell RG, Opperman HC, Brandeis WE: Skeletal lesions in Hodgkin's disease: review of literature and case reports. Pediatr Radiol 11:61, 1981.
Coles WC, Schulz M: Bone involvement in malignant lymphoma. Radiology 50:458, 1948.
Craver LF, Copeland MM: Lymphosarcoma in bone. Arch Surg 28:809, 1934.
Dresser R, Spencer J: AJR 36:809, 1936.
Forman GH, Wesson CM: Hodgkin's disease of the mandible. Br J Oral Surg 7:146, 1970.

Geschickter CF, Copeland MM: Tumors of Bone. 3rd Ed. Philadelphia:JB Lippincott, 1949, p. 538.
Granger W, Whitaker R: Hodgkin's disease in bone, with special reference to periosteal reaction. Br J Radiol 40:939, 1967.
Horan F: Bone involvement in Hodgkin's disease: a survey of 201 cases. Br J Surg 56:277, 1969.
Jackson H Jr, Parker F Jr: Hodgkin's Disease and Allied Disorders. New York:Oxford University Press, 1947, p. 25.
Kaplan HS: Hodgkin's Disease. 2nd Ed. Cambridge, MA:Harvard University Press, 1980, p. 1.
Lukes RJ, Butler JJ, Hicks EB: The natural history of Hodgkin's disease as related to its pathologic picture. Cancer 19:317, 1966a.
Lukes RJ, et al: Hodgkin's disease and report of nomenclature committee. Cancer Res 26:1311, 1966b.
Mayer D, Smalley RV: Hodgkin's disease and non-Hodgkin's lymphoma. In: Rose LF, Kaye D, eds. Internal Medicine for Dentistry. St. Louis: CV Mosby, 1983, p. 387.
Mirra JM: Bone Tumors. Vol 2. Philadelphia:Lea & Febiger, 1989, p. 1174.
Mussholf K: Prognostic and therapeutic implications of staging an extranodal Hodgkin's disease. Cancer Res 31:1814, 1971.
O'Carroll D, McKenna R, Brunning R: Bone marrow manifestations of Hodgkin's disease. Cancer 38:1717, 1976.
Parker BR, Marglin S, Castellino RA: Skeletal manifestations of leukemia, Hodgkin's disease and non-Hodgkin's lymphoma. Semin Roentgenol 15:302, 1980.
Patchefsky AS, et al: Hodgkin's disease: a clinical and pathologic study of 235 cases. Cancer 32:150, 1973.
Reed DM: On the pathologic changes in Hodgkin's disease with special reference to its relation to tuberculosis. Johns Hopkins Rep 10:133, 1903.
Steiner PE: Hodgkin's disease. Arch Pathol Lab Med 36:627, 1943.
Sternberg C: Ueber eine Eigerärtige unter dem Bilde der Pseudoleukamie varlaufende Tuberculose des lymphatischen Apparates. Ztschr Heilk 19:21, 1898.
Vieta JO, Friedell HL, Craver LF: A survey of Hodgkin's disease and lymphosarcoma in bone. Radiology 39:1, 1942.
Wilks S: Cases of lardaceous disease and some allied affections, with remarks. Guy's Hosp Rep 17(ser 11, vol. 2):103, 1856.

Leukemia

Becker MH, Engler GL, Klein M: Case report 93. Skeletal Radiol 4:111, 1979.
Bender IB: Bone changes in leukemia. Am J Orthod Surg 30:556, 1944.
Benz G, Brandeis WE, Willich E: Radiologic aspects of leukemia in childhood: an analysis of 89 children. Pediatr Radiol 31:201, 1976.
Brownstein EM, Hammond B, Schutzer B: Bone destruction in myelogenous marrow crisis. J Can Assoc Radiol 31:69, 1980.
Curtis AB: Childhood leukemias: osseous changes in jaws on panoramic dental radiographs. J Am Dent Assoc 83:844, 1971.
Epstein BS: Vertebral changes in childhood leukemia. Radiology 68:65, 1957.
Greenfield GB: Radiology of Bone Diseases. 4th Ed. Philadelphia:JB Lippincott, 1986, p. 491.
Lynch MA, Ship II: Initial oral manifestations of leukemia. J Am Dent Assoc 75:932, 1967.
Melhem RE, Saber TJ: Erosion of the medial cortex of the proximal humerus: a sign of leukemia on the chest film. Radiology 137:77, Oct 1980.
Nixon GW, Gwinn JL: The roentgen manifestations of leukemia in infancy. Radiology 107:603, 1973.
Parker BR, Marglin S, Castellino RA: Skeletal manifestations of leukemia, Hodgkin's disease and non-Hodgkin lymphoma. Semin Roentgenol 15: 302, 1980.
Peterson DE, Gerad H, Williams LT: An unusual instance of leukemic infiltrate. Cancer 51:1716, 1983.
Redmond J III, et al: Chronic lymphocytic leukemia with osteolytic bone lesions, hypercalcemia, and monoclonal protein. Am J Clin Pathol 79: 616, 1983.
Resnick D, Niwayama G: Diagnosis of Bone and Joint Disorders. 2nd Ed. Philadelphia:WB Saunders, 1988, p. 2461.
Schabel SI, Tyminski L, Holland RD, Rittenberg GM: The skeletal manifestations of chronic myelogenous leukemia. Skeletal Radiol 5:145, 1980.
Silverman FN: The skeletal lesions of leukemia: clinical and roentgenographic observations in 103 infants and children with review of the literature. AJR 59:519, 1948.
Simmons CR, Harle TS, Singleton EB: The osseous manifestation of leukemia in children. Radiol Clin North Am 6:115, 1968.
Stafford R, Sonis S, Lockhart P, Sonis A: Oral pathoses as diagnostic indicators in leukemia. Oral Surg Oral Med Oral Pathol 50:134, 1980.
Sullivan MP: Intracranial complications of leukemia in children. Pediatrics 209:757, 1957.
Thomas LB, et al: The skeletal lesions of acute leukemia. Cancer 14:608, 1961.
Van Slyck EJ: The bony changes in malignant hematologic diseases. Orthop Clin North Am 3:733, 1972.
Williams SA, Duggan MB, Varley CC: Jaw involvement in acute lymphoblastic leukemia. Br Dent J 155:164, 1983.
Wilson JKV: The bone lesions of childhood leukemia. Radiology 72:672, 1959.
Worth HM: Principles and Practice of Oral Radiologic Interpretation. Chicago:Year Book Medical Publishers, 1963, p. 370.

Chapter 15

Generalized Rarefactions

NORMAL BONE DENSITY

Bone density is maintained by a variety of interdependent metabolic mechanisms referred to as normal bone homeostasis. When an imbalance in homeostasis occurs, bone density may be affected in a generalized manner and may be increased or decreased. The following is a brief summary of the mechanisms involved in normal bone homeostasis:

Calcium is the primary mineral component of bone, with 99% of the supply being concentrated in bone. Serum calcium occurs in two primary forms: ionic and protein bound. Protein-bound calcium is pH dependent and decreases with acidosis. The protein consists primarily of albumin. Ionized calcium is more significant because parathormone responds to the level of ionized calcium in serum, not to the total serum calcium level. Approximately 3% of serum calcium is found in citrate and phosphate complexes. Calcium absorption varies with intake; thus, if intake is low, absorption is relatively higher. The converse is true if intake is high. Calcium is absorbed from the gastrointestinal tract by binding to a protein secreted by the mucosa of the small intestine and is controlled by vitamin D. Urinary excretion of calcium is directly proportional to dietary intake.

Phosphorus is absorbed by active transport across the intestinal wall and requires sodium. The serum phosphate level is controlled by a variety of factors that affect phosphate excretion. For example, phosphate excretion is decreased by vitamin D, glucocorticoids, and growth hormone; it is increased by parathormone and estrogens. Normally, 85 to 95% of the phosphorus is reabsorbed by the renal tubules, and a decrease in total reabsorption by the renal tubules is diagnostic of hyperparathyroidism. The serum phosphate level has no effect on the secretion of parathormone or thyrocalcitonin.

Vitamin D is necessary for the absorption of calcium because it is required for the synthesis of calcium binding protein by the mucosa of the small intestine. Vitamin D levels depend on dietary intake, stored as inert precursors. Sunlight activates the inert precursor (7-dehydrocholesterol) stored in the skin, and conversion occurs in the liver by hydroxylation to the metabolically active form (dihydroxyvitamin D_3). Vitamin D is necessary for parathormone to act on bone and stimulates osteoclastic resorption, thus liberating calcium from bone to serum.

Parathormone responds to low serum levels of calcium by causing a release of calcium from bone. There is controversy as to whether this occurs entirely by the action of osteoclasts or whether osteocytes themselves can exert an osteolytic action on bone mineral. Parathormone has a direct effect on the kidneys by stimulating tubular reabsorption of phosphorus.

Calcitonin, a polypeptide produced by the parafollicular cells of the thyroid gland, was discovered relatively recently. It inhibits bone resorption and has been effective in treating Paget's disease. Calcitonin causes persistence of bone sclerosis after parathyroid gland removal and may be responsible for the osteosclerosis seen in renal osteodystrophy.

Thyroid hormone has a general effect on metabolism and affects bone when its function is altered. Hyperthyroidism increases the release of calcium from bone, resulting in osteoid seams. Hypothyroidism diminishes bone modeling and decreases bone blood flow.

Growth hormone is produced in the anterior pituitary gland and stimulates bone formation, causing an increase in normal trabecular and cortical bone formation, resulting in an increase of skeletal mass. Thyroid hormone plays a permissive role in the action of growth hormone. For example, thyroid deficiency in childhood results in metabolic dwarfism.

Gonadal hormones, principally the androgens and estrogens, are responsible for epiphyseal closure. Thus, excessive gonadal hormones early in the adolescent growth spurt may result in stunting of growth, whereas inadequate production may result ultimately in a disproportionate growth of the long bones and small genitalia typical of eunuchoidism. In adults, the androgens, estrogens, and synthetic steroids depress bone resorption without influencing bone formation.

Adrenocortical steroids increase bone resorption and decrease bone formation.

Table 15–1 shows a classification whereby altered homeostasis of bone produces various diseases, all of which are characterized by rarefaction of bone at some stage. Although the problems are systemic or metabolic, some disorders target certain bones or even specific parts of a bone more than others. If the condition occurs during childhood, the teeth may be affected.

Table 15–2 shows the serum values for the key markers of these metabolic disorders.

Alkaline phosphatase levels are increased whenever bone turnover occurs; thus, they are elevated in most of these metabolic disorders. Exceptionally high values are seen in untreated Paget's disease during the active phases of the disease. All of the conditions listed in the table are described in this text, but not necessarily in this chapter.

◆ *RADIOLOGY*

The clear image of the jaws on the radiograph attests to their normalcy. On the panoramic radiograph, cortical bone is visualized especially well along the inferior border of the mandible, at the angle, at the posterior margin of the ramus, and on the head of the condyle.

TABLE 15–1
Generalized Rarefactions

A. Too little bone formation
   1. Too little formation of organic matrix (osteoid): osteoporosis
   2. Too little calcification of matrix: rickets (childhood), hypophosphatemia (childhood), osteomalacia (adults)

B. Too much bone resorption
   1. Too much resorption of matrix and mineral: hyperparathyroidism
   2. Paget's disease

TABLE 15–3
Thickness of Mandibular Angular Cortex (millimeters)

Age Intervals (years)	Men		Women	
	Mean	SD	Mean	SD
15–19	1.52	0.19	1.64	0.30
20–29	1.66	0.21	1.51	0.16
30–39	1.55	0.18	1.64	0.27
40–49	1.45	0.26	1.52	0.25
50–59	1.60	0.32	1.51	0.38
60–69	1.46	0.24	0.84	0.26

SD: Standard deviation.

(Adapted from Bras J, et al: Radiologic interpretation of the mandibular angular cortex: a diagnostic tool in metabolic bone loss. Part I. Normal state and postmenopausal osteoporosis. Oral Surg Oral Med Oral Pathol 53:544, 1982.)

Bras and colleagues (1982) observed that, after the fifteenth year, the thickness of the cortex at the mandible angle remains fairly constant, except in postmenopausal women 60 years of age and older, in whom the cortex is distinctly thinner. Their results are shown in Table 15–3.

Cortical bone cannot be seen well at the anterior margin of the ramus and in the maxilla and is minimal along the alveolar crest. In cross-sectional tomographic views and computed tomography images, the buccal and lingual cortical plates are well visualized. Generally speaking, the mandibular cortex may be three to four times thicker than in the maxilla. Cortex also may be studied in the walls of the sinuses, hard palate, walls of the nasal fossa, and orbital rims. The inner and outer tables of the skull are usually well imaged in a variety of views. In the normal state, the lamina dura is intact and well visualized. In the jaws, the trabecular pattern as imaged on periapical radiographs does not represent the loose spongy trabeculae of bone between the cortical plates and within the marrow space. Rather, the trabecular pattern represents the the buccal and lingual cortices. Thus, rarefactions of bone trabeculae within the marrow spaces cannot be detected on periapical radiographs. If there has been a 30% demineralization of the cortex, a change can be seen. When the demineralization is localized, the resulting radiolucent area is seen easily; however, when the demineralization is generalized, a much greater degree of rarefaction might be necessary for such to become apparent, or it might be necessary to use a previous radiograph to make a comparison. In addition, the trabecular pattern normally does not line up along particular lines of stress or in any particular pattern. It is described as loose when there are relatively fewer trabeculae and larger marrow spaces and dense when there are many trabeculae and smaller marrow spaces, which are all variations of normal.

When the teeth are lost, the alveolar bone in the edentulous area seems to become more radiolucent. This may be a relative change because the absence of teeth and lamina dura will contribute to the more radiolucent appearance of the remaining alveolar bone, without any real change in the bone itself. A frequently observed phenomenon, however, is the tendency of alveolar bone to resorb when teeth are lost, especially all of the natural teeth. This process is irreversible and is accelerated when the natural dentition in one arch opposes a complete denture in the opposite arch. Also, bone mass varies from one person to another; thus, radiographic exposure factors must be adjusted to achieve an ideal density, with sufficient contrast such that soft tissue outlines may be seen as well as good bony detail.

TABLE 15–2
Serum Values for Markers of Metabolic Disorders

Disorder	Calcium	Phosphorus	Alkaline Phosphatase
Osteoporosis	Normal	Normal	Normal
Rickets	Low	Low	High
Hypophosphatemia	Normal	Low	High
Osteomalacia	Low	Low	High
Hypophosphatasia	Normal	Normal	Low
Hyperparathyroidism			
Primary	High	Low	High
Secondary	Normal/low	High	High
Tertiary	High	Normal/high	High
Paget's disease	Normal	Normal	High

OSTEOPOROSIS

Osteoporosis is caused by a deficiency of organic bone matrix; however, there is normal mineralization of the remaining bone. This condition is one of the most common disorders affecting middle-aged and older women.

Pathologic Characteristics

According to Garn (1970), normal bone mass increases as a person progresses from infancy to 30 to 40 years of age and then decreases continuously at a rate of 8% per decade in women and 3% in men. This bone loss is particularly evident in the cortex and continues until a person dies. Fifty percent of men exhibit cortical bone osteoporosis by age 80; among women, 50% show cortical bone loss by age 70 and 100% by age 90. Trabecular bone is affected earlier than cortical bone, and the vertebral column is the prime site of involvement. In people 55 years of age and older and in advanced cases, the situation is reversed and cortical bone is affected more significantly. Riggs and colleagues (1981a). reported that women begin to lose vertebral bone within the third to fourth decades of life; according to Nordin (1983), the rate of bone loss is accelerated at menopause. There is a substantial loss in both sexes at middle age, but a new equilibrium is established at approximately 60 years of age, after which there is very little loss in the normal population.

A physiologic classification of osteoporosis has been suggested by Shapiro (1962) and appears in Table 15–4.

Clinical Features

Primary osteoporosis refers to a condition that is not associated with any of the diseases known to cause an osteoporotic state. No known causal condition has been established. Primary osteoporosis may be simple or accelerated. Simple primary osteoporosis occurs in men and women. At a 1984 Consensus Conference on osteoporosis, the condition was found to be more common in women. Additionally, Lachman (1955) reported that white women of Northern European ethnicity have a much higher incidence than those of Mediterranean descent. Lane and Vigorita (1983) and Farmer and co-workers (1984) found that black women rarely have osteoporosis. They also stated that osteoporosis is more common in women with the following characteristics: slender build, fair complexion, freckles, blonde hair, hypermobility of joints, and scoliosis. In women osteoporosis results from increased bone resorption that is associated with menopause. During menopause, there is diminished production of estrogens, which tend to protect the skeleton against the resorbing action of parathyroid hormone (PTH). Stevenson and colleagues (1981) and Slovik and co-workers (1981) pointed out that PTH levels increase with advancing age, whereas calcitonin levels and 1,25-dihydroxy-vitamin D production decrease; all these factors favor the development of osteoporosis. In men primary osteoporosis may develop from diminished androgen production. Mazzuoli and colleagues (1982) have shown that PTH levels increase in aging men, yet urinary excretion of calcium decreased with age. It is presumed that there is an increased tubular resorption of ionic calcium resulting from mild secondary hyperparathyroidism. This calcium-saving mechanism is missing in women. Accelerated primary osteoporosis is caused principally by calcium malabsorption. Various theories have been reviewed by Slovik and colleagues (1981) and Riggs and associates (1981b). A deficiency of 1,25-dihydroxy-vitamin D_3 secondary to functional depression of the renal enzyme 1a-hydroxylase has been proposed, or it may result from an end organ failure in the gastrointestinal tract. Affrim (1964) suggested that alcoholics are more susceptible to osteoporosis. Other factors include: cigarette smoking, gastrointestinal surgery, diabetes, low calcium intake, excessive protein consumption, family history of osteoporosis, small muscle mass, early menopause or oophorectomy, and liver disease. Regardless of the cause, osteoporosis results in an increase of fractures in the axial skeleton and possibly accelerated tooth loss and alveolar ridge resorption.

TABLE 15–4
Physiologic Classification of Osteoporosis Suggested by Shapiro

I. Defect in osteoblasts
   A. Congenital: osteogenesis imperfecta
   B. Lack of stress and strain: disuse atrophy
   C. Deficient estrogen: primary ovarian agenesis, postmenopausal osteoporosis

II. Defects in the matrix
   A. Deficient androgen: eunuchoidism, senile state in men
   B. Deficient protein: malnutrition—scurvy, anorexia nervosa; hyperthyroidism; uncontrolled diabetes; Cushing's syndrome; prolonged stress

III. Excessive utilization of calcium

(From Shapiro R: Metabolic bone disease: a basic review. Clin Radiol 13:238, 1962.)

Treatment/Prognosis

Heaney (1982) stated that the loss of bone mass resulting from osteoporosis generally is considered irreversible. Thus, prevention is preferred over treatment. Once the disease is present, supplying factors such as calcium and estrogen may be counterproductive, and here lies the controversy. As explained by Heaney (1983), calcium and estrogens stabilize bone mass by reducing remodeling. Thus, they not only impede additional bone loss, but also reversal and actual bone gain. Heaney (1983) recommended a preventive regimen for the young patient, consisting of a high calcium intake within the recommended daily allowance of 800 mg/day, regular and vigorous exercise, and avoidance of excess protein, alcohol, caffeine, and smoking. For the perimenopausal woman, loss should be prevented as much as possible. This is accomplished best by a high calcium intake of approximately 1.0 g/day or more. In the postmenopausal years, calcium intake should be increased to 1.5 g/day if no estrogens are used. Estrogens may be prescribed in a dose of 0.625 mg of conjugated equine estrogens given cyclically. Mechanical loading of the skeleton should be accomplished at as high a level as possible during all stages.

◆ RADIOLOGY (Figs. 15–1 to 15–3)

Radiologic Features

The radiology of osteoporosis is divided into two categories: (1) methods of measuring and quantifying bone mass, and (2) morphologic changes in the radiologic image of the bones. Then these findings usually are added to the results of other studies directed toward finding endocrine dysfunction, calcium imbalance, malabsorption, liver and renal dysfunction, and abnormalities in marrow status, usually by transiliac bone biopsy.

Assessment of Bone Mass by Morphometric Measurement

As reviewed by Benson (1986), there are many methods used to evaluate osteoporosis for which some aspect of radiology is used. A common morphologic method is the Singh index to evaluate the femoral head, where hip fractures commonly occur. Singh (1970) divided osteoporosis into seven grades, with grade 7 being normal. The grading system is based on the loss of parallel groups of trabeculae that line up in specific directions. Other simple noninvasive methods are termed radiomorphometric measurements, such as the Garn (1970) metacarpal or Benson (1986) mandibular indices. Other more complex methods include radiographic photodositometry, single-photon absorptiometry, dual-energy photon absorptiometry, local neutron activation of calcium, radionucleotide uptake, Compton scattering, computed tomography, and ultrasonics. Gordan and colleagues (1981) recommended morphometric measurement of cortical thickness or photon absorptiometry. In the latter method, the bone to be measured, usually a second metacarpal or radius, is placed over a radioactive isotope source, usually ^{125}I. A scintillation counter above the bone records the number of photons that pass through the bone: the higher the count, the less dense the bone. This technique is simple, safe, and reliable. Because it is highly automated, results are interpreted easily.

The most common macromorphometric method involves the Garn (1970) index of measuring the metacarpals. This method has been studied by Garn (1970), Garn and colleagues (1971), and Aloia and co-workers (1977). This technique uses a radiograph of the hand and is summarized as follows:

1. Selecting the second metacarpal (index finger) of the nondominant hand.
2. Obtaining calipers that measure to 0.1 mm.
3. Measuring at the midshaft.
4. Measuring the total diameter of the bone (T) at the subperiosteal surface.
5. Measuring the diameter of the medullary space (M) at the endosteal surface.
6. Determining the cortical area (CA) by using the following formula: $CA = 0.785\ (T^2 - M^2)$
7. Determining the percent cortical area (PCA) by using the following formula:

$$PCA = \frac{(T^2 M^2)}{T^2}\ 100$$

If a person is observed from year to year, the CAs are compared with previous values for that person. If the patient is compared with a similar population, the PCA is used to correct for differences in metacarpal size among people in a given population. Garn (1970) established normal values for various ages. His table (Table 15–5) uses the PCA for age 30 because this represents the time of maximum or near-

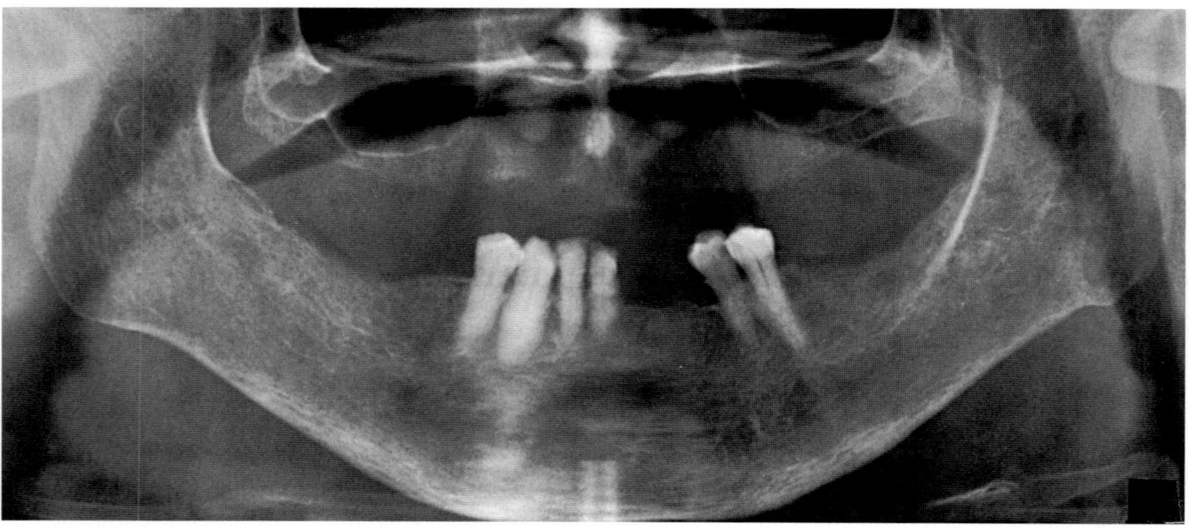

FIGURE 15–1.

Osteoporosis: Case in a 63-year-old white woman of British descent. Figure shows thinning of cortex at inferior border of mandible. The cortex is very thin at the angle. There are cortical lamellations with endosteal detachment. The alveolar bone is denser (darker) than normal, although the teeth are exposed correctly; trabeculae are fewer in number, coarser, and of reduced density (less radiopaque).

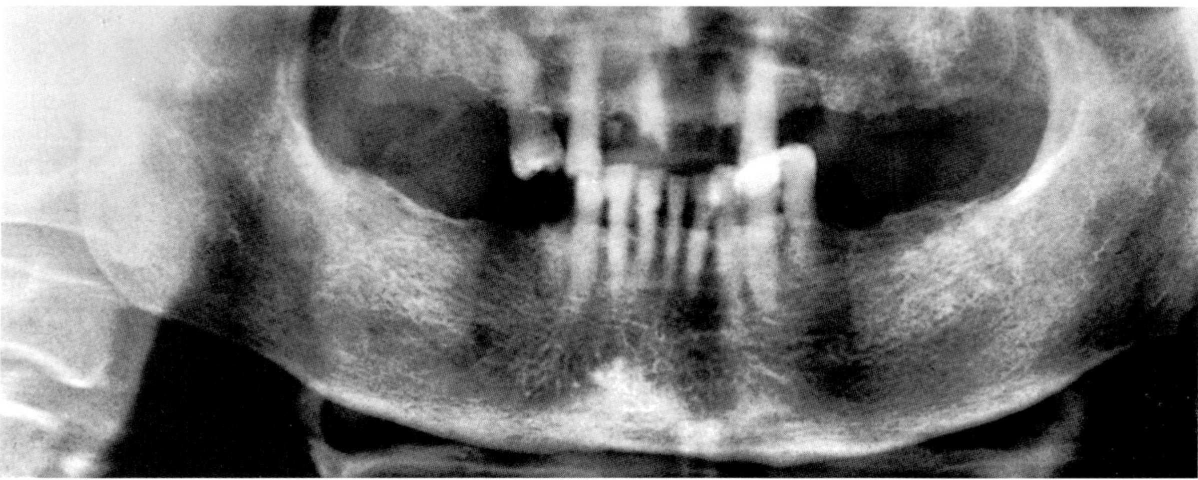

FIGURE 15–2.

Osteoporosis: Case in a 77-year-old woman of Mexican descent. The cortex is thinned and there are cortical lamellations with endosteal detachment. The trabecular pattern is coarser and denser. The figure is suggestive of a V-shaped deformity between the vertebrae and biconcave disks at the right angle of the mandible.

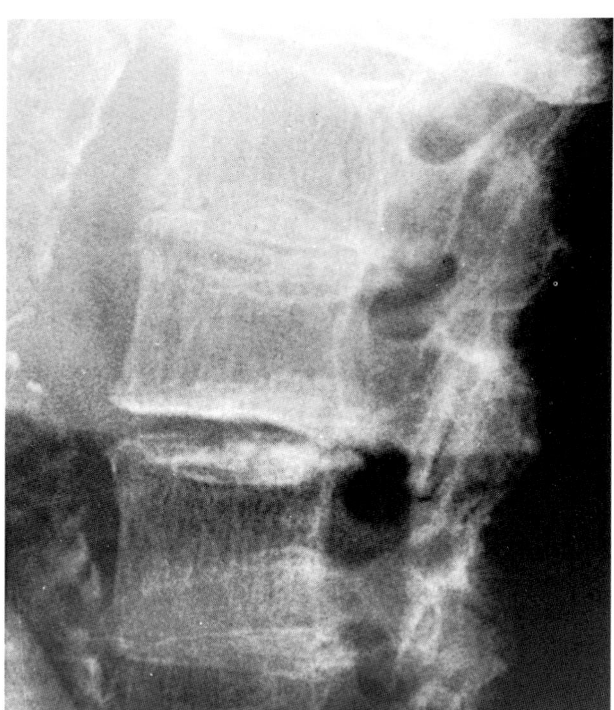

FIGURE 15–3.

Osteoporosis: Figure shows classic appearance in vertebral column: loss of horizontal trabeculae; thicker, more prominent vertical trabeculae; and more radiolucent vertebral body. The posterior vertebral plate is coarser, with an irregular endosteal surface. The intervertebral plates have become biconcave because of mass effect. There is a wedge-shaped deformity of the disk, as can be seen by the V-shape of the intervertebral space; in several places there is complete loss of the intervertebral space. (Courtesy of Dr. R. Cone, San Antonio, TX.)

maximum PCA. Statistically, osteoporosis is defined as a value for PCA plus or minus two standard deviations from the normal value.

Cortical bone loss in the mandible has been documented in a variety of macromorphometric studies, primarily by Bras and colleagues (1982a, 1982b) and Wovern and Stoltze (1979a, 1979b). These studies correlated well with measurements of the second metacarpal. Bones were measured in the area of the mental foramen or the cortical thickness at point gonion at the angle of the mandible. Benson (1986) developed the panoramic mandibular index or Benson index. The cortical bone along the inferior aspect of the mandible at the mental foramen was measured as a ratio of the cortical width to the distance between the inferior exosseous mandibular surface and the inferior border of the mental foramen. He found that the right side and inferior border of the mental foramen were more statistically representative and expedient than combinations using the left side or superior border of the mental foramen. He established normative values for

TABLE 15–5
Percent Cortical Area (PCA) in Patients Who Are 30 Years of Age

	Men		Women	
Subjects	**Mean PCA**	**SD**	**Mean PCA**	**SD**
United States (White people from Ohio)	86.1	4.4	89.1	5.7
United States (Texas-Mexican)	86.1	7.3	88.8	5.9

SD: Standard deviation.

(From Garn SM, Poznanski AK, Nagy JM: Bone measurement in the differential diagnosis of osteopenia and osteoporosis. Diagn Radiol 100:509, 1971.)

men and women between the ages of 30 and 79 years in three designated ethnic groups: Texas-black, Texas-Hispanic, and Texas-white. These useful normative values may be found in Benson's (1986) thesis.

Morphologic Changes

As reviewed by Benson (1986), bone is assessed for osteoporotic change by the following factors:

1. Degree of photographic blackening of the images on the radiograph.
2. Morphologic signs: thinning of cortex, diminished contrast between cortex and cancellous bone, rarefaction of the trabecular pattern, and lamellations in the cortex.
3. Manifestations of structural failure: wedge deformities of the vertebrae, biconcave disks, and fractures.

Radiology of the Jaws

Investigators such as Groen and colleagues (1968) and Krook and co-workers (1972) found that periodontal disease might result secondarily from disruption of the periodontal anatomy and physiology caused by a loss of bone mass. Worth (1963) observed that changes in the lamina dura might be the only osseous abnormality in the entire skeleton in early cases of osteoporosis because the film can be brought closer to teeth with minimal soft tissue intervening. This author also stated that, after tooth removal, the trabeculae become fewer and those that remain appear less dense than normal. Also, osteoporosis has been related to a more rapid resorption of the residual ridge, bone fracture during tooth removal, delayed healing after tooth removal, and referred dental pain from the thinned walls of the antrum, presumably when there are conditions such as maxillary sinusitis producing increased antral pressure.

Cortical changes are characteristic in osteoporotic bone but are seen only in advanced cases. Edeiken (1981) stated that an osteoporotic bone may have a thinned cortex, but, in many instances, the remaining cortex is of normal density. The endosteal surface of the cortex may appear irregular or lamellated because osteoporotic resorption occurs at the endosteal surface. Lamellations consist of horizontal lines of diminished density entirely within the cortex or as cortical remnants next to the endosteal surface. The most obvious appearance of osteoporosis in the jaws is seen in advanced cases, when the patient is edentulous. The cortex along the inferior border of the mandible is thinned or lamellated, and the alveolar bone is darker, as if the radiograph were overexposed. Bras and colleagues (1982a) suggested that the cortical thickness at the angle may be the most sensitive region for measurement. The medullary spaces may become enlarged and the remaining trabeculae appear coarser and fewer or they may become finer and less opacified. If teeth remain, periodontal disease may be present.

Vertebral Changes

The vertebrae contain very little cortical bone, thus osteoporotic changes often are observed first in this area, most certainly before those in the jaws. Vertebral changes are studied best in the lateral view. In extraoral radiographs such as the lateral cephalometric view, the cervical vertebrae are seen. One of the most important signs of osteoporosis in the axial skeleton is the loss of horizontal trabeculae in the vertebrae. The vertical trabeculae appear fewer in number and more pronounced, and the remainder of the vertebral body seems more radiolucent. The vertebral plates at the distal surface of the vertebrae may become thinned, with increased density and an irregular endosteal surface. As a result of compression, the disk between the vertebrae may become wedge shaped or biconcave, causing the intervertebral plates to appear concave.

Fractures

As reviewed by Garraway and colleagues (1979), age-related fractures are one of the most severe and debilitating consequences of osteoporosis. They found that 33% of women and 17% of men may experience fracture of the femoral neck by the time they are 90 years of age. The next most frequent fracture in this age group was a collar fracture, occurring at the lower end of the radius in 24% of women and 5% of men. Other fracture sites include the proximal humerus and pelvis. Melton and Riggs (1983) found that 21% of 70-year-old Danish women had compression fractures in the vertebrae. Jaw fractures may occur in association with tooth removal.

RICKETS/OSTEOMALACIA (Vitamin D-resistant rickets, hypophosphatemia, hypophosphatasia)

Rickets occurs in children and osteomalacia in adults; otherwise, the two conditions are closely related and may represent a continuum in some instances. Osteomalacia refers to bone softening. Both terms refer to any disorder in the vitamin D-phosphorus-calcium axis resulting in hypomineralized bone matrix. Other terms have been used; however, these are reserved for specific cases in which a certain etiologic factor further defines the cause. In all instances, there is delayed or inadequate calcification of bone matrix or osteoid.

Pathologic Characteristics

In rickets, the chondro-osseous complex or linear growth apparatus is affected. Instead of the normal orderly arrangement of cartilaginous growth-plate cells, there is a disorganized increase in unmineralized masses of cartilage cells. In osteomalacia, the problem arises after closure of the epiphyseal plates; thus, the amount of bone matrix in this region is normal but poorly calcified. Osteomalacia represents a disorder of lamellar bone (i.e., mature bone formation). This bone replaces the primary woven bone developing during initial bone formation; only lamellar bone is produced during adulthood. Thus, rickets and osteomalacia may co-exist during childhood and adolescence; however, in adulthood, the condition always is referred to as osteomalacia. During the nineteenth century, rickets and osteomalacia were found to be caused by a deficiency of vitamin D in childhood or adulthood. In parts of the world where nutritional deficiencies are prone to occur or strict vegetarianism is practiced, vitamin D deficiency is still the most common cause; however, in the Western world, inborn or acquired derangements of vitamin D and phosphate metabolism now are the most frequent cause.

Clinical Features

The classification shown in Table 15–6 was modified from the study of Arnstein and colleagues (1967). Although this table indicates that there are many conditions in which rickets/osteomalacia may develop, in most instances the condition results from one of two broad groups of circumstances: In the first there is insufficient entry of calcium or phosphate from the gastrointestinal tract, whereas in the second there is excessive loss of calcium or phosphate as a result of renal disease. The first group may consist of a dietary lack of calcium or vitamin D, a deficiency of endogenous vitamin D synthesis, or a lack of exposure to sufficient sunlight. In this instance, serum calcium and phosphorus levels often are low. The second group includes renal rickets, vitamin D-resistant rickets, de Toni-Franconi syndrome, and renal tubular acidosis. In this instance, hypophosphatemia (thus, the origin of the term) and elevated alkaline phosphatase levels occur; however, serum calcium levels are normal. Most of these conditions are resistant to vitamin D therapy. According to Jaworski (1972), the clinical manifestations of osteomalacia include three overlapping orders of change: (1) those of the primary disease (usually intestinal or renal) that cause vitamin D deficiency or hypophosphatemia (vitamin D-resistant rickets) and are the two main factors producing bone disease; (2) the manifestations of hypocalcemia or hypophosphatemia; and (3) the manifestations of the bone disease proper.

TABLE 15–6
Clinical Forms of Osteomalacia

I. Primary vitamin D deficiency—rickets/osteomalacia
II. Gastrointestinal malabsorption
   A. Partial gastrectomy
   B. Small intestinal disease
      1. Gluten-sensitive enteropathy
      2. Regional enteritis
   C. Hepatobiliary disease
      1. Chronic biliary obstruction
      2. Biliary cirrhosis
   D. Pancreatic disease: chronic pancreatitis
III. Primary hypophosphatemia; vitamin D–resistant rickets
IV. Renal disease
   A. Chronic renal insufficiency
   B. Renal tubular disorders
      1. Renal tubular acidosis
   C. Multiple renal defects
V. Hypophosphatasia; rickets and pseudohypophosphatasia in association with low alkaline phosphatase levels
VI. Fibrogenesis imperfecta osseum
VII. Axial osteomalacia
VIII. Miscellaneous diseases/problems
   A. Hypoparathyroidism
   B. Hyperparathyroidism
   C. Thyrotoxicosis
   D. Osteoporosis
   E. Paget's disease of bone
   F. Fluoride ingestion
   G. Ureterosismoidoscopy
   H. Neurofibromatosis
   I. Osteopetrosis
   J. Macroglobulinemia
   K. Malignancy

(Modified from Arnstein AR, Frame B, Frost HM: Recent progress in osteomalacia and rickets. Ann Intern Med 67:1296, 1967.)

◆ *RADIOLOGY (Figs. 15–4 to 15–6)*

The radiologic features of osteomalacia vary with age, anatomic location, and specific variants, depending on the cause and degree of advancement of the disease. The three main categories will be discussed separately.

Radiologic Features of Rickets

Many of the changes in this disease occur at the epiphysis, especially those undergoing the greatest degree of growth. These changes may be observed in hand-wrist radiographs used by oral surgeons, orthodontists, and pediatric dentists to assess skeletal age. According to Edeiken (1981), the normal epiphysis consists of four zones, proceeding from the epiphyseal ossification center toward the shaft: (1) the zone of resting cartilage, (2) the zone of proliferating cartilage, (3) the zone of maturing cartilage, and (4) the zone of degenerating cartilage.

The later zone of preparatory calcification appears as a radiodense transverse line where osteoblast and blood vessel invasion takes place, laying down osteoid on the calcified

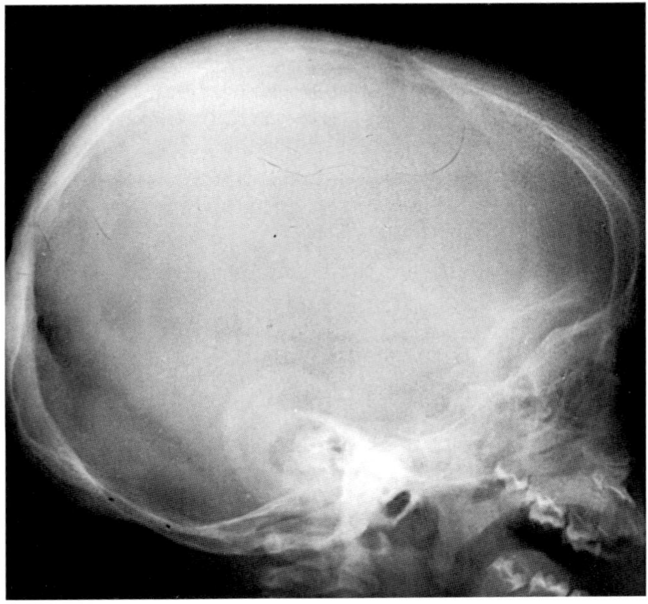

FIGURE 15–4.

Rickets: Case in a 3-year-old boy shows thinning of cranial tables and a bland appearance of the vault, lacking suture lines.

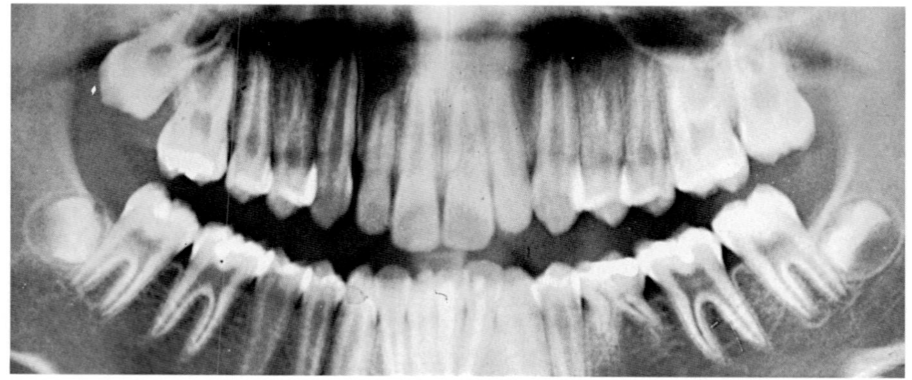

FIGURE 15–5.

Hypophosphatemia (Vitamin D-Resistant Rickets): Figure shows enlarged pulp chambers with nearly parallel root canal walls. (Courtesy of Dr. S. Matteson, University of Texas Dental School, San Antonio, TX, and Dr. J. Burkes, North Carolina School of Dentistry, Chapel Hill, NC.)

cartilage bridge. In rickets there is continued production of cartilage cells with little or no calcification, thus producing irregular widening of the epiphyseal plate, which tends to be radiolucent because of the lack of calcification. The epiphyseal line is irregular, and a zone of preparatory ossification does not form. The epiphysis appears widened, moth-eaten, and irregularly calcified, with thin, wispy, perpendicular trabeculae of bone extending into the epiphyseal area. The weight-bearing bones become bowed as a result of softening. Although greenstick fractures do occur in rare instances, the pseudofractures described by Milkman (1930) and later termed as Milkman's syndrome are pathognomonic of rickets and osteomalacia. Because of bone softening, the circumflex arteries create a depression in the surface resembling an incompletely calcified fracture callus. These lesions tend to be symmetrically bilateral. During healing, the changes are reversed. The zone of temporary calcification is the first to calcify. Temporary centers of ossification begin to appear, with progression to normal healing. Permanent bone deformities may remain.

According to Worth (1963), changes in the jaws are seen rarely. On such occasions, the tendency is toward deossification. The trabeculae are diminished in number and density and are narrower. In severe cases, no trabecular bone is seen and the teeth appear to be suspended in air. The cortex may be thinned or absent. This is not surprising because the trabeculae in jaw radiographs are cortical in origin. The cortical outlines of the inferior alveolar canal, antrum, and nasal fossa may be lost. In addition, the lamina dura and crypt walls of unerupted teeth may be lost. In some instances, enamel hypoplasia may occur, especially when the condition occurs in children between the ages of 3 months and 3 years, when the enamel is forming. Dentin dysplasia also may be seen. Eruption often is delayed, and this may be associated with deficient cementum formation. The pulp chambers appear to be normal in size.

Craniotabes is the descriptive term for the "square-head" appearance of the skull in patients with rickets; otherwise, the vault appears normal. When treatment is initiated, areas of bone thickening may be seen at the eminences of the frontal, parietal, and occipital bones during the healing phase.

Radiologic Features of Hypophosphatemia (Vitamin D-Resistant Rickets, Hypophosphatemic Osteomalacia)

Overall, the radiologic changes associated with hypophosphatemia are similar to those of rickets, except healing is difficult because the condition does not respond to therapeutic doses of vitamin D. Also, the condition persists into

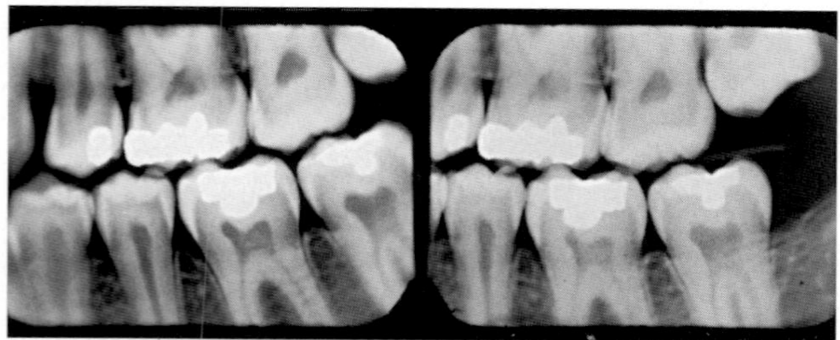

A

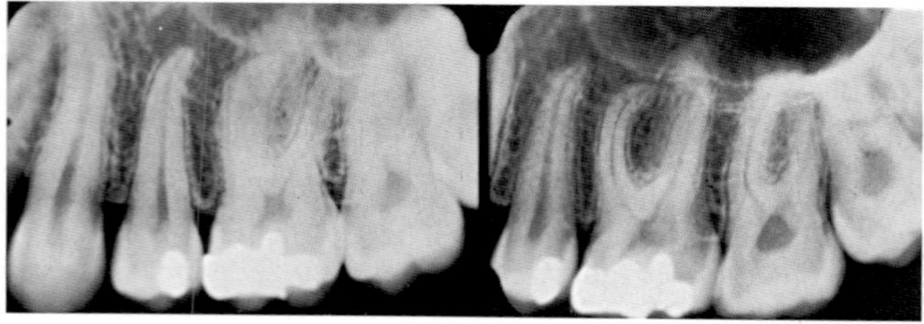

B

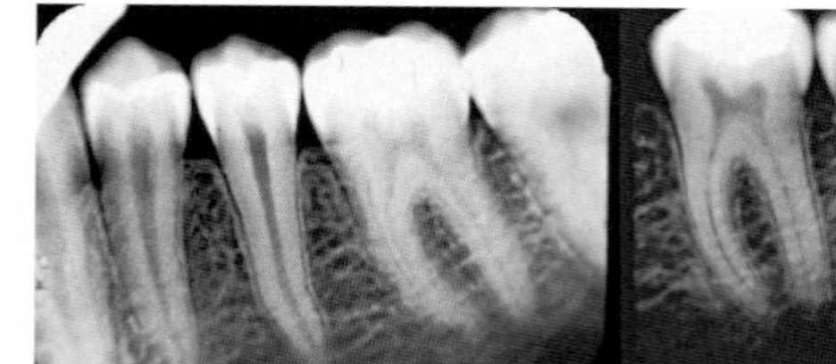

C

FIGURE 15–6.

Hypophosphatemia (Vitamin D-Resistant Rickets): A, B, and C, Large pulp chambers and root canal spaces with abnormally opaque dentinal walls, causing dentin immediately beneath enamel to appear relatively more radiolucent. This appearance results from intensive vitamin D therapy. (Courtesy of Dr. S. Matteson, University of Texas School of Dentistry, San Antonio, TX.)

adulthood, at which time it is known as hypophosphatemic osteomalacia. The dental changes are similar to those of rickets, with the following additional signs: abnormally large pulp chambers of the primary and permanent teeth, spontaneous periapical abscess formation without the presence of caries, and delayed closure of the apices of newly erupted teeth. The pulp chambers and root canal space become enlarged at the expense of dentin. Classically, the walls of the enlarged pulp and root canal spaces are nearly parallel; in other instances, the pulp chambers may appear normal. Although the dentin often looks normal, two abnormalities have been observed: Gibilisco (1985) stated that the dentinal walls of the pulp chambers become abnormally radiopaque after intensive vitamin D therapy, and Worth (1963) described a step effect at the apex of primary teeth, where the pulpal margin of dentin appears intact and the outside margin is resorbed. The cause of the idiopathic periapical rarefying osteitis is unknown, but it may result from the abnormally large pulp horns that, with minimal occlusal wear, result in pathologic pulp exposure, pulpitis, and periapical infection. Enamel hypoplasia also may be seen in many instances. Because the condition is hereditary, effects often occur before the patient is 3 years of age, when the enamel is forming.

Radiologic Features of Osteomalacia

Osteomalacia may occur with no radiologic changes. When changes occur, they may be nonspecific and usually are characterized by some form of deossification. The changes resemble those of osteoporosis and some of the findings in rickets. The deossification usually is generalized, with a loss of cortex and trabecular detail. Deossification may cause multiple compression fractures of the vertebrae, disappearance of trabeculation, and thinning of the cortex. In the phalanges, there is deossification of the cortex and spongiosum but no evidence of the lacelike subperiosteal bone resorption that occurs in hyperparathyroidism. Pseudofractures are present; they tend to be bilaterally symmetric and occur at right angles to the bone margin. They may extend all the way across the diameter of the bone or only part way into it.

Jaw changes are often minimal, and the teeth are not affected. When changes are seen, they are caused by deossification producing the following trabecular changes: a diminished number, diminished density, and narrowing. In more serious cases, no trabeculae may be seen, with the teeth apparently floating in air. Osteoporotic changes also may be found in the cortex. Worth (1963) reported a case of a 32-year-old woman with gross skeletal changes, who had a generalized loss of the lamina dura in the jaws and a pseudofracture through the mandible just anterior to the angle. In such pseudofractures, it is important to realize that, although there is a dark line across the bone simulating a fracture, there is no loss of bone continuity. Pseudofractures are seen most often in the pelvis and long bones and are rare in the jaws.

HYPOPHOSPHATASIA

The term hypophosphatasia was coined by Rathbun in 1948 in the first description of this inborn error in metabolism resulting in lowered levels of alkaline phosphatase. The first report in the dental literature was published in 1962 by Bruckner and colleagues. Fraser (1957) estimated a prevalence of 1/100,000 live births.

Pathologic Characteristics

The condition is hereditary and transmitted by an autosomal recessive gene. Occasionally it is transmitted by the autosomal dominant mode. Because the condition usually arises within the first 6 months of life, manifestations are present during childhood and resemble those of rickets. The symptoms include anorexia, irritability, persistent vomiting, low-grade fever, and failure to thrive. Hypophosphatasia sometimes may be associated with delayed manifestations that arise only during later childhood and sometimes during adulthood. As age of onset increases, the severity of symptoms decreases.

Clinical Features

Baer and colleagues (1964) reported that patients with hypophosphatasia have been divided into three groups, based on the age at which the condition first manifests: Group 1: infants in whom lesions were present at birth or within the first 6 months of life; Group 2: children and adolescents in whom lesions gradually became apparent after the age of 6 months; and Group 3: patients in whom hypophosphatasia first was diagnosed during the patient's adult life. The radiologic features of hypophosphatasia result from the continued proliferation of osteoid and cartilaginous tissue that does not calcify. This failure of calcification occurs in association with low levels of alkaline phosphatase. Also, increased levels of phosphorylethanolamine are found in the urine. When the condition arises during the first 6 months of life, the long bones and ribs are affected similarly to the manner in which they are affected in rickets, although in many instances the changes are less severe. If the condition occurs during childhood, club feet and genu valgum (knock knees) are the main features. The long bones may show a lack of remodeling, with the Erlenmyeyer flask deformity of the femur, in which the femoral neck appears abnormally wide.

Treatment/Prognosis

There is no treatment for hypophosphatasia. Spontaneous remission of the childhood form usually occurs. In adults, magnesium therapy may increase alkaline phosphatase levels.

◆ *RADIOLOGY (Fig. 15–7)*

Radiologic Features of the Jaws

In the jaws, the changes are similar to those of hypophosphatemia. The jaws appear osteoporotic. The trabeculae appear wispy, fewer in number, and somewhat elongated in some areas and completely absent in other regions. The cortical bone may be thinned or absent, and there may be varying degrees of loss of the lamina dura and crypt wall of developing teeth. According to Worth (1963), the most striking dental abnormality is premature loss of the primary teeth. Fung

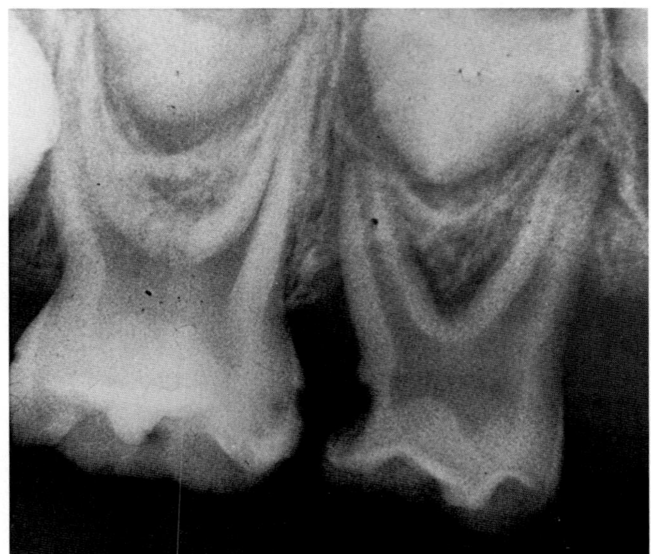
A

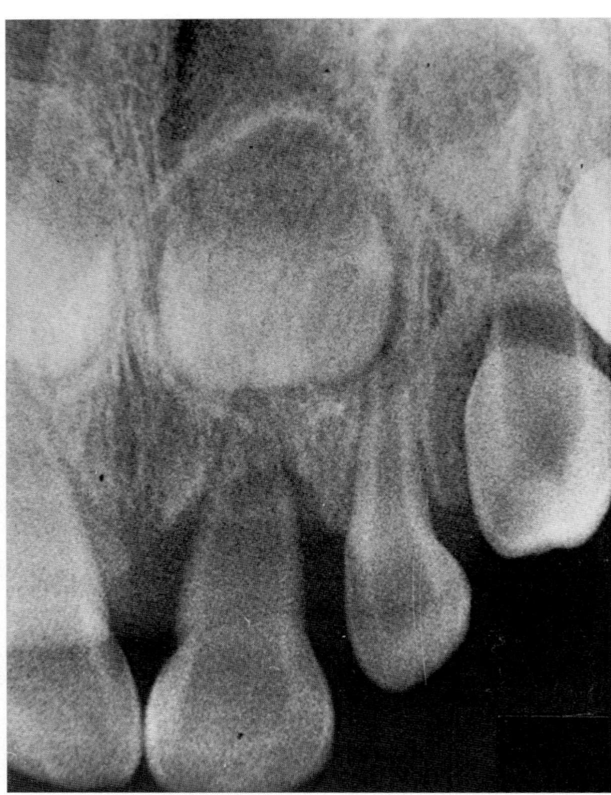
B

FIGURE 15–7.

Hypophosphatasia: Case in a 3 1/2-year-old child. A and B, Large pulps and almost parallel pulp walls. The primary central incisor is being exfoliated without root resorption, and the lamina dura is absent in many areas. The crypt walls of developing teeth appear poorly mineralized but slightly thicker and more diffuse. (From Beumer J, Trowbridge HO, Silverman S Jr, Eisenberg E: Childhood hypophosphatasia and premature loss of teeth: a clinical and laboratory study of 7 cases. Oral Surg Oral Med Oral Pathol 35:631, 1973.)

(1983) stated that premature exfoliation of the primary teeth occurs with little sign of root resorption, and more than 75% of childhood cases show this initial finding. The primary teeth may appear supraerupted or extruded. According to Beumer and colleagues (1973), almost all instances of premature exfoliation of primary teeth involved the anterior teeth, although this may occur in the posterior region. Fung (1983) also emphasized the importance of recognizing the absence of severe gingival inflammation, which helps to differentiate this condition clinically from Papillon-Lefebre syndrome. Deficient or cupped-out alveolar crests have been observed by Kjellman and associates (1973), Worth (1963), and others. This occurs after premature loss of the primary teeth and seems to be limited mainly to the anterior region. The primary teeth sometimes may be hypoplastic, with shortened roots resulting from failure to develop or from premature resorption; however, some root length usually remains when the teeth are exfoliated.

Beumer and colleagues (1973) found absent and poorly calcified cementum in the exfoliated primary teeth. They attributed the premature exfoliation to this cemental defect. The primary and permanent teeth may have abnormally large pulp chambers and root canal spaces. Fung (1983) stated that the primary teeth resemble "shell teeth." The pulp chambers appear to have parallel walls, perhaps less so than in hypophosphatemia. In many instances, the primary teeth all have been shed by the time a child is 3 years of age and, as reported by Dixon and Harrocks (1958), the eruption of the permanent dentition may be delayed. Enamel hypoplasia also may be present if the disease develops before a child is 3 years of age.

Radiologic Features of the Skull

Changes in the skull are characteristic and may show one of several appearances as described by Poyton (1982): (1) overall osteoporosis of the calvarium, with small, diffuse areas of normal density; (2) many intersecting curved lines of normal density in an osteoporotic skull, giving the appearance of "beaten copper"; (3) islands of normal bone density separated by wide bands of increased radiolucency; these resemble widened sutures but are actually zones of osteoid that merely have this appearance; and (4) premature closure of sutures, which may result in changes in skull shape such as dolichocephaly.

HYPERPARATHYROIDISM

Hyperparathyroidism first was described as a bone disease in 1891 by von Recklinghausen. In 1904, Askanazy was the first to describe a patient with a parathyroid tumor and osteitis fibrosa cystica; however, he made no correlation between the two conditions. Hyperparathyroidism now is a common disease. Jackson and Frame (1972) estimated that 1 in 1000 patients examined in a general diagnostic clinic will have hyperparathyroidism.

Pathologic Characteristics

Hyperparathyroidism occurs in three clinical forms: primary, secondary, and tertiary. In all instances, the disease is characterized by an increase in PTH levels and mobilization of calcium from bone. Primary hyperparathyroidism results from primary parathyroid hyperplasia, a benign parathyroid adenoma, or parathyroid carcinoma. Parathyroid adenomas in conjunction with the multiple mucosal neuroma syndrome of Sipple have been discussed by Sarosi and Doe (1968). Classically, increased production of PTH causes an increase in serum calcium levels by decreasing renal tubular reabsorption of phosphorus. Alkaline phosphatase levels are increased and serum phosphorus values are decreased. Bartter (1973) has found that 50% of patients with mild disease are normocalcemic.

Secondary hyperparathyroidism is a compensatory mechanism resulting from a primary condition producing hypocalcemia, such as rickets, osteomalacia, pregnancy, chronic renal insufficiency, calcium deprivation, or maternal hypoparathyroidism. Hypocalcemia prompts increased PTH production, with the liberation of calcium from bone. In association with the hypocalcemia, there is an increase in serum phosphorus and alkaline phosphatase levels. At times, the calcium level may approach low normal values; thus, multiple serum tests may be required or urinary calcium levels may be elevated even in patients on a low calcium diet.

In rare cases, tertiary hyperparathyroidism may occur after longstanding secondary hyperparathyroidism. It is characterized by the development of a functional parathyroid adenoma that causes excessive production of PTH; liberation of calcium from bone, producing hypercalcemia and elevated alkaline phosphatase levels. Increased serum phosphorus values may persist from the secondary hyperparathyroidism; however, increased levels of serum calcium bring the elevated levels of serum phosphorus down to normal in some cases. One of the most common causes of tertiary hyperparathyroidism is chronic renal failure, even if the patient is on dialysis. In 1985, Hutton reported that approximately 72,000 people in the United States were undergoing dialysis for end-stage renal disease.

Clinical Features

The clinical findings of hyperparathyroidism have been described by Jackson and Frame (1972) as the tetrad of "bones, stones, abdominal groans, and psychic moans with fatigue overtones," which is now classic. In their review of the literature, Terezhalmy and colleagues (1978) found that this condition occurs most commonly in women, with a peak incidence between the ages of 40 and 50 years. The most common sequel of the disease is renal calcification. The stones ultimately may cause renal damage and uremia. Hypercalcemia also may cause central nervous system manifestations ranging from mild personality problems to severe psychiatric disorders. Gastrointestinal disturbances may be associated with nausea, vomiting, anorexia, pancreatitis, and duodenal and peptic ulcers. Sometimes muscle weakness, hypotonia, and generalized achy tenderness may be the only symptoms. Hypercalcemia also may result in band keratopathy, a peculiar form of calcification occurring as a narrow band at the limbic margin of the cornea of the eye. Only the interpalpebral area is affected on the right and left sides of the cornea. The bone changes result in the liberation of calcium. The changes are generalized and will be described in the radiology section.

Treatment/Prognosis

Primary hyperparathyroidism usually is caused by a parathyroid adenoma; thus, surgical removal is the treatment of choice. Soon after surgery, symptoms of tetany develop, with a sensation of numbness and tingling in the fingers and lips. Tetany responds well to calcium gluconate or calcium lactate therapy, with vitamin D as an adjunct. With the return of normal serum calcium values, the brown tumors in the skeleton regress spontaneously and the appearance of the bone returns to normal. Pellegrino (1977) reported that, as the brown tumors begin to recalcify, a granular trabecular pattern appears and then is replaced by woven bone. According to Pellegrino (1977), surgical excision of the brown tumors is indicated under the following circumstances: (1) if the lesion is large and disfiguring, or (2) if the affected bone is weakened. This author stated that healing and remodeling are accelerated if the brown tumors are removed. The management of secondary hyperparathyroidism depends on successful treatment of the primary causative condition. In some instances, such as chronic renal insufficiency treated by renal dialysis, a parathyroid adenoma develops, necessitating surgical removal.

◆ *RADIOLOGY (Figs. 15–8 to 15–18)*

General Radiologic Features

The bony changes in hyperparathyroidism are identical, whether the cause is primary, secondary, or tertiary. According to Steinbach and colleagues (1961), the incidence of skeletal change is between 30 and 40%; however, with fine detail radiography, Weiss (1974) reported that subperiosteal resorption may be observed in as many as 60% of the cases. The classic radiologic features of hyperparathyroidism are as follows: (1) subperiosteal bone resorption; (2) generalized demineralization; (3) localized lytic bone lesions, known as brown tumors; and (4) metastatic calcification of soft tissues. Edeiken (1981) asserted that the earliest changes in hyperparathyroidism occur in the hands, calvaria, and alveolar bone of the jaws.

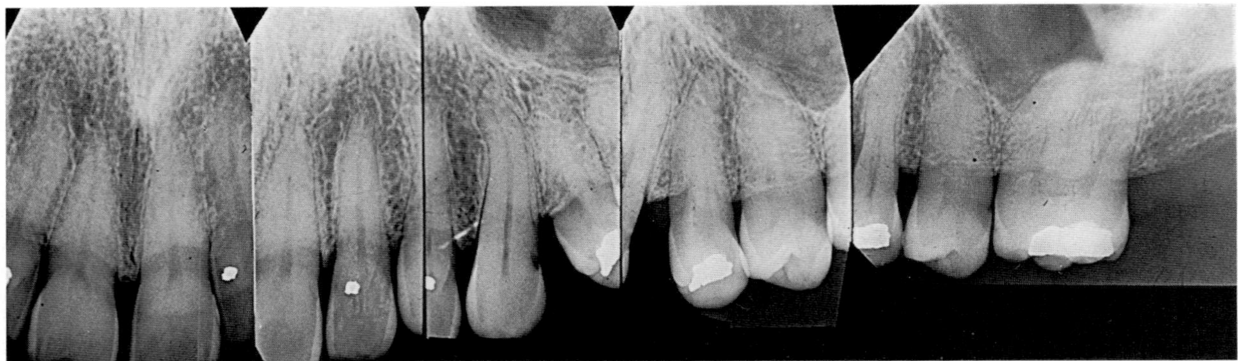

A

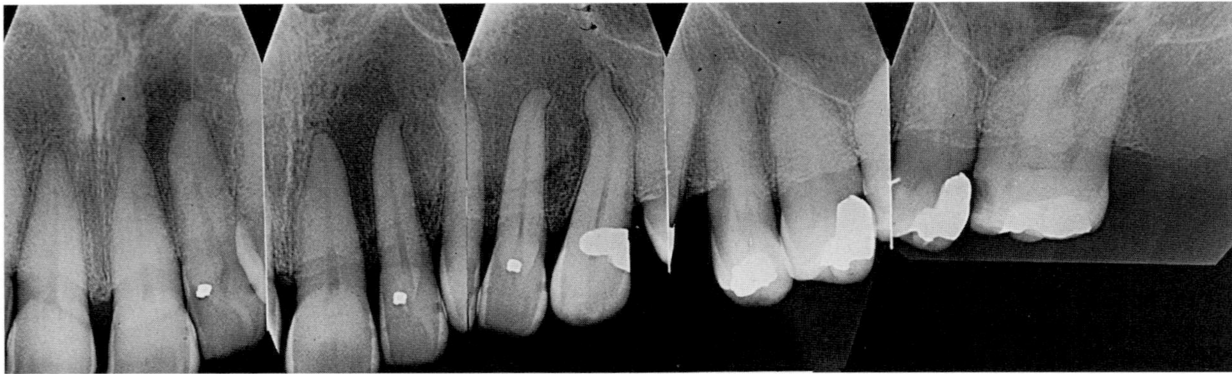

B

FIGURE 15–8.

Primary Hyperparathyroidism: Effects on jaws. A, Normal alveolar bone in 50-year-old woman. B, Same woman at 59 years of age, after development of parathyroid adenoma. Figure shows loss of the lamina dura, granular pattern of alveolar bone, and brown tumor in anterior region. (We received this case from the late Dr. Gordon Fitzgerald of San Francisco; it dates back to when intraoral radiographs were hand cut and packaged by the dentist.)

Radiology of the Jaws

Although this condition produces rarefaction of bone, Kelly and colleagues (1980), who studied 53 patients with end-stage renal disease, found that most observers associated the overall gray or white appearance of the radiographs with an increase in density (greater radiopacity). As the trabeculae become finer and more closely meshed, the overall appearance of the radiograph becomes more radiopaque. This is a paradoxic problem because this apparent increase in density is contradictory to the pathophysiologic events taking place, principally demineralization.

When the jaws are involved, the following tetrad of changes has been observed by Silverman and colleagues (1962, 1968) (1) generalized demineralization of bone, (2) resorption of the lamina dura, (3) subperiosteal erosion of the mandibular angle, and (4) brown tumors. When all four changes are present, they are highly suggestive of hyperparathyroidism. In addition, Spolnik and colleagues (1981) reported tooth abnormalities and extraosseous calcifications in association with end-stage renal disease.

Generalized Demineralization. Generalized demineralization is characterized by an overall lack of sharpness of the trabecular pattern, producing a uniform grayish density of the alveolar bone. This appearance has been described as granular and classically as osteoporosis fibrosa generalisata. It may look radiopaque to some observers and radiolucent to others. Demineralization in the jaws may begin in the lamina dura; then it may occur in the bone immediately surrounding the lamina dura and subsequently in the rest of the alveolar bone.

Resorption of Lamina Dura. Resorption of the lamina is the first sign of deossification in the jaws. In 220 patients studied by Rosenberg and Guralnick (1962), the lamina dura was absent in 40% of the cases. When the lamina dura was missing, they found that 62% exhibited classic bone disease, 27% had demineralization only, and 11% showed no apparent bone disease. When the lamina dura was present, the authors found that 74% had no bone disease, 17% had demineralization only, and 9% had classic bone disease. Thus, the presence or absence of the lamina dura is a good indicator of the degree of skeletal bone involvement. When the lamina dura is resorbed, Worth (1963) observed two relative changes: (1) thickening of the periodontal ligament space, and (2) a tapered appearance of the roots. The tapered appearance of the roots occurs because the lamina dura provides a definitive ''edge'' effect, accentuates the density of

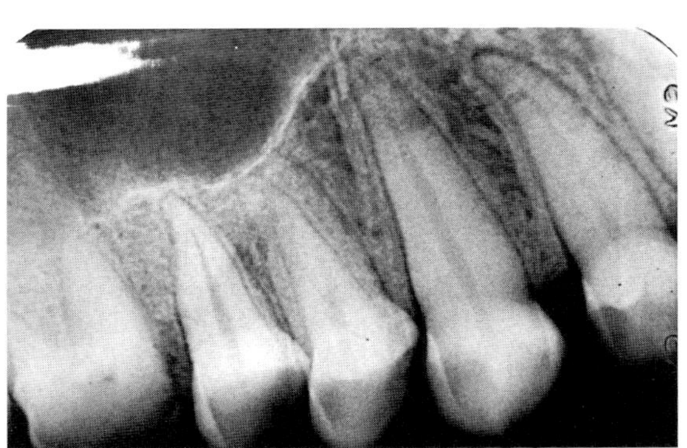

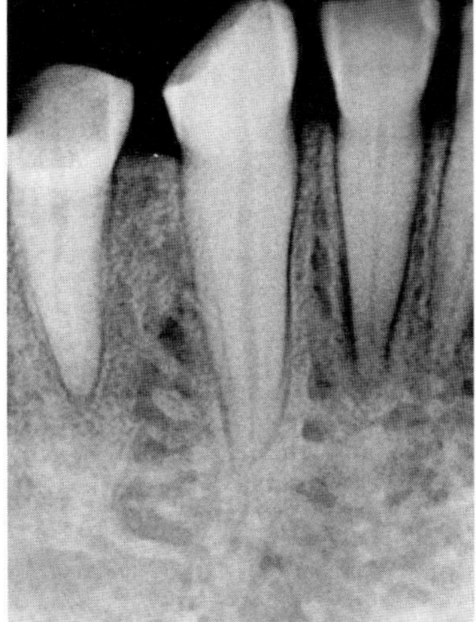

A B

FIGURE 15–9.

Secondary Hyperparathyroidism: Effects on jaws in a 19-year-old woman with a history of chronic renal failure and nausea. A and B, Deossification, which produces the granular pattern, begins in area of lamina dura and appears to extend to alveolar bone from this area outward.

the root, and usually is rounded at the tooth apex. The loss of the lamina dura may be generalized or localized. As the adjacent bone becomes demineralized, it takes on a ground glass appearance. Kelly and colleagues (1980) found that loss of the lamina dura and ground glass appearance of the alveolar bone occurred most frequently in the mandibular molar area above the mandibular canal. The lamina dura also may be absent in periodontitis, fibrous dysplasia, Paget's disease, Cushing's syndrome, and osteomalacia. The following conditions may show a loss of the lamina dura in combination with a ground glass pattern of the alveolar bone: hyperparathyroidism, fibrous dysplasia, Paget's disease, and dominant craniometaphyseal dysplasia.

Subperiosteal Erosion of Cortex. Subperiosteal erosion at the mandibular angle was studied by Bras and colleagues (1982). They used the thickness of cortical bone at the mandibular angle in panoramic radiographs as an index of bone demineralization in association with chronic end-stage renal failure. Their study included 12 patients whose mandibular angular cortex thickness was compared with the histologic grade of renal osteodystrophy, based on an undecalcified iliac crest biopsy specimen. In the normal population, the mean thickness of the point gonion cortex as seen in panoramic radiographs was established at 1.56 mm, and the value ranged from 1.0 to 2.5 mm, being calculated as the means of both sides. In their 12 patients with renal osteodystrophy, partial or complete loss of the mandibular angle cortex was an early radiologic finding because none of the patients showed other radiologic phenomena, such as loss of the lamina dura or a ground glass appearance of the bone. Their patients consisted of 7 men and 5 women, aged 23 to 56 years, with values ranging from 0.15 to 1.85 mm. Only 2 patients had values greater than 1.0 mm, and 7 had values of 0.55 mm or less.

Hyperparathyroidism also may cause resorption of the

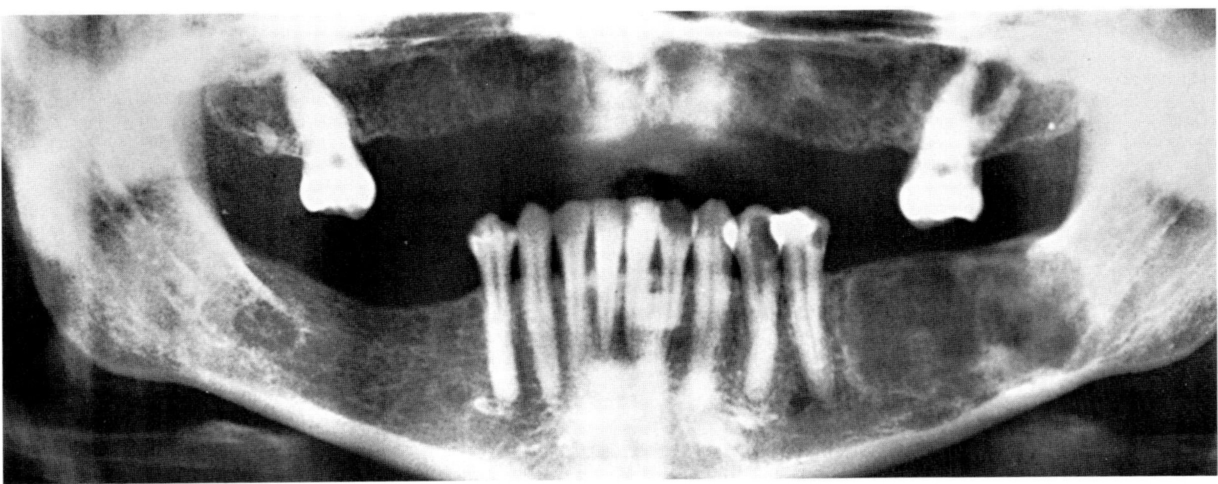

FIGURE 15–10.

Hyperparathyroidism: Effects on jaws. Figure shows moderate brown tumor formation in a 32-year-old woman. Small lesion in right mandible appears cystic; additional brown tumors may be seen in left mandible and maxilla. (From Farman AG, Nortjé CJ, Wood RE: Oral and Maxillofacial Diagnostic Imaging. Philadelphia:CV Mosby, 1993, p. 336.)

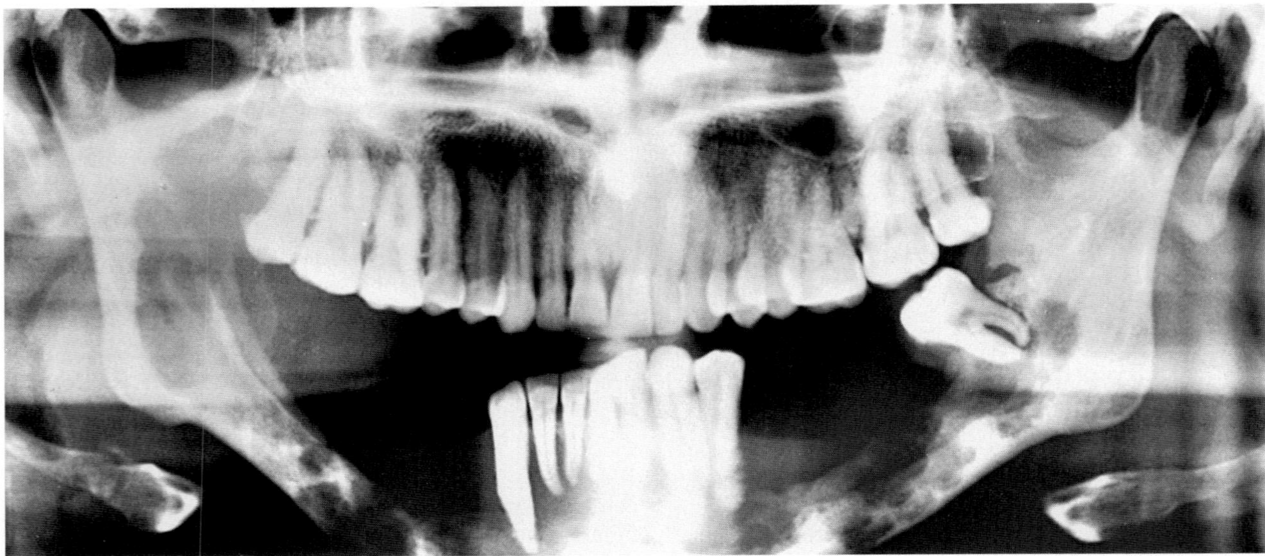

A

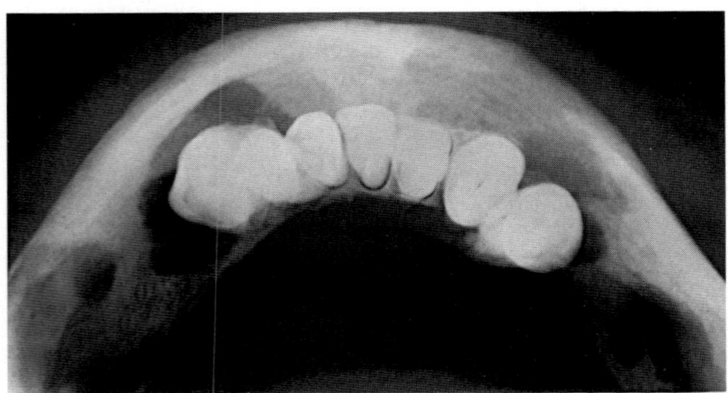

B

FIGURE 15–11.

Hyperparathyroidism: Effects on jaws. Severe brown tumor formation in 39-year-old woman with a history of primary hyperparathyroidism resulting from parathyroid adenoma. A, Multiple brown tumors throughout mandible and hyoid bone. B, Absence of host bone reaction, including expansion, periosteal reaction, and marginal sclerosis. (Courtesy of Professor L. Alfaro, University of Chile School of Dentistry, Chilean Referral Center for Pathology, Santiago, Chile.)

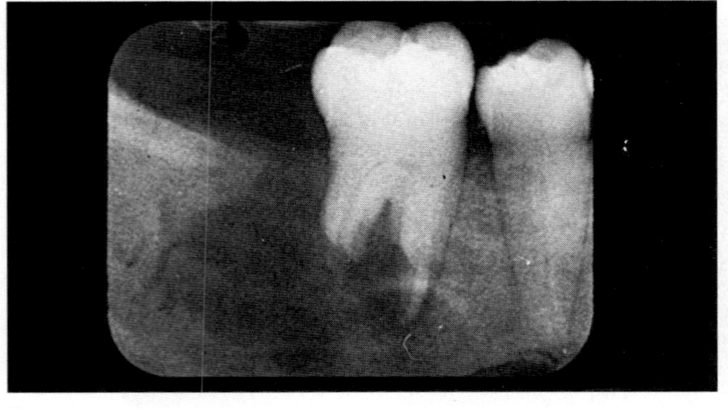

A

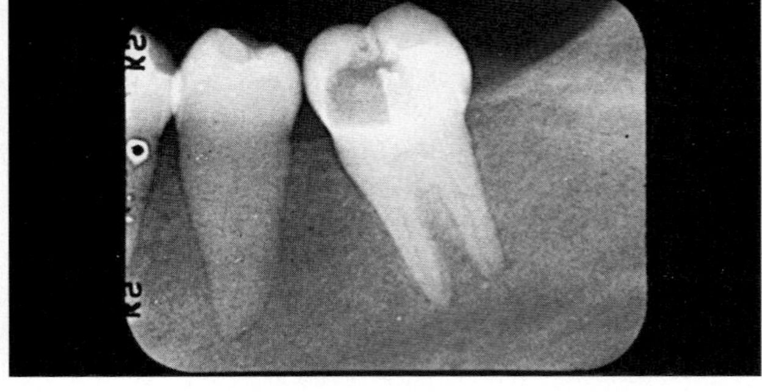

B

FIGURE 15–12.

Hyperparathyroidism: Effect on teeth of 26-year-old woman with a history of renal osteodystrophy. A, Brown tumor causes root resorption and extrusion of molar. B, Figure shows very small pulp chambers for a 26-year-old woman, loss of lamina dura, and tapered appearance of roots. The alveolar bone has a granular pattern.

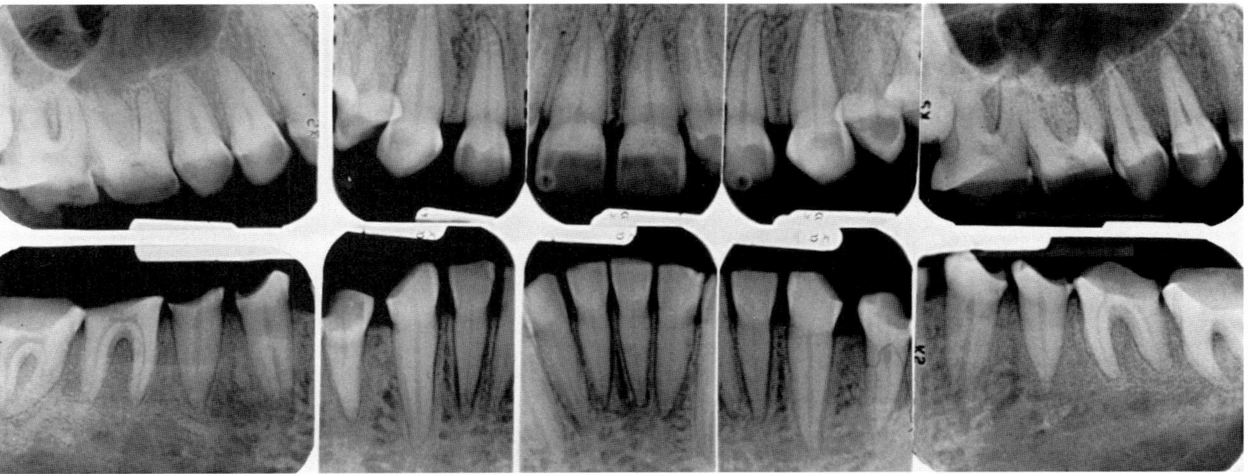

FIGURE 15–13.

Hyperparathyroidism: Effect on teeth of same patient in Figure 15–10. Prolonged hypercalcemia produces chronic nausea and vomiting, resulting in severe erosion of teeth. Figure shows relatively small pulp chambers for a 19-year-old woman.

inferior cortex of the mandible, the cortical lining of the inferior alveolar canal, and the walls of the antrum and nasal cavities.

Brown Tumors. Brown tumors are histologically identical to central giant cell granuloma; the surgical specimen appears brown. A histologic diagnosis of central giant cell granuloma always must be followed by a workup for hyperparathyroidism, especially when the following conditions are evident: (1) the lesion is posterior to the first molars in the mandible or anywhere in the maxilla, (2) the lesion is in the ramus, (3) several lesions are present, or (4) there are multiple recurrences. In a review of 300 patients with parathyroid tumors, Watson and Faccini (1976) found brown

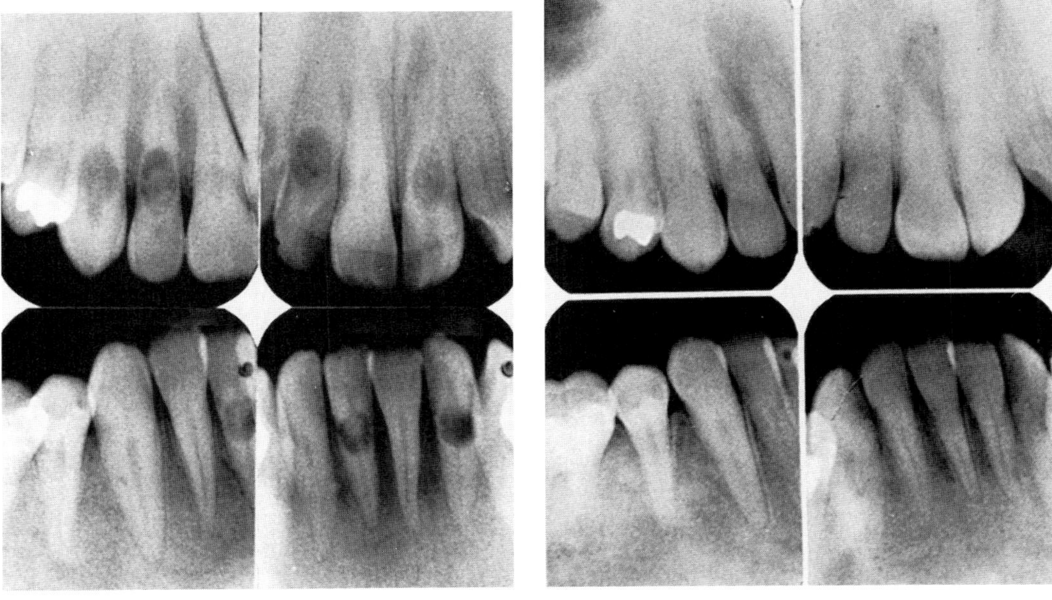

A B

FIGURE 15–14.

Hyperparathyroidism: Effect on teeth. A, A 22-year-old patient with end-stage renal disease. Multiple areas of internal resorption are present. B, Patient at 32 years of age, after successful treatment. There is apparent regeneration of internal elements of affected teeth. (From Hutton CE: Intradental lesions and their reversal in a patient being treated for end-stage renal disease. Oral Surg Oral Med Oral Pathol 60:258, 1985.)

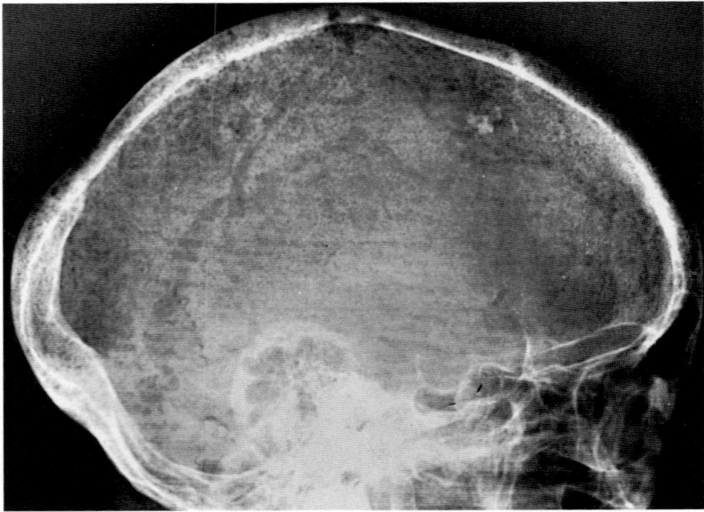

A

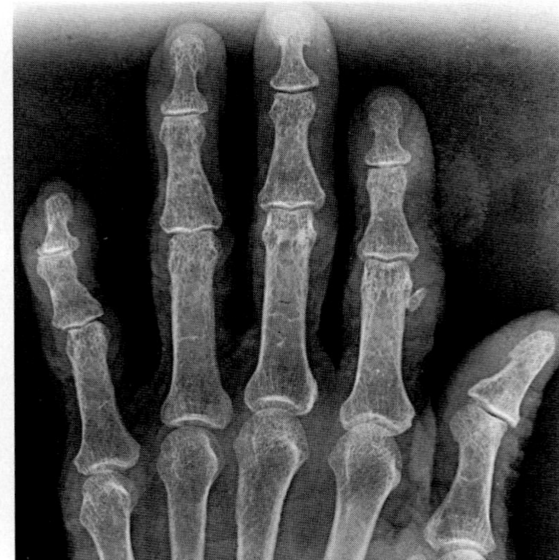

B

FIGURE 15–15.

Hyperparathyroidism: Effect on skull and hands of an 83-year-old man. A, Deossification of skull, producing granular appearance more toward outer third; almost complete effacement of outer table. B, Hand shows mild changes, principally subperiosteal erosion of cortex, especially in middle phalanges. (Courtesy of Dr. R. Cone, San Antonio, TX.)

tumors in 67 patients (22%), and 10 of these (15%) occurred in the jaws; Rosenberg and Guralnick (1962) found an incidence of 5% in the jaws. Brown tumors tend to be monocystic, without marginal scalloping, although internal septa may be seen rarely. The borders may be poorly defined, and there may appear to be a zone of reactive bone outlining the lesion. In addition, some may resemble cystic lesions.

Relationship to Teeth

Dental changes have been described in detail by Worth (1963). In developing or erupting teeth, (1) there may be a loss of the crypt wall; (2) eruption appears too far advanced for the degree of root development; (3) the roots appear very pointed and tapered, especially at the apical third; and (4) the pulp chambers appear to be abnormally large. In erupted teeth, the pulp chambers may appear abnormally large in younger people; however, pulp chambers in adults may be narrower than expected in correlation with the patient's age. Kelly and colleagues (1980) found two previous reports of pulpal narrowing with respect to age and reported pulp space narrowing in 11% of their dentate patients with end-stage renal disease; pulpal narrowing was observed most easily in the mandibular incisor area.

Hutton (1985) reported a remarkable case that is shown in Figure 15–14. A white man began hemodialysis at 22 years of age because of chronic renal failure; by the time he reached 25 years of age, he had rejected a kidney transplant and had severe difficulty in regulation of calcium-phosphorus levels. He underwent a subtotal parathyroidectomy and was given vitamin D and calcium, after which he began to improve. During this period, large, oval-shaped radiolucent areas, resembling internal resorption, developed in the cervical third of the root canal spaces of several anterior teeth; the patient responded well to treatment, and within 4 years the affected incisors appeared normal, with pulp and root canal spaces possibly narrower than normal for a 32-year-old person. Other findings associated less frequently with teeth include infrequent resorption of root tips and extrusion of the tooth in association with a brown tumor. Although root resorption is a relatively uncommon finding in hyperparathyroidism, it is more common in central giant cell granuloma.

Calculi and Metastatic Calcification

According to Wood and Goaz (1985), ectopic calcification of soft tissues is the most common feature of hyperparathyroidism; 45 to 80% of patients will have nephrolithiasis or nephrocalcinosis. Albright and Reifenstein (1948) stated that 5% of patients with urinary calculi have hyperparathyroidism. Bywaters and Dixon (1963) discussed calcification in joints and found an incidence between 10 and 20%, with fibrocartilage and the meniscus being the most common sites. According to Dodds and Steinbach (1968), a common site is the triangular cartilage of the wrist. Other affected tissues are the walls of blood vessels and subcutaneous tissues. Wood and Goaz (1985) stated that calculi frequently develop in the salivary glands. In their extensive review of the literature, Kelly and colleagues (1980) found two reports associating pulpal calcifications with hyperparathyroidism. In their study, Spolnik and colleagues (1981) found pulpal calcification in 10 of the 20 patients with teeth; these calcifications were mainly in the pulp chambers and resembled pulp stones. However, pulp calcifications are a common finding in the normal population.

Radiologic Features of the Skull

According to Worth (1963), the skull may appear osteoporotic, and this change may occur before jaw changes. Edeiken (1981) stated that the deossification appears granular and is most prominent in the outer third of the skull, and

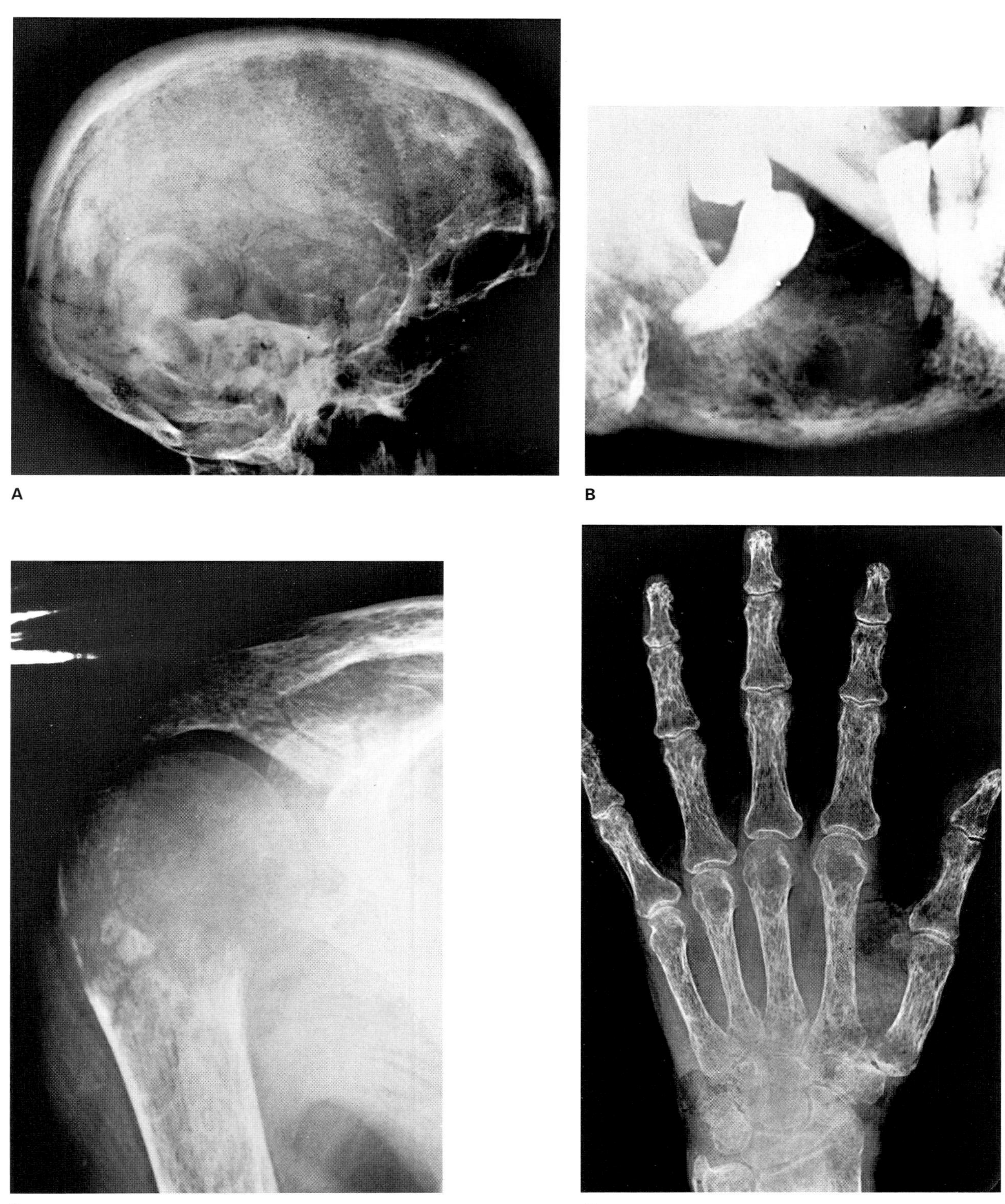

A B C D

FIGURE 15–16.

Hyperparathyroidism: Findings in a 52-year-old woman with primary hyperparathyroidism. A. Skull: granular appearance resulting from deossification; there are multiple small brown tumors, especially in the frontal, temporal, and occipital areas. B, Mandible: brown tumor and severe deossification producing permeative appearance. C, Humerus: brown tumor in epiphysis. D, Hand: significant deossification with coarse trabeculae, subperiosteal erosion of the cortices of phalanges, and erosion of the terminal tufts. (Courtesy of Dr. R. Cone, San Antonio, TX.)

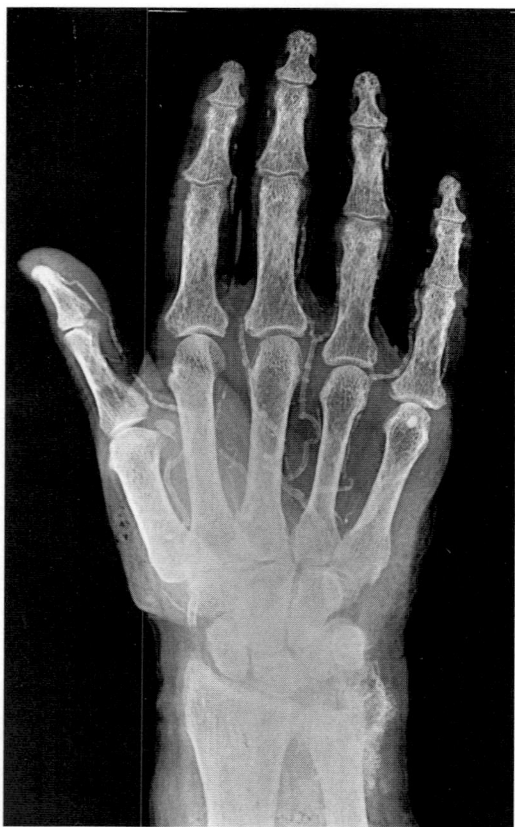

FIGURE 15–17.

Hyperparathyroidism: In a patient with primary hyperparathyroidism, hand shows subperiosteal erosion of cortex of all phalanges, resorption of terminal tufts, metastatic calcification of blood vessel walls, and soft tissue calcinosis producing "brushfire sign" at ulnar (little finger) side of wrist. (Courtesy of Dr. R. Cone, San Antonio, TX.)

this granularity may appear subtle at times. The granular pattern may be interrupted by one or many cystic areas representing brown tumors. These cystic areas often may appear roundish, with smooth or slightly irregular borders marginated with sclerotic reactive bone. In the lateral view, the outer table may appear to be completely effaced, whereas the inner table may appear significantly thinned. After resolution, the skull assumes a more normal appearance; however, the healed brown tumors appear as sclerotic islands, giving the skull a somewhat pagetoid appearance.

Radiologic Features of the Hand

According to Pugh (1951), the most important and reliable sign of hyperparathyroidism is subperiosteal erosion along the radial margin (toward the thumb) of the middle phalanges; this is accompanied occasionally by the same change on the ulnar side (toward the little finger). Immediately beneath the periosteum, the outer surface of the cortex appears lacelike. The endosteal margin of the cortex is unaffected until the disease becomes advanced. At this stage, the affected phalanx appears to have no cortex. Ultimately, all of the phalanges and long bones may be affected.

Other hand changes include the following: (1) destruction of the midportions of the terminal phalanges with a telescoped appearance, (2) formation of brown tumors, and (3) resorption of the terminal tufts. When the midportion of the terminal tufts is destroyed, there is a radiolucent band that appears to divide the terminal tuft into two parts. Clinically, this shortens the distal portion of the involved fingers, and the skin appears to be telescoped or in folds. The brown tumors appear as cystlike lesions in the bones of the hand. Internal trabeculations sometimes may develop within a brown tumor, the phalanx may appear expanded, and the finger may be swollen clinically. When the terminal tufts are resorbed, they lose their platypus beaklike appearance distally and assume a more pointed shape, with narrowing occurring toward the distal end. Clinically, this may cause the finger to appear clubbed, with the nail curving over the tip of the finger. If the serum calcium level has been elevated for a sufficient time, metastatic calcification may be observed in the walls of the blood vessels in the adjacent soft tissues of the fingers.

Radiologic Follow-up

Radiographic follow-up is directed toward evaluating the efficacy of treatment with a return of normal radiographic features. In some instances, healed areas may show an increased density.

MASSIVE OSTEOLYSIS (Essential osteolysis, progressive atrophy of bone, acute spontaneous absorption of bone, disappearing bone disease, phantom bone disease, progressive osteolysis, Gorham's massive osteolysis, Gorham's disease)

Massive osteolysis first was reported by Jackson in 1838 and later in 1872 when he reported a patient with a disappearing

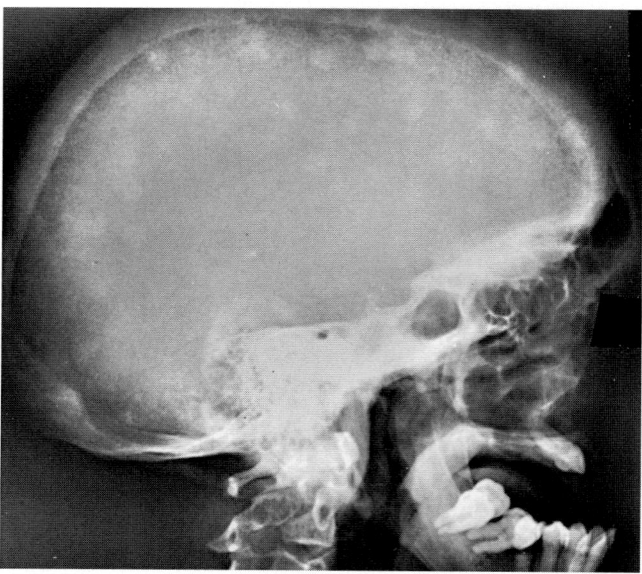

FIGURE 15–18.

Hyperparathyroidism: Skull: pagetoid appearance of healed brown tumors in a treated patient.

humerus. In 1955, Gorham and Stout first defined the condition as a specific pathologic process. Romer (1924) reported the first case in the jaws. In 1983, Frederiksen and colleagues and Heffez and co-authors (1983) published reviews. This disease is characterized by progressive resorption of contiguous osseous structures. Approximately 70 cases have been reported in the skeleton; among these, 14 were in the jaws.

Pathologic Characteristics

Histologically, there is a proliferation of thin-walled blood and lymphatic vessels at the site of bone destruction. Invariably, osteoclasts are present and the destroyed bone is replaced by fibrous connective tissue. Stout (1944) suggested the term hemangiomatosis to describe the histologic findings. Frederiksen and colleagues (1983) studied the electron microscopic features and concluded that the process is nonneoplastic in nature and shows features of an exuberant proliferative response of vascular and supportive elements.

Clinical Features

Frederiksen and colleagues (1983) and Heffez and co-authors (1983) found approximately 60 to 70 cases in the literature. Heffez and colleagues (1983) established the following eight histopathologic and clinical criteria for the diagnosis of massive osteolysis and reviewed the 42 cases meeting these criteria: (1) positive biopsy findings; (2) absence of cellular atypia; (3) minimal or no osteoblastic response and absence of dystrophic calcification; (4) evidence of local, progressive osseous resorption; (5) nonexpansile, nonulcerative lesion; (6) absence of visceral involvement; (7) osteolytic radiographic pattern; and (8) negative findings for a hereditary, metabolic, neoplastic, immunologic, or infectious origin.

Frederiksen and colleagues (1983) found no sex or racial predilection and reported that the disease usually develops before a person reaches the fourth decade of life. Heffez and colleagues (1983) found that the average age was 27 years when the patient was seen initially. The age range was 1.5 to 72 years. Applying their criteria, Heffez and colleagues (1983) found an equal distribution among male and female patients. These authors reported a history of slight to moderate trauma 2 months to 6 years before discovery of the disease in 17 of their 42 accepted cases. There appear to be 2 sequential phases of the disease clinically. In the first phase there is active bone destruction and lysis. This may be associated with mild to moderate pain; however, Frederiksen and colleagues (1983) stated that pain is not a feature unless there is an associated pathologic fracture. There may be slight soft tissue swelling and varying degrees of erythema, ultimately followed by radiographic evidence of progressive bone destruction. These changes occur slowly and insidiously over a period of years. The second phase is the quiescent stage, without swelling, pain, bone destruction, or radiographic evidence of bone repair. Multiple bones may be affected and, although death is not a usual sequel, several deaths have been reported, occurring most often with chest wall or clavicular involvement. In one case there was extension of mandibular disease to the cervical vertebrae, with severance of the spinal cord.

Treatment/Prognosis

Some ineffective treatments include pharmacotherapeutic regimens of all sorts aimed at stabilizing the lytic process, radiation therapy, and bone grafting, with the graft undergoing lysis. It appears that intraperiosteal or extraperiosteal resection of the affected area with adequate margins of uninvolved bone may arrest the process permanently. Curettage or incomplete resection are rarely effective. Once the osteolysis has been arrested, the use of autogenous grafts may be effective in reconstruction of the defect. Aston (1958) successfully grafted a left femur with an autogenous tibial graft after subperiosteal resection of the affected area. Ross (1978) and Butler and co-workers (1958) successfully grafted autogenous bone in sites of inactive disease.

◆ *RADIOLOGY (Figs. 15–19 and 15–20)*

General Radiologic Features

Johnson and McClure (1958) described the radiologic findings as follows: (1) The earliest evidence of disease consists of one or more intramedullary and subcortical radiolucent foci of varying sizes, usually with indistinct margins and sometimes with very thin radiopaque borders. (2) These foci enlarge, coalesce, and eventually involve the cortex. (3) A periosteal reaction is notably absent. (4) The cortex is destroyed, after which there is continued intraosseous and extraosseous resorption. (5) In the tubular bones, a tapering effect produces a conelike spicule of bone, and there is usually no expansion. Osteolysis does not respect joints and spreads to contiguous bones. According to Heffez and colleagues (1983), the following sites are affected most commonly (in order of frequency): (1) maxillofacial region, (2) lower extremities and pelvis, and (3) shoulder, girdle, rib cage, and vertebrae. Pathologic fractures may be observed, and they rarely heal.

Radiology of the Jaws

Frederiksen and colleagues (1983) found 14 cases involving the jaws and presented a review of these. It would appear that the mandible is involved most frequently because it was affected in all 14 cases and in the case described by Heffez and associates (1983). Frederiksen and colleagues (1983) observed that only the mandible was involved in 7 of 14 cases. The next most frequent combination was the mandible and maxilla, with varying degrees of involvement of contiguous structures, including the hard palate, sphenoid bone, zygomatic bone, and cervical vertebrae. Frederiksen and colleagues (1983) reported that there was no formation of focal lytic areas in the reported cases of jaw involvement, with progressive resorption and thinning of the mandible being the characteristic process. Lysis appears to progress until wispy remnants of bone remain, and then there is a complete absence of bone roentgenographically. In their review of the literature, Heffez and colleagues (1983) found that the

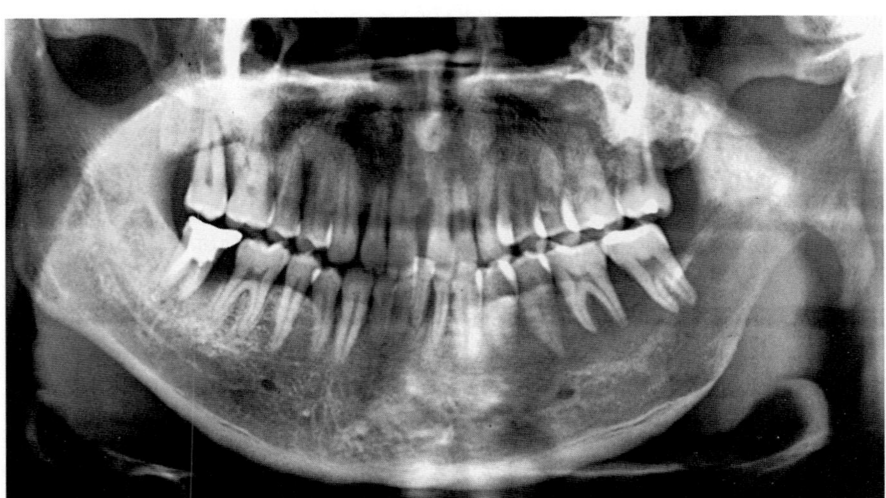
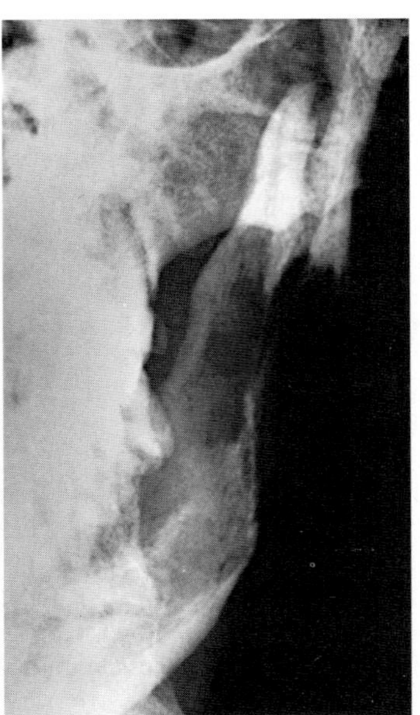

A B

FIGURE 15–19.

Massive Osteolysis: Case in a 47-year-old man. A, Conelike spur of remaining bone in left ramus. B, No periosteal reaction; lesion is entirely lytic with no evidence of reactive sclerosis at margins. (Courtesy of Professor H. Fuchihata, Dean, Osaka University School of Dentistry, Osaka, Japan.)

process crossed the midline in 5 cases. One case occurred in the cervical spine, 2 in the symphysis pubis, and 2 in the mandible.

The importance of computed tomography cannot be overemphasized because more involvement of the facial bones, base of the skull, and skull may occur than has been reported previously.

SICKLE CELL ANEMIA

Sickle cell anemia (SCA) first was described by Herrick in 1910. It is a hereditary form of chronic hemolytic anemia and mainly affects North Americans of African origin; however, other groups also may have the disease. The sickle cell trait is a dominant asymptomatic finding. Mourshed and Tuckson

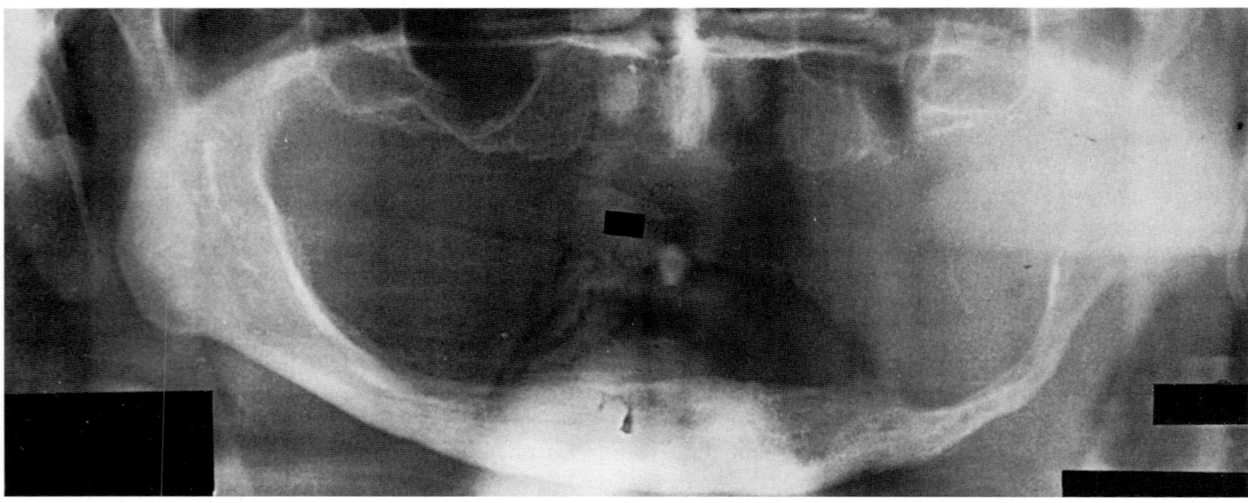

A

FIGURE 15–20.

Massive Osteolysis: Progression of disease in mandible and continued osteolysis in rib graft. A, August 12, 1976.

(*continued*)

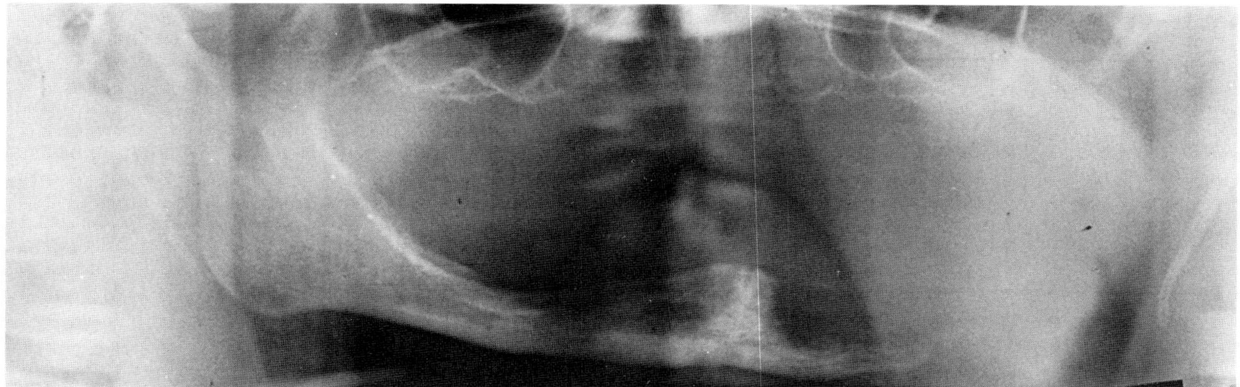

B

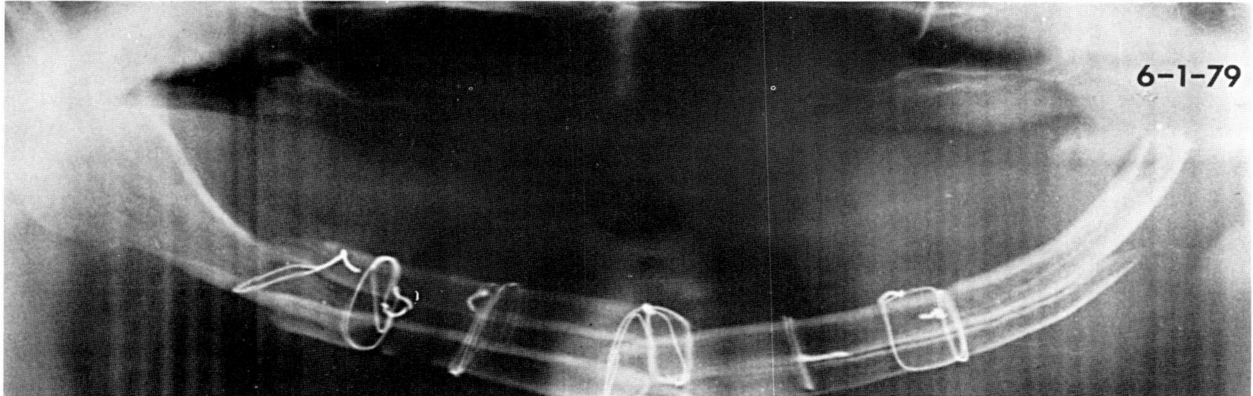

C

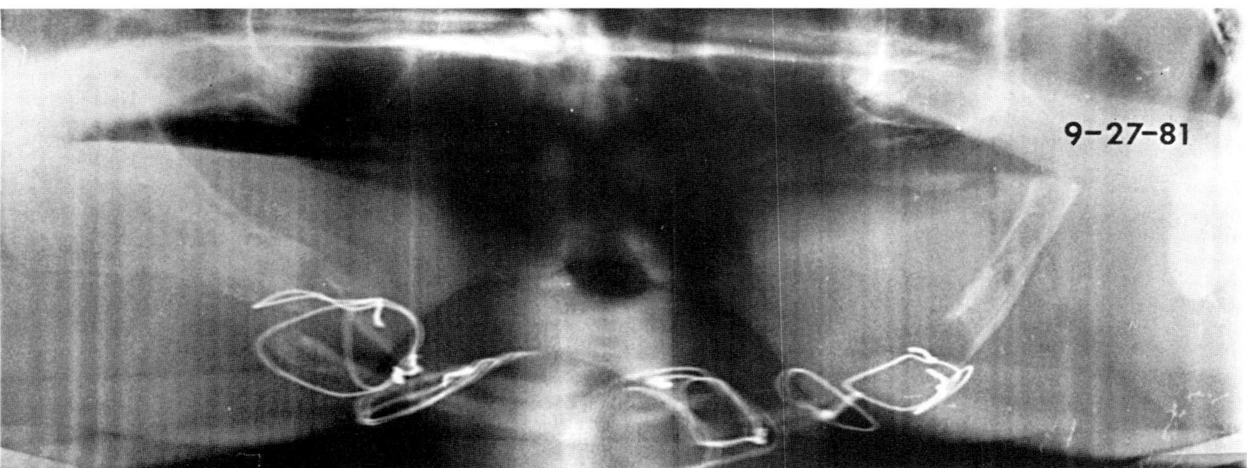

D

FIGURE 15–20.

(*continued*) B, September 15, 1977. C, June 1, 1979. D, September 27, 1981. (From Frederiksen NL, Wesley RK, Sciubbas JJ, Helfrick J: Massive osteolysis of the maxillofacial skeleton: a clinical, radiographic, histologic and ultrastructural study. Oral Surg Oral Med Oral Pathol 55:470, 1983.)

(1974) found that 1 in 10 Americans of African origin carries the sickle cell trait, and 1 in 500 black people has the disease. In a study of 8000 black Americans, Diggs (1933) found that 1 of 40 people carrying the trait manifested the disease. Some white people of Mediterranean origin also may have this disease, a condition distinct and separate from thalassemia. Heterozygotes carry the trait, but only homozygotes manifest the disease.

Pathologic Characteristics

In SCA, glutamic acid, normally present on the sixth position of the beta chain of hemoglobin, is replaced by valine. This alteration, according to Manning Cox (1984) and Cox (1977), increases the hemoglobin's sensitivity to lowered oxygen tension, even within normal physiologic ranges, causing elongation and distortion of the normally discoid erythrocyte into the characteristic sickled or crescent-shaped cell, which is 15 μm in length. Normal red blood cells are approximately 7 μm in diameter. The elongated and distorted sickle cells are less able to carry oxygen and are destroyed much more rapidly than normal red blood cells. The condition also results in stasis of blood flow, increased viscosity of the blood, and thrombosis. According to Manning Cox (1984) and Cox (1977), the decreased blood flow creates an acidotic environment, thus causing additional sickling, and initiates the sickle cell crisis.

Clinical Features

Mourshed and Tuckson (1974) stated that SCA is accompanied by recurrent attacks of pain in the abdomen and limbs, weakness, bone pain, shortness of breath, fever, jaundice, pallor, cardiomegaly, and leg ulcers. Manning Cox (1984) and Cox (1977) studied pain in the maxillofacial complex in SCA. In these reviews, there were reports of mental nerve paresthesia as a result of the sickle cell crisis. Konotey-Ahulu (1972) found moderate to severe mandibular pain, followed by paresthesia of the lower lip, in 4% of patients admitted to the hospital in acute crisis. In a study of 25 patients with homozygous SCA, Manning Cox (1984) and Cox (1977) found that oral and maxillofacial pain occurred in 36% and consisted of the following: (1) frontal headaches, (2) pain in the lower jaw, and (3) sensitivity or pain in the teeth. In this study, it was found that most patients had pain in several locations, with episodes lasting from a few hours to several days and recurring at least 2 to 3 times per year. It also was observed that painful attacks occurred in patients with mild and severe forms of the disease. Mourshed and Tuckson (1974) reported no sex predilection.

Treatment/Prognosis

According to Mourshed and Tuckson (1974), most patients are children and adolescents, and the life expectancy of most patients does not exceed 40 years. Because the sickle cell crisis results from decreased oxygenation of the tissues, it may be triggered by a general anesthetic, exercise, or infection. Patients with SCA may be more prone to osteomyelitis in the jaws, often as a complication of periodontal disease or pulpal infection.

◆ *RADIOLOGY (Figs. 15–21 and 15–22)*

First, the radiologic features of SCA result from one of the following characteristics of the disease: (1) marrow hyperplasia producing bone resorption and prominence and rearrangement of trabeculae, (2) thrombosis and infarction causing mainly sclerotic change, and (3) secondary osteomyelitis resulting in bone rarefaction. Second, the radiologic findings also depend on the age at which changes are observed: (1) children manifest alterations in bone resulting from marrow hyperplasia and growth defects, (2) adults are affected by marrow hyperplasia and thrombosis, and (3) the radiologic changes vary with anatomic location, showing significant differences from one region to another. Finally, the specificity of the radiologic changes varies greatly, and, in some instances, there is no appreciable difference from the normal population.

Radiology of the Jaws

In 1952, Robinson and Sarnat published the first descriptions of bony changes affecting the jaws. They reported that 18 of their 22 patients (82%) showed significant bone changes in periapical radiographs, which were characterized as osteoporotic in nature, with a decrease in the number of trabeculae and more sharply defined remaining trabeculae. The trabeculae appeared to be lined up in horizontal rows, with a stepladderlike effect between the roots of teeth. This parallel arrangement of the trabeculae was not found in edentulous areas. The lamina dura usually was not affected. Only 3 of Robinson and Sarnat's patients had significant findings in the long bones and only one displayed dramatic skull findings. This led the authors to conclude that periapical and lateral jaw radiographs were the strongest indicators of bony changes.

In 1974, Mourshed and Tuckson published the definitive study involving radiographs from 80 patients with SCA. They divided their study into three parts. The first involved the finding of increased radiolucency of bone and the formation of a coarse trabecular pattern, including a horizontal arrangement of the trabeculae between the roots of the teeth in a stepladder pattern in the jaws of patients with SCA. Although 85% had increased radiolucency and a coarse trabecular pattern, these authors found similar findings in a random sample of 20 patients without SCA, proven by hemoglobin electrophoresis. One in 16 young children had a stepladder trabecular pattern between the roots of teeth. In older children over 11 years of age, and adults, the stepladder interradicular trabecular pattern was observed in 47%; however, there were similar findings in regular clinic patients.

The second finding studied by Moushed and Tuckson (1974) related to thinning of the inferior cortex of the mandible. Reynolds (1962) reported that, in patients with SCA, the mandibular cortex is thinned to 4 mm or less; in contrast, the normal thickness is 6 mm. In their series of 80 cases, Mourshed and Tuckson (1974) measured the thickness of the mandibular cortex in the region of the mandibular first molar on panoramic radiographs, finding a thickness ranging from 1.5 to 4 mm; the cortex was 5 mm in only two cases. In 68% the thickness ranged from 3 to 4 mm, and in 30% it ranged from 1.5 to 2.5 mm. They compared these data with a random sample of 50 panoramic radiographs from the dental clinic and found that 68% were 3 to 4 mm and 24% were smaller than 3 mm. They concluded that thinning of the mandibular cortex is not a reliable radiologic criterion for SCA.

The third criterion studied by Mourshed and Tuckson (1974) was based on the data reported by Prowler and Smith

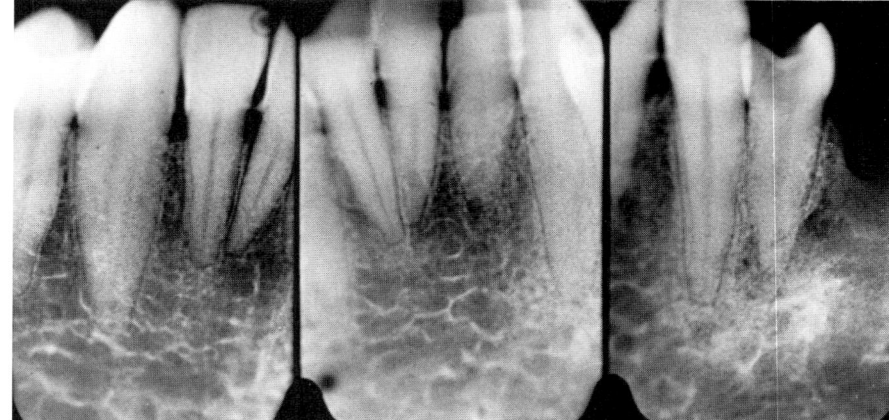

A

FIGURE 15–21.

Sickle Cell Anemia: A, B, and C, Young African-American man has enlarged marrow spaces and coarse trabeculae. Lamina dura is unaffected. (Courtesy of Dr. S. Matteson, University of Texas Dental School, San Antonio, TX.)

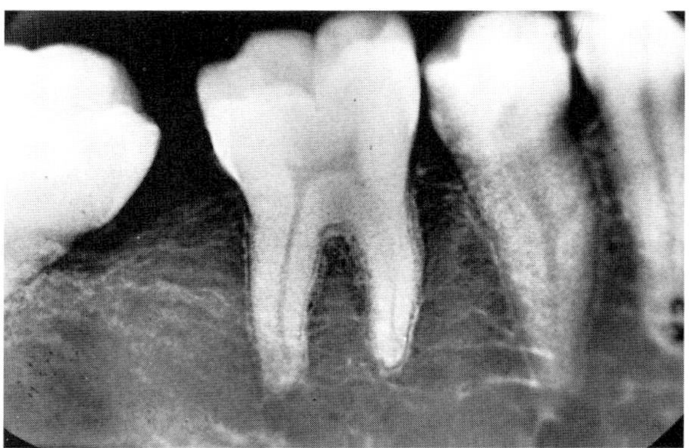

B

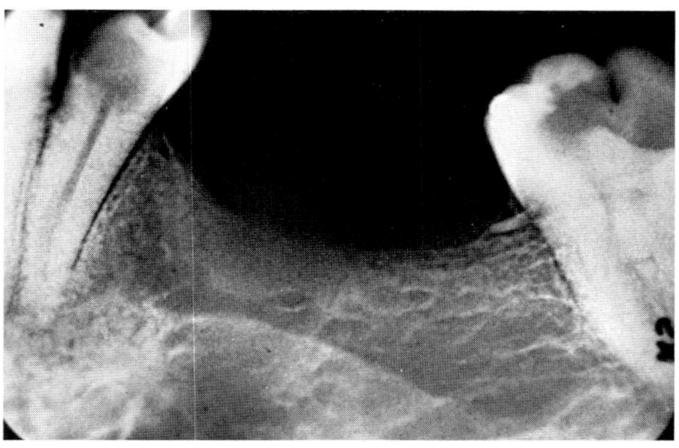

C

(1955), showing that 4 of 23 patients had distinct areas of increased radiopacity representing healed infarcts. Although infarctions are rare in children with SCA, they occur in the long bones of adults, especially in the subchondral portion of the head of the humerus. Infarction is characterized by juxta-articular sclerosis, dystrophic medullary calcification, a periosteal reaction producing a bone-within-a-bone appearance, and osteolysis. According to Edeiken (1981) and Sanger and colleagues (1977), the radiologic changes associated with infarction are indistinguishable from those caused by infection. To our knowledge, the possibility of bone infarction in the jaws has not been established. Mourshed and Tuckson (1974) found areas of increased opacity in the jaws in association with chronic infection; however, they believed there were no cases of healed infarct among their 80 patients. They concluded that SCA is not necessarily associated with healed infarcts in the jaws and that healed infarcts are not a reliable radiographic criterion for SCA in the jaws. More recently, Sanger and colleagues (1977) reported the cases of three patients with SCA who had radiopaque lesions in the jaws. One case resembled condensing osteitis, and two other cases looked like osteosclerosis. The authors emphasized the difficulty of making a definitive diagnosis without histologic analysis.

Despite the study by Mourshed and Tuckson (1974), we are convinced that some patients do manifest changes in the jaws. These may be summarized as follows: (1) generalized osteoporotic changes, (2) larger marrow spaces, (3) altered trabeculae, and (4) thinning of the cortex. It is important to maintain a high level of suspicion of this disease because infection prevention can save these patients' lives.

Radiology of the Skull

Robinson and Sarnat (1952), reviewed the following skull changes: (1) increased thickness of the vault; (2) perpendicular trabeculae radiating outward from the inner table, giving a "hair-on-end" appearance; (3) a thick, partially resorbed outer table, giving the skull a ground glass appearance; and (4) generalized osteoporosis. Sebes and Diggs (1979) reviewed skull radiographs of 194 patients whose ages ranged from 4 months to 55 years. The most common finding was osteoporosis (25%); widening of the diploe, with a decreased thickness of the outer table (22%); and perpendicular hair-on-end trabeculations (5%). The hair-on-end effect was seen in patients between the ages of 5 and 39 years. The authors also found that once the hair-on-end effect appeared, it did not regress with age. According to Robinson and Sarnat (1952), thickening of the diploe is seen most frequently in the parietal bone, followed by the frontal and temporal bones; it is bilaterally symmetric, is maximal toward the vertex, and tapers to normal in the temporal region. According to Edeiken (1981), the hair-on-end appearance is not as significant as in thalassemia. Infarcts have been described rarely in the skull.

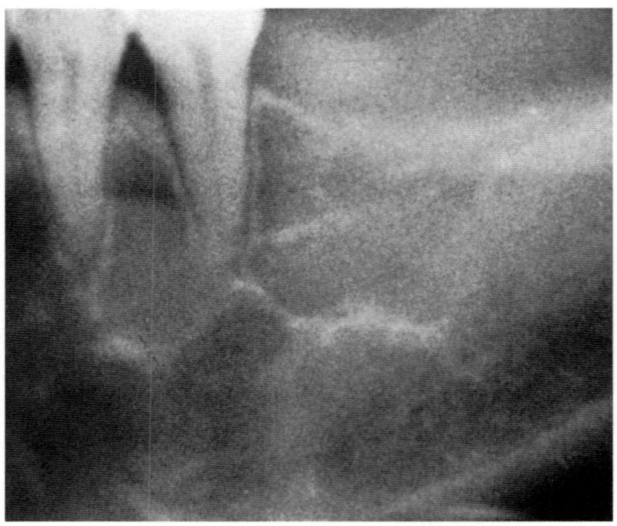

FIGURE 15–22.

Sickle Cell Anemia: Significant osteoporotic change showing several large, coarse trabeculae only.

THALASSEMIA (Mediterranean anemia, Cooley's anemia, familial erythroblastic anemia, hereditary leptocytosis)

Thalassemias were reviewed recently by Van Dis and Langlais (1986). In general, thalassemia may be classified as a hereditary blood disease transmitted by a recessive gene.

Pathologic Characteristics

There are homozygous and heterozygous subtypes of thalassemia. A patient with the heterozygous type exhibits minimal manifestations, whereas the homozygous subtype produces varying degrees of clinical expression. Van Dis and Langlais (1986) discussed these and other subtypes in some detail. According to these authors, thalassemias are classified according to the chain produced at the reduced rate. The most severe condition is a homozygous deletion defect, which results in excessive gamma chain production in the fetus and usually is fatal before or shortly after birth. A less severe homozygous defect, in which each of two different genes is defective, produces hemoglobin H disease. Patients with this disorder may reach adulthood and have varying degrees of anemia and splenomegaly. Hemoglobin values may range from 7 to 10 g/dl, and the erythrocytes show significant hypochromia and variations in size and shape. The heterozygous state is termed δ-thalassemia and may produce erythrocytes with a reduced mean corpuscular hemoglobin level of 20 to 25 picograms (pg) (normal range, 27 to 32 pg) and a mean corpuscular volume of 60 to 70 cubic microns (μm^3) (normal range, 80 to 94 μm^3). In other instances, heterozygotes may show only minimal evidence of hypochromic microcytic anemia. The δ-thalassemias are found most frequently in people from southeast Asia and parts of the Middle East and in some Mediterranean populations.

The β-thalassemias also result from a variety of genetic defects and produce diverse clinical and hematologic findings. The terms ''major'' and ''minor'' used in conjunction with β-thalassemia usually refer to the degree of severity of signs and symptoms, but several different genotypes may produce similar clinical presentations. In general, homozygous states result in the severe anemia of thalassemia major. The peripheral blood smear shows significant anisocytosis, poikilocytosis, reticulocytosis, hypochromia, and basophilic stippling. The bone marrow studies often show erythroid hyperplasia. The heterozygous states of β-thalassemia produce a milder degree of anemia, referred to as thalassemia minor. Hemoglobin values for men may range from 9 to 15 g/dl (normal range, 14 to 18 g/dl), and values for women may be 8 to 13 g/dl (normal range, 12 to 16 g/dl). The mild anemia of heterozygous β-thalassemia may be confused with iron deficiency anemia unless electrophoresis or other specific hemoglobin analyses are performed.

Clinical Features

Poyton and Davey (1968) stated that patients with thalassemia minor usually do not manifest clinical abnormalities; however, in their series of 16 children with thalassemia major, their patients exhibited some or all of the following clinical manifestations: (1) sallow complexion, sometimes accompanied by jaundice; (2) a prominent maxilla and short upper lip; (3) frontal bossing and occasionally exophthalmos; (4) frequent splenomegaly, and hepatomegaly often producing a protuberant abdomen; (5) pathologic fractures; and (6) spontaneous hemorrhage of the mucous membranes and purpura. Other features include a short stature, Down's syndrome-like facies, and abnormal menstruation.

Treatment/Prognosis

The treatment of thalassemia major includes multiple blood transfusions, and the primary complication of this treatment is iron overloading. Three factors may contribute to the deposition of iron in the tissues: (1) ineffective erythropoiesis with increased erythrocyte breakdown, (2) repeated transfusions, and (3) excessive iron absorption from the gut induced by chronic hypoxemia. Excessive iron deposition in tissues may result in damage to the myocardium, liver, spleen, pancreas, thyroid, parathyroids, and gastrointestinal mucosa. To reduce iron overload, splenectomy, transfusion with young red blood cells, and chelation therapy with deferoxamine have been used.

Patients with nontransfusion-dependent thalassemia minor also have complications from their condition. They appear to be at increased risk for chronic inflammatory liver disease, including viral hepatitis, typhoid fever, gastroduodenal ulcers, arthropathies, and possibly rheumatoid arthritis. Folic acid deficiency is common in heterozygotes because of the increased demand associated with chronic hyperactivity of the marrow. Ocular lesions are more common in patients with thalassemia minor versus thalassemia major.

◆ *RADIOLOGY (Fig. 15–23)*

General Radiologic Features

Patients with thalassemia minor do not manifest significant radiologic changes except in rare instances. Radiologic changes are seen mostly in thalassemia major, especially in the most severely affected patients. The radiologic findings result from hemolysis of red blood cells and compensatory erythroid hyperplasia of the red marrow. Marrow hypertrophy produces enlargement of the medullary spaces, fewer but coarser trabeculae, thinned cortices, and a widened dimension of the involved bone. The earliest findings are seen in the small bones of the hands and feet. Worth (1963) summarized these changes as follows: (1) increased width of the shafts with less constriction in the midportion, (2) thinning of the cortices, and (3) a thickened or coarse trabecular pattern. These changes regress completely at puberty.

Radiologic Features of the Jaws and Facial Bones

In their review of 16 cases of thalassemia major, Poyton and Davey (1968) found the following changes:

1. Small paranasal sinuses were found in 10 of the patients, particularly in the frontal and maxillary sinuses. Caffey originally described the classic changes in the frontal, temporal, and facial bones in 1957. Marrow hyperplasia in these bones prevents pneumatization of the paranasal and mastoid sinuses. The exception is the ethmoid sinuses because they lack red marrow. These changes are unique to thalassemia and are not seen in other anemias.
2. Osteoporosis was observed in seven patients; all of their patients were younger than 13 years of age.
3. A prominent anterior maxilla was present in 12 patients.
4. A thin cortex at the posterior and inferior margins of the ramus was obvious in 14 patients; in some instances, the abnormal thinning of the cortex extended along the lower border of the mandible.
5. The alveolar bone was characterized by blurring or effacement of the trabeculae, most commonly in the posterior regions. Marrow space enlargement with pronounced trabeculae was found in the anterior regions of the mandible and maxilla and occurred in seven of their patients.
6. Thinning of the lamina dura and crypts of developing teeth was observed easily in 14 patients, and in 2 patients the lamina dura and both crypts were not visible. The radiopaque outline of the crypts of developing teeth appeared to be separated from the teeth, with an enlarged space between the crypt and tooth. This finding was limited to the posterior regions only and was seen less frequently than the thinning of the lamina dura and tooth crypts.
7. The roots of the teeth appeared short and spike shaped. This was particularly apparent in the mandibular first molars and central incisors and occurred in 9 of their 16 patients.

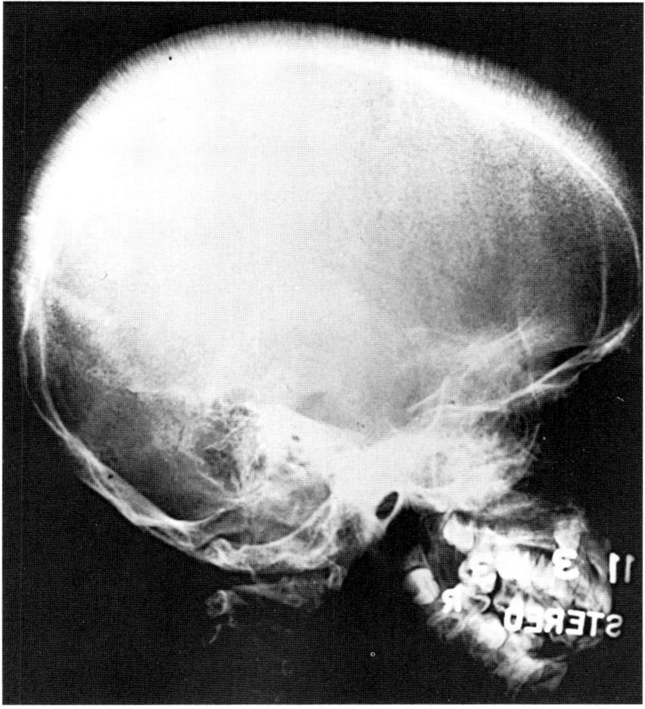

A

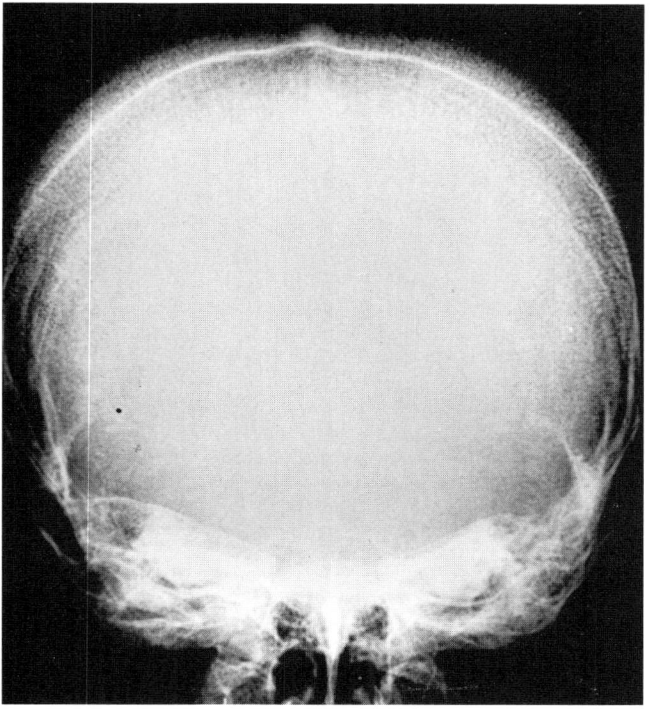

B

FIGURE 15–23.

Thalassemia: A and B, Figures show thinning of inner table, effacement of outer table, hair-on-end appearance of trabeculae, and granular appearance of most of the remaining skull.

Radiology of the Skull

In their review of 16 cases of thalassemia major in children, Poyton and Davey (1968), found the following changes:

1. Thickening of the calvarium, mostly in the anterior region, was found in 14 of their patients, and according to Caffey (1957), the frontal bones show the earliest and most striking changes. The result is a widened diploic space with displacement and thinning of the outer table.
2. A fine granular pattern, which was obvious and pronounced.
3. Circular holes in the diploe were observed in 15 of their patients and were thought to represent blood vessel spaces. These appear as vascular notches, which are normal, but are more prominent. Worth (1963) and Poyton and Davey (1968) postulated that these blood vessels play a role in the development of the widened diploe.
4. A condensed inner table of the calvarium was found. This accentuated inner plate was present in all of their patients. The thinned outer table adds to the prominence of this finding.
5. Striations of the calvarium were observed. Worth (1963) described this finding as a hair-on-end effect, caused by an alignment of the diploic trabeculae in a position perpendicular to the tables and a relative absence of the thinned outer table because of radiologic burnout.
6. In 12 of their patients, the shape of the pituitary fossa was altered; however, these authors found that such changes may be seen in normal patients. The change is characterized by a lobular enlargement of the pituitary fossa in the anterior region. They postulated that this finding may be associated with the stunted growth observed in many of these patients.

References

Normal Bone Density

Bras J, et al: Radiographic interpretation of the mandibular angular cortex: a diagnostic tool in metabolic bone loss. Part I. Normal state and postmenopausal osteoporosis. Oral Surg Oral Med Oral Pathol 53:545, 1982.

Osteoporosis

Affrim PA: An epidemiological study of clinical and trochanteric fractures of the femur in an unborn population: analysis of 1,664 cases with special reference to etiologic factors. Acta Orthop Scand [Suppl] 65:1, 1964.

Aloia JF, et al: Radiographic morphometry and osteopenia in spinal osteoporosis. J Nucl Med 18:425, 1977.

Benson BW: Age Related Changes in a Panoramic Mandibular Index of Cortical Bone Mass as Observed in Three Different Populations. Thesis, University of Texas Health Science Center School of Dentistry, 1986.

Bras J, et al: Radiologic interpretation of the mandibular angular cortex: a diagnostic tool in metabolic bone loss. Part I. Normal state and postmenopausal osteoporosis. Oral Surg Oral Med Oral Pathol 53:541, 1982a.

Bras J, et al: Radiologic interpretation of the mandibular angular cortex. Part II. Renal osteodystrophy. Oral Surg Oral Med Oral Pathol 53:647, 1982b.

Edeiken J: Roentgen Diagnosis of Diseases of Bone. 3rd Ed. Baltimore: Williams & Wilkins, 1981, p. 830.

Farmer HE, White LR, Brady JA, Bailey KR: Race and sex differences in hip fracture incidence. Am J Public Health 74:1374, 1984.

Garn SM: The Earlier Gain and the Later Losses of Cortical Bone in Nutritional Perspective. Springfield, IL:Charles C Thomas, 1970, p. 231.

Garn SM, Poznanski AK, Nagy JM: Bone measurement in the differential diagnosis of osteopenia and osteoporosis. Diagn Radiol 100:509, 1971.

Garraway WM, Stauffer RN, Kurland LT, O'Fallen WM: Limb fractures in a defined population: 1. Frequency and distribution. Mayo Clin Proc 54:701, 1979.

Gordan GS, Halden A, Vaughan C: Early detection of osteoporosis and prevention of hip fractures in elderly women. Med Times 21:104, 1981.

Groen JJ, Menczel J, Shapiros S: Chronic destructive periodontal disease in patients with pre-senile osteoporosis. J Periodontol 39:19, 1968.

Heaney RP: Paradox of irreversibility of age-related bone loss. In: Menczel J, Robin GC, Makin M, Steinberg R, eds. Osteoporosis. New York: John Wiley & Sons, 1982, p. 15.

Heaney RP: Prevention of age-related osteoporosis in women. In: Avioli LV, ed. The Osteoporotic Syndrome: Detection, Prevention, and Treatment. New York:Grune & Stratton, 1983, p. 124.

Krook L, Lutwak L, Whalen JP, et al: Human periodontal disease: morphology and response to calcium therapy. Cornell Vet 62:32, 1972.

Lachman E: Osteoporosis: the potentialities and limitations of its roentgenologic diagnosis. AJR Am J Roentgenol 74:712, 1955.

Lane SM, Vigorita VJ: Current concepts: review. Osteoporosis. J Bone Joint Surg (Am) 65:274, 1983.

Mazzuoli G, et al: Mechanisms involved in the loss of bone mass with age. In: Menczel J, Robin GC, Makin M, Steinberg R, eds. Osteoporosis. New York:John Wiley & Sons, 1982, p. 26.

Melton LJ, Riggs BL: Epidemiology of age related fractures. In: Avioli LV, ed. The Osteoporotic Syndrome: Detection, Prevention, and Treatment. New York:Grune & Stratton, 1983, p. 45.

Nordin BEC: In: Avioli LV, ed. The Osteoporotic Syndrome: Detection, Prevention, and Treatment. New York:Grune & Stratton, 1983, p. 30.

Riggs BL, et al: Differential changes in bone mineral density of the appendicular and axial skeleton with aging. J Clin Invest 67:328, 1981a.

Riggs BL, Hamstra A, DeLuca HF: Assessment of 25 hydroxyvitamin D 1a-hydroxylase reserve in postmenopausal osteoporosis by administration of parathyroid extract. J Clin Endocrinol Metab 53:833, 1981b.

Shapiro R: Metabolic bone disease: a basic review. Clin Radiol 13:238, 1962.

Singh M, Nagrath AR, Maimi PS: Changes in trabecular pattern of the upper end of the femur as an index of osteoporosis. J Bone Joint Surg (Am) 52:457, 1970.

Slovik D, et al: Deficient production of 1,25-dihydroxyvitamin D in elderly osteoporotic patients. N Engl J Med 305:372, 1981.

Stevenson J, et al: Calcitonin and the calcium regulating hormones in postmenopausal women: effect of estrogens. Lancet 1:693, 1981.

Worth HM: Principles and Practice of Oral Radiologic Interpretation. Chicago:Year Book Medical Publishers, 1963, pp. 181, 318.

Wovern NV: Variations in bone mass within the cortices of the mandible. Scand J Dent Res 85:444, 1977.

Wovern NV, Stoltze K: Sex and age differences in bone morphology of mandibles. Scand J Dent Res 86:478, 1978.

Wovern NV, Stoltze K: Age differences in cortical width of mandibles determined by histoquantification. Scand J Dent Res 87:225, 1979a.

Wovern NV, Stoltze K: Comparative bone morphometric analysis of mandibles and second metacarpals. Scand J Dent Res 87:358, 1979b.

Wovern NV, Stoltze K: Pattern of age related bone loss in mandibles. Scand J Dent Res 88:134, 1980.

Rickets/Osteomalacia

Arnstein AR, Frame B, Frost HM: Recent progress in osteomalacia and rickets. Ann Intern Med 67:1296, 1967.

Edeiken J: Roentgen Diagnosis of Diseases of Bone. 3rd Ed. Baltimore: Williams & Wilkins, 1981, p. 852.

Gibilisco JA: Stafne's Oral Radiographic Diagnosis. 5th Ed. Philadelphia: WB Saunders, 1985, p. 277.

Jaworski ZFG: Pathophysiology, diagnosis, and treatment of osteomalacia. Orthop Clin North Am 3:623, 1972.

Milkman LA: Pseudofractures (hunger osteopathy, late rickets, osteomalacia): report of a case. AJR Am J Roentgenol 24:29, 1930.

Worth HM: Principles and Practice of Oral Radiologic Interpretation. Chicago:Year Book Medical Publishers, 1963, p. 341.

Hypophosphatasia

Baer PN, Brown NC, Hamner JE III: Hypophosphatasia: report of two cases with dental findings. Periodontics 2:209, 1964.

Beumer J, Trowbridge HO, Silverman S Jr, Eisenberg E: Childhood hypophosphatasia and premature loss of teeth: a clinical and laboratory study of 7 cases. Oral Surg Oral Med Oral Pathol 35:631, 1973.

Bruckner RJ, Rickles NH, Porter DR: Hypophosphatasia with premature shedding of teeth and aplasia of cementum. Oral Surg Oral Med Oral Pathol 15:1351, 1962.

Dickson W, Harrocks RH: Hypophosphatasia in children. J Bone Joint Surg (Br) 40:64, 1958.

Fraser D: Hypophosphatasia. Am J Med 22:730, 1957.

Fung DE: Hypophosphatasia. Br Dent J 154:49, 1983.

Kjellman M, Oldfelt V, Nordenram A, Olow-Nordenram M: Five cases of hypophosphatasia with dental findings. Int J Oral Surg 2:152, 1973.

Poyton HB: Oral Radiology. Baltimore:Williams & Wilkins, 1982, p. 251.

Rathbun JC: Hypophosphatasia: a new developmental anomaly. Am J Dis Child 75:822, 1948.

Worth HM: Principles and Practice of Oral Radiologic Interpretation. Chicago:Year Book Medical Publishers, 1963, p. 341.

Hyperparathyroidism

Albright F, Reifenstein EC: The Parathyroid Glands and Metabolic Bone Disease. Baltimore:Williams & Wilkins, 1948, p. 175.

Askanazy M: Über Ostitis deformans ohne osteides Gewebe. Arb Geb Pathol Anat Inst Tübing 4:398, 1904.

Bartter FC: Bone as a target organ toward a better definition of osteoporosis. Perspect Biol Med 16:215, 1973.

Bras J, et al: Radiographic interpretation of the mandibular angular cortex: a diagnostic tool in metabolic bone loss. Part II. Renal osteodystrophy. Oral Surg Oral Med Oral Pathol 53:647, 1982.

Bywaters EGL, Dixon AS, Scott JT: Joint lesions of hyperparathyroidism. Ann Rheum Dis 22:171, 1963.

Dodds WT, Steinbach HI: Primary hyperparathyroidism and articular cartilage calcification. AJR 104:281, 1968.

Edeiken J: Roentgen Diagnosis of Disease of Bone. Baltimore, Williams & Wilkins, 1981.

Hutton CE: Intradental lesions and their reversal in a patient being treated for end-stage renal disease. Oral Surg Oral Med Oral Pathol 60:258, 1985.

Jackson CE, Frame B: Diagnosis and management of parathyroid disorders: symposium on metabolic bone disease. Orthop Clin North Am 3:699, 1972.

Kelly WH, Mirahmadi MK, Simon JH, Gorman JT: Radiographic changes in the jawbones in end stage renal disease. Oral Surg Oral Med Oral Pathol 50:372, 1980.

Pellegrino SV: Primary hyperparathyroidism exacerbated by pregnancy. Oral Surg Oral Med Oral Pathol 35:915, 1977.

Pugh DG: Subperiosteal resorption of bone: roentgenologic manifestations of primary hyperparathyroidism and renal osteodystrophy. AJR 66:577, 1951.

Rosenberg EH, Guralnick WC: Hyperparathyroidism: a review of 220 proved cases, with special emphasis on findings in the jaws. Oral Surg Oral Med Oral Pathol 15:84, 1962.

Sarosi G, Doe RP: Familial occurrence of parathyroid adenomas, pheochromocytoma and medullary carcinoma of the thyroid with amyloid stroma (Sipple's syndrome). Ann Intern Med 68:1305, 1968.

Silverman S, et al: The dental structures in primary hyperparathyroidism. Oral Surg Oral Med Oral Pathol 15:426, 1962.

Silverman S, Ware W, Gillooly C: Dental aspects of hyperparathyroidism. Oral Surg Oral Med Oral Pathol 26:184, 1968.

Spolnik KJ, et al: Dental radiographic manifestations of end-stage renal disease. Dent Radiogr Photogr 54:21, 1981.

Steinbach HL, et al: Primary hyperparathyroidism: a correlation of roentgen, clinical and pathologic features. AJR Am J Roentgenol 86:329, 1961.

Terezhalmy GT, Feltman R, Bottomley WK: Initial evidence of primary hyperparathyroidism presenting in the mouth: a case report. J Oral Med 33:4, 1978.

von Recklinghausen FD: Die fibrose oder deformirende Ostitis, die Osteomalacie und die osteoplastiche Carcinose in ihren gegenseitigen. Beziehungen, Festschrift. Berlin:Rudolf Virchow, 1891, p. 89.

Watson L, Faccini JM: Metabolic diseases in the jaws. In: Cohen B, Kramer RH, eds. Scientific Foundations in Dentistry. London:William Heinemann, 1976, p. 573.

Weiss A: Incidence of subperiosteal bone resorption in hyperparathyroidism studies by fine detail bone radiography. Clin Radiol 25:273, 1974.

Wood NK, Goaz PW: Differential Diagnosis of Oral Lesions. St. Louis: CV Mosby, 1985, p. 487.

Worth HM: Principles and Practice of Oral Radiologic Interpretation. Chicago:Year Book Medical Publishers, 1963, p. 354.

Massive Osteolysis

Aston JN: A case of massive osteolysis of the femur. J Bone Joint Surg (Am) 40:514, 1958.

Butler RW, McCance RA, Barret AM: Unexplained destruction of the shaft of the femur in a child. J Bone Joint Surg (Br) 40:487, 1958.

Frederiksen NL, Wesley RK, Sciubbas JJ, Helfrick J: Massive osteolysis of the maxillofacial skeleton: a clinical, radiographic, histologic and ultrastructural study. Oral Surg Oral Med Oral Pathol 55:470, 1983.

Gorham LW, Stout AP: Massive osteolysis (acute spontaneous absorption of bone, phantom bone, disappearing bone): its relation to hemangiomatosis. J Bone Joint Surg (Am) 37:985, 1955.

Heffez L, Doku HC, Carter BL, Feeney JE: Perspectives on massive osteolysis: report of a case and review of the literature. Oral Surg Oral Med Oral Pathol 55:331, 1983.

Jackson JBS: A boneless arm. Boston Med Surg J 18:368, 1838.

Jackson JBS: Absorption of humerus after fracture: reported to the Boston Society for Medical Improvement by the various gentlemen under whose observation the case had fallen. Boston Med Surg J 87:245, 1872.

Johnson PM, McClure JG: Observations of massive osteolysis radiology. Radiology 71:28, 1958.

Romer O: Die pathologie der Zahne. In: Henke F, Lubarsh O, eds. Handbuch der speziellen patologischen Anatomie und Histologie. Berlin:Springer-Verlag, 1924, p. 135.

Ross JL, Schinella R, Shenkman L: Massive osteolysis: an unusual cause of bone destruction. Am J Med 65:367, 1978.

Stout AP: Tumors of blood vessels. Tex Med 40:362, 1944.

Sickle Cell Anemia

Cox G: Pathological effects of sickle cell anemia on the pulp. Dent Res 56-B:B243 (abstr no. 767), 1977.

Diggs LW, Ahmann CF, Bibb J: Incidence and significance of the sickle-cell trait. Ann Intern Med 7:769, 1933.

Edeiken J: Roentgen Diagnosis of Diseases of Bone. 3rd Ed. Baltimore: Williams & Wilkins, 1981, p. 1047.

Herrick JB: Peculiar elongated and sickle shaped red blood corpuscles in a state of severe anemia. Arch Intern Med 6:517, 1910.

Konotey-Ahulu F: Mental nerve neuropathy: a complication of sickle cell crisis. Lancet 2:388, 1972.

Manning CG: A study of oral pain experience in sickle cell patients. Oral Surg Oral Med Oral Pathol 58:39, 1984.

Mourshed F, Tuckson CR: A study of the radiographic features of the jaws in sickle-cell anemia. Oral Surg Oral Med Oral Pathol 37:812, 1974.

Prowler JR, Smith GW: Dental bone changes occurring in sickle-cell diseases and abnormal hemoglobin traits. Radiology 65:762, 1955.

Reynolds J: An evaluation of some roentgenography signs in sickle-cell anemia and its variants. South Med J 55:1123, 1962.

Robinson IB, Sarnat BG: Roentgen studies of the maxillae and mandible in sickle-cell anemia. Radiology 58:517, 1952.

Sanger RG, Greer RO, Averbach RE: Differential diagnosis of some simple osseous lesions associated with sickle-cell anemia. Oral Surg Oral Med Oral Pathol 43:538, 1977.

Sebes JI, Diggs LW: Radiographic changes of the skull in sickle-cell anemia. AJR Am J Roentgenol 132:373, 1979.

Thalassemia

Caffey J: Cooley's anemia: a review of the roentgenographic findings in the skeleton. AJR Am J Roentgenol 78:381, 1957.

Poyton HB, Davey KW: Thalassemia: changes visible in radiographs used in dentistry. Oral Surg Oral Med Oral Pathol 25:564, 1968.

Van Dis ML, Langlais RP: The thalassemias: oral manifestations and complications. Oral Surg Oral Med Oral Pathol 62:229, 1986.

Worth HM: Principals and Practice of Oral Radiologic Interpretation. Chicago:Year Book Medical Publishers, 1963, p. 367.

Chapter 16

Focal Radiopacities

PERIOSTITIS OSSIFICANS OF GARRÈ

(Garrè's osteomyelitis, proliferative periostitis of Garrè, nonsuppurative ossifying periostitis, osteomyelitis sicca, osteomyelitis with proliferative periostitis, Garrè's chronic nonsuppurative sclerosing osteitis, periostitis ossificans, mandibular subperiosteal swellings in children, perimandibular ossification)

According to Shafer and colleagues (1983), periostitis ossificans of Garrè is a periosteal reaction characterized by a focal gross thickening of the periosteum with exuberant peripheral reactive bone formation in response to an attenuated infection. Many credit Carl Garrè (1893) as the first to describe this condition in 1893, 2 years before the discovery of x-rays. Garrè apparently reported a bony swelling of the jaw adjacent to a retained root of a lower first molar. He contended that the disease consisted of bone production but did not recognize it as a periosteal reaction.

Wood and colleagues (1988) reported that the condition is most common in the femur, not along the anterior surface of the tibia, in people younger than 25 years of age. According to Eversole and associates (1979), many orthopedic surgeons doubt that the condition exists as a discrete entity because a variety of orthopedic diseases may manifest a neoperiostosis, and although it may be controversial whether the entity exists in the long bones, it now seems that its existence in the jaws is unequivocal. In the more recent literature, this condition in the jaws probably was reported first by Lovemann in 1941, who discussed mandibular subperiosteal swellings in children. In 1948, Berger reported a case with all of the typical characteristics of periostitis ossificans and discussed a possible traumatic origin. In 1955, Pell and co-workers introduced the term Garrè's osteomyelitis of the mandible and described the definitive features. The term "periostitis ossificans" first was used by Gorman in 1957. Nortjé and colleagues reviewed the literature in 1988 and found 35 reported cases since Lovemann's article (1941). The condition is more common than this number of cases would indicate.

Pathologic Characteristics

Eversole and colleagues (1979) and Lichty and co-workers (1980) believed that periostitis ossificans is a reactive lesion of the periosteum. Eversole and colleagues (1979) classified the etiologic factors into two categories: odontogenic and nonodontogenic. The odontogenic group consists mainly of a carious tooth, pericoronal inflammation, and the inflammatory paradental cyst, especially those associated with mandibular first permanent molars. In reports by Gorman (1957), Lichty and colleagues (1980), Eversole and co-workers (1979), Mattison and co-authors (1981), Nortjé and co-investigators (1988), and Worth and Stoneman (1972), the inflammatory paradental cyst was not always recognized. Clinically evident osteomyelitis may or may not be present. When present, it may be of odontogenic origin. When the etiologic factor is eliminated, the condition resolves. In some documented cases, no etiologic factor can be found, such as mentioned by Ellis and colleagues (1977) and Eisenbud and co-authors (1981).

Histologically, the lesions are supracortical but subperiosteal and are composed of reactive trabecular bone and osteoid with an associated cellular fibrovascular connective tissue matrix. The osseous trabeculae are lined with numerous osteoblasts and manifest prominent reversal lines. Eversole and colleagues (1979) recognized three distinct patterns for the arrangement of the trabeculae: (1) parallel, showing a linear orientation of the trabeculae; however, these were perpendicular to the cortex; (2) retiform, showing a network or meshwork appearance; and (3) fibrous dysplasia-like, with irregular trabeculae that did not show anastomotic interconnections. The presence of inflammatory cells is a variable feature; however, some acute and mainly chronic inflammatory cells have been reported in the surrounding tissues.

Clinical Features

Nortjé and colleagues (1988) reviewed 35 reported cases. The mean patient age was 11 years, and the age range was 17 months to 31 years. Among their 93 new cases, the mean patient age was 13 years, with a range from 2 to 69 years. There was a predilection for male patients, with a ratio of 1.3:1 over female patients. Other clinical features have been reviewed by Lichty and co-authors (1980), Eversole and co-workers (1979), and Nortjé and co-investigators (1988). Facial asymmetry is invariably present. Usually, a focal nontender bony enlargement of the mandible is palpable; sometimes, this area is tender, and the mucobuccal fold may be lost. The swelling is of a "bony hardness," and the overlying skin and mucosa usually appear normal. Monteleone and colleagues (1962) reported that an extraoral fistula was present on the skin in their patient. Although pain usually is not a complaint, a history of antecedent pain may be elicited. Nortjé and colleagues (1988) observed that 75% of their cases were associated with a carious tooth, usually the mandibular first permanent molar; 10% occurred in association with untreated fractures; 2 of their cases (2%) were associated with inflammatory paradental cysts; and 1 patient (1%) had primary tuberculosis.

Treatment/Prognosis

The most common treatment has been removal of the causative tooth. Concurrent antibiotic coverage often is administered, although the utility of this therapy has not been proven. Mattison and colleagues (1981) were the first to treat the affected teeth by endodontic therapy in combination with antibiotics, which resulted in complete resolution. When an inflammatory paradental cyst is present, curettage of the area and antibiotic coverage produced resolution. The swelling usually disappears within 2 to 6 months, with a return of the normal bone architecture. At times, resolution is protracted over a 1-year period.

◆ *RADIOLOGY (Figs. 16–1 to 16–6)*

Periostitis ossificans evolves through three stages. The first consists of an apparent thickening of the periosteum, without radiologic evidence of new bone formation; however, when this tissue is examined histologically, osteoid and bone trabeculae are present. In the second stage, a single layer followed by multiple laminations of new bone are formed between the periosteum and cortex. The third stage occurs during resolution and is characterized as a gross thickening without laminations.

Nortjé and colleagues (1988) found that lateral views of the mandible consisting principally of panoramic and lateral oblique projections showed this condition best. In 84% of their cases, the lateral projection showed the periosteal reaction; 28% were visible on the posteroanterior views, and 25% were seen on the occlusal views. In 11% of patients, the reaction was solely visible on the occlusal view, and in 5% the condition could be seen only on the posteroanterior view. If lateral views alone were used, 16% (15 cases) would have gone undetected.

Location

Nortjé and colleagues (1988) found lesions in the following locations: lower first permanent molar, 51%; lower second permanent molar, 13%; lower primary second molar, lower premolar, lower third molar, and angle of the mandible, 9% each. Two percent occurred adjacent to fractures and in one instance adjacent to an upper premolar. The periosteal reaction was observed at three main sites: the inferior border of the mandible, 83%; buccal cortex, 43%; and lingual cortex, 7%. A single site occurred in 69% of the cases, 2 sites in 29%, and all 3 sites in 2% (2 cases). The condition was limited to the lingual side in only 2 patients. Periostitis ossificans is usually unilateral; however, in 2 cases the periosteal reaction crossed the midline. Seventy-five percent occurred on the left side. In 21 of the 93 cases in which periapical pathosis was equal bilaterally, 76% had periostitis ossificans on the left side and 24% on the right side. They also observed a case in the sigmoid notch area. Eisenbud and colleagues (1981) reported a case affecting all 4 quadrants in an 11-year-old girl with chronic rarefying osteomyelitis.

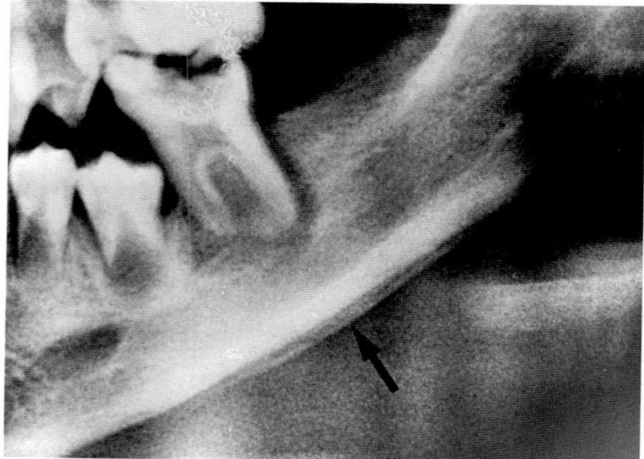

FIGURE 16–1.

Periostitis Ossificans of Garrè: Early reaction showing periosteal thickening and beginning of calcification of first lamination (arrow).

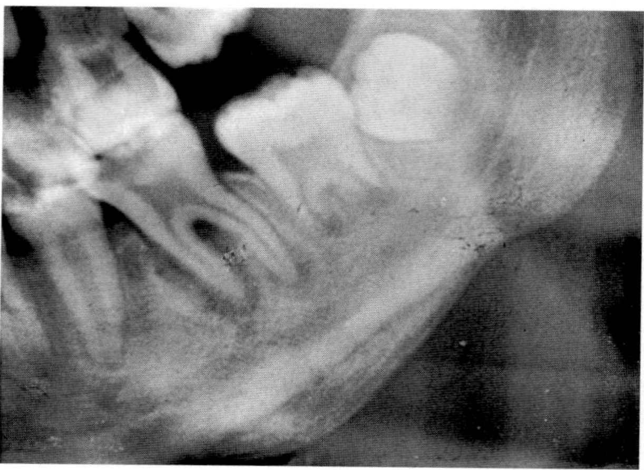

A

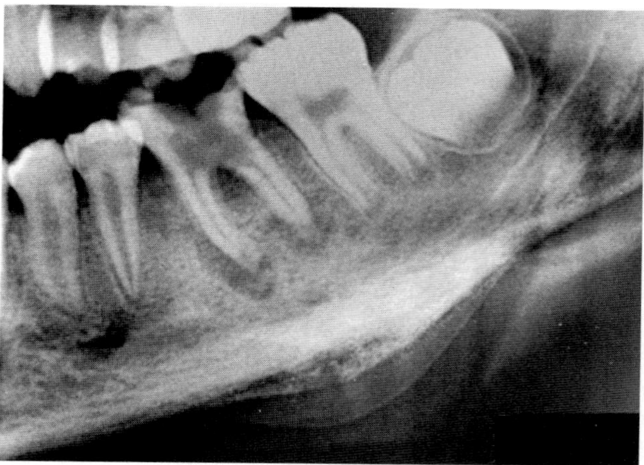

B

FIGURE 16–2.

Periostitis Ossificans of Garrè: In acute phase, distinct laminations are seen. A, Multiple laminations are present and inferior cortex is intact. B, Thickened area adjacent to cortex indicates previous resolution. New layers represent reactivation of untreated infection.

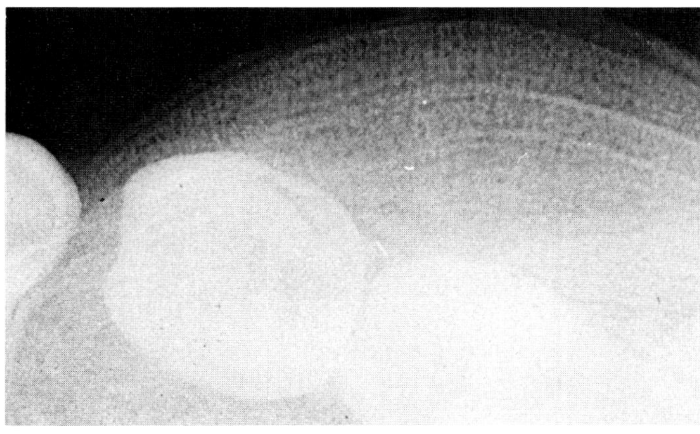

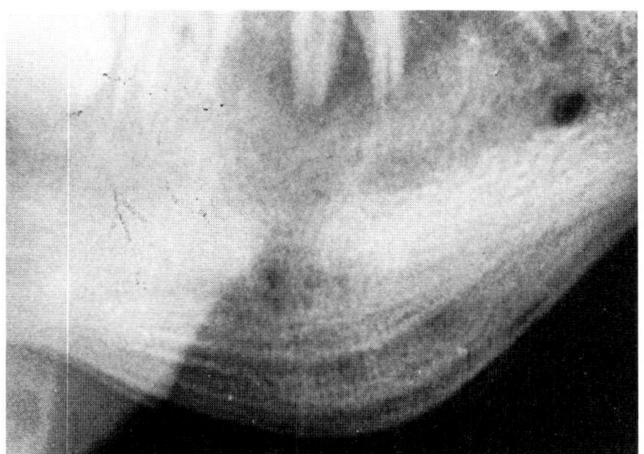

A B

FIGURE 16–3.

Periostitis Ossificans of Garrè: A and B, Fine radiaform striations perpendicular to laminations and cortex. (A, From Farman AG, Nortjé CJ, Wood RE: Oral and Maxillofacial Diagnostic Imaging. Philadelphia:Mosby-Year Book, 1993, p. 200; B, Courtesy of Drs. L. and I. Chilvarquer, São Paulo, Brazil.)

"Onion Skin" Pattern

A single or several layers of subperiosteal new bone are seen. The underlying cortex is usually visible and intact. The development of these laminations has been discussed by Smith and Farman (1977) and Nortjé and colleagues (1988). In the initial stage, the periosteum becomes elevated and appears thickened radiologically, but there is no evidence of calcification. The thickening consists of periosteum, uncalcified bone matrix, and poorly calcified bone. Calcification immediately beneath the periosteum becomes evident as a single curved line of cortex-like bone. Ultimately, inflammatory elements penetrate through this newly formed bone, and the same process is reinitiated and results in a second lamination of subperiosteal new bone. Multiple laminations give the reaction an onion skin appearance. During the phase in which laminations are being formed, radiolucent material may be seen separating the laminations and the outermost unmineralized layer is apparent. As resolution begins, the areas between the laminations appear more radiopaque and the outermost unmineralized layer disappears. The absence of such lucent zones indicates resolution of the disease. As healing progresses, the subperiosteal new bone is remodeled and resorbed until finally all evidence of the pre-existing periosteal reaction disappears, leaving normal cortical bone.

Nortjé and colleagues (1988) found that the number of

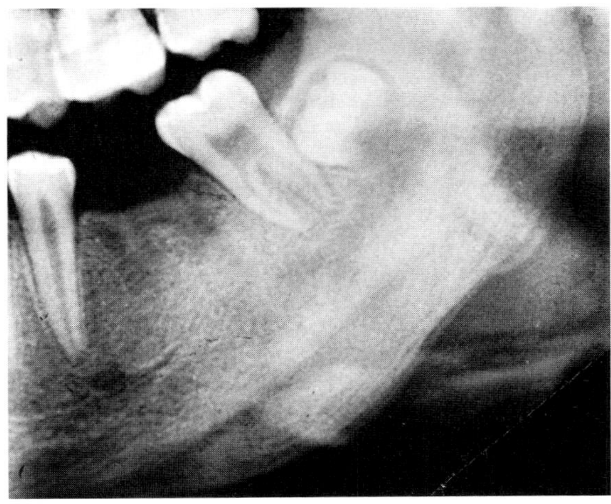

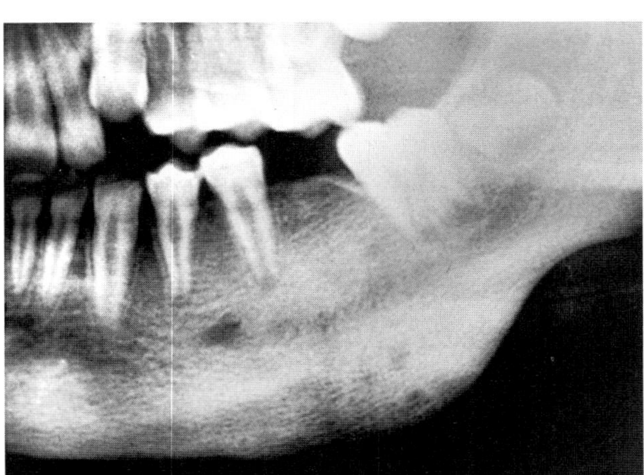

A B

FIGURE 16–4.

Periostitis Ossificans of Garrè: During resolution, laminations become less distinct. The inferior cortex blends with remodeling periosteal bone. A, Several months after tooth extraction. (Courtesy of Dr. P. Dhiravarangkura, Chulalonghorn University School of Dentistry, Bangkok, Thailand.) B, Five months after tooth extraction.

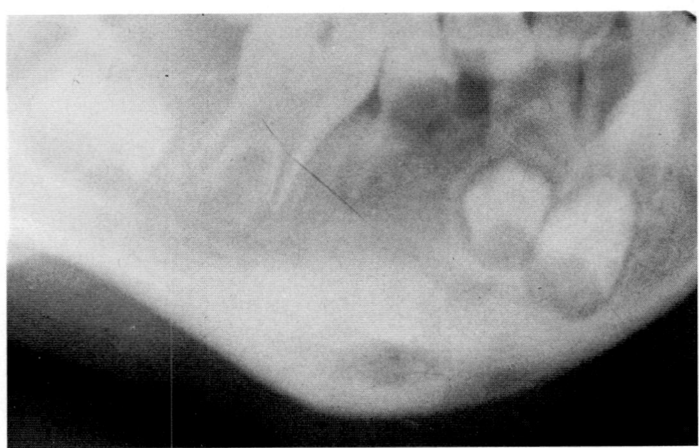

A

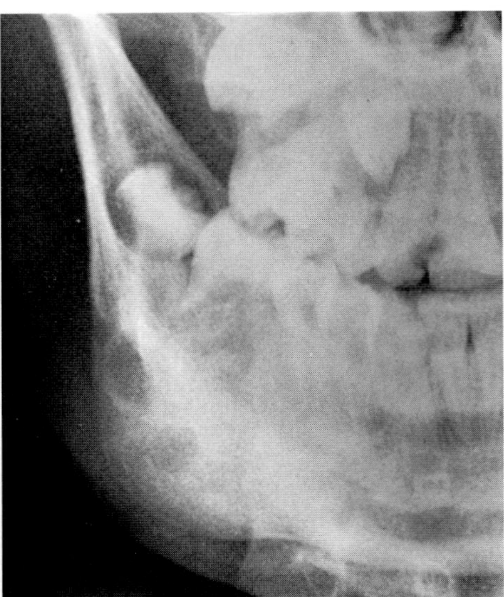

B

FIGURE 16–5.

Periostitis Ossificans of Garrè: Radiolucent areas are seen in acute and resolving cases. A, Lateral view. (Courtesy of Lilian and Israel Chilvarquer, São Paulo, Brazil.) B, Posteroanterior view. (Courtesy of Professor M.E. Parker, University of the Western Cape, Tygerberg, Republic of South Africa.)

laminations could be counted in 86 of 93 cases. In 58% a single lamination was observed, 2 laminations in 22%, 3 laminations in 8%, and 4 laminations in 4%. Five or more laminations were seen in only 7 cases, and the maximum number of laminations was 12. No factors predictive of the number of laminations could be found; however, in younger patients the periosteal response was wide and short, whereas in older patients it was longer and narrower.

Nortjé and colleagues (1988) observed areas of patchy increased density overlying the mandible in cases involving the buccal cortex. This increased density resembles osteosclerosis or focal sclerosing osteomyelitis; however, it is actually the result of attenuation of the x-ray beam as it passes through the layers of reactive subperiosteal buccal bone.

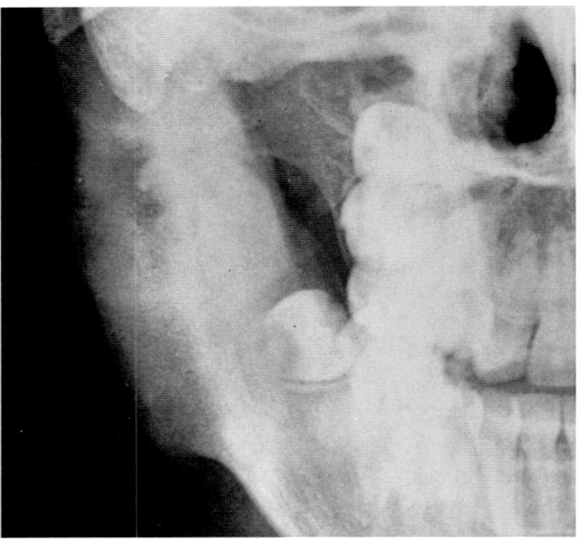

FIGURE 16–6.

Periostitis Ossificans of Garrè: Case involves the ramus.

"Radial" Pattern

In the occlusal view, a radial pattern of bony trabeculae may be seen perpendicular to the long axis of the mandibular body and cortex and perpendicular to the laminations of subperiosteal new bone. To our knowledge, this finding has not been reported. These radiaform trabeculae are fine, of uniform thickness, equidistant from each other, and separated by a thin band of radiolucent material and appear less calcified toward the periphery. At the outer surface, the periosteum and newly elaborated uncalcified matrix form the outermost layer, with the bands of radiolucent material extending into this most peripheral zone. These radiolucent bands probably represent the fibrovascular connective tissue seen histologically. Radiologically, it appears that outgrowths of this fibrovascular connective tissue may be associated in some way with the continued stimulation of the periosteal reaction and the radiaform pattern of the fine bony trabeculae. This radiaform pattern may be absent in some cases. Other patterns include a more disorganized arrangement of crisscrossing trabeculae and a ground glass-like appearance of the osseous material.

Other Radiologic Features

Nortjé and co-workers (1988) observed a number of other findings within the periosteal new bone and underlying cortex. In lateral-view radiographs, the cortex was well defined in 77%, moderately well defined in 14%, and poorly defined in 9%. Destruction of the shadow of the former cortex and within the periosteal new bone may be seen in association with some malignant conditions such as Ewing's sarcoma, osteosarcoma, and chondrosarcoma. In 21% of cases, irregular, or circular areas of lysis were seen within the periosteal new bone. These areas are presumed to be inflammatory in origin. In 66% of the cases, sequestrum formation was radiologically detectable. Among these cases, 62% were less than 1 mm in diameter, 20% were 1 to 2 mm, and 18% were larger than 2 mm. The size of the sequestra was age dependent, with smaller sequestra present in younger patients. Among those with sequestra, 82% had fewer than five sequestra, whereas the remainder had more than five radiologically detectable sequestra. These appear as small separate radiopaque flecks within the subperiosteal new bone. There are very few reports concerning the presence of sequestra in association with proliferative periostitis, although they were observed by Worth (1963).

Other findings include effacement of the crypt walls of developing teeth, a common finding, and more advanced eruption of developing teeth in the area as compared with the same teeth on the opposite side. Nortjé and colleagues (1988) postulated that when the radiologic features are pathognomonic, biopsy is unnecessary. If there is destruction of the underlying cortex, destruction within the periosteal new bone, or movement of teeth or tooth buds, a biopsy is highly recommended. After treatment, complete resolution is determined radiologically and characterized by the presence of a normal cortex and an absence of periosteal thickening. Although periostitis ossificans usually is diagnosed radiologically, it shows a fibro-osseous pattern histologically. Therefore, Eversole and colleagues (1979) emphasized that the histopathologic diagnosis of periostitis ossificans requires a review of the combined clinical, radiologic, and histologic features.

ROOT FRAGMENTS

Root fragments are seen in areas previously occupied by teeth. They may be seen occasionally in the maxillary sinus and paragnathic soft tissues. They result most often from neglect, iatrogenic dentistry, or trauma. Root fragments of primary teeth may occur idiopathically in one, several, or all four quadrants in the same person. Nyyssonen and colleagues (1983) examined 8000 Finnish adults who were 30 years or older; 15% had retained root tips. The male-to-female ratio was 2:1. It was surmised that this was because women receive more dental services. Although there were no significant age-related differences, the peak incidence was in the fifth decade. Older patients had relatively more retained roots with respect to remaining teeth because of previous extractions. City dwellers had slightly more retained roots than did rural populations. The mean number of retained roots was 0.4 per subject. Nyyssonen and colleagues (1983) obtained their data by visual inspection only and did not use radiographs; Makila and Suoranta (1978) and Wolf (1969) performed similar studies in Finnish population groups, but they used radiographs. The prevalence of retained roots was 14 to 19%; however, the mean number of roots per person increased from 0.4 to a mean of 1.4 to 1.5 per person. Thus, it seems prudent to at least take a panoramic radiograph for any new patient with missing teeth. Most retained root tips should be removed. If a root tip is buried in bone and there is no radiographic or clinical evidence of an associated abnormality, it may be left alone and observed periodically.

◆ RADIOLOGY (Figs. 16–7 to 16–10)

When root tips are observed radiographically, the following information should be obtained:

1. Root morphologic characteristics, including bulbous versus tapered, dilaceration, resorption, or ankylosis as evidenced by an absence of the periodontal membrane space.
2. Multiple roots as indicated by a "double" periodontal membrane space along one side of the root and an abrupt narrowing of the root canal space. These indicate either a "bell-shaped" root with a bifurcated root canal space or two roots, one superimposed on the other. An off-angle periapical view is useful in separating superimposed roots.
3. The relationship to the crest of the ridge, recorded as completely embedded in bone, contiguous with the crest of the ridge and covered by soft tissue, or projecting into the oral cavity. Because panoramic radiographs are produced with much less radiation than periapical films, they usually have sufficient latitude to show hard and soft tissue outlines, a feature often absent in intraoral films.
4. The relationship to anatomic structures such as the inferior alveolar canal, nasal fossa, and maxillary sinus. When an intimate relationship exists between a root and the inferior alveolar canal, there may be resorption of the cortical wall of the canal as it crosses the root, a horizontal dark band limited to the root area intersected by the canal, and a narrowing of the portion of the canal that intersects the root. In the first instance, the canal wall is resorbed by pressure from the adjacent root. In the second, the root is thinned and notched by the canal; therefore, it is relatively more radiolucent. In the last case the canal is narrowed because it is surrounded partly or completely by the adjacent root. One or more of these findings may be present. At times a root tip may appear to intrude into the maxillary sinus on a panoramic radiograph. The lingual object is projected upward and the buccal object downward with respect to objects in the central plane of the layer. Thus, apparent intrusion of a root tip into the maxillary sinus may represent panoramic projection geometry and not a true relationship. Corrected axial tomography through the root will show its position clearly with respect to adjacent structures such as the inferior alveolar canal or antrum.
5. The presence of an abnormality such as inflammatory disease, cyst formation, or a mass.

Root tips normally have a root canal space, lamina dura, and periodontal membrane space; however, when these are absent it may be difficult to distinguish a root tip from osteosclerosis and socket sclerosis. On close examination, os-

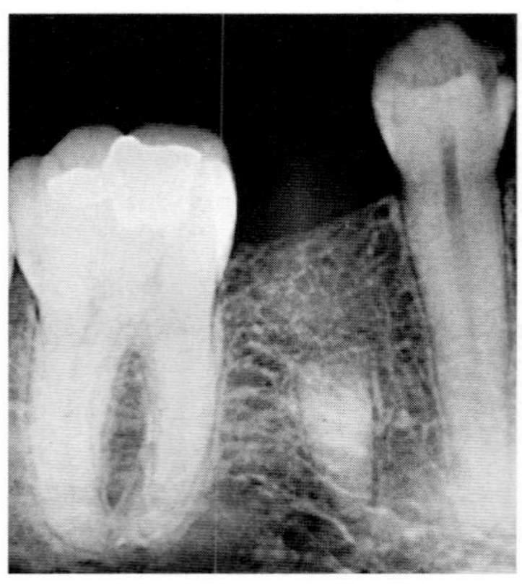
A

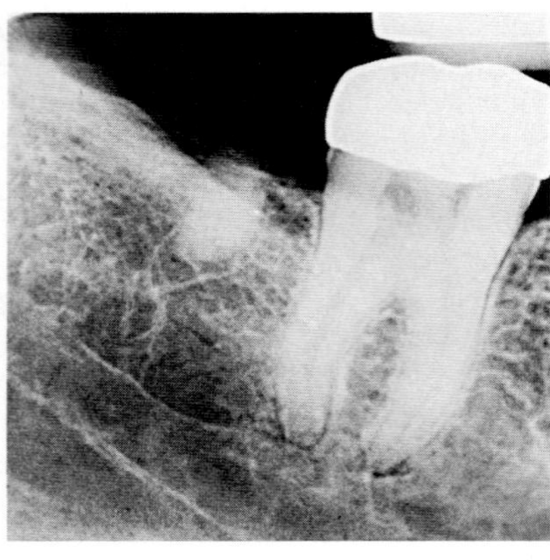
B

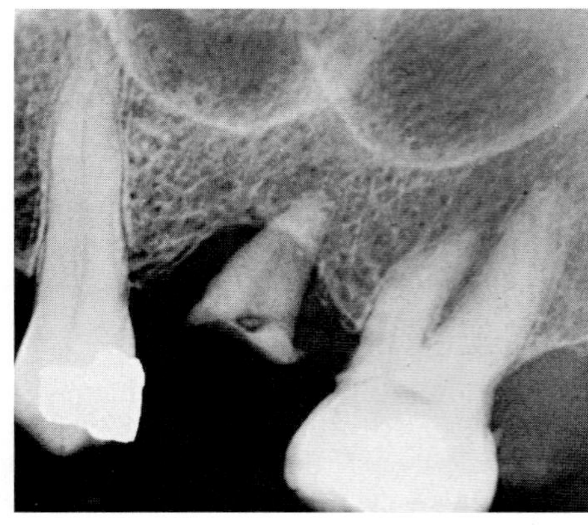
C

FIGURE 16–7.

Retained Root Tips: A, Entirely within bone. Lamina dura, periodontal membrane, and root canal spaces are seen. B, Covered by soft tissue. C, Open into the oral cavity.

teosclerosis may have small spurs along the margin, whereas in socket sclerosis the lamina dura is usually present. Also, root tips are retained purposely to stabilize a prosthesis and preserve the alveolar ridge; such root tips often are treated endodontically and may contain a gold or alloy restoration. In the maxillary sinus the root tip may resemble an antrolith or antral exostosis.

SOCKET SCLEROSIS (Localized osteosclerosis)

Socket sclerosis first was reported by Burrell and Geopp in 1973. It is a form of osteosclerosis occurring uniquely in the socket area of previously extracted teeth. Burrel and Goepp (1973) found an incidence of approximately 3% in a population of hospital patients.

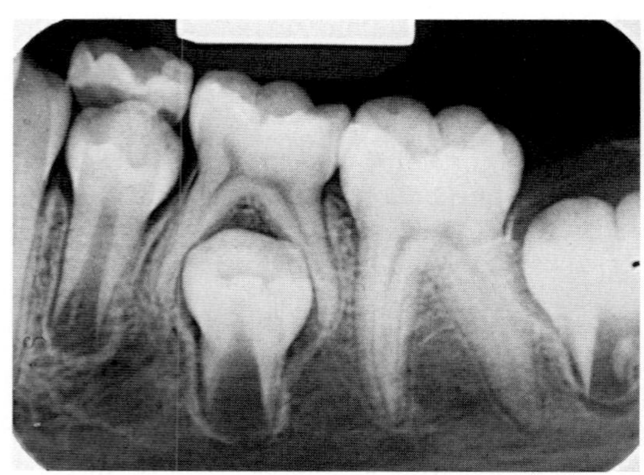
A

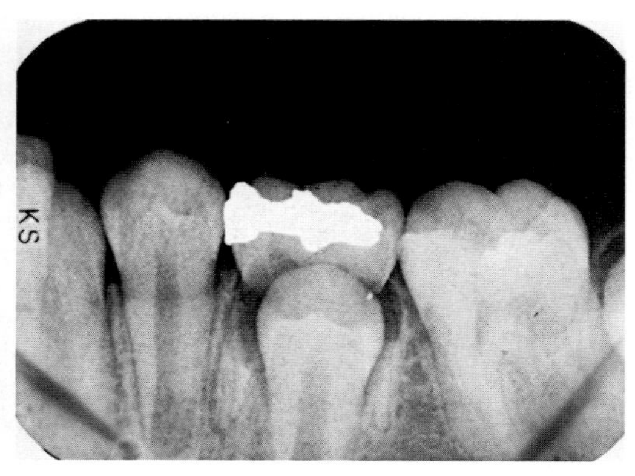
B

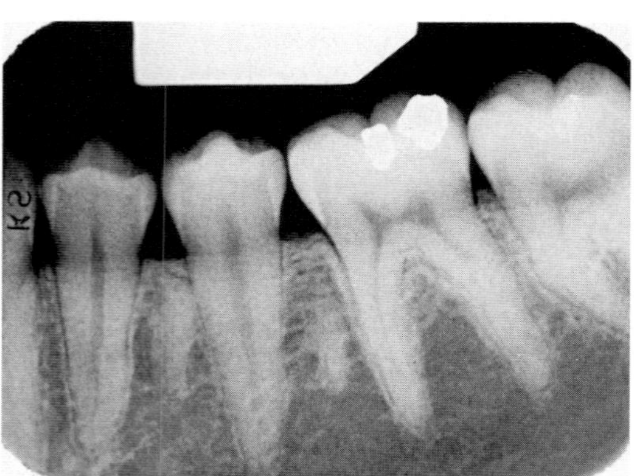
C

FIGURE 16–8.

Retained Root Tip: A, B, and C, Simulated chronology: development of noniatrogenically induced retained roots of primary first molar.

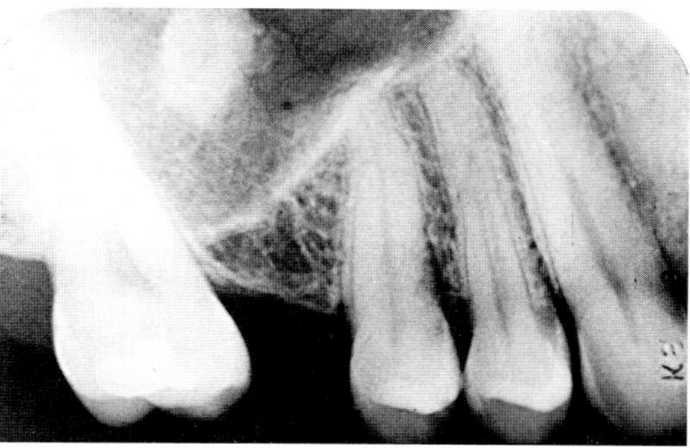

FIGURE 16–9.

Retained Root Tip: Shown in maxillary sinus. Differential diagnosis is antrolith or antral wall exostosis.

Pathologic Characteristics

Normal Socket Healing

Normal healing of the socket wound has been reviewed by Boyne (1966) and by Shafer and colleagues (1983). The histologic stages of healing are as follows:

1. There is an immediate reaction, during which a blood clot forms and fills the socket.
2. During the first week, the clot begins to organize as it starts to be replaced by young proliferating connective tissue (granulation tissue), which originates from remnants of the periodontal ligament at the periphery and proliferates toward the center of the clot.
3. During the second week, the organization process continues. The periodontal ligament remnants degenerate and are said to result in osteoblasts, which lay down trabeculae of osteoid extending out from the wall of the socket. From the edge of the soft tissue wound, epithelium begins to migrate across the top of the healing socket.
4. During the third week, trabeculae of uncalcified osteoid begin to replace the granulation tissue from the periphery inward. The lamina dura and crestal portions of the socket begin to be resorbed by prominent osteoclastic action, and a thin layer of epithelium covers the healing socket completely.
5. During the fourth week, the osteoid begins to calcify, forming a meshwork of coarse fibrillar bone throughout the socket.
6. During the final maturation process, there is progressive remodeling and replacement of immature bone by mature bone.

In an interesting study, Boyne (1966) injected patients with oxytetracycline at regular intervals, beginning on the fifth and sixth days after extraction. All patients were to receive maxillary complete dentures. In each patient, the healing maxillary premolar socket was excised surgically at 1-week intervals after two injections of oxytetracycline, 24 hours apart. Using fluorescence microscopy, Boyne (1966) could trace the origins of new bone formation. Minimal amounts of bone labeled on the fifth and sixth days were seen in the marrow vascular spaces of the bone surrounding the socket, with no new bone formation in the socket; however, on the seventh and eighth days, fluorescent new bone was observed in the marrow vascular spaces adjacent to and along the entire length of the lamina dura. Beginning on the ninth and tenth days, fluorescent new bone was present in the adjacent marrow vascular spaces and the socket proper along the peripheral aspect of the alveolus. By the thirteenth and fourteenth days, there was evidence of tagged new bone along the lateral wall of the socket and in the fundus, with approximately one third of the socket occupied by tagged bone. In summary, Boyne (1966) concluded that bone repair begins in the surrounding marrow, followed by the deposition of new bone along the wall of the socket and then filling

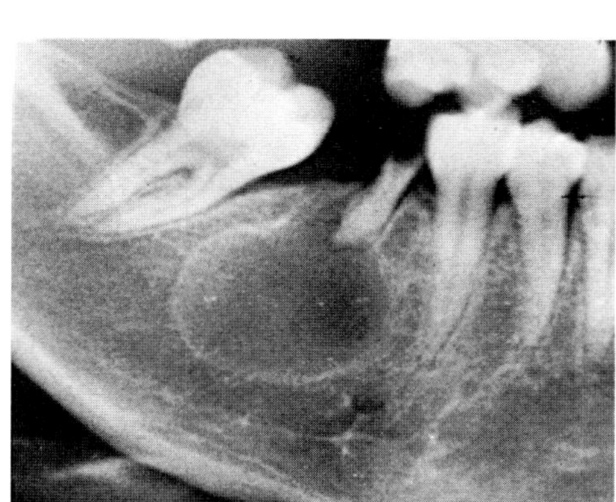

A

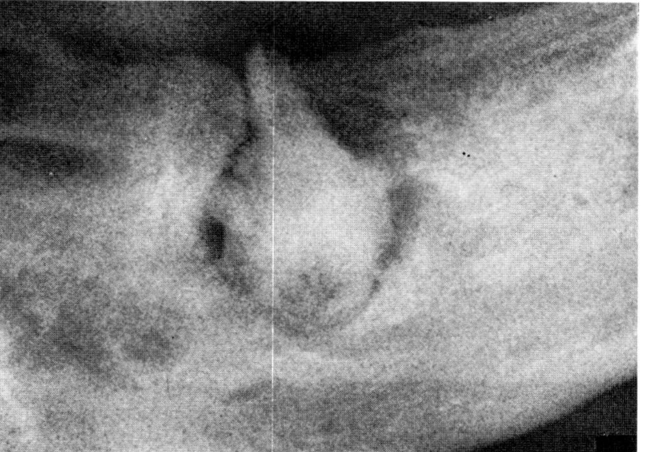

B

FIGURE 16–10.

Retained Root Tip: A, Associated with radicular cyst (apical periodontal cyst). B, Associated with benign cementoblastoma.

of the fundus. Even 2 weeks after surgery, Boyne (1966) observed new bone formation in the endosteal spaces adjacent to the socket. This study seems to indicate that the cells ultimately responsible for new bone formation originate in the adjacent marrow and not necessarily from multipotential cells of the periodontal ligament. The cells may originate from the adjacent periosteum and migrate to the socket through the surrounding marrow spaces.

Socket Sclerosis

Microscopically, socket sclerosis is seen as dense trabeculae of sclerotic bone. In a study of postextraction healing in vitamin A-deficient rats, Frandsen (1963) observed socket sclerosis radiologically identical to that observed by Burrell and Goepp (1973). Although Burrell and Goepp (1973) observed socket sclerosis in a number of patients with a variety of disorders, its presence correlated especially well with diseases of the gastrointestinal system and renal disorders. Additionally, 68% of patients with socket sclerosis had abdominal surgery. The gastrointestinal disorders affected the utilization of food products, especially inflammatory bowel, liver, and pancreatic diseases. The group with renal disorders had nephritis and nephrosis. Among these groups, Burrell and Goepp (1973) found normal serum calcium and phosphorus levels; however, the alkaline phosphatase levels were elevated slightly. Kaye and associates (1960) extensively analyzed 12 patients with chronic renal failure resulting from chronic pyelonephritis and found associated osteosclerosis, primarily in the lumbar vertebrae, but also at multiple other skeletal sites. Ball and Garner (1966) observed abnormal calcification at fracture sites in patients with malabsorption and azotemic forms of osteomalacia. Skoczylas and colleagues (1985) reviewed the literature and reported a case of myotonic dystrophy, a disorder associated with slow and insufficient intestinal absorption. These authors observed generalized osteosclerotic changes in the jaws and multiple areas of socket sclerosis.

Clinical Features

The patients had a median and average age of 40 years when socket sclerosis was discovered (age range, 16 to 76 years). Cases were distributed equally among men and women, and there was no racial predilection. Socket sclerosis is asymptomatic.

Treatment/Prognosis

We are are unaware of any studies determining whether socket sclerosis retrogresses on treatment of the systemic condition. Burrell and Goepp (1973) observed patients with socket sclerosis over many years and saw no change in bone density. The time period of disease onset can be estimated when the extraction histories of adjacent normally healed dentulous areas are compared with those of affected areas. Socket sclerosis also may be significant in forensic odontology because its presence in the absence of teeth may indicate past medical illness.

◆ RADIOLOGY (Figs. 16–11 to 16–13)

Radiologic Features of Normal Socket Healing

According to radiologic studies by Dalitz (1964), the first evidence of healing is the dissolution of the lamina dura, which can be observed between the eighth and sixteenth weeks. This may not be seen if the lamina dura was absent because of periodontal disease, other local disorders such as fibrous dysplasia, or a systemic disease such as hyperparathyroidism or Paget's disease. If there is sufficient film latitude, gingival tissue can cover the radiolucent socket during the fourth and fifth weeks. According to Shafer and colleagues (1983), radiologic evidence of calcification of the bone matrix does not occur until the sixth or eighth week after extraction, and there are still differences between the new bone of the healing socket and the surrounding alveolar bone for 4 to 6 months after extraction. Dalitz (1964) found that the socket disappeared after 17 to 34 weeks. There may be subtle changes for as long as 1 year and sometimes longer after extraction.

Radiologic Features of Socket Sclerosis

The radiologic features of socket sclerosis are unique. They are characterized by a lack of resorption of the lamina dura and deposition of sclerotic bone within the confines of the socket. The lack of lamina dura resorption is the earliest detectable sign of socket sclerosis. After this, there is an equal deposition of sclerotic bone longitudinally along the walls of the socket. Because the deposition along the walls is equal and the socket is narrower at the apex, the fundus is filled first. Finally, a thin radiolucent line of uncalcified

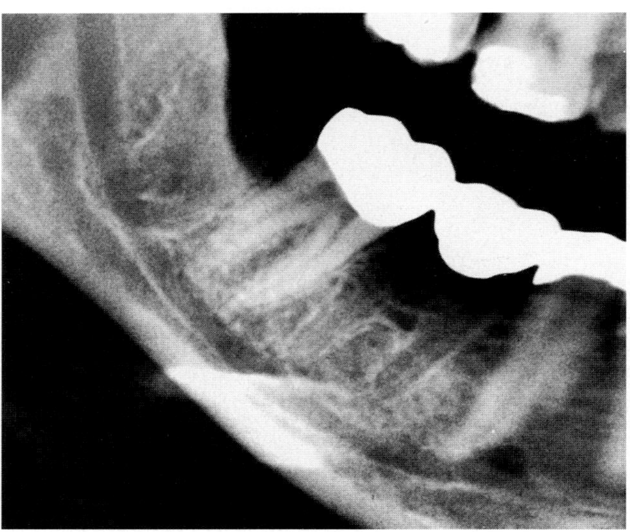

FIGURE 16–11.

Socket Sclerosis: First and third molar sockets are affected.

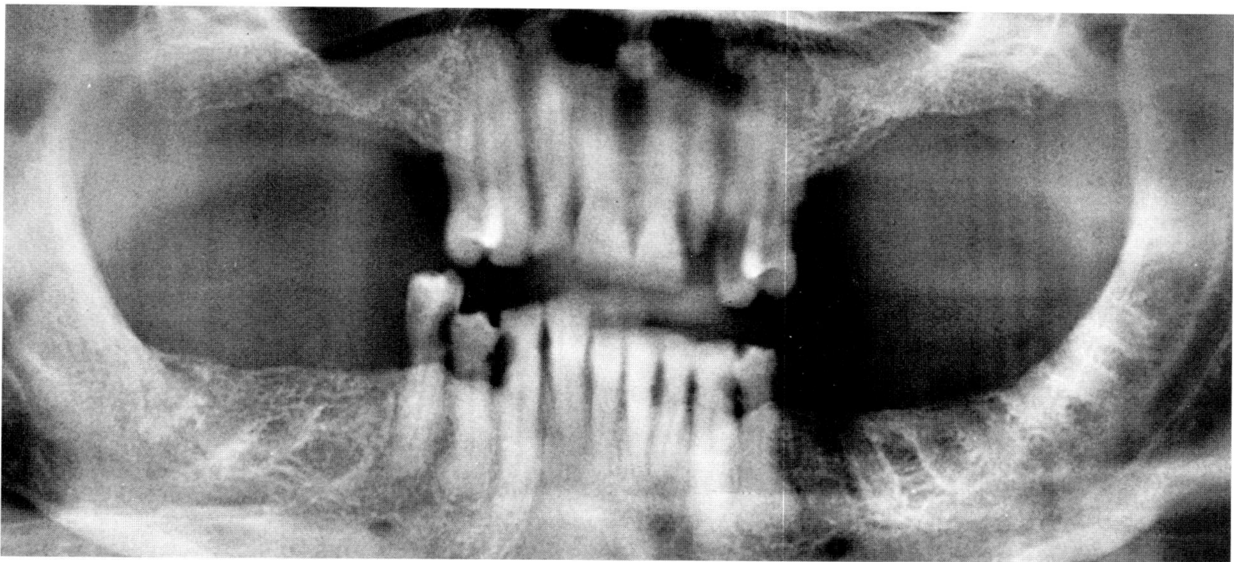

FIGURE 16–12.

Socket Sclerosis: Shown in a 63-year-old man receiving renal dialysis. Mandibular teeth were extracted after onset of renal disease, and maxillary teeth were removed before kidney problems occurred.

matrix is seen in the upper half of the socket. Ultimately all of the matrix calcifies and the thin line disappears, with the socket being filled completely with sclerotic bone. During these later two stages, socket sclerosis may be mistaken for an ankylosed root tip. The bone within the socket is denser than the surrounding bone. Eventually some trabeculation may crisscross the sclerotic socket; in some instances the trabeculation may be observed to be coarser, thicker, and denser than normal. Variations include an apparent disappearance of the lamina dura because of the extreme density of the sclerotic bone within the socket. Also, other cases may show a very prominent lamina dura but a much less dense material filling the socket area. In all instances, a return of trabeculation crisscrossing the affected socket indicates that the abnormal healing reaction is complete.

EXOSTOSIS

Exostoses are bony outgrowths from the outer cortex of the mandible and maxilla. Their cause is unknown; however, because they tend to occur in some families, a possible ge-

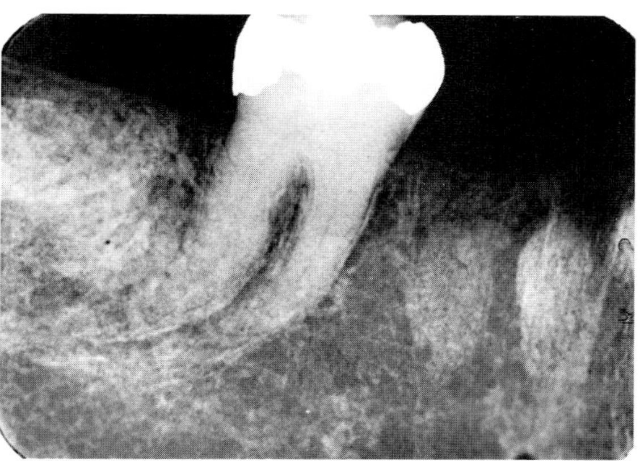

A

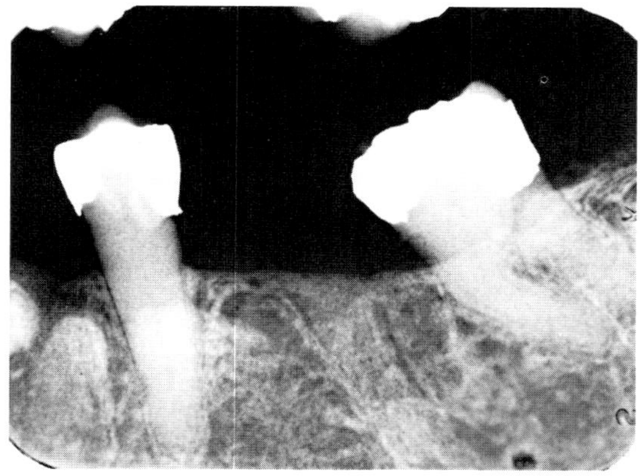

B

FIGURE 16–13.

Socket Sclerosis: A and B, A 47-year-old man with myotonic dystrophy. Progressive involvement of the smooth muscles of the gastrointestinal tract caused him to have ever-increasing malabsorption problems.

netic origin is suggested. Histologically, exostoses are indistinguishable from osteomas, with the distinction being based on clinical appearance and location. Exostoses may be very small, almost pinpoint in size, or they may occupy an entire quadrant. They may be nodular in shape and are sometimes lobulated. Exostoses usually are seen in adults; they begin to develop during the young adult years and reach their full size during the middle years. Most exostoses have a limited growth potential, reaching a certain size and remaining stable thereafter. The overlying tissue often has a normal color, although it may appear paler when the exostosis is pinpoint in size or when it is large. Overlying tissue does not tend to become traumatized in most patients. On palpation, exostoses are bony and hard, and pain should not be elicited. They are usually asymptomatic, although there may be pain if an area has been traumatized. Exostoses usually are diagnosed clinically and are not treated. They may be removed surgically for esthetics or if they interfere with a prosthesis. Exostoses usually do not grow again after complete removal.

◆ *RADIOLOGY (Figs. 16–14 and 16–15)*

The radiologic diagnosis of exostosis excludes the following more specific variants: lingual tori, palatal tori, subpontic hyperostosis, distal pseudohyperostosis, and osteoma. Exostoses usually are located on the periosteal surface of alveolar bone. They may be located on the buccal or lingual sides and may be single, multiple, or confluent. They are usually symmetrically bilateral. Radiologically, they appear as diffuse radiopacities in the region of the alveolar bone. An outer cortical margin may or may not be evident. Generally, those consisting of compact bone tend to have a uniform density, whereas those exhibiting an outer cortical rim may show a trabecular pattern with marrow spaces within.

TORI (Mandibular tori, lingual tori, palatal tori)

Tori are variants of exostosis occurring in a specifically defined location. In the jaws, tori are found in only two locations, with the specific nomenclature defining the location.

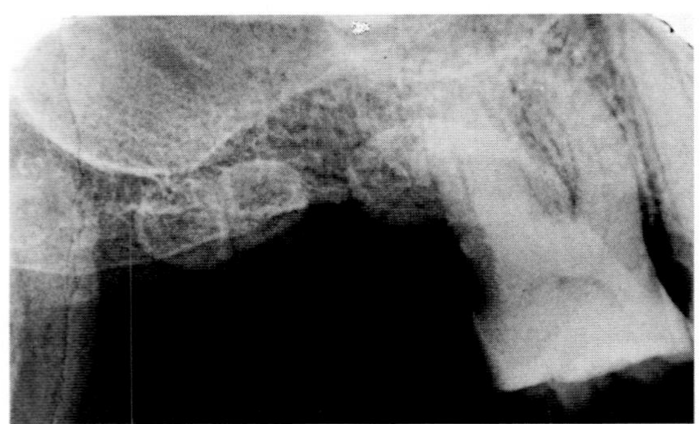

FIGURE 16–14.

Exostoses: Shown in a 55-year-old man. There are several small buccal exostoses in maxilla.

Mandibular or lingual tori occur on the lingual cortex of the mandible, whereas palatal tori are seen on the hard palate in the midline. Histologically, tori are identical to osteomas. They may be composed entirely of cortexlike compact bone, or there may be a central nidus of spongy bone surrounded by an outer layer of cortical bone. In a study of the Eskimo, Woo (1950) found torus palatinus in 65% of that population. Yaacob and colleagues (1983) reported an incidence of 25% in Malays, 23% in Chinese, and 6% in East Indian groups living in Malaysia. King and King (1981) cited an incidence of 36% among North Americans of African origin and 31% in white North Americans. King and Moore (1976) reported a much lower incidence in white people living in England. Although the differences between racial groups appear to be significant, Witkop and Barros (1963) found that the incidence of torus palatinus diminishes with more southerly latitudes, regardless of race. In Chile the incidence of maxillary torus was less than 1%.

The incidence of mandibular tori also varies among different racial groups. Yaacob and colleagues (1983) found an almost equal incidence of 2% among the Malays, Chinese, and East Indians studied. King and King (1981) reported an incidence of 14% among North Americans of African origin and 25% among white North Americans.

Suzuki and Sakai (1960) showed a strong hereditary pattern for palatal and mandibular tori. If either parent had tori, the minimum incidence in their children was 40%; if both parents had tori, the incidence in their offspring increased to 64%; and when neither parent had a torus, the incidence in the children was 5 to 8%.

Most studies show that women are affected by tori more often than men, particularly palatal tori. King and King (1981) found an incidence of 2:1, indicating a female prevalence of palatal tori, whereas the distribution of mandibular tori was equal among male and female patients. Yaacob and colleagues (1983) reported a female prevalence among those with palatal tori, with a ratio of 2.3:1 for Malays, 1.7:1 for Chinese, and 1.5:1 for East Indians. Among their 2400 patients in these ethnic groups, the incidence of torus mandibularis was approximately 1%, and all cases occurred in female patients.

Tori arise during adolescence, and the peak incidence occurs at age 30 in most studies. Palatal tori begin as small excretions and may achieve a diameter of approximately 4 cm. They may have one, two, four, or more lobes. Smaller tori tend to be attached on a broad base; however, larger palatal tori may be pedunculated. Mandibular tori are generally bilateral and may consist of a single nodule or three or four lobes. They tend to be symmetrical in form, number, and size. The lobes are side-by-side, causing the mandibular tori to extend more anteriorly or posteriorly, sometimes as far back as the second or third molar area. As they enlarge, they may meet in the midline, obscuring the anterior portion of the floor of the mouth. The soft tissue covering tori tends to be normal unless it has been traumatized. Pipe smoking and playing some wind instruments may cause chronic trauma of palatal tori. Usually tori are not treated, although they may be removed surgically if they interfere with function or a prosthesis.

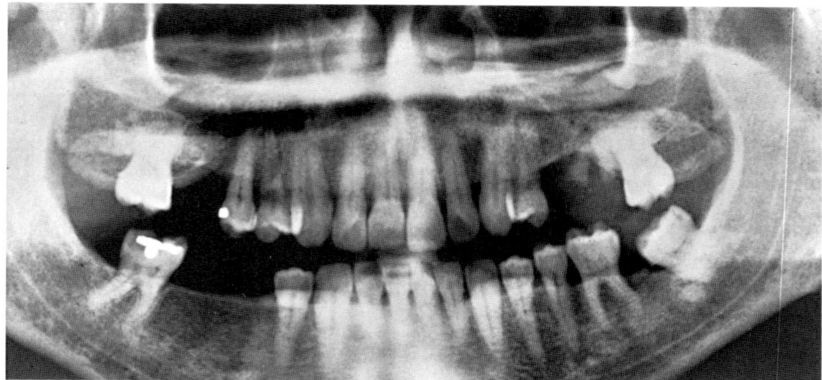

A

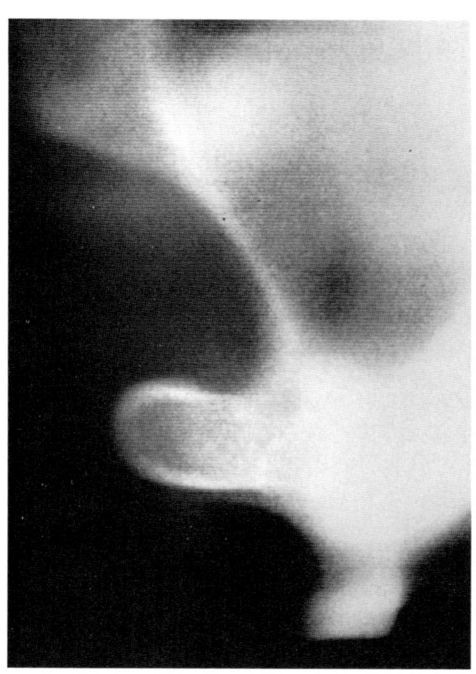

B

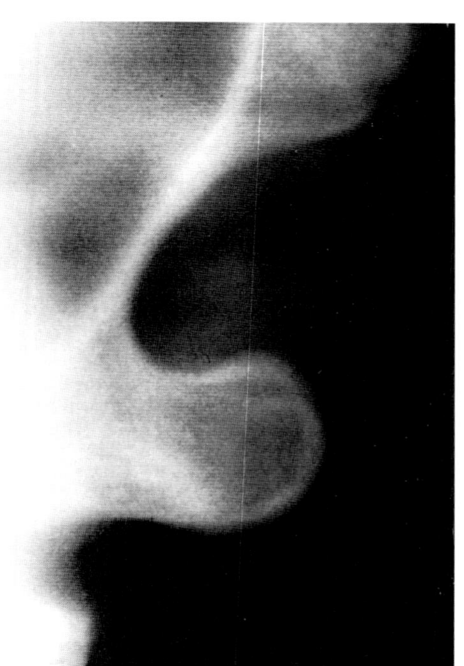

C

FIGURE 16–15.

Exostoses: A, Large bilateral buccal exostoses in the maxilla; outer cortex and medullary bone within. B and C, Coronal linear tomograms of similar case. Sinus and root of zygoma are shown above, and the maxilla and teeth are shown beside and below, respectively. (B and C, Courtesy of Dr. R. Monahan, Chicago, IL.)

◆ RADIOLOGY (Figs. 16–16 to 16–21)

The radiologic features of tori are similar to those of exostoses except tori are seen in specific locations. Tori may consist of a uniform radiodense area, or there may be an outer cortical rim with an inner core of medullary bone. They usually have smooth marginal contours, and bosselation may be evident when two or more lobes are present. Because tori increase in size by appositional bone growth, with incremental rings of new bone being laid down, this pattern sometimes can be seen radiologically. Although the torus appears to consist of a uniform radiodense mass, close scrutiny shows concentric rings of more dense bone within the sclerotic mass. Also, because tori are located on the outer cortex, they may extend beyond the limits of the alveolar bone in the image. This observation is important because excrescences of endosteal origin do not extend beyond the limits of the affected bone. In rare instances, mandibular and palatal tori may co-exist in the same patient; such instances have been documented by Suzuki and Sakai (1960). Occlusal films are useful in studying tori, especially mandibular tori.

Mandibular Tori

On periapical radiographs, mandibular tori tend to be projected in a superior direction if a negative projection angle of the beam is used. In panoramic radiographs they invariably are projected upward and may be superimposed on the cervical portion of the mandibular canine or bicuspid teeth. This upward projection results from the negative projection angle of the panoramic beam. Mandibular tori may not be seen in panoramic radiographs if they do not fall within the layer of the machine used. When they are imaged, they are disproportionately wide because of the horizontal magnification that occurs on the lingual side of the layer. Mandibular tori are in the canine-bicuspid area, above the mylohyoid ridge.

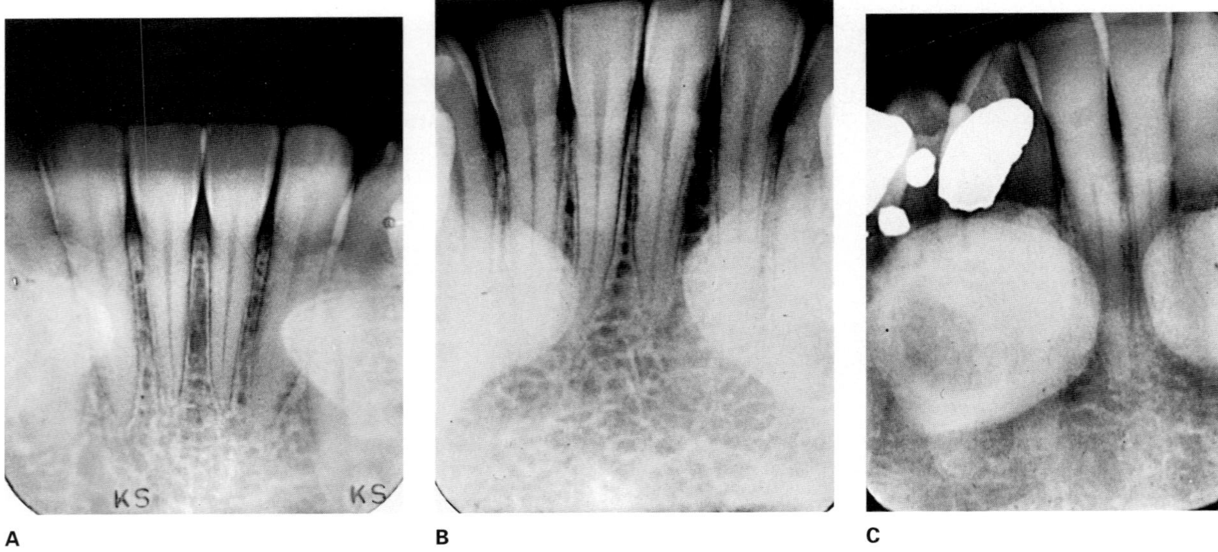

FIGURE 16–16.

Mandibular Tori: A, B, and C, Small, medium, and large bilateral mandibular tori, respectively.

Palatal Tori

On periapical radiographs, palatal tori tend to be projected downward and appear within the region of the maxillary sinus. When palatal tori are large and the film is placed sufficiently far back enough into the mouth, they may be superimposed at the apical region of anterior periapical views as well. On panoramic radiographs the palatal torus is seen as a double image bilaterally. The base of the torus is always continuous with the real image of the hard palate, and the torus may be seen to extend down into the sinus area or be superimposed on the apical portion of some of the maxillary anterior and posterior teeth. Depending on patient positioning and the machine design, the palatal torus will not be imaged if it does not fall within the diamond-shaped double-image zone as described by Langland and co-authors (1989).

SUBPONTIC HYPEROSTOSIS (Subpontic osseous hyperplasia, subpontic osseous proliferation, localized hyperostosis of the mandible, hyperostosis alveolaris externa)

Subpontic hyperostosis is a proliferation of bone on the alveolar ridge beneath a fixed bridge pontic. The condition probably is common, but we found only 6 reports of approximately 35 cases in the recent literature.

Pathologic Characteristics

The term hyperostosis implies an increased amount of normal bone. From reviews by Burkes and colleagues (1985), the cause is unknown. According to Wolfe's law, bone is laid down and remodeled in lines corresponding to the directions of stress, thus affecting the shape and dimensions of

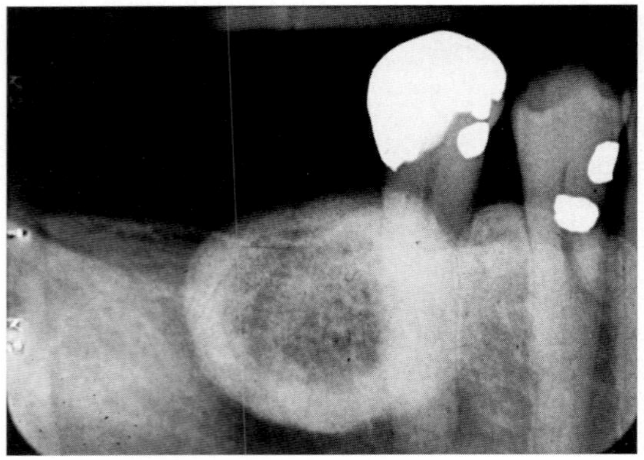

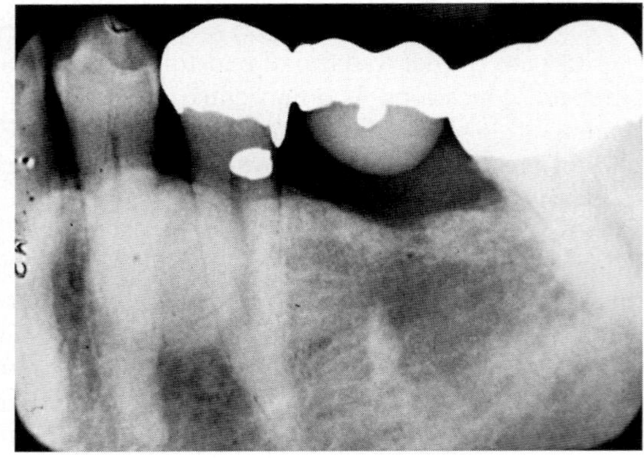

FIGURE 16–17.

Mandibular Tori: A and B, Large tori from Figure 16–16C. Right torus is composed of cortical bone and medullary bone within. Left side appears to consist solely of cortical bone.

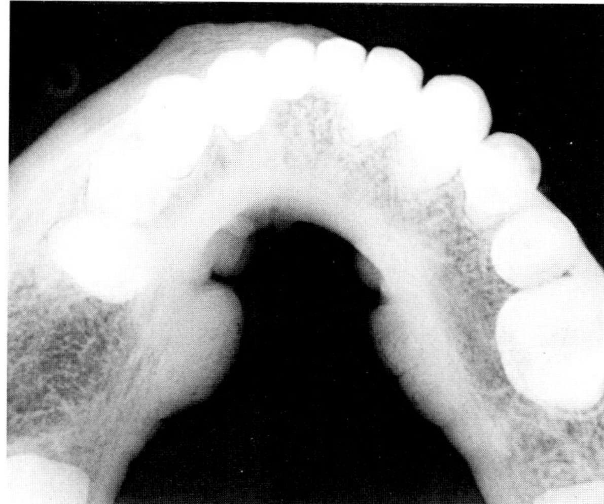

FIGURE 16–18.

Mandibular Tori: Occlusal view: multiple bilateral mandibular tori. (Courtesy of Professor L. Alfaro, University of Chile School of Dentistry, Pathology Referral Center, Santiago, Chile.)

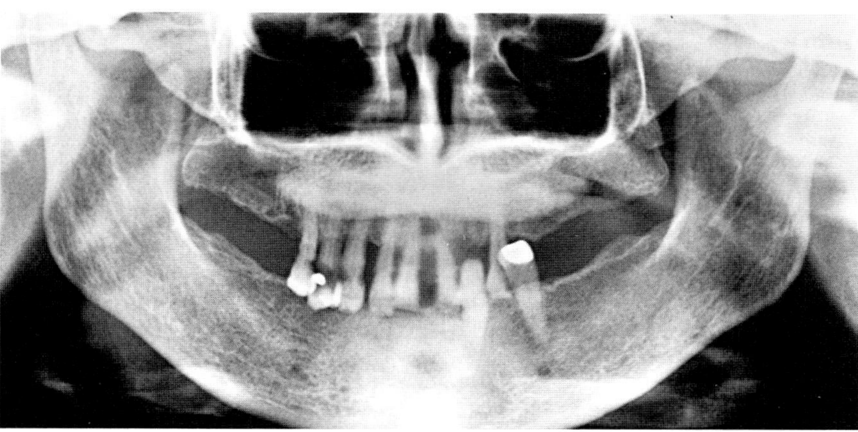

FIGURE 16–19.

Palatal Torus: The torus is seen as a single image in the maxillary midline because it is located anterior to the diamond-shaped area where double images occur.

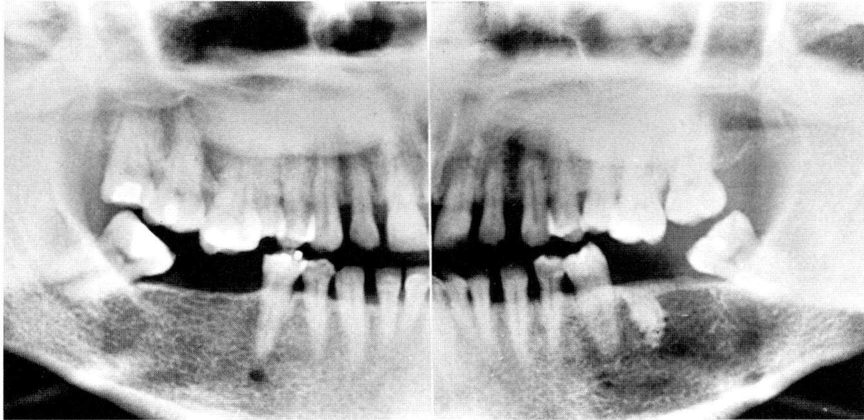

FIGURE 16–20.

Palatal Torus: The torus is seen as a double image in maxillary posterior regions bilaterally because it is located within the diamond-shaped area where double images are generated.

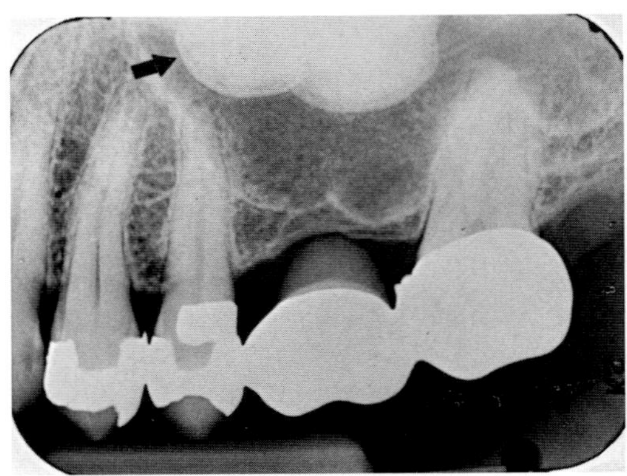

A

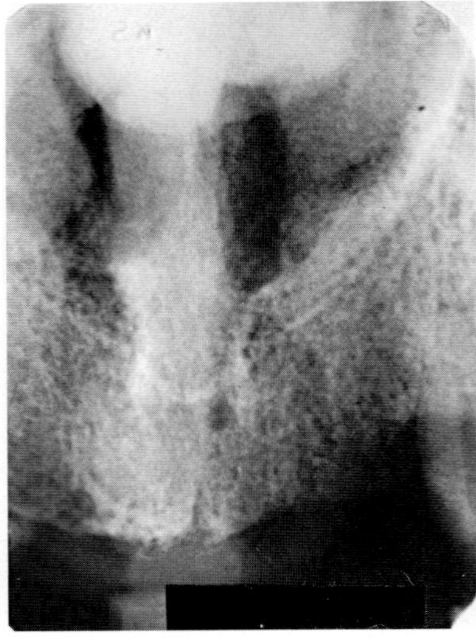

B

FIGURE 16–21.

Palatal Torus: A and B, Appearance of palatal tori in periapical views.

a bone. In hyperostosis alveolaris externa, these stresses may cause the crestal alveolar bone to grow along a vector opposing the forces of occlusion. There does not appear to be any association with the pontic design or material used; however, there may be some correlation with the presence of mandibular tori or buccal exostoses. Burkes and colleagues (1985) studied nine cases and found mandibular tori or buccal exostoses in six of nine patients. In reports by Morton and Nankin (1990) and Takeda and co-authors (1988), subpontic hyperostosis consists histologically of normal lamellar bone, occasional reversal lines may be seen, and an inflammatory cell infiltrate typically is absent. These findings are similar to those seen in tori, exostoses, and osteomas.

Clinical Features

After placement of a fixed prosthesis, hyperostosis develops months or many years later in a limited number of cases. In a case illustrated by Gibilisco (1985), the hyperostotic bone completely filled the space beneath the sanitary pontic within 4 years. Morton and Natkin studied 16 patients with 19 subpontic hyperostoses. Their sample included 10 men and 6 women with a mean age of 54 years. Most of the cases were asymptomatic, but one lesion was associated with dislodgement of the bridge. The overlying soft tissue usually appears normal; however, when the hyperostotic alveolar bone impinges on the pontic, the overlying gingiva may become inflamed, causing mild pain, food impaction, and occasional redness or bleeding. Appleby (1991), Calman and colleagues (1971), and Strassler (1981) have provided other reports. The shape, size, and height of the hyperostoses are related to the size of the edentulous space and the shape and height of the pontics.

Treatment/Prognosis

If the hyperostosis results in food impaction, gingival bleeding, compromised home care around the abutments, pain, or other related signs or symptoms, the hyperostotic bone should be removed.

In the report by Appleby, a subpontic hyperostosis was removed surgically and recurred later; conversely, when the patient's bridge became dislodged and was not replaced immediately, the hyperostotic area regressed spontaneously and a normal ridge contour was seen.

◆ *RADIOLOGY (Figs. 16–22 and 16–23)*

When antecedent radiographs have been available, the edentulous area appears normal, with no evidence of abnormal trabeculation or hyperostotic change. In some cases, mandibular tori or buccal exostoses may be observed. In the few published cases, including those of Gibilisco (1985), Langland and colleagues (1989), and Calman and colleagues (1971), the most frequent location was in the mandibular premolar-molar region. In some instances a single tooth is missing—often the mandibular first molar; in other cases the hyperostosis overlies an area previously occupied by several teeth. At least four bilateral cases have been reported. To our knowledge, no cases have been reported in the anterior mandible or anywhere in the maxilla.

The hyperostosis appears to manifest in two distinct morphologic patterns. In the first, the hyperostotic bone develops in the middle of the edentulous space and extends up toward the pontic in a mound-like fashion as its base broadens; thus, the hyperostotic bone is cone shaped, with the tip of the cone extending toward the pontic. The surface is usually smooth, but it may be slightly nodular. In the second morphologic pattern, the hyperostotic bone appears to extend up toward the pontic at the same rate as its base broadens; in this instance, the hyperostotic bone completely fills the space beneath the pontic, with the most superior aspect of the hyperostotic bone conforming to the shape of the base of the overlying pontic. The superior surface is either flat, referred to as "plateauization" by Strassler (1981), or it may be saucer shaped, depending on the shape of the pontic. It is possible that this second morphologic pattern represents a more mature form of the first mound-shaped pattern.

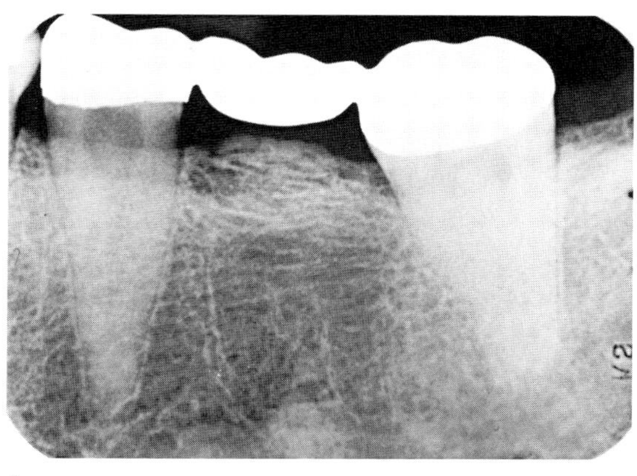

A

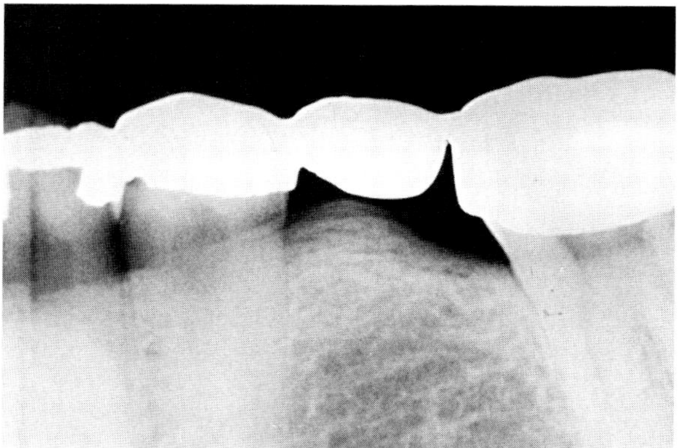

B

FIGURE 16–22.

Subpontic Hyperostosis: Dome shaped. A, Small hyperostosis. Trabeculae are more horizontal than is usual, with an increase in number, density, and thickness toward the pontic. B, Horizontal lamellae within the hyperostotic area.

The hyperostotic bone may consist entirely of bone, having the same density as alveolar bone without evidence of an overlying cortex. At times a thin layer of cortical bone overlies the hyperostotic outgrowth, and in other instances the entire hyperostotic excrescence may consist of a uniform density resembling cortical bone. In several cases described by Morton and Nankin (1990), a sclerotic reaction was observed in the adjacent alveolar bone, sometimes extending inferiorly to the level of the apices of the adjacent teeth. In several of our cases, we noticed a more horizontal arrangement of the trabecular pattern in the alveolar bone immediately subadjacent to the pontic. Toward the surface of the ridge, these horizontal trabeculae become coarser and more numerous, to become a distinct thickening at the crest of the ridge. These are incorporated into the hyperostotic area as distinct horizontal lamellations. There is a distinct absence of vertical trabeculations.

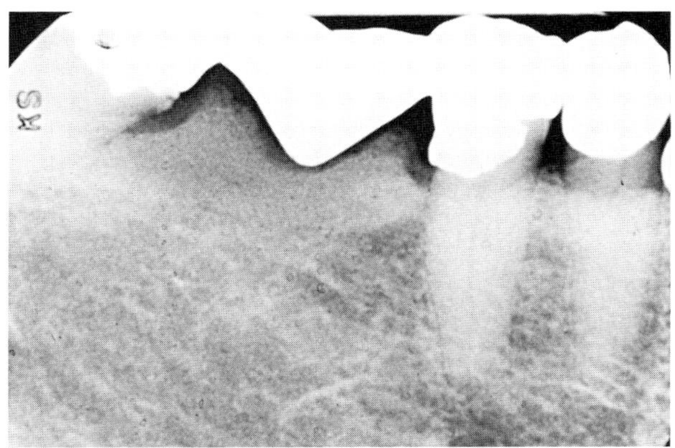

FIGURE 16–23.

Subpontic Hyperostosis: Saddle shaped. Hyperostotic area is very dense, like cortical bone. Fine, tightly arranged, slightly curved horizontal lamellae could be seen in the original radiograph.

DISTAL MANDIBULAR PSEUDOHYPEROSTOSIS

Distal mandibular pseudohyperostosis first was described by Langlais and Kastle in 1978. The case was recognized and provided by Dr. Monique Michaud, Université de Montréal, Québec, Canada. This condition represents an anatomic variant characterized by an apparent increase in the height of the alveolar bone seen on the distal of the last molar in the mandibular arch. The condition develops in all cases after removal of a tooth; however, there are two separate and distinct circumstances in which it occurs:

1. In the first instance, a molar immediately distal to the tooth in question has been extracted. The alveolar bone immediately distal to this tooth remains high relative to the remainder of the ridge previously occupied by the tooth or teeth.
2. In the second situation, a tooth immediately mesial to the molar in question has been extracted. The molar in question is tilted to the mesial, where a pseudopocket is observed; however, on the distal or tension side, an apparent ''build-up'' of alveolar bone is seen.

In both of the above etiologic circumstances, several common features are almost invariably present:

1. A missing tooth, either mesial or distal to the molar in question.
2. An excellent periodontal status at the interface between the apparently hyperostotic bone and root of the molar in question.
3. A small bony protuberance distal to the molar in question.
4. A mandibular molar location.

As with hyperostosis beneath a bridge pontic, very little is known regarding the demographics of the condition. Most patients have no symptoms; however, several of our patients have had pain resulting from trauma from food. No treatment is recommended.

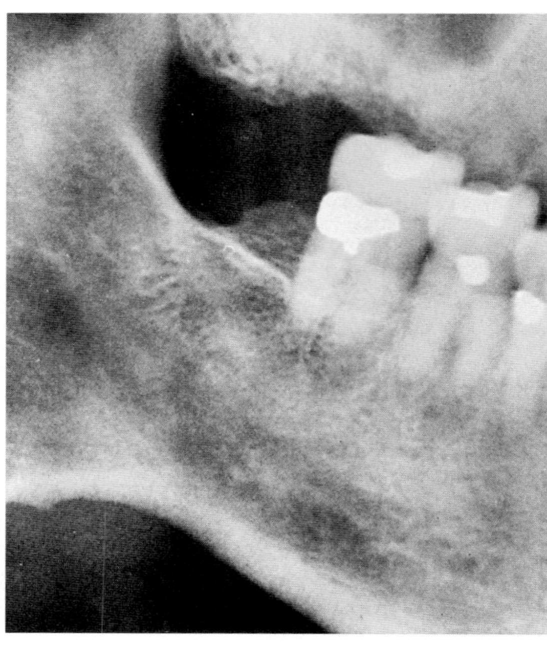

A

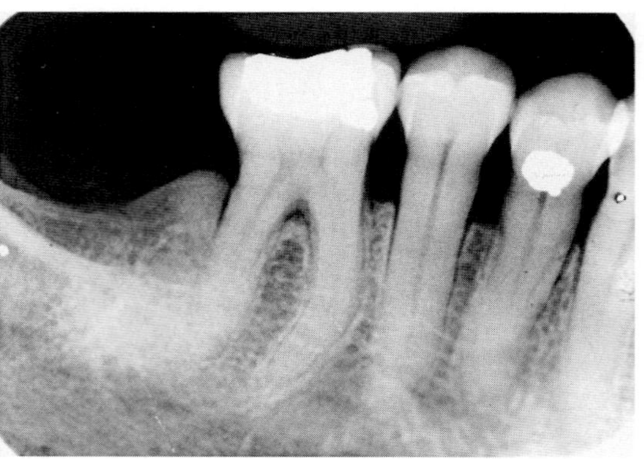

B

FIGURE 16–24.

Distal Mandibular Pseudohyperostosis: Extracted distal tooth with remaining teeth in place on mesial. A, Horizontal trabeculae within pseudohyperostotic area. B, Pseudohyperostotic bone appears more condensed, with greatest density toward the crestal area and lamina dura.

◆ *RADIOLOGY (Figs. 16–24 and 16–25)*

In all our cases, the condition occurred in the mandibular molar region; however, to our knowledge, no extensive studies have been performed to identify other locations. The term pseudohyperostosis is appropriate because the apparent increase in bone height is relative. In no instance does the bone appear to proliferate beyond the height of the normal cervical region of the tooth in question. The pseudohyperostotic bone may have the same density as the remaining alveo-

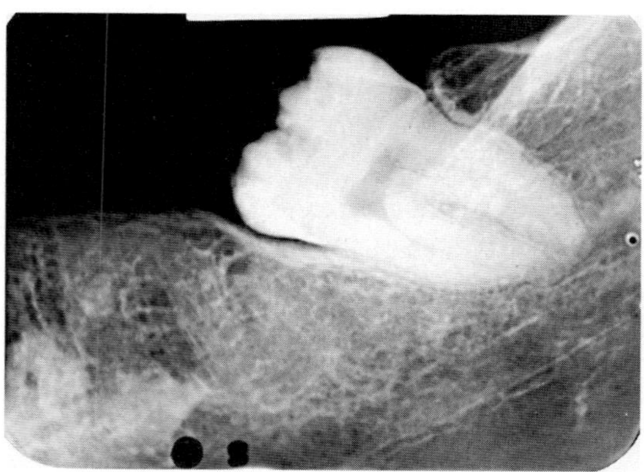

A

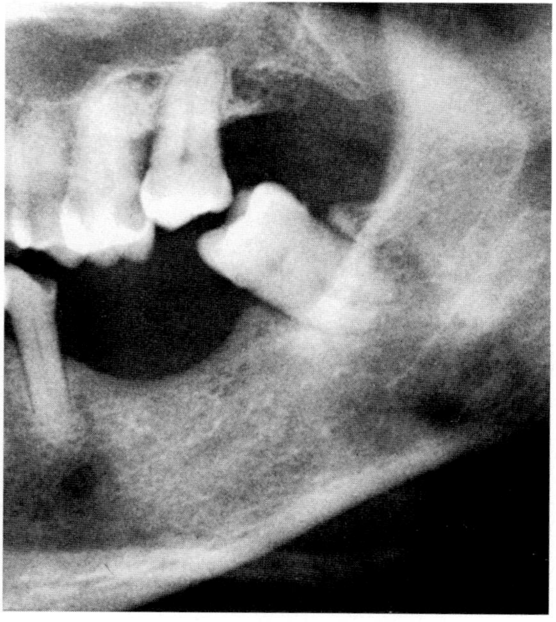

B

FIGURE 16–25.

Distal Mandibular Pseudohyperostosis: Tooth extracted on mesial of tooth in question, edentulous space not restored, and tooth tipped mesially. A, Original classic case. Trabeculae parallel to crest of ridge. (Courtesy of Dr. M. Michaud, Université de Montréal, Québec, Canada.) B, Pseudohyperostotic bone appears more condensed, with the greatest density toward the crest of ridge and lamina dura.

lar bone with trabeculae within, or it may appear more radiodense with an appearance more like that of a cortex. In most instances, the lamina dura forms the mesial wall of the pseudohyperostotic mass. Immediately adjacent to this area, the periodontal membrane space may be observed, and it may be slightly widened as is seen in orthodontic movement. Signs of periodontal disease such as "funneling" or a "V" shape of the crestal periodontal membrane space, loss or thinning of the lamina dura, "ramping" of the crestal bone, and tooth mobility usually are absent. The crestal portion of the pseudohyperostotic mass is usually smooth and lightly rounded, with a sloping distal surface toward the edentulous ridge. This sloping surface tends to be more steep in an upright tooth and less steep in a mesially tipped tooth.

ENOSTOSIS

Although the existence of enostosis as a separate entity is questioned by some people who consider it to be synonymous with idiopathic osteosclerosis, it is mentioned here for the sake of completeness. Enostosis refers to an inward growth of compact bone or a mixture of compact and cancellous bone from the endosteal surface of the buccal or lingual cortical plate. According to Worth (1963), it occurs more frequently in the mandibular canine-premolar area, below the apices of these teeth. We suggest that the term enostosis be reserved for the condition as we have defined it, which, simply stated, may be considered as the endosteal variant of exostosis. According to Worth (1963), enostosis should be considered a normal anatomic variant occurring in many other bones as well as the jaws. No treatment is necessary.

◆ *RADIOLOGY (Fig. 16–26)*

The radiographic features of enostosis are indistinguishable from those of idiopathic osteosclerosis. The distinction is academic because neither condition requires treatment, nor is there any histologic difference between them. In some circumstances the osteosclerotic area arises from the endosteal surface of the cortex, in which case the term enostosis may be considered more appropriate by some. Several enostoses may occur in one patient.

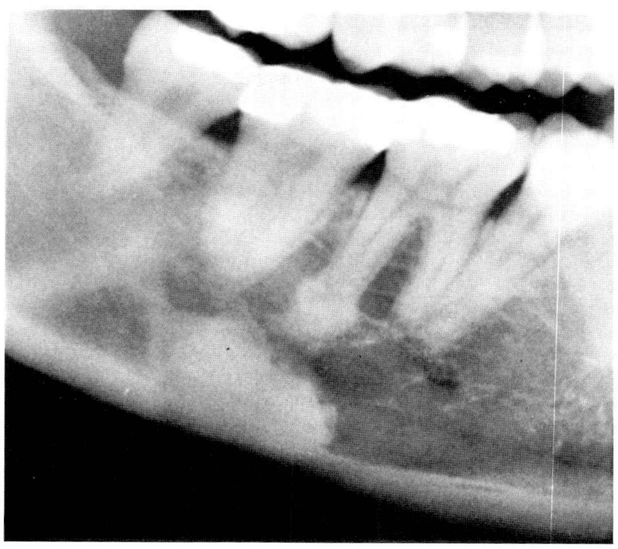

FIGURE 16–26.

Enostosis: Blending of osteosclerotic bone with inferior cortex. Adjacent area of idiopathic osteosclerosis at apex of first molar.

OSTEOMA (Peripheral osteoma; central or endosteal osteoma; soft tissue osteoma, osteoma cutis, osteoma mucosae, or osseous choristoma; compact osteoma, ivory osteoma, or osteoma ebernum; cancellous osteoma or osteoma spongiosum)

Shafer and colleagues (1983) have defined the osteoma as follows: "A benign neoplasm characterized by proliferation of compact or cancellous bone, usually in an endosteal or periosteal location and uncommonly entirely within soft tissue." Some pathologists postulate that the osteoma is not a true neoplasm and represents an osseous choristoma. Multiple osteomas are associated with Gardner's syndrome.

Pathologic Characteristics

Histologically the osteoma is composed of normal bone that is cancellous or compact. According to Shafer and colleagues (1983), the osteoma is well defined histologically but not encapsulated. Because the osteoma is histologically identical to mandibular tori, palatal tori, exostosis, hyperostosis, enostosis, and idiopathic osteosclerosis, the ultimate separation of osteoma from these variants is based on the clinical and radiologic features and the location.

Clinical Features

Based on location, osteomas may be classified as peripheral, central, or within soft tissue. When the internal architecture is determined clinically by radiographs, osteomas may be designated as compact or cancellous. Our discussion is limited primarily to the features of peripheral and central osteomas, whereas the soft tissue osteoma will be discussed in the chapter covering soft tissue opacities. Multiple osteomas of any type may be a sign of Gardner's syndrome, which consists of the following features: (1) potentially malignant polyposis of the large intestine, (2) multiple sebaceous or epidermoid cysts of the skin, (3) occasional desmoid tumors, (4) multiple osteomas, (5) unerupted normal or supernumerary teeth, and (6) odontomas.

Peripheral Osteoma

According to Schneider and colleagues (1980), the first case was reported by Messerly in 1939. They could find only 12 previously reported cases in the jaws and added a new case. Peripheral osteoma probably is not as rare as the small number of reported cases would indicate; the cases simply are not reported. Seven of their 13 cases occurred in female patients and 6 in male patients. Five of the 7 female patients had the compact type, whereas the cases of peripheral osteoma were divided evenly between the compact and cancellous subtypes in the male patients. Most peripheral osteomas are diagnosed after cessation of skeletal growth; 10 of the 13 reported cases occurred in the third, fourth, and fifth decades. The average patient's age was 38 years, with a range of 16 to 65 years. The peripheral osteoma usually is pedunculated or it may be sessile. The overlying mucosa and other soft tissues are usually normal unless trauma has occurred. They are usually asymptomatic and are easily palpated as bony-hard nodules or masses. Peripheral osteomas are slow growing; however, they may become egg sized.

Central Osteoma

Data on central osteoma in the jaws have been difficult to find. Central osteomas occur as localized or diffuse variants. They are slow growing and may be discovered initially as a result of asymmetry caused by expansion of the central lesion. Because this expansion is painless and slow to develop, the lesion often may be present for a considerable time before it is noticed.

Soft Tissue Osteoma

The soft tissue osteoma has been reviewed by Krolls and colleagues (1971) and more recently by Mesa and co-workers (1982). The first case was reported by Monserrat in 1913. Since then, an additional 30 cases have been reported. Most occurred in female patients (76%), and the patient's ages ranged from 8 to 73 years. Soft tissue osteomas are hard masses, usually in the tongue and rarely in the buccal mucosa. They are asymptomatic and treated by surgical removal; usually they do not recur. An additional discussion of soft tissue osteoma may be found in the chapter on soft tissue radiopacities.

Treatment/Prognosis

Peripheral osteomas often are removed surgically for cosmetic reasons. They usually do not recur. According to Schneider and colleagues (1980), only a single documented case of recurrent peripheral osteoma has been reported (Bosshardt and co-workers, 1971). The lesion recurred in a 32-year-old woman who observed its regrowth 3 years after surgery; she waited another 6 years to have the osteoma retreated. The central osteoma usually is not removed unless there is extensive asymmetry or interference with function. Although osteomas usually do not recur after complete surgical removal, the more diffuse type of central osteoma may be difficult to remove in toto. A case of recurrent soft tissue osteoma has been reported.

Osteomas do not show a tendency for malignant transformation. Some believe they are not true neoplasms, stating that they are either hamartomas or, in the case of soft tissue osteomas, choristomas.

◆ RADIOLOGY (Figs. 16–27 to 16–31)

The following is a summary of the radiologic features:

1. The most common site for all osteomas is in the calvaria of the skull and walls of the paranasal sinuses. They are considered rare in the jaws.

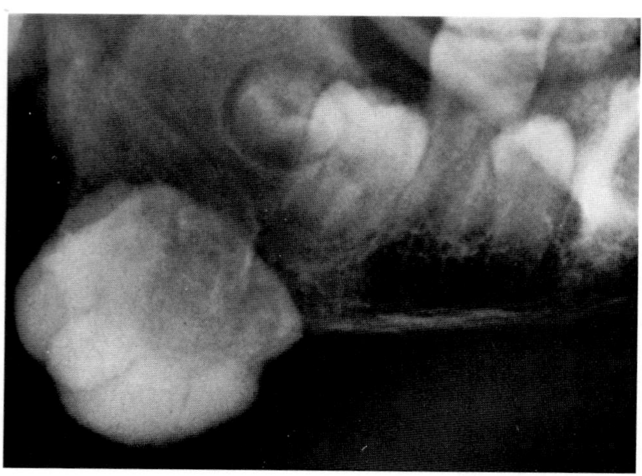

FIGURE 16–27.

Osteoma: Posterior mandible. Peripheral osteoma, compact type. It is bosselated (lumpy) and attached to lingual cortex on sessile (broad) base.

2. Osteomas are divided into peripheral, central, and soft tissue types.
3. The peripheral osteoma is divided into compact and cancellous subtypes. The outline may be smooth or lobulated. Some are pedunculated, and others are sessile.
4. The central osteoma may be focal and resembles osteosclerosis, or it may be diffuse with a mottled pattern. In the latter case the mottling may result from many individual small central osteomas or a heavy trabecular appearance.
5. Soft tissue osteomas are seen in the tongue and buccal mucosa. Compact and cancellous subtypes may be seen.

Osteoma in the Skull

According to Worth (1963), the skull is the most frequent site for the osteoma to develop, with the calvaria and paranasal sinuses being the most common areas. The frontal sinus is the most commonly affected paranasal sinus. The bony margins of the sinus may be expanded by the osteoma. When the calvaria are affected, the outer table is the most common site. When an osteoma arises from the inner table, it may be indistinguishable from hyperostosis secondary to meningioma. According to Worth (1963), osteomas may arise between the inner and outer tables of the skull within the diploic space.

Osteoma in the Jaws

According to Schneider and colleagues (1980), who reviewed the 13 reported cases of peripheral osteoma of the jaws, the most common location is the mandible, toward the buccal side. In fact, they could not find cases involving the maxilla proper; however, they did find a case reported by Leopard (1972) in which the osteoma was located in the maxillary antrum. According to Worth (1963), the most common location is in the mandibular molar region; however, he stated that any region of the mandible or maxilla may be affected. He illustrated several examples of maxil-

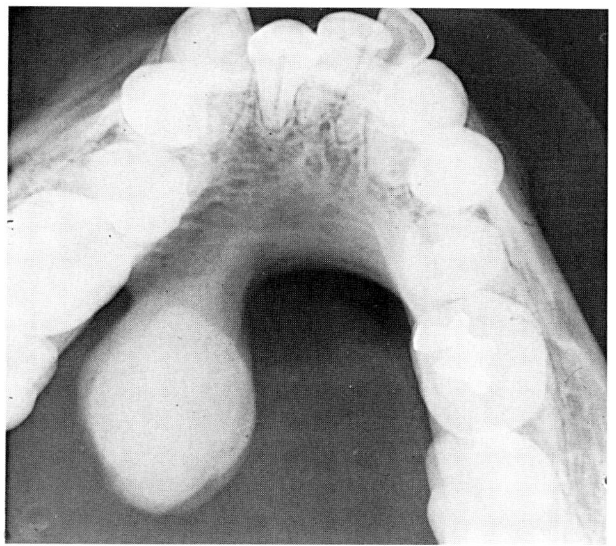

FIGURE 16–28.

Osteoma: Anterior mandible in a 14-year-old girl. Peripheral osteoma, compact type. It is nonbosselated (smooth) and attached to the mandible by a stalk (pedunculated). (Courtesy of Dr. M. Kasle, Indianapolis, IN.)

lary osteomas, providing almost as many examples as have been reported in the remainder of the literature. Of the 12 mandibular cases reported by Schneider and associates (1980), 3 involved the condyle. Of the remaining nine, six were on the buccal side of the mandible including one on the ramus, three at or near the angle, and two in the body, buccal to the molar. The remaining three cases were lingual to the mandibular molars.

Radiologic Features of Peripheral Osteoma in the Jaws

The peripheral osteoma usually does not exceed 2 cm, but some osteomas may reach massive proportions. Uhler (1957) reported an 8-cm-long intraoral osteoma; the patient died after surgery as a result of severe antecedent malnutrition. Richards and co-authors (1986) reported a large peripheral osteoma arising from the mandibular cortex, extending from the mandibular second molar to the midline anteriorly, occupying approximately two thirds of the floor of the mouth.

Radiologically and histologically, peripheral osteomas may be divided into compact and cancellous subtypes. Worth (1963) offered the best discussion on the radiologic features of these two lesions. The peripheral osteoma consists of a well-defined area of increased density projecting beyond the confines of the parent bone, but it also may be partially within the normal confines of the bone. Most peripheral osteomas are the cancellous type. The compact type is almost always sessile and rarely pedunculated. When the lesion is sessile, it usually has the same density as the cortex; thus, the original cortical outline of the mandible cannot be seen. In rare cases of pedunculated compact osteoma, the original normal bony cortex can be seen at the base of the lesion. The compact osteoma consists of a well-defined area of increased density. When the margins are superimposed on the subadjacent bone, they are usually well defined and rounded and sometimes are slightly lobulated. Within the bony mass, no trabecular pattern can be seen, but a granular or ground glass appearance sometimes can be identified. According to Worth (1963), some larger compact osteomas show an area of diminished density in one portion of the surface. In this area, perpendicular bony striae may be seen. These are fine and very closely set, resembling the margins of a feather.

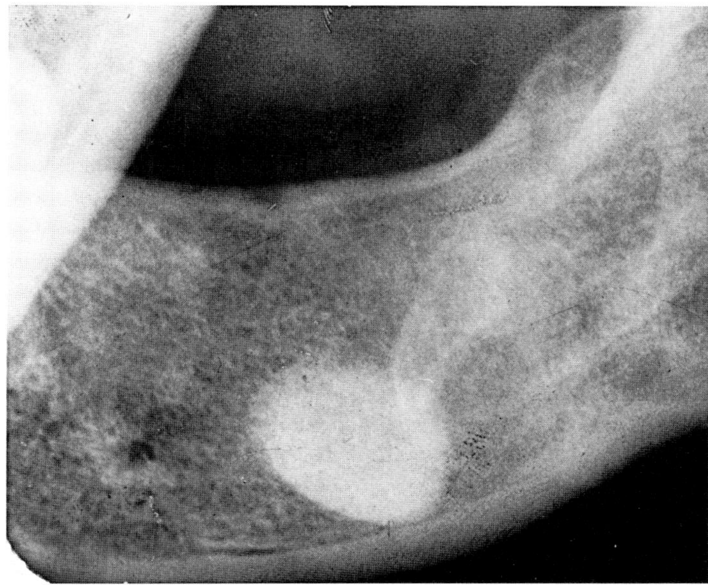

A

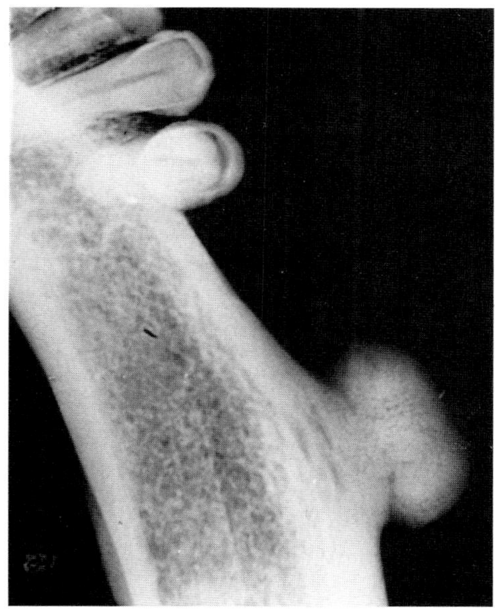

B

FIGURE 16–29.

Osteoma: Body of mandible. A, This peripheral osteoma resembles a central lesion, compact type. B, Occlusal view shows peripheral location. It is compact and sessile. (Courtesy of Dr. P. Dhiravarangkura, Chulalonghorn University School of Dentistry, Bangkok, Thailand.)

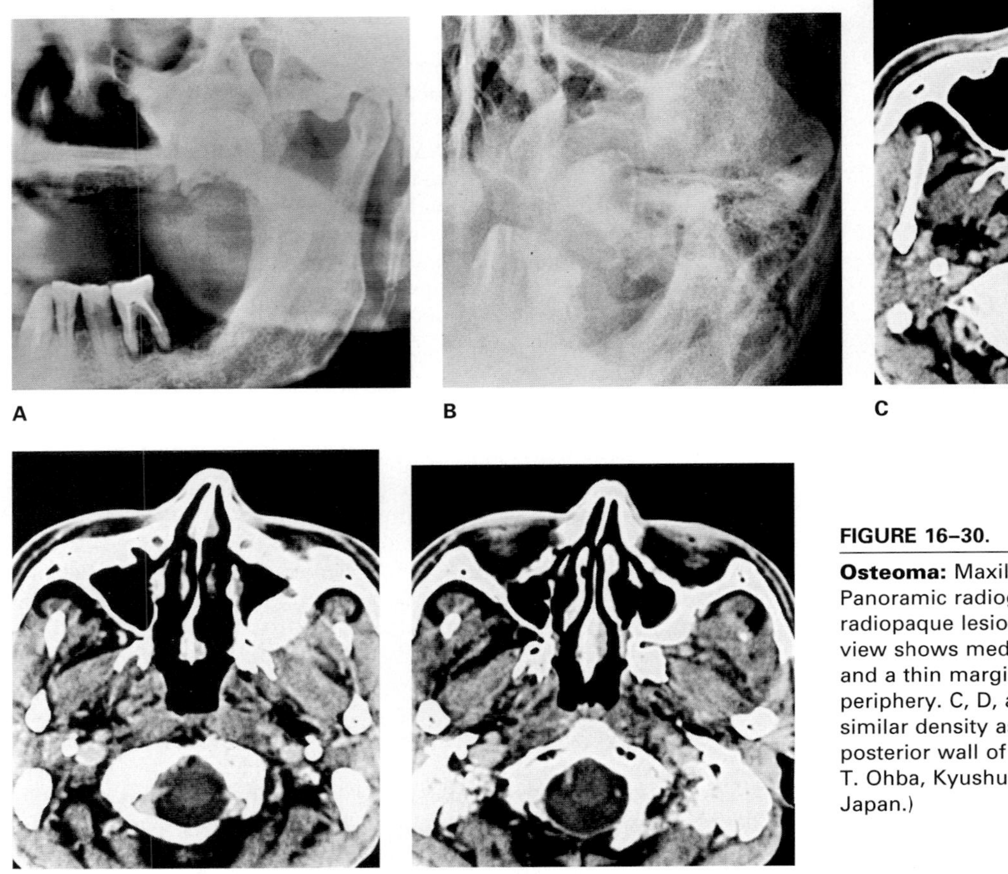

FIGURE 16–30.

Osteoma: Maxilla of a 69-year-old man. A, Panoramic radiograph shows smooth radiopaque lesion in the left maxilla. B, Waters view shows medial bowing of wall of antrum and a thin margin of compact bone at periphery. C, D, and E, CT images show mass of similar density as bone, and medial bowing of posterior wall of antrum. (Courtesy of Professor T. Ohba, Kyushu Dental College, Kitakyushu, Japan.)

According to Worth (1963), the cancellous type of peripheral osteoma usually is pedunculated, although it may have a broad base. He stated that this type usually arises from the alveolar process. The bone structure within the lesion is continuous with that of the underlying parent bone, with no intervening original cortex. The trabecular pattern within resembles that of the underlying bone; however, when the lesion is large, superimposition of trabeculae may cause the marrow spaces to appear relatively smaller. The outer margin of the cancellous peripheral osteoma usually consists of a well-defined layer of cortical bone, although this may be absent in rare instances. The outer margin is invariably smooth and rounded; however, slight lobulation may be present infrequently.

Radiologic Features of Central Osteoma in the Jaws

There is some doubt as to whether central osteomas occur in the jaws. According to Worth (1963), the evidence of their existence is not convincing, and he has stated the absence of any mass on the surface of the bone excludes osteoma. We believe central osteomas can be found in the jaws and manifest two patterns. We are especially impressed with such lesions in Gardner's syndrome, although they may occur in the absence of the syndrome.

The first pattern of the central osteoma consists of a well-defined localized area of more radiodense bone. The margins tend to be well defined and continuous with the adjacent bone. Because the osteoma is **not encapsulated,** a radiolucent line representing a soft tissue capsule is absent at the periphery. Rarely it may cause expansion of the bone within which it lies. The internal appearance of the lesion is usually densely sclerotic; a degree of irregular mottling of the bone sometimes may be seen. The margins are usually smooth and rounded, without bony spurs, which helps distinguish this lesion from idiopathic osteosclerosis, which may have irregular margins, with pointed bony spicules. Small central osteomas may be indistinguishable from small enostoses.

The second pattern of the central osteoma has been described by Langland and co-authors (1989) and consists of a diffuse radiopaque mottling of the parent bone over a localized area, a whole quadrant, or even an entire arch. Because of the diffuse mottling, the margins are much more indistinct than those of the localized type. The mottled pattern results from adjacent areas of increased density intermingled with areas of normal density, which appear relatively more radiolucent. Additionally, within the mottled areas, two distinct variations appear to affect the denser bonelike component. In the first instance, each of the radiopaque areas appears to resemble individual small central osteomas with well-

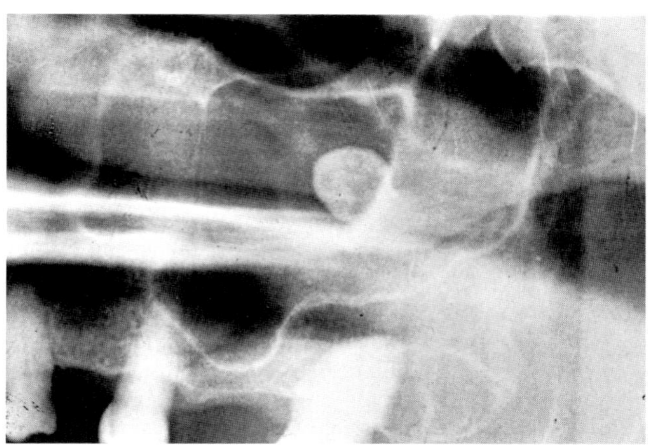

FIGURE 16–31.

Osteoma: On antral wall there is a thin rim of compact bone that is sessile. It is attached to lateral wall of antrum as indicated by focal thickening of panoramic innominate line at its base. Alterations in panoramic innominate line morphology and density locate lesion to lateral wall of antrum, near maxillary root of zygomatic arch. Distinction between osteoma and large antral exostosis is academic.

defined, rounded margins with a slight tendency toward lobulation in some instances. Together, the hundreds of more radiodense areas and adjacent normal bone form the mottled appearance. In the second instance, each of the radiopaque areas appear more irregular, in some instances resembling heavy trabeculae or focal areas of osteosclerosis admixed with areas with a coarse granular appearance. Collectively, the hundreds of more radiodense areas and adjacent normal bone form the mottled appearance.

We have observed the simultaneous occurrence of mottled central osteomas with peripheral osteomas bilaterally, suggesting the hamartomatous nature of some osteomas.

Radiologic Features of Soft Tissue Osteoma

Soft tissue osteomas are rare. From a review of some reported cases, it appears that both cancellous and compact subtypes may be seen. They rarely exceed 2 cm in diameter. Soft tissue osteomas also are discussed in Chapter 19, ''Soft Tissue Opacities.''

OSTEOID OSTEOMA

The osteoid osteoma first was described as a separate entity by Jaffe in 1935. In the series of 6221 bone tumors reviewed by Dahlin (1978), the 158 osteoid osteomas constituted 11% of the benign tumors. Enigmatically, the lesion is extremely rare in the jaws. Dahlin (1978) found that 1% of all osteoid osteomas occurred in the jaws. In 1968, Greene and associates found only seven cases of osteoid osteoma in the jaws.

Pathologic Characteristics

Although most investigators currently believe these lesions are neoplastic, some assert that they are reactive or inflammatory in nature. Histologically, osteoid osteoma closely resembles osteoblastoma. According to Smith and colleagues (1982) and Greer and Berman (1978), the two conditions are best differentiated on the basis of clinical and radiologic characteristics. Osteoid osteoma is rare in the jaws, and osteoblastoma is relatively more common. Osteoid osteoma occurs mainly in the major tubular bones, whereas osteoblastoma affects flat bones and tubular bones. With the exception of the condylar area, the jaws more closely resemble the flat bones—thus the greater frequency of osteoblastoma. Histologically, it consists of a central nidus that is demarcated distinctly from the surrounding bone. The nidus consists of an interlacing network of osteoid trabeculae rimmed with osteoblasts. There are varying amounts of mineralization; however, the central part of the nidus is the most mineralized. The trabeculae lie in a vascular fibrous connective tissue stroma, and bone marrow is absent. The surrounding bone tends to be compact if a small en bloc resection was performed to obtain the specimen.

Clinical Features

Most osteoid osteomas occur during the second decade of life, and although they are rare after 30 years of age, they may occur in people of any age. Males almost always are affected more frequently than females, with a ratio of 2 to 3:1. The most significant presenting complaint is pain. In the 158 cases reviewed by Dahlin (1978), only two lesions were painless. Classically, the pain is described as disproportionately severe with respect to the size of the lesion, yet relief is obtained easily with ordinary salicylates. The osteoid osteoma is a slow-growing lesion. Thus, the pain is initially mild and increases in severity with time; it is characterized as a dull, gnawing, unremitting ache that is worse in the evening. Some patients have periods of partial remission, followed by episodes of acute exacerbation. According to Dahlin (1978), pain may be related to nerves within the nidus that can be identified by special axon strains. Other clinical features include swelling, tenderness, and local erythema.

Treatment/Prognosis

Successful treatment of osteoid osteoma is predicated on complete surgical excision of the nidus. In the extragnathic skeleton, Gitelis and Schajowicz (1989) advocated conservative en bloc excision of the nidus, including some of the surrounding bone, to avoid recurrence. Dahlin (1978) emphasized the importance of including part of this surrounding bone. Greer and Berman (1978) recommended conservative excision in the jaws. The remaining reactive bone will resolve spontaneously if the entire nidus is removed. A few osteoid osteomas have been reported to undergo spontaneous remission. Osteoid osteoma is thought to have a limited growth potential, whereas osteoblastoma is prone to continue growing if left untreated. Also, some larger osteoblastomas have been classified as aggressive and have malignant potential.

◆ *RADIOLOGY (Fig. 16–32)*

The two most critical features in the definitive diagnosis of osteoid osteoma are the radiologic identification of the radiolucent nidus and the assessment of its size; osteoid osteoma is usually less than 1 cm in diameter.

Location

In the review presented by Gitelis and Schajowicz (1989), 57% of all osteoid osteomas occurred in the femur and tibia and 71% in the long bones. The usual site is the diaphysis toward the proximal end, often within or involving the cortex; the joint surface also may be involved, but much less frequently. In a series of seven jaw lesions reviewed by Greene and associates (1968), four occurred in the mandible; of these, three were in the body and one in the condyle. In the remaining three maxillary lesions, one involved the antrum.

Identification of the Nidus

The unique clinical profile—a teenage boy with severe unremitting pain that worsens at night and is eliminated with an aspirin—alerts the radiologist to the possibility of osteoid osteoma. The lesional tissue consists of a round or ovoid radiolucent nidus, surrounded by reactive bone. The nidus usually is located within or near the cortex. Within the radiolucent nidus, there may be a small central calcification. Subperiosteal layering may be observed adjacent to the area. The reactive bone surrounding the nidus may be thick and sufficiently dense to obscure the nidus. Thus, explained Worth (1963), overexposed radiographs may be necessary. At other times, the central calcification may enlarge to obscure the nidus; on such occasions radiographs in several planes may be necessary. Tomography and computed tomography (CT) are useful in localizing the nidus. When it is located within the spongy bone between the buccal and lingual cortical plates, it is difficult to detect. Occasionally it is surrounded by a sclerotic rim, which can be very prominent; however, this feature often is missing, thus causing difficulty in finding the nidus. A useful adjunct in locating the nidus is radioisotope imaging. Osteoid osteoma takes up ^{99m}technetium diphosphonate avidly because of the intense osteoblastic activity within the nidus. The surrounding reactive bone also takes up the radioactive isotope, but less so than the nidus. This results in a double-density hot spot, which is highly suggestive of osteoid osteoma but is not pathognomonic.

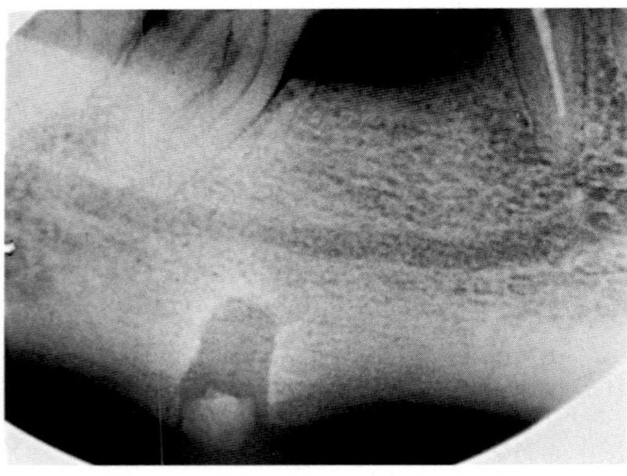

FIGURE 16–32.

Osteoid Osteoma: Nidus is radiolucent and located partially within cortex; it is approximately 6 to 8 mm in diameter. There is a zone of dense reactive bone surrounding nidus and focal thickening of the cortex. The cause of the fracture at the inferior margin of the cortex is not known. (Courtesy of Professor L. Alfaro, University of Chile School of Dentistry, Pathology Referral Center, Santiago, Chile.)

Size of the Nidus

The size of the nidus is an important factor because many physicians use size to differentiate osteoid osteoma from osteoblastoma. Most universally accept the diagnosis of osteoid osteoma if the nidus is 1 cm or smaller, and most radiologists accept the diagnosis of osteoblastoma if the radiolucent core is larger than 2 cm. The controversy lies with lesions between 1 and 2 cm. Some include lesions as large as 2 cm in the acceptable category of osteoid osteoma. Greer and Berman (1978) reviewed 12 documented osteoblastomas in the jaws, and only 2 of the 12 (17%) were greater than 2 cm in diameter. Others have suggested that when the typical clinical findings are present, osteoid osteoma can be diagnosed if the nidus is 2 cm or smaller; when the typical clinical profile is absent, lesions between 1 and 2 cm may be classified as "circumscribed osteoblastoma." All lesions larger than 2 cm should be considered "true osteoblastomas."

BENIGN OSTEOBLASTOMA (Osteogenic fibroma, giant osteoid osteoma, osteoblastoma)

Benign osteoblastoma, which occurs in many parts of the bony skeleton, represents approximately 1% of all primary bone tumors. It probably was reported initially by Jaffe and Mayer in 1932. In 1956, Jaffe and Lichtenstein, in independent articles, introduced the current term benign osteoblastoma. Because the word benign is redundant, some prefer the term osteoblastoma. Borello and Sedano reported the first case in the jaws in 1967. A periosteal counterpart was described first by Goldman in 1971, and in 1976 Farman and co-workers found reports of three periosteal benign osteoblastomas in the jaws, including their own case.

Pathologic Characteristics

According to Shafer and colleagues (1983), the histologic criteria for microscopically diagnosing benign osteoblastoma are as follows: (1) vascularity of the lesion, with many dilated capillaries throughout the tissue; (2) moderate numbers of multinucleated giant cells resembling osteoclasts throughout the tissue; and (3) irregular trabeculae of new bone paired with actively proliferating osteoblasts forming osteoid. The histologic findings of osteoid osteoma are sometimes identical. Some authors, such as Steiner (1976, 1977) Schajowicz and Lemos (1970), and Farman and colleagues (1976), suggested that osteoid osteoma and benign osteoblastoma are variations of the same lesion, with differing anatomicoclinical forms; however, the two lesions are regarded as separate entities primarily because of their characteristic radiologic differences. According to Shafer and colleagues (1983), the osteoblasts are so active and numerous that this lesion has been misdiagnosed as osteosarcoma. Smith and colleagues (1982) found three possibilities in which this can occur:

1. An osteoblastoma is overdiagnosed as an osteosarcoma.
2. An osteoblastoma subsequently becomes malignant because it was initially a well-differentiated osteosarcoma underdiagnosed as a benign osteoblastoma.
3. A benign osteoblastoma develops malignant histologic features, and its behavior becomes locally aggressive.

This latter group has been discussed by Schajowicz and Lemos (1970), who suggested the term "malignant osteoblastoma." The prognosis is better than that of conventional osteosarcomas.

Clinical Features

Benign osteoblastoma is relatively rare in the skeleton and even more uncommon in the jaws. Smith and colleagues (1982) compiled an excellent review of osteoblastoma in gnathic and extragnathic sites. They found 360 cases in the world literature and only 24 cases affecting the jaws. In jaw lesions there is a male predilection, with a male-to-female ratio of approximately 2:1. The patients' ages ranged from 15 to 37 years; however, the average age was 17 years. Almost 90% of the patients were younger than 30 years, and nearly 75% of cases occurred in patients in the second and third decades. In the axial skeleton, paresthesia and scoliosis occur in spinal lesions and atrophy occurs in limbs with functional impairment. In the 24 jaw lesions, pain and swelling were common findings. The oral pain is characterized as low grade; however, there are occasional reports of severe pain and, in a few instances, no pain. There was facial swelling in the tumor area in 79% of the cases. Ninety percent of the lesions with facial swelling were also painful; 8% of the lesions produced pain without swelling. Only one case was found with neither swelling or pain, located in the coronoid process. Other interesting findings in some cases of jaw lesions include a tendency for the swollen area to be very tender to palpation, redness of the overlying mucosa, and tooth mobility and tenderness to percussion. The symptoms lasted 2 weeks to 2 years before the jaw lesions were diagnosed.

Treatment/Prognosis

The treatment for jaw lesions should be limited to curettage or local excision. Radiation therapy along with surgery has been used in some cases of vertebral involvement; however, this was done only because the whole lesion could not be removed because of anatomic factors. Because jaw lesions respond well to conservative treatment and access has not been a problem, radiation therapy is not warranted because there is a risk of stimulating an anaplastic change. Because benign osteoblastoma is a relatively vascular lesion, significant hemorrhage may occur at surgery. Smith (1972) reported free bleeding, with 200 ml blood lost, whereas Farman and colleagues (1976) found a highly vascular bed, and replacement of 1500 ml whole blood was required. The tumor is described as reddish-brown with a gritty or a granular texture resulting from its mineralized component. Conservative treatment of jaw lesions usually results in healing.

In a review of recurrent osteoblastomas in the skeleton, Jackson (1978) found a recurrence rate of 10%. Smith and colleagues (1982) reported a similar rate for jaw lesions, with recurrence in 2 of the 24 reported cases. In the case described by Smith (1972), incomplete removal still resulted in resolution and complete healing. Merryweather and colleagues (1980) reported a case of malignant transformation of osteoblastoma to osteosarcoma.

◆ *RADIOLOGY (Figs. 16–33 to 16–36)*

Location

According to Smith and colleagues (1982), the most common locations are as follows: the vertebral column, 34%; long bones, 30%; hands and feet, 14%; and skull and mandible, 15%. Among the 24 jaw lesions, 15 (63%) were in the mandible and 8 (33%) in the maxilla; in one case the location was not reported. Farman and colleagues (1976) found a similar distribution, with 8 of 13 lesions (62%) in the mandible. The lesions occur primarily in the molar-premolar areas and other tooth-bearing regions. To our knowledge, no lesions have been reported in the ramus; however, there were two cases in the coronoid process.

Perplexing Features of Jaw Lesions

In our review of the literature, we found the following reported appearances: (1) a benign osteoblastoma-like appearance, as occurs in classic skeletal lesions; (2) an osteoid osteoma-like appearance, as occurs in the jaws and bony skeleton; (3) a benign cementoblastoma-like appearance, occurring only in the jaws; and (4) a resemblance to other fibro-osseous lesions. Some of the following factors relate to the problem: It is eminently apparent that benign cementoblastoma and benign osteoblastoma are difficult to diagnose definitively on a solely histologic basis in some instances; benign osteoblastoma and osteoid osteoma are so similar histologically that some believe them to be variants

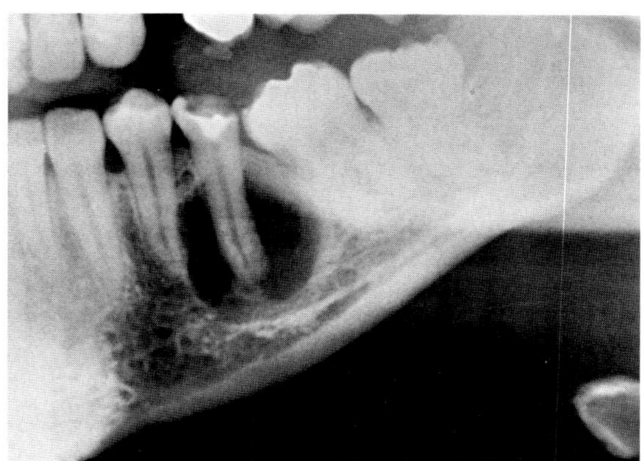

FIGURE 16–33.

Benign Osteoblastoma: A 36-year-old woman has a case in the early radiolucent stage, when lesion is well defined. (Courtesy of Dr. M. Van Dis, Indiana University, Indianapolis, IN.)

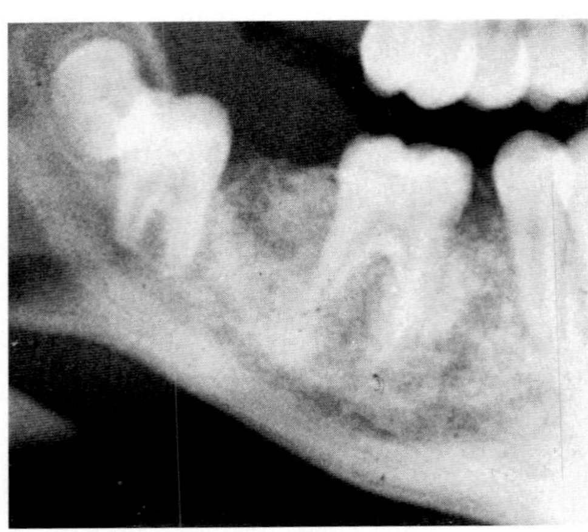

A

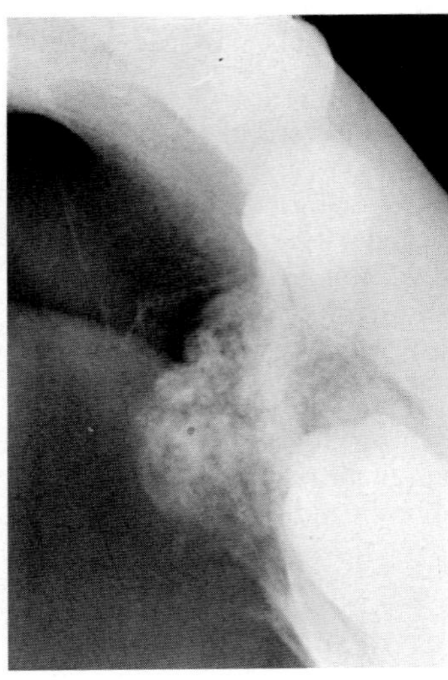

B

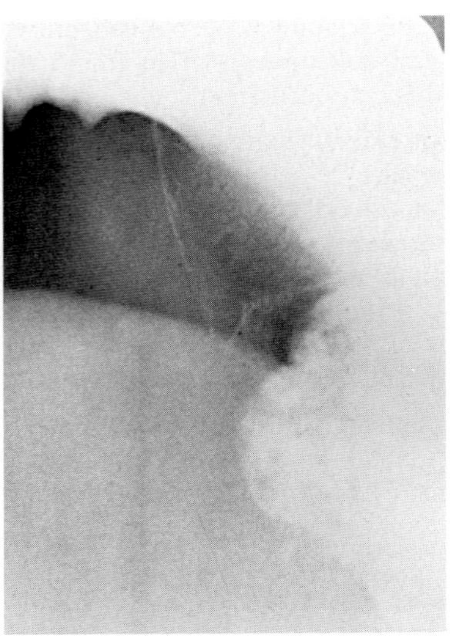

C

FIGURE 16–34.

Benign Osteoblastoma: Simulated case from two patients. A, Diffuse mottled radiopacity produced by moderate degree of tumor matrix calcification. Margins are somewhat indistinct, and there is displacement of adjacent teeth. A perplexing aspect of this case was the histologic diagnosis of benign cementoblastoma. (Courtesy of Dr. S. Lovestedt, Rochester, MN.) B and C, Peripheral extension of tumor mass, showing very thin expanded lingual cortex that is perforated posteriorly (B) and intact anteriorly (C). (B and C, Courtesy of Professor L. Alfaro, University of Chile School of Dentistry, Pathology Referral Center, Santiago, Chile.)

of the same lesion; and, finally, there is a remarkable histologic resemblance between all fibro-osseous lesions, especially at certain stages of development. Among the reports we reviewed, authors followed one of two possible approaches to determine the final diagnosis of their cases: The authors recognized convincing histologic evidence suggesting one diagnosis, but the clinical and radiographic findings were more suggestive of another diagnosis; as a result, some of the cases were diagnosed primarily on the basis of histologic criteria, whereas others were diagnosed with more weight placed on the clinical information. This perplexing problem with regard to osteoblastomas in the jaws has been discussed by Greer and Berman (1978). They have suggested that once the histologic features are known, the most reliable differential diagnostic measure is assessment of the radiographic appearance. The following are examples of perplexing cases reported as difficult diagnoses because of disparity between the clinical findings and histologic features:

1. A benign cementoblastoma-like radiologic appearance was illustrated by Remagen and Prein (1975). The lesion resembled cementoblastoma in all respects radiologically except the involved mandibular second molar was not attached to the mass, although both roots appeared to project into the mass. Their final diagnosis was benign osteoblastoma, although this was done with reluctance because of the clinical picture.
2. Greer and Berman (1978) found 12 documented osteoblastomas in the jaws for which size was specified. Only 2 of the 12 jaw lesions exceeded 2 cm in diameter. This is surprising because a size greater than 2 cm is the most important criterion for distinguishing osteoblastoma from the smaller osteoid osteoma.
3. An osteoid osteoma-like radiologic appearance was illustrated by Shatz and colleagues (1986). The lesion was at the angle of the mandible and was described as radiopaque, with a central radiolucent area measuring 1.5 cm in diameter. The histologic features were equivocal and could represent osteoid osteoma or benign cementoblastoma. In this case, Shatz and co-authors (1986) diagnosed benign osteoblastoma, mostly because the nidus was greater than 1 cm in diameter.

Radiologic Features of Jaw Lesions

In its classic presentation, benign osteoblastoma can be completely radiolucent or it may contain flecks of calcification. These flecks may be focal and few in number, or they may be dispersed throughout the lesion. They may coalesce to form focal larger areas of calcific material, or the lesion may appear completely radiopaque. According to Smith (1972), benign osteoblastoma may cause expansion of the cortex. At times the cortex may appear to be completely absent with an outgrowth of a soft tissue mass, and in other instances there is a thin rim of expanded cortical bone encasing the lesion. In the classic lesion, especially in the mandible, the margins appear somewhat indistinct because of a lack of reactive sclerosis but still can be distinguished from the surrounding bone. The margins of maxillary lesions and in some aggressive variants are less well defined. A radiolucent halo or outer sclerotic rim is not a usual feature of the classic benign osteoblastoma. Aggressive lesions have been discussed by Marsh and co-authors (1975), Schajowicz and Lemos (1970), and Ohkubo and colleagues (1989). These are characterized by rapid growth, more poorly defined margins, more severe bone destruction, and spread to adjacent atomic

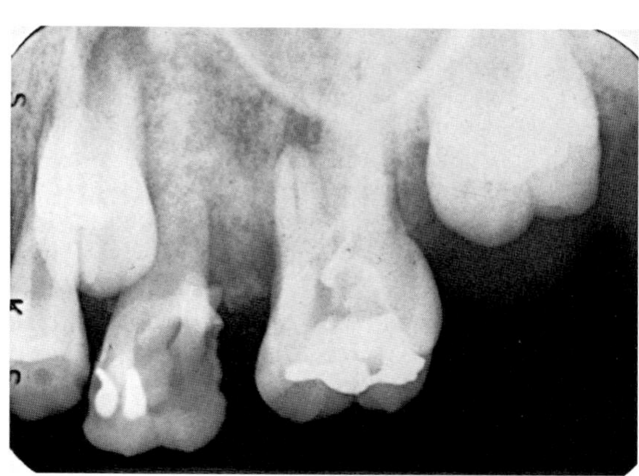
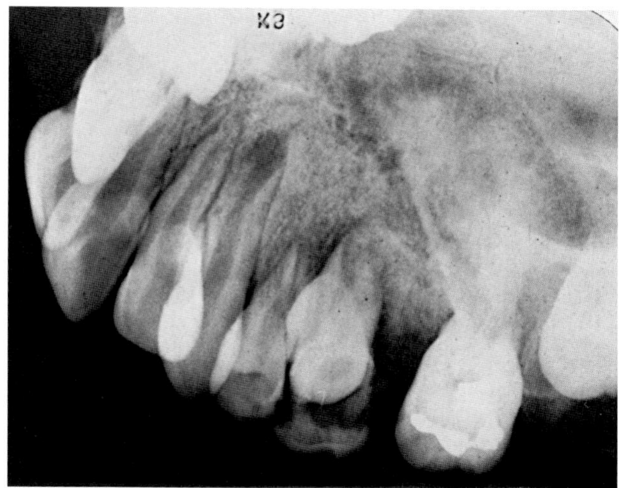

A B

FIGURE 16–35.

Benign Osteoblastoma: Case in a 9-year-old girl. A and B, Mottled appearance of radiopaque area. Margins are difficult to define, and extension into antrum is likely. Separation of erupted and unerupted teeth is a characteristic feature. (Courtesy of Professor H. Fuchihata, Dean, Osaka University School of Dentistry, Osaka, Japan.)

regions. In this instance, these authors caution the clinician to suspect the malignant counterpart of this lesion.

Relationship with Teeth

The benign osteoblastoma may extend up between the roots of adjacent teeth; however, the roots are usually apparent within the mass. Root resorption may be present, and there may be displacement and tipping of adjacent teeth. The teeth are not attached to the mass.

The **periosteal benign osteoblastoma** may show all of the features within the spectrum described. In the case of Farman and colleagues (1976), the lesion was entirely radiolucent, with the involved primary mandibular canine appearing as a floating tooth. The mass can be seen projecting beyond the mandible or maxilla, with focal involvement of the affected jaw at the base of the lesion.

CHONDROMA (Enchondroma, ecchondroma, periosteal chondroma)

The chondroma is a benign tumor of cartilage. In the series of 6221 tumors examined by Dahlin (1978), 11% were chondromas. Despite their frequency in the extragnathic skeleton,

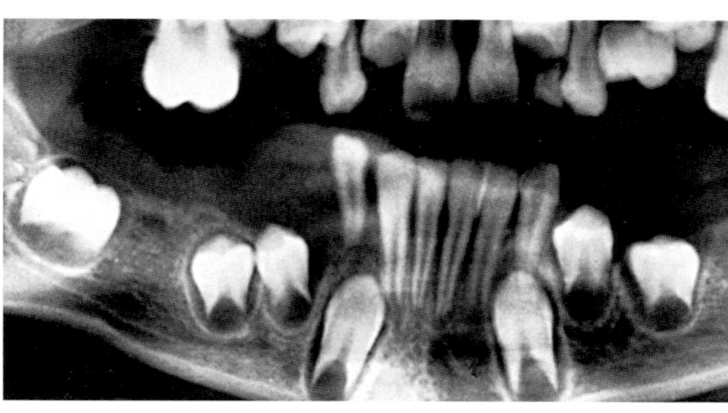
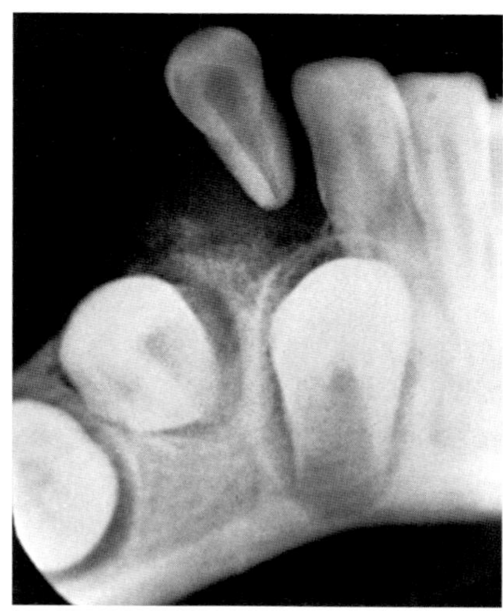

A B

FIGURE 16–36.

Benign Osteoblastoma: Periosteal variant in a 6-year-old boy. A, Peripheral mass resembles epulislike lesion on gingiva. B, Floating tooth appearance. Margin is irregular without reactive sclerosis.

they are very rare in the jaws. In 1961, Chaudhry and colleagues (1961) reviewed the English literature to 1912 and could find only 52 reported cartilaginous lesions in the jaws. Of these, 35% were benign, 19% were benign at the first diagnosis but later recurred as chondrosarcomas, and 46% were malignant from the beginning. Among the 18 benign cartilaginous lesions identified by Chaudhry and colleagues (1961), the diagnoses included chondroma, enchondroma, osteochondromas, myxochondroma, and fibro-osteochondroma. The number of true chondromas occurring in the jaws must be considered very small.

Pathologic Characteristics

Cartilaginous tumors may arise at the sites of cartilaginous rests in the jaws. Although the maxilla is a membranous bone, cartilaginous rests are located in the incisive canal and nasal fossa. In the mandible, Meckel's cartilage may result in cartilage rests in the posterior body; rests also are found in the coronoid process and condyle. Extraosseous chondromas may be seen, especially in the tongue. Gardner and Patterson (1968) reported one in the soft palate. Histologically, the chondroma is composed of a mature hyaline cartilage. These may give rise to some foci of endochondral ossification. Also, the cartilage may degenerate to be replaced with a calcific substance. A myxomatous ground substance also may be observed.

Clinical Features

Clinically, chondromas are divided into central and peripheral variants and thus are referred to as enchondromas or periosteal chondromas, respectively. Additionally, chondromas may be solitary or multiple. In the series of Dahlin (1978), 136 (84%) were solitary and the remainder were multiple. Multiple chondromas of bone represent a dysplastic condition in which there is failure of endochondral ossification, resulting in the development of tumefactive cartilaginous masses. This condition sometimes is called Ollier's disease and is called Maffucci's syndrome when associated with multiple hemangiomas. Although none of the chondromas in Dahlin's (1978) series were located in the jaws, the few reported gnathic lesions we have examined have been solitary. Men and women are affected equally. Chondromas may occur in people at any age. Chaudhry and colleagues (1961) found no reported cases in the jaws in the first decade of life and only one benign cartilaginous tumor developed in a person older than 60 years. Chondromas are slow growing and are most likely to be asymptomatic until they become large enough to cause noticeable swelling or interfere with function. If swelling is present, the overlying mucosa will appear normal and intact. The area will feel bony-hard on palpation in some instances or firm and slightly yielding in other cases. Pain is not a feature.

Treatment/Prognosis

Chondroma is treated by thorough excision. There is little tendency for recurrence; however, 19% of the 52 cartilaginous jaw lesions reported by Chaudhry and colleagues (1961) were diagnosed as benign on first removal but recurred in a more anaplastic form. Dahlin (1978) observed this phenomenon with respect to chondromas in the extragnathic skeleton; the author stated that such cases result from a failure to interpret the original specimen correctly and recommended the preparation of sufficient microscopic sections to completely evaluate the original specimen. Cartilaginous jaw lesions have a strong tendency toward malignancy, thus a diagnosis of chondroma should be viewed with cautious optimism and the patient should be observed closely for signs of recurrence. In the series of Chaudhry and coworkers (1961), chondroma recurred as chondrosarcoma within 1 month to 3 years, with the median being 18 months. Incising into the lesional tissue or otherwise contaminating instruments such as retractors with lesional tissue should be avoided because if the lesion is a well-differentiated chondrosarcoma, it is subject to recurrence by implantation with contaminated instruments. Because chondrosarcoma may recur late, long-term follow-up is especially important in cases of chondroma treated in this later fashion.

◆ *RADIOLOGY*

It is important to recognize the features of cartilaginous lesions radiologically before biopsy or surgery. Malignant cartilaginous lesions may appear benign histologically and radiologically. Incision into a malignant cartilaginous lesion can result in recurrence and a diminished prognosis.

Location

Chondromas occur most frequently in the small tubular bones of the hands. They also are seen in the epiphyses of the femur and humerus, much less frequently in the flat bones, and probably least frequently in the skull and jaws. In the maxilla, Chaudhry and co-workers (1961) found chondromas most frequently in the anterior alveolar ridge with extension into the sinuses; in the mandible, the common locations were in the body posterior to the canine teeth, coronoid process, and condyle. There may be a slight predilection for the mandible. In the jaws, central and peripheral lesions have been reported; however, there are so few that authors find it difficult to ascribe features that would typify jaw chondromas. Worth (1963), Gibilisco (1985), and Poyton (1982) have presented several cases. Several of these were located in the coronoid process and condyle and may have represented osteochondromas.

Radiologic Features of Jaw Lesions

In the jaws, chondromas are most likely to be central, although they may be placed eccentrically so that they localize toward an edge of the bone. The lesions are lytic and may contain calcific foci. These represent mineralization in degenerating cartilage or endochondral ossification and impart a flocculent or snowflake-like appearance to the lesional tissue in the radiograph. The margins may be sclerotic, and in several instances they have a scalloped appearance. They also tend to appear well delineated from the surrounding bone. When the lesion is close to the edge of the bone, saucerization of its surface may be observed. In this instance the outer margin of the tumor may not be evident because of an apparent absence of a bony wall. In other instances a very even thin rim of subperiosteal new bone representing an expanded cortex surrounds the lesion. Some central chondromas in the jaws have been described as locally destructive in appearance. Chondromas have the potential to destroy a large segment of the involved jaw. Chaudhry and colleagues (1961) observed root resorption in association with some chondromas. Such a finding is consistent with a slow-growing, locally destructive benign lesion.

The most important aspect in the radiologic evaluation of a chondroma in the jaws lies with the postoperative phase. During this period continuing efforts should be made to rule out recurrence, even 10 years after surgery.

OSTEOCHONDROMA (Osteocartilaginous exostosis)

The osteochondroma is the most common benign bone tumor in the extragnathic skeleton. Parenthetically, it is extremely uncommon in the jaws, but it does occur at this site. In a review of 6221 bone tumors at the Mayo Clinic, Dahlin (1978) found that osteochondromas accounted for 40% of all benign tumors and 9% of the total. Osteochondromas usually are seen as a solitary lesion. In rare instances there are multiple osteochondromas affecting many bones, which are referred to as hereditary multiple exostoses; however, this condition is unrelated to exostoses, which occur in the jaws. According to Worth (1963), the jaws are not affected when multiple osteochondromas are present. In Dahlin's (1978) series of 570 osteochondromas, 89% were solitary and none of the lesions in the series was located in the jaws.

Pathologic Characteristics

According to Dahlin (1978), osteochondromas usually arise at the site of tendon insertions and grow along the same line as the tendon's pull. In the jaws, osteochondromas arise in locations where there are cartilaginous foci, including the mandibular symphysis, condyle, and coronoid process. Shafer and co-authors (1983) stated that osteochondromas in the jaws are simply osteomas with foci of cartilage. In the extragnathic skeleton, they are believed to arise from aberrant cartilage of the growth plate in an endochondral bone in the region of the growth plate toward the metaphysis. The osteochondroma usually stops growing when the nearest epiphyseal plate fuses. According to Edeiken (1981), growth after this point suggests malignancy.

Clinical Features

Dahlin (1978) found that 60% of the patients were male. Because most osteochondromas arise during periods of active bone growth, approximately 57% of patients were younger than 20 years old at the time of excision, and most of these patients were in the second decade of life. Some patients are asymptomatic and the lesion is discovered during a routine radiographic examination. Others have swelling that is noticed by the patient or by the dentist during the examination. Those with involvement of the coronoid process may complain of limited opening and sometimes swelling in the region of the zygoma. They also may hear an audible "thump" at the point of maximum opening. Although pain may be present, it is not a usual feature.

Treatment/Prognosis

Osteochondromas are best treated by surgical excision with complete removal of the cartilaginous cap and overlying periosteum in peripheral lesions. Central lesions should be excised completely. Recurrence is rare, although 2% of cases recurred within 2 to 26 years in Dahlin's (1978) series. The second operation was curative in all instances.

In patients with multiple osteochondromas, approximately 10% will have malignant transformation to chondrosarcoma. In their reviews of the English literature, Loftus and co-authors (1986) and Schweber and Frensilli (1986) found no report of malignant transformation occurring in cases of osteochondroma of the facial skeleton or jaws.

◆ *RADIOLOGY (Fig. 16–37)*

Worth (1963) has stated that osteochondromas in the jaws may be central or peripheral. The central variety is much like the chondroma, with the following two exceptions: (1) osteochondromas tend to be localized more sharply, with a corticated margin; and (2) bone is present within the lesion. If there is expansion, the cortex overlying the expanded area will be intact and continuous. Jaw lesions tend to be round or ovoid. The radiopaque component within the lesion may show one of two patterns: (1) trabeculations, produced by osseous elements in the tumor matrix; or (2) irregularly shaped amorphous calcific masses, elaborated by the cartilaginous part of the tumor matrix. Worth (1963) observed that cystlike spaces in the region of the coronoid process or base of the condyle have been diagnosed as osteochondromas. This author illustrated a lesion in the body of the mandible that was predominantly radiolucent, with elongated trabeculae, and there was resorption of the apices of the first molar.

According to Worth (1963), the peripheral variety of osteochondroma may be found most commonly in the coronoid process. In this instance, the coronoid process may appear enlarged and more radiodense and may have an altered shape.

BENIGN CHONDROBLASTOMA (Codman tumor, chondroblastoma, calcifying giant cell tumor, epiphyseal chondromatous giant cell tumor)

Jaffe and Lichtenstein coined the term benign chondroblastoma in 1942 and established the distinctive features of this neoplasm. Earlier, in 1931, Codman recognized some of the features, and the lesion often still is referred to as a Codman tumor. According to Brecher and Simon (1988), approximately 800 cases have been reported in the literature. In the series of 6221 bone tumors reviewed by Dahlin (1978), less than 1% (44 cases) were benign chondroblastomas and only

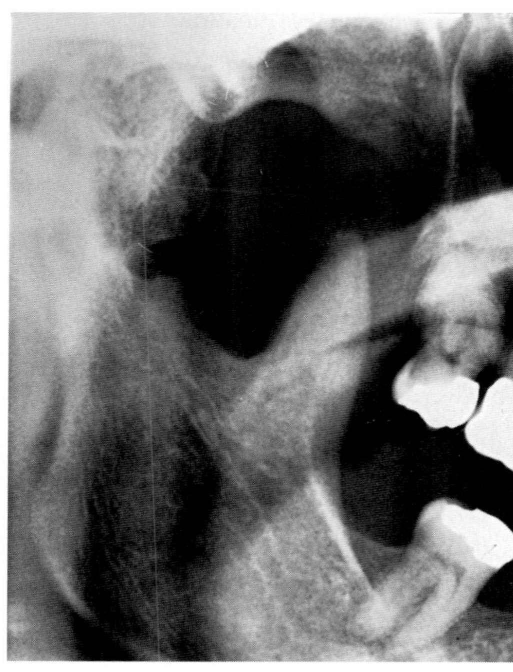

A

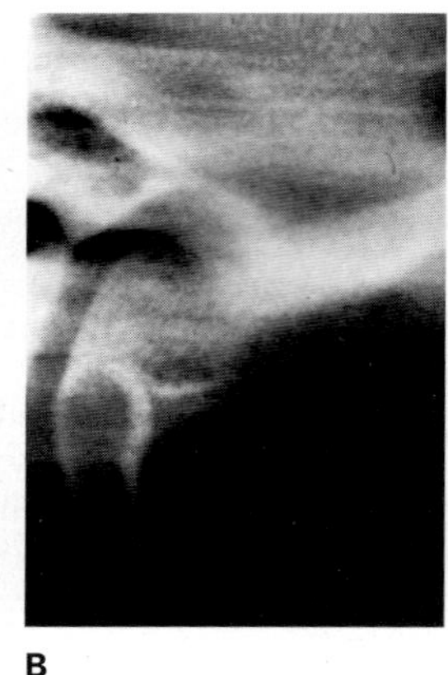

B

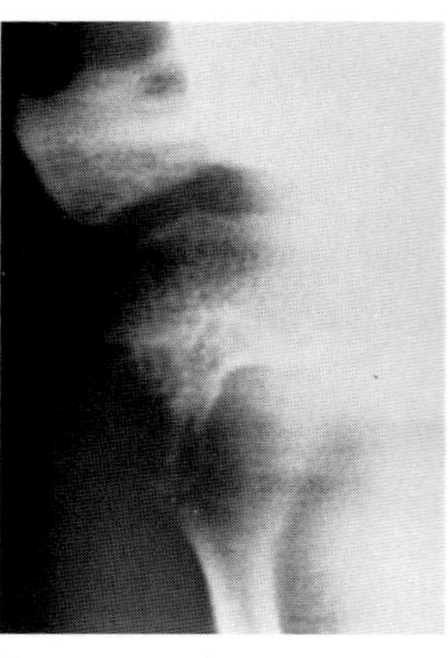

C

FIGURE 16–37.

Osteochondroma: Shown on head of condyle. A, Panoramic view. B, Corrected lateral tomogram shows lesion on head of condyle. C, Anteroposterior tomogram shows stalk and mushroom-like appearance.

1 occurred in the jaws. In a review of 465 chondroblastomas, Mirra (1980) reported an incidence of only 1% in the mandible. In a report of 30 chondroblastomas in the skull and facial bones, Bertoni and colleagues (1987) found 6 cases in the mandible and 2 in the temporomandibular joint areas.

Pathologic Characteristics

Histologically, the lesional tissue consists of proliferating chondroblasts producing zones of chondroid material; these zones may degenerate and calcify. Among the proliferating chondroblasts, multinucleated giant cells can be seen.

Clinical Features

Schajowicz and Gallardo (1970) reviewed the features of this tumor in their analysis of 69 cases; Bertoni and colleagues (1987) reviewed 30 chondroblastomas of the skull and facial bones. These tumors are seen more frequently in male patients, with a 2:1 ratio over female patients. Most patients are younger than 20 years of age at diagnosis; however, Bertoni and co-authors (1987) found a mean age of 44 years, with a range from 3 to 70 years. Most patients with temporal bone and jaw lesions were older than 30 years, making this group older than those with lesions in the long bones. The most frequent presenting symptom is pain, which may have existed for several years before the patient sought care. Bertoni and co-authors (1987) also observed that the duration of symptoms was known for 19 of their 30 cases and ranged from 1 month to 30 years. In 10 cases the symptoms had been present for more than 1 year. Other symptoms included a plugged sensation in the ear or hearing loss when the temporal bone was involved. Pain and swelling may occur in the temporomandibular joint area.

Treatment/Prognosis

This tumor usually is treated by thorough curettage, and recurrence is possible but rare. As with other cartilaginous tumors, surgical implantation of tumor cells with contaminated instruments is possible. In such instances, there has been recurrence in an adjacent bone or in soft tissues. Dahlin (1978) has recommended that, when possible, benign chondroblastomas should be excised with a surrounding shell of bone. In the cases reported by Bertoni and colleagues (1987), approximately 50% recurred after curettage; however, conservative re-excisions were usually curative.

On extremely rare occasions, a benign chondroblastoma with totally benign features metastasizes, usually to the lungs. Green and Whittaker (1975) reported such a case. The lesional tissue in the lungs appears benign and nonaggressive, although its management with radiation therapy and chemotherapy has been debated.

◆ *RADIOLOGY (Fig 16–38)*

General Radiologic Features

In most parts of the skeleton the radiologic features are characteristic; this is partially because of the patients' ages and the characteristic radiologic signs. According to Edeiken (1981), the benign chondroblastoma is almost always in the epiphysis of a long bone and the epiphyseal line is usually evident. The lesions tend to be smaller than 2 cm. They are usually well defined and surrounded by a sclerotic rim. Punctate or irregular calcifications representing calcified cartilaginous areas are found in more than 50% of the tumors; these are tiny, perhaps 1 mm in size, and are often in little clusters, with a density somewhat less than that of the surrounding bone. In other areas, a much greater degree of

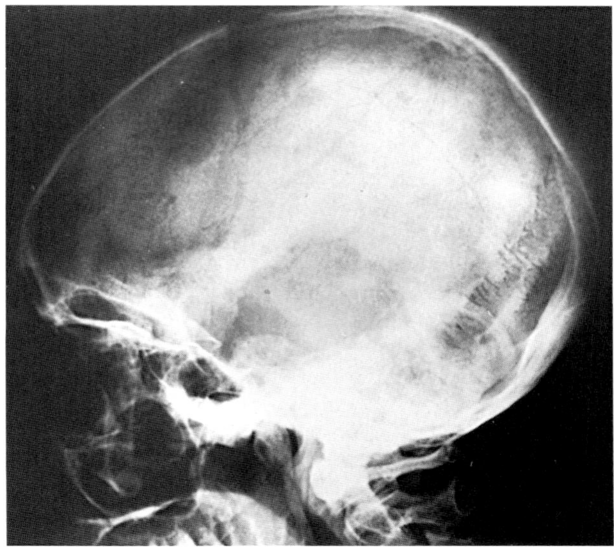

A

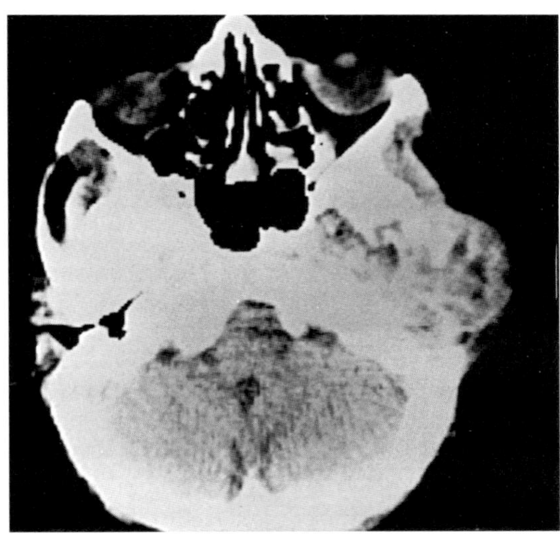

B

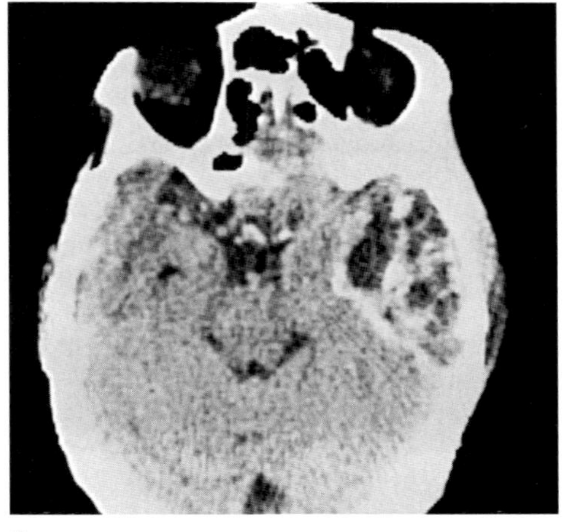

C

FIGURE 16–38.

Benign Chondroblastoma: A, B, and C, Benign chondroblastoma in temporal bone with tumor mass and intracranial extension. (From Anim JT, Baraka ME: Chondroblastoma of the temporal bone: unusual histologic features. Ann Otol Rhinol Laryngol 95:260, 1986.)

calcification produces a more flocculent appearance, with a much greater radiodensity than that of the punctate calcifications. At times, expansion may be present, but in chondroblastomas this is exceedingly rare. Internal trabeculation is not a feature, although the margins may be loculated on rare occasions.

Radiologic Features of the Jaws and Skull

Al-Dewachi and co-workers (1980) reviewed 13 craniofacial benign chondroblastomas. Of these, 9 were located in the temporal bone, 1 in the parietal bone, 2 in the mandible, and 1 in the anterior maxilla in a 13-year-old girl. The condyle is a common site, and cases have been reported by Goodsell and Hubinger (1964) and Dahlin and Ivins (1972). In a series of 30 chondroblastomas in the skull and facial bones, Bertoni and colleagues (1987) observed that 21 occurred in the temporal bone. Among these, 16 were confined to the temporal bone only and 5 extended to adjacent bones. Among those with extension, 1 extended to the parietal bone, 2 extended to the base of the skull, and 2 extended to the temporomandibular joint. Six patients had primary involvement in the jaws; among these, 3 cases were in the condyle, 1 in the coronoid process, 1 in the angle, and 1 in the body. Bertoni and colleagues (1987) obtained preoperative radiographs in 17 cases. Of these, 16 were essentially radiolucent and only 1 case had clumps of calcific foci within the lytic area. The margins were usually well defined, and expansion was a common finding. Although the radiologic findings were rarely diagnostic, the general impression was that of a benign but aggressive lesion.

OSTEOSARCOMA (Osteogenic sarcoma)

According to Dahlin (1978), osteosarcoma is the most frequent primary malignant bone tumor when multiple myeloma is excluded. The tumor affects 1 person per 100,000 people per year in the United States. Large series of osteosarcoma of the jaws included 56 cases from the Armed Forces Institute of Pathology (AFIP) reported by Garrington and co-authors (1967) and 66 cases from the Mayo Clinic reported by Clark and co-workers (1983). According to Forteza and colleagues (1986), more than 400 cases of osteosarcoma of the maxilla and mandible have been described in the world literature. Garrington and co-authors (1967) estimated that osteogenic sarcoma of the jaws affects 1 person per 1,500,000 people per year in the United States. They also estimated that approximately 65% of all osteosarcomas arise in the jaws. Osteosarcomas have been subclassified into 5 types: (1) central osteosarcoma, (2) multicentric osteosarcoma, (3) periosteal osteosarcoma, (4) parosteal osteosarcoma, and (5) extraosseous osteosarcoma. Our discussion focuses primarily on central osteosarcoma, but several other subtypes are outlined briefly. The authors are not aware of a case of multicentric osteosarcoma affecting the jaws.

Pathologic Characteristics

Although the cause is poorly understood, three main etiologic factors have been identified: (1) radiation therapy, mainly for fibrous dysplasia; (2) pre-existing benign bone disorders, especially fibrous dysplasia, cartilaginous lesions, and Paget's disease; and (3) trauma such as caused by an automobile or bicycle accident, being struck by a baseball, a hard blow to the mandible while fighting, and a hard bump on the chin that loosened two teeth. These factors have been discussed by Clark and co-workers (1983), Boutouras and Goodsitt (1963), Rosenmertz and Schare (1969), and Garrington and colleagues (1967). Histologically, the diagnostic feature of osteosarcoma is the presence of osteoid produced by malignant cells with three histologic variants. In the series of 66 jaw tumors reported by Clark and colleagues (1983), 48% showed a predominantly chondroid differentiation and were termed "chondrogenic osteosarcoma," 29% showed abundant osteoid production and were termed "osteoblastic osteosarcoma," and 23% showed a pattern resembling fibrosarcoma with malignant spindle cells arranged in a herringbone pattern and were designated "fibroblastic osteosarcoma." Dahlin (1978) stated that there is a slightly better survival rate with chondroblastic osteosarcoma, and, according to Garrington and co-workers (1967), this holds true for osteogenic sarcoma in the jaws. Osteogenic sarcoma is graded by the method of Broders (1925), with the most differentiated designated as grade 1 and the least differentiated, grade 4. According to Dahlin (1978), 80% of osteosarcomas of the long bones are grade 3 or 4. Osteosarcomas of the jaws are better differentiated; Clark and colleagues (1983) found that none was grade 1; 44%, grade 2; 41%, grade 3; and 15%, grade 4.

Serum alkaline phosphatase levels often are increased in cases of osteogenic sarcoma. When the tumor is removed, the serum alkaline phosphatase level slowly returns to normal; with recurrence or metastasis, the alkaline phosphatase level increases. Alkaline phosphatase levels may be helpful in distinguishing chondroblastic osteosarcoma from chondrosarcoma, in which the alkaline phosphatase levels are usually lower.

Clinical Features

In the long bones osteogenic sarcoma usually arises during the second and third decades of life, with a slight male predilection. For osteogenic sarcoma in the jaws, the mean patient age is 30 to 34 years, with cases occurring approximately 10 years later than in the long bones. Krolls and colleagues (1980) reviewed 141 cases of osteogenic sarcoma in the jaws from the AFIP, including the earlier 66 cases of Garrington and co-authors (1967), and reported that the average age was 30 years for women and 36 years for men (age range, 4 to 84 years). Garrington and colleagues (1967) found a sharp age peak for maxillary osteosarcomas, with 41% occurring in people between the ages of 20 and 29 years; by comparison, there was no sharp peak in the mandible, and lesions were just as likely to occur in the young as the elderly. With regard to the sex distribution for osteosarcoma in the jaws, 56 to 64% of these lesions occur in male patients. In the AFIP series of Garrington and colleagues (1967), however, 44% of patients were female; this is notably high because the sex ratio at the AFIP almost always favors men, presumably because there are more men in the Armed Forces. Garrington and co-workers (1967) found that 22 of the 24 female patients (92%) had mandibular lesions, whereas in male patients the tumors were distributed equally between the maxilla and mandible.

The most common presenting findings in osteosarcoma of the long bones are swelling and pain, which are invariably present. Although 93 to 94% of patients with jaw lesions have swelling, only 25 to 43% of cases are painful. All patients with maxillary lesions complained of swelling, and most observed a recent increase in size. Krolls and colleagues (1980) estimated that the potential doubling time of osteogenic sarcoma is 32 days. In the long bones, the lesion often measures 10 cm when it is discovered. In the jaws, swelling is observed earlier, often before the onset of pain; thus, jaw lesions are much smaller than 10 cm when discovered. Other reported symptoms, in decreasing order of frequency, include loose teeth (17%), paresthesia (13%), toothache (7%), bleeding (6%), and nasal obstruction (6%). Other less frequent findings include separated teeth, headache, a watery eye associated with exophthalmia, a buzzing sensation in the ear, a burning tongue, and cacogeusia. Jaw lesions usually are covered by normal-appearing mucosa, but redness and bleeding may be present. The average interval from the first symptom was 3 to 4 months.

Treatment/Prognosis

When planning treatment for osteosarcoma, it is important to recall that this disease spreads hematogenously, often early in its course. Whenever possible, definitive treatment should be planned on the day of biopsy. In other words, as much of the workup as possible should be completed before the biopsy, including the identification of metastatic lesions. According to Dahlin (1978), good fresh frozen sections are adequate for the definitive diagnosis, especially because nearly all osteosarcomas contain small or large foci that require no decalcification before sectioning, and delayed study of heavily ossified portions of the tumor or adjacent cortical bone is not necessary in establishing the correct diagnosis. As stated by Dahlin (1978): "Some patients must pay with their lives when treatment is delayed unnecessarily." Surgical incision into the tumor should be avoided during the definitive procedure. The best treatment method appears to be ablative radical surgical excision. In osteogenic sarcoma of the jaws, the recurrence rate is high. Of all cases, 70% will recur at least once. In the maxilla the recurrence rate is 74% and in the mandible, 66%. When patients with radical resections are excluded, 80% of the remainder had recurrences. In patients with maxillary and mandibular recurrences, the mortality rates were 72% and 71%, respectively.

Garrington and co-workers (1967) found metastasis in 51% of the cases with follow-up information. Among these, the most common metastatic sites, in descending order of frequency, were the lung (49%), lymph nodes (17%), brain (9%), and liver, adrenal gland, dermis, small intestine, pericardium, and perirenal fat (each 4%). Metastasis occurred within 1 to 3 years after the onset of symptoms.

As reported by Krolls and colleagues (1980), the 5-year survival rate for osteogenic sarcoma in the long bones is 5 to 23%. According to McKenna and colleagues (1964), the 5-year survival rate in patients with osteosarcoma developing in Paget's disease is 2%. Clark and colleagues (1983) found an overall survival rate of 40% for osteogenic sarcoma in the jaws. Garrington and colleagues (1967) stated that the 5-year survival rate for osteogenic sarcoma in the maxilla is 25% and 41% for that in the mandible; the 10-year survival rate was 20% for cases in the maxilla and 38% for those in the mandible; and the 15-year survival rate was 0% for cases in the maxilla and 33% for those in the mandible. Mandibular anterior lesions had the best prognosis. Clark and colleagues (1983) found that those who received ablative radical surgery had a 60% 5-year survival rate; less aggressive surgery combined with radiation therapy or radiation therapy alone resulted in death in most of these patients. Clark and colleagues (1983) reported that, of the patients who died, 50% did so within the first year and 78% within 2 years.

◆ RADIOLOGY (Figs. 16–39 to 16–47)

Radiologically, osteogenic sarcomas are seen in three broad categories: (1) most commonly as a central lesion in bone; (2) rarely in a juxtacortical relationship with the affected bone, as discussed later; and (3) in very exceptional cases, in the extraskeletal soft tissues, including the lip.

Location

Central osteosarcoma may be located in either jaw. Depending on the study, 31 to 51% may be found in the maxilla and 49 to 68% in the mandible. In the maxilla, 75% arise in the alveolar bone, one third of which occur in the anterior region, and 25% in the antrum. In the mandible, 61% occur in the body; 17%, the angle; 14%, the symphysis; and 8%, the ramus. Other reported sites include the temporomandibular joint, juxtacortical locations, and soft tissue.

General Radiologic Features of Central Osteogenic Sarcoma

Central osteogenic sarcoma usually arises in the metaphysis of a long bone, especially the femur and tibia toward the knee. It also may be found at the proximal end of the humerus. Regardless of which bone is affected, central osteosarcoma begins within the bone and later may break out. In general, all bone reacts to irritants whether they are inflammatory or neoplastic. These reactions tend to be osteolytic or osteoblastic. Osteoblastic responses often are referred to as reactive bone, new bone formation, sclerotic bone, or increased bone density. Benign bone responses may be iden-

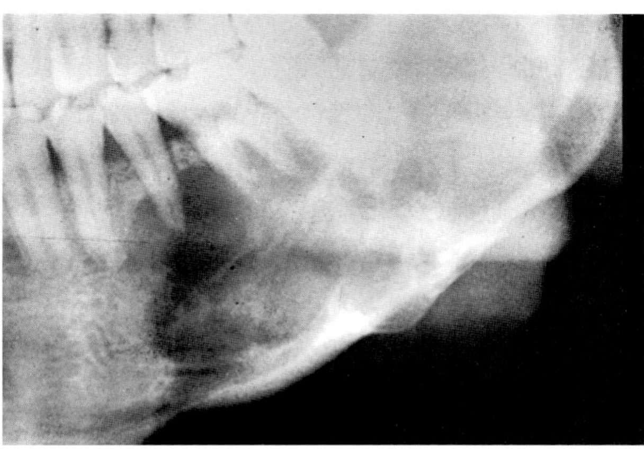

A

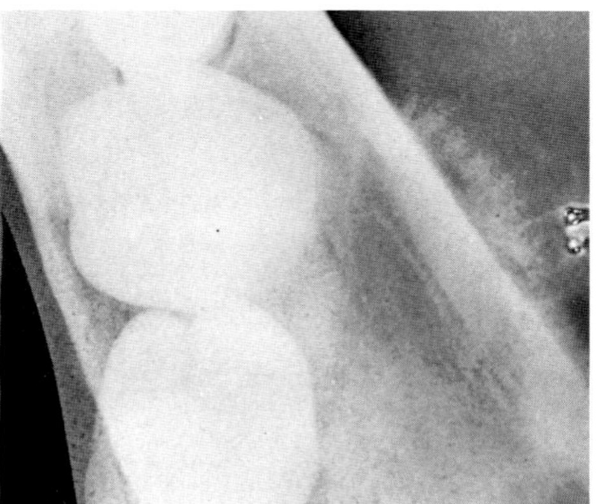

B

FIGURE 16–39.

Osteogenic Sarcoma: Mixed osteolytic/osteoblastic response in a 29-year-old man. A, Geographic area of bone destruction within which there are several strands of bone and a small island of bone anteriorly. There is erosion of the inferior cortex and a periosteal reaction. B, Occlusal view shows periosteal reaction with sunburst pattern, with zig-zagging striae within. (Courtesy of M. Araki and K. Hashimoto, Nihon University School of Dentistry, Tokyo, Japan.)

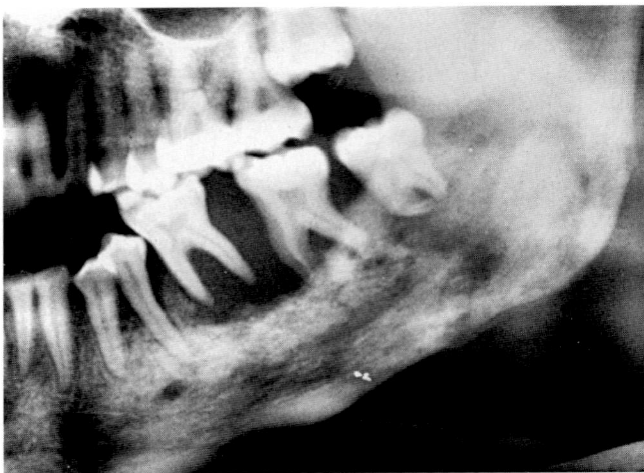

FIGURE 16–40.

Osteogenic Sarcoma: Mixed osteolytic/osteoblastic response in a 21-year-old man. Floating tooth in lytic area with malignant bone beneath resembling benign reactive response. There are permeative changes throughout and a large island of neoplastic bone in the angle area. The inferior cortex is eroded, and a faint periosteal reaction is present.

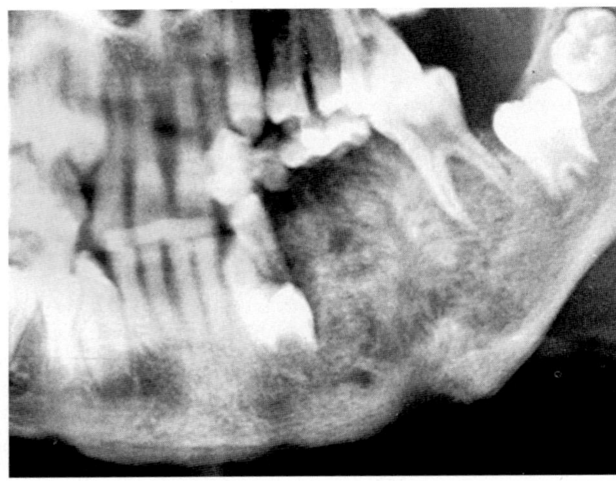

FIGURE 16–41.

Osteogenic Sarcoma: Blastic response in a 10-year-old boy. There is resorption of the primary root tips, displacement of developing permanent teeth, destruction of the inferior cortex, and a periosteal reaction producing a Codman's triangle.

tified by the uniformity of their density and distinctness of their margins; the less uniform the density and the less definite the margin, the greater is the likelihood of malignancy. The sclerotic changes associated with osteogenic sarcoma represent neoplastic proliferation of malignant new bone replacing healthy bone. In the jaws, variants of three basic patterns are seen: (1) an osteolytic pattern, in which no bone is formed; (2) a mixed pattern, in which some bone is formed; and (3) a sclerotic pattern, which is almost entirely bone forming. According to Garrington and co-workers (1967), each of these patterns was observed with approximately equal frequency. Clark and colleagues (1983) found there is no correlation between the radiologic appearance and histologic subtype; however, they found differences in the radiologic appearance based on location. In the maxilla, 50% were sclerotic, 38% lytic, and 12% mixed; in the mandible, 43% were lytic, 29% sclerotic, and 29% mixed. In general, most observers agree that the bony changes are suggestive of malignancy, and in rare instances these are sufficiently typical to suggest osteogenic sarcoma specifically. Occasionally, the changes also may mimic benign dis-

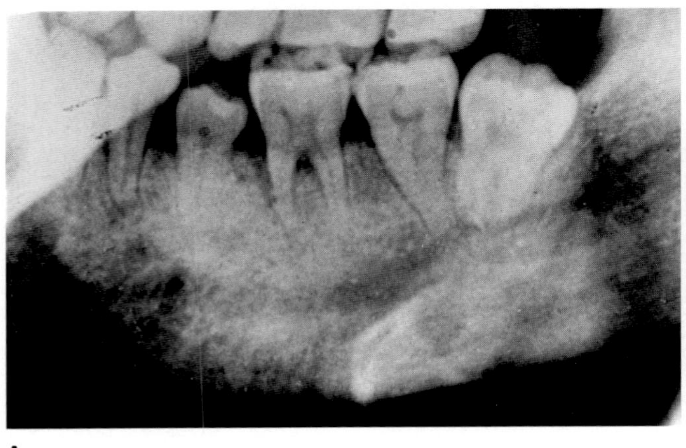

A

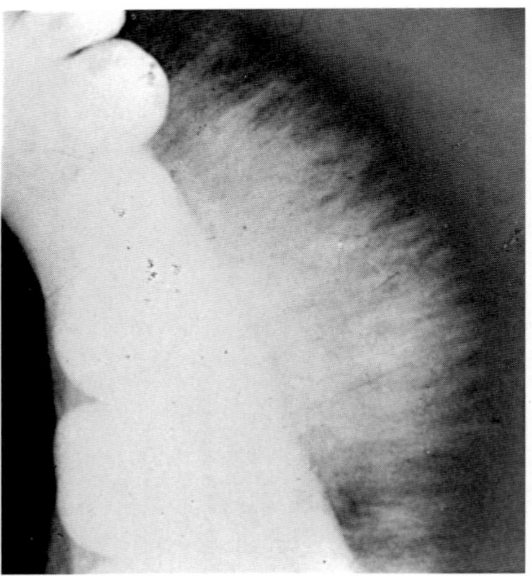

B

FIGURE 16–42.

Osteogenic Sarcoma: Apparent blastic response. A, Widened periodontal membrane space associated with pathologic fracture. B, Exuberant sunray response masks changes in body of mandible. (Courtesy of Dr. P. Dhiravarangkura, Chulalonghorn University School of Dentistry, Bangkok, Thailand.)

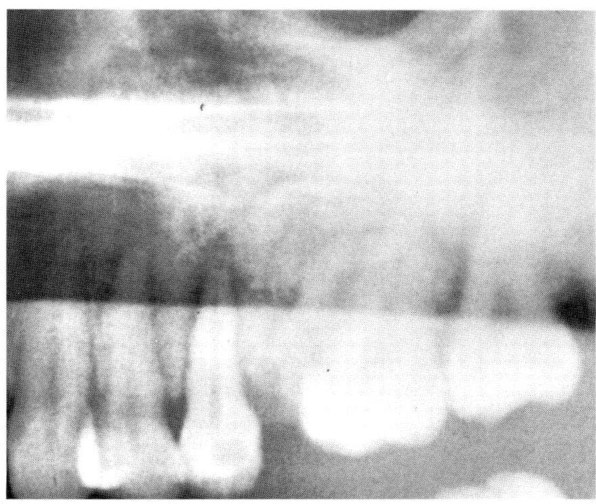

A

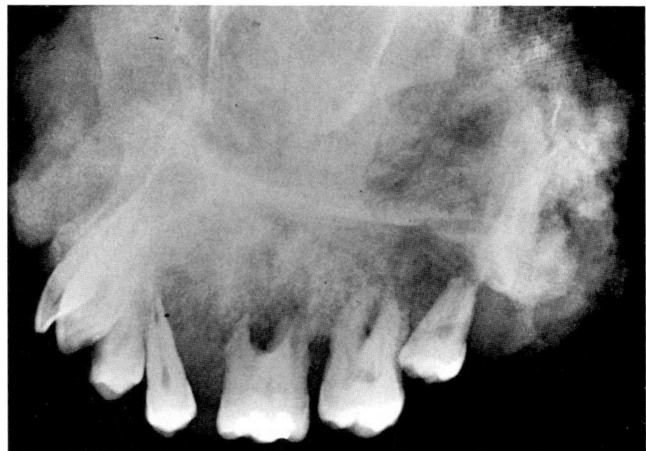

B

FIGURE 16–43.

Osteogenic Sarcoma: Effect on teeth. A, Widened periodontal ligament space, premolars, and molars. There is an increased interseptal bone height distal to the second premolar resulting from neoplastic bone. B, Surgical specimen with spiked pattern of root resorption on first molar.

ease. In the series of Clark and co-workers (1983), 22 cases had radiographs of the jaws. Of these, 82% (18 cases) were considered to have radiologic evidence of malignancy; among this subset, a specific diagnosis of osteosarcoma was suggested for 56% (10 cases).

Worth's Descriptions of Central Osteosarcoma of the Jaws

Osteolytic Osteosarcoma. According to Worth (1963), the osteolytic type may have one of the following appearances:

1. Resembling that of central squamous cell carcinoma, characterized as a poorly defined lytic area, except that osteosarcoma may extend more deeply into the bone, be more susceptible to pathologic fracture, and have a more clearly defined margin that may be corticated and intact, although there is usually some evidence of breakthrough by the tumor. Squamous cell carcinoma rarely produces corticated margins, except in early disease arising in a dentigerous cyst or ameloblastoma.
2. Resembling that of acute osteomyelitis, characterized by a motheaten pattern, except that osteosarcoma may destroy the surface of a bone, break through, and stimulate a periosteal reaction. In this case, the new bone follows the contour of the tumor, thus expanding the outline of the jaw in an irregular fashion; this new bone is not parallel to the original bone margin, and it usually has defects in which new tumor growth has broken through. In osteomyelitis the surface of the bone may be destroyed and a layer of subperiosteal new bone is produced. Although it may be irregular, it is parallel to the original margin of the bone and tends to remain intact.
3. A poorly defined lytic area in the maxilla that breaks through into the antrum. In this instance, there is either complete destruction of the maxilla and antral floor with no osseous tissue separating the tumor from the remainder of the sinus, or a portion of intact cortex lining the floor or wall of the antrum remains attached to the tumor mass as it invades the sinus above.
4. A significant early lytic finding in osteogenic sarcoma first was described by Garrington and colleagues in 1967. It consists of a symmetrically widened periodontal membrane space along the length of a root of one or several adjacent teeth. The widened periodontal membrane space characteristically is limited to one side of the root, even if several roots of a multirooted tooth are affected or if several adjacent teeth are involved. There also may be evidence of displacement of the affected tooth away from the widened periodontal membrane space. Alternately, the entire periodontal membrane space around one or several teeth may be widened. Clinically, such teeth may be very painful, mobile, and associated with altered occlusion. Gardner and Mills (1976) have shown that the cause of this widening is infiltration by tumor into the periodontal ligament. Focal thickening of the periodontal membrane space also may be seen in periodontal disease, metastatic disease, early primary squamous cell carcinoma, and chondrosarcoma.

Mixed Osteolytic/Osteoblastic Osteosarcoma. According to Worth (1963), the mixed osteolytic/osteoblastic type may have one of the following appearances:

1. There may be a well-defined geographic area of bone destruction with partially sclerotic margins, with some bone within the rarefied area. This bone may consist of strands forming trabeculae, which may be few or many, and they may intersect or produce a honeycomb pattern, thus greatly resembling a central giant cell granuloma.

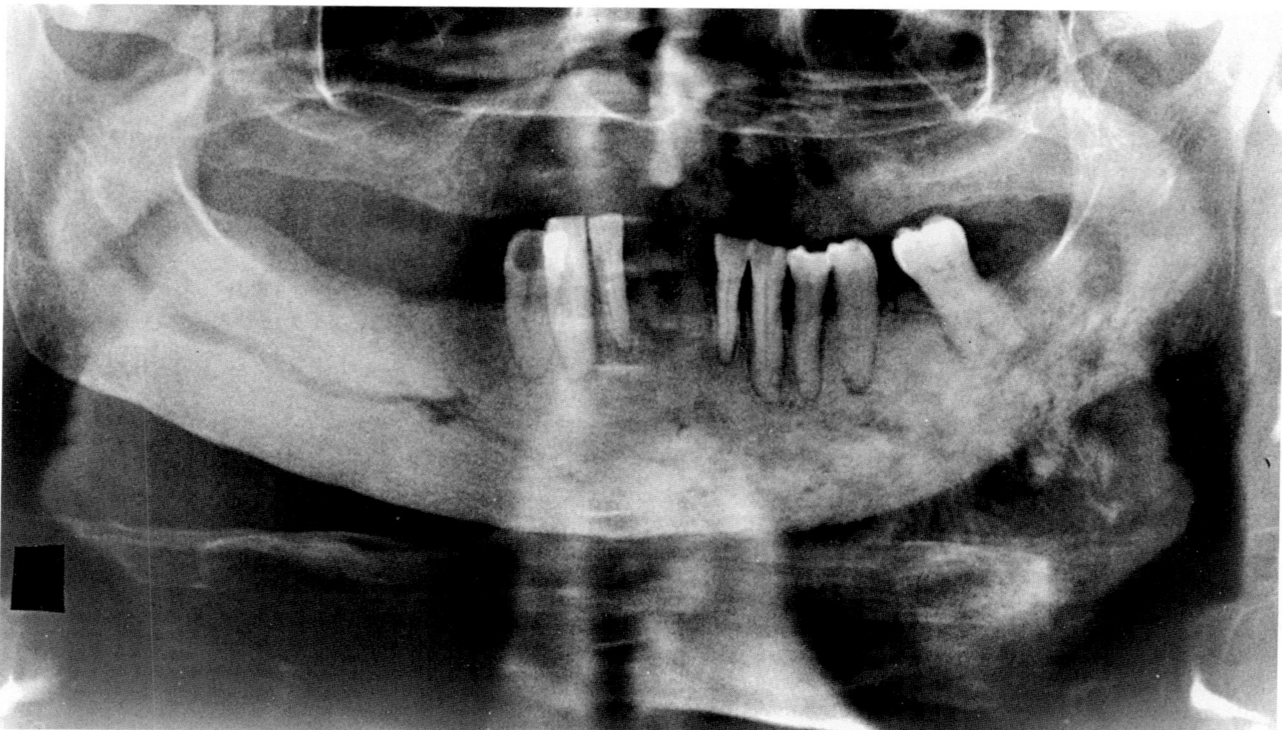

FIGURE 16–44.

Osteogenic Sarcoma: Diffuse sclerotic appearance in 70-year-old woman. There is bilateral cortex destruction, and the right mandible greatly resembles diffuse sclerosing osteomyelitis. The left side is mixed with motheaten and permeative changes and a sunray periosteal reaction. (Courtesy of Professor T. Noikura, Second Oral Surgery Department, Kagoshima University, Kagoshima, Japan.)

2. There may be a well-defined area of bone destruction with partially sclerotic margins, showing solid islands of bone within the rarefied area. These may be single or multiple, small or large, irregular in outline, and of a uniform density without internal structure. These bone masses tend to resemble each other vaguely and are different from the original healthy bone.
3. The smaller the amount of new bone formation, the more likely the margins will be poorly defined. Additionally, irregular projections of tumor produce little "bays" extending into normal bone, are interpreted as infiltration, and are strongly suggestive of malignancy.
4. A pattern of perpendicular bony striae that radiate from the surface of the bone has been termed a sunburst or sunray pattern. The peripheral margin of the striae often has a semicircular arrangement with respect to the surface of the underlying host bone, within which varying degrees of destruction are present. The striae may be few or many, short or long, thick and coarse, or sparse and thin. On close inspection, they form tiny zigzags along their length, a highly suggestive sign of osteosarcoma. The bony striae sometimes are observed only in a right-angle view of the tumor. Although the sunray appearance is regarded by some as a periosteal reaction, Worth (1963) has stated that it is usually a change within the tumor itself. Even though the sunray pattern is highly suggestive of osteosarcoma, it has been found in some hemangiomas, other vascular tumors, thalassemia, sickle cell anemia, meningioma, odontoma, myeloma in the jaw, and chondrosarcoma.

Sclerotic Osteosarcoma. According to Worth (1963), the sclerotic variety may have one of the following appearances:

1. The whole area may consist of a single solid mass of dense bone that may affect a large portion of the mandible or maxilla.
2. In other cases, the dense sclerotic area is limited to a small section of involved bone.
3. Many sclerotic lesions are only partially sclerotic, with other affected portions being partly or totally osteolytic. There is a great tendency for the sclerotic mass to break down and become lytic to some degree.
4. This type has the greatest propensity for a benign appearance; thus, multiple views should be used to scrutinize these carefully for subtle signs suggestive of malignancy.
5. A subtle but highly suggestive sign of malignancy in the sclerotic variant occurs when the sclerotic area is between the teeth and involves the intercrestal bone. It will be observed that there is a buildup of intercrestal sclerotic bone in such a way that the alveolar process is higher than the normal unaffected adjacent areas. This buildup may be so slight that it is detected only by the wariest of observers. At other times, this change

1

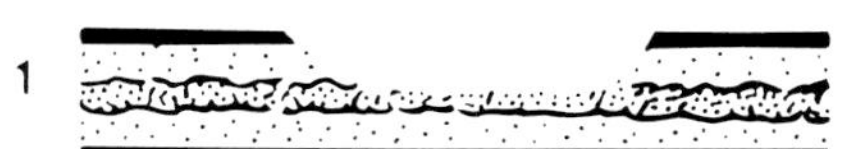

Bone destruction with no periosteal new bone formation.

2

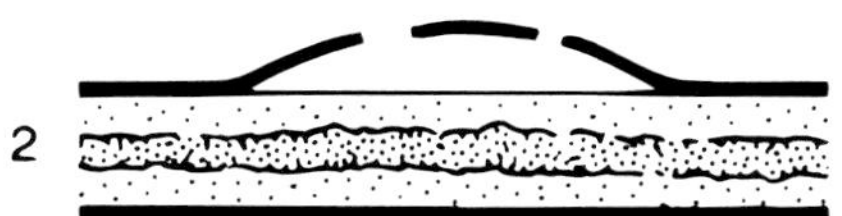

Thin layer of new bone deep to periosteum, but with discontinuities. This is usual, but not invariable; no bone destruction here, but usually present.

3

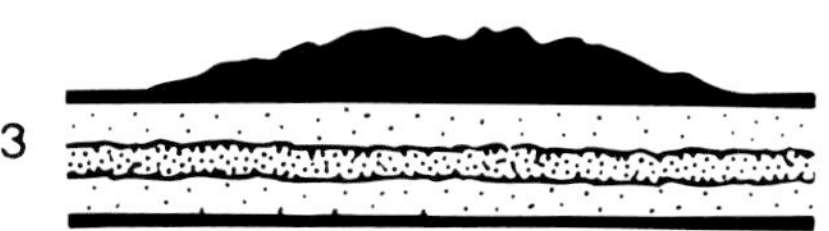

Irregular mass of subperiosteal new bone, usually associated with some bone loss.

4

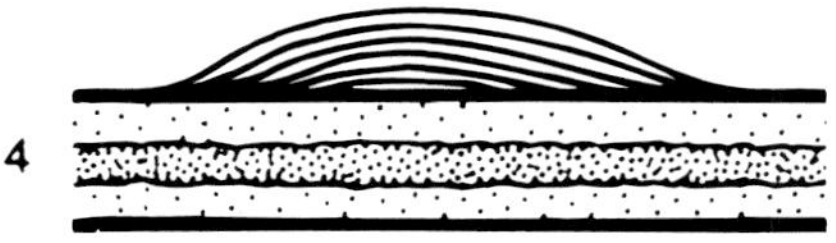

Laminated subperiosteal new bone formation, as is found often in inflammatory conditions.

5

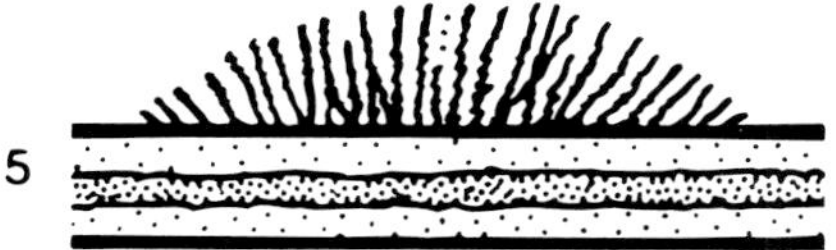

Radiating bony spicules, often regarded as periosteal reaction, but actually a change within tumor itself.

6

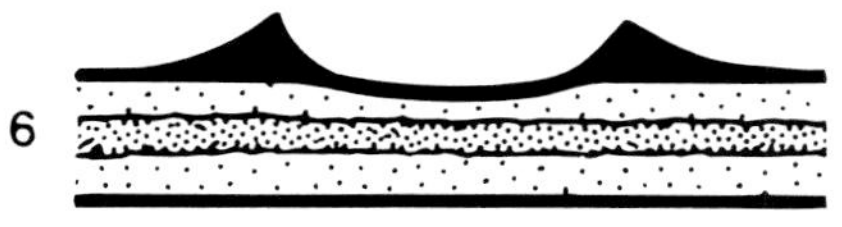

Codman's triangle, an appearance highly suggestive of osteogenic sarcoma. Tumor strips periosteum from bone and new bone is laid down between tumor and attachment of periosteum to bone.

FIGURE 16–45.

Osteogenic Sarcoma: Various periosteal reactions in osteogenic sarcoma. (Courtesy of H. M. Worth, Vancouver, Canada.)

is found in conjunction with a symmetric widening of the periodontal membrane space in an adjacent area. The only other circumstance in which this change has been observed is in chondrosarcoma.

Periosteal Reactions in Osteosarcomas of the Jaws. Osteogenic sarcoma often provokes a periosteal reaction when the long bones are affected. These also may be observed in the jaws, and they have been described in detail by Worth (1963). He has classified six possible changes, as can be seen in Figure 16–45:

1. Bone destruction with no periosteal new bone formation.
2. Formation of a thin discontinuous layer of new bone beneath the periosteum. Usually the underlying bone has been destroyed.
3. An irregular mass of subperiosteal new bone, usually associated with some loss of underlying bone.
4. Successive laminations of subperiosteal new bone formation. In the jaws, this is seen in Garrè's osteomyelitis, chronic rarifying osteomyelitis, Ewing's sarcoma, and chondrosarcoma.
5. Radiating striae forming a sunburst or sunray pattern as previously described.
6. Codman's triangle, which occurs when the tumor breaks through the surface of the bone, separating the periosteum from the underlying bone as it perforates through, and subsequent ossification of the space between the periosteum and underlying bone.

Variants of Osteogenic Sarcoma

Additional variants of osteogenic sarcoma include juxtacortical osteogenic sarcoma, a discussion of which immediately follows, extraosseous osteogenic sarcoma, and multicentric osteogenic sarcoma. Extraosseous osteogenic sarcoma occurs entirely within soft tissue, especially in the thighs; however, cases have been reported in the neck, face, orbit, submental region, and lip. Their behavior and prognosis are similar to those of central osteosarcoma. Some may contain calcified material, whereas others appear as nonspecific soft tissue masses. Multicentric osteosarcoma, also known as osteosarcomatosis, is extremely rare. It occurs in children between the ages of 6 and 9 years and almost never affects adults. Lesions occur in the metaphyses of multiple long bones and are symmetrically bilateral. The prognosis is extremely poor because the condition is invariably fatal. Multiple lung metastases are often present at diagnosis. According to Worth (1963), the various tumors look very similar and are invariably osteoblastic, although a few osteolytic cases have been reported. There is some controversy as to whether multicentric osteogenic sarcoma is a specific variant or whether it simply represents multiple metastases from a single primary tumor. We are not aware of any case affecting the jaws.

JUXTACORTICAL OSTEOSARCOMA

(Parosteal osteogenic sarcoma and periosteal osteogenic sarcoma)

Parosteal and Periosteal Osteosarcoma

Parosteal osteogenic sarcoma first was described in 1949 and 1951 by Geschickter and Copeland and had seemingly benign clinical and histologic features, yet some lesions re-

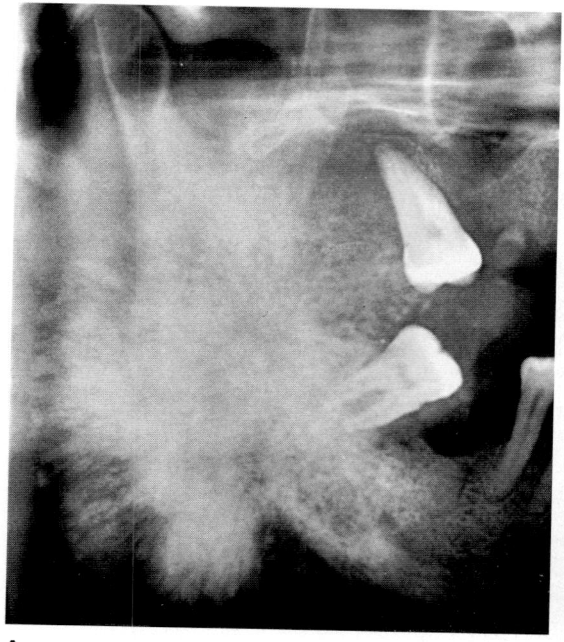

A

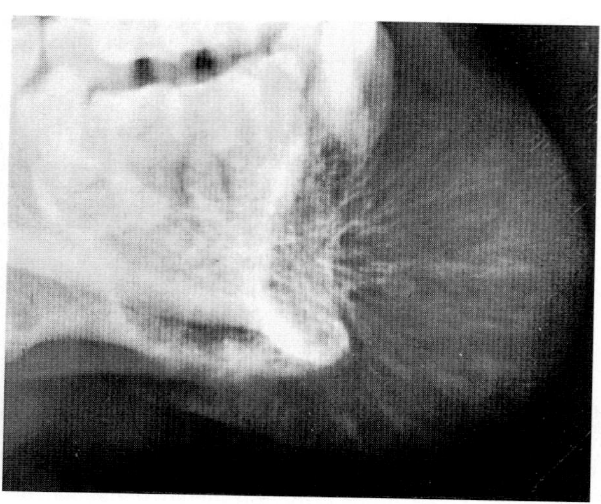

B

FIGURE 16–46.

Osteogenic Sarcoma: Periosteal reactions. A, There is a sunburst pattern, underlying bone destruction, and large snowflakelike pattern between upper and lower molars. The flocculent nature of spicules suggests a cartilaginous component. (Courtesy of Professor L. Alfaro, University of Chile School of Dentistry, Pathology Referral Center, Santiago, Chile.) B, Irregular spicules in sunburst-like pattern; destruction underlying bone and cortex.

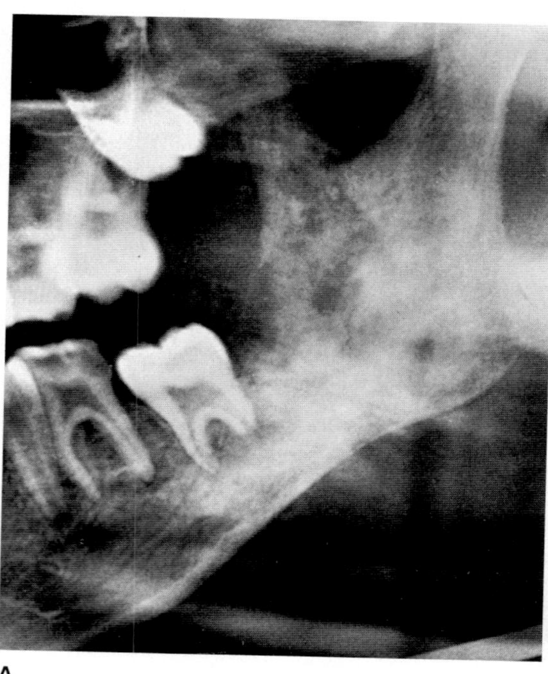

A

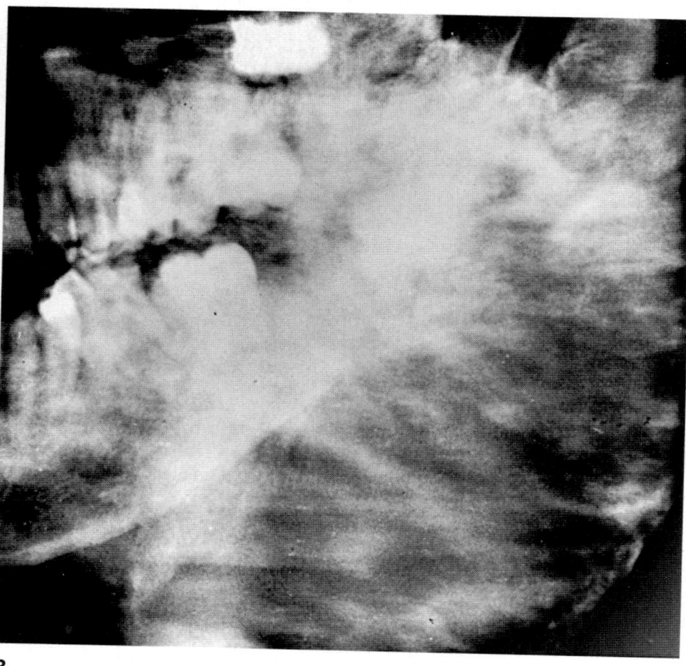

B

FIGURE 16–47.

Osteogenic Sarcoma: Case in a 13-year-old boy. A, Lesion shows mixed reaction, destruction of the inferior cortex, and irregular spicules of periosteal reaction. (From Farman AG, Nortjé CJ, Wood RE: Oral and Maxillofacial Diagnostic Imaging. Philadelphia:Mosby-Year Book, 1993, p. 283.) B, Two months after initiation of a full course of radiation therapy.

curred and others metastasized. According to Edeiken (1981), the term **parosteal** osteosarcoma has become synonymous with juxtacortical osteogenic sarcoma, a term coined by Jaffe (1958). It refers to an osteogenic sarcoma that develops in the periosteum, grows outward from the bone, and tends to surround the host bone rather than invade it. In most instances, it has a better prognosis than other osteogenic sarcomas. According to Dahlin (1978), **periosteal** osteosarcoma should be considered a separate entity, distinct from parosteal osteosarcoma, because it is more aggressive and has a poorer prognosis, although the prognosis is better than that of central osteogenic sarcoma. Huvos (1970) stated that parosteal and periosteal osteosarcomas represent variations of the same condition. He suggested that both should be referred to as **juxtacortical** osteogenic sarcoma, which he defines as a separate and distinct variation of osteogenic sarcoma that originates on the external surface of a bone specifically from the periosteum or underlying connective tissue. Although juxtacortical osteosarcomas account for approximately 5% of all osteosarcomas, Bras and colleagues (1980), using the definition of Huvos (1970), could find only six cases involving the jaws and added a seventh.

Pathologic Characteristics

Histologically, two groups of tumors have been identified. Approximately 75% are low-grade malignant tumors, with chondroid differentiation in roughly half; as the grade of malignancy increases, so does the incidence of recurrence within this first group. The remaining 25% are poorly differentiated from the beginning and carry a poorer prognosis.

Clinical Features

Bras and co-workers (1980) found 56 reported cases of extragnathic juxtacortical osteosarcoma in the literature and compared these with the 7 cases affecting the jaws. The male-to-female ratio is 2:3 in favor of female patients, and the peak incidence occurs in patients between the ages of 20 and 30 years. Six male patients and one female patient had cases affecting the jaws; the average age of these patients was 35 years (age range, 17 to 63 years). The initial complaints are swelling and, in approximately half of the patients, pain. The swelling often consists of an exophytic mass on the buccal or lingual side of the jaw. The exophytic mass is an integral part of the clinical picture because of the juxtacortical nature of the lesion.

Treatment/Prognosis

Extragnathic juxtacortical osteosarcomas are treated based on the histologic grading of the tumor. Low- and intermediate-grade tumors are treated only by ablative surgical resection, and the 5-year survival rate is approximately 50 to 75%. High-grade or poorly differentiated lesions often are treated by ablative surgical resection, followed by high-dose, multidrug, multicycle chemotherapy after surgery; the 5-year survival rate is approximately 15 to 25%. The seven cases involving the jaws initially were treated as follows: curettage (one case), local excision (three cases), partial maxillary resection (two cases), hemimandibulectomy (one case), and hemimandibulectomy plus chemotherapy (one case). One to three recurrences were reported in five of the seven cases, a recurrence rate of 71%. Only the cases treated by partial maxillary resection and hemimandibulectomy plus chemotherapy did not recur, but the former had only a 6-month follow-up. The follow-up period ranged from 6 months to 11 years, and all patients were alive at follow-up. Three of these were observed for 1 year or less, and the other four had follow-up periods of 6, 8, 10, and 11 years.

◆ *RADIOLOGY (Figs. 16–48 and 16–49)*

General Radiologic Features

According to Bras and co-workers (1980), juxtacortical osteosarcoma is found most commonly in the long bones in the metaphysis at the distal end of the femur, either end of the tibia, and the proximal humerus. It usually is seen as a dense mass of new bone with varying degrees of opacification within; the densest portion is usually at the base, where a central stalk attaches to the cortex. Early in the disease, a characteristic radiolucent line parallel to the long axis of the bone separates the dense tumor mass from the parent bone. This is observed in 30% of the cases. This radiolucent line is interrupted by the small radiopaque stalk attaching the tumor mass to the cortex. As the lesion matures, the radiodense stalk broadens at its base and eventually obliterates the radiolucent line. The peripheral portion of the lesion is usually more radiolucent and is often lobulated because of the fusion of several radiopaque masses. When the peripheral masses are detached from the main tumor mass, they are referred to as ''satellite'' lesions. Sometimes trabeculation may be seen in some portion of the mass, and a sunburst pattern of the trabeculae may be apparent. Approximately 25% show a peculiar tendency to encircle the parent bone. It is important to study the underlying cortex for involvement of the spongiosa within. According to Ahuja and colleagues (1977), medullary involvement in patients with low-grade tumors does not necessarily imply a worse prognosis; however, it may in people with high-grade lesions. Others, such as Unni and colleagues (1975), found that medullary infiltration indicated a poorer prognosis. A sunburst pattern usually is not seen unless there has been cortical invasion by the tumor.

Radiologic Features of the Jaws

According to Bras and co-authors (1980), juxtacortical osteogenic sarcoma of the jaws has a similar radiographic appearance to that in the skeleton, although their material is based on the seven reported cases. The periapical projection shows areas of mottled density diffusely involving much of the region covered by the radiograph; however, the occlusal film of the same region showed the characteristic features. In the posterior areas, occlusal and anteroposterior views were helpful, and in the anterior region, occlusal and lateral views were best. In their case, Bras and colleagues (1980) emphasized that medullary involvement could not be seen from the radiographs; however, it was observed on the gross and histologic sections.

The differential diagnosis consists of peripheral osteoma and myositis ossificans. The peripheral osteoma tends to

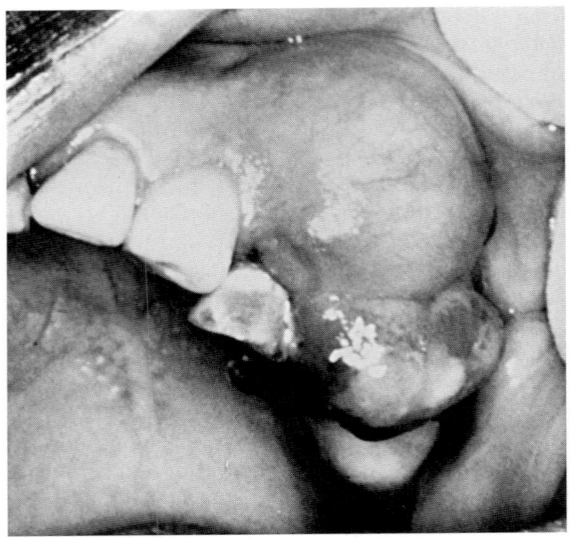

A

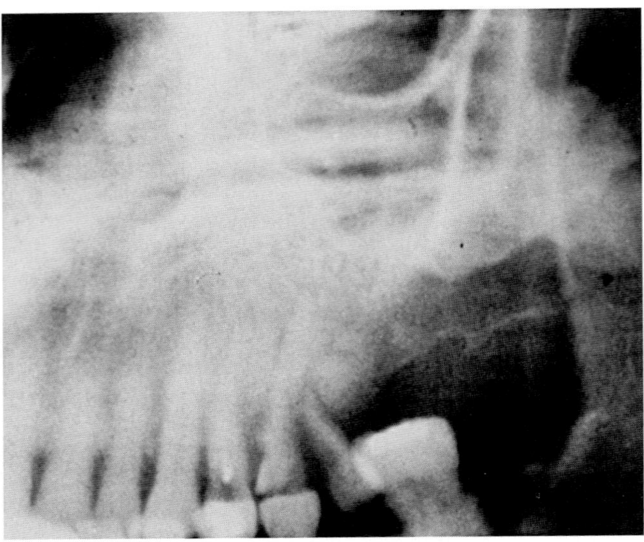

B

FIGURE 16–48.

Juxtacortical Osteosarcoma: A, Exophytic mass is typically present. B, Diffuse radiopaque lesion in left maxilla. (From Patterson A, Greer RO, Howard D: The periosteal osteosarcoma of the maxilla: a case report and review of the literature. J Oral Maxillofac Surg 48:522, 1990.)

be more radiodense because of the absence of cartilaginous areas, and in osteoma the rare striae tend to be fine and closer together, like the edge of a feather. Myositis ossificans consists of two radiologic variations: (1) a feathery type caused by ossification of a hematoma in muscle fascia, and (2) an irregular solid structure resulting from a calcified solitary hematoma. Myositis ossificans tends to show the great-

CHONDROSARCOMA (Chondrogenic sarcoma)

Chondrosarcoma was considered a form of osteosarcoma until 1930, when Phemister first described its clinically different behavior. In 1943, Lichtenstein and Jaffe provided definitive evidence that chondrosarcoma is a separate clinicopathologic entity. Chondrosarcoma remains poorly under-

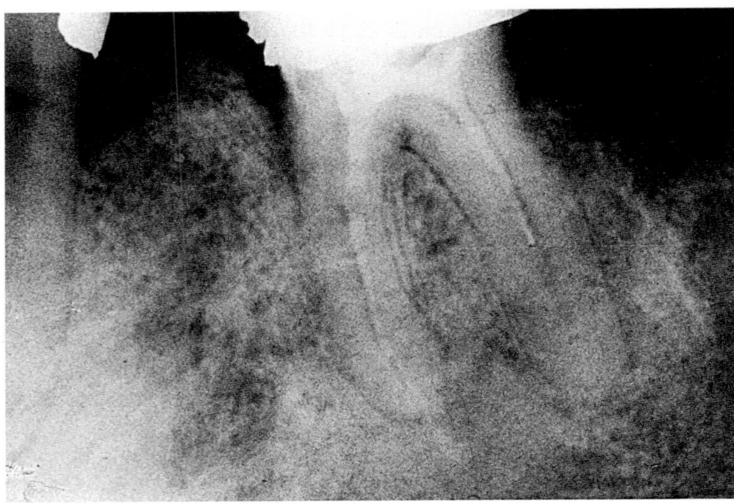

A

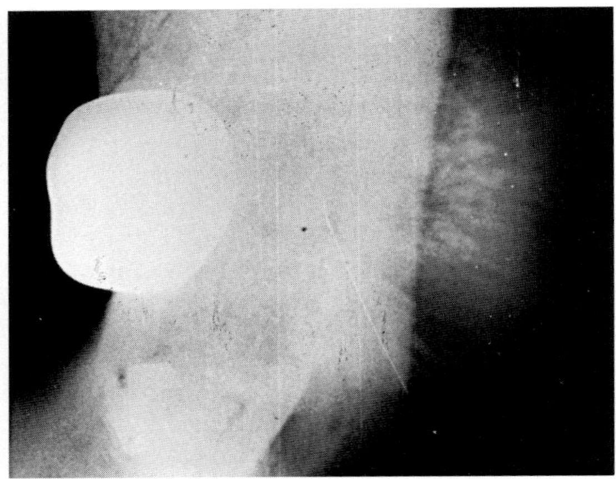

B

FIGURE 16–49.

Juxtacortical Osteosarcoma: A, Mottled radiopacity. B, Occlusal view shows sunburst pattern of zig-zagging striae. A feature is a radiolucent line at base of striae separating them from the cortex. On resection, this lesion showed intramedullary extension. (From Bras JM, et al: Juxtacortical osteogenic sarcoma of the jaws: review of the literature and report of a case. Oral Surg Oral Med Oral Pathol 50:535, 1980.)

stood. The literature is replete with conflicting reports leading to confusion and uncertainty with respect to a clear delineation of its characteristics. Christensen (1982) pointed out that mesenchymal chondrosarcoma was not mentioned in any of the major reviews of chondrosarcoma of the jaws. According to Dahlin (1978), chondrosarcoma is one of the most difficult of the malignant tumors from the histopathologic viewpoint. It may be mistaken easily for a chondroma or chondroblastic osteosarcoma. When there is spindling of cells at the periphery, it may be misinterpreted as a mesenchymal chondrosarcoma; conversely, in older reports mesenchymal chondrosarcoma simply would be classified as a dedifferentiated chondrosarcoma. Dahlin (1978) analyzed 470 cases at the Mayo Clinic and found that chondrosarcoma accounted for 10% of all malignant bone tumors. Excluding multiple myeloma, Krolls and colleagues (1980) determined that chondrosarcoma is the second most common primary malignant tumor of bone after osteogenic sarcoma, including that in the jaws. According to Chaudhry and colleagues (1961), 65% of all cartilaginous tumors occurring in the jaws represent chondrosarcomas. In 1974, 60 cases of chondrosarcoma of the jaws were reported at the AFIP. In 1979, Buchner and co-workers estimated that approximately 80 cases of chondrosarcoma of the jaws were reported in the literature.

Pathologic Characteristics

The pathogenesis of chondrosarcomas in the jaws has been discussed by Chaudhry and co-workers (1961). The premaxilla and maxilla are primarily membranous bones; however, cartilage from the developing nasal septum may become entrapped between the palatal shelves, and cartilage cell rests have been observed in the incisive canal region. Thus, chondrogenic tumors of all types are prone to occur in the anterior maxilla. In the mandible, tumors may originate from remnants of Meckel's cartilage in the body and the secondary cartilage that forms in the mental region, coronoid process, and condyle. Other sources of cartilage in the jaws include undifferentiated mesenchymal cells and metaplasia of connective tissue into cartilage. There is little fundamental difference between a chondroblast and osteoblast because either one may be transformed into the other.

According to Dahlin (1978), chondrosarcoma can be categorized into four basic types:

1. Primary chondrosarcoma was the most common type, accounting for 76% of the group. It arises de novo within the host bone and is composed of malignant cartilaginous tissue throughout. This cartilaginous tissue may differentiate to form trabeculae of bone; however, if the malignant cells are forming osteoid, even in minute quantities, the pathologist should classify the lesion as a chondrogenic osteosarcoma. Undoubtedly, a number of chondrogenic osteosarcomas have been reported as chondrosarcomas. Osteosarcoma occurs twice as frequently as chondrosarcoma, has a strong peak of incidence during the second decade of life, grows rapidly, and is prone to metastasize early. Chondrosarcoma evolves slowly, with a peak incidence in the sixth decade of life; metastasis is rare and occurs later in the disease.
2. Secondary chondrosarcomas accounted for 11% of all chondrosarcomas. They are said to arise from a previously existing benign cartilaginous tumor. Most of these benign cartilaginous tumors were multiple (44%) or solitary osteochondromas (41%), and a few were multiple chondromas.
3. Dedifferentiated chondrosarcomas accounted for 11% of the chondrosarcomas. In this instance, a primary, secondary, or clear cell chondrosarcoma gives rise to a more malignant tumor, either fibrosarcoma or osteosarcoma, often Broders' grade 3 or 4.
4. Clear cell chondrosarcomas constituted 2% of the sample. They resemble osteoblastoma or chondroblastoma histologically and occur mainly on the femur and humerus, sometimes affecting the joint. To our knowledge, none have been identified in the head and neck region or jaws.

In 1961, Chaudhry and colleagues reviewed the literature for chondrogenic tumors in the jaws; they found 52 well-documented cases and added 2 cases of their own. They divided these into three groups:

Group 1 consisted of 18 patients (35%) with a diagnosis of chondroma, osteochondroma, myxochondroma, fibro-osteochondroma, and enchondroma. The peak age of incidence was the sixth decade.

Group 2 consisted of 10 patients (19%) whose cartilaginous tumors were diagnosed as benign at the first microscopic examination and rediagnosed subsequently as chondrosarcoma. These represent secondary chondrosarcomas as classified by Dahlin (1978).

Group 3 consisted of 24 patients (46%) with an original diagnosis of chondrosarcoma. They had primary chondrosarcomas according to the classification of Dahlin (1978).

In Dahlin's (1978) series of 470 cases of **chondrosarcoma**, 90% were classified as Broders' grades 1 and 2. Long bone **osteosarcomas** are most often Broders' grades 3 and 4, whereas **osteosarcomas** in the jaws are most often Broders' grades 2 and 3. It is easy to conceive how a grade 2 chondrogenic osteosarcoma in the jaws might strongly resemble a grade 2 chondrosarcoma. According to Chaudhry and co-workers (1961), 19% of malignant chondrogenic tumors of the jaws were underdiagnosed inadvertently at the first microscopic interpretation. Sanerkin (1980) proposed measurement of alkaline phosphatase levels in the constituent tumor cells; chondrosarcoma would have negative results for alkaline phosphatase, and osteosarcoma, including chondroblastic osteosarcoma, would have positive results.

Clinical Features

According to Dahlin (1978), the peak incidence occurred in the sixth decade, with a normal distribution curve between the third to eighth decades. Only 4% of cases were diagnosed in the second decade of life, the peak decade of incidence of osteosarcoma. Secondary chondrosarcomas occurred in younger patients, with most cases developing in the third, fourth, and fifth decades, in descending order of frequency. In the 36 cases of chondrosarcoma in the jaws reviewed by Chaudhry and colleagues (1961), the peak age of incidence occurred in the sixth decade; however, 36% of cases developed in the first three decades. Of the 18 primary chondrosarcomas of the head and neck reported by Arlen and co-workers, 14 occurred in the jaws; 33% occurred in the first two decades of life, and 66% arose in patients younger than 40 years. According to Dahlin (1978), any large series on chondrosarcoma that includes a relatively large number of patients in the first two decades of life probably includes patients with chondroblastic osteosarcoma. Dahlin (1978) reported that 60% of his patients were male. Chaudhry and associates (1961) found that 54% of primary chondrosarcomas in the jaws occurred in men; however, in secondary chondrosarcomas, the male-to-female ratio was 2:1. In the series of Arlen and colleagues (1970), the overall male-to-female ratio was 2:1.

Terezhalmy and Bottomley (1977) reviewed the literature for the clinical signs of chondrosarcoma in the jaws. The most common presenting sign is swelling, and, in the series of Arlen and co-workers (1970), 12 patients (66%) had a painless mass. The mass usually is associated with expansion of the buccal or lingual cortical plates, or both; in the maxilla, a mass may occur on the palate. The overlying mucosa may be normal, show an increased number of telangiectatic surface vessels, or be ulcerated, or spontaneous bleeding may be present. Pain is a late feature, often appearing in the later stages. There also may be signs of involvement of the antrum, nasal cavity, and orbit. According to Chaudhry and co-workers (1961), the teeth often were affected, showing extrusion and root resorption. Characteristically, regional lymphadenopathy is absent. Other symptoms include nasal obstruction, epistaxis, proptosis, blurred vision, headache, toothache, and a feeling of numbness. When the temporomandibular joint is involved, there may be swelling in front of the ear, deviation to the opposite side, and disarticulation of the teeth on the affected side. In the series of Arlen and associates (1970), the lesion was present 6 to 8 weeks before diagnosis. In general, chondrosarcoma of the jaws behaves in an insidious manner, such that the disease may be advanced before the patient or clinician notices clinical changes.

Treatment/Prognosis

Early investigators originally thought that chondrosarcoma had a better prognosis than osteosarcoma because it tends to grow slowly and metastasize less rapidly. In the following 20 years, it became evident that chondrosarcoma had a fatal outcome more often than osteosarcoma when adequate resection was not performed. Currently, surgeons radically resect all chondrosarcomas and avoid delays between biopsy and definitive treatment; under these circumstances, chondrosarcoma may have a better prognosis than osteosarcoma. Dahlin (1978) recommended early radical resection and the use of definitive therapy at the time of biopsy. He emphasized the importance of referring to the radiograph in selecting the biopsy site; this may show the most aggressive and infiltrative portion of the tumor, which should be included in the specimen. The biopsy instruments should not be reused for the definitive procedure because chondrosarcoma is notorious for recurring after implantation. The excision should be wide and complete the first time around because some chondrosarcomas recur as a more anaplastic, dedifferentiated, and aggressive lesion.

Varying combinations of radiation therapy and, more recently, chemotherapy have been used in combination with radical surgery with varying degrees of success. These have been used more frequently in controlling recurrent lesions. In a study of 288 cases of chondrosarcoma in 1963, Henderson and Dahlin found that the 10-year survival rate was only 20% because of inadequate resection. In recent years, when radical excision has become more common, long-term survival could be achieved in more than 50%. Dahlin (1978) emphasized that late recurrences are so prone to occur that 5-year survival rates are not very significant as a criterion for cure. Evans and colleagues (1977) found that low-grade chondrosarcomas were locally aggressive and nonmetastasizing, whereas high-grade chondrosarcomas had a high metastatic potential; however, they concluded that the incidence of local recurrence depended most on the adequacy of surgical removal, rather than on histologic grading. The ultimate prognosis for jaw lesions depends on the following factors: (1) the site and extent of the tumor, (2) adequacy of surgical margins, and (3) tumor differentiation. The patient should be observed radiologically for at least 10 years, after which there should be awareness that recurrence is still a viable possibility. In one case reported by Arlen and colleagues (1970), the patient had recurrence 13 years after surgery.

◆ RADIOLOGY (Figs. 16–50 to 16–55)

Location

In general, central chondrosarcoma may occur in any bone preformed in cartilage. It is seen most frequently in the long bones, usually at the metaphysis and occasionally in the midshaft. It may be seen in the flat bones; however, the hands, feet, and vertebrae rarely are affected. In the skull the most common location is the sphenoid bone (70%), followed by the cerebellopontine angle (17%), occipital bone (5%), and frontal, parietal, and temporal bones (2%). The lesion also may be observed intracranially in almost any location; however, the falx and intercerebellar areas are the most frequent.

In the jaws, Chaudhry and colleagues (1961) found a slight predilection for the maxilla, in which 58% of the cases occurred. In their 14 cases involving the jaws, Arlen and associates (1970) found that 71% of these occurred in the maxilla. Kragh and colleagues (1960) found 10 cases of chondrosarcoma involving the maxilla; however, only 2 were thought to have arisen within the maxilla itself, whereas the remainder were thought to have originated in the nasal cavity and involved the maxilla secondarily. Chaudhry and co-workers (1961) stated that the anterior alveolar ridge was the predominant site, often with extension of the tumor into the palate, nasal fossa, and paranasal sinuses; this held true for primary and secondary chondrosarcomas in the maxilla. Chaudhry and co-workers (1961) found 9 cases in the mandible. Of these, 44% occurred in the body in the premolar-molar area, 33% in the symphysis region, and one case each

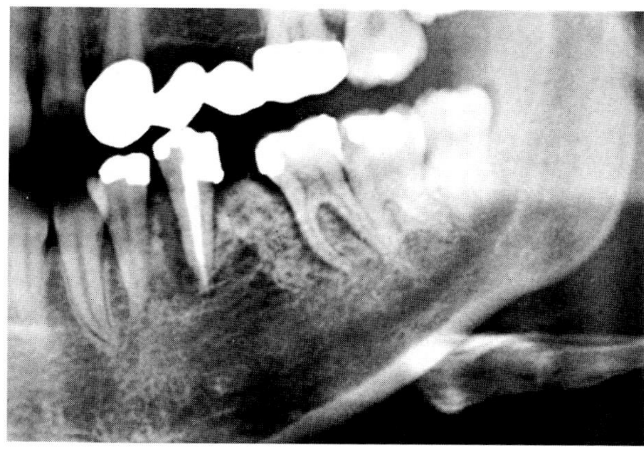

A

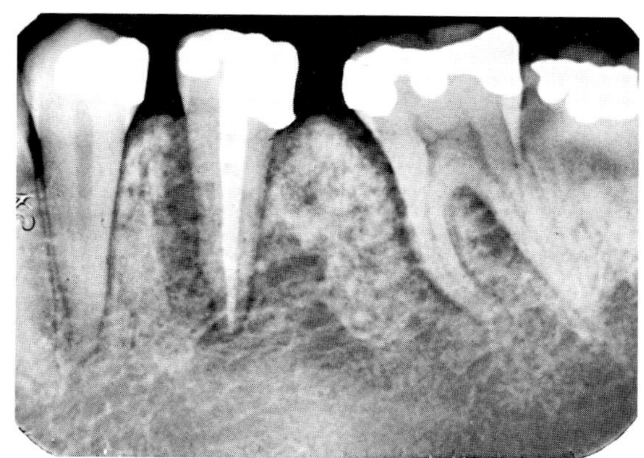

B

FIGURE 16–50.

Chondrosarcoma: Case in a 32-year-old woman. A, Shows widened periodontal ligament space, punctate radiopaque area, separation of teeth, and apparent extrusion of second premolar. B, The level of crestal bone is higher than normal. There are permeative changes within radiolucent areas, and premolar is at a normal height. Lingually placed objects are projected upward in panoramic image. (Courtesy of B. Glass, University of Texas, San Antonio, TX.)

in the coronoid process and condyle. In the mandible, secondary chondrosarcomas were seen only in the body, in the molar-premolar region.

Radiologic Features

Dahlin (1978) stated "the radiograph is nearly always helpful and often affords almost pathognomonic evidence of chondrosarcoma." According to Edeiken (1981), "when the distinctive punctate or snowflake cartilaginous calcifications (calcific foci) are found within this tumor, the diagnosis radiographically is not too difficult...it usually proves to be chondrosarcoma." In the jaws, Worth (1963) had very little confidence in the utility of radiographs in the diagnosis of chondrosarcoma; in most instances, chondrosarcomas appeared malignant, although they may show any of the features of osteosarcoma.

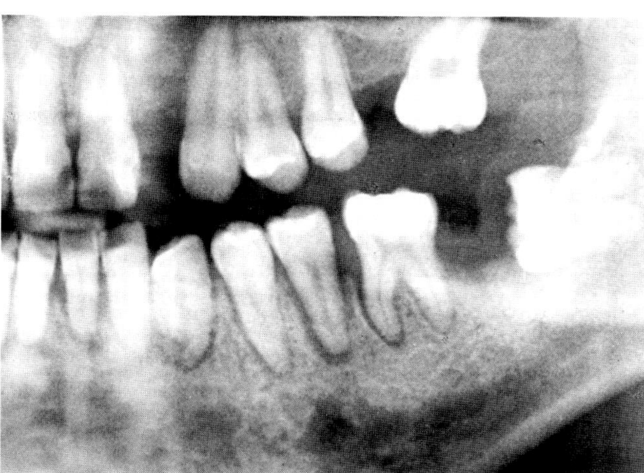

FIGURE 16–51.

Chondrosarcoma: Left mandible shows areas of increased and decreased density, and there is widening of the periodontal membrane space of most teeth in quadrant. (Courtesy of Drs. L. Archila, F. Erales, and R. Carlos, Guatemala City, Guatemala.)

Edeiken (1981) stated that central chondrosarcomas have two distinct radiologic appearances:

1. The first is an osteolytic lesion with a relatively benign appearance. The lesions tend to be small, ranging from 1 cm to several centimeters in diameter. The margins are well defined, with a short transitional zone, and sometimes there is a sclerotic margin. Small, irregular, calcified foci are distributed throughout the lesion and usually do not coalesce. According to Edeiken (1981), their density is much less than the tumor bone density in osteosarcoma. The cortex sometimes is expanded and thickened. Edeiken (1981) emphasized that, up to this point, chondrosarcoma is the one malignant bone tumor that may appear perfectly benign radiologically. If the lesion progresses, however, it will become less well defined and ultimately will perforate the cortex and assume the appearance of a rapidly growing malignant bone lesion.
2. The second type of central chondrosarcoma may be a later phase of the first. The lesions are predominantly osteolytic, blend imperceptibly with the adjacent normal bone, and lack any evidence of a sclerotic margin. They may be as small as 1 cm in diameter; however, they may replace large portions of the host bone. Characteristically this type contains the irregular punctate snowflake type of calcified chondroid matrix. These calcific foci are usually of low density, somewhat less than bone; however, the density may increase when many are present. Edeiken (1981) emphasized that when these calcifications are absent, chondrosarcoma hardly can be distinguished from fibrosarcoma and osteolytic osteosarcoma. Periosteal reactions are seen commonly with chondrosarcoma.

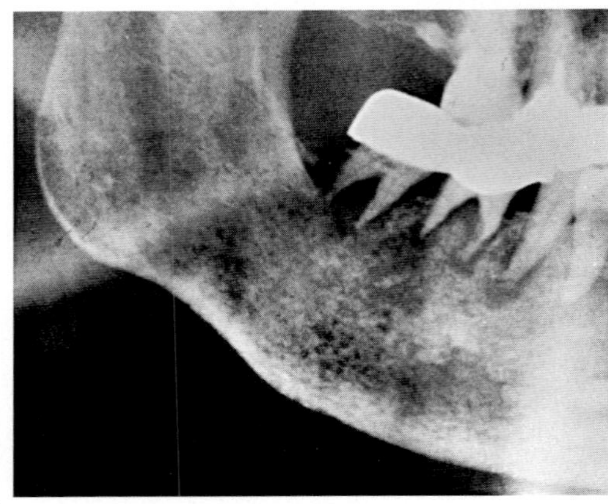

A

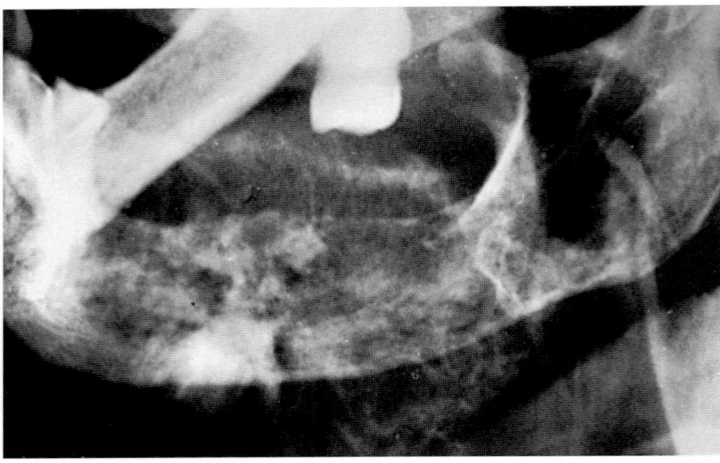

B

FIGURE 16–52.

Chondrosarcoma: A, Case in a 66-year-old woman shows spiked apices, a widened periodontal membrane space, and permeative changes admixed with calcific foci. (Courtesy of Professor H. Fuchihata, Osaka University School of Dentistry, Osaka, Japan.) B, Case in a 65-year-old woman shows blastic and lytic changes and a periosteal reaction with irregular striae. The most characteristic feature is small flocculent calcific foci, especially in the premolar area.

Some jaw lesions are well defined and lytic and contain varying amounts of flocculent calcific material appearing as tiny punctate flecks or larger granules. They have a density less than that of the surrounding bone, but this must be assessed at the periphery, where more details can be seen. There is no tendency for calcific foci to coalesce in a benign cartilaginous lesion, whereas in chondrosarcoma coalescence may be present. The calcific foci may aggregate to form snowflake-like patterns, although the patterns are more bizarre and the size of the individual foci may vary greatly. As the tumor mass enlarges, the calcific foci become superimposed on one another, appear denser than bone, and may obscure lytic changes within the host bone. A short transition zone usually is seen between the tumor mass and normal bone. These lesions often have a benign appearance.

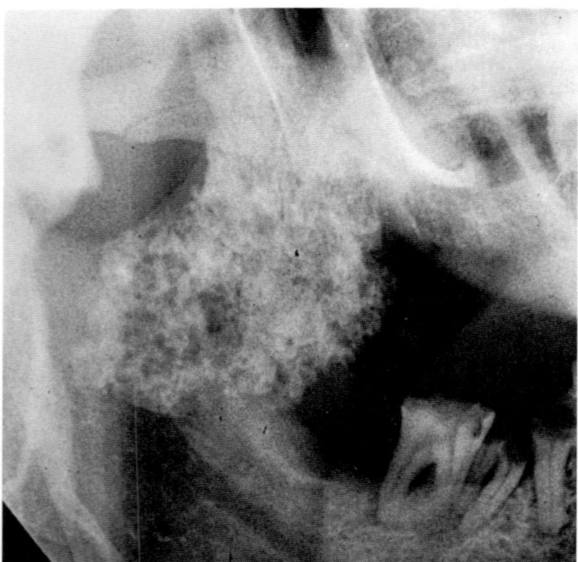

FIGURE 16–53.

Chondrosarcoma: Case in a 21-year-old woman. Several loose maxillary molars were extracted, after which this mass grew rapidly in the maxillary tuberosity area. The calcific foci are more granular in size and form doughnutlike and snowflakelike shapes; their density is usually somewhat less than that of bone. (Courtesy of Dr. M. Kasle, Indianapolis, IN.)

In addition, the following are specific characteristics in the jaws: (1) projection of the crestal portion of the tumor beyond the normal height of alveolar bone; (2) a uniform thickening of the periodontal membrane space along one side of the root of one or more teeth in the region; (3) evidence of a sclerotic or partially sclerotic margin; (4) root resorption (5) evidence of long-standing tooth displacement; (6) discovery as an incidental finding on routine radiologic examination; and (7) small localized lesions on the coronoid process or condyle.

Additional features include expansion, with perforation of the cortex by the tumor mass. The entire hemimandible or maxilla may be involved. In the mandible, there may be extension into the ramus. The maxilla may have extension into the palate, antrum, or nasal cavity with additional involvement of the paranasal sinuses and orbit. The involved teeth may be painful, especially if they are in traumatic occlusion. Periosteal reactions may be seen, including the sunburst pattern.

Cohen and co-authors (1984) pointed out the advantages of axial and coronal CT with respect to maxillary chondrosarcomas, reporting the case of a 51-year-old man with a large soft tissue mass extending from the left maxilla. The authors indicated the particular value of CT in detecting the telltale characteristic soft tissue calcifications, which may

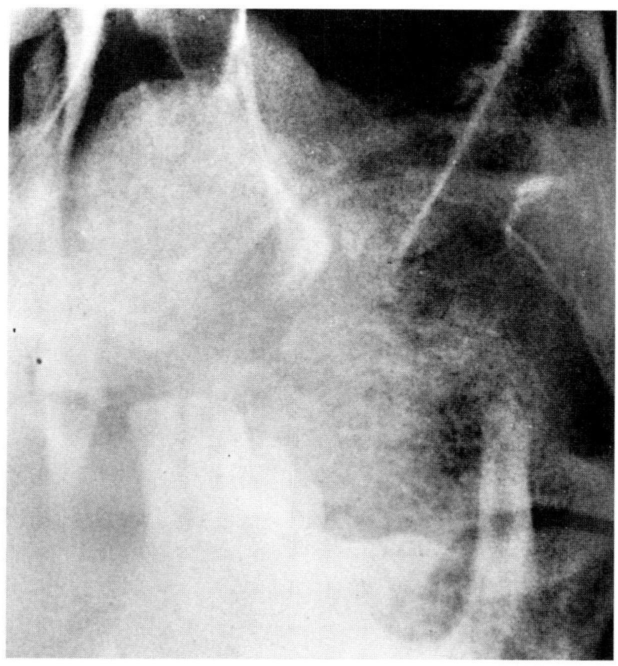

A

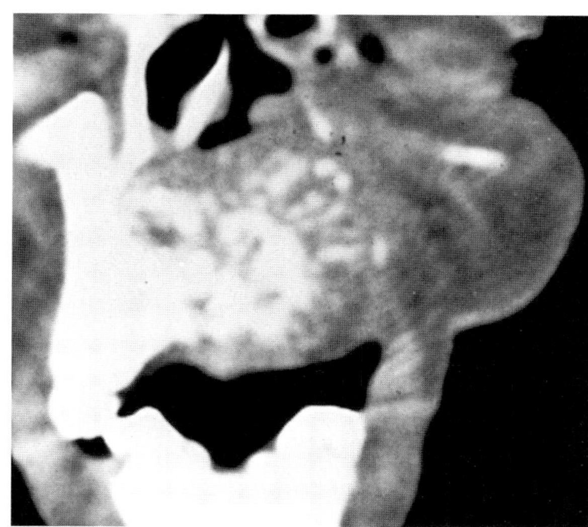

B

FIGURE 16–54.

Chondrosarcoma: A, Plain radiograph shows large mass in left maxilla. Calcific foci are difficult to characterize, although doughnut-like shapes, with a density less than that of bone, can be seen toward the periphery. (From Farman AG, Nortjé CJ, Wood RE: Oral and Maxillofacial Diagnostic Imaging. Philadelphia:Mosby-Year Book, 1993, p. 287.) B, CT image of this lesion. Calcific foci appear to have formed granules and masses. The entire lesion resembles a huge bizarre snowflake.

be ''burned out'' in routine radiographs. They also emphasized the utility of CT when the histologic diagnosis of malignancy is questionable.

Peripheral Chondrosarcoma

Peripheral chondrosarcomas occur primarily in the flat bones and on the ends of the femur and humerus. They are rare in the vertebrae, skull, and jaws, as well as the other long bones and small tubular bones of the hands and feet. They arise in the cartilaginous cap of an osteochondroma, especially in patients with multiple hereditary exostoses. They are seen as a soft tissue mass apparently attached to the bone, containing minute or massive telltale calcific masses. Often the underlying cortex is intact. In more advanced stages, there may be considerable destruction of the underlying bone.

Extraskeletal Chondrosarcomas

Extraskeletal chondrosarcomas occur entirely in soft tissue and have been reviewed by Edeiken (1981). Cases may occur in patients at any age. They may be found in the gluteal region and lower extremities, including the feet, although this is quite rare. Extraskeletal chondrosarcomas have been seen in the shoulder, upper extremities, and hands. Vassar (1958) reported a case of extraosseous chondrosarcoma in the tongue. The recurrence rate may be as high as 40%, and metastasis may occur in 15% of cases. According to Edeiken (1981), the characteristic cartilaginous calcifications occur in 30%.

MESENCHYMAL CHONDROSARCOMA

Mesenchymal chondrosarcoma first was reported as a separate entity by Lichtenstein and Bernstein in 1959. It was recognized later by the World Health Organization in 1972. The mesenchymal chondrosarcoma has two interesting characteristics: (1) the most common site of occurrence is the head and neck region, including the jaws; and (2) one third of these tumors occur in the extraskeletal soft tissue, including the paraoral regions. In Dahlin's 1978 series of 6221 bone tumors at the Mayo Clinic, only 15 mesenchymal chondrosarcomas could be identified. These accounted for less than 1% of the malignant bone tumors in the series. In 1982, Christensen found 22 reported cases involving the jaws and added a new case.

Pathologic Characteristics

The tumor is believed to originate from primitive cartilage forming mesenchyme, with some cells undergoing differentiation into cartilage and others remaining in an undifferentiated state. This produces a characteristic histologic picture. As described by Christensen (1982), the lesion shows a bimorphic pattern consisting of small or large well-demarcated

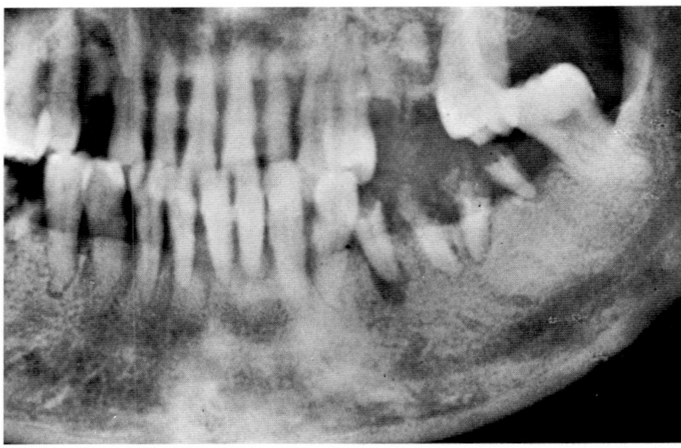

A

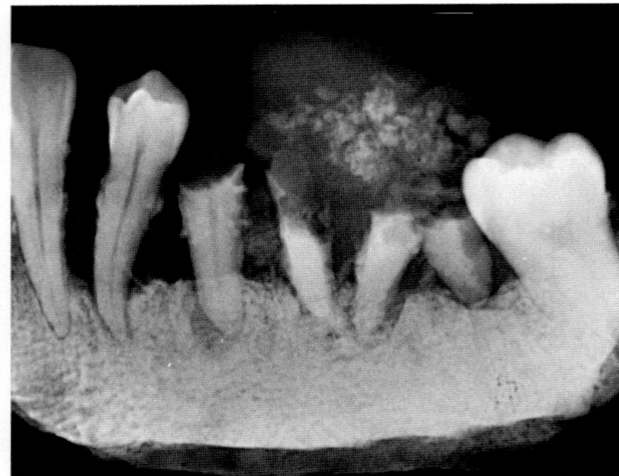

B

FIGURE 16–55.

Chondrosarcoma: Case in a 38-year-old woman. A and B, Possible peripheral variant. A large exophytic mass was superimposed on retained root tips and alveolar ridge. There are calcific granules within mass and some are doughnut shaped. (Courtesy of Drs. M. Araki and K. Hashimoto, Nihon University School of Dentistry, Tokyo, Japan.)

zones of well-differentiated chondroid material adjacent to sheets or clusters of highly undifferentiated oval or round cells, arranged around numerous slitlike spaces or capillaries. According to Dahlin (1978), it may resemble Ewing's sarcoma, and he recommended a radiograph to ensure that the biopsy specimen represents a mineralized portion of the tumor.

Clinical Features

In the extragnathic sites, Chavez (1966) found a dramatic peak in the second and third decades of life. Christensen (1982) reported that, among the 23 cases involving the jaws, only 2 occurred in patients outside this age range; one patient was 32 years and the other was 46 years. Male and female patients were affected equally. The most common initial complaint is swelling, often painless, although pain has been reported in a few cases. Other findings include epistaxis, hearing loss, paresthesia, gingival bleeding, and loose teeth. The average delay between the onset of symptoms and treatment was approximately 6 months, and all but one patient had a delay of 6 weeks to 1 year. In one patient there was a 10-year delay.

Treatment/Prognosis

This tumor is treated by radical surgical resection with a wide margin. Although the tumor is considered radioresistant, radiation therapy and chemotherapy have been used in conjunction with surgery. Among the 15 patients reported by Dahlin (1978), 12 (80%) died, usually with metastases. Six of these 12 survived 5 to 10 years; however, all 6 died several years later of multiple lung or bone metastases or recurrent local disease. Batsakis (1979) stated that jaw lesions may have a more rapidly fatal course. Christensen (1982) found 8 cases of mesenchymal chondrosarcoma of the jaws for which there was follow-up for 5 or more years; 5 of the patients were dead, 1 was alive with metastasis at 14 years, and the remaining 2 were free of disease.

◆ RADIOLOGY (Fig. 16–56)

Location

Dahlin (1978) found that one third of all the skeletal cases occurred in the jaws. Other skeletal sites include the flat bones, especially the ribs, ilium, scapula, vertebral column, and calvarium of the skull. An additional one third of the cases were found in extraskeletal soft tissue sites. Christensen (1982) found a slight predilection for the maxilla, with 61% occurring in this location and the remainder in the mandible.

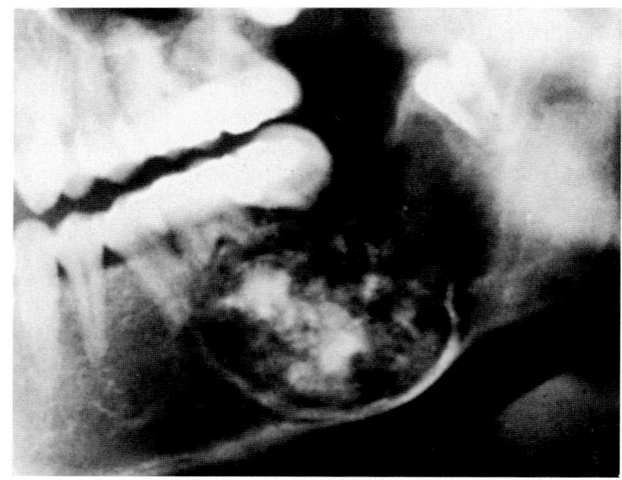

FIGURE 16–56.

Mesenchymal Chondrosarcoma: Case in a 16-year-old girl. The lesion is described in detail in text. (Courtesy of Dr. S. Lovestedt, Rochester, MN.)

Radiologic Features

Christensen (1982) reviewed the radiologic features mentioned for the 22 cases affecting the jaws. He stated that most jaw lesions showed nonspecific osteolytic areas. The lesions may be small or large, with well-defined margins and especially sclerosis, which may be present in some areas and absent in others within the same lesion. There may be perforation of the cortex and herniation of a soft tissue tumor mass. Mazabraud (1974) used arteriography and showed hypervascularization in the area of the tumor. In the maxilla, Christensen (1982) found that there is often involvement of the sinuses, with expanded and displaced antral walls, perforation of antral walls, and complete tumefaction of the sinus. In one of the cases in the antrum, calcific material was observed within the tumor mass. In another case, the lesion resembled a cyst between the maxillary canine and premolar teeth.

Dr. Stanley Lovestedt from the Mayo Clinic provided us with a case that may be seen in Figure 16–56. A 16-year-old girl had a lesion that seemed to have a bimorphic appearance in the mandibular left molar-ramus area. The anterior portion of the tumor appeared strikingly benign and circular in shape, measuring approximately 3 cm in diameter. Although there were lytic areas, there were numerous calcific foci, some of which appeared to have coalesced. The most radiodense calcific material was toward the center of the lesion. Superiorly, there was almost complete resorption of the roots of the second premolar and first and second molars. The inferior cortex of the mandible was thinned and expanded very slightly. The superior, anterior, and inferior margins were surrounded by a thick, almost continuous sclerotic margin. The posterior half of the tumor showed some features of malignancy, and the tumor extended into the ramus, displacing the developing third molar to a level approximately 2.0 cm below the sigmoid notch. This area was primarily lytic, with less defined margins and perforation at the anterior border of the ramus. Within the lytic area, several poorly calcified foci were present. Root resorption is an indication of a locally aggressive benign lesion and almost never is seen in malignant diseases; one of the rare exceptions is chondrosarcoma. Tooth displacement within bone is also a relatively benign feature because most malignant tumors grow around teeth without any tendency to displace them within the jawbone. The thickened sclerotic margin is a deceptively benign feature; however, this may be seen in osteosarcoma and chondrosarcoma. The lytic posterior area has margins that appear infiltrating in some parts without evidence of expansion, and a portion of the mandible has been perforated in an irregular manner. Perforation in the absence of expansion is strongly suggestive of malignancy.

In summary, the lesion appeared to have a bimorphic appearance with locally aggressive benign features in one part and features suggestive of malignancy in the other part.

"BLASTIC" METASTATIC TUMORS

(Secondary carcinoma)

Most metastatic tumors to the jaws are lytic in nature, and these have been discussed in Chapter 14, "Poorly Defined Radiolucencies." The classic report with respect to metastatic bone disease was published by Geschickter and Copeland in their 1936 monograph of 334 cases. The primary sites as reviewed by Clausen and Poulsen, in descending order of frequency, were the breast (33%); lung (18%); kidney (16%); thyroid, colon, rectum, and prostate (7% each); melanocarcinoma of skin and stomach (5% each); and, rarely, the testes, bladder, liver, uterine cervix, and ovary. Bhaskar (1973) stated that only 1% of malignant tumors in the body metastasize to the jaws and, of all oral malignant neoplasms, only 1% represent metastatic foci. The group of 25 cases reported by Meyer and Shklar (1965), represented approximately 1% of the 2400 malignant oral tumors in their files. According to van der Kwast and van der Waal (1974), the rarity of metastatic spread to the jaws may result from the relative lack of red marrow, which is replaced with fatty marrow with advancing age. Metastatic bone lesions occur preferentially in sites of greater red marrow concentrations. Because the marrow lacks a system of lymphatic vessels, metastatic spread to the jaws is usually hematogenous. In 1963, Clausen and Poulsen reviewed the literature from 1884 to 1961 and found 92 cases of metastatic tumors to the jaws, and in 1982 Bucin and colleagues identified 424 reported cases. Thompson and colleagues (1986) stated that 90% of all oral metastases occur in the jawbones, principally the mandible, whereas the remaining 10% are to the oral soft tissues, including the tongue (5%), buccal mucosa (3%), and all other sites (1 to 2%).

Pathologic Characteristics

To classify a lesion as metastatic, the following criteria have been established by Clausen and Poulsen (1963): (1) a primary tumor must be identified conclusively; (2) there must be histologic and radiologic evidence of jawbone metastasis; (3) the metastatic oral lesion must be correlated histologically with the primary lesion; and (4) when the primary lesion is anatomically close to the metastatic lesion, direct extension must be ruled out by a wide, clear margin around the primary site, with no tumor present between the two foci. These criteria hold true for lytic and blastic metastases. Meyer and Shklar (1965) found that 70% of their 25 cases represented adenocarcinomas. Oikarinen and colleagues (1975) reported that 84% of all jaw metastases consisted of carcinoma and adenocarcinoma; neuroblastomas were seen in 9% and sarcomas in 6%, and the least common was melanoma (1%).

Carcinomas and adenocarcinomas spread mainly through the lymphatics, whereas sarcomas spread hematogenously. Lymphogenous spread consists of a phased transfer from gland to gland; hematogenous spread is a phased transfer from organ to organ. Breakthough into an organ usually occurs at the capillary level; once this capillary filter is broken, dissemination to the next organ takes place. Hematogenous spread usually results from invasion into a venous lumen but also can occur when lymph containing metastatic tumor cells is effused into the bloodstream. According to van der Kwast and van der Waal (1974), metastatic spread usually is characterized by a standard sequence consisting of the liver first, followed by bone marrow and kidney; however, primary disease of the breast, thyroid, and prostate was more likely to disseminate to the skeleton than to the liver.

Clinical Features

In most series, older men and women were affected equally, although the primary site varied between sexes. In men, Bucin and colleagues (1982) observed that metastases to the oral cavity originated most often from primary tumors in the lungs, kidneys, prostate, colon, and rectum. In women, the breast, kidneys, colon, and rectum were the most common primary sites. In the series of 25 jaw metastases reported by Meyer and Shklar (1965), 52% of the patients were older than 50 years of age, 32% were between 40 and 60 years of age, and 12% were younger than 40 years of age; two were children. In children with metastatic tumors to the jaws, the most common primary lesions are bone sarcomas. Meyer and Shklar (1965) reported that pain was the most striking symptom, affecting the bone, teeth, and soft tissues. The most significant sign was loosening of one or more teeth without obvious periodontal disease. Other reported findings included swelling, paresthesia, anesthesia, toothache, pathologic fracture, and secondary infection. The onset is usually rapid, with the patient noticing a change in the size of the swelling. In rare instances, metastatic disease is asymptomatic and found on routine radiologic examination. According to Bhaskar (1973), approximately one third of oral metastases represent the first clinical indication of malignancy. Swollen neck nodes are a variable finding.

Treatment/Prognosis

Treatment depends on the type of tumor, degree of spread, and protocol developed by the tumor board of the treating institution. Chemotherapy and sometimes hormone therapy are used with varying combinations of surgery and radiation therapy for the primary tumor and metastatic lesion. The objective of therapy may be curative in some instances and palliative on other occasions, depending on how advanced the disease. Meyer and Shklar (1965) stated that the prognosis is very grave. In their series, other metastases were present in 52% of the patients at diagnosis; in those free of other metastases, many soon had them develop. According to Bucin and colleagues (1982), approximately 70% of patients with oral metastases die within 1 year of diagnosis.

◆ *RADIOLOGY (Figs. 16–57 and 16–58)*

General Radiologic Features

According to Schreiber (1981), metastatic bone tumors occur in locations rich in red marrow, including the axial skeleton, rib cage and sternum, femur, and humerus. Radiologically, they may mimic almost any other lesion; however, when multiple lesions are present in a middle-aged or older person, a diagnosis of metastatic disease is strongly suggested. According to Schreiber (1981), metastatic lesions are either erosive or reactive. Erosive lesions are lytic and occur in four patterns:

1. Geographic, characterized by a large solitary hole in the bone with a sharply demarcated edge; these are slow growing and less aggressive.
2. Motheaten, typified by multiple medium-sized holes in medullary or cortical bone; these sometimes coalesce to form larger confluent areas and represent moderately aggressive disease.
3. Permeative, consisting of multiple tiny holes, often seen in cortical bone, representing a rapidly destructive, aggressive process.
4. With multifocal areas of bone destruction when varying combinations of the foregoing three patterns are seen.

In bone, Schreiber (1981) reported that the restricting or restraining response consists of a laying down of new bone. Generally, malignant tumors grow too rapidly for this restricting process to occur. Blastic lesions may be located endosteally or at the periosteal surface, and they may consist of tumor bone or active new bone. In the endosteal location, blastic tumor bone that replaces normal bone is seen mainly in metastatic osteosarcoma; however, reactive new bone may be seen as a zone of sclerosis around a lytic focus, or reactive new bone may be only seen without osteolysis, as is especially prone to occur in metastatic prostate lesions. Periosteal new bone formation also may be seen, and it may be parallel or perpendicular to the cortex; it may be unilayered or multilayered. When the lesion is slowly progressive, the cortex is thickened gradually as periosteal new bone is laid down. When there is simultaneous erosion of the underside of the cortex and subperiosteal new bone formation on the outside of the cortex, the cortex takes on a bulging or expanded appearance. As stated by Schreiber (1981), metastatic lesions only rarely tend to evoke periosteal reactions, as compared with those seen in primary bone neoplasms; however, in osteoblastic metastases a periosteal reaction may be observed, especially in metastatic lesions of the prostate. New bone at angles to the cortex, referred to as spiculation, is very rare in metastatic disease; however, it does occur.

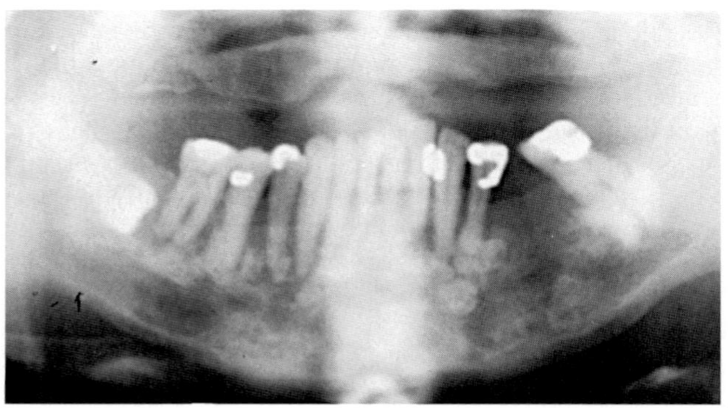

FIGURE 16–57.

Blastic Metastatic Tumor: A 72-year-old man with metastatic adenocarcinoma of prostate. There are well-defined radiopaque areas throughout the mandible. (Courtesy of Dr. H. Schwartz, Kaiser Permanente Medical Group, Los Angeles, CA.)

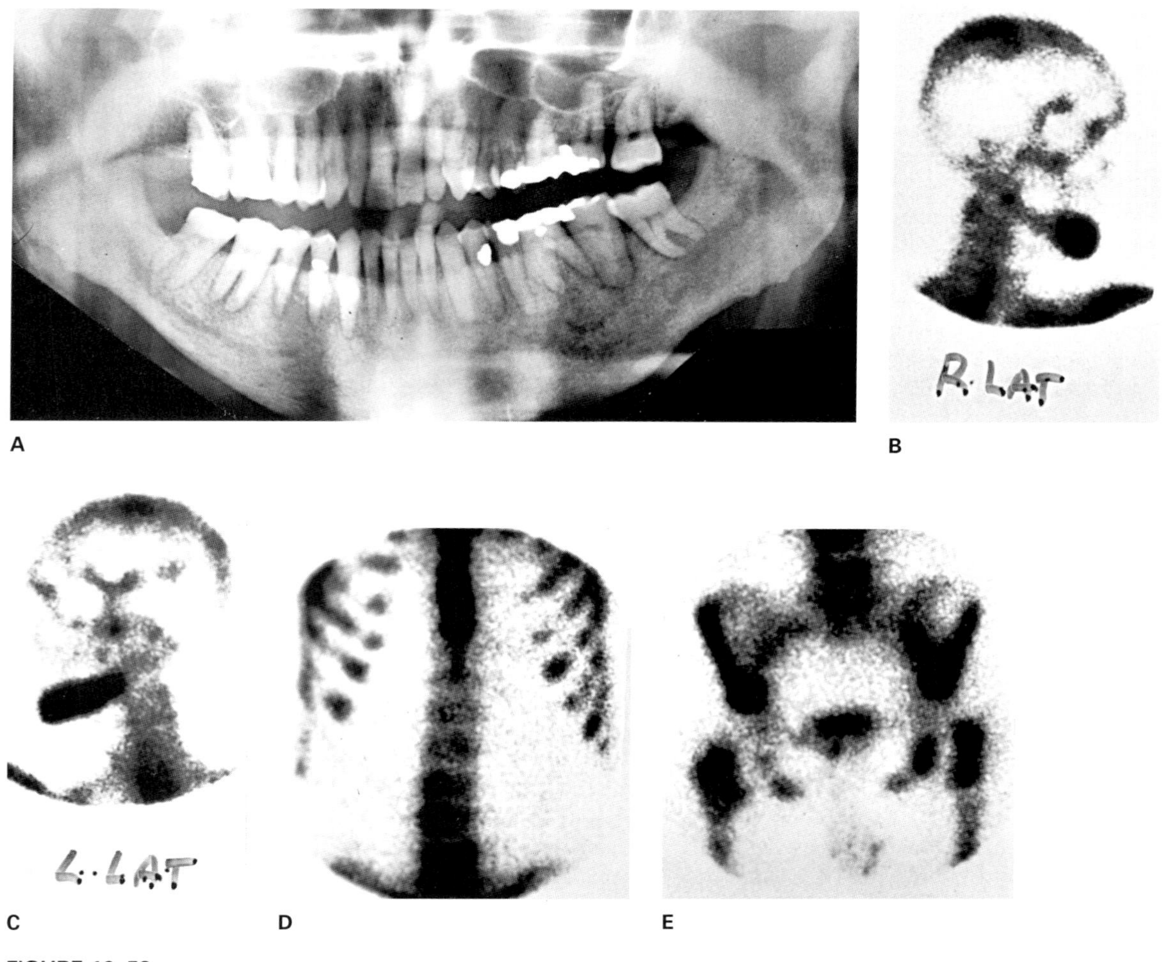

A B
C D E

FIGURE 16–58.

Blastic Metastatic Tumor: Case in a 75-year-old man. A, Widening of periodontal ligament space around multiple mandibular teeth, and diffuse radiopaque appearance of mandible. B, C, D, and E, Bone scan shows extent of jaw metastases and metastatic disease in multiple other skeletal sites. (Courtesy of Dr. B. Ciola, Westhaven, CT.)

As reviewed by Schreiber (1981), osteoblastic metastases are seen most often in carcinoma of the prostate, breast, and gastrointestinal tract, including the colon, gallbladder, and pancreas. Mixed lytic and blastic metastases may arise from carcinoma of the breast, prostate, thyroid, and gastrointestinal tract. Breast carcinoma, although usually lytic, is especially prone to be blastic after therapy. Even though carcinoma of the prostate is predominantly blastic, lytic lesions may be seen in older patients; when a periosteal reaction occurs, the bone may appear larger than normal. Lymphomas also may provoke a blastic response, especially Hodgkin's disease. Lung carcinoma usually produces lytic metastatic lesions; however, if the patient is known to have primary lung cancer and osteoblastic metastases occur, the primary lesion is most likely an adenocarcinoma. Carcinoids of the lung also produce predominantly blastic bone metastases. Although most gastrointestinal metastases are lytic, most stomach cancers and occasional colonic carcinomas produce predominantly blastic metastatic bone lesions. Of the gynecologic malignant neoplasms principally involving the uterus, ovaries, and vulva, only the uterine cervix occasionally may show a mixed lytic and blastic metastasis; almost all tend to be lytic. When the prostate is involved by carcinoma of the urinary bladder, blastic metastases may occur, although they are usually lytic. At times, testicular metastases are blastic; however, they also are usually lytic. The most common intracranial neoplasm that metastasizes extracranially is the cerebellar medulloblastoma; these metastases arise only after surgery, and the lesions may be lytic, mixed, or blastic.

Radiologic Features of Jaw Lesions

According to Meyer and Shklar (1965), metastatic lesions to the jaws occur most frequently in the mandible. Approximately 85% are seen in this location, whereas 15% occur in the maxilla. In two cases, metastatic lesions were found in both jaws. The posterior mandible is the most frequent site, especially in the molar and premolar regions. Notably, these areas contain hematopoietic marrow. Cash and associates (1961) reviewed 20 jaw metastases, and only one was osteoblastic and represented cancer of the prostate.

Worth (1963) discussed osteoblastic metastases in the jaws and stated that their appearance is similar to that in other bones. The increased density in the area results from bone laid down in the marrow spaces. The marrow spaces may be obliterated completely, and there may be a loss of any trabecular pattern or some coarse trabeculae may persist. There may be a lytic component and it may be within the radiopaque mass or adjacent to it. Some cases may appear as more or less rounded radiopacities, greatly resembling the lesions in Paget's disease. In rare instances, an osteoblastic lesion may be present in association with a uniform widening of the periodontal membrane space along one side of a root or several roots of one or more teeth. Although this appearance is associated most frequently with primary osteosarcoma and primary chondrosarcoma, it is especially prone to occur in metastatic disease; tumor invasion along the periodontal membrane space ultimately may surround the entire tooth, producing a floating tooth appearance. This widening may be seen along with lytic, blastic, or mixed lesions in the jaws. Metastatic disease in the jaws has a tendency to mimic many other disorders. Yagan and colleagues (1984) indicated that the bone scan is normal in approximately 5% of bone metastases with a radiologically demonstrable destructive lesion. According to Alazraki (1981), this is believed to be related to the fact that there is no significant difference in the degree of osteogenesis and blood supply in the tumor and normal surrounding bone. Decreased uptake in malignant bone disease is rare.

Spott (1985) and Wheaton (1985) reported a case of metastatic breast carcinoma. The lesion was seen in the maxillary premolar region and consisted of a widening of the periodontal membrane space along one side of the root and apex and resembled periodontal or periapical disease; the tooth appeared vital and sound and had never been restored.

In Ciola's (1981) case of metastatic carcinoma of the prostate to the left mandibular molar region, the lesion consisted of a diffuse area of increased lucency with multiple motheaten radiolucent holes in the bone. The cortex and teeth were uninvolved. The area showed prominent increased radionuclide uptake. Mesa (1977) reported a case of metastatic carcinoma of the prostate to the edentulous mandibular molar region. Initially the lesion resembled nonspecific osteitis; however, approximately 1 month later clinical swelling and pain occurred in the area and there was a periosteal reaction along the inferior margin of the mandibular cortex. The lesion was radiodense and caused a distinct downward bulge at the inferior margin of the mandible.

Kaugars and Svirsky (1981) found 37 acceptable cases of jaw metastasis from primary tumors of the lung and reported a new case. In most metastatic tumors to the jaws, the mandible-to-maxilla ratio is 5:1, whereas for lung tumors it is only 3:1. Most jaw metastases from the lung consisted of squamous cell carcinoma (11 cases), poorly differentiated carcinoma and anaplastic carcinoma (7 cases each), oat cell carcinoma (5 cases), adenocarcinoma (3 cases), and large cell carcinoma (1 case). Kaugers and Svirsky (1981) found that 49% of the cases were discovered in the jaws before the primary lung tumors. In the case of metastatic lung carcinoma reported by Ciola and Yesner (1977), the location was the anterior maxilla. Radiologically, the lesion consisted of an ill-defined lytic area encompassing the central, lateral, and canine teeth. Scattered remnants of incompletely resorbed trabeculate could be seen within the area. The peripheral margin was poorly defined; however, saber-like extensions of alveolar bone appeared to extend into the lytic defect.

Mast and Nissenblatt (1987) found only 19 reported cases of colon and rectal carcinoma metastatic to the jaws and added a new case, an adenocarcinoma of the cecum. Only one other case of cecal adenocarcinoma metastatic to the jaws has been reported. Among the 20 cases, 45% consisted of rectal adenocarcinoma, 30% colon carcinoma of an unspecified site, 15% sigmoid colon carcinoma, and 10% right colon or cecal adenocarcinoma. According to Mast and Nissenblatt (1987), rectal carcinoma is more likely to spread to bone than colon carcinoma. Although most jaw lesions have been lytic, Castigliano and Rominger (1965) reported a jaw metastasis to the ramus, from a rectal carcinoma, that appeared as a large expansile mass with osteolytic and osteoblastic components.

Welch and colleagues (1985) reviewed metastatic melanoma to the jaws and found only 12 reported cases and added a new case. Of the cases reviewed, 6 (50%) were to the mandible, 3 (25%) to the maxilla, 1 to the pulp of a maxillary incisor tooth, and 2 to unspecified sites in the jawbones. The other 2 maxillary lesions involved the maxillary sinus. The 6 mandibular lesions were distributed equally among the premolar, molar, and ramus regions. The case of Welch and co-authors was an apical periodontal cyst of the maxillary right lateral incisor. The tooth appeared to be floating within a poorly defined lytic area. Other soft tissue sites also were affected, including the tongue, maxillary gingiva in the incisor and premolar regions, and mandibular gingiva in the molar region.

Carter and colleagues (1977) reviewed the literature with respect to malignant renal tumors metastatic to the jaws; they found only 12 reported cases since 1920 and added a new case. According to these authors, 85% of all malignant renal tumors consist of renal cell carcinomas, also known as clear cell carcinoma, Grawitz tumor, adenocarcinoma, and hypernephroma. Carter and colleagues (1977) indicated that 34% of renal malignant neoplasms metastasize to bone and, of these, 20% metastasize to the skull and facial bones. Their case consisted of a clear cell carcinoma producing a lytic lesion in the angle ramus region. Jaw lesions tend to be osteolytic, with expansion or perforation of the cortical plates. Florine and colleagues (1988) reported a clear cell sarcoma of the kidney metastatic to the mandible that mimicked a benign myxomatous lesion. Clear cell sarcoma is one of the variations of Wilms' tumor, a renal malignant neoplasm occurring primarily in children. The mandibular lesion occurred in the body and angle and appeared multilocular, with thinning and expansion of the inferior cortex. The individual cystic spaces appeared well corticated. The technetium uptake was increased notably in the area of the lesion.

References

Periostitis Ossificans of Garrè

Berger A: Perimandibular ossification of possible traumatic origin: report of a case. J Oral Surg 6:353, 1948.

Eisenbud L, Miller J, Roberts IL: Garrè's proliferative periostitis occurring simultaneously in four quadrants of the jaws. Oral Surg Oral Med Oral Pathol 51:172, 1981.

Ellis DJ, Winslow SR, Indovina AA: Garrè's osteomyelitis of the mandible: report of a case. Oral Surg Oral Med Oral Pathol 44:183, 1977.

Eversole LR, Leider AS, Corwin JD, Karian B: Proliferative periostitis of Garrè: its differentiation from other neoperiostosis. J Oral Surg 37:725, 1979.

Garrè C: Uber besondere formen und folgezustände der akuten infektiösen osteomyelitis. Beitrz Klin Chir 10:241, 1893.

Gorman JM: Periostitis ossificans: report of a case. Oral Surg Oral Med Oral Pathol 10:129, 1957.

Lichty G, Langlais RP, Aufdermorte T: Garrè's osteomyelitis literature review and case report. Oral Surg Oral Med Oral Pathol 50:309, 1980.

Lovemann CE: Mandibular subperiosteal swellings in children. J Am Dent Assoc 28:1230, 1941.

Mattison GD, Gould AR, George DI, Neb JL: Garrè's osteomyelitis of the mandible: the role of endodontic therapy in patient management. J Endod 7:559 1981.

Monteleone L, Hagy DM, Hernandez A: Garrè's osteomyelitis. J Oral Surg 20:423, 1962.

Nortjé CJ, Wood RE, Grotepass F: Periostitis ossificans versus Garrè's osteomyelitis: part II. Radiologic analysis of 93 cases in the jaws. Oral Surg Oral Med Oral Pathol 66:249, 1988.

Pell GJ, et al: Garrè's osteomyelitis of the mandible: report of a case. J Oral Surg 13:248, 1955.

Shafer WG, Hine MK, Levy BM: A Textbook of Oral Pathology. 3rd Ed. Philadelphia:WB Saunders, 1983, p. 506.

Smith SN, Forman AG: Osteomyelitis with proliferative periostitis (Garrè's osteomyelitis): report of case affecting the mandible. Oral Surg Oral Med Oral Pathol 43:315, 1977.

Wood RC, et al: Periostitis ossificans versus Garrè's osteomyelitis: part I. What did Garrè really say? Oral Surg Oral Med Oral Pathol 65:773, 1988.

Worth HM: Principles and Practice of Oral Radiologic Interpretation. Chicago:Year Book Medical Publishers, 1963, p. 226.

Worth HM, Stoneman DW: Radiographic interpretation of antral mucosal changes due to localized dental infections. J Can Dent Assoc 38:111, 1972.

Root Fragments

Makila E, Suoranta K: Oral health among the inmates of old people's homes. Proc Finn Dent Soc 74:11, 1978.

Nyyssonen V, Paumio I, Rajala M: Prevalence of retained roots in the Finnish adult population. Community Dent Oral Epidemiol 11:117, 1983.

Wolf J: An orthopantomographic preprosthetic study of pathologic findings in the edentulous jaws (English summary). Proc Finn Dent Soc 65:240, 1969.

Socket Sclerosis

Ball J, Garner A: Mineralization of woven bone in osteomalacia. J Pathol Bacteriol 91:563, 1966.

Boyne PJ: Osseous repair of the post extraction alveolus in man. Oral Surg Oral Med Oral Pathol 21:805, 1966.

Burrell KH, Goepp RA: Abnormal bone repair in jaws, socket sclerosis: a sign of systemic disease. J Am Dent Assoc 87:1206, 1973.

Dalitz GD: A radiographic study of the rate at which human extraction wounds heal. Aust Dent J 9:466, 1964.

Frandsen AM: Experimental investigations of socket healing and periodontal disease in rats: effects of local roentgen irradiation; effects of vitamin A deficiency. Acta Odontol Scand 21(Suppl 37):13, 1963.

Kaye M, Pritchard JE, Halpenny GW, Light W: Bone disease in chronic renal failure with particular reference to osteosclerosis. Medicine 39: 157, 1960.

Shafer WG, Hime MK, Levy BM: A Textbook of Oral Pathology. 4th Ed. Philadelphia:WB Saunders, 1983, p. 601.

Skoczylas LJ, Langlais RP, Young KS: Myotonic dystrophy: review of the literature and new radiographic findings. Dentomaxillofac Radiol 14: 101, 1985.

Tori

Gibilisco JA: Stafne's Oral Radiographic Diagnosis. 5th Ed. Philadelphia: WB Saunders, 1985, p. 210.

King D, Moore GE: An analysis of torus palatines in a transatlantic study. J Oral Med 31:44, 1976.

King DR, King AC: Incidence of tori in three population groups. J Oral Med 36:21, 1981.

Langland OE, Langlais RP, McDavid WD, Del Balso AM: Panoramic Radiology. 2nd Ed. Philadelphia:Lea & Febiger, 1989, p. 183.

Suzuki M, Sakai T: A familial study of torus palatines and torus mandibularis. Am J Phys Anthropol 18:263, 1960.

Witkop CJ, Barros L: Oral and genetic studies of children: 1960. Oral anomalies. Am J Phys Anthropol 21:15, 1963.

Woo J: Torus palatines. Am J Phys Anthropol 8:81, 1950.

Yaacob H, Tirmzi H, Ismail K: The prevalence of oral tori in Malaysians. J Oral Med 38:40, 1983.

Subpontic Hyperostosis

Appleby DC: Investigating incidental remission of subpontic hyperostosis. J Am Dent Assoc 122:61, 1991.

Burkes EJ, Marby DL, Brooks RE: Subpontic osseous proliferation. J Prosthet Dent 53:780, 1985.

Calman HI, Eisenberg M, Grodjesk JE, Szerlip L: Shades of white, interpretation of radiopacities. Dent Radiogr Photogr 94:3, 1971.

Gibilisco JA: Stafne's Oral Radiographic Diagnosis. 5th Ed. Philadelphia: WB Saunders, 1985, p. 145.

Langland OE, Langlais RP, McDavid WD, Del Balso AM: Panoramic Radiology. 2nd Ed. Philadelphia:Lea & Febiger, 1989, p. 315.

Morton TH, Nankin E: Hyperostosis and fixed partial denture pontics: report of 16 patients and review of the literature. J Prosthet Dent 64:539, 1990.

Strassler HE: Bilateral plateauization. Oral Surg Oral Med Oral Pathol 52: 222, 1981.

Takeda Y, Itagaki M, Ishibashi K: Bilateral subpontic hyperplasia. J Periodontol 59:311, 1988.

Distal Mandibular Pseudohyperostosis

Langlais RP, Kasle MJ: Exercises in Dental Radiology. Vol. 1. Intra-oral Radiographic Interpretation. Philadelphia:WB Saunders, 1978, pp. 82, 138.

Enostosis

Worth HM: Principles and Practice of Oral Radiologic Interpretation. Chicago:Year Book Medical Publishers, 1963, p. 271.

Osteoma

Bosshardt L, et al: Recurrent peripheral osteoma of the mandible. J Oral Surg 29:446, 1971.

Krolls SO, Jacoway JR, Alexander WN: Osseous choristomas (osteomas of intraoral soft tissues). Oral Surg Oral Med Oral Pathol 32:588, 1971.

Langland OE, Langlais RP, McDavid WD, Del Balso AM: Panoramic Radiology. 2nd Ed. Philadelphia:Lea & Febiger, 1989, p. 319.

Leopard PJ: Osteoma of the maxillary antrum. Br J Oral Surg 10:73, 1972.

Mesa ML, Schneider LC, Northington L: Osteoma of the buccal mucosa. J Oral Maxillofac Surg 40:684, 1982.

Messerly CD: Osteoma of the mandible. Am J Orthod 25:1224, 1939.

Monserrat M: Opsteome de la langue. Bull Soc Anat 88:282, 1913.

Richards HE, et al: Large peripheral osteoma arising from the gerrial tubercle area. Oral Surg Oral Med Oral Pathol 61:268, 1986.

Schneider LC, Dolinsky HB, Grodjesk JE: Solitary peripheral osteoma of the jaws: report of a case and review of the literature. J Oral Surg 38: 452, 1980.

Shafer WG, Hine MK, Levy BM: A Textbook of Oral Pathology. 4th Ed. Philadelphia:WB Saunders, 1983, p. 163.

Uhler IV: Massive osteoma of the mandible. Oral Surg Oral Med Oral Pathol 10:143, 1957.

Worth HM: Principles and Practice of Oral Radiologic Interpretation. Chicago:Year Book Medical Publishers, 1963, p. 534.

Osteoid Osteoma

Dahlin DC: Bone Tumors: General Aspects and Data on 6,221 Cases. 3rd Ed. Springfield, IL: Charles C Thomas, 1978, p. 75.
Gitelis S, Schajowicz F: Osteoid osteoma and osteoblastoma. Orthop Clin North Am 20:313, 1989.
Greene GW Jr, Natiella JR, Spring PN Jr: Osteoid osteoma of the jaws: report of a case. Oral Surg Oral Med Oral Pathol 26:342, 1968.
Greer RO, Berman DN: Osteoblastoma of the jaws: current concepts and differential diagnosis. J Oral Surg 36:304, 1978.
Jaffe HL: Osteoid osteoma: a benign osteoblastic tumor composed of osteoid and atypical bone. Arch Surg 31:709, 1935.
Smith RA, Hansen LS, Resnick D, Chan W: Comparison of the osteoblastoma in gnathic and extragnathic sites. Oral Surg Oral Med Oral Pathol 54:285, 1982.
Worth HM: Principles and Practice of Oral Radiologic Interpretation. Chicago:Year Book Medical Publishers, 1963, p. 539.

Benign Osteoblastoma

Borello ED, Sedano HO: Giant osteoid osteoma in the maxilla. Oral Surg Oral Med Oral Pathol 23:563, 1967.
Farman AG, Nortjé CJ, Grotepass F: Periosteal benign osteoblastoma of the mandible: report of a case and review of the literature pertaining to benign osteoblastic neoplasms of the jaws. Br J Oral Surg 14:12, 1976.
Goldman RL: Periosteal benign osteoblastoma. Am J Clin Pathol 56:73, 1971.
Greer RO Jr, Berman DN: Osteoblastoma of the jaws: current concepts and differential diagnosis. J Oral Surg 36:304, 1978.
Jackson RP: Recurrent osteoblastoma: a review. Clin Orthop 131:229, 1978.
Jaffe HL, Mayer L: An osteoblastic tissue forming tumor of a metacarpal bone. Arch Surg 24:500, 1932.
Jaffe HL: Benign osteoblastoma. Bull Hosp Jt Dis 17:141, 1956.
Lichtenstein L: Benign osteoblastoma: a category of osteoid and bone forming tumors other than classical osteoid osteoma which may be mistaken for giant cell tumor or osteogenic sarcoma. Cancer 9:1044, 1956.
Marsh BW, Bonfiglio M, Brady LP, Enneking WF: Benign osteoblastoma: range of manifestations. J Bone Joint Surg (Am) 57:1, 1975.
Merryweather R, Middlemiss JH, Sanerkin NG: Malignant transformation of osteoblastoma. J Bone Joint Surg (Br) 62:381, 1980.
Ohkubo T, Hernandez JC, Ooya K, Krutchkoff DJ: Aggressive osteoblastoma of the maxilla. Oral Surg Oral Med Oral Pathol 68:69, 1989.
Remagen W, Prein J: Benign osteoblastoma. Oral Surg Oral Med Oral Pathol 39:279, 1975.
Schajowicz F, Lemos C: Osteoid osteoma and osteoblastoma. Acta Orthop Scand 41:272, 1970.
Shafer WG, Hine MK, Levy BM: A Textbook of Oral Pathology. 4th Ed. Philadelphia:WB Saunders, 1983, p. 165.
Shatz A, Calderon S, Mintz S: Benign osteoblastoma of the mandible. Oral Surg Oral Med Oral Pathol 35:191, 1986.
Smith NHH: Benign osteoblastoma of the mandible: report of a case. J Oral Surg Oral Med Oral Pathol 30:288, 1972.
Smith RA, Hansen LS, Resnick D, Chan W: Comparison of the osteoblastoma in the gnathic and extragnathic sites. Oral Surg Oral Med Oral Pathol 54:285, 1982.
Steiner GC: Ultrastructure of osteoid osteoma. Hum Pathol 7:309, 1976.
Steiner GC: Ultrastructure of osteoblastoma. Cancer 39:2127, 1977.

Chondroma

Chaudhry AP, Rosinovitch MR, Mitchell DF, Vickers RA: Chondrogenic tumors of the jaws. Am J Surg 102:403, 1961.
Dahlin DC: Bone Tumors: General Aspects and Data on 6,221 Cases. 3rd Ed. Springfield, IL: Charles C Thomas, 1978, p. 28.
Gardner DG, Patterson JC: Chondroma or metaplastic chondrosis of the soft palate. Oral Surg Oral Med Oral Pathol 26:601, 1968.
Gibilisco SA: Stafne's Oral Radiographic Diagnosis. 5th Ed. Philadelphia: WB Saunders, 1985, p. 217.
Poyton HG: Oral Radiology. Baltimore:Williams & Wilkins, 1982, p. 291.
Worth HM: Principles and Practice of Oral Radiologic Interpretation. Chicago:Year Book Medical Publishers, 1963, p. 529.

Osteochondroma

Dahlin DC: Bone Tumors: General Aspects and Data on 6,221 Cases. 3rd Ed. Springfield, IL:Charles C Thomas, 1978, p. 17.
Edeiken J: Roentgen Diagnosis of Diseases of Bone. 3rd Ed. Baltimore: Williams & Wilkins, 1981, p. 70.
Loftus MJ, Bennett JA, Fantasia JE: Osteochondroma of the mandibular condyles: report of three cases and review of the literature. Oral Surg Oral Med Oral Pathol 61:221, 1986.
Schweber SJ, Frensilli JA: Osteochondroma of the mandibular condyle: report of a case and review of the literature. J Am Dent Assoc 113: 269, 1986.
Shafer WG, Hine MK, Levy BM: A Textbook of Oral Pathology. 4th Ed. Philadelphia:WB Saunders, 1983, p. 163.
Worth HM: Principles and Practice of Oral Radiologic Interpretation. Chicago:Year Book Medical Publishers, 1963, p. 531.

Benign Chondroblastoma

Al-Dewachi HS, Al-Naib N, Sangal BC: Benign chondroblastoma of the maxilla: a case report and review of chondroblastomas in the cranial bones. Br J Oral Surg 18:150, 1980.
Bertoni F, et al: Chondroblastoma of the skull and facial bones. Am J Clin Pathol 88:1, 1987.
Brecher ME, Simon MA: Chondroblastoma: an immunohistochemical study. Hum Pathol 19:1043, 1988.
Codman EA: Epiphyseal chondromatous giant cell tumors of the upper end of the humerus. Surg Gynecol Obstet 52:543, 1931.
Dahlin DC, Ivins JC: Benign chondroblastoma: a study of 125 cases. Cancer 30:401, 1972.
Dahlin DC: Bone Tumors: General Aspects and Data on 6,221 Cases. 3rd Ed. Springfield:Charles C Thomas, 1978, p. 43.
Edeiken J: Roentgen Diagnosis of Diseases of Bone. 3rd Ed. Baltimore: Williams & Wilkins, 1981, p. 83.
Goodsell JD, Hubinger HL: Benign chondroblastoma of the mandibular condyle: report of a case. J Oral Surg 22:355, 1964.
Green P, Whittaker RP: Case report with pulmonary metastasis. J Bone Joint Surg (Am) 57:418, 1975.
Jaffe HL, Lichtenstein L: Benign chondroblastoma of bone: a reinterpretation of the so-called calcifying or chondromatous giant cell tumor. Am J Pathol 18:969, 1942.
Mirra JM: Bone Tumors: Diagnosis and Treatment. Philadelphia: JB Lippincott, 1980, p. 219.
Schajowicz F, Gallardo H: Epiphyseal chondroblastoma of bone. J Bone Joint Surg (Br) 52:205, 1970.

Osteosarcoma

Boutouras GD, Goodsitt E: Sarcoma arising in Paget's disease: report of two cases and review of the literature. J Int Coll Surg 40:380, 1963.
Broders AC: The grading of carcinoma. Minn Med 8:726, 1925.
Clark JL, Unnik K, Dahlin KDC, Denine KD: Osteosarcoma of the jaw. Cancer 51:2311, 1983.
Dahlin DC: Bone Tumors: General Aspects and Data on 6,221 Cases. 3rd Ed. Springfield, IL: Charles C Thomas, 1978, p. 226.
Forteza G, Colmenero B, Lopez-Barea F: Osteogenic sarcoma of the maxilla and mandible. Oral Surg Oral Med Oral Pathol 62:179, 1986.
Gardner DG, Mills DM: The widened periodontal ligament of osteosarcoma of the jaws. Oral Surg Oral Med Oral Pathol 41:652, 1976.
Garrington GE, Schofield HH, Cornyn J, Hooker SP: Osteosarcoma of the jaws. Cancer 20:377, 1967.
Krolls SO, Schaffer RC, O'Rear JW: Chondrosarcoma and osteosarcoma of the jaws in the same patient. Oral Surg Oral Med Oral Pathol 50: 146, 1980.
McKenna RJ, Schwinn CP, Soong KY, Higinbotham NL: Osteogenic sarcoma arising in Paget's disease. Cancer 17:42, 1964.
Rosenmertz SK, Schare HJ: Osteogenic sarcoma arising in Paget's disease of the mandible. Oral Surg Oral Med Oral Pathol 28:304, 1969.
Worth HM: Principles and Practice of Oral Radiologic Interpretation. Chicago:Year Book Medical Publishers, 1963, p. 563.

Juxtacortical Osteosarcoma

Ahuja SC, et al: Juxtacortical (parosteal) osteogenic sarcoma: histological grading and prognosis. J Bone Joint Surg (Am) 59:632, 1977.

Bras JM, et al: Juxtacortical osteogenic sarcoma of the jaws: review of the literature and report of a case. Oral Surg Oral Med Oral Pathol 50:535, 1980.

Dahlin DC: Bone Tumors: General Aspects and Data on 6,211 Cases. 3rd Ed. Springfield, IL: Charles C Thomas, 1978, p. 261.

Edeiken J: Roentgen Diagnosis of Diseases of Bone. 3rd Ed. Baltimore: Williams & Wilkins, 1981, p. 209.

Geschickter CF, Copeland MM: Parosteal osteoma of bone: a new entity. Ann Surg 133:790, 1951.

Geschickter CF, Copeland MM: Tumors of Bone. 3rd Ed. Philadelphia:JB Lippincott, 1949, p. 367.

Huvos AG: Bone Tumors: Diagnosis Treatment and Prognosis. Philadelphia:WB Saunders, 1970, p. 94.

Jaffe HL: Tumors and Tumorous Conditions of the Bones and Joints. Philadelphia:Lea & Febiger, 1958, p. 274.

Unni KK, Dahlin DC, Beabout JW: Periosteal osteogenic sarcoma: an entity distinct from parosteal osteogenic sarcoma [abstract]. Lab Invest 32: 438, 1975.

Chondrosarcoma

Arlen M, Tollefsen HR, Huros AG, Marcove RC: Chondrosarcoma of the head and neck. Am J Surg 120:456, 1970.

Buchner A, Ramon Y, Begleiter A: Chondrosarcoma of the maxilla: report of a case. J Oral Surg 37:822, 1979.

Chaudhry AP, Robinovitch MR, Mitchell DF, Vickers RA: Chondrogenic tumors of the jaws. Am J Surg 102:403, 1961.

Christensen R: Mesenchymal chondrosarcoma of the jaws. Oral Surg Oral Med Oral Pathol 54:197, 1982.

Cohen MA, Mendelsohn DB, Hertzanu Y: Chondrosarcoma of the maxilla. Int J Oral Surg 13:528, 1984.

Dahlin DC: Bone Tumors: General Aspects and Data on 6,221 Cases. 3rd Ed. Springfield, IL: Charles C Thomas, 1978, p. 190.

Edeiken J: Roentgen Diagnosis of Diseases of Bone. 3rd Ed. Baltimore: William & Wilkins, 1981, p. 223.

Evans HL, Ayala AG, Romsdahl MM: Prognostic factors in chondrosarcoma of bone. Cancer 40:818, 1977.

Henderson ED, Dahlin DC: Chondrosarcoma of bone: a study of 288 cases. J Bone Joint Surg (Am) 45:1450, 1963.

Kragh LV, Dahlin DC, Erich JB: Cartilaginous tumors of the jaws and facial regions. Am J Surg 99:852, 1960.

Krolls SO, Schaffer RC, O'Rear JW: Chondrosarcoma and osteosarcoma of the jaws in the same patient. Oral Surg Oral Med Oral Pathol 50: 146, 1980.

Lichtenstein L, Jaffe HL: Chondrosarcoma of bone. Am J Pathol 19:553, 1943.

Phemister DB: Chondrosarcoma of bone. Surg Gynecol Obstet 50:216, 1930.

Sanerkin NB: Definitions of osteosarcoma, chondrosarcoma and fibrosarcoma of bone. Cancer 46:178, 1980.

Terezhalmy GT, Bottomley WK: Maxillary chondrogenic sarcoma: management of a case. Oral Surg Oral Med Oral Pathol 44:539, 1977.

Vassar PS: Chondrosarcoma of the tongue: a case report. Arch Pathol 65: 261, 1958.

Worth HM: Principles and Practice of Oral Radiologic Interpretation. Chicago:Year Book Medical Publishers, 1963, p. 576.

Mesenchymal Chondrosarcoma

Batsakis JG: Tumors of the Head and Neck: Clinical and Pathological Considerations. 2nd Ed. Baltimore:Williams & Wilkins, 1979, p. 385.

Chavez E: Mesenchymal chondrosarcoma. Arch Ital Pathol Clin Tumor 9: 97, 1966.

Christensen RE: Mesenchymal chondrosarcoma of the jaws. Oral Surg Oral Med Oral Pathol 54:197, 1982.

Dahlin DC: Bone Tumors: General Aspects and Data on 6,221 Cases. 3rd Ed. Springfield, IL: Charles C Thomas, 1978, p. 218.

Lichtenstein L, Bernstein D: Unusual benign and malignant chondroid tumors of bone: a survey of some mesenchymal cartilage tumors and malignant chondroblastic tumors, including a few multicentric ones as well as many atypical benign chondroblastomas and chondromyxoid fibromas. Cancer 12:1142, 1959.

Mazabraud A: Le chondrosarcome mésenchymateux: à propos de six observations. Rev Chir Orthop 60:197, 1974.

"Blastic" Metastatic Tumors

Alazraki N: Bone Imaging by radionuclide techniques. In: Resnick D, Niwayama G, eds. Diagnosis of Bone and Joint Disorders. Philadelphia: WB Saunders, 1981, p. 639.

Bhaskar SN: Synopsis of Oral Pathology. 4th Ed. St. Louis: CV Mosby, 1973, p. 304.

Bucin EWA, Andreasson L, Bjorlin G: Metastases in the oral cavity: case reports. Int J Oral Surg 11:321, 1982.

Carter DG, Anderson EE, Currie DP: Renal cell carcinoma metastatic to the mandible. J Oral Surg 35:992, 1977.

Cash CD, Royer RQ, Dahlin DC: Metastatic tumors to the jaws. Oral Surg Oral Med Oral Pathol 14:897, 1961.

Castigliano SG, Rominger CJ: Metastatic malignancy of the jaws. Am J Surg 87:496, 1954.

Ciola B, Yesner R: Radiographic manifestations of a lung carcinoma with metastases to the anterior maxilla. Oral Surg Oral Med Oral Pathol 44: 811, 1977.

Ciola B: Oral radiographic manifestations of a metastatic prostatic carcinoma. Oral Surg Oral Med Oral Pathol 51:105, 1981.

Clausen F, Poulsen H: Metastatic carcinoma to the jaws. Acta Pathol Microbiol Scand 57:361, 1963.

Florine BL, et al: Clear cell sarcoma of the kidney: report of a case with mandibular metastasis simulating a benign myxomatous tumor. Oral Surg Oral Med Oral Pathol 65:567, 1988.

Geschickter CF, Copeland MM: Tumors of Bone (Including Jaws and Joints). 3rd Ed. Philadelphia:JB Lippincott, 1949. p. 220.

Kaugars GE, Svirsky JA: Lung malignancies metastatic to the oral cavity. Oral Surg Oral Med Oral Pathol 51:179, 1981.

Mast HL, Nissenblast MJ: Metastatic colon carcinoma to the jaw: a case report and review of the literature. J Surg Oncol 34:202, 1987.

Mesa ML: Metastatic prostate carcinoma to the mandible: report of a case. J Oral Surg 35:133, 1977.

Meyer I, Shklar G: Malignant tumors metastatic to mouth and jaws. Oral Surg Oral Med Oral Pathol 20:350, 1965.

Oikarinen VJ, Calonius PEP, Saino P: Metastatic tumors to the oral region: an analysis of cases in the literature. Proc Finn Dent Soc 71:58, 1975.

Schreiber RR: The radiologist and the diagnosis of bone metastasis. In: Weiss L, Gilbert HA, eds. Bone Metastasis. Boston:GK Hall Medical Publishers, 1981, p. 190.

Spott RJ, Wheaton D: Metastatic breast carcinoma disguised as periapical disease in the maxilla. Oral Surg Oral Med Oral Pathol 60:327, 1985.

Thompson CC, Bartley MH, Woolley LH: Metastatic tumors of the head and neck: a 20 year oral tumor registry report. J Oral Med 41:175, 1986.

van der Kwast WAM, van der Waal I: Jaw metastases. Oral Surg Oral Med Oral Pathol 37:850, 1974.

Welch RD, Hirsch SA, Danis RG: Melanoma with metastasis to an apical periodontal cyst. Oral Surg Oral Med Oral Pathol 59:189, 1985.

Worth HM: Principles and Practice of Oral Radiologic Interpretation. Chicago:Year Book Medical Publishers, 1963, p. 562.

Yagan R, Bellon EM, Radivoyevitch M: Breast carcinoma metastatic to the mandible mimicking ameloblastoma. Oral Surg Oral Med Oral Pathol 57:189, 1984.

Chapter 17

Periapical Radiopacities

IDIOPATHIC OSTEOSCLEROSIS (Focal periapical osteopetrosis, osteosclerosis, bone sclerosis, enostosis, compact bone islands, bone scar, bone whorls, eburnated bone)

Assessment of the literature for idiopathic osteosclerosis and condensing osteitis has been difficult and somewhat inconclusive. Although many pathologists can find no difference between the two conditions, most radiologists and other clinicians believe pragmatically that the two problems are different. Therefore, many investigators such as Boyne (1960) prefer the term ''osteosclerotic areas,'' without distinguishing the two disorders. We believe the two disorders are different, although at this time they are believed to be histologically similar and at times identical. The importance of distinguishing between them is based on our belief that they differ with regard to clinical presentation, natural history, treatment and perhaps histologic characteristics.

As stated by Austin and Moule (1984), osteosclerosis refers to localized regions of abnormally dense bone that apparently do not result directly from infection or systemic disease. In a study of 1921 patients, Geist and Katz (1990) found an incidence of 5%; thus, the condition may be considered common. These areas may be seen at the apex of vital teeth, beyond the apices of vital teeth, between vital teeth, and in edentulous areas. In the latter instance, they may represent healed areas of condensing osteitis. Our discussions of idiopathic osteosclerosis and condensing osteitis have been phrased, so identical text is used to describe areas of commonality between the two conditions, and variations in the text highlight differences in the two disorders.

Pathologic Characteristics

As stated by Eversole and colleagues (1984) in their review of 41 histologically documented cases of condensing osteitis and idiopathic periapical osteosclerosis, no etiologic factors have been confirmed in the latter instance. All of the cases of idiopathic periapical osteosclerosis were found at the apices of posterior teeth that were clinically sound or with small carious lesions or restorations. Eversole and colleagues (1984) found no instances in which pulp vitality was proven by biopsy in association with idiopathic osteosclerosis. Histologically, idiopathic osteosclerosis is characterized by an obliteration of the normal marrow spaces by heavy trabeculation or dense compact bone. With the reduced marrow channels, inflammatory elements are minimal or nonexistent. Clinically, Eversole and colleagues (1984) observed that homogeneous radiopaque lesions lacking a perilesional radiolucent halo were most prevalent in cases classified as idiopathic osteosclerosis and lacked any significant hypercellular fibrous marrow elements histologically; however, in condensing osteitis a radiopacity with a radiolucent halo was the most frequent pattern observed and was characterized by the presence of hypercellular fibrous marrow elements. The clue to the histologic distinction between idiopathic osteosclerosis and condensing osteitis might be the presence of hypercellular fibrous marrow elements, whereas inflammation appears to be minimal or lacking in both conditions.

Clinical Features

In their review of 600 European dental outpatients and 600 dental outpatients from the racially mixed group in South Africa known as Cape Coloured, Farman and colleagues (1978) observed an equal distribution among men and women of both races for lesions at the apices of vital teeth and those in edentulous areas. In their study of 100 Chinese and Indochinese patients and 100 white patients, Austin and Moule (1984) found no sex difference between the Asian men and women and found too few cases among the white patients to allow them to draw any conclusions. They did find that osteosclerosis was much more prevalent in the Asian group, with an incidence of 31% compared with 8% among white people. Farman and colleagues (1978) observed no difference in incidence between white people and ''Cape Coloureds'' for idiopathic periapical osteosclerosis and osteosclerosis in edentulous areas. They also observed no age differences among people younger than 25 years of age and those older than 25 years with idiopathic periapical osteosclerosis; however, there was a much greater occurrence of idiopathic osteosclerosis in edentulous areas in those older than 25 years.

In their study of 1921 North American patients, Geist and Katz (1990) found an equal distribution among male and female patients for the overall sample; however, they observed a slight but significant predilection for Americans of African origin. Within these people, this condition was especially prone to develop in women. Most lesions occurred in people between the ages of 21 and 40 years (range, 14 to 77 years). No cases of idiopathic osteosclerosis were found in children during the primary dentition or mixed dentition stages of development. Idiopathic osteosclerosis is asymptomatic. It is diagnosed as an incidental finding on a radiograph or after pulpal inflammation is ruled out when the condition is located at the apex of a tooth. Because expansion is not a feature, idiopathic osteosclerosis does not tend to affect the fit of prostheses. Some people have postulated that trauma from prostheses is an etiologic factor; however, no study has proven this.

Treatment/Prognosis

Once discovered, idiopathic osteosclerosis rarely progresses or regresses. No treatment is required.

◆ *RADIOLOGY (Figs. 17–1 and 17–2)*

Location

Idiopathic osteosclerosis is more common in the mandible than the maxilla. In their study of 600 Europeans and 600 "Cape Coloureds," Farman and colleagues (1978) found 6 cases of idiopathic periapical osteosclerosis in the maxilla and 23 cases in the mandible in the "Cape Coloured" group; however, in the Europeans there were only 2 lesions in the maxilla and 20 in the mandible. A similar distribution was found in edentulous areas, with 46 maxillary lesions and 109 mandibular lesions among "Cape Coloured" patients; among the Europeans there were 8 maxillary and 28 mandibular lesions. Using the data of Farman and colleagues (1978), one can conclude that idiopathic osteosclerosis occurs five times more frequently in edentulous regions than at the apices of vital teeth, and the condition is seen 2.5 times more frequently in the mandible than in the maxilla. Also, maxillary lesions were more common in the "Cape Coloured" group than in Europeans. According to Farman and colleagues (1978), the teeth most commonly affected by idiopathic periapical osteosclerosis were as follows (in descending order of frequency): mandibular first premolar (26%), mandibular molars (24%), and mandibular canine teeth (20%). There were very few lesions in the maxilla of white patients; the molar area was the most frequent site in the "Cape Coloured" group (8%). Idiopathic osteosclerosis occurred in the following edentulous regions: mandibular first molar (17%), mandibular third molar (11%), and mandibular premolars (13%). In the maxilla, lesions in the posterior area were more common than those in the anterior region. Lesions also may occur in the inter-radicular space; Austin and Moule (1984) found that this was the least frequent location.

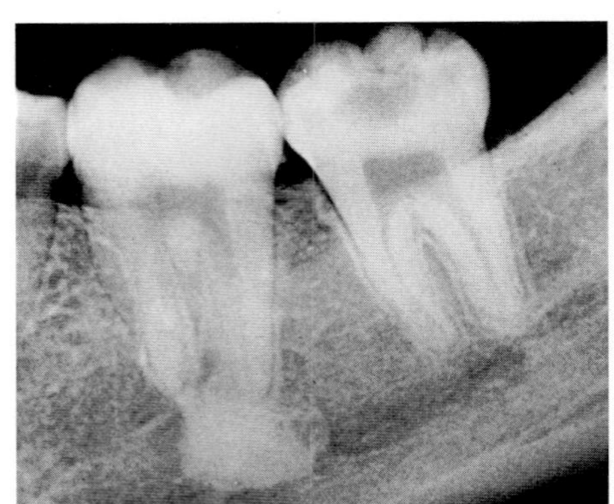

A

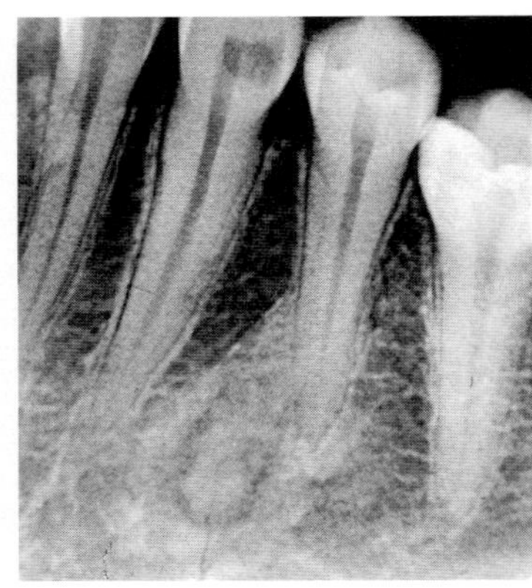

B

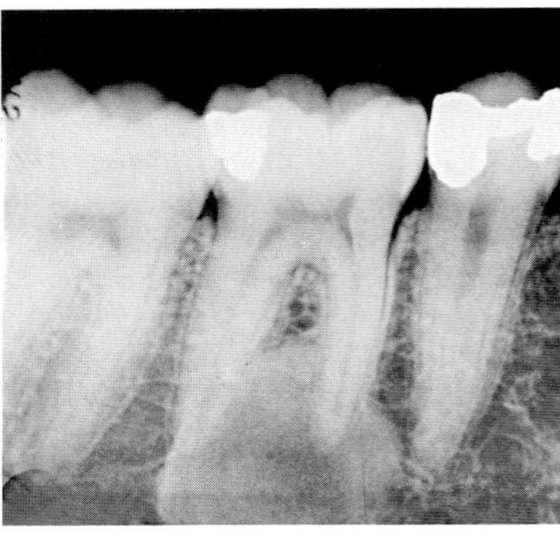

C

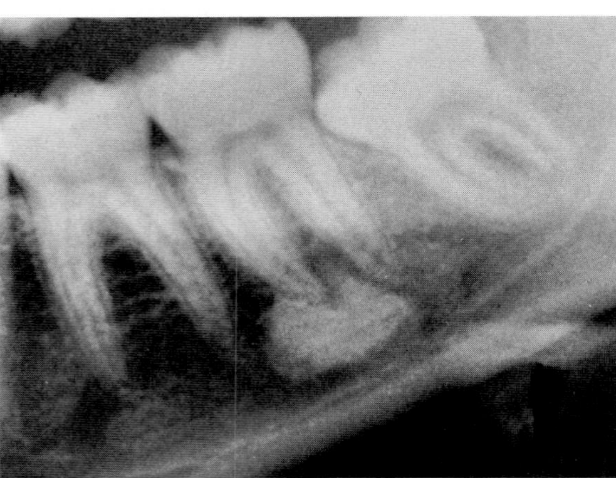

D

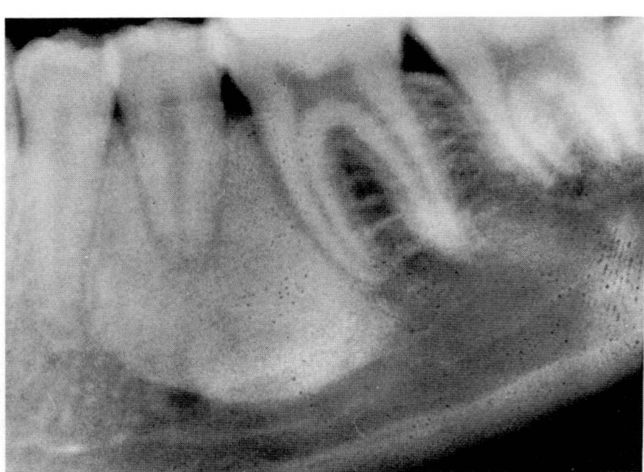

E

FIGURE 17–1:

Idiopathic Osteosclerosis: Five types as classified by Eversole and associates (1984). A, Focal type, with obscuring of the periodontal ligament space and lamina dura. B, Target type in a 28-year-old white man. C, Ground glass type, which is fibro-osseous histologically. D, Multiconfluent type, with second area forming at distal apex. There is relative widening of the periodontal ligament space mesial and distal roots. E, Root resorption type with large focal pattern occupying interdental spaces, relative enlargement of periodontal ligament space, and resorption of involved root.

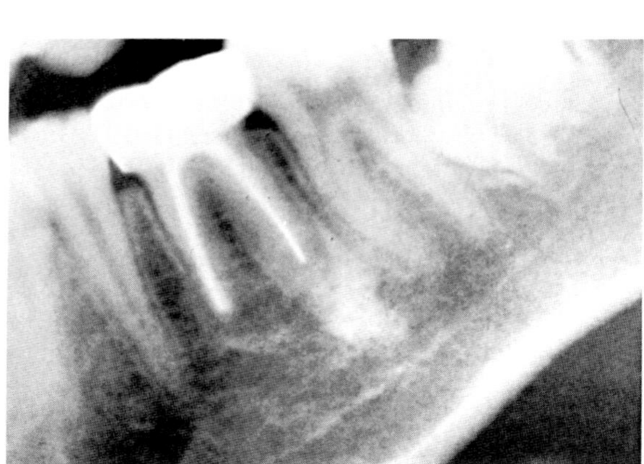

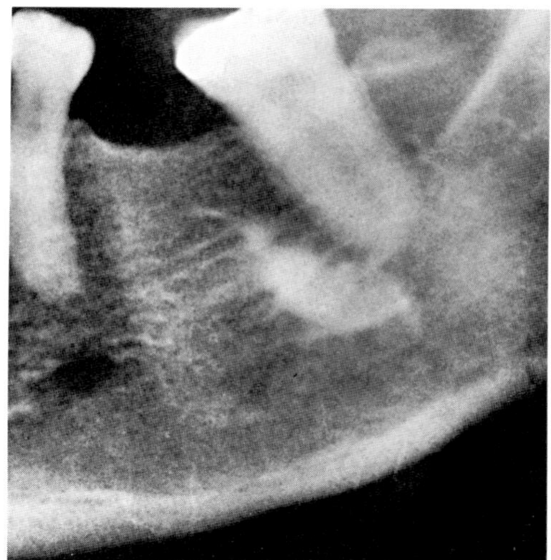

A B

FIGURE 17–2:

Idiopathic Osteosclerosis: A, Apical scar after successful root canal therapy. B, Edentulous area with irregular peripheral contour and pointed spicules at margin.

Geist and Katz (1990) observed that 89% of the cases occurred in the mandible. Approximately 71% involved the premolars only or the premolars and the adjacent first molar or canine; 88% were in the posterior quadrants, whereas 12% occurred anterior to the canine teeth.

Relationship to Teeth

Geist and Katz (1990) separated their cases into four categories with respect to association with teeth:

1. Limited to the tooth apex (42%).
2. Limited to the inter-radicular area (28%).
3. Involving the apical region with extension into the inter-radicular area (13%).
4. No apparent connection to the teeth (27%).

Eversole and associates (1984) reported root resorption in 12% of the cases; although most of these were at the apex, resorption of the lateral aspect of the root was seen when the location of the idiopathic osteosclerosis was inter-radicular.

Radiologic Features

Lesions may vary from a few millimeters to more than 2 cm in diameter. The area of increased density often is rounded or ovoid; however, it may be quite irregular. The margins are sometimes smooth, although they often may be irregular, with spicules radiating from the margin. The borders also are well defined, with distinct boundaries. The apical periodontal ligament space sometimes may be obliterated by the radiopaque mass; when present, it may be of a normal dimension or widened, a feature that has not been explained adequately. In the inter-radicular location, the lesion often occupies the entire space, extending up to the crest of the ridge, but does not extend beyond the normal level of bone and does not encroach on the embrasure space. The lamina dura may disappear within the sclerotic mass, which may extend beyond the apices of the adjacent teeth and occupy the inter-radicular space on both sides of a single tooth. In this instance, the root outline and periodontal ligament space usually can be seen within the radiopaque area, although a small portion of the root may be obscured at times. The mass itself usually is densely homogeneous, especially when it is significantly radiodense. In less dense lesions, a few coarse trabeculae, some of which may extend beyond the area of increased density, may be seen. A radiolucent component is rare in idiopathic osteosclerosis, although it may be present in some cases.

Eversole and co-workers (1984) identified 5 distinct radiographic patterns in idiopathic periapical osteosclerosis: (1) a "focal" pattern characterized as a homogeneous radiopaque mass lacking a perilesional radiolucent halo; (2) a "target" pattern consisting of a central radiopacity with a circumferential radiolucent band; (3) a "lucent" or granular pattern described as a nonexpansile periapical radiolucency displaying a fibro-osseous pattern histologically; (4) a "multiconfluent" pattern, in which several target lesions at the apices of a single multirooted tooth become closely apposed; and (5) a "resorption" pattern, characterized by external root resorption in association with any of the previous patterns. The sample reported by Eversole and associates (1984) included 41 histologically documented cases consisting of idiopathic periapical osteosclerosis or condensing osteitis. In the idiopathic periapical osteosclerosis group, the most common finding was the focal pattern; however, there were documented examples of the target, lucent, and multiconfluent variations. Root resorption was observed with equal frequency (12%) in idiopathic periapical osteosclerosis and condensing osteitis. Resorption may be at the root apex when the lesion is periapical or along the lateral aspect of the root when the lesion is inter-radicular. In this instance, the periodontal ligament space may be focally absent, with partial resorption of the affected tooth.

Austin and Moule (1984) observed a target pattern in two

of the Asian patients in their study. Both lesions were found in the mandibular first premolar region at the apices of vital teeth and were approximately 1 cm in diameter, with a central radiopacity surrounded by a radiolucent zone that was encompassed by a prominent band of sclerotic bone. In both cases, the teeth were sound and had never been restored.

CONDENSING OSTEITIS (Chronic focal sclerosing osteomyelitis, chronic sclerosing osteomyelitis, sclerosing osteitis, bone eburnation, chronic productive osteitis, focal sclerosing osteomyelitis)

Assessment of the literature for idiopathic osteosclerosis and condensing osteitis has been difficult and somewhat inconclusive. Although many pathologists can find no difference between the two conditions, most radiologists and other clinicians believe pragmatically that the two problems are different. Therefore, many investigators, such as Boyne (1960), prefer the term "osteosclerotic areas" without distinguishing the two disorders. We believe that the two disorders are different, although at this time many pathologists believe that they are histologically identical. The importance of distinguishing between them is based on our belief that they differ with regard to clinical presentation, natural history, and treatment. Our discussions of condensing osteitis and idiopathic osteosclerosis have been phrased such that identical text is used to describe areas of commonality between the two conditions and variations in the text highlight differences in the two disorders.

Pathologic Characteristics

As Austin and Moule (1984) stated, condensing osteitis refers to lesions that have resulted directly from infection. These lesions are seen almost exclusively at the apices of teeth with pulpal infection. According to Eversole and colleagues (1984), the condition is thought to represent a reactive hyperplasia of osteoblasts whereby a pulpal insult can be observed. Clinically, this means a deep carious lesion or large restoration is seen, including failed endodontic restorations. One may observe a deep periodontal pocket that may give rise to pulpal inflammation. As Eversole and associates stated (1984), very little has been done to prove histologically that such pulpal inflammation exists, but he and his co-workers performed biopsies on several cases in their 1972 study and found vital pulps with histologic evidence of mild chronic inflammation in association with condensing osteitis. Thus, pulpal inflammation may result in a periapical radiolucency or periapical radiopacity. In their study of 1149 roots treated by endodontic therapy, Eliasson and colleagues (1984) found a periapical radiolucency in 28%, whereas condensing osteitis was observed in 2%. In his series of 21 patients with osteosclerotic areas for which biopsy was performed, Boyne (1960) did not attempt to distinguish the biopsy specimens from cases with periapical abnormalities of pulpal origin from those from the apical region of vital teeth.

Histologically, condensing osteitis has been separated into two groups by Eversole (1984) and associates. In radiodense lesions, there is an obliteration of the normal marrow spaces by dense lamellar bone, with small marrow channels occupied by alveolar fibrovascular tissue. Predominantly lucent lesions and those with a radiolucent halo surrounding a central opacification consisted of irregular lamellar osseous trabeculae within a hypercellular fibrous marrow element. In either instance, inflammatory cell infiltration usually was lacking or minimal. Waldron and colleagues (1975) recognized condensing osteitis on a histologic basis; both cases were symptomatic, and biopsies were performed after extraction of the involved teeth.

Clinical Features

In their review of 600 European and 600 "Cape Coloured" dental outpatients, Farman and colleagues (1978) observed an equal distribution between men and women in both racial groups. In addition, they observed an equal incidence of 4% among the two racial groups, and there was also an equal distribution among those younger than 25 years of age and those older. Other authors, such as Shafer and colleagues (1983) and Bhaskar (1981), have stated that condensing osteitis occurs almost exclusively in people younger than 20 years of age. Condensing osteitis usually is asymptomatic, although the associated low-grade chronic pulpal infection may produce mild symptoms from time to time. According to Eliasson and colleagues (1984), part of the pulp will be nonvital; however, Eversole and associates (1972) have shown by biopsy that a mildly inflamed vital pulp also may produce condensing osteitis.

Treatment/Prognosis

We believe endodontic therapy will be necessary in most cases. On radiographic follow-up, approximately 75% of the cases of condensing osteitis can be expected to regress totally, whereas the remainder may remain as "bone scar." In an analysis by Eliasson and co-authors (1984), condensing osteitis did not progress in any instance after endodontic treatment. The persistence of a radiolucent component sometimes may indicate endodontic failure.

◆ *RADIOLOGY (Figs. 17–3 to 17–5)*

Location

Condensing osteitis is more common in the mandible than the maxilla. In their study of 600 European and 600 "Cape Coloured" patients, Farman and colleagues (1978) found 13 cases of condensing osteitis in the maxilla and 24 in the mandible in the "Cape Coloured" patients, whereas in the Europeans there were only 2 maxillary and 50 mandibular lesions. From these data, it may be concluded that condensing osteitis occurs 25 times more frequently in the mandible than the maxilla of Europeans, whereas in the "Cape Coloured" group the ratio was only 2:1, with a greater predominance in the mandible compared with the maxilla. Farman and colleagues (1978) found that the most common locations were as follows: mandibular first molar (41%), mandibular second molar (20%), and mandibular second premolar (16%). Only one case was found at the apex of a third molar

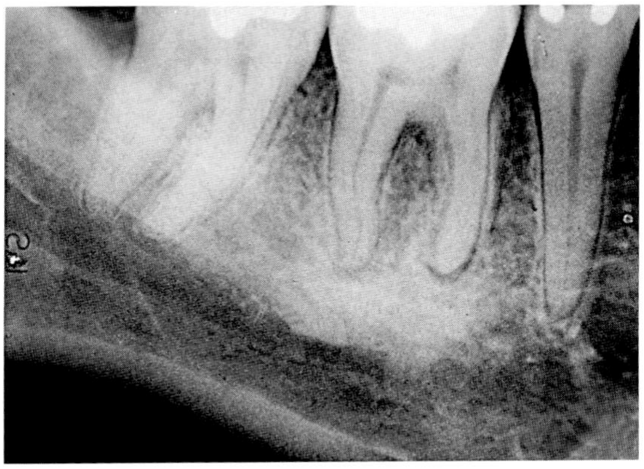

A

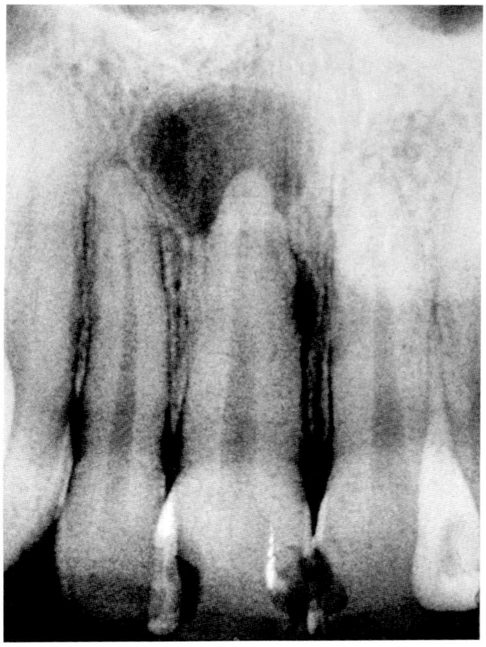

B

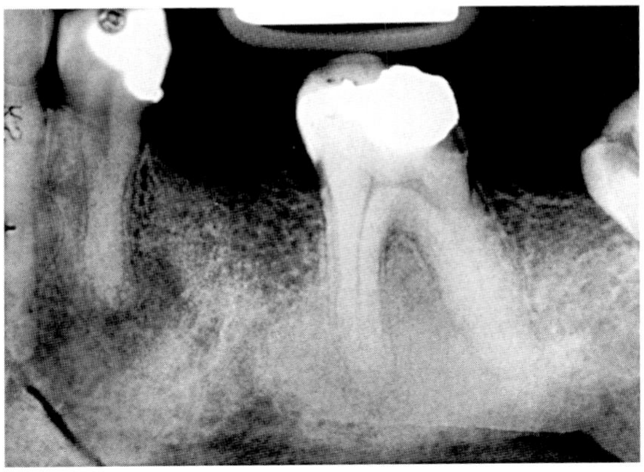

C

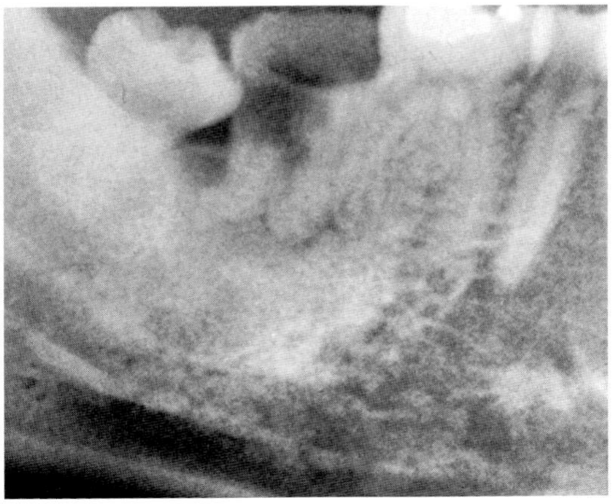

D

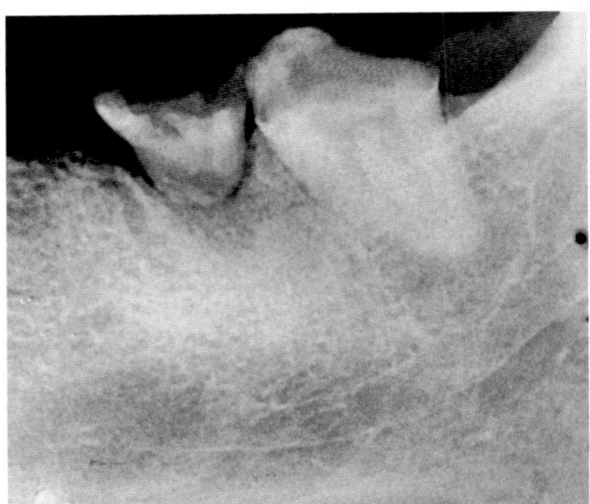

E

FIGURE 17–3.

Condensing Osteitis: Five types as classified by Eversole and associates (1984). A, Focal type showing widening of periodontal ligament space and destruction of lamina dura at both apices; clinically, the tooth appeared sound. B, Target type, with central radiopacity within radiolucent area. C, Radiolucent/granular type; radiolucent area at premolar contains tiny granular radiopacities; molar resembles ground glass. D, Multiconfluent type, with three radiopaque foci surrounded by radiolucent area. E, Focal pattern with root resorption; widened periodontal ligament space containing cementicles.

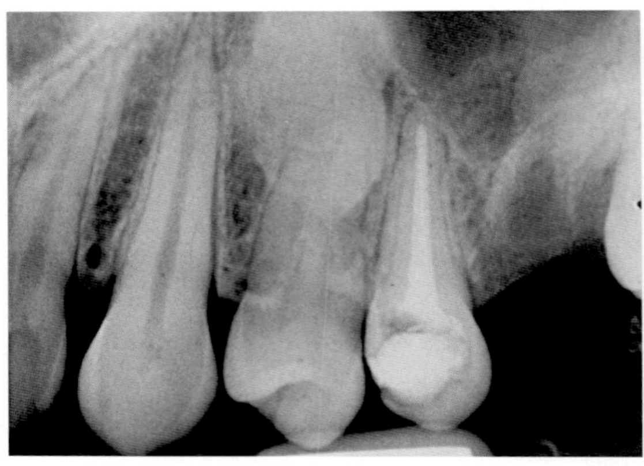

A

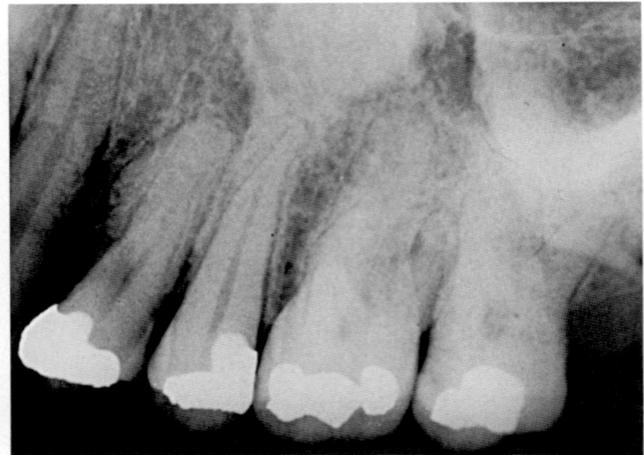

B

FIGURE 17–4.

Condensing Osteitis Versus Idiopathic Osteosclerosis: A, Idiopathic osteosclerosis. The patient had pain in the left maxilla. The first premolar was vital and the second premolar caused the pain. B, Condensing osteitis. A 28-year-old woman had a history of tic douloureux. The second premolar was nonvital on testing. The pulp was extirpated, and tic douloureux symptoms disappeared.

in the mandible of a European. Eversole and associates (1984) found a similar site predilection for condensing osteitis: mandibular first molar (56%), mandibular second molar (20%), and mandibular second premolars (15%). Thus, approximately 60 to 75% of the cases involve the mandibular first or second molars, whereas idiopathic osteosclerosis primarily involves the mandibular premolars and canine teeth, with only 24% in the molar areas.

Relationship to Teeth

The most common location is the apex of a nonvital mandibular first or second molar. The apex almost always is involved; however, there is little tendency to locate in the inter-radicular area or regions separate from the apex. Both Eversole (1984) and associates and Eliasson and colleagues (1984) found root resorption in 12% of the cases.

Radiologic Features

Eversole and colleagues (1984) identified five distinct radiographic patterns in condensing osteitis: (1) a focal pattern characterized as a homogeneous radiopaque mass lacking a perilesional radiolucent halo, (2) a target pattern consisting of a central radiopacity with a circumferential radiolucent band, (3) a lucent or granular pattern described as a nonexpansile periapical radiolucency displaying a fibro-osseous pattern histologically, (4) a multiconfluent pattern where several target lesions at the apices of a single multirooted tooth become closely apposed, and (5) a resorption pattern

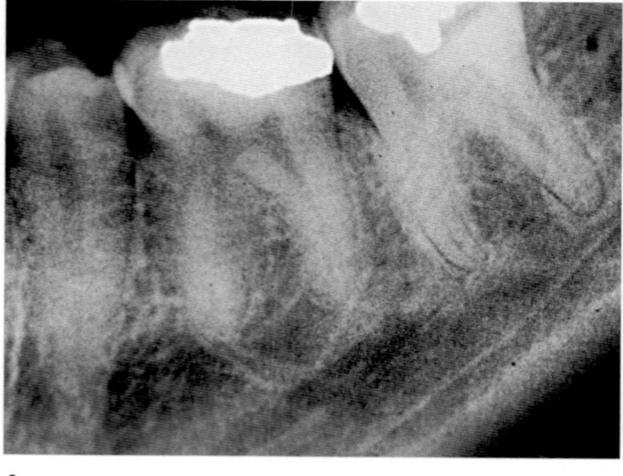

A

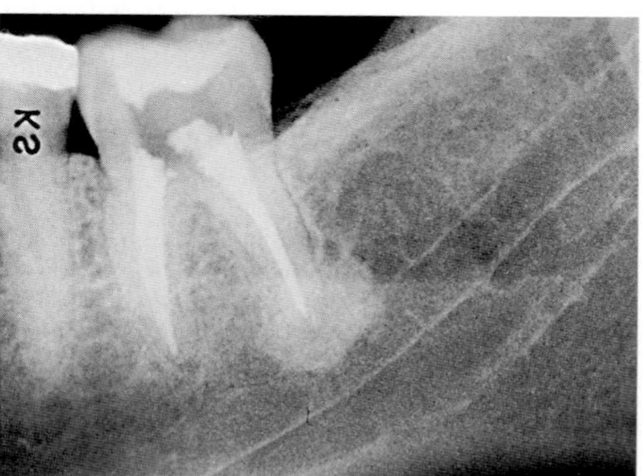

B

FIGURE 17–5.

Condensing Osteitis: A, Patient had paresthesia in left lower lip. The nuclear scan had negative results. The dental radiologist recognized early condensing osteitis at distal apex of second molar. B, Paresthesia disappeared with endodontic treatment, but condensing osteitis continued to develop during endodontic therapy and now remains stable as a periapical scar. (Courtesy of Dr. L. Otis, University of California at San Francisco, CA.)

characterized by external root resorption in association with any of the previous patterns. The sample reported by Eversole and associates (1984) consisted of 41 histologically documented cases consisting of idiopathic periapical osteosclerosis or condensing osteitis. In the condensing osteitis group, the most common finding was the target pattern. In addition, the radiolucent pattern was far more common in condensing osteitis than in idiopathic periapical osteosclerosis. The focal and multiconfluent patterns were seen in a few cases. Root resorption occurred with equal frequency (12%) in condensing osteitis and idiopathic periapical osteosclerosis and usually occurs at the root apex. Eliasson and colleagues (1984) also observed root resorption, with 12% of cases occurring in association with condensing osteitis.

In condensing osteitis, the focal pattern appears to be similar to that described for idiopathic periapical osteosclerosis in all aspects except the apical periodontal ligament space, which may be obliterated; it may be widened very slightly but more prominently radiolucent than the remainder of the periodontal ligament space, or it may be grossly widened within a lytic area up to several millimeters in diameter, separating the root apex from the subadjacent osteosclerotic area.

The target pattern greatly resembles periapical cemental dysplasia (PCD). It consists of a single, usually rounded or ovoid, homogeneous, central radiopaque mass with a radiolucent band of uniform diameter (up to several millimeters in thickness) surrounding the mass. The apical periodontal ligament space may be widened. Beyond the radiolucent band there may be a zone of reactive sclerotic bone.

The multiconfluent pattern is especially prone to occur when both apices of a mandibular molar have lesions resembling the target pattern. In this instance, the central portion of the lesion contains several distinct radiopaque masses separated by the radiolucent band interwoven between them. The outer margins of the radiopaque mass are scalloped because of the confluence of several masses. Beyond this, a radiolucent band of uniform thickness surrounds the outer contours of the radiopaque masses and anastomoses with the radiolucent bands interwoven between the central radiopaque masses. Beyond the outer radiolucent band, a zone of reactive sclerotic bone may be seen.

The radiolucent pattern as described by Eversole and associates (1984) is interesting. The apical region of the tooth, usually a mandibular first molar, is surrounded by a well-defined radiolucent area. On closer examination, the radiolucent zone may contain tiny radiopaque flecks, giving the rarefied area a slightly more radiopaque haze or granular appearance. The apical radiolucent area may be surrounded by a thin band of reactive sclerotic bone. This pattern was seen with much greater frequency among the condensing osteitis group. Thus, when a periapical radiolucency of pulpal origin is suspected, the histologic diagnosis might be one of the following: (1) periapical abscess, (2) apical periodontal cyst, (3) periapical granuloma, (4) periapical cholesteatoma, and (5) condensing osteitis.

In their study of 49 roots on 36 teeth with condensing osteitis, Eliasson and colleagues (1984) observed regression to normal after endodontic treatment in 73% of the roots, with a normal radiographic appearance. The remaining 27% did not return to normal after endodontic treatment. Although the mean observation period was 4.3 years, the range was 7 months to 12 years. After root canal therapy, condensing osteitis did not reveal progression in any case.

HYPERCEMENTOSIS (Cementum hyperplasia, exostosis of the root)

According to Shafer and colleagues (1983), hypercementosis is a regressive change that sometimes occurs in some or all of the teeth. It may result from local factors, from systemic disease, as an inherited disorder, or idiopathically. The local factors include the following: (1) tooth mobility, including supraeruption, periodontal disease, hyperocclusion, and autogenous transplants of partially developed teeth; (2) inflammation around the tooth as may be seen in periodontal disease and periapical infection; and (3) trauma from the occlusion and as a repair mechanism in vital root fractures. The systemic disorders include Paget's disease and hyperpituitarism, including gigantism and acromegaly. The mechanism by which excess cementum production occurs is poorly understood. As Worth (1963) explained, cementum is not a static tissue and, like bone, it is resorbed and replaced constantly; thus, a variety of stimuli are associated with cementum resorption, replacement, and proliferation. In hypercementosis, this process is limited to cementum, which remains attached to the dentin of the root surface. According to Wood and Goaz (1985), the excess cementum may be primary or acellular and more often secondary or cellular. It usually is deposited in layers; however, it may be irregular with fibrovascular inclusions. Hypercementosis is asymptomatic, although some of the conditions with which it is associated may be symptomatic. Hypercementosis does not require treatment or justify tooth removal; however, if a tooth with hypercementosis must be removed, the extraction may be more difficult than normal because of the bulbous shape of the root. Cementum is unique in that it is the only tissue in the human body that does not have a known malignant counterpart.

◆ *RADIOLOGY (Figs. 17–6 to 17–12)*

The radiologic features of hypercementosis consist of an area of increased density surrounding the root of a tooth through which the dentinal outline can be seen. The periodontal ligament space and lamina dura usually are present and of normal proportions. Hypercementosis may be seen only in the root of a tooth and never occurs within the jaws in locations separate from the teeth. This disorder may be focal or generalized; when generalized, it may be a marker of a systemic disease or genetic disorder.

Location

According to Gibilisco (1985), hypercementosis is associated most often with the premolars, and Worth (1963) has stated that the upper premolars are the favored site. The premolars are affected with a frequency of 6:1 over other teeth; according to Gibilisco (1985), the second most likely

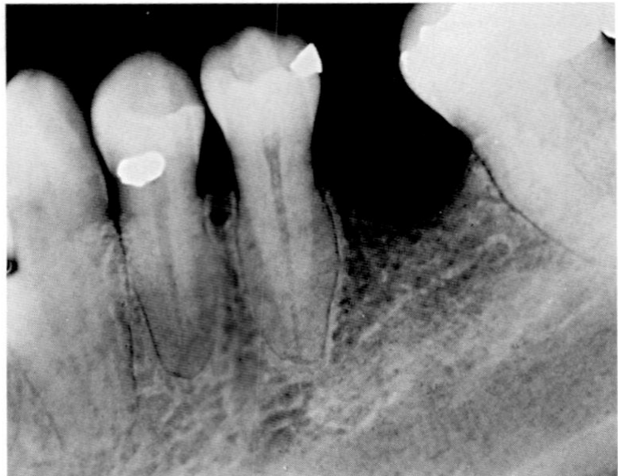

FIGURE 17–6.

Hypercementosis: Typical appearance of hypercementosis in a common location, showing dentinal outline within excess cementum and normal periodontal ligament space and lamina dura.

sites are the first and second molars and, according to Worth (1963), the lower first molars. Permanent teeth are affected much more often than primary teeth. When local factors are responsible, only one tooth may be affected; at other times the condition may be symmetrically bilateral. When systemic or genetic factors are the cause, the condition may be generalized.

Radiologic Features

Classic Hypercementosis. Hypercementosis is characterized by the deposition of excess cementum about the root. The hyperplastic cementum is less dense than the adjacent dentin; thus, the dentinal root outline can be seen within the cemental enlargement. Three distinct patterns can be seen within the excess cementum: (1) homogeneous, whereby the excess cementum exhibits no internal structure; (2) mottled, wherein the cementum exhibits an admixture of more and less dense areas throughout; and (3) feather-like, whereby the cementum exhibits regularly spaced, often fine horizontal bands of more radiopaque cementum laid down at right angles to the dentinal surface. The significance of these three patterns is not known. The outline of the excess cementum usually follows the shape of the underlying root; however, it may be deposited focally anywhere on the root. The outer periphery of the excess cementum is usually smooth; however, it may be wavy. Beyond the cementum, there is the periodontal ligament space, which is of normal dimensions. The lamina dura usually is seen in the absence of periodontal disease, except in some cases of Paget's disease. When associated with a supraerupting tooth, periodontal disease and the lost antagonist combine to accelerate movement of the affected tooth out of the socket. As this occurs, cementum first is deposited around the apical region of the tooth, then along the root surface, and tapers off toward the cervical part of the root. In periodontal disease, particularly when there has been horizontal bone loss and increased tooth mobility, hypercementosis may be seen about the remainder of the root within the alveolar bone. Presumably this is a reactive mechanism to increase the area of attachment and thus stabilize the tooth. Hypercementosis usually is not seen in an ankylosed tooth, although there are exceptions. In most instances, the presence of a periodontal ligament space is integral to the diagnosis of hypercementosis.

Spherical Hypercementosis. In the anterior region, hypercementosis may be laid down in a spherical pattern centered on the apex or off to one side. Although the upper and lower incisors are the most common site for this variant, other teeth may be affected. This spherical growth of cementum rarely exceeds 0.5 cm in diameter, and because it may achieve a density that approximates that of dentin, the apical portion of the root may be obscured.

Concrescence. In some instances, hypercementosis is sufficiently extensive to cause two adjacent teeth to become attached to each other, which is best described as "concrescence." Concrescence is defined as the union of two teeth

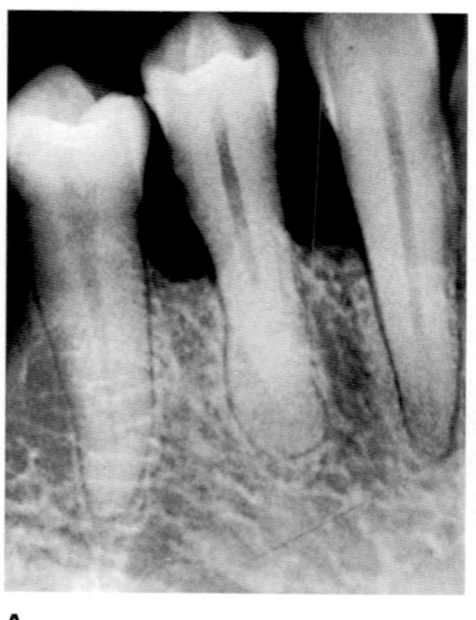

A

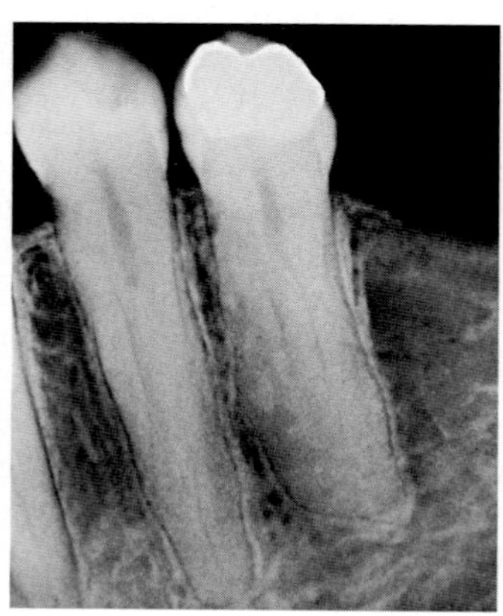

B

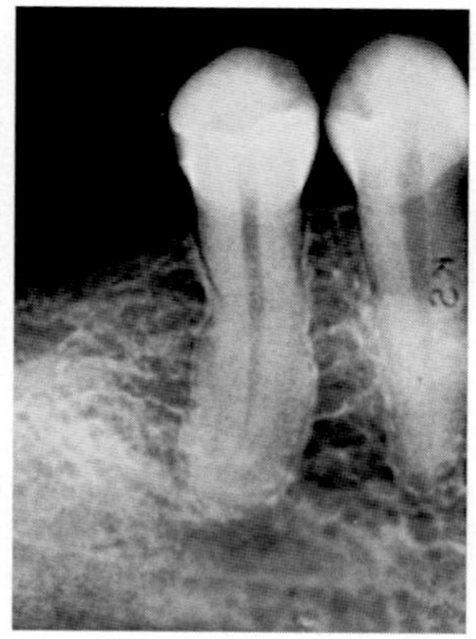

C

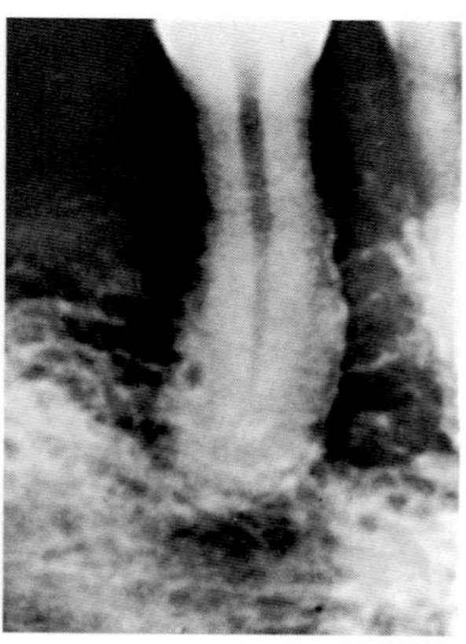

D

FIGURE 17–7.

Hypercementosis: Patterns. A, Homogeneous. B, Mottled; mesial of second premolar. C and D, Feather-like; C is actual radiograph, and D is digitally processed image of C.

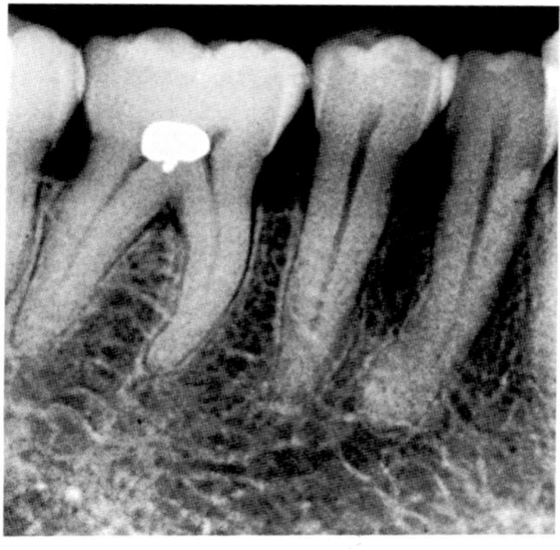

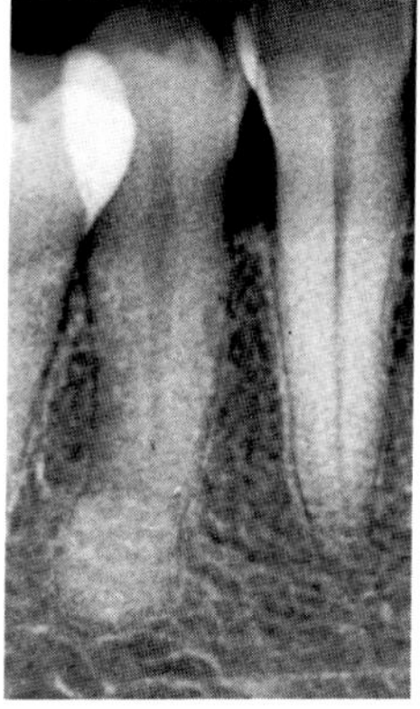

A B

FIGURE 17–8.

Hypercementosis: Spheric variant. A and B, At apex of first premolar. Excess cementum has mottled appearance and periodontal ligament space and lamina dura are present.

by cementum only. The term fusion should be reserved for two teeth joined by dentin and one other dental tissue. In two fused teeth there may be a common root canal space in some portion of the root or union of the coronal portion of the teeth; in concrescence there are always two separate root canal spaces and the coronal portion is never joined because no cementum occurs in this area.

Hypercementosis in Transplanted Teeth. When partially developed teeth are transplanted within the same person, a number of events occur that defy explanation and disrupt current theories of tooth development and eruption. In our experience, a common situation is the replacement of an extracted permanent first molar with a developing third molar. The most desirable time for transplantation is before root formation in the transplanted tooth. The recipient transplant site is prepared by opening into and curetting the surface of the alveolar bone. The developing third molar and papilla are positioned in the prepared cryptlike cavity, in infraocclusion, and stabilized. In time, root formation occurs, with the root, periodontal ligament space, and lamina dura growing into the previously healed alveolar bone. Root development often is stunted with a poor crown-to-root ratio. We have observed the development of hypercementosis about the cervical region of the root, presumably to increase the area of attachment and stabilize the transplanted tooth. We have used the term "fat man girth" to describe this appearance of the hypercementosis. Worth (1963) also observed this pattern in nontransplanted normal-sized teeth. In view of the case of Israel (1984), as discussed later, it is possible that this pattern of hypercementosis develops in association with the eruption of a tooth.

Hypercementosis in Periapical Infection. When hypercementosis is seen with periapical infection, the tooth usually is nonvital. This is the only instance in which hypercementosis occurs with a nonvital tooth. The cementum is laid down on the root surface at a distance from the apex; during this stage, the root is said to acquire an hourglass shape. In the apical region, there may be resorption of the root apex, including cementum and dentin. Ultimately the hyperplastic cementum is deposited apically. Although there is no possibility for the replacement of resorbed dentin at the apex of the root, it may be replaced with cementum. The hyperplastic cementum is surrounded by a radiolucent area that is wider than the normal periodontal ligament space, and the lamina

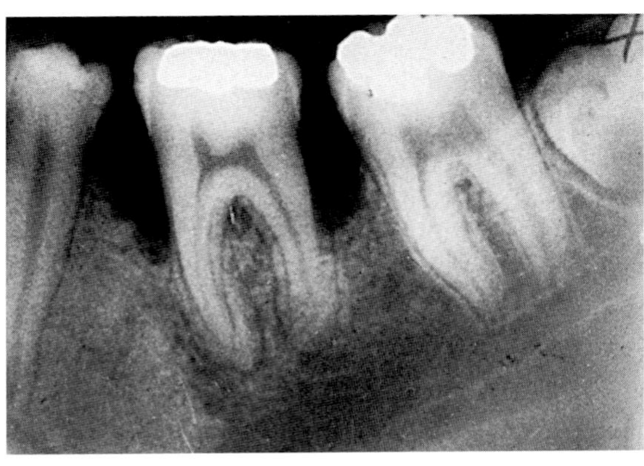

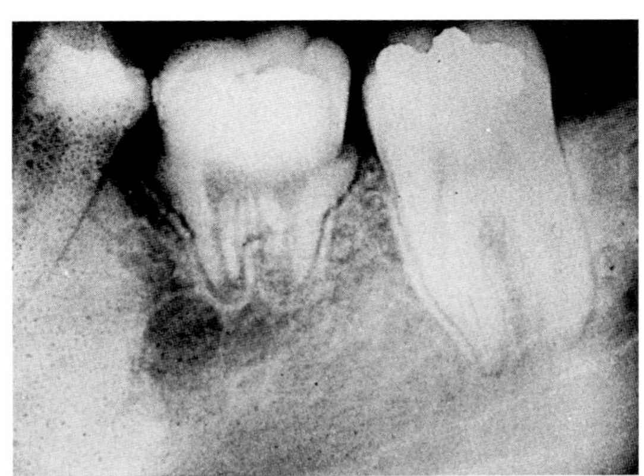

A B

FIGURE 17–9.

Hypercementosis: Vertical variant. A, Juvenile periodontitis affecting first molar. Developing third molar can be seen. B, Transplanted third molar with "fat man girth" appearance of excess cervical cementum.

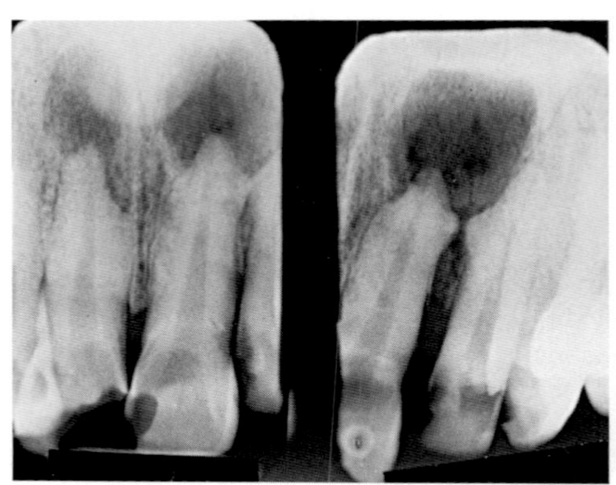
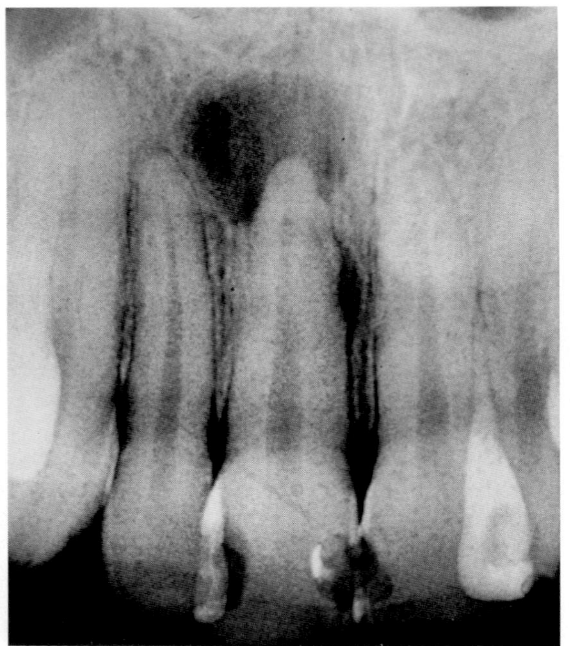

A B

FIGURE 17–10.

Hypercementosis: A, Associated with periapical infection. Triangular mass of excess cementum is cervical to root apex of central and lateral incisors at margin of apical inflammatory lesion. B, Associated with traumatic occlusion. Fine, almost indiscernible 2-mm-long spikelike radiations of cementum at apex of left central incisor (crowding can be seen); inflammatory hypercementosis on mesial surface of root.

dura is absent in the region. This form of hypercementosis is characterized by a widening of the periodontal ligament space and absence of the lamina dura.

Hypercementosis Associated with Occlusal Trauma. A variant of hypercementosis occurs in a spikelike manner in some cases of excessive occlusal trauma. Very fine, almost feathery spikelike areas of excess cementum may radiate from the tooth's surface, often at the apex. In this instance, the periodontal ligament space and lamina dura may be thickened to approximately double the normal thickness.

Hypercementosis and Fractured Roots. When a root is fractured, the tooth sometimes may remain vital. In this in-

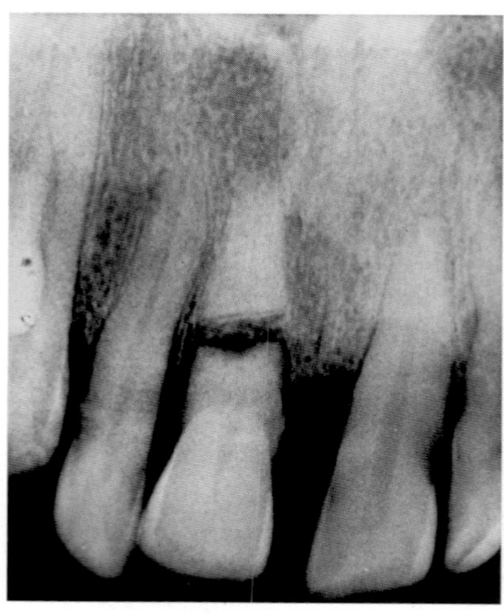
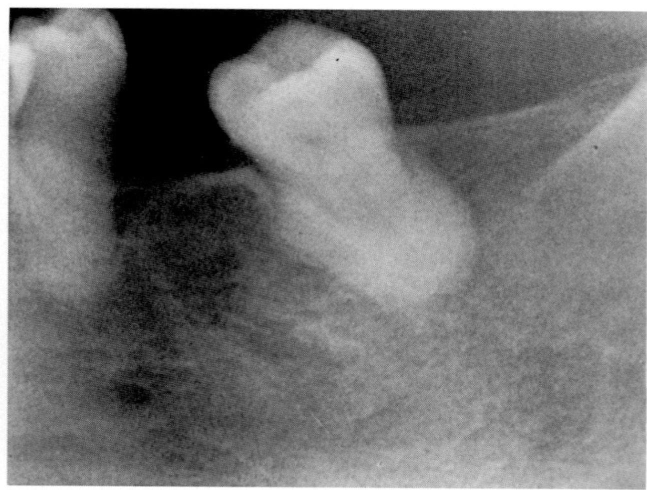

A B

FIGURE 17–11.

Hypercementosis: A, Representing attempt of cementum to bridge between two fracture segments. B, Unusual case associated with apparent ankylosis.

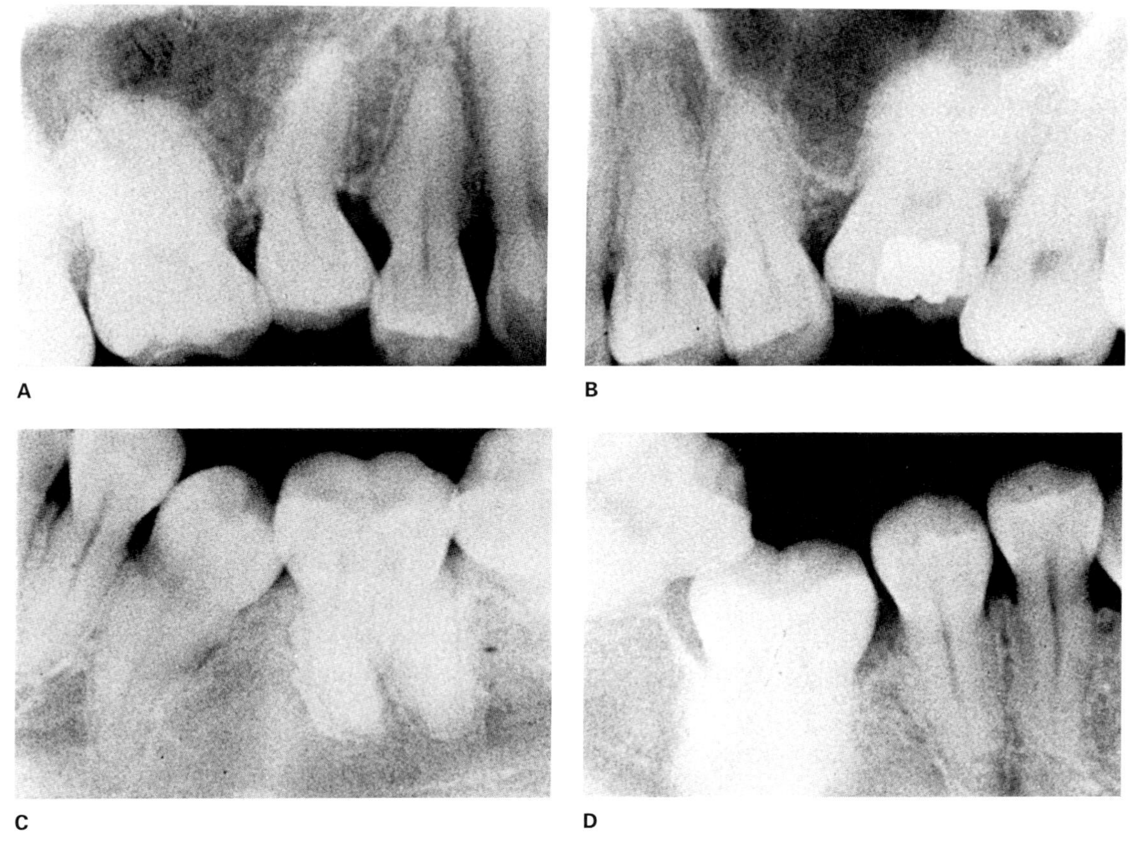

FIGURE 17–12.

Hypercementosis: A to D, Inheritable form affects partially erupted premolars in all four quadrants of the same patient. (From Israel H: Early hypercementosis and arrested dental eruption: heritable multiple ankylodontia. J Craniofac Genet Dev Biol 4:243, 1984.)

stance, cementum may be laid down between the two fragments to effect a cementum bridge. Sometimes a space of several millimeters develops between the root fragments. The cementum between the fragments is less dense and sometimes extends beyond the root outline as it attaches to the two segments. In other instances, normal alveolar bone fills the gap between the two fractured root elements.

Generalized Hypercementosis. Generalized hypercementosis has been observed in patients with Paget's disease, although in various cases only some teeth are affected. Hypercementosis may be independent of jaw involvement with the typical bony changes, or it may be seen along with these bony changes. The hypercementosis tends to extend along the full length of the involved teeth, tapering off toward the cervical portion of the root. Some authors in the medical literature erroneously interpreted the sclerotic masses in the jaws as hypercementosis. When Paget's disease affects the alveolar bone, it is possible that, in some instances, the hypercementosis will occur in association with loss of the lamina dura. Except in cases of periodontal disease and periapical infection, a normal lamina dura is present in hypercementosis. This disorder also has been observed as a variable feature of Gardner's syndrome, which is inherited as an autosomal dominant trait. In these cases, the hypercementosis tends to be generalized, may be severe, and may be associated with radiopaque osteomatous changes in the jaws. Generalized hypercementosis also has been reported with hyperpituitarism, in the pituitary giant and acromegaly.

Hereditary Hypercementosis. An inheritable form of hypercementosis has been reported by Israel (1984) in association with heritable multiple ankylodontia. He studied four affected members of the same family over three generations and concluded that the pattern of inheritance is autosomal dominant. The condition is enigmatic for two reasons: It occurs early in the permanent dentition before eruption, and there is a concomitant loss of the periodontal ligament space, ankylosis, and incomplete eruption of the affected teeth. Involved teeth consisted principally of the second premolars and first molars in all four quadrants. Clinically, the affected teeth sounded dull to percussion, and malocclusion resulted from a collapse of the occlusion.

Hypercementosis and Traumatic Cyst. The association of cemental lesions, such as florid cemento-osseous dysplasia (FCOD) and periapical cemental dysplasia (PCD), with traumatic cysts has been reported. To our knowledge, no cases of hypercementosis have been seen with a traumatic cyst. The case in this text (in the discussion on traumatic cyst) may be the first such case.

CEMENTICLES

According to Shafer and colleagues (1983), cementicles are small foci of calcified tissue within the periodontal ligament. Although these are spherical and resemble cementum histologically, they are thought to represent dystrophic calcification resulting from degenerative change. Mikola and Bauer (1949) stated that these are analogous to phleboliths. They are found throughout the periodontal ligament and may be in the apical region. Cementicles produce no symptoms and, according to Shafer and colleagues (1983), are not associated with any known abnormality of the teeth. We have seen changes that may be consistent with cementicle formation in association with infection, especially apical periodontitis. In most instances, cementicles remain undetected clinically and do not require treatment.

◆ *RADIOLOGY (Figs. 17–13 and 17–14)*

According to Shafer and colleagues (1983), cementicles are found within the periodontal ligament space. They may be located anywhere along the root or at the apex. Because they are 0.2 to 0.3 mm in diameter, they are thought to be too small to be seen in the radiograph. We believe that the threshold of visual perception in a well-exposed and processed radiograph is 0.2 mm under the magnifying lens. Shafer and colleagues (1983) also stated that clusters of cementicles may form and, when this occurs at the apex of a tooth, they may resemble a cementoma. If this is true, smaller clusters of cementicles also may be assumed to be visible to the keen observer. In addition, it is possible that the radiolucent pattern of condensing osteitis and idiopathic osteosclerosis classified by Eversole (1984) as producing a fibro-osseous pattern histologically, represents proliferation of cementicles.

If cementicles can be seen, they enter the threshold of visibility as very tiny flecks that cause the widened periodontal ligament space to become more radiopaque. On close inspection with the magnifying lens, the area of increased opacity consists of tiny calcified bodies. These eventually coalesce to form discernible granules. In this early stage of apical periodontitis, these are contained and restrained within the periodontal ligament, which is still intact. At this point the cementicles line up as a more or less single row of granular structures within the periodontal ligament space radiologically. As infection continues, the periodontal ligament breaks down, as does the alveolar bone surrounding it. In some circumstances there may be proliferation of connective tissue, possibly of periodontal ligament origin, and more cementicles are formed. Radiologically the cementicles no longer form a single row and may occupy much of the area of apical bone destruction. It might be that the granular appearance within an area of periapical bone destruction, as described by Eversole and colleagues (1984), represents a fibro-osseous response by cementicles and the periodontal ligament to pulpal infection.

In the discussion of Shafer and co-authors (1983), there was no radiograph to illustrate the radiologic appearance because it was assumed that cementicles are invisible. With more scrupulous scrutiny of our radiographs and further correlation with histologic studies, the radiologic description of cementicles may become more precise; that is why they have been included in this text.

PERIAPICAL CEMENTAL DYSPLASIA

(Cementoma, periapical cementifying dysplasia, periapical osteofibrosis, periapical fibrous dysplasia, sclerotic cemental masses, focal cemento-osseous dysplasia)

PCD is common, but its cause remains unknown. One of the earliest large surveys was reported by Stafne in 1934, when the condition was known as periapical osteofibrosis.

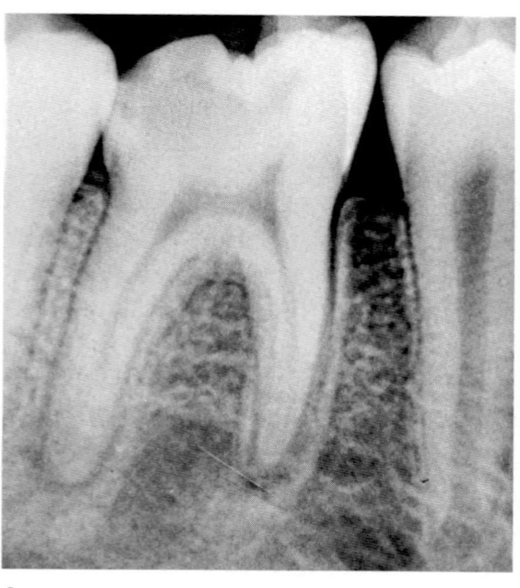

A

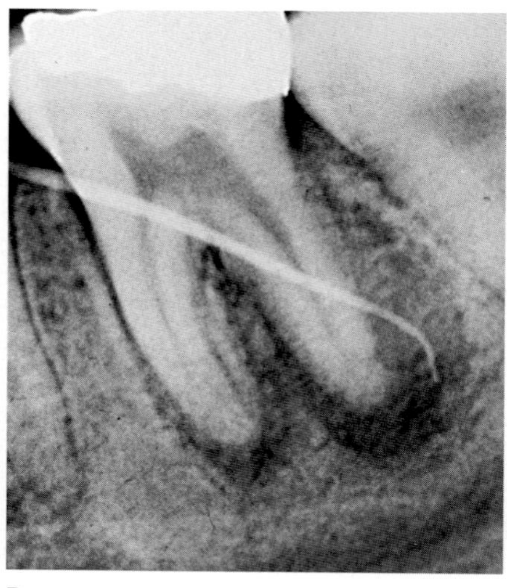

B

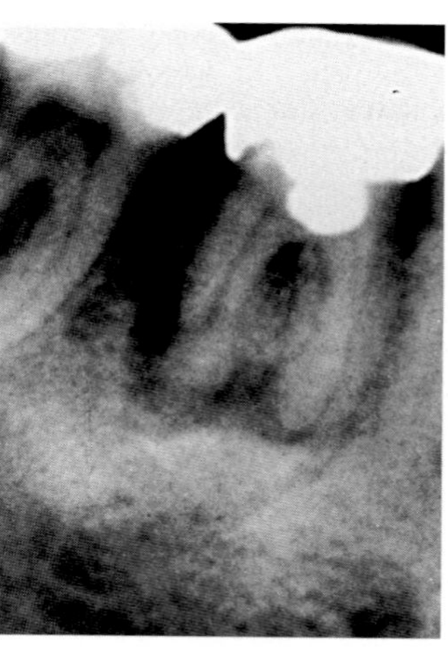

C

FIGURE 17–13.

Cementicles: A, Within periodontal ligament space, mesial root of molar. B, Single row of spheric structures around mesial root of molar. C, Clustered at distal apex, resembling cementoma.

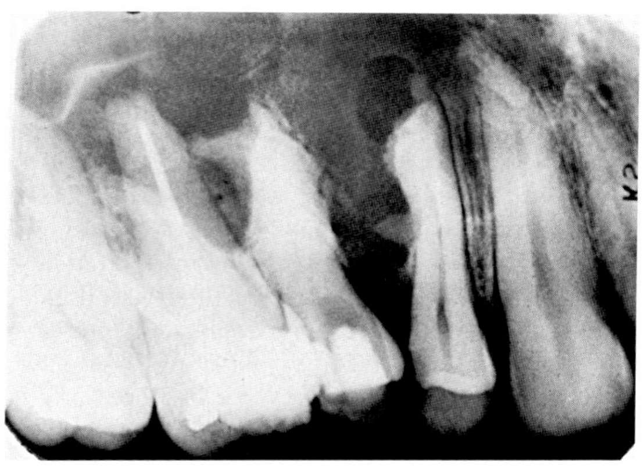

FIGURE 17–14.

Cementicles: Lesion is odontogenic keratocyst with secondary infection. Triangular masses of hypercementosis on roots of premolars may result from infection or tooth mobility. There is fine radial spiking of cementum at apex of palatal root of molar and canine, possibly resulting from hyperocclusion. A single row of cementicles is seen at distal apex of first premolar and along mesial of root of second premolar, perhaps resulting from infection.

Waldron (1985) presented one of the most recent reviews. In their series of 706 cases sent for biopsy, Regezi and colleagues (1978) found that PCD was the third most common diagnosis after odontoma and ameloblastoma. Because PCD is recognized most often by its clinical and radiologic features and biopsies rarely are performed, it is more common than these data indicate; Stafne (1934) found an incidence of 24 in 10,000 patients. It is also the most common of the cementifying lesions: In their series of 166 cementifying lesions sent for biopsy, Hamner and colleagues (1968) found that 49% were PCD, 40% cementifying fibroma, 9% cementoblastoma, and 2% FCOD.

Some American pathologists believe that cementomas occur only in the mandibular incisor region; therefore, the condition is termed periapical cemental dysplasia. In the posterior region, we believe that histopathologically identical lesions are seen clinically as focal or florid variants. The focal variant sometimes is termed "sclerotic cemental masses" or "focal osseous dysplasia" and only involves individual teeth. The florid variant most frequently is termed "florid osseous dysplasia," "chronic diffuse sclerosing osteomyelitis," or, our preferred term, "florid cemento-osseous dysplasia," characterized by the coalescence of cemental masses to involve a whole quadrant or more. We believe that the anterior and focal posterior variants represent the same condition, and these are the subject of this discussion under Periapical Cemental Dysplasia. FCOD may represent a more exuberant form of PCD and will be discussed in the chapter titled Generalized Radiopacities.

Pathologic Characteristics

Currently, most investigators believe PCD is a reactive disorder rather than a neoplastic process. The reactive elements consist of the periodontal ligament, cementum, and bone. The possibility that cementicles play a role generally has not been considered. The stimulus for this presumed reactive process remains a mystery, but trauma and infection are implicated most frequently. Microscopically, the diagnosis of PCD can be difficult because the tissue resembles other separate and distinct ossifying and cementifying lesions. Because the condition is distinct radiologically, many pathologists will not diagnose PCD without radiographs. Histologically, PCD is a solid, well-calcified, "cementoid" mass with few cementocytes; few or many trabeculae of woven bone also may be present, usually at the periphery. At the periphery of the cemental mass, droplet cementum and hypercellular fibrous tissue may be evident and often contains chronic inflammatory cells. Although mature lamellar bone polarizes light well, in a mature PCD the parallel birefringent lines are finer and more delicate than those in lamellar bone. It is not known whether PCD can arise de novo in an edentulous area; those occurring in such areas are presumed to have been at the apex of a tooth before extraction.

Clinical Features

Zegarelli and colleagues (1964a) reviewed the cases of 230 patients with 435 individual lesions of PCD. These were associated with 554 existing teeth, and 82 (19%) were in edentulous areas. Most (52%) were diagnosed in patients between the ages of 31 and 45 years, and approximately 20% each were discovered in patients between the ages of 21 and 30 and between 45 and 60 years. The youngest patient was 20 years old. Zegerelli and colleagues (1964a) found 83% in African-American patients and 17% in white patients, even though the ratio of white-to-black people was 1.6:1 in the sample. The authors also reported that 91% were seen in women, for a female-to-male ratio of 10:1. Zegerelli and colleagues (1964a) specifically looked for trauma and infection. Only 9% of the patients could recall episodes of trauma in the general region of PCD involvement, and none of the teeth submitted to pulp vitality studies were nonvital. There was periodontitis of varying degrees of severity: 37% had mild cases; 29%, moderate cases; 8%, significant cases; and 1%, severe cases. There was no periodontal disease in 26% of the teeth with PCD. Clinically the affected teeth appear normal in color. Because PCD resembles a periapical radiolucency of pulpal origin during the early stage, pulp vitality tests are essential in ruling out this possibility.

Treatment/Prognosis

PCD usually requires no treatment, although infection, sequestration, and traumatic cysts are complicating factors in rare instances. Notably, when PCD is excised, it tends to be removed in fragments that are somewhat bloody. This gross finding is helpful to the pathologist because ossifying fibroma (cementifying variant) usually shells out in a single solid avascular mass. If an associated tooth is extracted, the cementoma will be retained within the bone, whereas benign cementoblastoma remains fixed to the associated root. Cementomas normally do not retrogress after tooth extraction; however, progression may be expected in the future. With resorption of the alveolar ridge, the lesion may contact the surface. Osteomyelitis may affect the adjacent bone, and the entire cemental mass may be sequestered, after which the area heals. Traumatic cysts associated with PCD may fill in with lesional tissue postoperatively and be more prone to recurrence in this group of patients.

◆ RADIOLOGY (Figs. 17–15 to 17–25)

General Radiologic Features

In any cemental lesion, the following radiologic features should be assessed. These 12 features are based on the assumption that PCD is the archetypical lesion within the group and that all others retain some features with variations that help to suggest the diagnosis or separate cementum-containing lesions from those with other forms of mineralized matrix:

1. Development is in phases characterized by an early osteoporotic stage, followed by a lytic radiolucent stage, an intermediate cementoblastic stage in which radiopaque calcific spherules are elaborated, and, finally, a mature stage in which a radiopaque cemental mass is formed.
2. Cemental lesions are characterized by active and quiescent periods. Evidence of a quiescent period is indicated by the lack of a peripheral radiolucent zone and the absence of an outer sclerotic margin. In this instance the central cemental mass appears to be in direct apposition with the adjacent bone. In active periods, the peripheral radiolucent zone reappears first, followed by the outer reactive sclerotic margin. The thicker and more diffuse the sclerotic margin, the greater is the degree of metabolic activity within the lesion.
3. With a magnifying lens, small clusters of tiny speck-like calcific spherules, which may be derived from cementicles within the periodontal ligament, can be seen within the radiolucent zone. These usually are circular and may represent droplet cementum. The most immature calcific spherules are located toward the outer margin of the radiolucent zone; these are doughnut shaped, with a radiolucent center and an outer radiopaque rim. Their density is less radiopaque than that of mature cementum. Toward the central portion of the radiolucent zone, the calcific spherules tend to be more radiopaque without the radiolucent center. In this instance, calcific spherules coalesce to form small massules, which are larger. Near the inner margin of the radiolucent zone next to the central cemental mass, there is evidence of coalescence of individual calcific spherules with each other, forming massules that coalesce with the central cemental mass. Individual calcific spherules tend to be almost perfectly round; several coalesced spherules known as massules may have a more linear curvoid or globular appearance. Ultimately, a more radiopaque central cemental mass appears that enlarges equally in all directions at its periphery. When a root apex is present, a crescent-shaped central cemental mass may develop as it molds itself around the apex. Cemental masses approximately 1 cm in diameter also may coalesce to form a large mass, and several large masses may coalesce to involve an entire quadrant or arch.
4. Cementogenesis occurs within the peripheral radiolucent zone, which is divided into three parts: In the outer or blastic portion, lysis of host bone and genesis of the calcific spherules occurs; the midportion is the zone of cemental spherule mineralization and coalescence; and the inner portion consists of the growth zone of the central cemental mass.
5. Calcific spherules are strongly suggestive that the mineralized tumor matrix consists of cementum.
6. Cemental lesions tend to produce a mineralized mass in the center of the lesion, thus creating a targetlike appearance. A lack of centricity of the mineralized

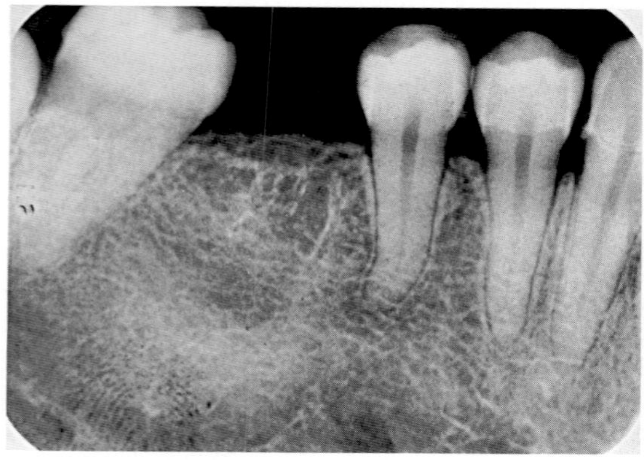

A

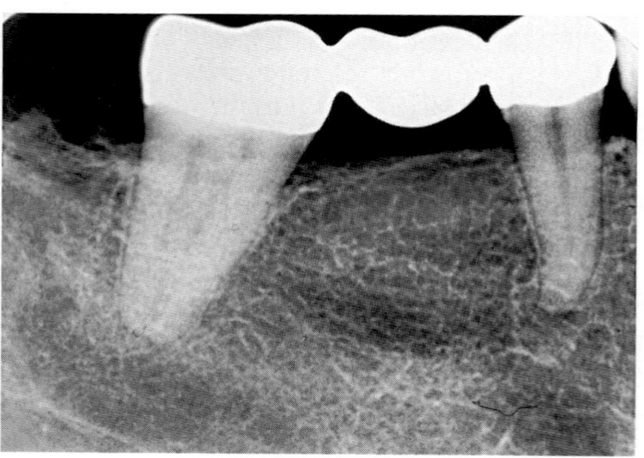

B

FIGURE 17–15.

Periapical Cemental Dysplasia: mandibular second premolar. A, First osteoporotic stage in 25-year-old Hispanic woman; loss of lamina dura, more radiolucent marrow spaces, and more prominent but fewer trabeculae. B, Same patient at age 45. There is more rarefaction, fewer trabeculae, and a thin radiopaque sclerotic rim. Typical cementomas occurred in other areas.

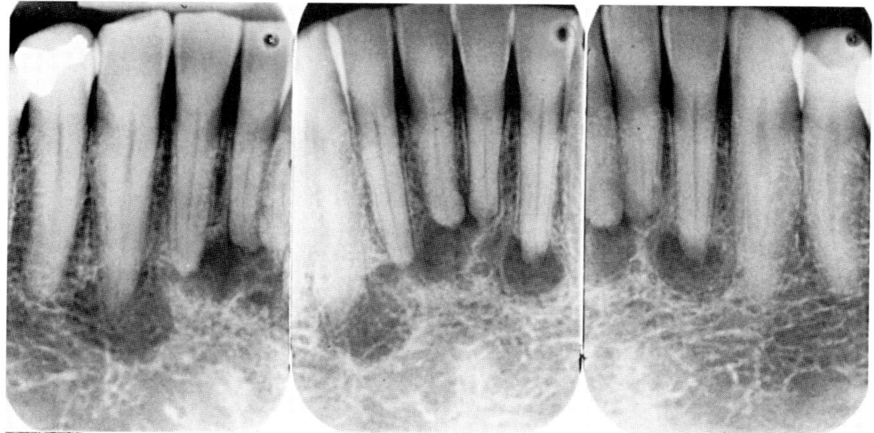

FIGURE 17–16.

Periapical Cemental Dysplasia: First osteoporotic stage in right canine (trabeculation is still present); second osteolytic stage in other teeth. The lesions appear inactive.

product contradicts the diagnosis of a purely cemental lesion. A noncentric cemental mass or several noncentric cemental masses with nearby calcific spherules are suggestive of a mixed cemento-osseous lesion.

7. Cemental masses, whether they are large or small, centric or eccentric, tend to have rounded margins, even though they may be irregular in shape. Additionally, small excrescences at the surface will be rounded and not spiked or pointed, as occurs in osseous foci.
8. Calcific spherules representing cementum are radiologically distinct from the snowflakelike or flocculent calcific foci in calcified cartilaginous matrix and the spiked or trabecular osseous foci occurring in bone lesions.
9. Cementum tends to be homogeneous in density, though radiolucent areas may intervene within a single mass or between several masses.
10. Cementum is coalescent by nature, and although several separate lesions may exist, there may be evidence of coalescence of two or more larger masses in the same patient.
11. Cemental lesions appear only in the tooth-bearing areas of the jaws and are not seen in any other part of the jaws or extragnathic skeleton. They are especially prone to occur in the mandible, although they may be seen in the maxilla.
12. Because cementum is the only human tissue that does not produce malignant tumors, radiologic evidence of malignant transformation or outright malignancy is not seen. Such features, when present, rule out the diagnosis of a cemental lesion.

Location

Most cementomas occur in the mandible. In their large series of 435 cementomas in 230 patients, Zegarelli and colleagues (1964b) found 94% in the mandible and 6% in the maxilla. Among the mandibular lesions, 77% occurred in the incisor region between the canine teeth and 71% had multiple individual lesions. In their review of 148 patients with cementomas, Hamner and co-workers (1968) found 81% in the mandible and 60% of patients had multiple lesions. Notably, in female Japanese patients, Tanaka and colleagues (1987) found that the mandibular premolar and molar areas were the preferred sites.

Radiologic Features

In a study of 67 lesions of PCD observed in 30 patients (28 women and 2 men) who were 25 to 68 years of age, Zegerelli and colleagues (1964a) made some interesting observations concerning the progression of cementomas through the three classic stages of maturation:

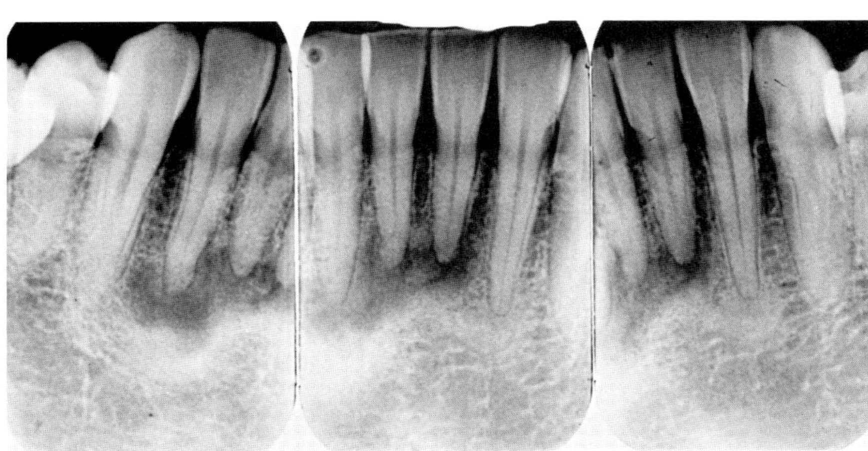

FIGURE 17–17.

Periapical Cemental Dysplasia: Third cementoblastic stage; lesions are very active.

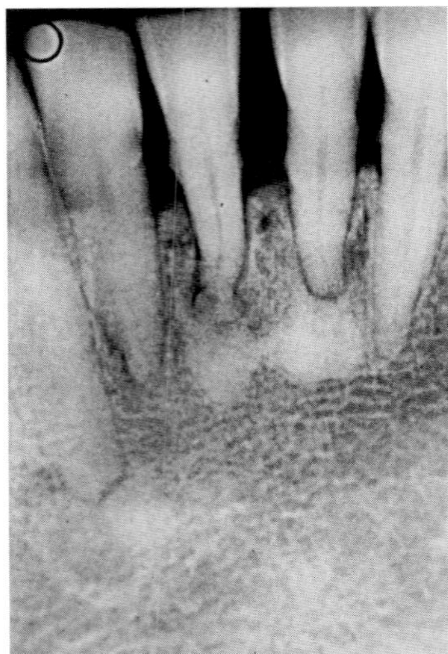

FIGURE 17–18.

Periapical Cemental Dysplasia: Fourth mature stage; the lesion in the left central incisor area is inactive, and lesions in the right central incisor and canine areas have reactivated.

1. The maturation rate of PCD is slow, with evidence of mineralizing activity over periods longer than 20 years.
2. No mature cementoma developed in less than 11 years after its prior discovery as an early-stage osteolytic lesion.
3. During a period of 6 to 10 years after the initial diagnosis as a radiolucent-stage PCD, at least five lesions disappeared, apparently resolving completely. The authors' findings suggested that some lesions of PCD may retrogress; according to Worth (1963), cementomas do not retrogress. We believe that the mechanism by which some lesions disappeared is sequestration of the cemental mass, followed by healing.

Traditionally, the lesions of PCD have been described in one of three stages: (1) osteolytic, (2) cementoblastic, and (3) mature. We believe there are two additional stages: an earlier osteoporotic stage in all cases and a later florid stage in some cases. Because the literature and data are based on the three classic stages, we will describe the earlier osteoporotic stage now and present our discussion on the florid stage under the condition titled Florid Cemento-Osseous Dysplasia, in the chapter titled Generalized Radiopacities.

Osteoporotic Stage. The early osteoporotic stage consists of the following radiologic features:

1. Loss of the lamina dura in the apical region, extending cervically some 2 to 4 mm on each side of the root; the periodontal ligament may appear more prominent.
2. A focal region of osteoporosis in the alveolar bone immediately apical to the root apex. This zone may range from several millimeters to 1 cm in diameter. The osteoporotic region appears more radiolucent than the surrounding alveolar bone. At times the marrow spaces appear slightly enlarged, whereas the trabeculae appear thinned, diminished in number, or, in some cases, slightly thicker. The most osteoporotic zone is more toward the root apex. The osteoporotic zone may be delineated by a very thin margin of reactive bone.
3. At the end of the osteoporotic phase there is a thickening of the apical periodontal ligament space and disappearance of trabeculation within the osteoporotic area, signaling the beginning of the osteolytic phase.
4. Because the osteoporotic stage has not been recognized previously, it is possible that the changes in this stage are very subtle but now will be recognized more frequently in younger susceptible patients.

Osteolytic Stage. The osteolytic stage is characterized by a circular area of rarefaction at the apex of a vital tooth. The lamina dura is usually absent in the apical region of the adjacent tooth. The radiolucent area is well demarcated from the surrounding alveolar bone and a sclerotic rim may be present, which is thicker, more irregular, and more diffuse than the margin of a cystic lesion. The average lesion is approximately 0.5 to 1 cm in diameter during this stage; in rare instances, the lesion may be larger than 1 cm, in which case it is most likely that multiple teeth will be involved. The lesion is usually round when it is smaller than 1 cm; it spreads laterally as it enlarges, eventually losing its circular configuration.

Cementoblastic Stage. The cementoblastic stage is characterized by the appearance of a radiodense cemental mass toward the center of the lesion. Initially, a single mass develops that may be very faint. The radiolucent component re-

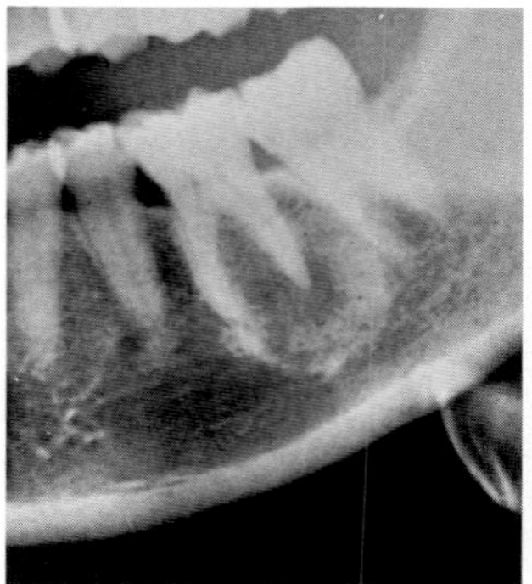

A

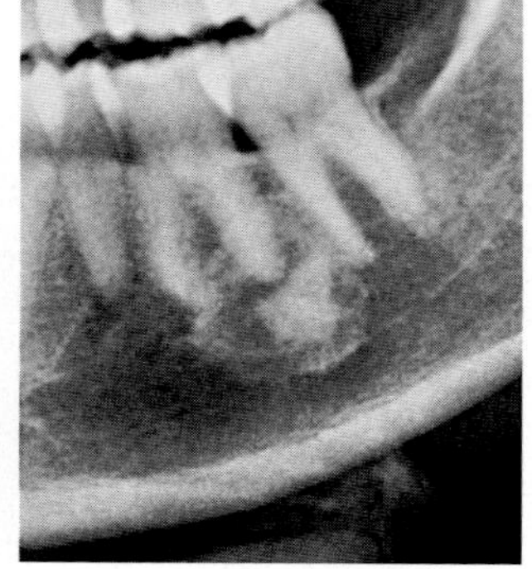

B

FIGURE 17–19.

Periapical Cemental Dysplasia: American woman of African origin. A, At 31 years of age, cementoblastic stage. B, At 37 years of age, mature stage. (Courtesy of Dr. B. Pass, Dalhousie University, Halifax, Nova Scotia, Canada.)

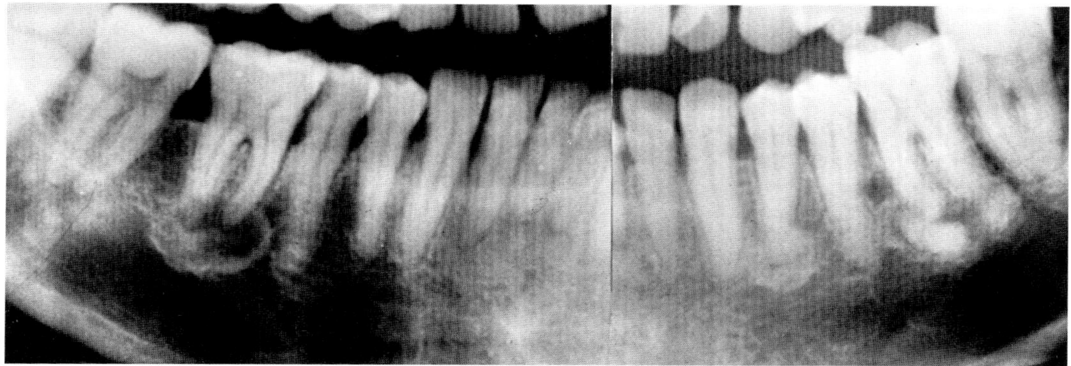

FIGURE 17–20.

Periapical Cemental Dysplasia: Right first molar: cementoblastic stage 3, active. Left first molar: mature stage 4, active. Anterior lesions in florid stage 5, inactive. Lesions at other sites in various stages.

mains prominent. An outer rim of sclerotic bone may be present, especially if active lysis of host bone is in progress. The radiolucent zone between the central mass and sclerotic rim is divided into three radiologically distinct bands. The outer band is the region in which calcific spherules of cementum-like material are formed. In the intermediate band, one can see individual calcific spherules coalescing with each other to form calcific massules. In the inner band, which is adjacent to the central mass, individual massules are seen that coalesce with the central mass.

Mature Stage. In the mature stage a single central mass develops. In some instances the mass envelops the apex of the involved tooth, causing it to have a crescent shape. The periphery of the mass tends to have a smooth surface, although it may be irregular or even lobulated as a result of coalesced massules. During periods of dormancy, the cemental mass is in direct apposition with the adjacent bone and may be mistaken easily for idiopathic osteosclerosis. During active periods, an outer radiolucent fibrocemento-osseous band and radiopaque margin of reactive bone reappear. The radiolucent band is usually several millimeters wide; however, it may be as thin as a normal periodontal ligament space or as wide as 0.5 cm. In some instances, especially on panoramic radiographs, the lingual aspect of the radiolucent outer rim may appear to extend up onto the root of a tooth; however, this may represent projection artifact. The cemental mass may grow to either side of the root, but it usually does not attach to the root apex. The outer rim of sclerotic bone is a variable feature. Zegerelli and colleagues (1964b) found a partial or complete sclerotic rim in only 2% of their cases. When it is present, the lesion may be thought to be active or growing; when absent, the lesion is most likely in a dormant stage. Active stages probably are brief, whereas dormant or inactive stages predominate.

PCD evolves through its developmental stages and eventually enters a dormant stage; the lesion may become dormant during one or more of its stages of development, and at any time the lesion may reactivate and re-enter dormant periods. A dormant, completely inactive lesion is in close

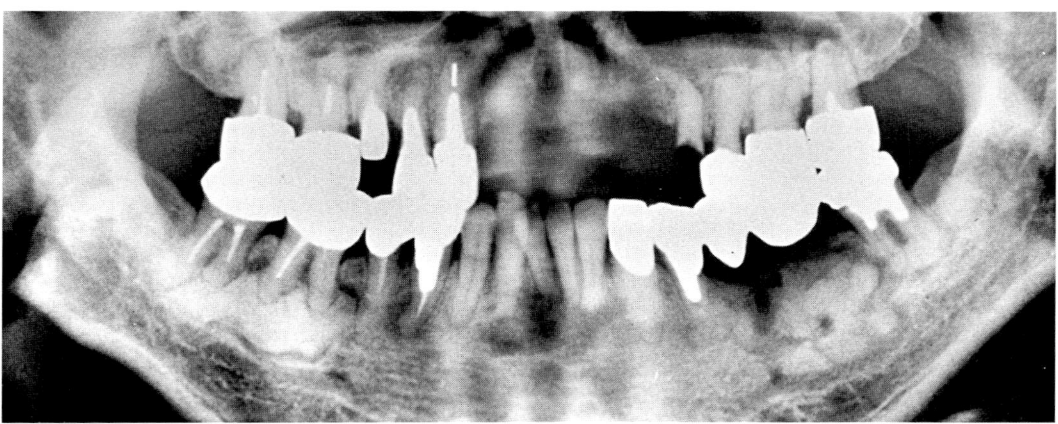

FIGURE 17–21.

Periapical Cemental Dysplasia: Florid stage 5. In left mandible, multiple masses are coalescing with each other. In right side, coalescence is complete. Other areas in mandible and maxilla are affected. (Courtesy of Drs. M. Araki, K. Hashimoto, and K. Honda, Nihon University School of Dentistry, Tokyo, Japan.)

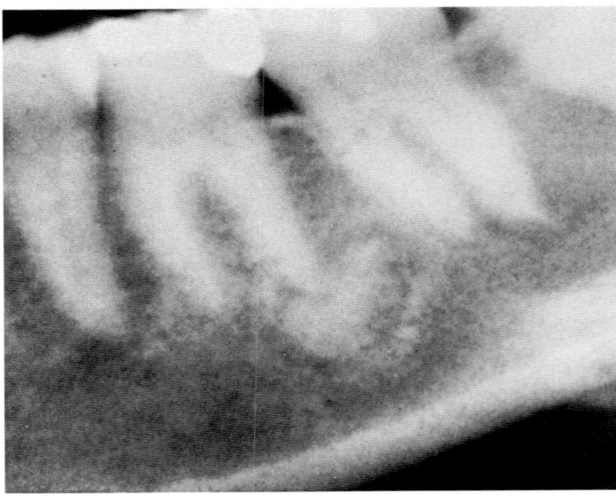

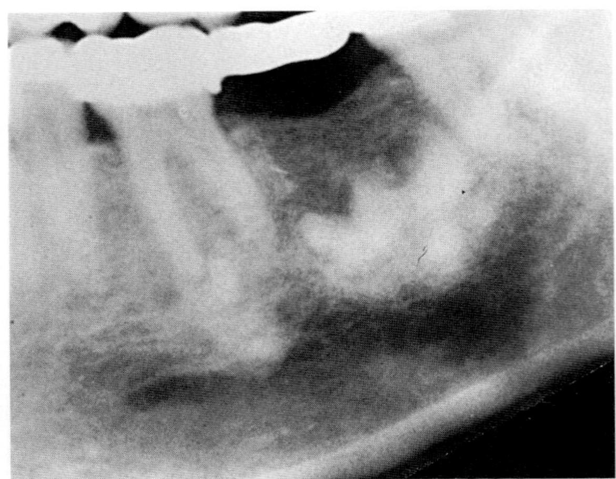

A B

FIGURE 17–22.

Periapical Cemental Dysplasia: Crescent shape. A, Multiple punctate calcific spherules, larger massules, and central mass; calcific spherules and massules aggregate to form circular structures with radiolucent center. B, Persistence of crescent shape after extraction of associated tooth.

apposition with the adjacent bone. A reactivating or deactivating lesion probably has a radiolucent rim without evidence of reactive sclerosis. The most active lesion has the target appearance with a radiopaque central mass surrounded by a radiolucent fibrocemento-osseous zone with an outer margin of sclerotic reactive bone. In their series of 435 cementomas in all stages, Zegerelli and colleagues (1964b) reported the following size distribution: 1 to 3 mm, 36%; 4 to 9 mm, 39%; 10 to 19 mm, 19%; and larger than 20 mm, 8%. Most lesions are smaller than 1 cm in diameter. Additionally, these authors observed that 29% of cases were in the first stage (osteolytic), 54% were in the second stage (cementoblastic), and 18% were in the third stage (mature). The initial osteoporotic stage had not yet been considered in 1964.

PCD in Edentulous Areas. When PCD occurs in edentulous areas, the lesions tend to be circular or ovoid. It is not clear whether PCD can develop de novo in an edentulous area or whether the lesions begin to develop before extraction of the teeth. In some instances, the central cemental mass retains its crescent shape; PCD is the only lesion that may produce a crescent-shaped radiopaque mass. In other cases the cemental masses are round or ovoid, with a variable radiolucent rim and outer sclerotic margin. When multiple lesions are present, different stages may be seen in the same quadrant. Zegerelli and colleagues (1964b) reported that expansion was not observed in any of their cases, but mild expansion does occur; the occlusal view must be taken to show expansion.

Association with Traumatic Cysts. Higuchi and colleagues (1988) published the first report of traumatic cysts in association with lesions that they termed cemento-osseous dysplasia. These lesions represent sclerotic cemental masses as we have defined them here as the synonym for PCD in the posterior region and representing the focal variant of FCOD. Their series consisted of four cases; the average pa-

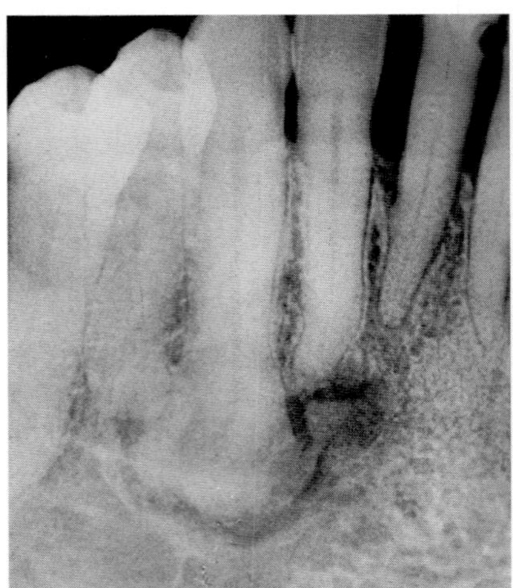

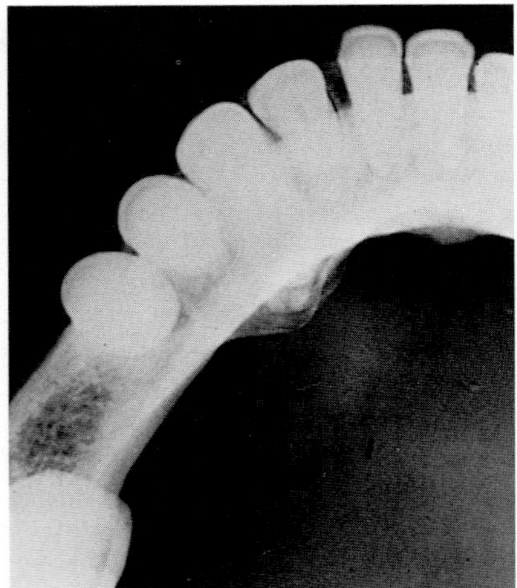

A B

FIGURE 17–23.

Periapical Cemental Dysplasia: A, Lateral incisor: calcific spherules within radiolucent area surrounding small central mass. Canine: calcific spherules coalescing with mass. B, Expansion of lingual cortex in same patient; several massules within expanded area.

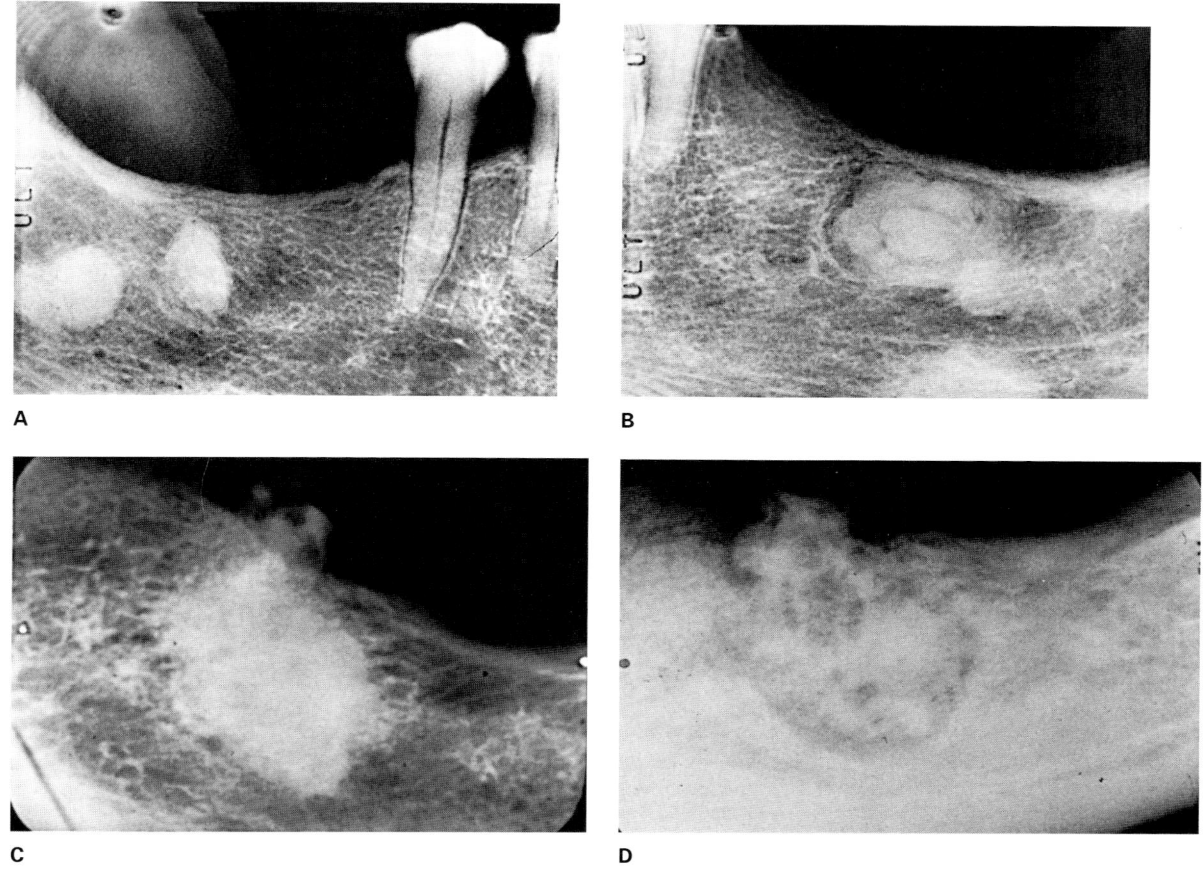

FIGURE 17–24.

Periapical Cemental Dysplasia: Active versus inactive lesions. A and B, A 61-year-old American woman of Hispanic origin. Right side: two cemental masses in dormant stage; tiny calcific spherules on mesioinferior surface of most distal mass. Left side: active lesion consisting of multiple smaller masses coalescing with each other and central mass. (Courtesy of Dr. A. Jainkittavong, University of Texas School of Dentistry, San Antonio, TX.) C and D, A 55-year-old American of African origin: C, Sclerosing cemental mass in dormant phase. D, Same mass sequestered 4 years later.

tient age was 41 years (age range, 31 to 49 years). All of the patients were women, presumably Japanese. Every lesion occurred in the mandible; one each was associated with the canine, second premolar-first molar, second molar, and third molar. The cystic lesions ranged from approximately 2 to 4 cm in diameter, and the cemental mass was centered within the cyst. Three of the cases showed a sclerotic rim, whereas the other cyst margin was lytic. One of the cysts was scalloped at the margin, whereas the other three were roughly circular in shape, with distinct but irregular margins.

BENIGN CEMENTOBLASTOMA (True cementoma, attached cementoma, cementoblastoma)

Benign cementoblastoma first was reported by Norberg in 1930 and was termed true cementoma. According to Pindborg (1970), the term benign cementoblastoma originally was suggested by I.R.H. Kramer in London. The lesion remained obscure, however, until the 1974 report of Cherrick and colleagues, who established the following definitive clinical and histologic criteria for the lesion: (1) a bulbous growth of cementum on the root of a tooth; (2) its tendency to expand the bony plates of the jaw; and (3) its active histologic appearance. The benign cementoblastoma is one of four cemental lesions categorized by the World Health Organization (WHO); the other three are PCD, cementifying fibroma, and gigantiform (familial) cementoma (florid osseous dysplasia). Hamner and colleagues (1968) found 166 lesions in 148 patients with cemental lesions as classified by the WHO. The distribution was as follows: (1) PCD, 49%; (2) cementifying fibroma, 40%; (3) benign cementoblastoma, 9%; and (4) gigantiform cementoma, 2%. The benign cementoblastoma is unique in two ways: it is the only true neoplasm of cementum and the only cemental lesion (excluding hypercementosis) that is attached routinely to an involved tooth. The benign cementoblastoma is an uncommon lesion, with approximately 75 cases reported, some of which have not been accepted universally as sufficiently documented. In the series of 706 odontogenic tumors sent for biopsy, Regezi and colleagues (1978) found only one case.

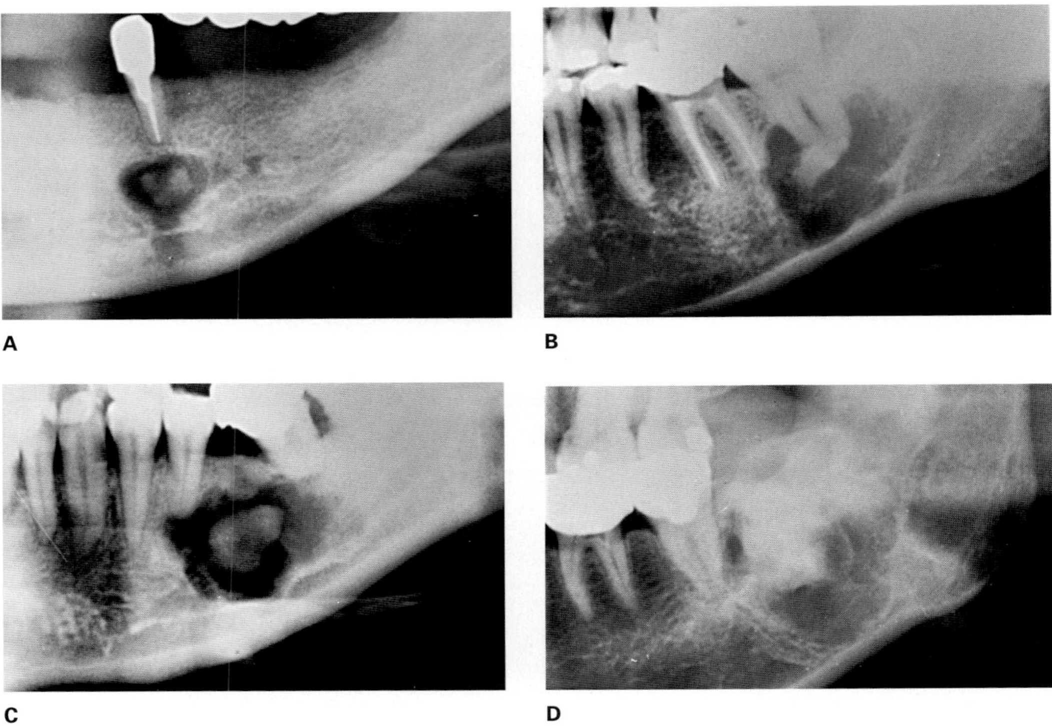

FIGURE 17–25.

Periapical Cemental Dysplasia: Associated with traumatic cysts. A, B, C, and D, Cases reported by Higuchi and colleagues and described in text. (From Higushi U, Nakamura N, Tashiro H: Clinicopathologic study of cemento-osseous dysplasia producing cysts of the mandible: report of 4 cases. J Oral Maxillofac Surg 16:757, 1987.)

Pathologic Characteristics

According to Gingell and colleagues (1984), the benign cementoblastoma probably is derived from root cementum or the connective tissue of the periodontal ligament. Histologically, the central portion of the lesion is a solid sheet of cementum with numerous reversal lines, suggesting a mosaic design. Gingell and colleagues (1984) reported that there are peripherally radiating columns of a cementum-like substance. In the peripheral area there are trabeculae of cementum with prominent cementoblastic and cementoclastic activity. Shafer and associates (1983) maintained that this activity causes the lesion to resemble osteosarcoma histologically; more often, there is difficulty distinguishing this lesion from osteoid osteoma and osteoblastoma when it is viewed under a microscope. The peripheral area is said to be surrounded by a connective tissue capsule. Other histologic features described by Corio and colleagues (1976) included root resorption, attachment of the mass to the root, replacement of pulp tissue by tumor, and lesional tissue within the root canal.

There are several areas of contention with respect to the histopathologic characteristics of the lesion:

1. It has been debated whether the lesional tissue is cementum, cementum-like, or osseous. Discussions have been presented by Fujita and colleagues (1989), Larsson and co-authors (1978), and Eversole and co-workers (1973). These authors concluded that because there was attachment to the roots along with a characteristic radiographic appearance, the lesions were benign cementoblastomas.
2. Larsson and colleagues (1978) proposed that the radiolucent area at the periphery of the lesion corresponds mainly to unmineralized tumor matrix and proliferating cells, rather than a thick layer of capsular fibrous connective tissue.

Clinical Features

Reviews have been presented by Corio and colleagues (1976), Farman and associates (1979), and Makek and Lello (1982). In 1982, Makek and Lello accepted only 33 cases as sufficiently documented to be included in their series. Unlike others who have found a male predilection, Makek and Lello (1982) and Farman and colleagues (1979) concluded that male and female patients were affected equally. According to Farman and colleagues (1979), the patients' ages ranged from 10 to 72 years; however, the average age at detection was 26 years. These authors also reported that more than half of the tumors were detected in people younger than 20 years. The most common sign was swelling, observed in 73% of the cases. Pain was the most frequent symptom and occurred in 53% of the patients; it was usually low grade and often intermittent. Mader and Wendelburg (1979) believed that the pain in their patient was caused by occlusal pressure resulting from extrusion of the tooth caused by pressure from the tumor; however, in the case of Forsslund and colleagues (1988), the pain persisted several years after incomplete removal of the lesion. The remaining segment was not in occlusion, and the pain resolved with complete excision. In the case of Cherrick and colleagues (1974), only the tooth was removed because the lesion was radiolucent; the pain persisted and increased until the lesion was removed in toto. Mader and Wendelburg (1979) discussed pulp testing in the affected teeth and expressed caution in regard to interpretation of the results. Although most accept the fact that the affected teeth have vital pulps when examined histologically, clinical pulp testing may produce variable results. In one instance, the tested tooth was nonvital on electric pulp tests but vital to drilling.

Treatment/Prognosis

Most authors still espouse the concept originated by Cherrick and colleagues (1974) that this lesion appears to have unlimited growth potential. Thus, immediate surgical extraction of the involved tooth and attached mass is the usual treatment. Goerig and colleagues (1984) successfully treated a case by completing endodontic procedures on the involved mandibular first molar and then completely removing the mass surgically through a window in the buccal cortex. Although there are no reported cases of recurrence, pain has persisted after surgery when the lesion was removed incompletely. Forsslund and colleagues (1988) showed that pulpectomy alone will not arrest continued development of the lesion.

◆ *RADIOLOGY (Figs. 17–26 to 17–31)*

The radiologic features of benign cementoblastoma are as follows:

1. Intimate involvement with a whole tooth root, usually the mandibular first molar.
2. An early, contentious, radiolucent stage, followed by a radiopaque stage, with an obscured root outline within the lesion.

Location

In the series of 34 cases reviewed by Makek and Lello (1982), 85% of the tumors were located in the mandible, and 60% were associated with the mandibular first molar. According to Gingell and colleagues (1984), the mandibular premolars are the second most common location; these authors also found reports of involvement of the mandibular canine and multiple teeth. Chaput and Mark (1965) reported the only case involving a primary tooth, occurring in the right mandibular second primary molar in a 10-year-old girl; Farman and colleagues (1979) and Makek and Lello (1982) accepted this case as sufficiently documented.

Radiologic Features

The benign cementoblastoma probably develops in three radiologically distinct stages: (1) uncalcified matrix stage, (2) calcified blastic stage, and (3) a possible mature stage.

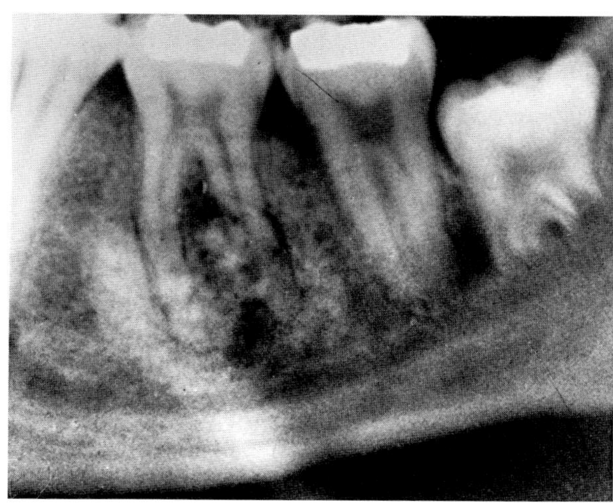

FIGURE 17–26.

Benign Cementoblastoma: Early lesion: mesial root obscured, distal root resorbed. Observe the rounded calcific spherule and massulelike structures. (Courtesy of Dr. G. Terezhalmy, Case Western University School of Dentistry, Cleveland, OH.)

Uncalcified Matrix Stage. Although there are reports describing a first radiolucent stage, including those of Cherrick and colleagues (1974), Gingell and co-authors (1984), Raveh (1980), and Eversole and co-workers (1973), others such as Abrams (1974) do not accept this position, stating that such cases probably represent other conditions such as PCD. The uncalcified matrix stage is characterized by development of a circular radiolucent area at the apex of a vital tooth. In some cases the apical third of the root may be seen within the area; in others, as much as half of the root length may be resorbed by the radiolucent mass. In some instances the radiolucent area is surrounded by a thick band of reactive sclerotic bone, which may be 1 to 3 mm in thickness and

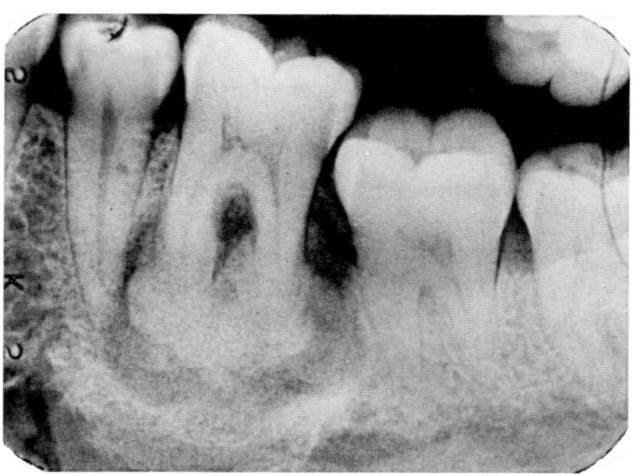

FIGURE 17–27.

Benign Cementoblastoma: Case in a 29-year-old woman. Affected tooth is extruded because of lack of opposing occlusion. Peripheral margin of reactive bone is shown. Proliferating and mineralizing tumor matrix is within radiolucent area.

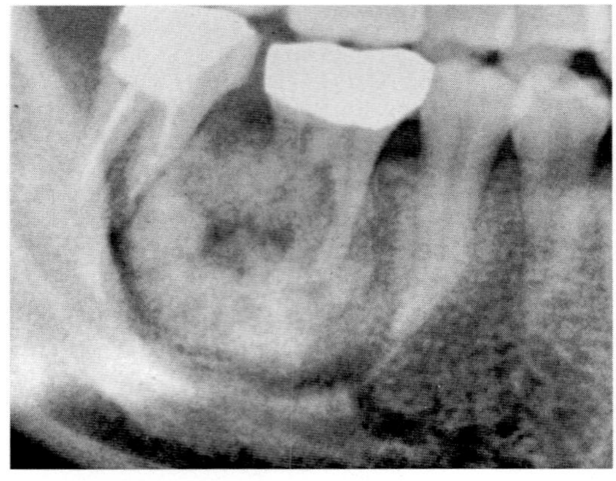

A

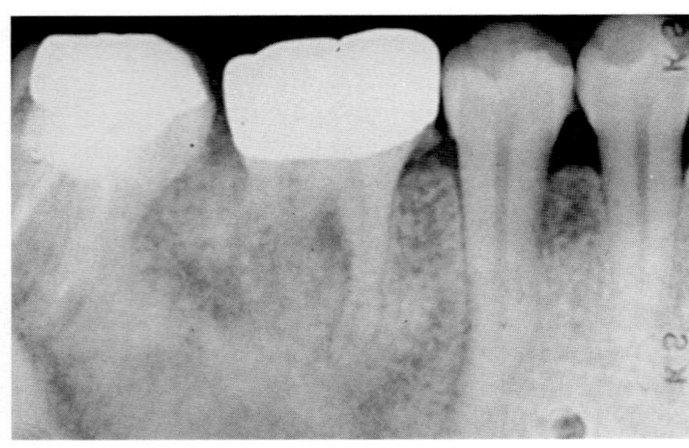

B

FIGURE 17–28.

Benign Cementoblastoma: Case in a 30-year-old woman. A, Mass well delineated by peripheral radiolucent zone. B, Multiple calcific spherulelike bodies throughout. Significance of central radiolucency not known; it may be a previous biopsy site. (Courtesy of Drs. M. Araki, K. Hashimoto, and K. Honda, Nihon University School of Dentistry, Tokyo, Japan.)

rather diffuse in appearance. The lesion may reach a diameter of approximately 1.5 cm during this stage, which is brief and may only last several weeks.

Cementoblastic Stage. Radiographic evidence of the cementoblastic stage begins with the appearance of radiodense material in the center of the lesion. As the lesion mineralizes, additional cementum-like material appears to coalesce with the central mass, with more mineralization usually developing toward the periphery. In the case illustrated by Cherrick and colleagues (1974), the initial lesion consisted of a predominantly radiolucent mass that was approximately 1.5 cm in diameter with a small radiopaque mass in the central area. The affected tooth was removed; however, the mass remained in the mandible. Two weeks later, the mass was completely mineralized. The developing lesion remains circular until it reaches a diameter of approximately 3 cm, when it becomes more ovoid in shape, with an egglike appearance. The lesion invariably is surrounded by a distinct and prominent radiolucent band that is approximately 2 mm wide. An outer rim of sclerotic bone is a variable finding; however, it is possible that it may be present more frequently during the early stages rather than later.

Mature Stage. Most investigators do not believe that a mature stage exists because the lesion is said to have unlimited growth potential; however, from studying reports of very large lesions greater than 3 cm in diameter, we have observed the following signs of diminished growth potential: As the lesion approaches the inferior cortex of the mandible, it becomes ovoid and enlarges along the length of the body, with minimal expansion of the inferior cortex. In larger lesions, the outer radiolucent rim and sclerotic margin are variable features; when these become indistinct, the lesion enters a more quiescent phase.

Growth Rate and Size. In the case of Forsslund and colleagues (1988), the lesion had become radiodense when it reached only 0.5 cm in diameter, with an obscured root outline and radiolucent rim. After 2 years, the lesion had reached approximately 1 cm in diameter. In the case of Makek and Lello (1982), the presenting lesion was approximately 3 cm and enlarged to approximately 6 cm within almost 3 years. Reported sizes have varied from 0.5 to 8 cm in diameter, and according to Vindenes and colleagues (1974), the diameter expands by approximately 0.5 cm per year. In most cases in which the lesion was observed over several years, only the tooth was removed or it was treated endodontically.

Other Radiologic Features. The mass should be examined from a lateral and occlusal aspect. In the lateral view, the radiopacity has a mottled appearance, with multiple radiolucent areas within the radiodense mass. The mass may have a more radiolucent center, a finding we have observed but cannot explain adequately in light of current studies. The roots of the involved tooth are partially obscured toward the apex, either because of resorption of the roots or the density of the mass; most agree there is a combination of both factors. There is infrequent slight displacement of the roots of adjacent erupted teeth without resorption of the displaced roots. In the occlusal view, both buccal and lingual expansion of the cortex occurs; however, the thinned cortex is rarely apparent. The expanding lesion may be directed more toward the buccal or lingual side. A characteristic finding sometimes observed in the occlusal view consists of radiating spicules of cementoid material emanating from the central area and radiating toward the periphery, giving a sunray appearance; the spicules are more mineralized toward the center of the lesion, with individual spicules appearing thinner and less radiodense toward the periphery. In rare instances, the radiating spicules may be seen in the lateral view. The lesion usually does not extend to involve the crestal portion of the alveolar bone, although this may occur in rare cases.

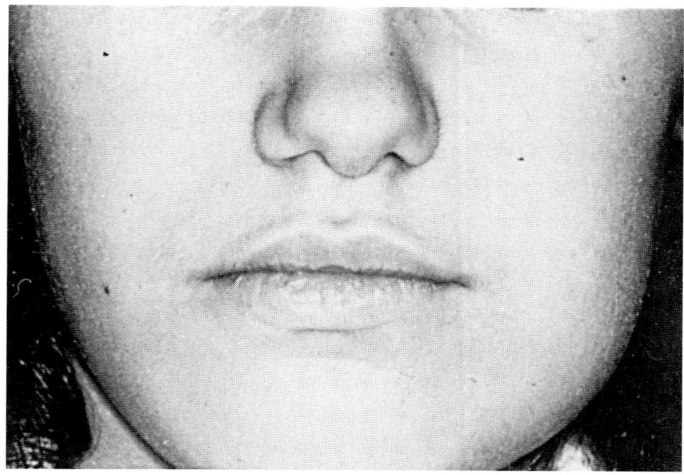

A

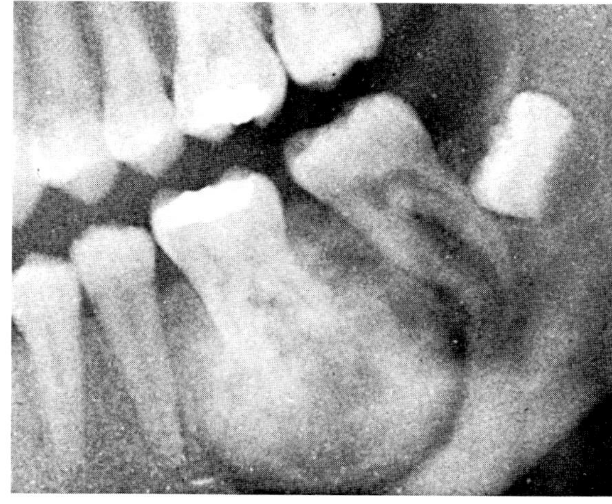

B

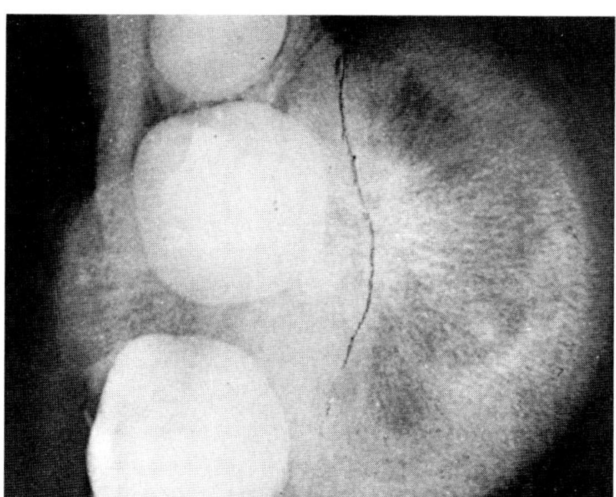

C

FIGURE 17–29.

Benign Cementoblastoma: A, Facial swelling caused by lesion. B, Round radiolucent periphery, absent marginal sclerosis. C, radiating striae are less dense and more delicate toward periphery. Lesion is denser toward the periphery and more radiolucent centrally. (From Larsson A, Forsberg O, Sjögren S: Benign cementoblastoma: cementum analogue of benign osteoblastoma. J Oral Surg 36:299, 1978.)

Although buccal and lingual expansion of the cortex usually occurs, significant expansion of the inferior cortex of the mandible usually is not seen. Only slight bowing of the inferior border of the mandible is a late feature in huge lesions; Makek and Lello (1982) reported a large lesion extending from the distal of the mandibular canine to the distal root of the tipped second molar, with only minimal bowing of the inferior border of the mandible. Downward displacement of the inferior alveolar canal may be seen. In rare instances the lesion may contain an inner radiolucent band because of its egg shape in a buccal-lingual direction.

OSSIFYING FIBROMA (Cementifying fibroma, cemento-ossifying fibroma, fibro-osteoma, osteofibroma, benign fibro-osseous lesion of periodontal ligament origin, benign periodontoma)

Ossifying fibroma first was reported in the jaws by Montgomery in 1927. Since then, cementifying fibroma and cemento-ossifying fibroma have been reported as histologic variants. Most authors now agree that all three conditions probably represent variants of the same disorder and have suggested that the term ossifying fibroma be used, regardless of the histologic subtype. Most recently, Makek (1983) suggested the term benign periodontoma.

Pathologic Characteristics

In 1968, Hamner and colleagues proposed that all three histologic variants originate from the periodontal ligament; the WHO designates the cementifying fibroma as odontogenic and the ossifying fibroma as nonodontogenic in origin and suggests that they are separate entities. Reviews have been presented by Waldron and Giansanti (1973), who studied 65 cases; Eversole and colleagues (1985a), who reviewed 64 cases; and Waldron (1985). These and others, such as Hamner and co-authors (1968), concluded that separation of the three conditions is arbitrary and unnecessary because the clinical, radiologic, and prognostic features of the lesions are identical. These authors theorized that mesenchymal progenitor cells of the periodontal ligament can elaborate bone and cementum and they represent histologic variants of the same neoplastic process. Eversole and colleagues (1985) dis-

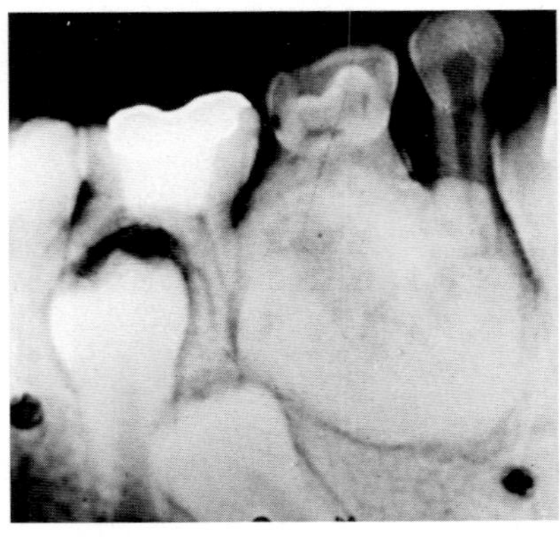

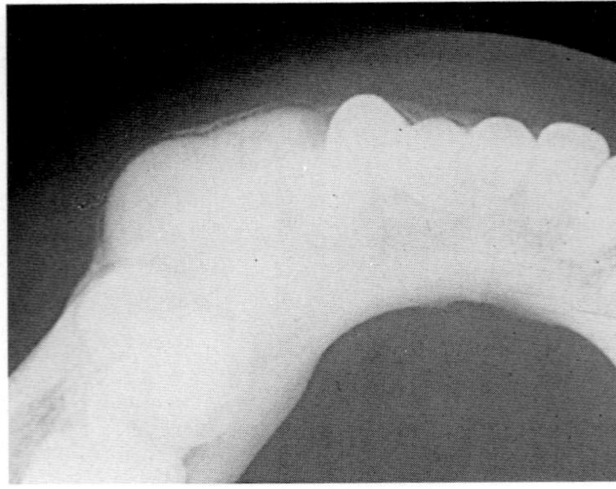

A B

FIGURE 17–30.

Benign Cementoblastoma: Case in a 10-year-old girl. A, Radiolucent central area. B, Periosteal reaction: single thin layer of subperiosteal new bone becoming inapparent at area of greatest expansion. (Courtesy of Drs. M. Araki, K. Hasimoto, and K. Honda, Nihon University School of Dentistry, Tokyo, Japan.)

cussed the histologic features of this neoplasm. A mineralized matrix is seen within a fibrous connective tissue stroma with large numbers of active proliferating fibroblasts. Four basic hard tissue configurations were described: (1) woven bone trabeculae, (2) lamellar bone trabeculae, (3) ovoid-curvoid deposits, and (4) anastomosing curvilinear trabeculae. A single matrix type was seen in 53% of the cases; of these, 31% consisted of bone only, 11% were spheroid-curvoid only, and 11% were curvilinear only. The remaining 47% of the lesions contained varying admixtures of two or three of the four basic matrix types. The lesion usually is surrounded by a connective tissue capsule.

Clinical Features

The average patient age is 36 years, with 56% of patients in the third and fourth decades at diagnosis. In the series reported by Eversole and co-workers (1985a), 15% of cases occurred in patients younger than 20 years of age, with only two cases seen in those in the first decade of life; 85% of patients were older than 40 years old. There is a striking predilection for female patients, with a ratio of 5:1 over male patients. The distribution among races was as follows: white patients, 47%; Hispanic patients, 24%; African-American patients, 16%; Asian patients, 11%; and Native American patients, 2%. The proportion of Hispanic patients exceeded the normal Hispanic population ratio in the region. In the series of Waldron and Giansanti (1973), all the African-Americans were female. The authors reported that the clinical symptoms were minimal in their series of 65 cases. According to these authors, as well as others, such as Sweet and colleagues (1981), Eversole and colleagues (1985a), and Miller (1979), most cases were detected incidentally during a routine radiographic survey. In the series of Waldron and Giansanti (1973), 20% showed facial asymmetry at diagnosis. Other findings included pain in four patients and numbness in two patients. It was surmised that the probable duration was less than 5 years in 90% of the cases.

Treatment/Prognosis

Waldron (1985) emphasized the importance of the surgical findings when a pathologist is separating ossifying fibroma from fibrous dysplasia histologically, especially when a definitive capsule is not seen. At surgery, ossifying fibromas tend to enucleate out with relative ease, often as a single,

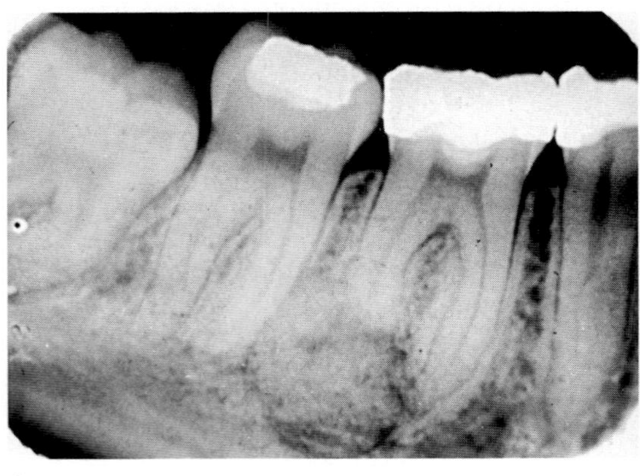

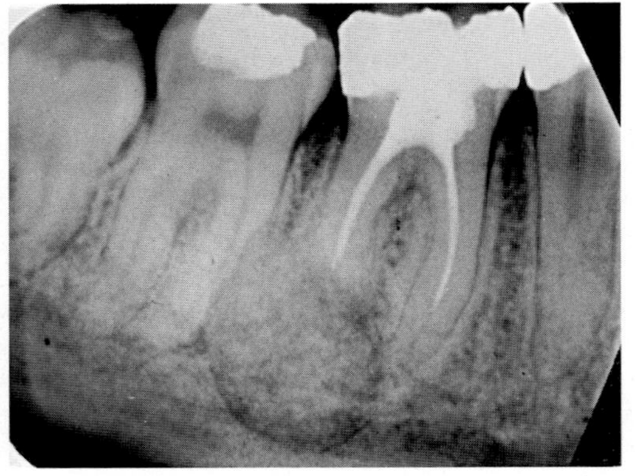

A B

FIGURE 17–31.

Benign Cementoblastoma: Simulated history. A, There was pain in region. Pulp testing indicated diminished or questionable vitality, and radiopaque area was interpreted as condensing osteitis. Endodontic therapy completed. B, Persistence of pain after endodontic therapy; case referred to radiologist for interpretation. (Courtesy of Dr. D. Stoneman, Toronto, Ontario, Canada.)

solid, whitish, avascular mass; this ease of enucleation is the single most important factor in differentiating this lesion from monostotic fibrous dysplasia. This is true even when the clinical, radiologic, and biopsy findings strongly suggest a diagnosis of fibrous dysplasia. There is also a problem with the histologic differentiation of cementifying fibroma from PCD and its variants. PCD not only is distinct radiologically, but it tends to be removed in fragments, which may be somewhat reddish or bloody in appearance. In the series of Eversole and colleagues (1985a), the postoperative follow-up period was available for 23 of the cases and ranged from 12 to 120 months, with a mean follow-up of 38 months. The initial recurrence rate was 28%. At least half of the recurring lesions did so twice. Eversole and colleagues (1985) could not find histologic evidence predictive of recurrence. Others, such as Waldron (1985), implied that recurrence is seen less frequently with complete enucleation, stating that recurrence is unusual. Taylor and colleagues (1973) reported a recurrent maxillary lesion appearing 24 years after the initial enucleation.

◆ *RADIOLOGY (Figs. 17–32 to 17–41)*

Almost all the authors we studied emphasized the importance of the radiomorphologic features in differentiating fibrous dysplasia from ossifying fibroma of the jaw bones. One of the primary differences between the two conditions is that ossifying fibroma exhibits a well-demarcated margin whereas fibrous dysplasia does not.

Location

Most authors report a striking predilection for the mandible, ranging from 70 to 89%. In addition, the lesions appear to be limited to the tooth-bearing areas, with an intimate relationship to the roots of teeth or the periapical region. A few have extended into the angle-ramus area or encroached on the maxillary sinus. Eversole and colleagues (1985b) reported the following locations: molar region (52%), premolar area (25%), incisor area (13%), and cuspid region (11%). Although Waldron and Giansanti (1973) found no lesions in the anterior maxilla, Eversole and associates (1985b) found 4 cases in this location; thus, any tooth-bearing site within the jaws may be affected.

Although most ossifying fibromas are solitary, Hamner and colleagues (1968) found multiple lesions in some of their patients. The osteoid type had the lowest occurrence of multiple lesions, with an incidence of 3 in 57 cases (5%); multiple cemento-osteoid lesions occurred in 7 of 42 cases (17%); and cementoid lesions were the most frequent, with an incidence of 27 of 148 cases (18%). In several instances, multiple lesions were observed in both the maxilla and mandible. Only 4% of multiple cementoid lesions occurred in the maxilla, multiple cemento-osteoid types were seen in the maxilla in 24%, and the multiple osteoid type occurred in 1 of 3 cases (33%) in the maxilla. Among solitary lesions, Hamner and colleagues (1968) saw much less of a difference with regard to tissue type and location. Solitary cementoid lesions were observed in the maxilla in 21%, cemento-osteoid in 24%, and osteoid in 30%. Several conclusions can be drawn from these data: (1) when osteoid is the dominant matrix type, there is little tendency for multiple lesions; (2) multiple lesions are seen most often in association with a cementoid or cemento-osteoid matrix; (3) osteoid and cemento-osteoid matrices are more likely to be associated with maxillary lesions than cementum; and (4) cementum seems to influence a mandibular location and multiple lesions; osteoid influences a maxillary location and solitary lesions.

Radiologic Features of Jaw Lesions

Waldron and Giansanti (1973) discussed the radiographic appearance of 43 of their cases. Most lesions were predominantly lytic, with varying amounts of mineralized matrix and a well-circumscribed margin. They reported that 26% were

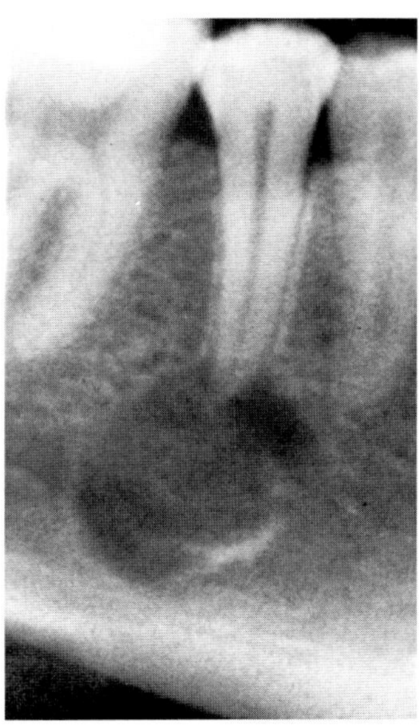

A

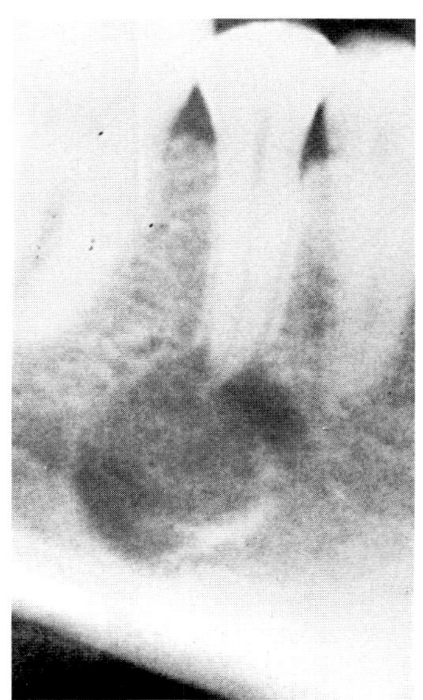

B

FIGURE 17–32.

Ossifying Fibroma: Eversole type 1. A, Panoramic view. B, Bright light image. Single, thick, y-shaped structure resembling bone. Other foci resemble calcific spherules seen in cemental lesions. Histopathologic diagnosis was periapical cemental dysplasia.

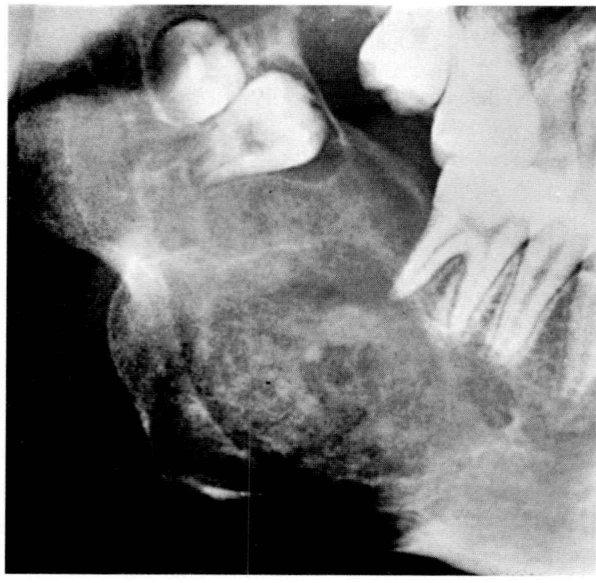

A

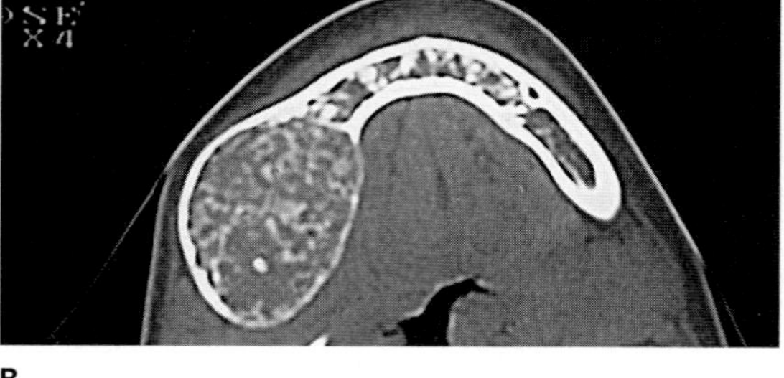

B

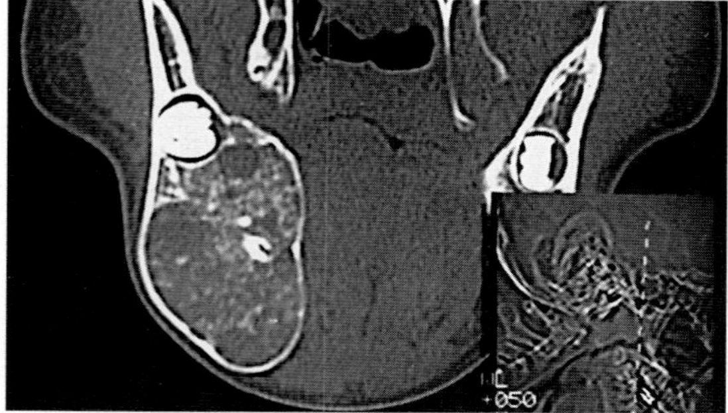

C

FIGURE 17–33.

Ossifying Fibroma: Eversole type 3. A, Tiny round punctate flecks and doughnutlike shapes resemble calcific spherules. There is downward displacement of the inferior alveolar canal, and the inferior cortex is expanded. B and C, Computed tomography images show typical equidirectional expansion, intact margins, and noncoalescing foci of mineralization. The case was labeled ossifying fibroma. (Courtesy of Drs. M. Araki and K. Hashimoto, Nihon University, Tokyo, Japan.)

lytic only, 63% were lytic with radiopaque foci, and 12% consisted of a diffuse, homogeneous appearance that was mildly radiopaque, described as a ground glass appearance by others. These authors observed that the marginal area of the mass was radiolucent in all of the cases with radiopaque foci. A sclerotic rim sometimes is present within the host bone at the margin; it may be smooth and delicate or it may be slightly irregular, more diffuse, and of varying thicknesses (up to approximately 3 mm). Waldron and Giansanti (1973) found this feature in 53% of their cases; the remainder appeared "punched out," with no sclerosis at the margin. Some smaller lesions may be less well defined; a few were observed to blend with the surrounding bone but did so within a transitional zone of several millimeters. The expanded cortex characteristically is very thin and may seem to disappear on plain radiographs. The reported diameter of the lesions ranges from 1 to 7 cm. Eversole and colleagues (1985b) reported divergence of adjacent roots in 17% of the cases and root resorption in 11%; displacement of developing teeth also may be seen, and 35% of cases occurred in edentulous areas.

Eversole and colleagues (1985b) studied 43 cases of ossifying fibroma in which radiographs were available and found 6 variations:

1. A unilocular radiolucency containing radiopaque foci without root divergence or root resorption. The radiopaque foci yielded a target appearance with dense foci, ground glass opacification, or irregular opacification. This was the most prevalent pattern; it was observed in 42% of the sample, and 40% of these cases occurred in edentulous areas.
2. A well-delineated unilocular radiolucency without radiopaque foci superimposed over intact roots without divergence or resorption. This pattern occurred in 28% of the cases, and 25% of these cases arose in edentulous areas.
3. A radiolucency with central opacifications, root divergence, and/or root resorption. The radiopaque foci yielded a target appearance with dense foci, ground glass opacification, or irregular opacification. This pattern was seen in 9% of the cases.
4. Massive, expansile lesions larger than 5 cm, occurring in 9% of the sample. These exhibited well-defined margins with ground glass or mottled radiopacities. These were classified as active or aggressive ossifying fibromas (AOFs).
5. A multilocular radiolucency with or without root resorption. This was observed in 7% of the sample.

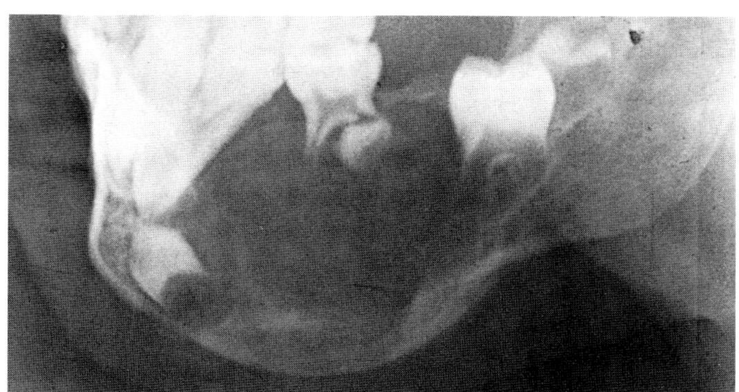

A

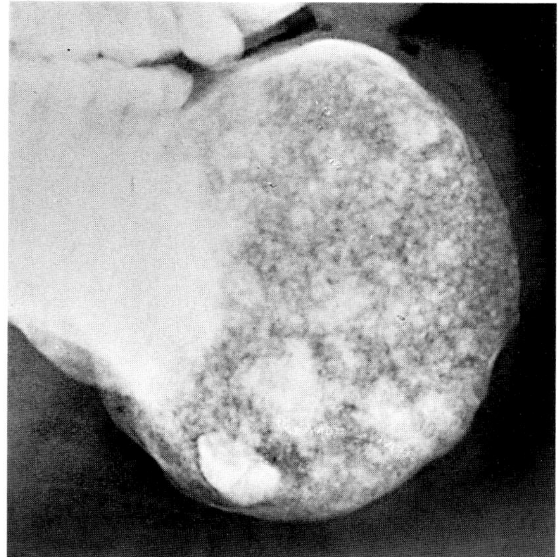

B

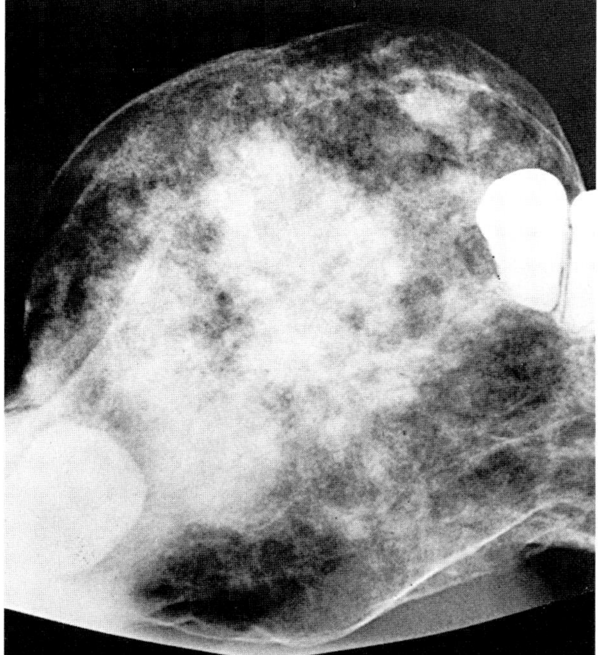

C

FIGURE 17–34.

Ossifying Fibroma: Eversole type 4. A, Mostly radiolucent, with bowing of inferior cortex and displacement of unerupted teeth. (Courtesy of Israel and Lilian Chilvarquer, São Paulo, Brazil.) B, Tiny punctate flecks, doughnut shapes, and masses. C, Thin but intact expanded cortex; coalesced mass in center suggests a cemental component. (Courtesy of Dr. P. Dhiravarangkura, Chulalonghorn University, Bangkok, Thailand.)

6. A unilocular radiolucency interposed between divergent or resorbed roots. This was the least prevalent pattern, being observed in 5% of the cases. All of the lesions in this sample had well-circumscribed margins.

It has been emphasized by Shafer and co-authors (1983) that the typical ossifying fibroma grows in a centrifugal fashion, producing a ball-like circular lesion. The lesion enlarges equally in all directions, producing expansion of the buccal and lingual cortical plates and, most notably, the inferior cortex of the mandible. The expanded inferior cortex is exactly parallel to the margin of the tumor mass above. Other lesions such as fibrous dysplasia cause a linear expansion of the cortex; thus, the expanded cortex cannot be in this exact parallel relationship to the tumor mass. Inferior bowing of the lower border of the mandible is almost a constant feature in larger lesions.

A variation of ossifying fibroma is seen when the lesion resembles a coiled worm. This pattern is rare and appears more frequently in the mandible. In this instance, the radiopaque component appears to be coiled in circles, with the coils separated by a thin radiolucent area. It is possible that

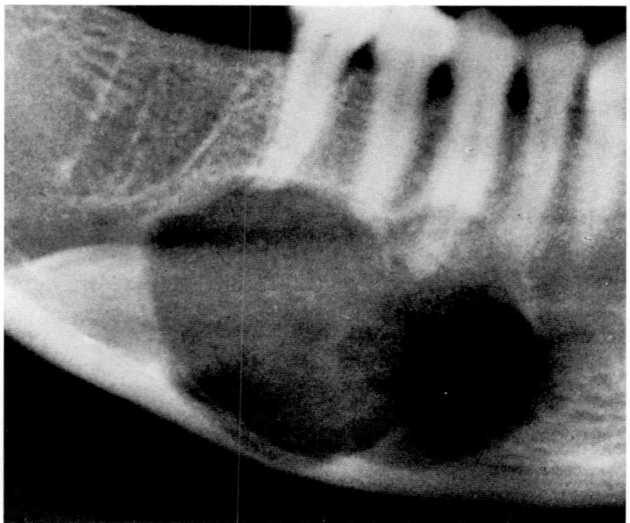

FIGURE 17–35.

Ossifying Fibroma: Eversole type 5. Tendency toward multilocularity. Figure shows endosteal scalloping of cortex and punctate and doughnut-shaped calcified tumor matrix. Lesion appears punched out.

this appearance suggests a predominantly cementifying tumor matrix, but this remains to be proven. This appearance should not be mistaken for a variation of the "thumb print" pattern of fibrous dysplasia, which has a blending margin with the adjacent normal host bone.

Some ossifying fibromas, especially maxillary lesions, have behaved more aggressively. We have included a separate discussion on these in the section on aggressive ossifying fibroma.

Radiologic Features of Extragnathic Ossifying Fibroma

Ossifying fibroma has been reported in other parts of the bony skeleton. In this regard, there appear to be two distinctly different lesions, and we refer to them as psammous desmo-osteoblastomas of the maxillofacial region and ossifying fibroma of the tubular bones.

Psammous Desmo-osteoblastoma. Psammous desmo-osteoblastomas have been discussed by Waldron (1985) and Eversole and co-workers (1985a), and especially by Makek (1983), who has suggested the term psammous desmo-osteoblastomas for these lesions. They are histologically identical to the variant of ossifying fibroma characterized by a spheroid-curvoid product resembling a cementicle; others have designated this variant as cementifying fibroma or cemento-ossifying fibroma. These lesions have been found in the non-tooth-bearing areas of the jaws, maxillary antrum, and ethmoid, sphenoid, frontal, and temporal bones. This finding prompted Eversole and colleagues (1985a) to question the origin of the spheroid-curvoid product in jaw lesions and propose that it is not related to cementogenesis. Rather, the spheroid-curvoid deposits are somehow unique to membranous bones such as the jaws and craniofacial complex. According to Makek (1983), jaw lesions in nondental sites and those in the bones of the craniofacial complex are more aggressive than the usual ossifying fibroma and are also distinct from and perhaps less destructive than the aggressive ossifying fibroma, which is discussed in the next section. Radiologically, the psammous desmo-osteoblastoma is usually well circumscribed; however, the margin may be poorly defined. Frontoethmoid lesions sometimes encroach on the medial wall of the orbit, causing proptosis and exophthalmos on the affected side. There is a tendency for recurrence, and,

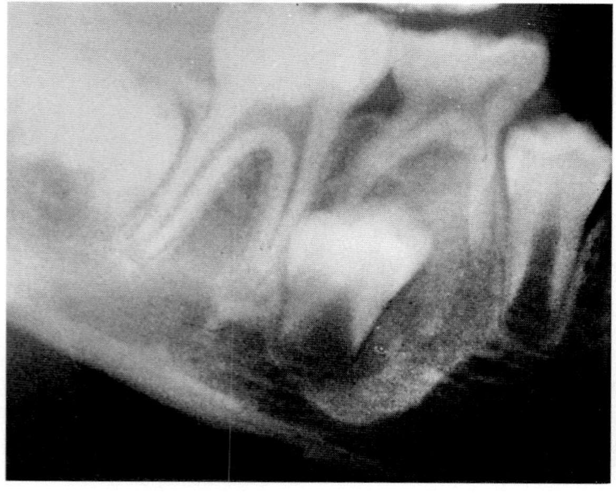

A

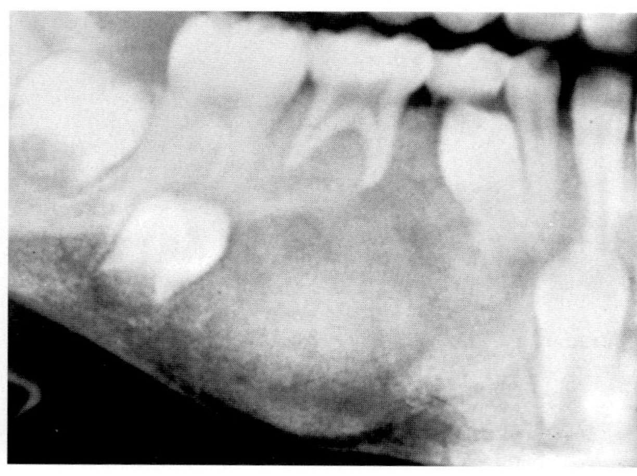

B

FIGURE 17–36.

Ossifying Fibroma: A and B, Granular, ground glass, or homogeneous appearance of mineralized tumor matrix. (B, Courtesy of Dr. H. Schwartz, Kaiser Permanente Medical Group, Los Angeles, CA.)

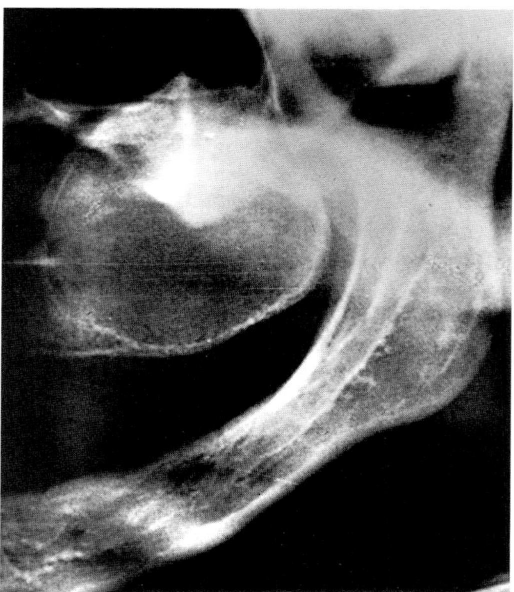

A

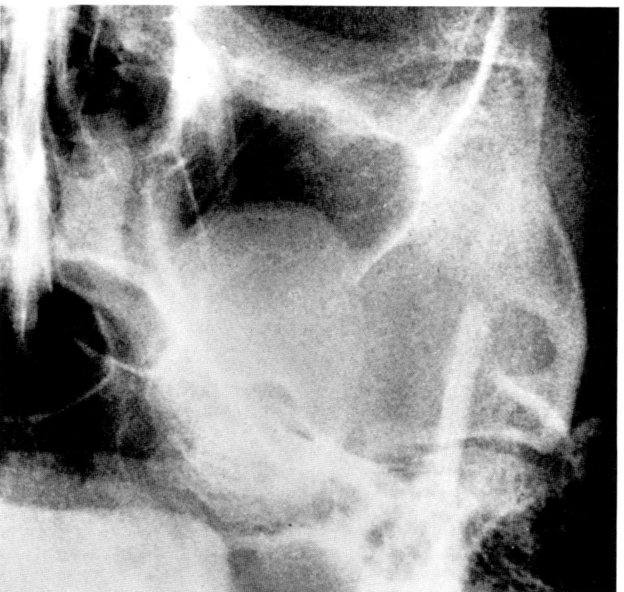

B

FIGURE 17–37.

Ossifying fibroma: Small maxillary lesion. A, Sinus floor thin but intact; lesion shelled out in a single avascular mass. B, Waters' view shows egglike shape of mass, with lateral and medial expansion.

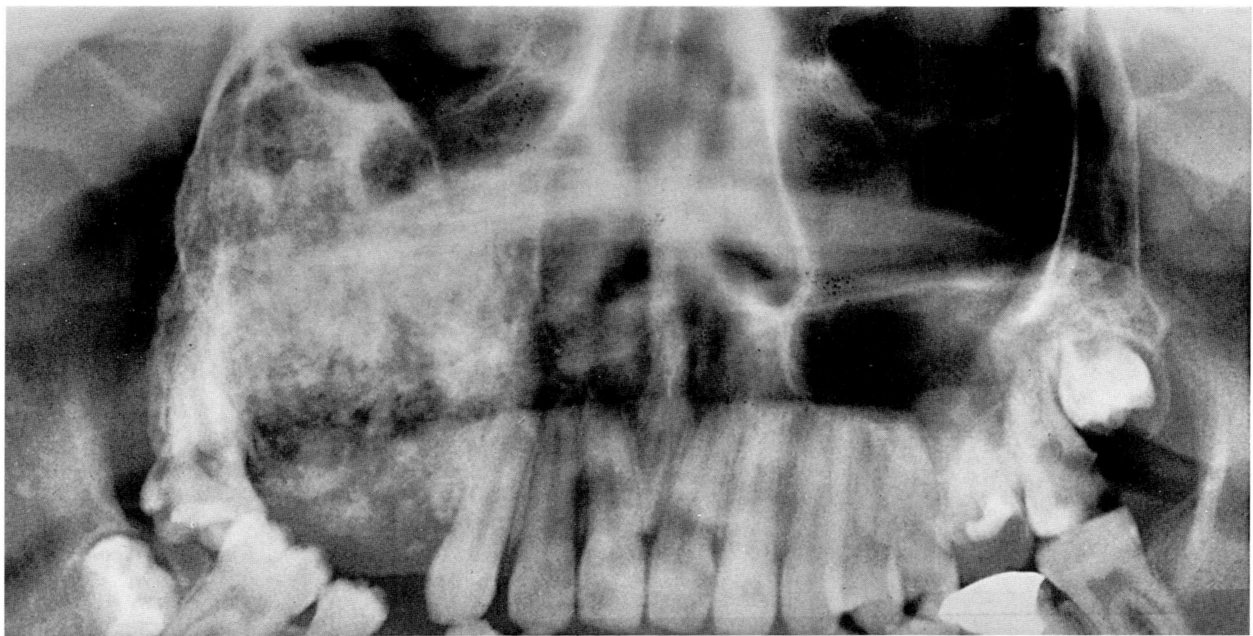

FIGURE 17–38.

Ossifying Fibroma: Large maxillary lesion, with upward bowing of sinus floor and tooth displacement. (Courtesy of Professor T. Noikura, First Oral Surgery Department, Kagoshima University School of Dentistry, Kagoshima, Japan.)

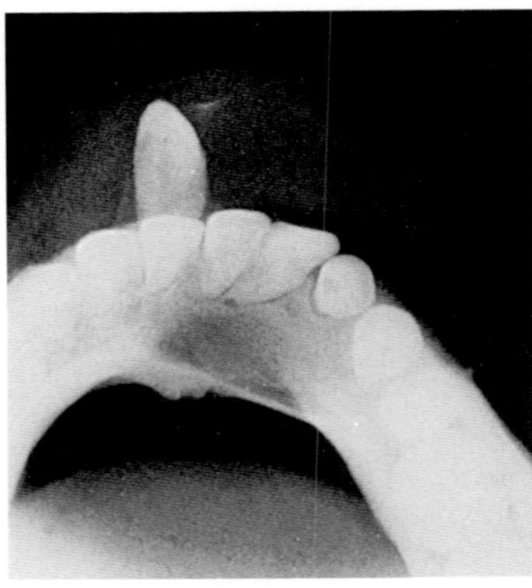
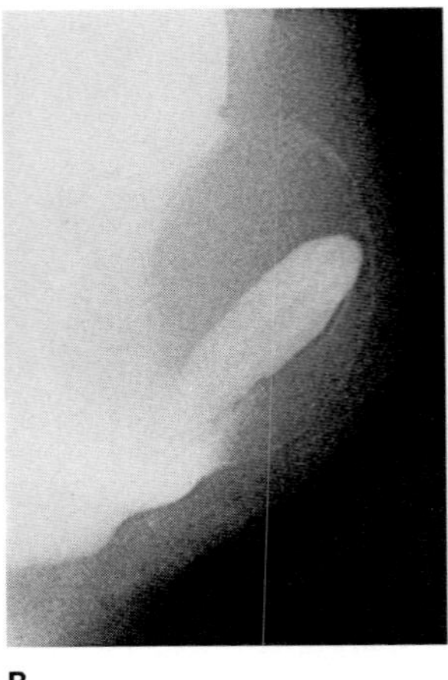
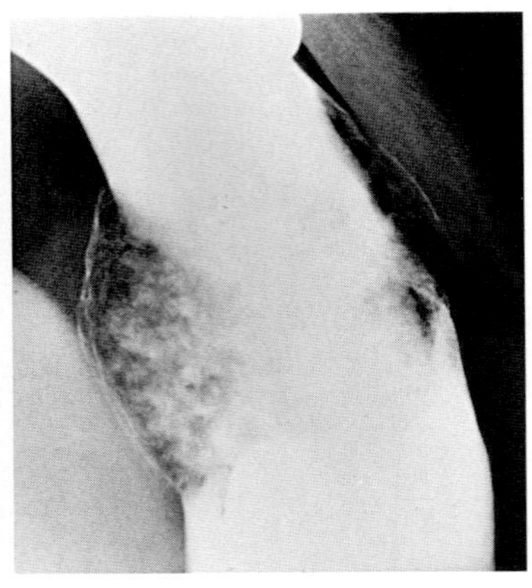

A B C

FIGURE 17–39.

Ossifying Fibroma: Thin, almost-disappearing expanded cortex. A and B, Case 1: buccal displacement of adjacent canine. (Courtesy of Professor L. Alfaro, University of Chile Dental School, Pathology Referral Center, Santiago, Chile.) C, Case 2: occlusal view showing thin intact cortex. (Courtesy of Drs. M. Araki, K. Hashimoto, and K. Honda, Nihon University School of Dentistry, Tokyo, Japan.)

according to Waldron (1985), lesions involving the craniofacial complex recur more than jaw lesions.

Ossifying Fibroma of Tubular Bones (Osteofibrous Dysplasia). Waldron (1985) stated that this lesion is almost identical to monostotic fibrous dysplasia histologically. It occurs during the first and second decades of life, and the male-to-female ratio is equal. Once present, the lesions are usually stable; however, they may regress spontaneously, progress, or recur after curettage. The most common location is the tibia, but lesions also may occur in the fibula, radius, humerus, metatarsals, and phalanges. The most characteristic radiologic feature of this radiolucency is its multilocular appearance. Other patterns include a diffuse homogeneous ground glass appearance, and occasionally the lesion is entirely osteosclerotic. The size ranges from 1 to 10 cm.

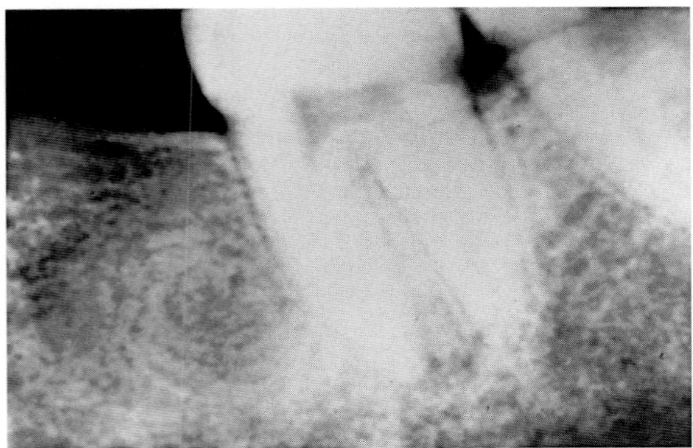

FIGURE 17–40.

Ossifying Fibroma: Digitally processed periapical radiograph. We believe the coiled pattern represents a manifestation of a cementifying variant of ossifying fibroma distinct from the fingerprint pattern of fibrous dysplasia.

AGGRESSIVE OSSIFYING FIBROMA

(Juvenile active ossifying fibroma, active ossifying fibroma, trabecular desmo-osteoblastoma)

Some explanation is needed to justify this separate discussion of AOF. Although it is agreed universally that some ossifying fibromas behave in an aggressive fashion clinically, investigators such as Eversole and colleagues (1985a, 1985b) could find no histopathologic features unique to this group. Among 43 cases of ossifying fibroma in which radiographs were available, Eversole and associates (1985b) classified nearly 1 in 10 as active or aggressive. According to Waldron (1985), this tumor is more cellular than the usual ossifying fibroma and relatively little collagen is produced. Thin streams of osteoid are formed that may resemble the osteoid produced in osteosarcoma; plump osteoblastlike cells surround the osteoid. Giant cells resembling osteoclasts are often present, sometimes in large numbers. Reed and Hagy (1965) stated that AOF and osteoblastoma are variants of the same lesion.

A separate discussion is presented here because there are distinct clinical differences characterized principally by location, behavior, and patient age. Because, to our knowledge, no author of a large series has reviewed this lesion, it is difficult to describe the clinical features accurately. According to Waldron (1985), most patients are in the first or second decade of life, but a number of cases have been reported in older groups. Information about sex, racial predilection, and clinical symptoms is sparse. Many patients have facial swelling in the maxillary region, suborbital swelling,

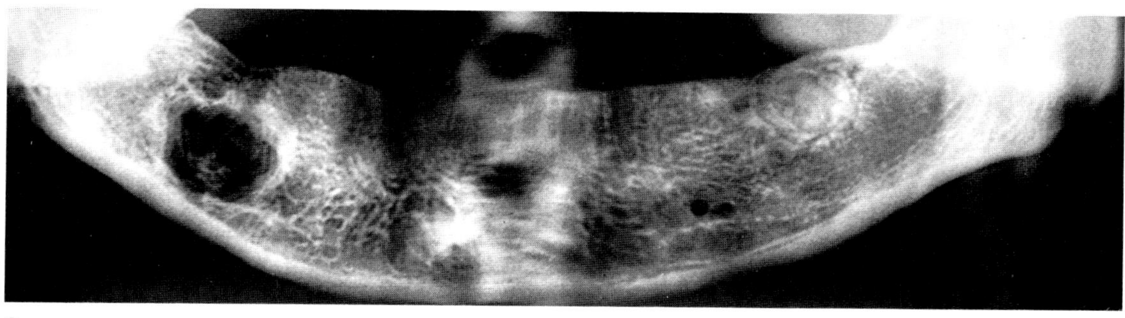

A

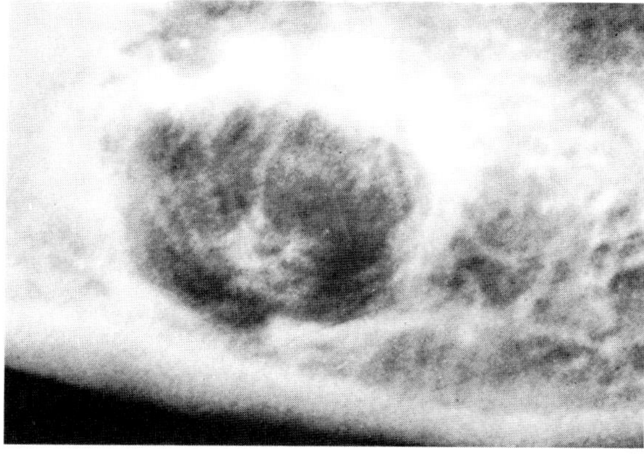

B

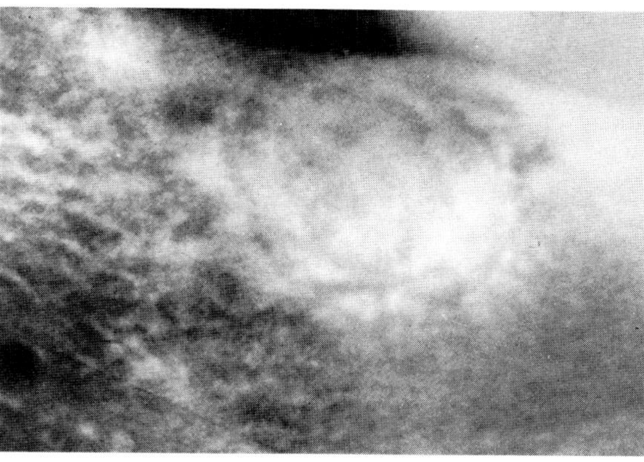

C

FIGURE 17–41.

Ossifying Fibroma: A, Multiple coiled type. B and C, Magnified views show coiled appearance. The histologic diagnosis was cementifying fibromas.

and palatal swelling intraorally; there may be tenderness associated with the swelling. Sometimes exophthalmos, proptosis, diplopia, and epiphora are associated findings. The AOF is more likely to be painful than is the ossifying fibroma. This lesion tends to grow more rapidly; therefore, the interval since onset may be described more in terms of weeks or months, rather than as 1 year or more.

At the time of initial surgery, there are very few clinical and radiologic indicators that a given lesion is aggressive. Many classic nonaggressive ossifying fibromas occur in the maxilla in young people, and although incisional biopsy is diagnostic of ossifying fibroma, it may not provide a clue as to its aggressiveness. Therefore, large maxillary lesions should not be assumed to be aggressive, but it is prudent to treat maxillary lesions by thorough enucleation, followed by careful curettage of the walls of the tumor cavity. The patient should be observed very carefully to verify complete resolution. Because recurrence is the most important distinguishing feature of AOF, patients with maxillary lesions should be observed very closely with radiologic examinations. Recurrent lesions, especially those showing rapid regrowth, should be considered for more aggressive surgical retreatment. Radiation therapy is contraindicated. It should be emphasized that AOFs have been reported in the mandible, as in the case of Reaume and colleagues (1985). According to Waldron (1985), some AOFs may undergo anaplastic change to osteogenic sarcoma.

◆ *RADIOLOGY (Figs. 17–42 to 17–46)*

These are some of the signs suggestive of AOF:

1. Occurrence of a lesion in a child or adolescent.
2. History of a rapid increase in swelling reported by the patient.
3. Pain reported by the patient or occurring on palpation.
4. Occurrence of a lesion in a maxillary location.
5. Large size of the lesion radiologically (greater than 5 cm in diameter).
6. Expanded cortex visibly perforated on computed tomography, but not the burnt-out appearance commonly seen in plain radiographs.
7. Recurrence of the lesion; many cases reported as aggressive actually did not recur.

Although the information specific to AOF is mostly anecdotal, it appears that there may be a predilection for the maxilla, although mandibular lesions do exist. In addition, many will have extended into the antrum, nasal fossa, and orbit at the time of initial diagnosis. The mandible also may be affected; however, there is no specific location. Eversole

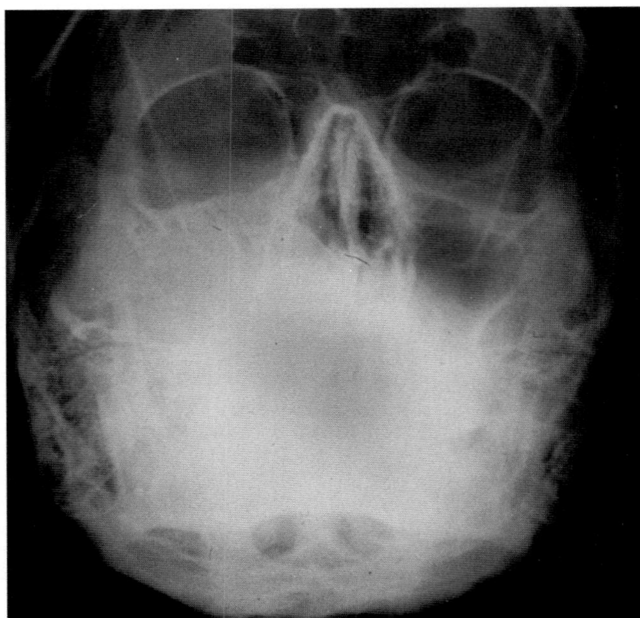

A

FIGURE 17–42.

Aggressive Ossifying Fibroma: A to C, Maxillary lesion reported by Wenig and colleagues is described in text. Margins are not intact, a sign of aggressiveness. (From Wenig B, et al: A destructive maxillary cemento-ossifying fibroma following maxillofacial trauma. Laryngoscope 94:810, 1984.)

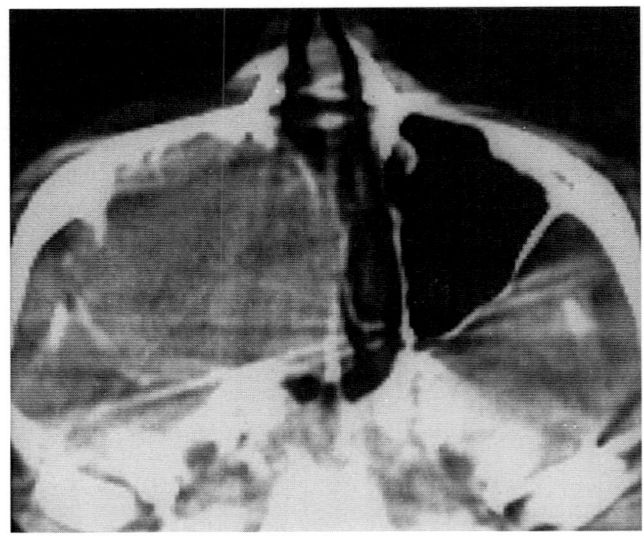

B

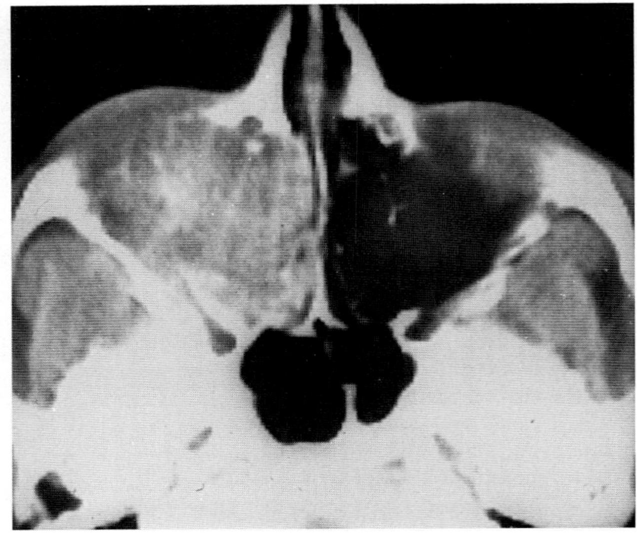

C

and colleagues (1985a) classified all lesions larger than 5 cm on radiographs as active or aggressive; these tended to contain ground glass or mottled radiopacities. So-called aggressive cases have been reported by Wenig and colleagues (1984) in the maxilla and antrum of a 26-year-old Hispanic man, by Walter and co-workers (1979) in the maxilla of a 14-year-old boy, and by Reaume and associates in the mandible of a 10-year-old American boy of African origin. The lesions were described as easily removed, easily shelled out, or excised, and none recurred, with follow-up periods from 9 months to 1 year.

In a case that Dale Miles shared with us, a 12-year-old boy had a mandibular lesion with multiple recurrences. There was a very intense uptake of technetium, producing a well-defined distinct hot spot in all of the area occupied by the tumor. Radiologically, the lesion appeared as an ovoid radiolucency in the body of the mandible, approximately 5 cm in diameter, with bowing of the inferior border and expansion of the buccal and lingual cortices.

We believe recurrence should be the most important criterion for classifying a lesion as aggressive; however, we and many others have not been able to define a single feature that is consistently predictive of recurrence. We recommend thorough curettage as the initial treatment of choice for all ossifying fibromas and very careful follow-up of all cases. Even when there are features suggestive of aggressiveness as listed here, we do not believe that radical ablative disfiguring surgery should be the initial treatment of choice.

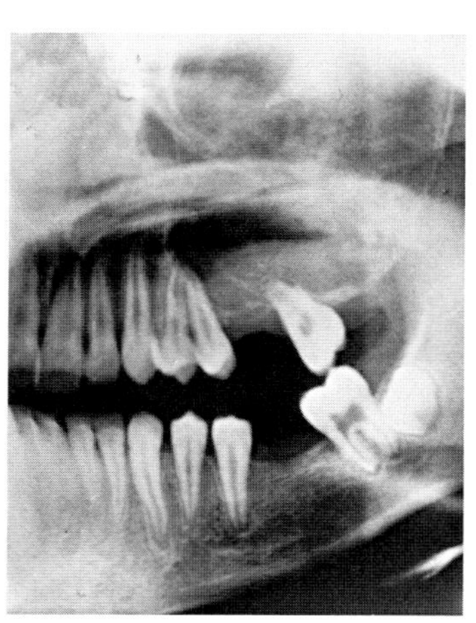
A

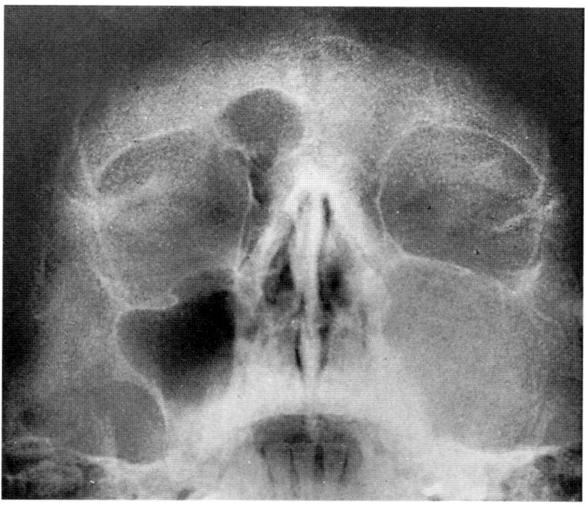
B

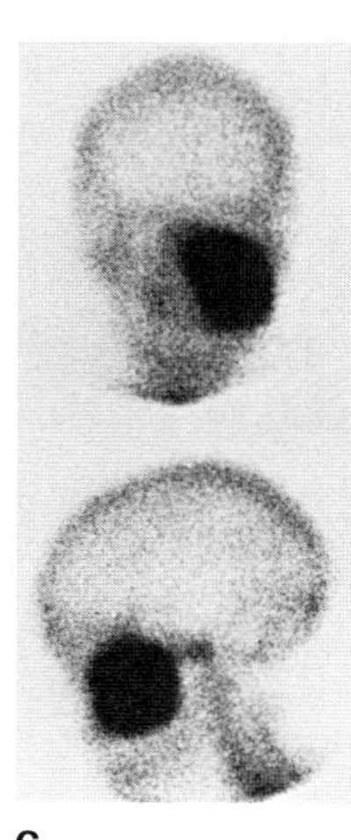
C

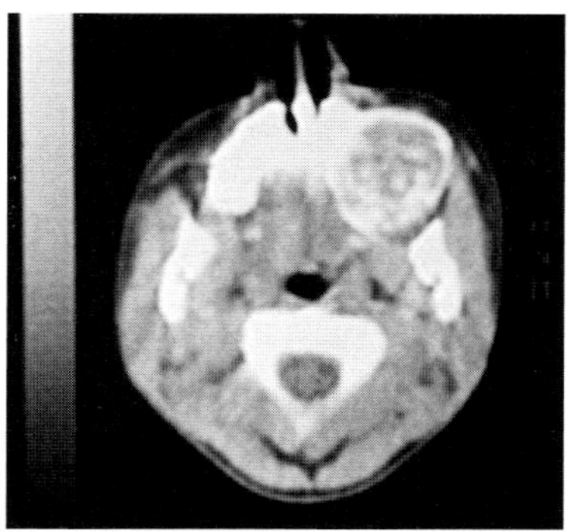
D

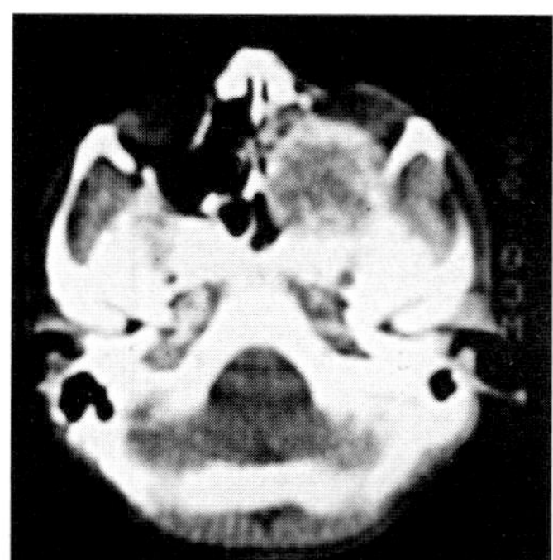
E

FIGURE 17–43.

Aggressive Ossifying Fibroma: Maxillary lesion reported by Walter and colleagues (1979) was discussed in text. A, Soft tissue density in upper part of left antrum. B, Opacification of left antrum, anterior ethmoids, and frontal sinus on left side. C, Significant uptake in region of antrum and nasal cavity but not in frontal sinus. D and E, Computed tomographic images show involvement of maxilla, antrum, and nasal fossa; opacification of frontal and ethmoid sinuses probably resulted from tumor obstruction of ostea and subsequent accumulation of fluid. (From Walter J, et al: Aggressive ossifying fibroma of the maxilla: a review of the literature and report of a case. J Oral Surg 37:276, 1979.)

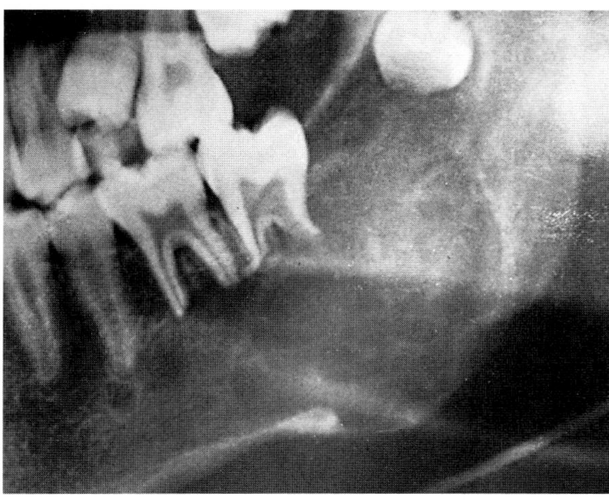
A

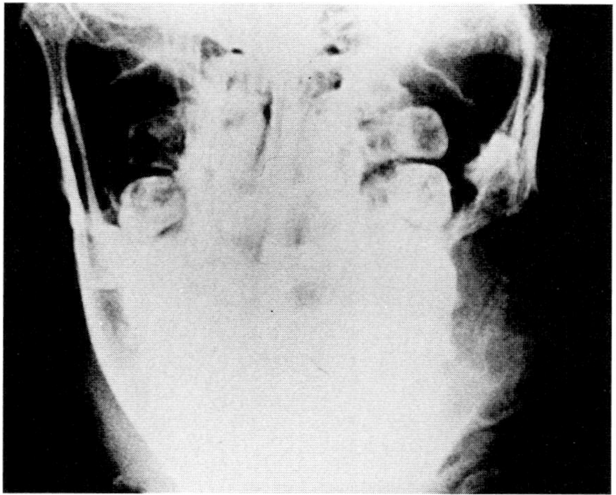
B

FIGURE 17–44.

Aggressive Ossifying Fibroma: Mandibular lesion reported by Reaume and colleagues (1985), discussed in text. A, Typical features. B, Expanded cortex is inapparent on plain radiograph. (From Reaume C, Schmid R, Wesley R: Aggressive ossifying fibroma of the mandible. J Oral Maxillofac Surg 43:631, 1985.)

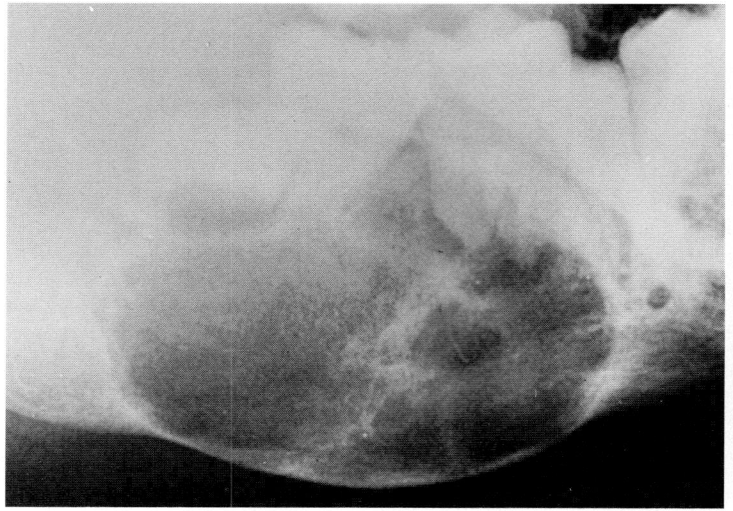
A

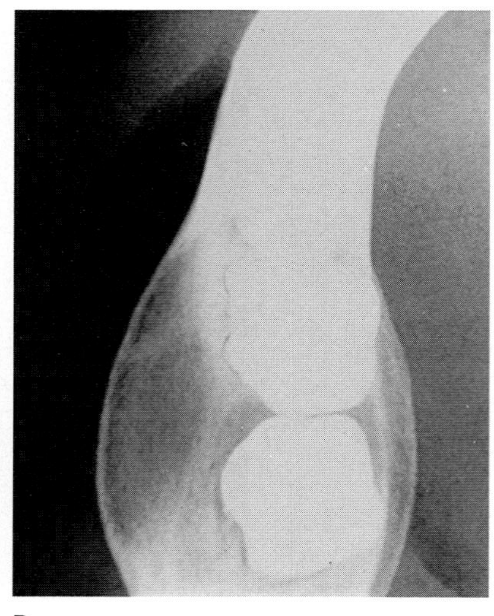
B

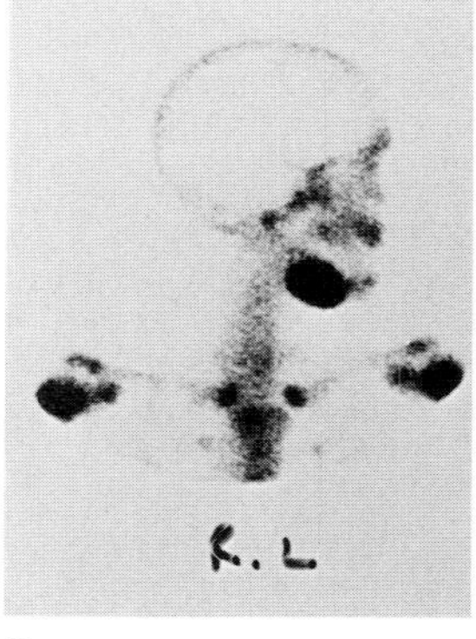

C

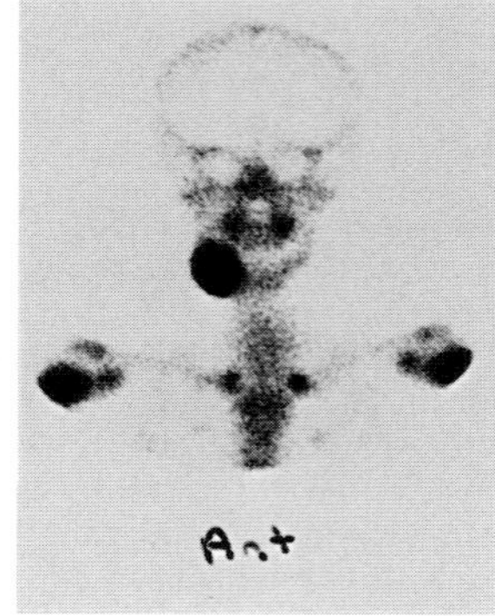

D

FIGURE 17–45.

Aggressive Ossifying Fibroma: Mandibular lesion was described in text. A and B, Recurrent lesion in a 12-year-old boy. C and D, Increased uptake in lesion and at growth plates of humerus and clavicles. (Courtesy of Dr. D. Miles, Indiana University, Indianapolis, IN.)

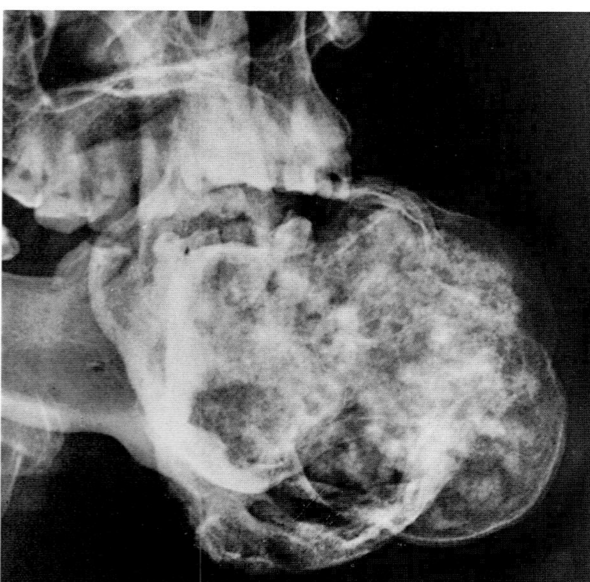
A

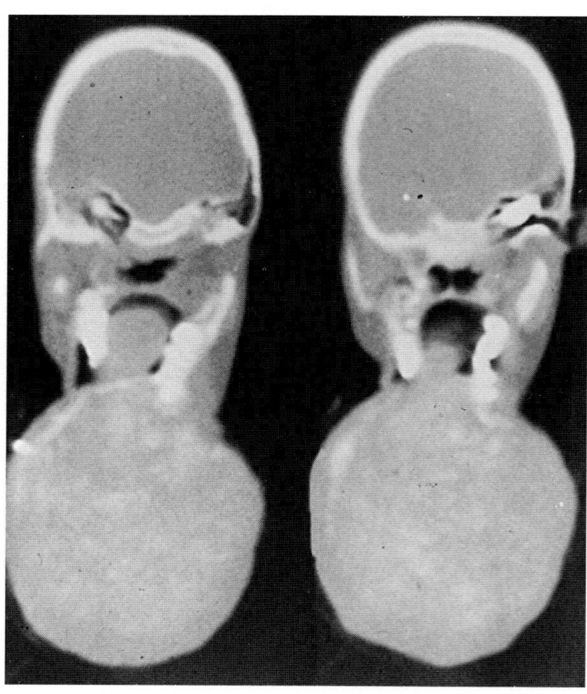
B

FIGURE 17–46.

Aggressive Ossifying Fibroma: A, Large ossifying fibroma in mandible of an adult. (Courtesy of Dr. P. Dhirravarangkura, Chulalonghorn University School of Dentistry, Bangkok, Thailand.) B, Large ossifying fibroma in mandible of a 14-year-old boy. (Courtesy of Dr. Neil Hodges, Durban, Republic of South Africa.)

References

Idiopathic Osteosclerosis

Austin BW, Moule AJ: A comparative study of the prevalence of mandibular osteosclerosis in patients of Asiatic and Caucasian origin. Aust Dent J 29:36, 1984.

Boyne PJ: Incidence of osteosclerotic areas in the mandible and maxilla. J Oral Surg 18:486, 1960.

Eversole LR, Stone CE, Strub D: Focal sclerosing osteomyelitis/focal periapical osteopetrosis: radiographic patterns. Oral Surg Oral Med Oral Pathol 58:456, 1984.

Farman AG, Joubert JJD, Nortjé CJ: Focal osteosclerosis and apical periodontal pathoses in "European" and Cape Coloured dental outpatients. Int J Oral Surg 7:549, 1978.

Geist JR, Katz JO: The frequency and distribution of idiopathic osteosclerosis. Oral Surg Oral Med Oral Pathol 69:388, 1990.

Condensing Osteitis

Austin BW, Moule AJ: A comparative study of the prevalence of mandibular osteosclerosis in patients of Asiatic and Caucasian origin. Aust Dent J 29:36, 1984.

Bhaskar SN: Synopsis of Oral Pathology. 6th Ed. St. Louis:CV Mosby, 1981, p. 350.

Boyne PJ: Incidence of osteosclerotic areas in the mandible and maxilla. J Oral Surg 18:486, 1960.

Eliasson S, Halvarsson C, Ljunsheimer G: Periapical condensing osteitis and endodontic treatment. Oral Surg Oral Med Oral Pathol 57:195, 1984.

Eversole LR, Sabes WR, Rovin S: Fibrous dysplasia: a nosologic problem in the diagnosis of fibro-osseous lesions of the jaws. J Oral Pathol 1: 189, 1972.

Eversole LR, Stone CE, Strub D: Focal sclerosing osteomyelitis/focal periapical osteopetrosis: radiographic patterns. Oral Surg Oral Med Oral Pathol 58:456, 1984.

Farman AG, Joubert JJD, Nortjé CJ: Focal osteosclerosis and apical periodontal pathoses in "European" and Cape Coloured dental outpatients. Int J Oral Surg 7:549, 1978.

Shafer WG, Hine MK, Levy BM: A Textbook of Oral Pathology. 4th Ed. Philadelphia:WB Saunders, 1983, p. 502.

Waldron CA, Giansanti JS, Browland BC: Sclerosing cemental masses of the jaws (so-called chronic sclerosing osteomyelitis, sclerosing osteitis, multiple enostosis and gigantiform cementoma). Oral Surg Oral Med Oral Pathol 39:590, 1975.

Hypercementosis

Gibilisco JA (ed): Stafne's Oral Radiographic Diagnosis. 5th Ed. Philadelphia:WB Saunders, 1985, p. 28.

Israel H: Early hypercementosis and arrested dental eruption: heritable multiple ankylodontia. J Craniofac Genet Dev Biol 4:243, 1984.

Shafer WG, Hine MK, Levy BM: A Textbook of Oral Pathology. 4th Ed. Philadelphia:WB Saunders, 1983, p. 333.

Wood NK, Goaz PW: Differential Diagnosis of Oral Lesions. 3rd Ed. St. Louis:CV Mosby, 1985, p. 572.

Worth HM: Principles and Practice of Oral Radiologic Interpretation. Chicago:Year Book Medical Publishers, 1963, p. 178.

Cementicles

Mikola OJ, Bauer WH: Cementicles and fragments of cementum in the periodontal membrane. Oral Surg Oral Med Oral Pathol 2:1063, 1949.

Shafer WG, Hine MK, Levy BM: A Textbook of Oral Pathology. 4th Ed. Philadelphia:WB Saunders, 1983, p. 336.

Periapical Cemental Dysplasia

Hamner JE, Scofield HH, Cornyn J: Benign fibro-osseous lesions of periodontal membrane origin. Cancer 22:861, 1968.

Higuchi U, Nakamura N, Tashiro H: Clinicopathologic study of cemento-osseous dysplasia producing cysts of the mandible: report of 4 cases. Oral Surg Oral Med Oral Pathol 65:339, 1988.

Regezi JA, Kerr DA, Courtney RM: Odontogenic tumors: analysis of 706 cases. J Oral Surg 36:771, 1978.

Stafne ED: Periapical osteofibrosis with formation of cementoma. J Am Dent Assoc 21:1822, 1934.

Tanaka H, et al: Periapical cemental dysplasia with multiple lesions. J Oral Maxillofac Surg 16:757, 1987.

Waldron CA: Fibro-osseous lesions of the jaws. J Oral Maxillofac Surg 43:249, 1985.

Worth HM: Principles and Practice of Oral Radiologic Interpretation. Chicago:Year Book Medical Publishers, 1963, p. 596.

Zegerelli EV, et al: The cementoma: a study of 230 patients with 435 cementomas. Oral Surg Oral Med Oral Pathol 17:219, 1964a.

Zegarelli EV, Kutscher AH, Budowsky J, Hoffman PJ: The progressive calcification of the cementoma: a roentgenographic study. Oral Surg Oral Med Oral Pathol 18:180, 1964b.

Benign Cementoblastoma

Abrams AM, Kirby JW, Melrose RJ: Cementoblastoma. Oral Surg Oral Med Oral Pathol 38:394, 1974.

Chaput A, Marc A: Un cas de cémentome localisé sur une molaire temporaire. Schweiz Monatsschr Zahnheilk 75:48, 1965.

Cherrick HM, King OH, Lacatorto FM, Suggs DM: Benign cementoblastoma. Oral Surg Oral Med Oral Pathol 37:54, 1974.

Corio RL, Crawford BE, Schaberg SJ: Benign cementoblastoma. Oral Surg Oral Med Oral Pathol 41:524, 1976.

Eversole LR, Sabes WR, Danchess VG: Benign cementoblastoma. Oral Surg Oral Med Oral Pathol 36:824, 1973.

Farman AG, Kohler WW, Nortjé CJ, Van Wyk CW: Cementoblastoma: report of a case. J Oral Surg 37:198, 1979.

Forsslund HG, Bodin T, Julin P: Undiagnosed benign cementoblastoma in a patient with a 6 year pain condition. Oral Surg Oral Med Oral Pathol 66:243, 1988.

Fujita S, et al: A case of benign cementoblastoma. Oral Surg Oral Med Oral Pathol 68:64, 1989.

Gingell JC, Lunin M, Beckerman T, Levy BM: Benign cementoblastoma. J Oral Med 39:8, 1984.

Goerig AC, Fay JT, King E: Endodontic treatment of a cementoblastoma. Oral Surg Oral Med Oral Pathol 58:133, 1984.

Hamner JE, Scofield HH, Cornyn J: Benign fibro-osseous jaw lesions of periodontal membrane origin: analysis of 249 cases. Cancer 22:861, 1968.

Larsson A, Forsberg O, Sjögren S: Benign cementoblastoma: cementum analogue of benign osteoblastoma. J Oral Surg 36:299, 1978.

Mader CL, Wendelberg L: Benign cementoblastoma. J Am Dent Assoc 99: 990, 1979.

Makek M, Lello G: Benign cementoblastoma: a case report and literature review. J Max Fac Surg 10:182, 1982.

Norberg O: Zun Kenntnis der dysodontogenetischen Geschwülste der Kieferknochen. Vjschr Zahnheilk 46:321, 1930.

Pindborg JJ: Pathology of the Dental Hard Tissues. Copenhagen:Munksgaard, 1970, p. 412.

Raveh J: Current forming tumors of the lower jaw. J Max Fac Surg 8:146, 1980.

Regezi JA, Kerr DA, Courtney RM: Odontogenic tumors analysis of 706 cases. J Oral Surg 36:771, 1978.

Shafer WG, Hine MK, Levy BM: A Textbook of Oral Pathology. 4th Ed. Philadelphia:WB Saunders, 1983, p. 302.

Vindenes H, Nilsen P, Gilhuus-Moe O: Benign cementoblastoma. Int J Oral Surg 8:318, 1974.

Ossifying Fibroma

Eversole LR, Leider AS, Nelson K: Ossifying fibroma: a clinicopathologic study of sixty-four cases. Oral Surg Oral Med Oral Pathol 60:505, 1985a.

Eversole LR, Merrell PW, Strub D: Radiographic characteristics of central ossifying fibroma. Oral Surg Oral Med Oral Pathol 59:522, 1985b.

Hamner JE, Scofield HH, Cornyn J: Benign fibro-osseous jaw lesions of periodontal membrane origin: an analysis of 249 cases. Cancer 22:861, 1968.

Makek M: Clinical Pathology of Fibro-Osteo-Cemental Lesions in the Cranio-Facial and Jaw Bones. Basel:S Karger, 1983, p. 38.

Miller SI: Pathologic quiz case 1. The resident's page. Arch Otolaryngol 105:742, 1979.

Montgomery AH: Ossifying fibroma of the jaws. Arch Surg 15:30, 1927.

Shafer WG, Hine MK, Levy BM: A Textbook of Oral Pathology. 4th Ed. Philadelphia:WB Saunders, 1983, p. 298.

Sweet RM, Bryarly RC, Kornblut AD: Recurrent cementifying fibroma of the jaws. Laryngoscope 91:1137, 1981.

Taylor ND, Watkins JP, Bear E: Recurrent cementifying fibroma of the maxilla: report of a case. J Oral Surg 35:204, 1973.

Waldron CA, Giansanti JS: Benign fibro-osseous lesions of the jaws: a clinical radiologic histologic review of sixty-five cases. Oral Surg Oral Med Oral Pathol 35:340, 1973.

Waldron CA: Fibro-osseous lesions of the jaws. J Maxillofac Surg 43:249, 1985.

Aggressive Ossifying Fibroma

Eversole L, Leider AS, Nelson K: Ossifying fibroma: a clinicopathologic study of 64 cases. Oral Surg Oral Med Oral Pathol 60:505, 1985a.

Eversole LR, Merrell PW, Strub D: Radiographic characteristics of central ossifying fibroma. Oral Surg Oral Med Oral Pathol 59:522, 1985b.

Miles DM: Aggressive ossifying fibroma, personal communication.

Reaume CE, Schmid RW, Wesley RK: Aggressive ossifying fibroma of the mandible. J Oral Maxillofac Surg 43:631, 1985.

Reed RJ, Hagy DM: Benign non-odontogenic fibro-osseous lesions of the skull. Oral Surg Oral Med Oral Pathol 19:214, 1965.

Waldron CA: Fibro-osseous lesions of the jaws. J Oral Maxillofac Surg 43:249, 1985.

Walter JM, et al: Aggressive fibroma of the maxilla: a review of the literature and report of a case. J Oral Surg 37:276, 1979.

Wenig BL, et al: A destructive maxillary cemento-ossifying fibroma following maxillofacial trauma. Laryngoscope 94:810, 1984.

Chapter 18

Generalized Radiopacities

GARDNER'S SYNDROME

In 1953, Gardner and Richards described this syndrome. Classically, it was characterized by the following triad of clinical features: (1) familial polyposis of the large intestine, (2) osteomas, and (3) skin lesions consisting of epidermoid cysts and fibromas. Earlier co-workers helped Gardner and Richards establish the features of the syndrome: Stephens and Gardner described the malignant potential of the familial polyposis in 1950, and Gardner and Plenk (1952) helped establish the presence of osteomas and the hereditary pattern, consisting of a non-sex-linked autosomal dominant gene. Reed and Neel (1955) estimated that the incidence of Gardner's syndrome in the United States is 1 in 8300 births, whereas Komatsu (1968) estimated the incidence to be 1 in 10,000 births in Japan. Bochetto and colleagues estimated that the incidence may be as low as 1 in 16,000 births in some regions.

Retrospectively, the first, though unrecognized, case of Gardner's syndrome was reported in 1912 by Devic and Bussy, who described a woman with cysts of the scalp, multiple lipomas, osteomas of the mandible, and multiple intestinal polyposis. The first case to appear in the dental literature was reported in 1943, by Gordon M. Fitzgerald, one of the pioneers of dental radiology in America. His patient was a 39-year-old woman with abdominal desmoid tumors, intraosseous osteomas, bony exostoses, multiple cystic odontomas, and multiple polyposis of the large bowel. The patient also had multiple rudimentary teeth, extensive hypercementosis, torus palatinus, and scoliosis. In 1955, O'Brien and Wels first reported the appearance of desmoid tumors in the syndrome. In 1962, Fader and colleagues added the finding of multiple impacted supernumerary and permanent teeth in the maxilla and mandible. By 1966, Jones and Cornell identified and reviewed 75 cases of Gardner's syndrome as reported in the literature. The features of Gardner's syndrome have been expanded to include the following:

1. Soft tissue surface tumors including fibromas, sebaceous cysts, leiomyomas, desmoid tumors, keloids, neurofibromas, lipomas, incisional fibromas, mesenteric and retroperitoneal fibrous tumors and occasional cases of fibrosarcoma and liposarcoma.
2. Bony lesions consisting of osseous and dental abnormalities, including peripheral osteomas, endosteal osteomas, cortical thickening, multiple unerupted supernumerary and permanent teeth, multiple compound odontomas, and hypercementosis. According to Small and colleagues (1980), fibrous dysplasia (FD) occurs in 8% of the cases and, in rare instances, osteosarcoma has been reported.
3. Multiple polyposis of the large intestine and rectum has a great propensity for malignant transformation. Many consider Gardner's syndrome a variation of familial polyposis coli.

Pathologic Characteristics

Although biopsies often are performed on peripheral osteomas of the syndrome and the lesions are confirmed as osteomas, the enostotic jaw lesions rarely are studied histologically. Ida and colleagues (1981) found two reports whereby nonexpansile enostotic mandibular bone was examined at autopsy and confirmed histologically as central osteoma consisting of mature lamellar bone. They propose that the enostotic changes in the syndrome have limited growth potential. A mandibular specimen examined histologically by Offerhaus and colleagues (1987) showed that the radiopaque lesions consisted of dense bone compatible with endosteoma.

Epidermoid cysts are the most common soft tissue lesions and are recognized by their excess numbers and unique distribution. They are especially prone to occur on the scalp and the skin of the back and are seen infrequently on the face and extremities; however, in the familial polyposis coli syndrome epidermoid cysts often are seen on the arms and legs. In a case reported by Marshall and colleagues (1985), a 28-year-old woman with Gardner's syndrome had 24 disfiguring facial epidermoid cysts. Over the previous 18 years she underwent 10 separate procedures to remove epidermal cysts from her face.

Desmoid tumors are locally aggressive fibrous lesions that may involve voluntary muscle and fascial structures. They often are seen on the shoulder, thigh, and buttocks; however, in Gardner's syndrome desmoid tumors may appear in the incisional scars of previous abdominal or rectal surgery.

According to Fader and colleagues (1962), intestinal polyposis first was recognized in 1721 by Menzel, was described in more detail by Virchow in 1863, and in 1881, Cripps first reported the inheritable quality of the disease and termed it familial adenomatosis. In the early 1950s, Gardner and several other co-workers observed familial adenomatosis with the syndrome bearing his name. Fader and colleagues (1962) stated that isolated adenomatous polyps are the most common tumors in the colon and rectum. They occur in 7 to 9% of the adult population, usually in people older than 30 years of age. They rarely are seen in children. Familial polyposis is characterized by the development of multiple adenomas in the rectum and colon. These infrequently involve the ileum, but sometimes the entire gastrointestinal tract may be affected. In 1981, Ida and colleagues studied the osteomatous and dental abnormalities in the jaws of patients with familial adenomatosis coli (AC), also known as familial polyposis coli, and hereditary intestinal polyposis. They found that 81% of patients with AC had osteomatous lesions in the jaws, along with lesser numbers of the various dental abnormalities associated with Gardner's syndrome.

Intestinal polyposis in Gardner's syndrome is inherited as an autosomal dominant trait with varying degrees of expressivity. The intestinal polyposis of the syndrome develops after the onset of osteomas and other dental abnormalities in the jaws. According to Ida and colleagues (1981), the intestinal polyposis may be of the carpeted or noncarpeted type. Patients with the carpeted type may have as many as 5000 adenomas in the colon and rectum and may develop colorectal adenocarcinoma earlier than patients with the noncarpeted type. Also, these authors stated that the onset of intestinal polyposis occurs earlier in patients with the carpeted type. In their study, 8 of 52 (15%) of their patients with familial polyposis had the carpeted type and all had osteomatous changes in the jaws, although 3 of the 8 had fewer than 2 lesions. Intestinal polyposis will develop in 50% of the patients with Gardner's syndrome by the time they reach the age of 30 years, and it ultimately will develop in most patients by the time they are 50 years of age.

Clinical Features

One of the most important features of Gardner's syndrome is the tendency for the osseous and dental abnormalities to develop before the intestinal polyposis; thus, bony hard swellings about the jaws, face, scalp, and neck areas, especially if they are multiple in a teenager or young adult, should alert the clinician to the possible diagnosis of Gardner's syndrome. Additionally, orbital osteomas may cause unilateral proptosis. According to Whitson and colleagues (1986), osteomas account for 0.6 to 2.5% of all orbital mass lesions in adults; however, they believe that orbital osteomas are rare in Gardner's syndrome. Their patient was a 30-year-old woman with Gardner's syndrome with gradual proptosis of the left eye over a period of at least 1 month. The cause was a medial orbital wall osteoma.

Also, multiple soft swellings, often of uniform size, about the face, neck, or arms should suggest the possibility of multiple epidermal cysts of the syndrome. Only approximately 30% of patients with intestinal polyposis have symptoms at the time of examination. Some symptoms include rectal bleeding, melena, persistent occult blood in the stools, cramplike abdominal pain, and diarrhea. The remainder presumably are discovered as a result of family history or a complaint referring to the other manifestations such as the osteomas or skin lesions. According to Fader and colleagues (1962), 75% of all benign polyps of the large intestine can be diagnosed by sigmoidoscopic examination and biopsy. Barium enema studies are also highly diagnostic.

Treatment/Prognosis

Marshall and colleagues (1985) described a rhytidectomy incision to remove multiple facial epidermal cysts; however, after removal, new cysts can be expected to develop. Their patient underwent 10 separate procedures to remove epidermal cysts from her face during an 18-year period. The osteomas are removed for cosmetic reasons only or if they interfere with function. There is no tendency for the osteomas to undergo malignant transformation.

Robbins (1957) stated that all adenomatous polyps of the large intestine have a high incidence of malignant degeneration; however, in this disease there is a virtual 100% chance of development into carcinoma if left untreated. Polyposis of the large intestine is treated by resection of the entire large bowel and rectum. In the early stages, the osseous and dental changes in the jaws are often sufficiently characteristic to suggest the presence of the syndrome. Many of the reported cases have been discovered because of the alertness of the dentist or oral surgeon on viewing routine dental radiographs. Early diagnosis is lifesaving for these patients because, without intervention, virtually all will develop malignant intestinal polyposis, many before the age of 30 years.

◆ *RADIOLOGY (Figs. 18–1 and 18–2)*

General Radiologic Features

An excellent review of the bone abnormalities in Gardner's syndrome has been presented by Chang and colleagues (1968). They examined 33 patients with the syndrome (age range of patients, 4 to 48 years). All 33 patients were from 2 families. The authors characterized the bone abnormalities as benign osteomatosis consisting of dense bony proliferations, from slight thickening of the cortex to large masses. Chang and colleagues (1968) found the following locations for the osteomatous changes: (1) long tubular bones, 48%; (2) mandible, 33%; (3) short tubular bones, 27%; (4) skull and facial bones, 21%; (5) flat bones, 21%; and (6) cuboid bones, 6%. Dental abnormalities were observed in 24% of the cases. They found no abnormalities in the vertebrae. In general, the osteomatous changes were described as localized cortical thickening producing no deformity of the bone, wavy cortical thickening producing a slight bulging of the cortex, exostoses and enostoses, and osteomas.

The most frequently affected site in the axial skeleton was the long tubular bones. Most changes consisted of localized cortical thickening (69%), wavy cortical thickening (56%), and exostoses (19%); pedunculated osteoma was seen in one case (6%). In the short tubular bones of the hands and feet, multiple exostoses were the most common findings, with a few instances of localized cortical thickening. The cuboid bones were involved very rarely; however, several small osteomas were observed. In the flat bones, both localized and wavy cortical thickening was found in the pelvis, whereas in the ribs only wavy cortical thickening was discovered.

Chang and colleagues (1968) also examined the skull, facial bones, mandible, and teeth and found these to be the most commonly affected areas in the bony skeleton. All the skull lesions consisted of dense osteomas, either arising from the outer table to cause a protuberant palpable bump or occurring near the paranasal sinuses or facial bones and projecting into the sinuses. Those arising from the outer table were seen most frequently in the occipital and frontal areas, whereas those affecting the sinuses were seen in the frontal, maxillary, and sphenoid sinuses. In the mandible, the authors

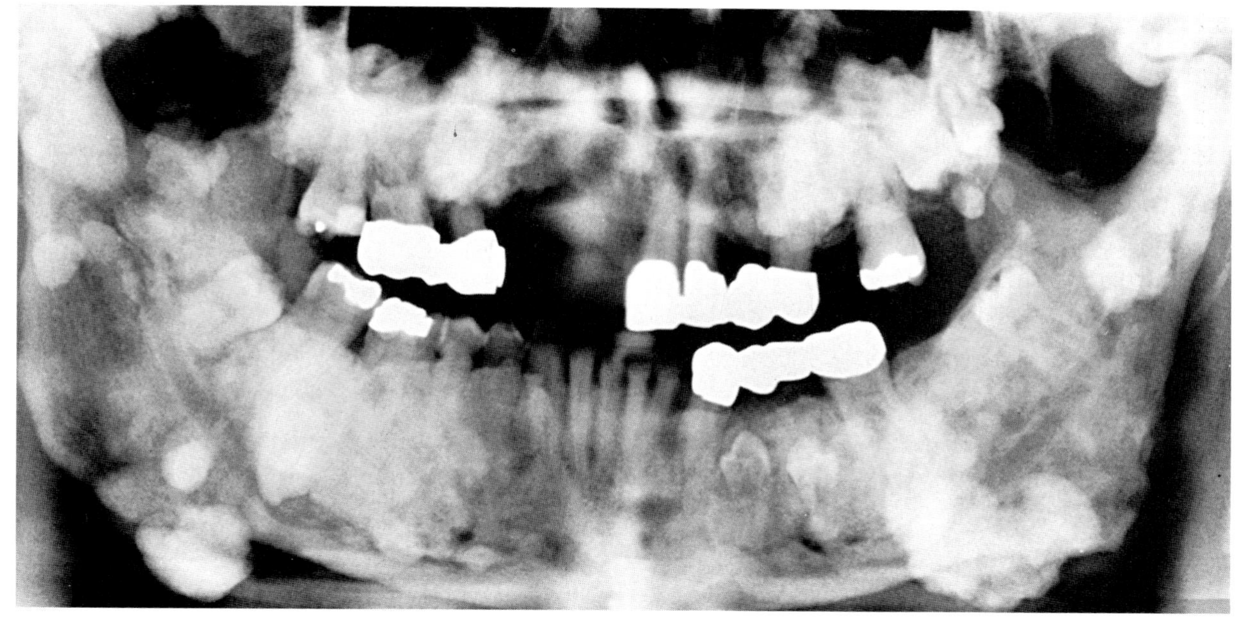

A

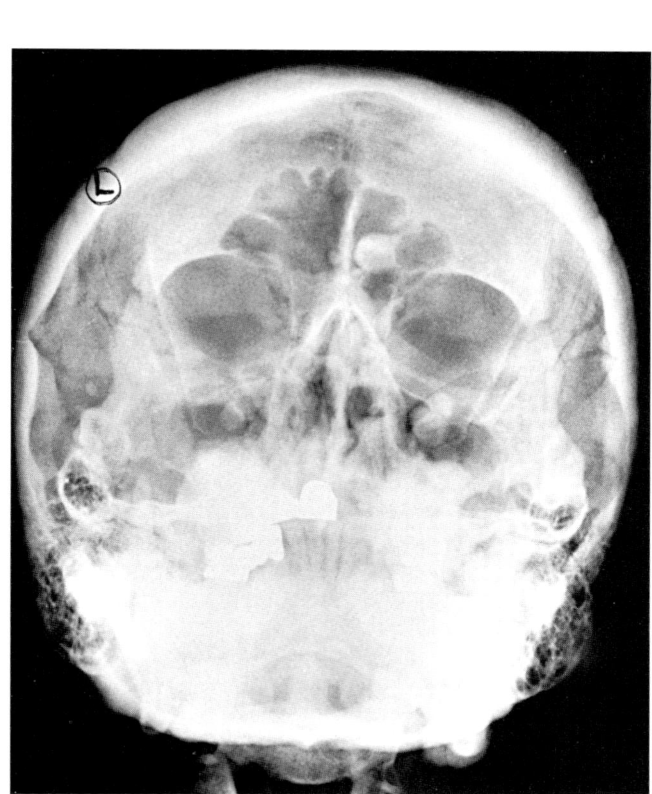

B

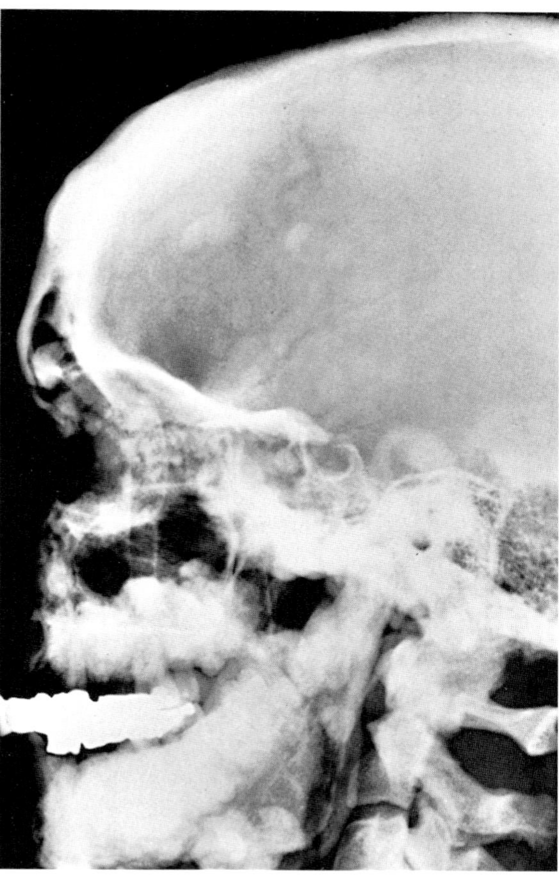

C

FIGURE 18–1.

Gardner's Syndrome: A, Multiple peripheral and enostotic osteomas. Endosteal osteomas consist of small round structures that form a more diffuse or mottled pattern. Multiple supernumerary and unerupted teeth are present, along with thickening of the walls of the right inferior alveolar canal. B and C, Cortical thickening of outer table of skull. Osteomas are seen in the skull, frontal and maxillary sinuses, and jaws. (Courtesy of Dr. D. Barnet, Oregon Health Sciences Center, Portland, OR.)

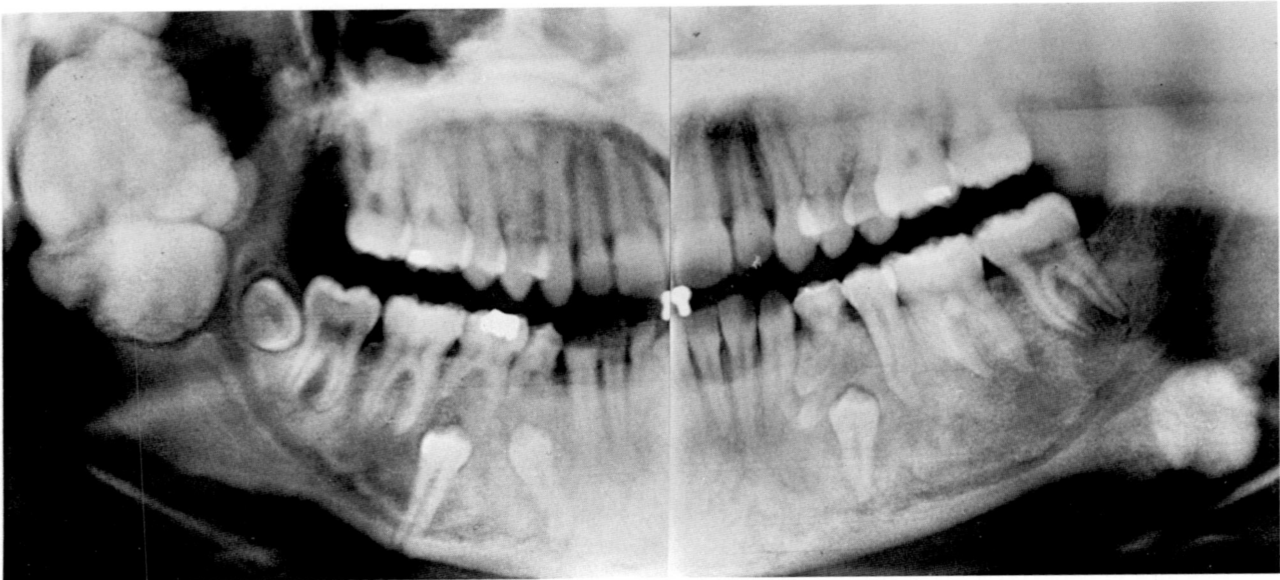

FIGURE 18–2.

Gardner's Syndrome: Several peripheral osteomas and multiple endosteal osteomas with a diffuse homogeneous appearance resembling that of fibrous dysplasia. Figure shows multiple unerupted teeth, compound odontoma in the left mandible, thickening of the walls of the right inferior alveolar canal, and downward displacement of the inferior alveolar canal.

observed 2 types of lesions: The first consisted of a protuberant, lobulated osteoma most often near the angle of the mandible, which seemed to increase in size with increasing age. The second type of lesion was centrally located. These consisted of irregular radiodense areas described as enostoses, which were seen in 9 of the 11 cases with mandibular involvement (82%) and often were associated with dental abnormalities. Eight of 9 (89%) patients with jaw enostoses had dental abnormalities consisting of supernumerary and unerupted teeth and hypercementosis. Chang and co-workers (1968) stated that the large, protuberant, lobulated osteomas arising from the buccal cortex at the angle of the mandible were characteristic of Gardner's syndrome.

Radiologic Features of the Jaws

Additional details concerning the osteomatous and dental changes in the jaws have been elaborated by Ida and co-workers, who studied the panoramic radiographs of four groups of patients:

1. This group was designated AC (+) and consisted of 52 patients with AC.
2. This group was designated AC (−) and consisted of 33 patients who were 13 years or older and came from affected families but were free of AC.
3. This group consisted of children and included 12 patients who were 12 years of age or younger. All were members of families affected by AC. Of these, 5 were found to have intestinal polyps and 7 were free of polyposis.
4. This group consisted of 892 normal adult panoramic radiographs from patients 13 years of age and older and 512 panoramic radiographs of normal children between the ages of 6 and 12 years.

Their osteomatous findings in the jaws were as follows:

1. Most patients with AC have one or more osteomatous lesions in the mandible or maxilla, measuring 5 mm or more in diameter.
2. The number of osteomatous lesions was significant for several factors: First, when four or more osteomatous lesions were present, there was a highly likely association with AC. Forty-six percent of patients with AC had four or more lesions, whereas only 1% of normal patients had two lesions and none had more than three. Secondly, in the patients with AC with four or fewer osteomatous lesions in the jaws, the type of lesion consisted of nonexpansile enostosis. Those with five or more osteomatous lesions had a more generalized multiple enostotic pattern involving the entire body of the mandible bilaterally.
3. In normal patients, the frequency of osteomatous lesions increases with age.
4. In the second group, identified as AC (−), the highest frequency of osteomatous changes occurred in the youngest patients. Thus, a positive family history of AC and osteomatous changes in the jaws at a young age are probably a strong indicator of future development of AC.

We believe that osteomatous bony lesions and intestinal polyposis probably represent a diagnosis of Gardner's syndrome with incomplete penetrance. Three types of osteomatous lesions were identified by Ida and colleagues (1981) as follows:

1. Nonexpansile enostosis, consisting of a well-defined radiopacity of a density similar to cortical bone with no radiolucent rim. It is limited to the tooth-bearing areas of the mandible and maxilla and usually is not superimposed on the apices of the adjacent teeth.
2. Multiple enostotic lesions throughout the body of the mandible, appearing to be linked irregularly. This pattern was observed in 23% of the AC (+) group.
3. Peripheral osteoma occurred only once in the entire sample. The lesion was located at the angle of the mandible and was lobulated and attached to the buccal cortex by a stalk; however, the patient was normal, as were other members of her family.

Although these types of osteomas have been documented in other studies, it would appear that the enostotic osteomatous changes in the jaws are the most suggestive of the syndrome, at least within the Japanese population studies.

Relationship to Teeth

Ida and colleagues (1981) reported dental findings as follows: In the AC (+) group, 12 of 52 patients (23%) had impacted teeth. Of these teeth, 39% were canines, 39% were incisors, and 22% were mandibular premolars. Additionally, 56% of these impacted teeth were associated intimately with either 1 or 2 supernumerary teeth or a compound odontoma. These supernumerary teeth were peg shaped, very small, and located in the interdental alveolar bone or in intimate contact with the follicular sac of an embedded tooth. Also, 5 of the 52 patients with AC (10%) had compound odontomas. Only 2% of the normal group had impacted teeth, of which 45% were canines and 55% were premolars; none of these was associated with a supernumerary tooth or odontoma. In the normal group, only 1% exhibited supernumerary teeth, of which 67% were maxillary mesiodens, 17% were maxillary fourth molars, and 17% had small peg-shaped supernumerary teeth in the alveolar bone. In the AC (+) and normal groups, impacted third molars were excluded.

Although hypercementosis has been mentioned in numerous reports, there is very little information as to its distribution and extent. Fitzgerald (1943) observed extensive hypercementosis that simulated concrescence. Although some reports have included increased susceptibility to caries in Gardner's syndrome, there is little evidence indicating that the caries history in Gardner's syndrome is different from that in a similar normal population.

FLORID CEMENTO-OSSEOUS DYSPLASIA (Florid osseous dysplasia, chronic diffuse sclerosing osteomyelitis, sclerosing cemental masses of the jaws, diffuse cementosis, multiple enostosis, gigantiform cementoma, familial dominant cemental dysplasia)

This condition probably was defined first as a clinicopathologic entity by Bhaskar and Cutright in 1968, although there were earlier reports of cases described as multiple cementomas, cementomatoses, sclerosing cementomas, and fibrocementomas. Although Bhaskar and Cutright (1968) suggested the term multiple enostosis, other authors have recommended a plethora of names since that time. We believe that the term florid cemento-osseous dysplasia (FCOD) as suggested by Waldron (1985) is the most accurate, whereas the term florid osseous dysplasia is probably the most popular. The plethora of terms for this condition probably indicates that a full understanding about its nature is yet to come. In our opinion, FCOD simply represents a more advanced stage of periapical cemental dysplasia in people predisposed to development of this last stage.

Pathologic Characteristics

Some authors believe that FCOD is a reactive fibro-osseous lesion of periodontal ligament origin. Regardless of its pathogenesis, we believe that it is the end point of a continuum beginning with periapical cemental dysplasia in the anterior region and/or sclerosing cemental masses in the posterior area that ultimately coalesce with each other to involve the anterior and posterior regions of one or both jaws. During this period of development, active and dormant phases are seen. As teeth are removed, the alveolar ridge heals, and then it resorbs slowly over many years. Because the mineralized masses have little tendency to resorb, they ultimately lie immediately beneath the soft tissue of the edentulous ridge. At this point, trauma may cause ulceration. Infection then spreads from the base of the ulcer around the periphery of the avascular mass, followed by fistula formation and sequestration of the mass. This is especially prone to occur when the missing teeth have been replaced by removable prostheses, either partial or complete. In other instances, traumatic cysts are found in association with the condition. There is nothing in the reported histologic features that contradicts the previously postulated pathophysiologic characteristics.

As stated by Melrose and colleagues (1976), most cases are composed of a mixture of cementum-like material and irregular trabeculae of bone. Mincer and colleagues (1977), using ultrastructural studies, found that the hard tissue component consisted of cementum. They used polarization microscopy and described 3 distinctive fiber patterns: parallel fiber, quiltlike, and coalescing globule. Although all 3 patterns were present in most lesions, approximately half of the cases consisted mainly of the coalescing globule pattern and half showed a predominance of the quiltlike pattern. According to Waldron and colleagues (1975), who examined specimens under the light microscope, the cemental mass tended to be solid with lobulated smooth margins. In 14 of the 34 cases there was a globular accretion pattern, and in 7 cases there was a thick trabecular pattern of cementum at the periphery of the mass. In two cases the cemental mass consisted mainly of thick, anastomosing trabeculae of secondary cementum with a sparse and loose connective tissue stroma. Waldron and colleagues (1975) reported woven or lamellar bone in 11 of the 34 specimens; in almost every instance this bone was peripheral to the dense cemental mass and distinguished easily from the cementum. In our opinion, this corresponds to host bone in intimate contact with the cemental mass in a dormant lesion. In 15 of the 34 cases, a zone of fibrocellular connective tissue was present peripheral to the dense cemental mass. We believe that this corresponds to the peripheral radiolucent zone within which cementogenesis occurs in an active lesion. In 13 of these 15 cases (87%), the connective tissue contained small amorphous droplet structures referred to as cementicles. These probably become visible radiologically when they reach 0.2 mm in diameter, at which time they form structures we have described as calcific spherules. In 5 of 13 cases containing cementicles (38%), trabeculae of woven bone were interspersed between the cementicles. This represents bone being replaced by cementum and occurs at the peripheral margin of the radiolucent layer in an active lesion. In 2 of the 15 cases (13%) with a zone of fibrocellular connective tissue, only woven bone was present in the fibrocellular stroma. This could denote the late osteoporotic or early lytic stage before cementogenesis. In 4 of 34 cases (27%), fusion of cementum and bone was evident. This would be the expected picture in a dormant lesion in which the cemental mass is in direct contact with host bone with no intervening radiolucent area.In 16 of the 34 specimens (47%), an inflammatory response was observed and consisted of polymorphonuclear leukocytes, lymphocytes, and plasma cells. This indicates that infection has spread from a superficial gingival ulcer to the underlying bone surrounding the cemental mass. Under these circumstances, the condition had been known as chronic diffuse sclerosing osteomyelitis with fistula formation and sequestration of the mass.

In 4 of the 38 cases analyzed by Waldron and colleagues (1975), the hard tissue component consisted only of bone. For the following reasons, we believe that none of these last 4 cases represented FCOD: Radiographs showing a florid distribution were not available in any of the cases; and 3 of the patients were white, with 2 being male and 2 younger than 30 years of age. In this particular instance, we have described the histologic features in detail because they will have some bearing on the radiographic description that follows and the various active stages, dormant periods, and complication of infection.

Clinical Features

This condition is seen mainly in black women more than 30 years of age. In the series of 15 cases reported by Bhaskar and Cutright (1968), 73% of the patients were female. In their series of 34 cases, Melrose and colleagues (1976) reported that 97% of the cases occurred in women, and in 14 cases for which complete radiographs of the jaws were available, Waldron and colleagues (1975) found that 100% occurred in women. Although most patients are Americans of African origin, rare cases have been reported in white patients. Cases also are seen frequently in Oriental patients. Melrose and colleagues (1976) found that patients' ages ranged from 26 to 59 years at diagnosis, with a mean of 42 years. In the series of Waldron and colleagues (1975), the two youngest women were white and both were 34 years of age. The oldest patient was 67 years.

The World Health Organization has recognized a familial variant of FCOD. In such instances, the terms gigantiform cementoma and familial multiple cementoma have been used. These are based on a few cases reported by Agazzie and Belloni in the Italian literature in 1953. Currently, there have been few other cases reported; thus, most authors consider these a variant of FCOD. In 1982, Sedano and colleagues reported one family with 10 members with autosomal dominant cemental dysplasia. They believed that this condition is different from gigantiform cementomas and FCOD.

Melrose and colleagues (1976) reported that 23 of their 34 patients (66%) had no symptoms, and the condition was discovered on routine radiographs. In the group of 14 patients with adequate radiographs, Waldron and colleagues (1975) found that 57% had symptoms, whereas Bhaskar and Cutright (1968) found that 40% had symptoms. The most common symptom is pain, which usually is described as dull and persistent. Other signs include redness and swelling over the affected area, ulceration, a fistulous tract with or without visible purulent drainage, and sequestration of a pale yellowish mineralized material. Most patients are completely or partially edentulous at diagnosis. In 67% of the cases of Bhashkar and Cutright (1968), the involved regions were edentulous. Notably, almost all patients with symptoms experienced pain in an edentulous area, especially when removable prostheses were being worn. Significantly, Waldron and colleagues (1975) observed that in every instance in which inflammation was present histologically, the history and radiographs indicated that the cemental mass was exposed to the oral cavity because of ulceration or the presence of a fistula. Waldron (1985) stated that the onset of symptoms usually is associated with exposure of the cemental mass to the oral environment from progressive alveolar atrophy under a denture, traumatically induced ulceration of the alveolar mucosa, tooth extraction, or biopsy. Other complaints include progressive loss of fit of the prosthesis, including tightness, looseness, and changes in occlusion. Vital signs and results of various laboratory investigations consistently have been reported to be normal.

Melrose and colleagues (1976) reported an increased tendency of traumatic cysts to develop in patients with FCOD. These occurred in 14 of their 34 patients (41%). Five of their patients (36%) had pain or a dull aching sensation at the site of a traumatic bone cyst. Only 4 of the 17 traumatic cysts found in these patients occurred in edentulous areas. Follow-up information was available for 9 of the 14 patients, with follow-up ranging from 1 to 29 years. In 6 of these 9 patients, resolution was observed after surgical treatment; however, the area filled with abnormal tissue similar to the tissue in the adjacent bone. In the other 3 patients, only partial resolution occurred and the cysts persisted or enlarged. In a period of 7 years, 1 patient had 3 traumatic cysts develop, each in different parts of the mandible. Two of these healed after surgery, and the third remained unchanged; a fourth traumatic cyst then developed in the anterior maxilla. Another patient had three separate traumatic cysts develop over a 22-year period; however, each healed after surgery.

In summary, the traumatic cysts associated with FCOD are essentially similar to other traumatic cysts with these differences: (1) a tendency to occur in adults; many traumatic cysts occur in children, but Kaugars and Cale (1987) observed that those in patients without FOCD who were older than 30 years occurred mostly in black women; (2) a tendency to occur in female patients; ordinary traumatic cysts occur with a ratio of 2:1, favoring male over female patients; (3) a tendency to be symptomatic; most traumatic cysts are asymptomatic; (4) a tendency to heal with the lesional tissue of FCOD after surgery; ordinary traumatic cysts heal with normal healthy bone; (5) a tendency to recur or enlarge after treatment; although the sample was small (three of nine cases), recurrence of ordinary traumatic cysts is rare but may occur, especially as found by Kaugars and Cale (1987) in women; and (6) a tendency toward multiple traumatic cysts in a single patient; ordinarily, multiple traumatic cysts are a rare occurrence, but Kaugars and Cale (1987) observed that when multiple traumatic cysts occur in the same patient, there is a greater tendency toward recurrence.

Mirra and co-workers (1978) reported that approximately 10% of traumatic cysts in the long bones contain a cementum-like substance within their walls. They cited several reports, including that of Friedman and Goldman (1969) and Mirra and colleagues (1978). They found that the largest proportion of these cases were in the neck of the femur, even though most traumatic cysts in the long bones occur in the humerus. Mirra and colleagues (1978) stated that this substance does not represent true cementum, but that it is a cementum-like substance consisting of hypocellular, cementum-like osteoid and bone that may represent ''ancient'' filled-in forms of the traumatic cyst. One wonders whether the cementum-like substance found in association with traumatic cysts in the long bones is similar to the cementum-like substance in FCOD. In the jaws, there is an association of some cases of FCOD with traumatic cysts,and in the long bones, there is an association of some traumatic cysts with a cementum-like substance in their walls. The similarity of the two tissues was so great that Friedman and Goldman (1969) reported these cases as ''cementoma of the long bones.''

Treatment/Prognosis

Waldron (1975) has discussed treatment methods for this condition. He stated that biopsy probably is not indicated for asymptomatic lesions discovered on routine radiographs; however, the patient should be examined radiographically periodically. In the patient with symptoms, the usual cause is infection, which produces chronic osteomyelitis. Because of this complication, some believe that this condition should be termed chronic diffuse sclerosing osteomyelitis. We do not favor the use of this term, but we do believe that chronic osteomyelitis should be diagnosed when signs and symptoms indicate that such a complication has occurred in a patient with FCOD. Waldron (1975) recommended the use of antibiotics for chronic osteomyelitis; however, antibiotic treatment alone has had limited success, perhaps because some of these infections are caused by anaerobes. Thus, culture (both aerobic and anaerobic) and sensitivity tests are useful. Drugs such as clindamycin have been effective for anaerobic infections in bone. Waldron (1975) also suggested that sequestration of the cemental mass should be allowed to occur slowly and healing will follow. He stated that attempts at saucerization or partial surgical removal of the large sclerotic masses have not been very beneficial, and total removal requires fairly extensive surgery. Such a case illustrating these points has been reported by Goldstein and colleagues (1979). Waldron (1975) recommended that all reasonable efforts should be made to preserve the teeth because a protracted clinical course of osteomyelitis and pain have followed elective extractions. Additionally, missing teeth should be replaced with fixed prostheses when circumstances permit.

◆ *RADIOLOGY (Figs. 18–3 to 18–7)*

In our experience, FCOD is the most common generalized radiopacity in the United States. In its mature form, it consists of multiple sclerotic masses usually involving the anterior and posterior regions of at least one jaw and sometimes both and is limited to the tooth-bearing areas. This condition appears to occur only in the jaws. Melrose and colleagues (1976) obtained skeletal radiographs for three patients with extensive four-quadrant jaw involvement and found no evidence of skeletal osseous disease. Before reviewing the detailed radiologic features of FCOD, one should check the radiologic description of periapical cemental dysplasia because this information is additive and in some cases applicable to periapical cemental dysplasia. To explain the radiologic characteristics of FCOD, we will study the radiologic details of a single sclerotic mass. Most of these details also may be seen in periapical cemental dysplasia.

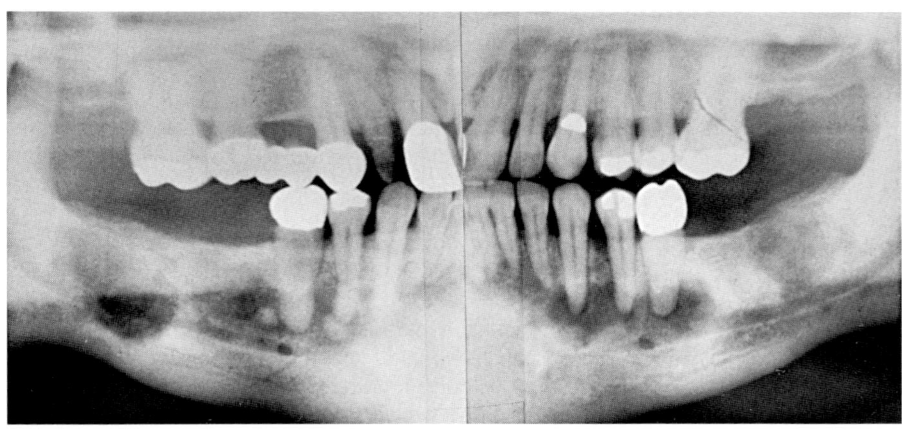

FIGURE 18–3.

Florid Cemento-osseous Dysplasia: Early osteolytic and cementoblastic stages involving mandible and parts of maxilla.

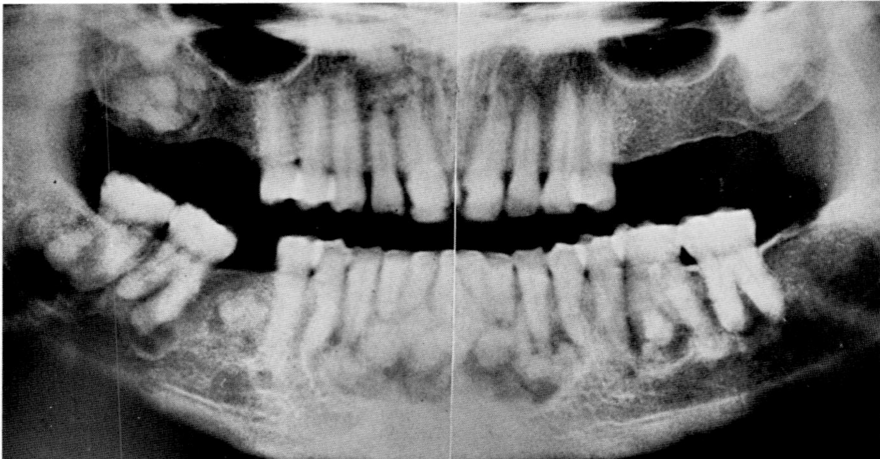

FIGURE 18–4.

Florid Cemento-osseous Dysplasia: Mature stage, with multiple cemental masses in all quadrants. Individual central masses are surrounded by more masses, forming a larger mass.

General Radiologic Features

Before studying the more intimate radiologic details of FCOD, one also should remember the following characteristics of most cemental lesions: (1) development in stages, with radiolucent, mixed, and radiopaque phases; (2) the simultaneous presence of lesions of varying maturity in the same patient; (3) the presence of multiple foci of lesional tissue; (4) the development of a radiopaque component toward the center of a radiolucent area, giving a ''targetlike'' appearance; (5) maturation through brief active phases and longer dormant periods, with the total minimum maturity time possibly exceeding 10 years; (6) smooth and rounded cemental masses, possibly with irregular or lobulated margins, that lack pointed spicules as are seen at the margins of bone masses; cemental masses tend to be of homogeneous density, but small islands of radiolucent material also may be seen within the mass; (7) possible disappearance of cemental masses without treatment, probably through chronic infection and sequestration; (8) possible retrogression of a mature lesion to an earlier stage during additive periods of reactivation; and (9) probable failure of the cemental mass to be resorbed, although it may be added to, it may coalesce with an adjacent mass, or it may sequestrate.

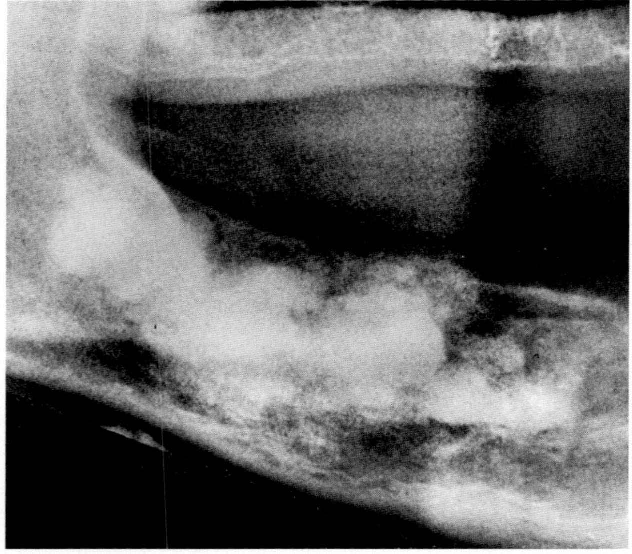

FIGURE 18–5.

Florid Cemento-osseous Dysplasia: In this instance, the mature stage consists of a continuous band of coalesced masses. There are calcific spherules and massules in the region of masses.

Location

FCOD occurs most frequently over a large expanse of the affected bone. Most lesions are seen in the mandible, and some patients also have maxillary lesions. In their series of 16 cases, Bhaskar and Cutright (1968) reported that 7 occurred in the mandible alone (44%), 7 in the mandible and maxilla (44%), and 2 in the maxilla only (12%).

Melrose and colleagues (1976) subdivided their 34 cases into those with traumatic bone cysts and those without. Of the 20 cases without traumatic bone cysts, all but one involved the anterior mandible and both posterior quadrants. The one case not involving the anterior mandible had bilateral involvement of the posterior quadrants only. Among the 19 cases involving the anterior mandible and both posterior quadrants, posterior quadrant involvement was symmetrically bilateral in most cases, extending at least as far back as the first molar and most often to the third molar. Among these 20 cases, 14 (70%) also had maxillary involvement. In 6 of these maxillary cases, involvement was as extensive and symmetrically bilateral as in the mandible, with anterior and posterior quadrants affected. In the remaining 8 maxillary cases, involvement was less extensive, with smaller anterior regions alone or smaller posterior regions alone being affected; in some instances, unilateral involvement occurred only in the posterior quadrants. The FCOD did not extend beyond the third molar regions in any case.

Among the 14 cases of FOCD with traumatic bone cysts reported by Melrose and colleagues (1976), all but 4 involved the anterior mandible and both posterior quadrants with sclerosing cemental masses. Among the 4 remaining cases, 1 involved the anterior mandible and 1 posterior quadrant only and the other 3 involved mandibular posterior

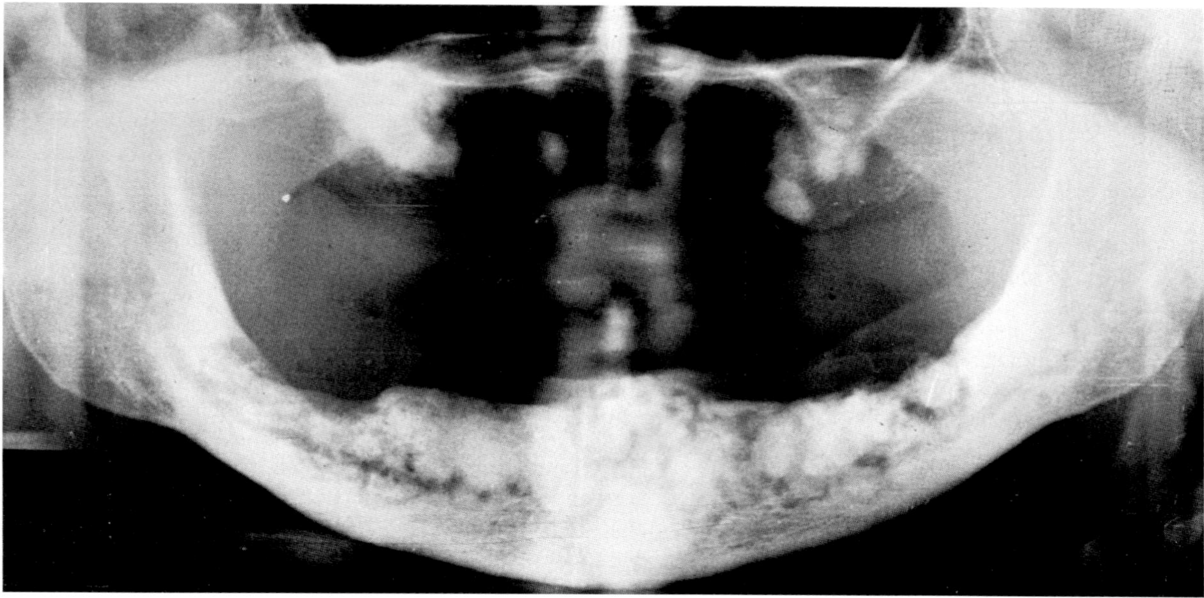

FIGURE 18–6.

Florid Cemento-osseous Dysplasia: Figure shows complication of chronic osteomyelitis in mandible, with some masses undergoing active sequestration. Masses are surrounded by a distinct radiolucent margin representing a zone of inflammation between reactive host bone and nonreactive cemental masses. Maxillary lesions are dormant.

quadrants only; however, all 3 of these cases also involved the maxilla (1 in the anterior region only, and 2 cases in the anterior and posterior regions). Among the 14 cases with traumatic cysts, 10 (71%) involved the mandible and maxilla. Although most of these cases extended back to the third molar region, the symmetric bilateralism of the involved regions was interrupted by the presence of traumatic cysts. The FCOD did not extend beyond the third molar regions in any case.

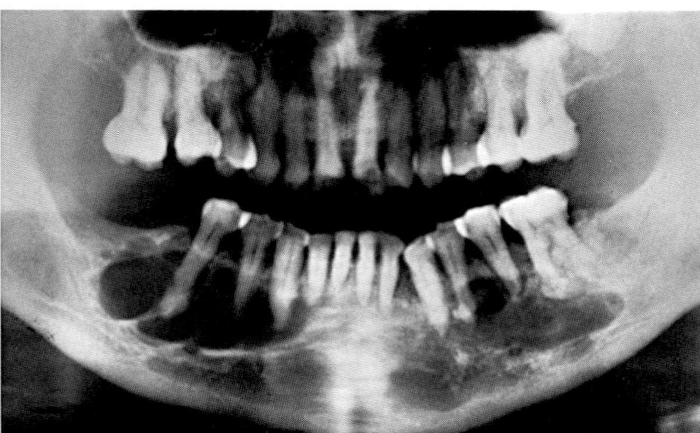

FIGURE 18–7.

Florid Cemento-osseous Dysplasia: Figure shows complication of traumatic cyst in the mandible of a 36-year-old black woman. A biopsy was performed on the lesion in the left mandible several weeks previously; it was found to be a traumatic cyst. The lesion in the right mandible represents a second traumatic cyst. (Courtesy of Dr. Linda L. Otis, University of California at San Francisco, San Francisco, CA.)

Radiologic Features

The radiologic characteristics of FCOD are identical to those of periapical cemental dysplasia, except that more areas are involved, more severely. It is a more mature and generalized manifestation—thus the term "florid." This florid form develops in four possible ways:

1. Initial involvement of the anterior region of the mandible, known as periapical cemental dysplasia during this stage, through to more advanced stages and subsequent involvement of the posterior quadrants in a bilateral and symmetric manner. This pattern is seen most frequently in Americans of African origin.
2. Initially, but much less frequently, involvement of the posterior regions of the mandible bilaterally, known as sclerosing cemental masses during this stage, through to more advanced stages and subsequent involvement of the anterior region. This pattern is seen more frequently in Japanese patients and possibly Americans of Mongoloid extraction.
3. Simultaneous initial involvement of the anterior and posterior regions of the mandible, with the entire arch progressing through the various stages.
4. In 70% of the cases, ultimate or simultaneous involvement of the maxilla in one of the following patterns: (a) in the anterior midline only; (b) symmetrically bilaterally in the posterior quadrants only; (c) unilaterally in one posterior quadrant only; or (d), in approximately half the maxillary cases, in a generalized manner involving the entire arch.

In studying the radiologic characteristics of FCOD, it is important to remember that the lesional tissue of FCOD is cementum or a cementum-like substance, identical to that of periapical cemental dysplasia. Thus, FCOD develops in stages: (1) osteoporotic, showing a focal more osteoporotic area at the apex of an affected vital tooth; (2) osteolytic, characterized by the development of radiolucent areas at the apices of vital teeth, representing lysis of bone and replacement with a fibrovascular connective tissue; (3) cementoblastic, with the development of a radiopaque component within the radiolucent areas representing bone trabeculae undergoing lysis, a fibrovascular connective tissue, proliferating cementum, and a small central cemental mass; (4) mature, characterized by cemental masses as large as 1.5 cm either surrounded by a radiolucent zone ranging from 1 to 3 mm in size or in direct apposition with normal alveolar bone; and (5) florid, consists of the coalescence of individual mature cemental masses that have reached a size of 1.5 cm or greater to form a more or less continuous, albeit irregular, band of radiopaque material extending throughout the jaws in the tooth-bearing portions.

Osteoporotic Stage. We have not observed the osteoporotic stage in a case of FCOD, but we surmise that such a stage exists. Because this finding is new with regard to periapical cemental dysplasia and remains to be confirmed by more definitive studies, we await additional information with regard to this stage in FCOD.

Osteolytic Stage. The lytic radiolucent stage usually is confined to the apical regions of one or several vital anterior or posterior teeth; however, in FCOD large regions of an entire arch or both arches may be so affected. A rather thick, irregular, sclerotic rim of reactive host bone may be seen at the margin of the radiolucent area. The apical portion of the lamina dura is usually absent around the involved teeth.

Cementoblastic Stage. The cementoblastic stage is most interesting and characteristic. Initially, there is a small central radiopaque cemental mass measuring 3 to 5 mm in diameter, surrounded by a radiolucent zone measuring 2 to 7 mm in width; the outer margin of the radiolucent zone may or may not be lined by a thick, irregular sclerotic rim of host bone. The central cemental mass consists of a homogeneous density, sometimes interspersed with small radiolucent islands, and the mass has smooth, rounded margins, although these may be irregular or granular.

The intermediate radiolucent zone is divided into three radiologically distinct "activity bands." The outer band is primarily lytic in nature and represents replacement of host bone with fibrous connective tissue and cementicles. In this band, trabeculae of bone and connective tissue may be seen histologically. In some regions of the middle band of the radiolucent zone, tiny clusters of radiopaque calcific spherules, with or without a radiolucent center, can be seen. These spherules are round or ovoid and consist of a very faint radiodensity, perhaps less than that of the bone initially. They are approximately 0.2 mm in diameter, and the clustering characteristic helps make them visible. These spherules represent partially or completely coalesced cementicles. They can be viewed best through the magnifying lens, and, in our experience, they seem to be seen more easily on panoramic radiographs than periapical radiographs; however, more details are apparent in the intraoral radiographs on occasions when the calcific spherules are readily seen. In other regions of the middle band, spherules can be seen to coalesce, forming small massules that have a granular appearance radiologically. These massules are more radiodense than spherules and measure 1 to 2 mm. Although the massules are often circular and droplet-like, they also may assume irregular shapes but with smooth contours. The inner activity band of the radiolucent zone lies in direct apposition with the central cemental mass. In this region, massules coalesce with each other and with the central cemental mass.

During the cementoblastic stage, the central cemental mass grows in a fairly circular fashion and sometimes in a crescent shape as it enlarges around the apices of teeth. As the central mass enlarges, the radiolucent zone narrows. In periapical cemental dysplasia (PCD), the growth of cementomas appears to be limited to approximately 1 or 1.5 cm in diameter. In FCOD, the cementoblastic stage is more persistent, with most cemental masses larger than 1.5 cm in diameter. Additionally, multiple foci of involvement may be seen throughout the jaws.

Mature Stage. In the mature stage, a central cemental mass is observed. The margins are smooth, although they may be irregular and granular. Spiculation is absent. The mass is most often densely homogeneous, without internal structure. At times, a slight whorl-like pattern may be observed or tiny islands of radiolucent material may be seen throughout the cemental mass. The cemental mass usually is surrounded by a thin radiolucent zone. In such instances a sclerotic rim may be present at the outer margin, but rarely so during this stage unless the lesion is reactivating. On rare occasions the cemental mass is in direct apposition with the surrounding bone, without a radiolucent halo, signifying a dormant state. In these cases the cemental mass greatly resembles sclerotic bone; however, the internal characteristics of the cemental mass, with smooth, rounded, or granular margins and the lack of pointed spicules at the margin help to indicate the diagnosis. Additionally, because cemental lesions are multifocal, other areas of the jaws may manifest more diagnostic lesions at different stages.

Florid Stage. In FCOD we mentioned that there is a florid (fully developed) stage. This is truly appropriate; whether the lesion is florid from inception or it becomes florid from a pre-existing PCD, it is this stage that distinguishes FCOD as separate from PCD. During this stage, small radiolucent zones representing earlier phases may appear adjacent to part of a large mass. These "additive zones" are 0.5 to 1 cm in diameter and show all of the features of the stages previously described. As the masses enlarge beyond 1.5 cm in diameter, they become less circular and more ovoid in appearance. During this period, one mass can be seen to coalesce with another as the additive zones evolve through the various stages. At this point, the multiple coalesced masses impart a pagetoid appearance to the jaws; however, one must remember the following differences between Paget's disease and FCOD: (1) FCOD is more severe in the mandible, with less severe or even no involvement of the maxilla in some cases, whereas Paget's disease involves primarily the maxilla and is seen rarely in the mandible; (2) FCOD is much more radiodense than Paget's disease; and (3) Paget's disease invariably shows zones of alveolar bone changes characterized by a ground glass appearance and loss of the lamina dura. The alveolar bone and cervical two thirds of the lamina dura are normal in FCOD. Occasionally a continuous band of homogeneous cementum-like material extends throughout the tooth-bearing areas; the appearance resembles a band more frequently when the teeth are present and may occur in people of Asian extraction.

Active/Quiescent Periods. Active and quiescent periods have been mentioned with respect to this condition. The outer sclerotic rim has been reported as a variable feature in PCD and FCOD. Because the sclerotic rim is seen in earlier stages, it probably represents an attempt to contain the lytic process by reactive host bone. Thus, when the outer sclerotic rim is present, bone lysis probably is occurring actively. Sometimes, during the cementoblastic stage, the outer sclerotic rim becomes nonexistent. This feature, along with narrowing of the radiolucent band and an absence of spherule and massule formation, indicates that the lesion has become quiescent. When the cemental mass can be found in direct apposition with bone, it may be considered absolutely inactive. If a narrow radiolucent band is seen along with a prominent sclerotic rim, the lesion may be determined to be undergoing reactivation.

Other Radiologic Features. Other features of FCOD include expansion, as seen on occlusal radiographs. Thus, prostheses tend to lose their fit. Also, hypercementosis has been observed in a few cases; however, we believe that hypercementosis is not a usual feature of FCOD. In other cases, the cemental masses appear to attach directly to the roots of some involved teeth, but tooth removal usually does not result in removal of the mass.

Complications/Sequelae: Chronic Osteomyelitis. One complication of FCOD is the development of chronic osteomyelitis and sequestration of a cemental mass. As previously mentioned, this complication usually occurs after tooth extraction over an involved area or in edentulous regions. With resorption of the alveolar ridge, eventually there is no alveolar bone between the soft tissue and the cemental mass. As infection develops, a radiolucent component may appear surrounding one of the cemental masses partially or completely. When infection is present, individual cemental masses become more evident. The affected mass will project into the oral cavity and ultimately may sequestrate. Usually, one area becomes infected at a time; however, patients with edentulous areas are subject to multiple episodes of infection and sequestration. Because of this complication, Shafer (1957) previously used the term chronic diffuse sclerosing osteomyelitis for FCOD.

Complications/Sequelae: Traumatic Cysts. One of the complications of FCOD is the development of traumatic cysts. Their frequency and distribution already have been discussed. Melrose and colleagues (1976) found a total of 17 traumatic cysts in 14 patients. Only one of the traumatic cysts did not occur in the mandible. The cysts were 0.5 to 3.5 cm except for one very large cyst involving almost the entire mandible. Four of the cysts were found in edentulous regions. The remaining 13 were associated with dentate areas, and 3 of these were limited to the area between the roots of mandibular molars. Smaller cysts were unilocular; however, larger cysts appeared multilocular, with internal septa and scalloped margins. Larger cysts appeared to extend up between the teeth and down to the inferior border of the mandible. Expansion was found in 4 patients with larger cysts; in these areas the cortex appeared intact but thinned. In 3 cases mineralized tissue attached to a root apex projected into the bony cavity. The larger multilocular cysts resembled other multilocular lesions; however, all of these showed involvement of other areas of the mandible and maxilla with FCOD, thus suggesting the diagnosis of traumatic cyst for the multilocular lesions.

DIFFUSE SCLEROSING OSTEOMYELITIS

In light of the previous discussion on FCOD, one is left in doubt as to whether diffuse sclerosing osteomyelitis remains a distinct entity. Shafer and colleagues (1983) stated that both conditions are almost identical clinically and radiologically, except in one instance the calcified product is bone, whereas in the other it is cementum. We believe that FCOD and the lesions identified by Shafer and colleagues as chronic diffuse sclerosing osteomyelitis are very similar, in that the latter represents FOCD with the complication of osteomyelitis. These two conditions are distinct from the condition we describe in this chapter as diffuse sclerosing osteomyelitis. We believe that diffuse sclerosing osteomyelitis as described here represents a distinct and separate entity. Therefore, we suggest that the term chronic diffuse sclerosing osteomyelitis as defined by Shafer and colleagues (1983) be discontinued. The 2 largest reported series of diffuse sclerosing osteomyelitis consisted of 21 Swedish patients reported by Jacobsson and Hollender (1980) and 27 Dutch patients studied by van Merkesteyn and colleagues (1988). Jacobsson and Hollender (1980) considered the condition rare because they found only 35 cases in the records of 18 Swedish clinics.

Pathologic Characteristics

Jacobsson and Hollender (1980) classified sclerosing osteomyelitis into focal and diffuse types. The focal type is known as condensing osteitis or focal sclerosing osteomyelitis, whereas the diffuse type is referred to as diffuse sclerosing osteomyelitis (DSO). The former condition is discussed in Chapter 17. According to their findings, the clinical symptoms, radiologic appearance, and histologic features of DSO are characteristic but not pathognomonic. When a diagnosis is made, treatment often is protracted, with many patients failing to respond or having multiple relapses, often over a lifetime. They believe that the condition is caused by the hematogenous spread of normal oral flora to the bone marrow, but with some local or systemic factor that predisposes the patient to a protracted clinical course. Other etiologic hypotheses, as discussed by van Merkesteyn and colleagues (1990), include the following: an immunologic reaction to bacterial toxins, endogenous bacterial infection, and hyperactive immunologic response. Additionally, occasional cases of spontaneous regression have been reported by Jacobsson (1984) and van Merkesteyn and colleagues (1988). In a study of 27 cases of diffuse sclerosing osteomyelitis, van Merkesteyn and co-authors (1990) found little evidence supporting an infectious origin of the disease. They also proposed that chronic tendoperiostitis of one or more of the masseter or digastric muscles is an etiologic factor in DSO of the mandible.

According to van Merkesteyn and colleagues (1988), the histologic characteristics consist of subperiosteal bone formation and remodeling of cortical and subcortical bone, which result in an increase in bone volume. Necrotic foci are a variable feature because they were present in the series of Jacobsson and Heyden (1977) and absent in the series of van Merkesteyn and colleagues (1988). The latter authors found small collections of granulocytes or lymphocytes in approximately 50% of the cases. They found that the bone and stromal pattern was suggestive of a reactive process, however; paradoxically, bacteriologic studies and treatment results did not show any evidence of a microbial cause. They suggested that the small foci of inflammatory cells could be explained by tissue breakdown.

Clinical Features

Jacobsson and Hollender (1980) studied a series of 21 patients. Five of these patients were excluded because of inadequate follow-up. The remaining 16 were observed for 3 to 19 years. The sample consisted of 12 female and 4 male patients, for a female-to-male ratio of 3:1. In comparison, in most studies of FCOD the female-to-male ratio is 10:1. The age at onset ranged from 8 to 53 years; the mean patient age was 25 years, and the average was 27 years. Only 3 patients were older than 40 years. Thus, the age was significantly lower than that of patients with FCOD. Additionally, all of the patients were white (personal communication). Van Merkesteyn and colleagues (1988) studied 27 Dutch patients over an 8-year period. Among these, 14 were female and 13 were male. The ages at diagnosis ranged from 10 to 72 years, and the median and mean ages were approximately equal (43 years). The onset of symptoms occurred approximately 4 years before diagnosis.

Diffuse sclerosing osteomyelitis is characterized by recurrent pain and swelling, usually in half of the mandible, and often is accompanied by limited opening of the mouth. During exacerbations, patients often have subfebrile temperatures and increased erythrocyte sedimentation rates. Hyperesthesia of the mental nerve is a rare finding. According to van Merkesteyn and colleagues (1988), sinus tract formation does not occur and is considered to be incompatible with a diagnosis of DSO. Jacobsson and Hollender (1980) reported symptoms including pain, swelling, and trismus for all of the patients. Additionally, severe ankylosis of the temporomandibular joint developed in 3 patients. Sometimes body temperatures were slightly elevated, with increased erythrocyte sedimentation rates. Van Merkesteyn and colleagues (1988) found that recurrent pain was the major complaint in most cases. The pain occurred in the mandible in all cases. In 2 of the 27 cases, the pain began in the temporomandibular joint. An additional 3 patients had pain in the temporal bone at a later stage of the disease. All but 1 patient reported recurrent swelling, which occurred most often at the inferior border of the mandible in the region of the body, angle, and ramus. Recurrent trismus was found in 18 patients (67%). In 7 patients (26%), slight changes in sensation in the chin or lower lip were noticed during acute exacerbations. In FCOD, the vital signs and laboratory values usually are normal, and approximately 50 to 70% of patients with FCOD had no symptoms at diagnosis.

Treatment/Prognosis

Jacobsson and Hollender (1980) recommended the following management regimen, with emphasis on early diagnosis and treatment for the best prognosis: (1) initially, penicillin should be administered, even if culture results are negative, and continued for at least 3 months unless culture and sensitivity tests indicate a more favorable antibiotic; (2) cortisone therapy has been especially helpful to those with prolonged, unresponsive pain and swelling during the initial phases; (3) the patient should be observed for several years, with routine physical and radiologic examinations; (4) in patients with trismus, stretch exercises should be avoided; (5) in those with trismus, dental extractions also should be avoided and, when absolutely necessary, should be performed with antibiotic prophylaxis; (6) on failure of the initial therapy and with progression of the clinical and radiographic findings, surgical debridement (decortication) may be performed; the prognosis is best when the condition extends minimally into the ramus; and (7) cortisone is an excellent adjunct to therapy in the late chronic stages.

◆ *RADIOLOGY (Figs. 18–8 and 18–9)*

Diffuse sclerosing osteomyelitis is characterized by progressive, diffuse sclerosis of the mandible and, in very rare instances, the maxilla in white patients.

Location

Diffuse sclerosing osteomyelitis is confined mainly to the mandible. Jacobsson and Hollender (1980) reported that several cases have been found in the maxilla. Additionally, Hardmeier and colleagues (1974) described a case affecting the elbow. In the 16 cases analyzed by Jacobsson and Hollender (1980), all were in the mandible. None was bilateral or limited to the midline. All of the cases involved the mandibular body most frequently in the premolar and molar regions, and some extended to the canine incisor area. All but one of the cases (94%) also extended posteriorly to involve part or all of the ramus. In 7 cases (44%) involvement of the ramus included the coronoid process, sigmoid notch, and mandibular condyle. One case showed sclerosis of the condylar fossa as well. Van Merkesteyn and colleagues (1988) found that the location could be divided into 4 patterns: (1) involvement of the mandibular angle, with some cases extending to the

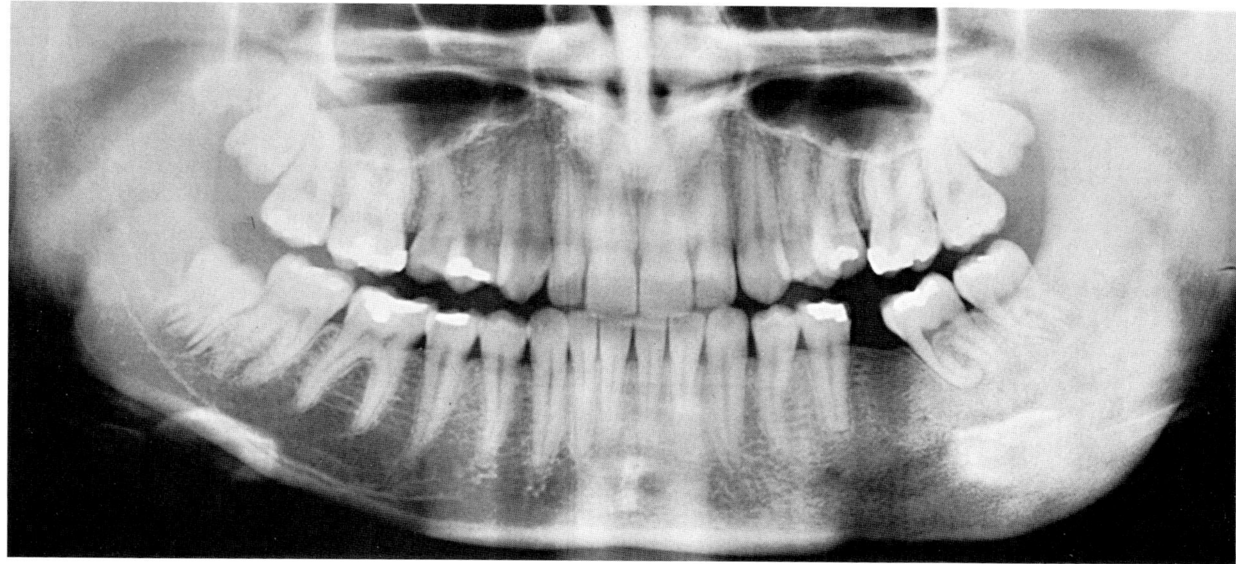

A

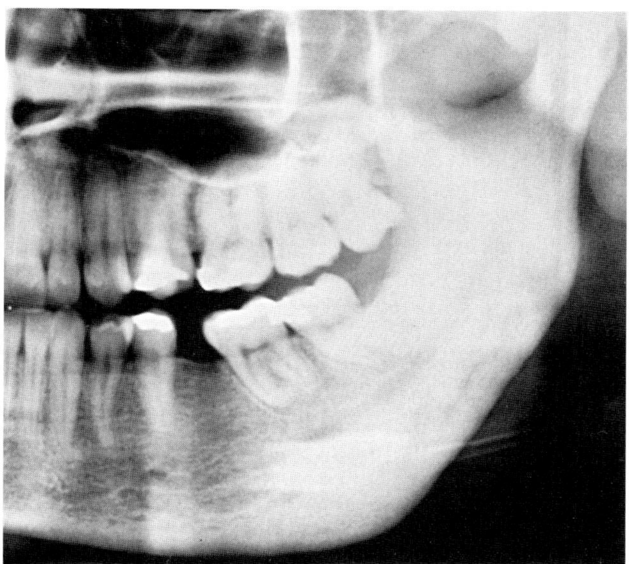

B

FIGURE 18–8.

Diffuse Sclerosing Osteomyelitis: Case in a Swedish woman. A, At age 18, there is more advanced eruption of the mandibular left third molar. The cortex appears thinned on the left, and there is diffuse sclerosis of the left angle and ramus. B, At age 22, the affected area is more diffusely homogeneous, and the canal within is more prominent. (Courtesy of L. Hollender, University of Washington School of Dentistry, Seattle, WA, and the Department of Dental Radiology, Göteborg University, Göteborg, Sweden.)

midline with or without ramus involvement including the condyle and coronoid process (41%); (2) involvement of the angle, with some cases extending beyond the midline to the contralateral side with or without ramus involvement including the condyle and coronoid process (41%); (3) involvement of the midline, including the angle bilaterally, with some cases extending part way up the ramus unilaterally or bilaterally (15%); and (4) involvement of the midline, with bilateral extension to the molar region only (7%).

Jacobsson and Hollender (1980) reported that 81% involved the right mandible, whereas van Merkesteyn and colleagues (1990) observed right side involvement in 74%, although some of these also included involvement of the left side. There were only 6 cases (22%) with involvement of the left side alone, whereas there were 11 cases (41%) with involvement of only the right side.

Radiologic Features

According to van Merkesteyn and associates (1988), lesions can be characterized as diffusely sclerotic (37%) or sclerotic with lytic areas intermingled (63%). The condition probably begins in the molar-ramus region and spreads anteriorly and posteriorly. Van Merkesteyn and associates (1988) believed there is a striking preference for involvement of the buccal portion of the distal mandibular body from the mandibular angle to molar region, with decreasing changes toward the ramus and canine regions. Teeth may or may not be present. According to Jacobsson and Hollender (1980), the sclerotic areas appear to be in direct apposition with normal bone, without any of the features of FCOD. Ultimately, the entire mandibular body becomes involved diffusely. The areas of increased density are diffuse, homogeneous, and much like the diffuse homogeneous pattern seen in some cases of fi-

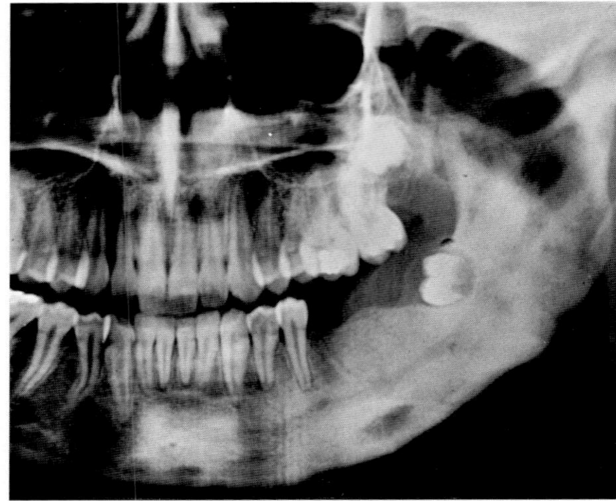

A

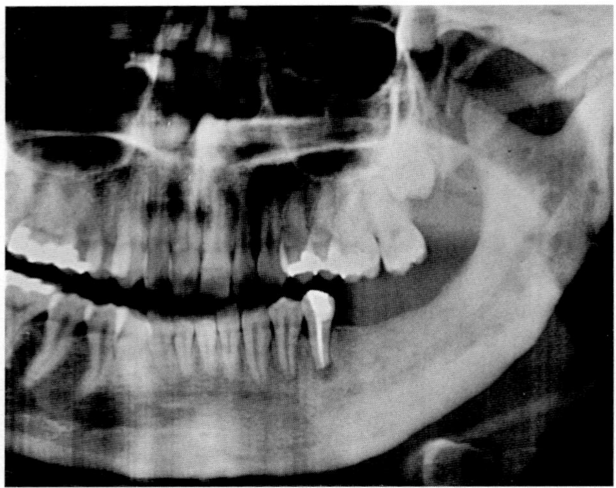

B

FIGURE 18–9.

Diffuse Sclerosing Osteomyelitis: Case in a Swedish woman. A, At age 13, there is diffuse sclerosis from the left ramus to right canine, radiolucent foci of inflammation, and a larger area of rarefaction including the cortex in ramus. The inferior alveolar canal is prominent. The left third molar is closer to the crest of the ridge, and the cortical outline of the crypt blends imperceptibly with surrounding bone. B, At age 18, affected area appears thinned. Some radiolucent foci have healed, and others remain in the upper ramus area. (Courtesy of L. Hollender, University of Washington, Seattle, WA; and the Department of Dental Radiology, Göteborg University, Göteborg, Sweden.)

brous dysplasia. The area does not appear pagetoid. The inferior alveolar canal may have a more pronounced appearance within the sclerotic bone. Rarely, there also may be deviation of the canal. The sclerotic changes spread slowly to involve the whole ramus, coronoid process, and condyle. The overall size of the mandible and ramus in affected areas, especially the angle, actually becomes smaller, even when surgery has not been performed. The condyles and coronoid process may become enlarged or deformed, with concomitant reduction in the depth of the sigmoid notch. Occasionally, one or several punched-out radiolucent areas of osteolysis appear within the sclerotic bone. Such changes often are associated with the onset of symptoms and vanish as the clinical symptoms improve.

With therapy and time, symptoms become less severe and less frequent, with the appearance of fewer osteolytic areas and a predominance of the homogeneous sclerotic pattern. Van Merkesteyn and associates (1990) found external resorption of the inferior border of the mandible in six patients. In four cases, the erosion was present at diagnosis; in one case it appeared before the radiologic signs of DSO; and in another case the erosion developed later. In some cases, the sclerosis may regress to a normal bone architecture.

Special Imaging Studies

On computed tomography scans, there is no endosteal destruction suggestive of abscess formation. Subperiosteal bone formation and endosteal sclerosis can be seen clearly in most cases. Presumably, preferential involvement of the buccal cortex also may be observed.

There is a strong uptake of radionuclide in the mandible in all cases reported in the series of van Merkesteyn and colleagues (1988). They also found increased uptake in the zygomatic arch in two patients, the mandibular fossa in one patient, and the mastoid process in one patient.

FIBROUS DYSPLASIA

According to Waldron (1985) and most other authorities, fibrous dysplasia (FD) is believed to be a non-neoplastic hamartomatous developmental lesion of bone of unknown origin. It is characterized by the replacement of bone with fibro-osseous tissue. In most instances, a certain diagnosis cannot be made on a histologic basis alone, nor can it be made without appropriate, quality radiographs. Mirra and colleagues (1989) stated that FD represents 1% of biopsy-analyzed primary bone conditions and is divided into two basic types: monostotic, in which only one bone is affected, and polyostotic, in which multiple bones are affected. These authors asserted that polyostotic FD is at least six times less frequent than the monostotic type. The polyostotic type may be divided into three subtypes: (1) craniofacial FD, in which only the bones of the craniofacial complex are affected, including the mandible and maxilla; (2) Lichtenstein-Jaffe type, in which multiple bones of the skeleton are involved and, in some instances, there are café au lait pigmentations on the skin and rare endocrinopathies; (3) Albright's syndrome, characterized by the triad of severe polyostotic FD (mostly unilateral), café au lait pigmentations on the skin, and various endocrinopathies, especially precocious puberty in girls.

Historically, polyostotic FD was recognized before the monostotic type. The first cases probably were reported by von Recklinghausen in 1891. Polyostotic FD with skin pigmentations and precocious puberty in girls was recognized independently in 1937 by Albright and colleagues, who suggested the term osteitis fibrosa disseminata, and by McCune and Burch (1937), who recommended the term osteodystrophia fibrosa. In 1938, Lichtenstein suggested the term fibrous dysplasia and described polyostotic FD affecting multiple bones but without skin or endocrine involvement. In 1942, Lichtenstein and Jaffe recognized that polyostotic and monostotic forms may occur. Finally, in 1957 Daves and Yardley recognized instances in which polyostotic FD is limited to the bones of the craniofacial complex, including the jaws, thus the term craniofacial FD.

Pathologic Characteristics

The histologic description of FD is important because jaw lesions are said to be more radiopaque than other skeletal lesions. Additionally, the histologic characteristics of jaw lesions vary somewhat from those reported for the other bones. Waldron (1985) stated that FD, especially in the axial skeleton, classically consists of cellular fibrous connective tissue often arranged in a whorled pattern and containing irregularly shaped trabeculae of immature woven (nonlamellar) bone with feathered margins, arranged in a pattern resembling the letter "C" or "Y" or Chinese characters. Classically, these trabeculae are said to be devoid of osteoid rims and plump appositional osteoblasts. Eversole and coworkers (1972) and Waldron and Giansanti reported that lamellar compact bone and trabecular bone with osteoblastic rimming often were seen in jaw lesions. Also, the incidence of lamellar bone seemed to increase with older lesions. In addition, Eversole and colleagues (1972) observed varying amounts of spheroidal amorphous calcifications that had a greater resemblance to cementum than bone. According to Waldron (1985), similar structures are seen occasionally in FD of the long bones, and Dahlin (1978) stated that these spheroid amorphous structures are the predominant or almost exclusive calcified component of FD involving the skull. In summary, FD involving the jaws may contain the following calcified products: (1) lamellar compact bone, (2) lamellar trabecular bone, (3) woven bone, and (4) cementum-like amorphous calcifications; this probably explains the increased opacity of some jaw lesions.

Clinical Features

Monostotic Fibrous Dysplasia

By definition, monostotic FD occurs in only one bone. In an analysis of 67 cases of monostotic FD, Schlumberger (1949) reported the locations listed in Table 18–1.

According to Mirra (1989), monostotic FD in the skeleton is at least 6 times more common than polyostotic FD. Waldron (1985) also asserted that monostotic FD of the jaws is considerably more common than polyostotic FD. In a series of 69 cases of jaw involvement reported by Zimmerman and colleagues (1958), only 1 patient had extracraniofacial lesions. Among 47 Nigerian patients with FD in the jaws

TABLE 18–1
Locations of 67 Cases of Monostotic Fibrous Dysplasia

Location	No. Cases	Percentage
Ribs	29	43
Femur	9	13
Tibia	8	12
Maxilla	7	10
Calvarium	5	7
Mandible	2	3
Humerus	2	3
Ulna	2	3
Vertebra	1	1.5
Pelvis	1	1.5
Fibula	1	1.5

(Data from Schlumberger HG: Monostotic fibrous dysplasia. Milit Surg 99: 504, 1946.)

reported by Daramola and colleagues (1976), 43 cases (91%) were monostotic, 3 cases (6%) were polyostotic and of the Lichtenstein-Jaffe type, and 1 case (2%) consisted of Albright's syndrome. In this series, 29 cases (62%) were located in the maxilla and 18 cases (38%) in the mandible. Invariably, most authors reported more frequent involvement of the maxilla compared with the mandible.

Polyostotic Fibrous Dysplasia: Craniofacial Type

Eversole and colleagues (1972) classified the craniofacial type as polyostotic because many bones of the craniofacial complex are involved that, except for the mandible, are separated from each other only by sutures. In their series of 25 patients with craniofacial FD, Obisesan and colleagues (1977) found 35 lesions at different sites. Among these, 16 (46%) were in the maxilla, 12 (34%) in the mandible, and 7 (20%) in the craniofacial bones. These latter included 3 in the zygoma, 2 in the orbital walls, and 1 each in the sphenoid and frontal bones. In this series, posterior lesions occurred two to four times more frequently than did anterior lesions. This was true for maxillary and mandibular lesions. In a series of 37 patients with polyostotic FD reported by Harris and colleagues (1962), 15 of the 37 had craniofacial FD, and among this latter group, 50% had thickening of the occiput and base of the skull. They believed these were the 2 most common locations when there is skull involvement.

Polyostotic Fibrous Dysplasia: Lichtenstein-Jaffe Type

Polyostotic FD of the Lichtenstein-Jaffe type involves multiple bones anywhere in the skeleton, including the craniofacial bones and jaws, although such involvement is considered rare. Some of the commonly affected bones include the clavicles, pelvic bones, scapulae, long bones, metacarpals, and metatarsals. The most common site of FD in the extragnathic skeleton is the neck of the femur; this is often the area where the disease first is seen. Café au lait skin pigmentations sometimes may occur in the Lichtenstein-Jaffe type. Mirra and co-workers (1989) estimated that it is present in approximately 50% of cases. Generally speaking, the degree of bone involvement is much milder in this type than in Albright's syndrome. Some authors such as Mirra and associates (1989) include patients with endocrinopathies among those with the Lichtenstein-Jaffe type when the polyostotic FD is not severe or disfiguring.

Polyostotic Fibrous Dysplasia: Albright's Syndrome

Albright's syndrome is the most severe, albeit least frequent, manifestation of FD. According to Mirra and associates (1989), approximately 1 in 30 to 40 patients with FD will have Albright's syndrome. It consists of the classic triad of polyostotic FD, café au lait pigmentation, and precocious puberty in girls. Since the original reports, certain features have been added to each of the basic elements of the classic triad.

Waldron (1985) reported that the extent of bone involvement in polyostotic FD ranges from 5 to 60% of the skeleton. In Albright's syndrome, more bones tend to be involved, individual bone lesions usually are larger and more disfiguring, and the craniofacial complex often is involved in severe cases. Additionally, skeletal involvement tends to be distributed significantly to one side of the skeleton, although the opposite side may be involved. Expansion causes disfigurement, and in the long bones pathologic fractures cause deformities.

The café au lait skin pigmentations tend to be rather large, with irregular margins showing a pattern described as the "coast of Maine.". These often are contrasted with the café au lait skin pigmentations of neurofibromatosis, which have smooth outlines, described as the "coast of California." Additionally, the skin pigmentations also tend to be confined to one side of the body because they often correspond to the locations of severe bone involvement. Skin pigmentations are not present at all sites of bone involvement, however.

The endocrinopathies include precocious puberty characterized by the onset of menses and development of the breasts and sexual organs, sometimes before the age of 3 years. In boys the genitals may be enlarged, and secondary sex characteristics are present. Other endocrinopathies seen much less frequently include hyperthyroidism, hyperparathyroidism, acromegaly, Cushing's syndrome, and diabetes mellitus. Accelerated skeletal growth sometimes is observed.

According to Mirra and colleagues (1989), who reviewed 344 cases of monostotic FD throughout the skeleton, including 6 cases in the mandible, 5 in the maxilla, and 6 in the skull, women were affected slightly more frequently than men, with a male-to-female ratio of 1:1.3. Eversole and colleagues (1972) reviewed 534 cases of FD affecting the jaws, including monostotic, polyostotic, and craniofacial types, and found that female patients were affected more commonly than male patients, depending on the type of FD. In monostotic FD, the ratio was 1.6:1; in polyostotic FD, 1.2:1; and in craniofacial FD, 1.9:1. In FD involving the jaws, authors such as Waldron (1985) reported an approximately equal frequency between male and female patients. Obisesan and colleagues (1977) reported a female-to-male ratio of 2.1:1 in their series of 25 Nigerian patients with FD involving the jaws. In a similar study of 47 Nigerian patients, Daramola and colleagues (1976) found a female-to-male ratio of 3:1.

Mirra and colleagues (1989) reported that FD has been diagnosed in patients 1 to 80 years of age or older, although it rarely is diagnosed before a patient is 2 years of age. According to these authors, 75% of the patients are younger than 30 years of age at diagnosis. The age at diagnosis often is based on the severity and extent of the disease. In a series of 25 patients with FD involving the jaws, Obisesan and colleagues (1977) found that 48% of cases were diagnosed in the second decade of life and 96% of patients were younger than 40 years of age. Eversole and colleagues (1972) reported the following average ages at admission for patients with the various types of FD: craniofacial, 21 years; polyostotic, 24 years; and monostotic, 25 years. All 534 cases that they reviewed from the literature showed jaw involvement, and most of these cases were diagnosed before the patient was 30 years of age. Although most FD cases involving the jaws were diagnosed in the second decade of life, the one exception was polyostotic FD, which had a peak incidence of 39% in the first decade, approximately 25% in the second decade, and only 5% in the third decade. The monostotic and craniofacial types had a peak incidence in the second decade of life, and approximately twice as many cases were diagnosed in the third decade as in the first decade. Thus, diagnosis of FD involving the jaws during the first decade is somewhat predictive of a polyostotic distribution. The literature has numerous reports of patients who were unaware of their disease until accidental discovery in the sixth or seventh decade of life, but these cases are atypical. Such a case was included in the series of Obisesan and colleagues (1977). Harris and colleagues (1962) reported a case that was not diagnosed until the man was 68 years of age, even though the patient had involvement of 30% of his skeleton.

In the axial skeleton FD may be associated with pain, limping, and pathologic fracture, especially when the neck of the femur is affected. Other cases are discovered because swelling is observed. In rare instances, FD is detected when radiographs are taken for other reasons. When Albright's syndrome is present, the initial sign may be vaginal bleeding in a child. In the jaws, pain or fracture is rarely present. The most common complaint is swelling, often toward the buccal side. On examination, the tissue overlying the swelling is a normal color. The teeth usually are not mobile, although in severe cases they may be displaced. With involvement of the maxilla, the nose may appear displaced and there may be nasal obstruction and exophthalmia. In more severe cases of craniofacial involvement, the patient's face may appear significantly asymmetric; with severe involvement, grotesque deformity may be present. The serum laboratory values in FD are usually within normal limits.

Treatment/Prognosis

The clinical course, treatment, and prognosis of FD have been discussed by El Deeb and colleagues (1979) and Waldron (1985). Enlargement is slow and insidious and usually persists until cessation of skeletal growth. In rare instances, enlargement continues into adulthood. The treatment of choice is surgery. When the lesion is small, it may be excised in toto. The goal of treatment for larger lesions should be correction of esthetic and functional disturbances. When surgery is planned in children, it must be remembered that FD is rather vascular, and bleeding problems may be encountered. The blood supply and extent of FD usually are verified by technetium scanning. According to Zimmerman and colleagues (1958), approximately 20% of the lesions continue to grow after therapy in younger patients; however, when the deformity is severe, treatment may be necessary at a younger age. In general, it is recommended that treatment be delayed until after a patient reaches puberty, when lesions tend to become static. In older patients, surgical treatment and tooth extraction may result in osteomyelitis, which may be difficult to manage and result in a protracted course of therapy. As reported by El Deeb and colleagues (1979), in older patients the affected bones in FD tend to become avascular, hard, and sclerotic, thus resulting in bone that is more susceptible to infections. Radiation therapy should not be used to manage any cases of FD. It may be tempting to use radiation therapy in severe cases because such therapy has met with some success; however, as explained by Shafer and colleagues (1983) and Waldron (1985), radiation therapy may result in radiation-induced sarcomas, especially osteogenic sarcoma. Such a case was reported by Slow and colleagues (1971), and many similar reports exist in the literature. Occasionally, however, FD may undergo malignant transformation to osteogenic sarcoma even when radiation therapy is not used. Schwartz and Alpert (1964) reviewed 16 such cases and observed that it occurred more frequently in polyostotic FD and the most common location was the craniofacial region.

◆ *RADIOLOGY (Figs. 18–10 to 18–23)*

The radiology of FD is divided into three main areas of discussion: (1) radiology of the jaws, (2) radiology of the skull and facial bones, and (3) radiology of the skeleton. Additionally, FD may produce radiolucent, radiopaque, or mixed-density lesions. Within these variations certain distinct patterns may be seen. Therefore, we divided our discussion into these topic areas.

Radiologic Features of the Jaws

Most authors agree that the radiographs do not always correlate with the histologic variations. In other words, when the radiograph is predominantly radiolucent, the histologic picture may not be dominated by the fibrous component. Such lesions may or may not contain vast amounts of calcified tissue. The same may be said for predominantly radiopaque manifestations of FD. Additionally, the radiographic variations in bone density do not depend on the age of the lesion or the patient, although we will comment on age with respect to some patterns. It also must be remembered that FD represents a fibrous replacement of bone and that the process occurs from within the bone rather than on the outside. Thus, if the jaws are enlarged it is because of a process occurring entirely within the jaws.

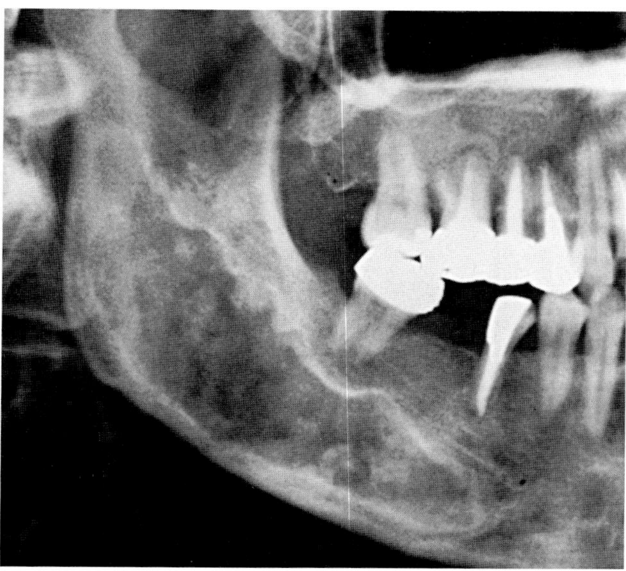

FIGURE 18–10.

Fibrous Dysplasia: Case in a 39-year-old woman shows unicystic radiolucency with rindlike sclerotic margin, containing opacities. The inferior cortex is affected minimally. (Courtesy of M. Araki and K. Hashimoto, Nihon University, School of Dentistry, Tokyo, Japan.)

Location. In the review of Eversole and colleagues (1972), most authors showed that when the jaws are affected by FD, the maxilla is involved more frequently than the mandible. Additionally, the posterior jaws are affected more frequently, although numerous cases have been reported in the anterior jaws. Jaw lesions tend to be monostotic. Involvement of other bones occurs in less than 2% of the cases of jaw FD. Daramola and associates (1976) reported that, among Nigerians, FD is more common in the jaws than in the long bones. In most populations, the most commonly reported site is the femoral neck.

Worth (1963) provided extensive information on the radiology of FD as it affects the jaws; thus, much of our discussion is based on his observations. For this description of FD in the jaws, we divided the radiologic manifestations of FD into three groups: (1) radiolucent, (2) radiopaque, and (3) mixed.

Radiolucent Lesions in the Jaws

The first appearance is that of a unicystic radiolucency. The lesion may be round, oval, or irregularly shaped, with a sclerotic margin. It may be 1 cm in diameter or involve a whole quadrant. In the long bones, the sclerotic margin is highly diagnostic and described as rindlike. In the jaws the sclerotic margin may show one of three appearances: (1) it may be smooth, thin, and sharply defined, exactly resembling a cyst; (2) more frequently, the sclerotic margin is thin but appears granular, suggesting that the lesion is not a cyst; or (3) the margin may consist of a wider band of increased density that is granular in appearance and, when present in a young person, suggests the diagnosis of FD. Worth (1963) emphasized that this sclerotic margin may not surround the radiolu-

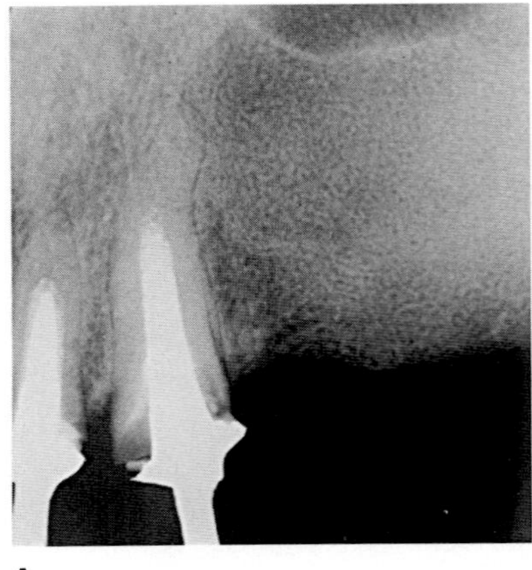

A

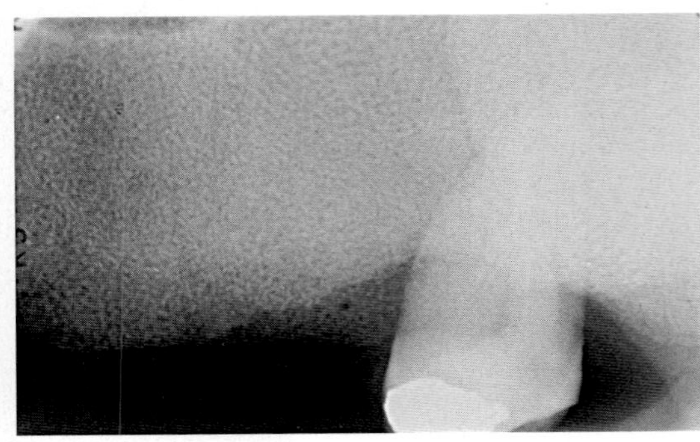

B

FIGURE 18–11.

Fibrous Dysplasia: Case in a 60-year-old man. A and B, Orange peel or stippled radiopaque pattern, distinct from ground glass pattern. (Courtesy of T. Noikura, First Department of Oral Surgery, Kagoshima University, Kagoshima, Japan.)

cent area completely, with only a portion of the periphery so affected. Obisesan and colleagues (1977) observed this pattern with a cystlike sclerotic rim in 1 of their 25 cases.

The second appearance is that of a unilocular radiolucent lesion without a sclerotic margin. In this instance, the margin may show one of two variations: (1) it may be sharply defined and punched-out, without cortication of any kind; or (2) it may be ill defined and trail off imperceptibly into normal bone, thus having a wide transitional zone. In some cases a slight irregularity of the margin can be detected where it abuts on normal bone.

The third appearance is that of a multilocular radiolucent lesion. In this instance, the trabeculae forming the locules may show one of two appearances: (1) they may be few in number, wispy, and of poor density, much like those in central giant cell granuloma; or (2) they may be coarse and thick and resemble those of an ameloblastoma at first glance; in FD, however, they do not tend to be curved or appear to conform to rounded cavities within the bone. The margins are as described for the unilocular variants. Obisesan and colleagues (1977) observed a multilocular pattern in three of their cases (12%).

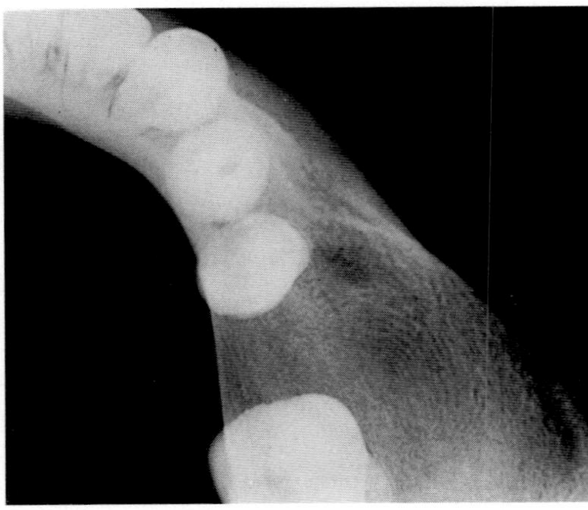

FIGURE 18–12.

Fibrous Dysplasia: Pathognomonic "thumbprintlike" granular radiopaque pattern. (Courtesy of L. Alfaro, University of Chile School of Dentistry, Pathology Referral Center, Santiago, Chile.)

In the study of radiolucent lesions of FD, Worth (1963) advised close scrutiny of the radiolucent area for evidence of opacities. Good-quality radiographs should be used or these can be missed. The opacities, which may be several or many, may show one of two appearances: (1) they may be very small, punctate opacities of poor density and easily go undetected; or (2) they may be larger and appear to be granular.

Radiopaque Lesions in the Jaws

The first variant is that of an "orange peel" or "fingerprint" appearance. This variant is more prone to occur in younger patients and in the maxilla, although it may be seen in the mandible. This bone is denser than normal and very homogeneous in appearance. The margins merge imperceptibly over a broad front with the adjacent bone in most cases. According to Worth (1963), no other lesion shows these changes, thus they are considered pathognomonic. This particular variant curettes out readily, in significant contrast to other varia-

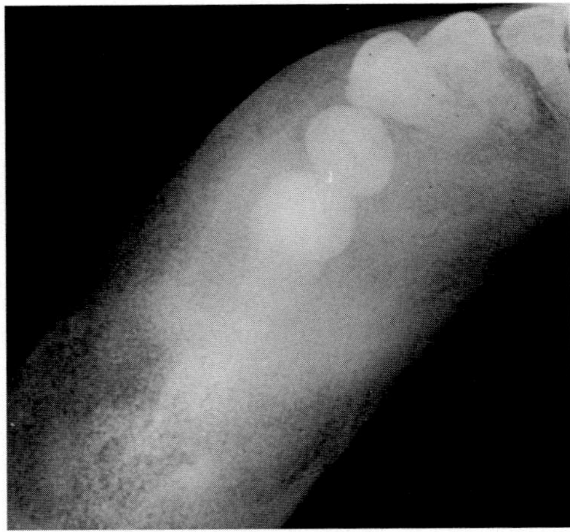

FIGURE 18–13.

Fibrous Dysplasia: There is a ground glass radiopaque pattern and a grayish homogeneous appearance. Cortices have been replaced by fibro-osseous tissue. Although the mandible is widened bucco-lingually, cortical expansion is absent. (Courtesy of L. Alfaro, University of Chile School of Dentistry, Pathology Referral Center, Santiago, Chile.)

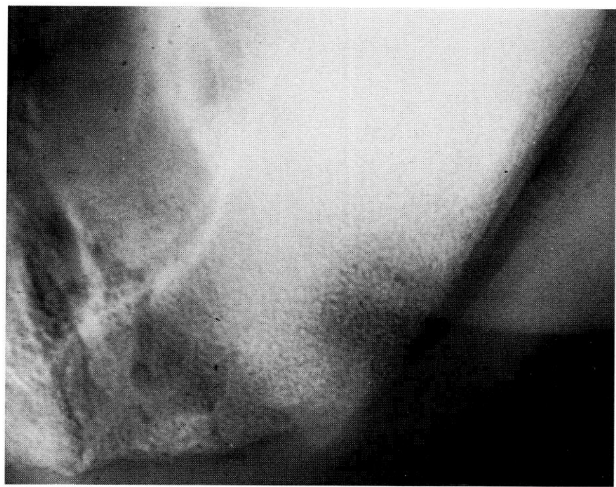

FIGURE 18–14.

Fibrous Dysplasia: Hyperostotic radiopaque pattern in posterior maxilla, with granular appearance anteriorly. (Courtesy of L. Alfaro, University of Chile School of Dentistry, Pathology Referral Center, Santiago, Chile.)

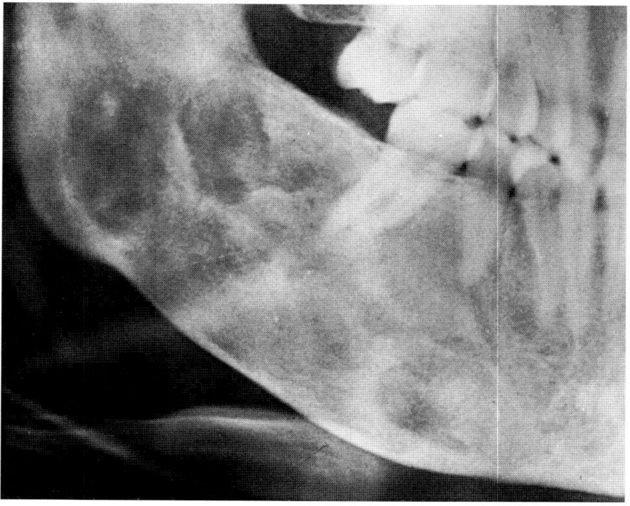

FIGURE 18–15.

Fibrous Dysplasia: Mixed radiolucent and radiopaque pattern in a 44-year-old woman. The molar-premolar area has a ground glass appearance. The angle area shows a multilocular radiolucent pattern with radiopaque masses within. Marginal sclerosis is variable; the inferior cortex is thinned significantly; and the mandible is widened superio-inferiorly.

tions. In the mandible, the stippled (fingerprint) pattern may be arranged more closely than in the maxilla. Also, enlargement may be present, so that the vertical height of the mandible is increased, especially toward the occlusal, and the mandible may increase in width. Although there may be expansion toward the lingual, the buccal side is affected most frequently and to the greatest degree.

Worth (1963) mentioned three additional observations with respect to the inferior cortex: (1) When the mandible is expanded by other diseases, the inferior cortex usually is thinned to some degree; however, when the mandible is enlarged as described by Worth (1963), but with little or no resorption of the inferior cortex, this combination of findings permits immediate recognition of FD. Thus, cortical persistence in combination with bone enlargement is a valuable observation. (2) In other cases, the cortex undergoes the same structural change as the adjacent bone; thus, it takes on an orange peel appearance. (3) The last variation consists of a localized loss of the inferior cortex, whereby it takes the appearance of a thumb print. It looks as though the cortex were soft and, when compressed beneath the thumb, there is a smooth projection downward, with the convexity in an inferior direction. The affected cortex has a stippled appearance, but when it is examined closely, the stippling actually looks like a fingerprint. This fingerprint appearance may be seen anywhere in the mandible and, when recognized, it stamps the diagnosis on the radiograph! In the series of Obisesan and co-workers (1977), the orange peel pattern was seen most frequently, occurring in 10 of the 25 patients (40%), whereas the fingerprint pattern described as whorled plaques was observed in 5 of the 25 cases (20%).

The second variant is that of a ground glass appearance. According to Worth (1963), this pattern is not likely in young patients and is more common in adults. Additionally, this abnormal osseous tissue tends to be extremely hard. It is difficult to remove surgically. The radiographic density of the ground glass appearance is the same as that of the orange peel pattern; however, in this instance the granularity is absent, so the affected area has a very homogeneous gray appearance. The ground glass pattern can be visualized by imagining the surface of a stopper in a large glass or crystal decanter. According to Worth (1963), this variant is more likely in the maxilla than the mandible. In the series of Obisesan and colleagues (1977), this pattern was referred to as chalky and was seen in 1 of the 25 cases.

The third variant is that of a dense structureless homogenous density sometimes referred to as hyperostosis. No stippling (fingerprint) or other pattern is apparent, and the lesional tissue is more or less homogeneously white. This variant is also, according to Worth (1963), more common in the maxilla and the base of the skull. Obisesan and colleagues (1977) termed this pattern ''diffuse sclerotic'' and found it in 4 of the 25 cases (16%). Hyperostosis is a descriptive term, and its use is not limited to the changes produced by FD.

Mixed Radiolucent-Radiopaque Lesions in the Jaws

According to Worth (1963), this is the most common manifestation of FD in the jaws. It simply consists of a mixture of the radiolucent and radiopaque patterns previously described. The most frequent site is the mandible, although it may be seen in the maxilla. When the anterior jaws are affected, this is the pattern that usually is seen. In the mandible, persistence of even a portion of the inferior cortex, in combination with the presence of bone enlargement and areas of bone loss, usually establishes the diagnosis. In other instances, there appears to be an admixture of very dense bone

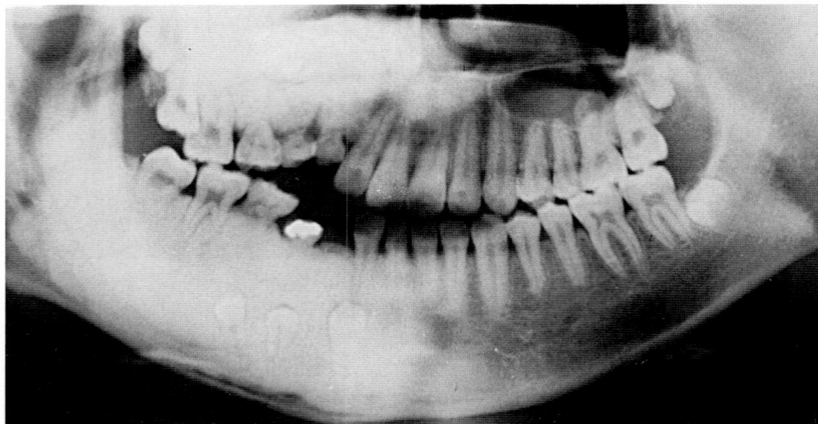

A

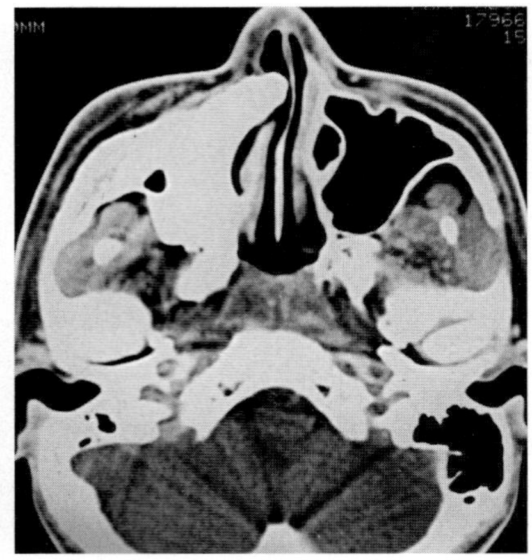

B

FIGURE 18–16.

Fibrous Dysplasia: Figure shows impaction of teeth (craniofacial polyostotic type) in a 16-year-old boy. A, Impaction of unerupted teeth indicates rare early onset and increased possibility of polyostotic distribution. B, Involvement of maxilla, sinus, nasal cavity, and zygoma. (Courtesy of C. S. Park, Department of Dental Radiology, Yonsei University, College of Dentistry, Seoul, Korea.)

in a generally rarefied area and, if a small area with ground glass or orange peel changes can be identified, the diagnosis is suggested. In this mixed type, the proportion of radiolucent versus radiopaque findings is variable, with either appearance predominating or a more or less equal amount of lucent and dense changes.

Worth (1963) described a peculiar pattern in which a wormlike radiodensity appears coiled up within an area of slightly increased radiolucency. There may be several such areas, inferior to the apices of the teeth, most often in the mandible. They usually reach a diameter of approximately 1 inch. It has been our experience that this pattern most often represents examples of central ossifying fibroma that often cannot be distinguished from FD histologically. We illustrate this appearance in Chapter 17. The coiled worm appearance of ossifying fibroma should not be confused with the thumbprint pattern of FD.

Relationship to Teeth. Unerupted teeth are rarely seen in FD, probably because most cases develop after tooth eruption. In rare instances, impacted unerupted teeth may be seen. More frequently, there is displacement of erupted teeth and subsequent alterations in the occlusion. In a series of 25 Nigerian patients reported by Obisesan and colleagues (1977), dental displacement occurred in 9 cases (36%). They found that tooth displacement correlated with lesion size and location. Larger lesions and involvement of incisor teeth resulted in the most displacements. When there is extension into the antrum, teeth may be displaced into the sinus along with the fibro-osseous tissue. Root resorption is not a usual

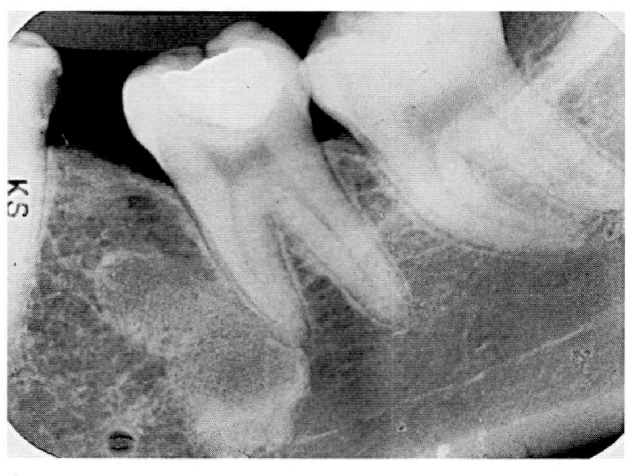

A

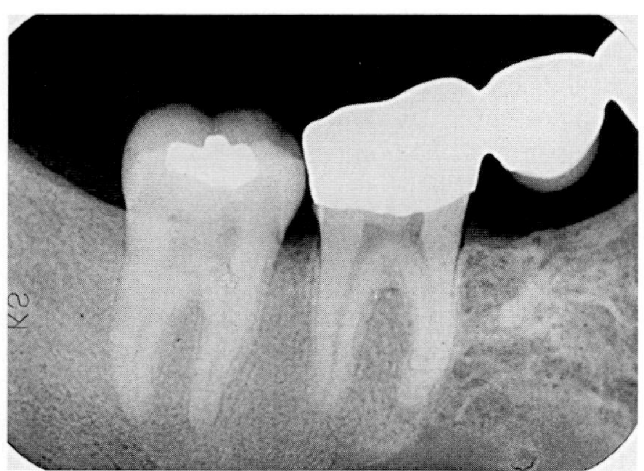

B

FIGURE 18–17.

Fibrous Dysplasia: A, Early lesion shows typical granular appearance and rindlike sclerotic margin; lamina dura is unaffected. B, Typical granular pattern in a 24-year-old woman with no symptoms. Although the lamina dura is resorbed in most areas, it remains intact along the distal root of molar abutment.

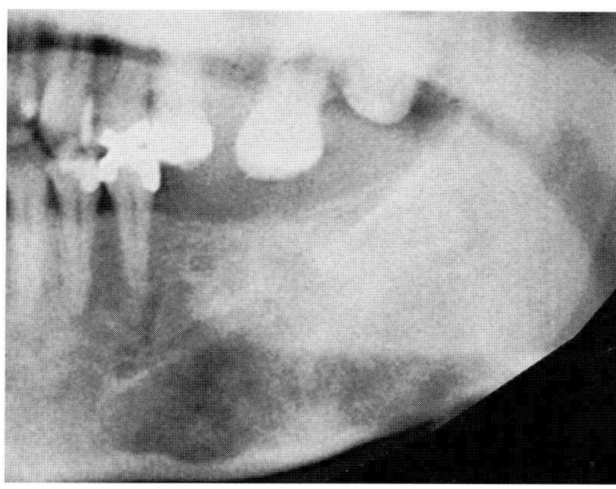

FIGURE 18–18.

Fibrous Dysplasia: Superior displacement of inferior alveolar canal. (From Giunta JL, Heffez L, Doku HC: Superior and buccal displacement of the mandibular canal in fibrous dysplasia. J Oral Maxillofac Surg 43:460, 1985.)

feature of FD. We have not observed this feature in any of our cases, but others, such as Stafne and Gibilisco (1975), reported resorption. Observation of the lamina dura is especially important if a diagnosis of FD is contemplated. Obisesan and colleagues (1977) described loss of the lamina dura in 13 of the 14 patients who had teeth within the areas of their lesions; however, Worth (1963) cautioned that he observed many cases in which the lamina dura persisted in areas affected by FD.

Other Radiologic Features of Jaw Lesions. Evidence of a periosteal reaction or pathologic fracture is not found in the jaws, although it is seen in the long bones. A periosteal reaction in the jaws may strongly suggest sarcomatous transformation.

In 1981 Goldberg and Sperling, and subsequently Giunta and colleagues (1985), described superior displacement of the inferior alveolar canal in association with FD. In the case of Giunta and colleagues (1985), there was a combined radiolucency and ground glass pattern with indistinct margins. The canal was displaced superiorly and laterally. This finding is important for two reasons: (1) it may be highly suggestive of a diagnosis of FD, and (2) it helps distinguish this condition from ossifying fibroma, which, as reported by Farman and associates (1977), causes inferior displacement of the inferior alveolar canal. An extensive discussion of this lesion is found in Chapter 17.

When the maxilla is involved, FD often is more difficult to manage. Extension into the antrum, nasal cavity, and orbit is a frequent development. Computed tomography images are needed to detect such changes. Additionally, involvement of the craniofacial complex occurs more frequently in maxillary cases. As such, the risk of malignant transformation is greater for these cases than for those in the mandible; thus, it is important for the radiologist to be vigilant of such changes.

There are several reports of aneurysmal bone cyst occurring in conjunction with FD in the jaws. In their review of the literature, El Deeb and colleagues (1980) found that, among 53 cases of aneurysmal bone cyst, 11 (21%) were associated with fibro-osseous lesions. These included central giant cell granuloma, cementifying fibroma, ossifying fibroma, and FD. The lesion in conjunction with aneurysmal bone cyst appeared to be localized to a portion of it.

Wannfors and colleagues (1985) reported a case of dentin dysplasia type 1 in association with FD. The FD involved the maxilla, mandible, frontal and occipital bones, ilium, proximal ulna, and ribs.

Radiologic Features of the Skull and Facial Bones

As previously stated, when FD affects the jaws, especially the maxilla, the skull and facial bones also may be affected. Such involvement helps indicate the diagnosis. All of the appearances previously described may affect the skull and facial bones, with one notable exception: According to Worth (1963), the orange peel variant does not affect the

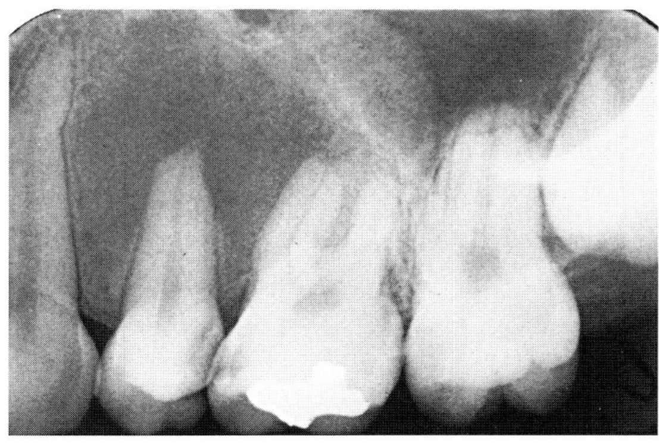

A

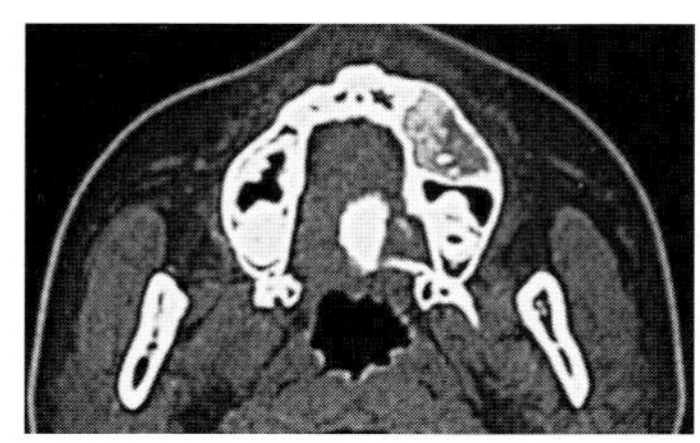

B

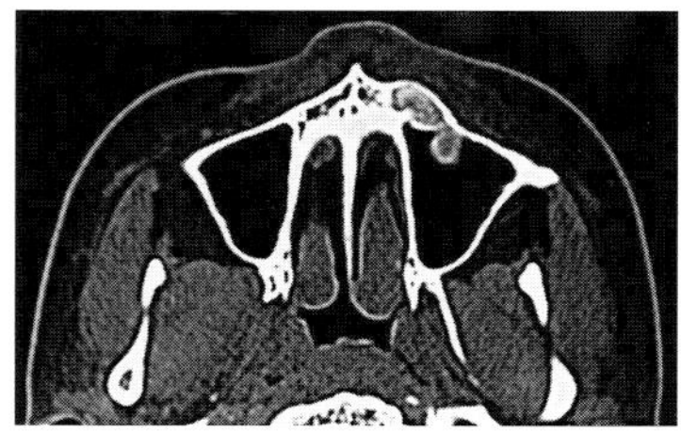

C

FIGURE 18–19.

Fibrous Dysplasia: Case in the maxilla, with slight extension into the antrum, in a 19-year-old woman. A, Grayish homogeneous ground glass appearance and rare root tip resorption. B and C, Widening of maxilla and sinus extension. (Courtesy of M. Araki and K. Hashimoto, Department of Dental Radiology, Nihon University, Tokyo, Japan.)

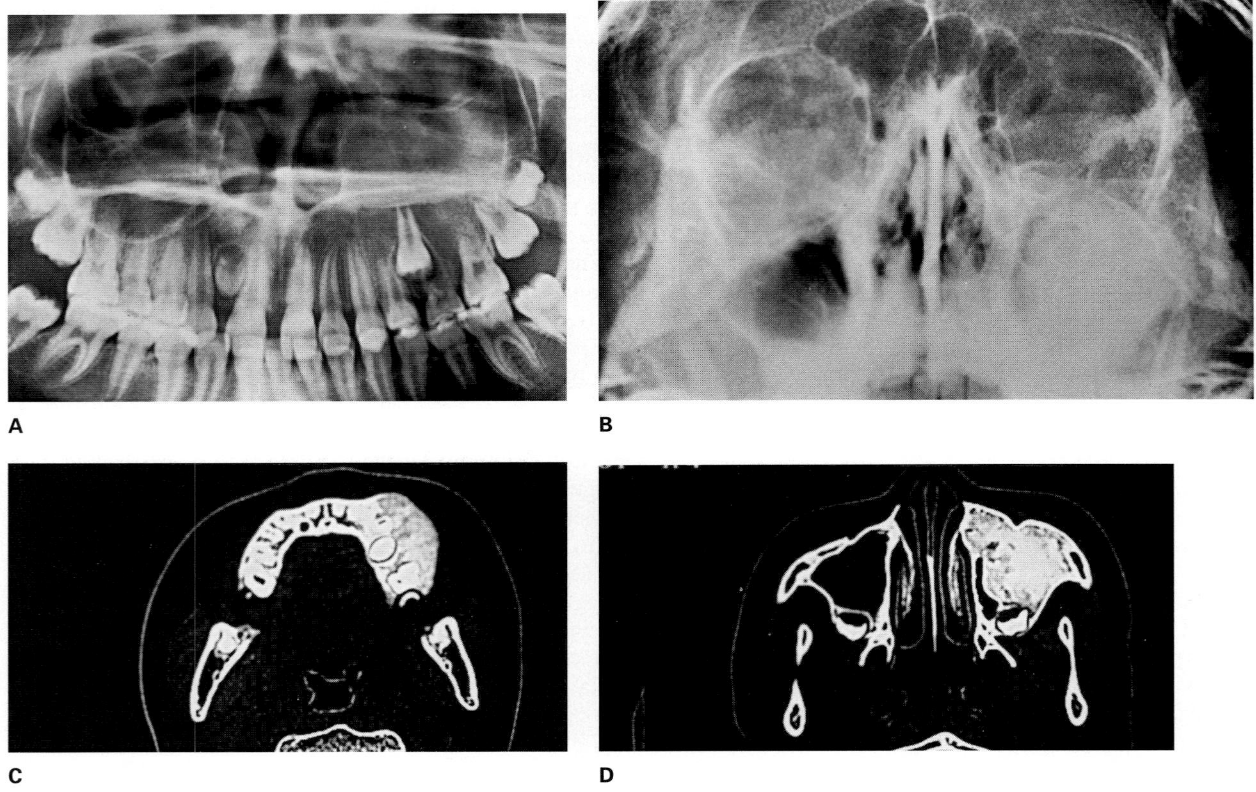

FIGURE 18–20.

Fibrous Dysplasia: Case in the maxilla, with extensive involvement of the antrum, in a 10-year-old girl. A, Delayed eruption of second premolar. B, Opacification of the antrum. C and D, Widening of maxilla buccally and extension into antrum. (Courtesy of M. Araki and K. Hashimoto, Dental Radiology Department, Nihon University School of Dentistry, Tokyo, Japan.)

skull. Additionally, when the skull or facial bones are affected along with the jaws, the radiographic appearance of the jaws usually will be different from that of the skull and facial bones, and rarely it may be identical. When the facial bones or base of the skull is involved, extension into the adjacent sinus cavities is common and helps suggest the diagnosis.

When the facial bones are involved, any of the appearances previously described may be seen; however, certain combinations of bone involvement, along with the radiographic pattern, are seen more frequently than others. These have been described in some detail by Worth (1963): A pattern described as ''leontiasis ossea'' occurs when the sites of involvement include the anterior maxilla with extension into the maxillary antrum and walls of the orbit. The distribution may be unilateral; however, when it is symmetrically bilateral, the patient may have a leonine appearance clinically. Involvement of the orbital walls may cause proptosis of the eyeball. The pattern is usually that of the dense structureless homogenous density, although granularity (orange peel) may be seen. Leontiasis ossea is a descriptive term that is not limited to FD.

The skull may be divided into two regions: (1) the base of the skull, and (2) the vault or calvarium proper.

As previously mentioned, the base of the skull may be the most common site of involvement in craniofacial FD. According to Worth (1963), the sphenoid bone is the most commonly affected. There is often extension to involve the basilar portion of the occipital bone. Extension anteriorly may cause involvement of the frontal bone and orbit. Spread into the paranasal sinuses along the base of the skull, including the sphenoidal and ethmoidal sinuses, is common. The pattern seen in the base of the skull consists of the hyperostotic variant, and some granularity may be observed rarely. At times, FD produces small or large localized protuberant masses on the sphenoid ridges and olfactory plate of the ethmoid bone, producing an appearance exactly the same as meningioma. In addition, both conditions can cause hyperostosis of the sphenoid and frontal bones, exophthalmos, and optic nerve involvement; however, as stated by Edeiken (1981), cerebral arteriography shows an absence of meningoarterial blood supply in FD, thus distinguishing the condition from meningioma.

When assessing the changes affecting the vault, there are certain general considerations. First, the granular pattern is not seen, but all of the others are. According to Worth (1963), the dominant pattern is that of the mixed radiolucent/radiopaque type. Additionally, the outer table and diploic space are affected most, with minimal involvement of the inner table. The most common site is the frontal bone, although

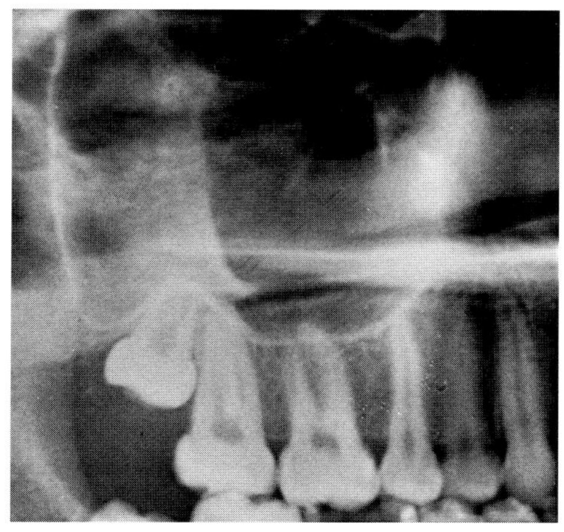

A

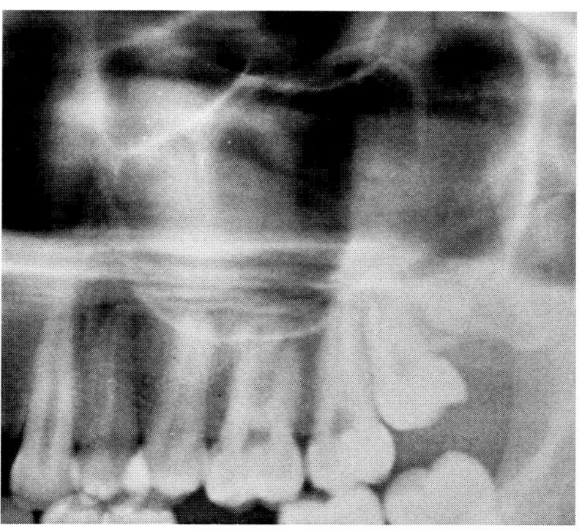

B

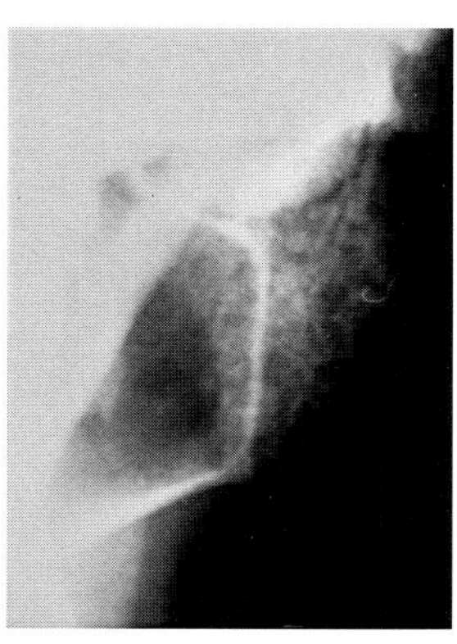

C

FIGURE 18–21.

Fibrous Dysplasia: Craniofacial type. A, Normal side. B, Destruction of panoramic innominate line in left maxillary sinus indicating involvement of lateral wall. C, Tomogram indicating involvement of left zygomatic process. (Courtesy of Drs. A. and G. Castro Delgado, Universidad Javeriana, Santa Fé de Bogotá, Colombia.)

any part of the calvarium may be affected. Worth (1963) described a highly characteristic manifestation in which the frontal bone, roof of the orbits, orbital plates, and ethmoids are involved and the nasal septum is dense, thickened, and grossly curved into an ''S'' shape. The bone changes are usually heterogeneous, although they may be hyperostotic. This finding is highly suggestive of FD, especially when there is extension into the antrum and involvement of the orbital walls. Very localized small or large lesions may arise from the calvarium and in some cases resemble osteoma. Because they are usually of the mixed variety and often present for a long time, FD can be suspected. When the changes involving the vault are purely osteolytic, they may resemble the early lytic stage of Paget's disease, which in Paget's disease is referred to specifically as ''osteoporosis circumscripta'' when it occurs in the skull. According to Worth (1963), the two conditions may be distinguished as follows: (1) The age factor is important, with Paget's disease occurring mainly in older people. (2) In FD there appears to be bone effacement as if there were a hole in the skull, whereas in osteoporosis circumscripta there is gross loss of density but no appearance of a hole in the skull. (3) FD may progress from radiolucent to contain radiopaque elements, even becoming totally hyperostotic; however, the inner table is rarely affected. In Paget's disease, sclerosis of the inner table occurs early, along with involvement of the diploe, to produce the characteristic cotton wool appearance. (4) When the base of the skull is involved with FD, there is no tendency for softening. In Paget's disease, the base of the skull invaginates, producing a ''tam-o'-shanter'' skull appearance.

Radiologic Features of the Skeleton

Because FD may involve any part of the skeleton, we will provide a brief discussion on how it affects other bones. First, it shows the same radiologic manifestations as previously described for the jaws, including radiolucent, radiodense, and mixed-density lesions. There is uptake of technetium in most skeletal lesions of FD. The primary site is the long bones in the metaphysis, and the epiphysis usually is spared. The most common location is the neck of the femur. In many instances the initial complaint is pain around the hip joint resulting from a stress fracture in an involved area in the femoral neck. Increased involvement of the upper femur results in softening and rounding of the bone, referred to as the ''shepherd's crook'' deformity. This is the most characteristic presentation in the long bones. It causes shortening of the leg, limping, and, ultimately, secondary spinal deformities and back pain. ''Bowing deformities'' also occur in other parts of the weight-bearing long bones and result from softening, stress fractures, and healing. Localized cortical thickening indicates healed fracture sites; sequestration may occur without osteomyelitis in the long bones.

In radiolucent lesions there is thinning of the cortex at the medullary margin, and the entire cortical outline may be lost. The radiolucent area often is marginated by a thick, well-defined, rindlike sclerotic margin, which is produced as a reactive process by the host bone. The inner surface of this rindlike area is the most dense, with the outer surface gradually effacing (disappearing) into the normal adjacent bone. The sclerotic rim may be absent. Punctate or flecklike calcifications may be seen within the radiolucent area. Unilocular and multilocular patterns are observed. The affected bone may be expanded. Expansion is common in the ribs.

In radiopaque lesions, the bone assumes a dense homogeneous appearance throughout its transverse diameter, causing the cortical definition to be lost. This appearance often is seen in the ribs and long bones.

Mixed lytic and sclerotic patterns also are seen. One is described as a ''candle flame'' pattern, in which the lesion appears more lytic distally and more sclerotic proximally. Within the more sclerotic proximal portion is a thin band of even greater density, thus giving the area a candle flame

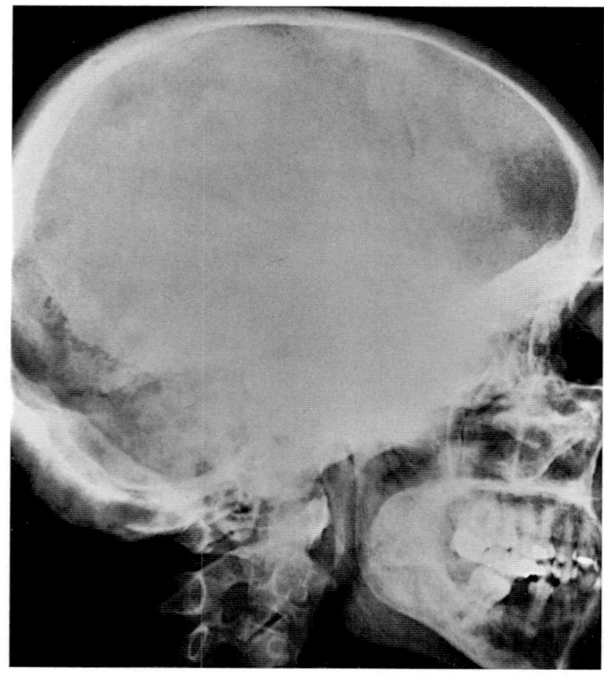

A

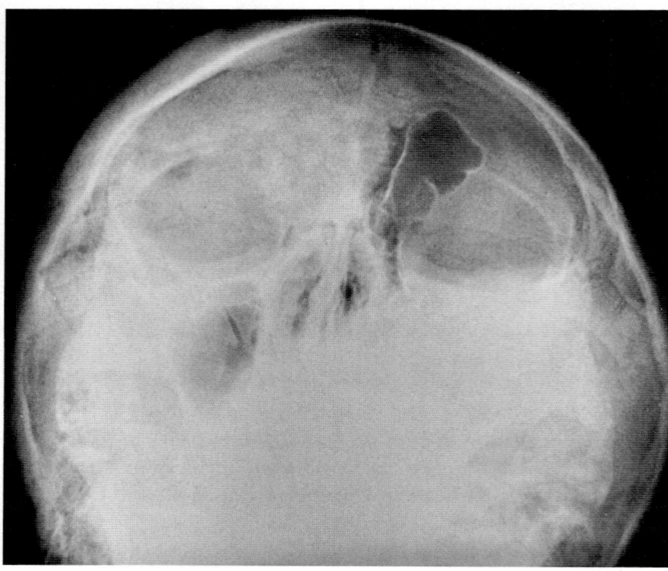

B

FIGURE 18–22.

Fibrous Dysplasia: Craniofacial polyostotic type in a 27-year-old man. A. Radiograph of base of the skull and vault shows hyperostosis of the base of the skull and thickening of the outer table, especially in occipital area. Entire vault appears pagetoid. B, Figure shows thickening of right parietal and frontal bones, with extension into frontal sinus; involvement of left maxilla; and extension into left antrum, zygoma, and nasal fossa. (Courtesy of R. Cone, San Antonio, TX.)

appearance. The other heterogeneous lesions show different combinations of lytic and sclerotic variants as were described previously for the jaws.

Malignant Transformation

Signs of malignant transformation include new areas of lysis after a long quiescent period, loss of a sclerotic margin, and the presence of a soft tissue mass. These changes may be accompanied by pain.

PAGET'S DISEASE (Osteitis deformans)

In 1877, Sir James Paget described a bone disease that he called osteitis deformans. Later, the disorder was designated Paget's disease. As reported by Smith and Eveson (1981), it was Czerny who first used the term osteitis deformans in 1873 to describe an acute inflammation in the tibia of a young man. Two other unrelated diseases have been named after Paget: Paget's disease of the breast and Paget's quiet necrosis of bone.

Pathologic Characteristics

Paget's disease is widely believed to consist of a noninflammatory condition of bone characterized by exuberant osteoclastic activity and subsequent faulty osteoblastic repair. It is purely a disease of bones, although secondary systemic disorders may develop, principally high-output cardiac failure. Although the cause is unknown, current data suggest that Paget's disease is an expression of a ''slow'' paramyxovirus infection that predominantly localizes to the nuclei of the osteoclast. Mirra and associates (1981) observed similar intranuclear cylindrofilamentous structures consistent with paramyxovirus within the nuclei of osteoclasts in giant cell tumors of bone that sometimes develop in association with Paget's disease. Vacher-Lavenu and colleagues (1981) found similar intranuclear inclusions in 6 of 31 cases of giant cell tumor of bone. If Paget's disease is caused by a virus, its mode of transmission remains a mystery. Sofaer (1984) surveyed a series of 360 patients with Paget's disease and no spouses were affected; however, in their review of the literature, Smith and Eveson (1981) found reports of familial clustering. They could not find evidence of a specific HLA antigen, ABO blood group, or secretor status in which affected families were studied.

In considering the radiology of Paget's disease, it is most important to realize that the variety of radiographic appearances results from and indicates one of three phrases through which Paget's disease progresses from incipience through maturity. The first or incipient phase is described as the active or destructive stage. There is pathologic activation of osteoclasts, followed by advancing lysis from a single focus. Maldague and Malghem (1987) stated that the lytic front

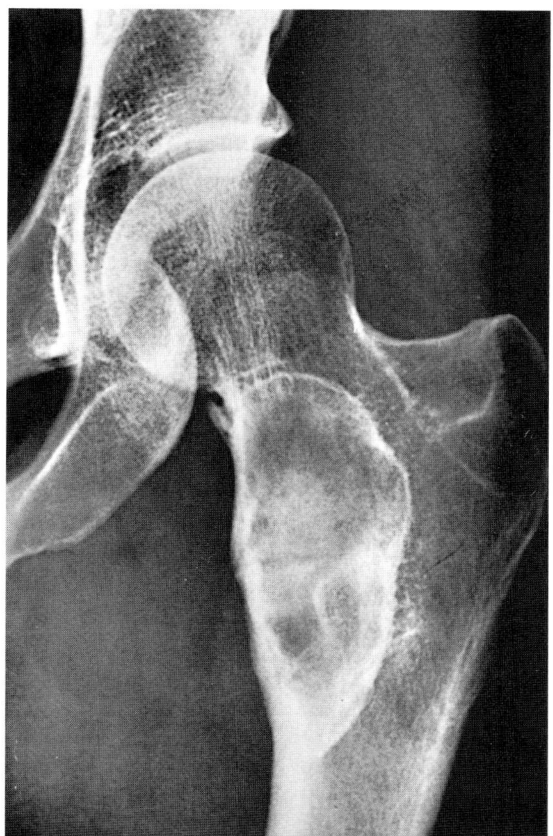

A

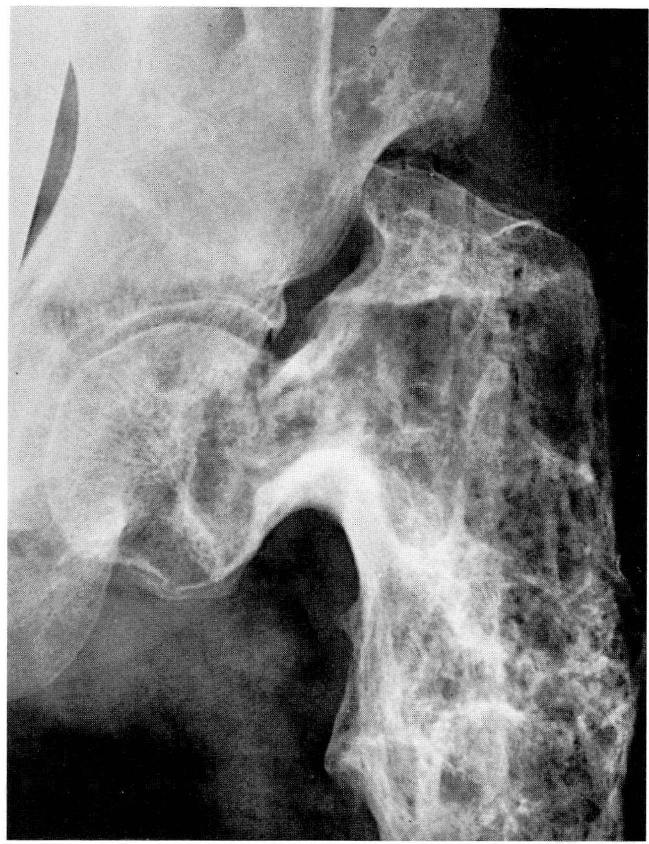

B

FIGURE 18–23.

Fibrous Dysplasia: Skeletal weight-bearing effects. A, Initial lesion in neck of left femur in a 32-year-old woman. Ground glass pattern and rindlike sclerotic margin are seen. Within the middle of the lesion, there is a pathologic stress fracture. B, "Shepherd's crook" deformity at femoral neck in a 20-year-old man. There is a multilocular pattern in the involved bone. (Courtesy of R. Cone, San Antonio, TX.)

advances at a rate of approximately 1 mm per month. The osteoclasts are large and irregularly shaped and, according to Krane (1977), may contain 100 or more nuclei. Mirra and colleagues asserted that more than one or two osteoclasts per square centimeter is suggestive of Paget's disease. The lysed bone is replaced with a cellular fibrovascular connective tissue. The second phase or midphase is characterized by destruction and repair. Thus, it is referred to as the biphasic stage. During this period, there is activation of osteoblasts by which reactive bone forms as a secondary phenomenon to resorption. As explained by Mirra and colleagues (1989), normal bone healing consists first of woven bone formation, then lamellar bone. Pagetic bone consists of an admixture of woven, woven-lamellar, and pure lamellar bone. Additionally, Smith and Eveson (1981) explained that the new bone is formed from disoriented collagen fibers running in many directions. Also, new bone is laid down within the fibrocellular marrow and on the walls of resorbed bone. The newly formed bone also may be resorbed. As described by Mirra and co-workers (1989), numerous large multinucleated osteoclasts are seen, and bone trabeculae are thinned. During this early midphase, the cement line can be seen within the trabeculae. Later, osteoblastic rimming with osteoid seams is seen along thicker trabeculae. Subsequently, the bone becomes quite thick, with less osteoblastic rimming and fewer osteoclasts. Throughout the biphasic stage, cement or reversal lines are seen within the bone trabeculae. The cement lines impart a "jigsaw puzzle" or "mosaic" pattern that is a classic histologic feature of pagetic bone. Hamdy (1977) estimated that the rate of bone turnover in Paget's disease may be 10 to 20 times that of normal bone. In the late or inactive stage, osteoblastic activity abates and may disappear in some areas. In this phase the bone trabeculae show their greatest thickness. The irregular hematoxylinophilic cement lines are prominent. According to Mirra and colleagues (1989), bone altered by Paget's disease rarely, if ever, returns to a normal architecture.

Clinical Features

In a review of the literature, Smith and Eveson (1981) found that people of Anglo-Saxon descent are particularly vulnerable. The disease is especially common in the United Kingdom, with an incidence of 3 to 5% among the population. It is relatively common in Germany and France but rare in Scandinavia, Spain, Italy, Central Europe, the Balkans, and Russia. It is also uncommon in North and South America and Australia. The incidence in the United States ranges from 0.006 to 0.12%, and in Australia it is 0.15%. It is rare in Africa, the Middle East, India, Japan, and China. The disease commonly is reported to affect men more than women, with a ratio of 1.8:1. In a series of 360 British patients with Paget's disease, Sofaer (1984) found a male-to-female ratio of 1.7:1. Approximately 90 to 95% of patients are older than 40 years of age at diagnosis. Schmorl (1932) found an incidence of 0.1% in people aged 40 to 50 years, 2 to 4% among those aged 50 to 90 years, and 10% in people older than 90 years. Although Schmorl (1932) found a rare incidence in people younger than 40 years, his data were derived from autopsies. Dickson and colleagues (1945), who used data based on radiologic evidence, found that 10% of people younger than 40 years of age in their sample were affected. In 1977, Greenspan and colleagues reviewed the literature and found 23 cases of Paget's disease in patients 11 to 35 years of age.

With respect to the clinical features, the following is reproduced from Paget's original 1877 report:

> It begins in middle age or later, is very slow in progress, may continue for many years without influence on the general health and may give no trouble other than those which are due to the changes of shape, size and direction of the diseased bones. The disease affects most frequently the long bones of the lower extremities and the skull, and is usually symmetric. The bones enlarge and soften and those bearing weight yield and become unnaturally curved and misshapen . . . and remain strong and fit to support the trunk. In its earlier periods and sometimes through all its course, the disease is attended with pains in the affected bones, pains widely various in severity, and variously described as rheumatic, gouty, or neuralgic, not especially nocturnal or periodic. It is not attended with fever or any other known constitutional disease, unless it be cancer.

This clinical description has held with remarkable consistency over the past century. In the early stages of the disease the patients have no symptoms. Later, symptoms arise as a result of the secondary effects of the disease and include bone pain, mostly from stress fractures; bowing of the legs; and kyphosis of the spine. As the cranial bones enlarge, patients complain of a need for an increasing hat size, and when dentures are worn they become too tight if the jaws are affected. With enlargement of the skull, attendant neurogenic disorders and symptoms develop and may include blindness, deafness, and facial paralysis. Because there is an enormously increased vascularity in pagetic bone, the bones (especially the skull and face) become warm to the touch. An audible bruit over the head may be detected with the stethoscope. The increased vascularity results in a high cardiac output, cardiac enlargement, and, ultimately, cardiac failure. Marks and Dunkelberger (1980) stated that high-output cardiac failure is most prone to occur after one third of the bony skeleton becomes affected.

Paget's disease is characterized by an increase in heat labile (bone origin) serum alkaline phosphatase levels. This disease is said to produce the highest levels of alkaline phosphatase, with levels as high as 100 Bodansky units (normal level in adults, 1.5 Bodansky units). Alkaline phosphatase levels may be expressed in other units that have different values. These levels may not be elevated during the early stage because they are primarily an indicator of osteoblastic activity. During bone lysis hydroxyproline is released, and some is excreted in the urine. Urinary levels of 1 g per 24 hours sometimes are measured during the osteolytic stage. Normal urinary hydroxyproline levels are approximately 40 mg per 24 hours. Urinary levels of hydroxyproline and serum levels of an alkaline phosphatase are used to stage the disease and determine the level of severity and response to treatment. During the osteolytic stage, there are elevated levels of serum calcium and phosphorous. Some of the calcium spills into the urine, resulting in hypercalciuria and the formation of renal calculi.

According to Smith and Eveson (1981), enlargement of the jaws is a common oral finding. The alveolar ridges may widen and the palate may flatten. The teeth may loosen or spaces may develop between them. The teeth may show any of the following: marrowed pulp and root canal spaces resulting from the deposition of atypical secondary dentin, pulp calcifications, hypercementosis, and ankylosis purportedly caused by fusion between pagetic bone and hyperplastic root cementum. According to Marks and Dunkelberger (1980), dentists may be the first to detect this disease because earlier asymptomatic and later symptomatic manifestations in the skull and jaws often precede those in other areas of the body. Additionally, Burket (1970) documented cases in which the only areas of involvement were in the maxilla and mandible.

Treatment/Prognosis

The main indications for treatment are pain, cardiac failure, and hypercalcemia. According to Smith and Eveson (1981), the most successful therapeutic agents in the management of Paget's disease have been calcitonin, diphosphonates, and mithramycin. Calcitonin is a polypeptide hormone secreted by the parafollicular or "c" cells of the thyroid gland. It is antagonistic to parathormone and thus suppresses bone resorption. This therapy may result in reversal of all of the signs and symptoms within a few weeks. Although calcitonin is derived from salmon and pigs, side effects usually are not a problem.

The diphosphonates, as outlined by Smith and Eveson (1981), suppress the growth of hydroxyapatite crystals and bone mineralization and inhibit bone resorption. Like thyrocalcitonin, the diphosphonates return serum alkaline phosphatase and urinary hydroxyproline levels to normal. One advantage of the diphosphonates is that they are administered orally, whereas calcitonin is given by injection. Therapy with calcitonin in combination with diphosphonates has been successful.

Mithramycin is a cytotoxic drug that acts directly on osteoclasts and causes a return to normal laboratory values in patients with Paget's disease. It relieves bone pain and congestive heart failure rapidly; however, it is toxic to the kidneys and liver and produces thrombocytopenia. Thus, its usefulness is limited.

Oral complications of Paget's disease are as follows:

1. There may be difficulty with endodontic procedures because of obstruction or reduction in size of the root canal space.
2. Tooth extractions may be more difficult than normal because of hypercementosis, ankylosis, or failure of pagetic bone to yield on tooth luxation. This was confirmed by Sofaer (1984), who studied 360 patients with Paget's disease. He also found that extractions occurred more frequently in the maxilla in patients with Paget's disease and correlated this with the greater frequency of involvement of the maxilla than the mandible.
3. There may be difficulty with hemostasis after tooth extraction or other surgery because of the increased vascularization of pagetic bone, especially in the earlier phases.
4. Osteomyelitis may develop as a complication of tooth extraction, periapical disease, periodontal disease, or surgical procedures within pagetic bone. This is especially so in the later stages. All patients with Paget's disease should be given antibiotics prophylactically when surgical procedures are being planned.
5. When prosthetic appliances are being made, patients should be told that the appliances may need to be replaced because of the additive nature of the disease. Poorly fitting prostheses may contribute to the acceleration of periodontal disease in abutment teeth or ulceration of the oral soft tissues, with either possibly leading to osteomyelitis. Patients with excessively large ridges may require surgical reduction. In a case reported by Welfare (1985), no additional growth occurred in the maxilla in his case 8 years after reduction.
6. Although pathologic fracture and bowing deformities are common sequelae of Paget's disease in the weight-bearing bones, pathologic fracture does not occur in the jaws.
7. The most common benign tumor that develops in association with Paget's disease in the axial skeleton is the giant cell tumor, usually in the epiphysis of a long bone. In the jaws, tumors indistinguishable from central giant cell granuloma have occurred. According to Mirra and associates (1989), approximately 100 such cases have been recorded; 50% of which were in the axial skeleton and 50% within the skull and jaws. These authors referred to these as osteoclastomas, stating that they are histologically indistinguishable from the giant cell lesion of bone and the brown tumor of hyperparathyroidism, presumably including central giant cell granuloma in the jaws. Benign giant cell tumors have been reported in the maxilla by Tillman (1962), Hutter and colleagues (1963), and Goldstein and Laskin (1974), whereas mandibular giant cell lesions have been reported by Hutter and colleagues (1963), Brooke (1970), Standish and Gorlin (1970), and Singer and co-authors (1978). When these lesions are excised, recurrences may be expected; however, their course is benign. A few cases of malignant giant cell tumors have been reported in the axial skeleton, but they are extremely rare.
8. The most severe consequence of Paget's disease is sarcomatous transformation. According to Mirra and co-authors (1989), approximately 347 cases of sarcomatous transformation were reported in association with Paget's disease during the 1980s alone. The incidence ranges from 1 to 6%, and Jaffe (1972) reported that it occurs in 5 to 10% of patients with extensive polyostotic involvement. The sarcomatous lesions included osteosarcoma (81%), fibrosarcoma (14%), chondrosarcoma (3%), malignant fibrous histiocytoma (1%), malignant giant cell tumor (0.5%), and lymphoma (0.5%). Mirra and colleagues (1989) reported that 25% occurred in the femur, 22% in the pelvis, 18% in the humerus, 11% in the tibia, 8% in the skull, 6% in the spine and sacrum, 5% in the jaw, and 2% in the clavicle. Multiple reports of sarcomatous transformation in the jaws have been reviewed by Smith and Eveson (1981). According to Marks and Dunkelberger (1980), sarcomas usually are associated with an increase in pain and swelling and sometimes an explosive increase in alkaline phosphatase, especially in large sarcomas. In a series of 128 cases of Paget's disease with concomitant sarcoma, Poretta (1957) found that 20% of patients in whom sarcoma developed gave a history of fracture at the site of subsequent malignant changes. When sarcomas develop in patients with Paget's disease, the prognosis is very poor, with a 5-year survival rate less than 10%.

◆ RADIOLOGY (Figs. 18–24 to 18–33)

In studying the radiology of Paget's disease, the radiomorphologic characteristics of the bone changes correlate very well with the stage of the disease; however, there are differences from one anatomic region to another. Although all three stages may be seen in the jaws, some anatomic regions show more pronounced changes than others. We will divide

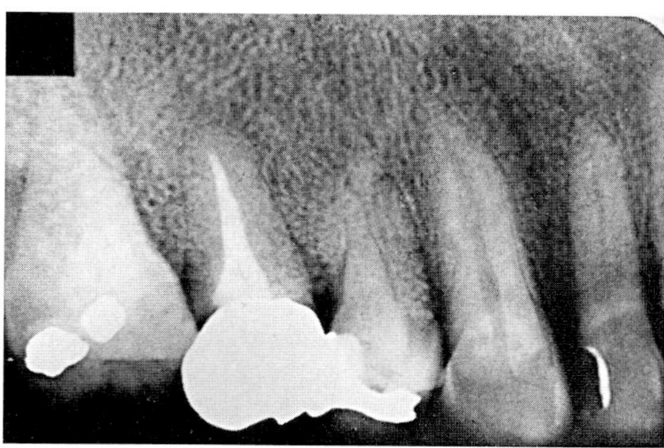

FIGURE 18–24.

Paget's Disease: Lytic phase in the jaw: alveolar bone is more radiolucent and has a granular appearance. The lamina dura is absent, but thin remnants remain. The periodontal ligament space is absent in some areas, indicating ankylosis. (Courtesy of the Eastman Kodak Company, Rochester, NY.)

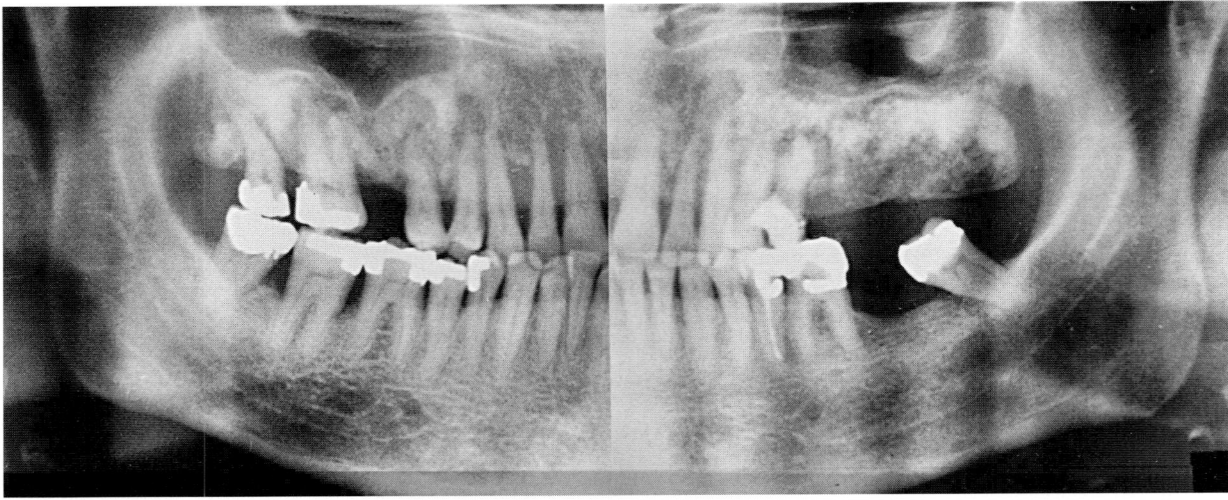

A

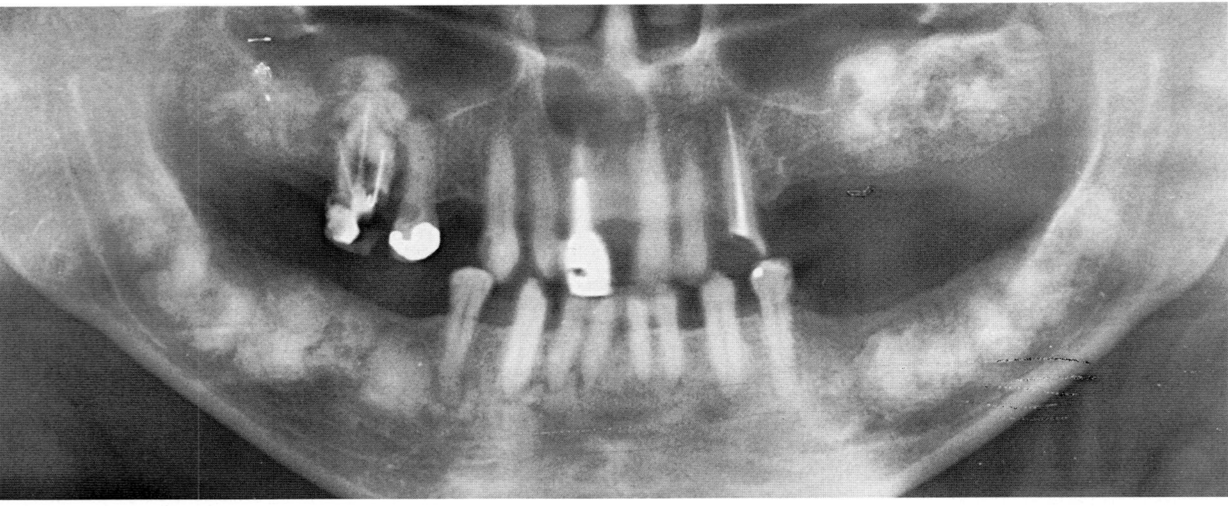

B

FIGURE 18–25.

Paget's Disease: Biphasic stage in the jaw is characterized by multiple radiopaque masses. A, Maxilla only. (Courtesy of D. Stoneman, University of Toronto, Toronto, Canada.) B, Maxilla and mandible. (Courtesy of Israel and Lilian Chilvarquer, São Paulo, Brazil.)

our discussion to include the jaws, skull and facial bones, and the remainder of the skeleton. Generally the initial stage is characterized by lysis and occurs most extensively in the skull. The biphasic stage is seen most frequently in the pelvis and long bones, and lytic and blastic elements may be seen. The inactive stage is characterized by sclerosis and is seen most frequently in the pelvis and clavicle. All of the stages may not be seen clearly in all of the bones; with treatment, bone changes are much less dramatic and sometimes may be absent. When the skull and jaws are involved, the skull changes usually precede jaw changes, and maxillary involvement tends to precede mandibular manifestations. Additionally, the changes tend to be progressive, with more advanced disease in the skull, earlier changes in the jaws, and maxillary changes preceding mandibular changes.

According to Worth (1963), "Biopsy is usually unnecessary in Paget's disease, for a confident diagnosis is possible in most cases from the radiographs alone." Smith and Eveson (1981) observed that there is increased uptake of radionuclides in Paget's disease even when there is no change in serum alkaline phosphatase and urinary hydroxyproline levels. Some of the radionuclides include gallium 67, strontium 85, strontium 87, fluorine 18, and ^{99}technetium methyl disphosphonate.

Radiologic Features of the Jaws

Location. There is no question that the maxilla is affected more frequently than the mandible. In a review of 152 cases affecting the jaws, Smith and Eveson (1981) found that the maxilla was affected twice as frequently as the mandible.

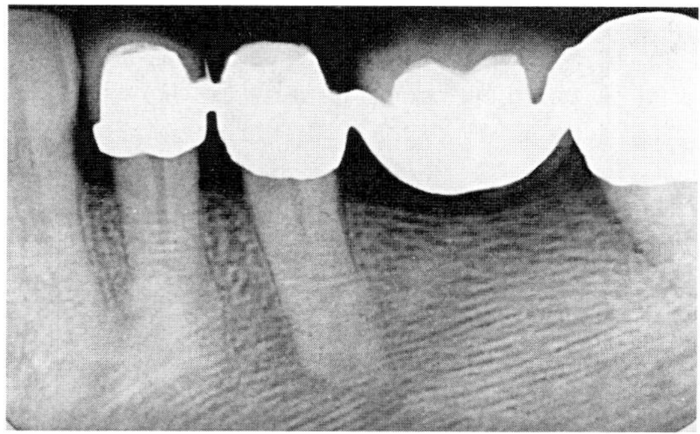

FIGURE 18–26.

Paget's Disease: Late mature phase in the jaw. Dense trabeculae are aligned along the long axis of the mandibular body, and the mandible appears diffusely radiodense. (Courtesy of the Eastman Kodak Company, Rochester, NY.)

Among those cases, 98 involved the maxilla; 28, the mandible; and 26, both jaws. In their classic study, Stafne and Austin (1938) reviewed 138 cases and found involvement of the jaws in 23 (17%) patients. Among these cases, 20 were in the maxilla and only 3 in the mandible. Guyer and Clough (1978) reviewed the radiographs of 1225 patients with Paget's disease. Among these, 27% showed skull involvement, but only two of these patients had involvement of the maxilla and one had involvement of the mandible only. Although the lesions of Paget's disease are most often polyostotic, monostotic forms do exist. The jaws usually are involved when the distribution is polyostotic or when the skull is affected. According to Smith and Eveson (1981), Paget's disease is never completely generalized.

General Radiologic Features of Jaw Lesions. With respect to the radiology of Paget's disease as it affects the jaws, Worth (1963) made the following general statements:

1. Although multiple patterns may be seen, it is more common for a single pattern to be observed in any patient.
2. When the jaw is affected, the whole bone shows evidence of the change, although at times to a lesser degree in the rami.
3. Jaw involvement tends to be symmetrically bilateral.
4. The lamina dura may be partially absent in association with many of these patterns; however, its absence is not generalized and remnants are found in various locations.
5. Changes can be staged as lytic, biphasic, or late, depending on the radiologic presentation.

Lytic Stage in the Jaws. There may be only one manifestation of the early lytic stage in the jaws. Worth (1963) described the changes as predominantly radiolucent in nature, with one of two variations:

1. The most common consists of radiolucent areas within a much greater area of dense bone, often with a granular (orange peel) appearance. Although the margins of the radiolucent areas are irregular, they are not infiltrative, as is seen in malignant disease.
2. The whole bone is radiolucent with added areas of even greater radiolucency. These changes are similar to those seen in osteoporosis circumscripta in the skull. There appear to be areas of complete bone destruction; however, this is not the case. The bone structure is simply reduced but present in a limited amount.

Biphasic Stage in the Jaws. In the jaws, evidence of the biphasic stage is often present. There are several patterns, each with different radiomorphologic features that may be seen during this stage:

1. One of the most common patterns consists of a replacement of normal trabeculae by a dense granular bone that appears more radiopaque. Such areas resemble an orange peel. The jaws are likely to be enlarged, especially in the mandible. In the maxilla these changes may be limited primarily to the alveolar bone or they may be more generalized.
2. Another pattern occurs in which the bone loses density and becomes significantly osteoporotic in appearance. It sometimes resembles an overexposed radiograph. The bone that can be seen appears granular; overall the jaw appears enlarged. Although these changes may be seen in some cases of hyperparathyroidism, in Paget's disease the jaws are enlarged and the lamina dura is visible but difficult to see.
3. In association with a more generalized, denser bone pattern (list item 1) or the osteoporotic appearance (list item 2), there may be rounded areas of greatly increased density. Within these denser areas, no bone structure can be seen. These densities may range from

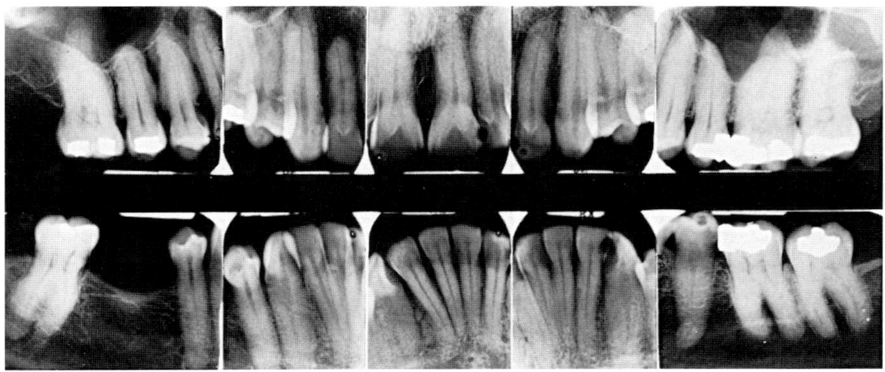

FIGURE 18–27.

Paget's Disease: Figure shows effect on teeth, with hypercementosis mainly affecting maxillary posterior teeth in a 55-year-old woman with no other jaw involvement. (Courtesy of L. Otis, University of California at San Francisco, San Francisco, CA.)

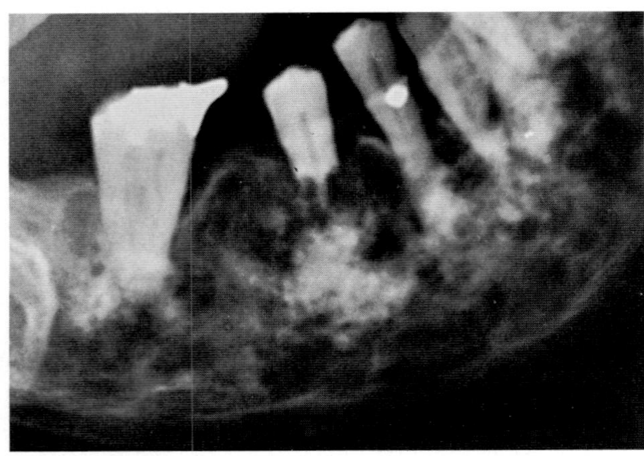

FIGURE 18–28.

Paget's Disease: Figure shows effect on teeth in early biphasic stage. The typical spacing that develops between teeth is seen, along with rare root resorption. (Courtesy of Eastman Kodak Company, Rochester, NY.)

1 cm to several centimeters and are observed most frequently in the mandible, although they can be seen in the maxilla. These changes resemble those of florid osseous dysplasia. This pattern is equivalent to the cotton wool arrangement in the skull.

Late Stage in the Jaws. In our experience, signs of the late phase are not seen as frequently in the jaws, but they are characteristic. Worth (1963), however, described several variations:

1. The trabeculae appear reduced in number, are more coarse, and tend to run in the direction of the bone with a minimum of intersections. This is most likely in the posterior and premolar regions. In the area anterior to this, the trabeculae are coarse and relatively straighter than normal but intersect to produce marrow spaces that are larger than normal and irregular in shape and size.
2. The trabeculae appear increased in number, are finer in texture, and assume the same tendency to run in the direction of the bone.
3. Coarse and sparse trabeculae tend to converge toward the midline; according to Worth (1963), this sign is highly suggestive of Paget's disease.
4. The inferior cortex loses density and assumes a laminated appearance.
5. In each of these instances (list items 1 to 4) the jaw shows slight or significant enlargement, which is a characteristic of Paget's disease. According to Sutton (1975), Paget's disease causes more bony enlargement than any other disease.
6. The mandible tends to assume a more sclerotic appearance, with the bone appearing densely homogenous, with a granular pattern, and enlarged overall. The inferior cortex may not be apparent, taking on the same appearance as the remainder of the mandible.
7. Encroachment on the antral cavity is almost a constant feature in Paget's disease, especially affecting the floor and sometimes the lateral wall. The antral floor and wall appear thickened and densely sclerotic. In comparing FD with Paget's, FD extends and fills the maxillary sinus (antrum) in a much more definitive manner than does Paget's disease.

Relationship to Teeth. Other changes in Paget's disease include hypercementosis of the teeth. According to Worth (1963), hypercementosis develops as a late feature and is generalized. In a woman with Paget's disease, we observed

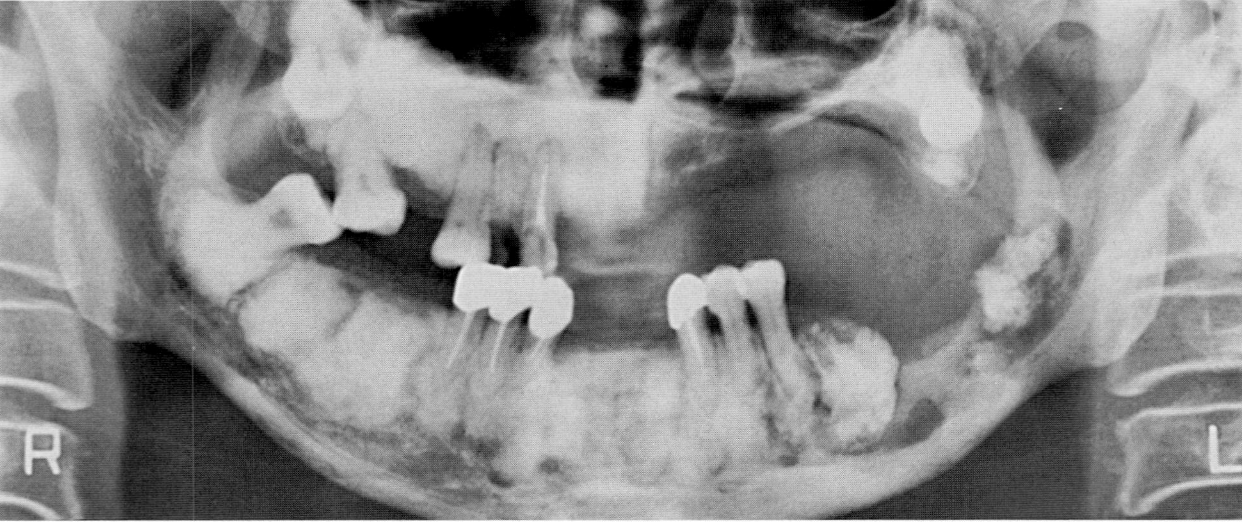

FIGURE 18–29.

Paget's Disease: Complications of the late phase in a 54-year-old woman. The left mandible shows osteomyelitis and sequestration of masses. In the left maxilla, a similar problem occurred, healed, and produced a defect. (Courtesy of T. Noikura, Kagoshima University, Kagoshima, Japan.)

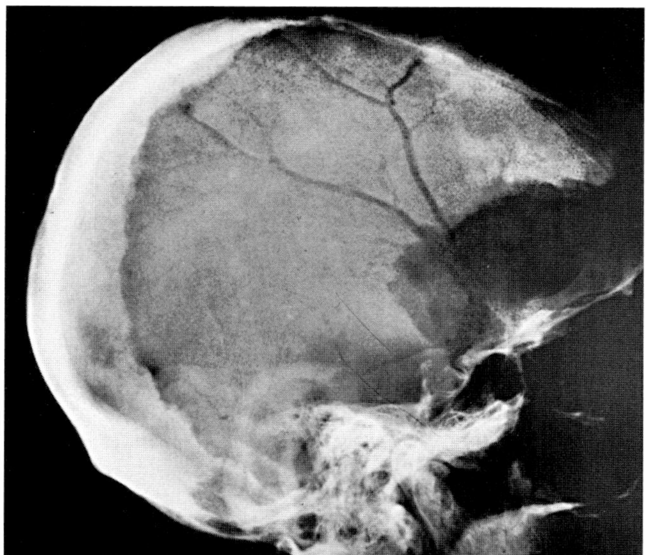

FIGURE 18–30.

Paget's Disease: Lytic stage in the skull shows osteoporosis circumscripta or geographic skull. First wave of lysis occurred in frontal area, and several successive waves are seen toward the posterior. The affected bone appears granular. Meningeal vascular impressions remain because the endosteal surface of the inner table is unaffected. (Courtesy of M. E. Parker, University of the Western Cape, Tygerberg, Republic of South Africa.)

hypercementosis as the primary manifestation of jaw involvement. The hypercementosis is said to ankylose with masses of pagetic bone and thus contribute to the difficulty in tooth extraction. We have found sclerotic masses of pagetic bone superimposed on the roots of teeth, especially in the posterior regions; however, in the anterior teeth hypercementosis may appear to be more limited to the apices and assume a more globular, massive appearance, somewhat reminiscent of benign cementoblastoma but smaller. When true hypercementosis exists, a periodontal membrane space and occasionally lamina dura remnants surround the mass. Such teeth may be difficult to extract. In the medical literature, many authors erroneously identify the dense sclerotic masses of pagetic bone as hypercementosis. Alternately, close examination with periapical radiographs may show that no hypercementosis is present; however, unaffected teeth also may be difficult to extract because pagetic bone may be more unyielding on tooth luxation. In other instances, frank evidence of ankylosis between a tooth, with or without hypercementosis, and pagetic bone may be seen. In such instances the periodontal ligament space is absent. Percussion may produce the characteristic hollow wooden sound. On auscultation of the mandible, ankylosed teeth transmit sound more clearly and audibly than nonankylosed teeth. Such teeth will be difficult to extract.

In summary, the following radiographic findings may be helpful in identifying teeth that will be difficult to extract in patients with Paget's disease: (1) teeth with classic hypercementosis along the roots, (2) those with the globular periapical variety of hypercementosis, (3) teeth in close proximity to or with superimposition of pagetic bone on the roots, and (4) ankylosed teeth.

Other Features of the Jaws. When infections develop in pagetic bone, they are characterized by large sequestra that form and separate from the surrounding bone.

Radiologic Features of the Skull

The skull is a frequent site of involvement in Paget's disease. Using quantitative bone scans in 170 untreated patients with

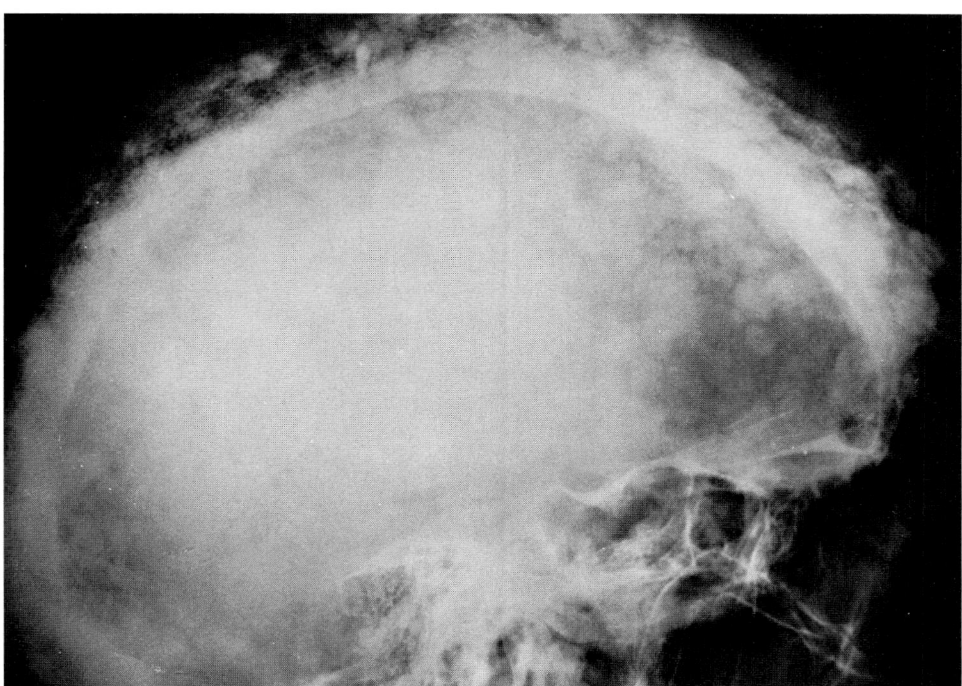

FIGURE 18–31.

Paget's Disease: Biphasic stage in the skull shows classic cotton wool appearance. Inner table is thickened, but not at the expense of the cranial cavity. At the top of the figure, masses of pagetoid bone lie within the diploic space and the outer table has not yet remineralized. (Courtesy of the Eastman Kodak Company, Rochester, NY.)

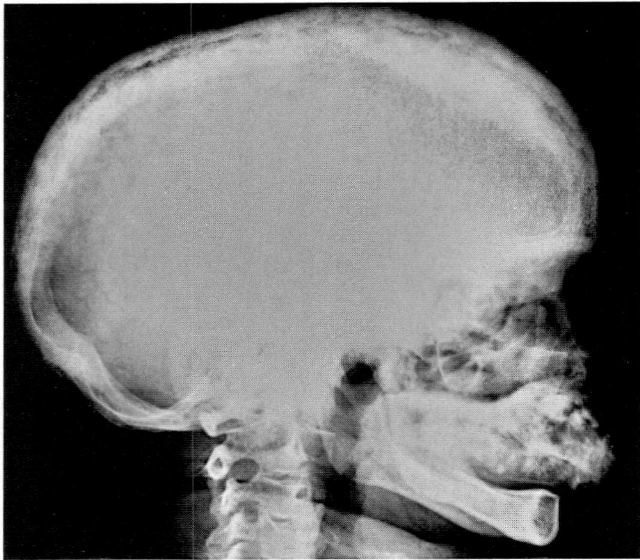

FIGURE 18–32.

Paget's Disease: Late stage in the skull. Vault appears densely homogeneous, with a lack of penetration. Inner table is thickened, diploic space is thin, and outer table has remineralized and appears fused with inner table in posterior area. Maxilla is in biphasic stage and is grossly enlarged. (From Farman AG, Nortjé CJ, Wood RE: Oral and Maxillofacial Diagnostic Imaging. Philadelphia:Mosby-Year Book, 1993, p. 326.)

863 skeletal lesions, Meunier and co-workers (1987) found that 42% of these sites were in the skull. Skull involvement may be somewhat predictive of jaw changes.

Lytic Stage in the Skull. The skull shows the most characteristic changes during the lytic stage of the disease. These changes have been called ''osteoporosis circumscripta,'' and the appearance is radiologically pathognomonic. This term was used first by Schuller in 1926; however, Sosman first applied it to Paget's disease in 1927. Others have used the term ''geographic skull'' or ''skull cap'' zone of rarefaction to describe the changes. Osteoporosis circumscripta consists of one or more circumscribed areas of diminished density, usually beginning in the outer table of the frontal bone and progressing posteriorly. At times the process begins in the occipital area. The loss of density seems to occur in waves, with the most anterior regions almost completely burned out and large zones of increasing density toward the most recent wave of deossification. The result is a geographic appearance of the vault, with the margins of each deossified area quite clearly seen, although irregular. Conversely, the entire deossified area may consist of a single area of diminished density. During this stage the outer table is deossified first, from within. Meningeal vascular grooves are not obliterated because the meningeal surface of the inner table has not been deossified. Worth (1963) emphasized that although the appearance is one of bone destruction, careful examination will show that the process is deossification, with the bone present but reduced in amount. During this stage, the skull is enlarged because of the replacement of bone with highly vascularized connective tissue. Mirra and associates (1989) characterized this stage as one of advancing lysis, and, as reported by Maldague and Malghem (1987), the lytic front advances at a rate of approximately 1 mm per month. Thus, the extent of the lytic front in osteoporosis circumscripta in the skull may be useful in determining the time of disease onset. In its most advanced stage, osteoporosis circumscripta is associated with the temporary radiologic absence of the inner and outer tables.

Biphasic Stage in the Skull. During the second or biphasic stage, replacement of the fibrous connective tissue with pagetic bone begins. New bone fills the deossified space from the inner table. The inner table becomes thickened and more sclerotic. Within the diploe, multiple sclerotic masses begin to appear in areas of rarefaction. These masses are said to have a fluffy appearance and are described classically as having a cotton wool or cotton ball appearance. At first the sclerotic masses are few and distributed to the area of earliest involvement. Ultimately, the sclerotic masses predominate and the outer table begins to reappear.

Late Stage in the Skull. The mature phase is characterized by thickening of the inner and outer tables and a widened diploic space. The entire skull is enlarged and thickened to two to five times its normal thickness, although the cranial cavity is not encroached upon; however, the foramina of the cranial nerves are diminished in size, a finding especially associated with deafness and blindness. In the mature phase, differentiation between the inner and outer tables may be lost, with the entire cranium appearing diffusely sclerotic and thickened.

Other Features in the Skull. In Paget's disease the bones are softened during the early phases and are subject to weight effects. If the base of the skull is involved, softening produces basilar invagination, a phenomenon referred to as ''platybasia.'' The appearance is described as a tam-o'-shanter skull, which is named after the floppy hat. The base of the skull is flattened and curves upward with the occipital region, appearing abnormally low with respect to the cervical spine. The complication of platybasia is encroachment upon the basilar foramina. At times, involvement of the maxilla and orbital and frontal areas of the skull produces a leonine appearance described as ''leontiasis ossea.'' Like osteoporosis circumscripta and other terms, leontiasis ossea is descriptive and does not represent a separate diagnosis.

Radiologic Features of the Skeleton

Location. The major sites of involvement have been determined by Meunier and co-workers (1987), who used quantitative bone scans in 170 untreated patients with Paget's disease. They found 863 bone lesions among these patients. The most common location was the pelvis, where involvement occurred in 72% of patients. Other common sites included the lumbar spine (58%), femur (55%), thoracic spine (45%), sacrum (43%), skull (42%), tibia (35%), humerus (31%), scapula (24%), cervical spine (14%), and clavicle (11%).

In the skeleton, the disease begins as a single focus of bone lysis, which spreads slowly to one end of the bone. It

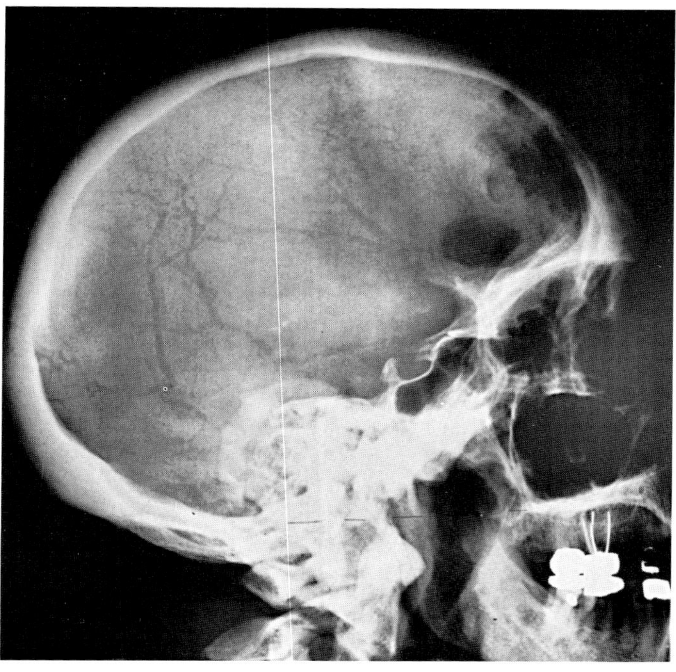

A

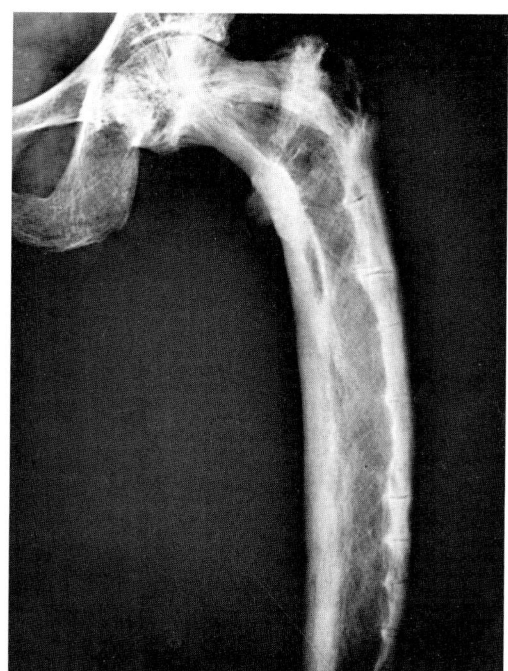

B

FIGURE 18–33.

Paget's Disease: Weight-bearing effects in a 52-year-old woman. A, Skull has osteoporosis circumscripta in frontal area. There is no basilar invagination. B, Femur in late phase, with cortical thickening, has widened bone diameter, lateral bowing deformity, and pseudofractures within lateral cortex with endosteal and periosteal healing. (Courtesy of R. Cone, San Antonio, TX.)

has been estimated that the lytic margin advances at a rate of 1 mm per month.

Lytic Stage in the Skeleton. The lytic stage begins at one end of the long bones; thus, the joints are involved early. During this phase there is usually a pathognomonic v-shaped wedge of rarefaction at the advancing edge; however, this edge may be rounded, with a sclerotic rim. There may be a bubbly or multilocular appearance in the smaller or flat bones. The cortices in the affected area may be partially or completely rarefied. If rarefaction is extensive, there may be pathologic fracture during this stage.

Biphasic Stage in the Skeleton. In the biphasic stage, the effects of softening can be noticed with the development of deforming curvatures. The weight produces lateral deformities in the femur and anterior deformities in the tibia. In this phase, the cortices are remineralized. There is widening of the transverse diameter without cortical thickening resulting from outer deposition and endosteal resorption. During this phase, the bone trabeculae along the lines of stress become prominent and sclerotic.

Late Stage in the Skeleton. The quiescent phase is characterized by cortical thickening. Although pathologic fractures are seen most frequently in the lytic stage, pagetic bone remains susceptible to pathologic fracture. The most common sites of such fractures are the femoral neck and subtrocanteric regions. Pagetic bone is also subject to fracture where normal bone does not (e.g., the so-called "banana fracture," where there is an incomplete transverse fracture in the widest part of the tibia). "Pseudofractures" also are seen. These are often multiple, are limited to the cortex, and heal only at the endosteal and periosteal surfaces.

Other Features of the Skeleton. When the spinal column is involved, changes usually are observed in the biphasic and sclerotic stages. A characteristic but infrequent finding is the picture frame or bone-within-a-bone appearance within the vertebral body, whereby the trabeculae become prominent, especially at the periphery. When a single vertebra is affected, a homogeneous densely sclerotic appearance usually is seen. The weight effect on the spine produces a molding result, whereby the vertebral body becomes shorter, with a decreased anteroposterior dimension. Paradoxically, such affected vertebrae may become more radiolucent. Such changes may be caused by focal circulatory or metabolic disturbances, resulting in resorption, especially in the presence of compression fractures. Similar changes have been observed in the long bones. Progressive lysis in the vertebral column has been discussed by Maldague and Malghem (1987).

Malignant Transformation in Any Location

With respect to malignant transformation, Mirra and colleagues (1989) recalled the "When you see...think" rule: "When you see any rounded to loculated lesion, lytic or blastic, with well or poorly circumscribed borders that arises as a new dominant mass in a chronically diseased pagetic bone, always think sarcoma, whether or not ominous periosteal reactions or a soft tissue mass is present.''

OSTEOPETROSIS (Albers-Schönberg disease, marble bone disease, osteosclerosis fragilis generalisata, osteopetrosis generalisata)

Osteopetrosis first was reported by Albers-Schönberg in 1904. In 1921, Schulze reviewed six cases from the German literature and observed their peculiar appearance on radiographs, designating them as resembling ''marmorknochen'' (marble bones). Subsequently, Karshner termed the disorder osteopetrosis (stonelike or petrified bone) in 1926. In his description, Karshner (1926) explained that the increased hardness more closely resembled that of limestone than marble. Subsequently, many surgical reports described the consistency of osteopetrotic bone as chalklike. Osteopetrosis is a rare, generalized disorder of bone characterized by a significant increase in the density of the skeletal tissues.

Pathologic Characteristics

Osteopetrosis has been reviewed extensively by Smith (1966) and, more recently, Steiner and colleagues (1983), who found that 450 cases of osteopetrosis were reported by 1978. In 1983, they presented an in-depth review of the 57 reported cases with jaw involvement and osteomyelitis. Ruprecht and colleagues also presented a review in 1988. Osteopetrosis is a hereditary disorder that usually is divided into two primary basic types: an autosomal dominant benign form and an autosomal recessive malignant form. Rubin (1964) designated the malignant type as osteopetrosis congenita and the benign type as osteopetrosis tarda. Hanhart (1948) suggested that each of the two basic types had monotropic and pleitropic forms that differed in severity, with the monotropic type being more benign than the pleitropic.

Sly and co-authors (1985) stated that a third type has been reported. It consists of a recessive intermediate form with an associated carbonic anhydrase II deficiency, renal tubular acidosis, and cerebral calcification. The radiologic manifestations are similar to those of moderate to severe osteopetrosis, without the hematopoietic complications. Cranial nerve neuropathies also have been reported.

Some authors, such as Zachariades and Koundouris (1984), asserted that osteopetrosis is the bone disorder in pyknodysostosis, a term derived from the Greek, meaning ''a condition of abnormally dense bone.'' It is autosomal recessive and characterized by benign osteopetrosis, dwarfism, shortened terminal phalanges, delayed closure of the fontanels, and, occasionally, open cranial sutures. The paranasal sinuses often are underdeveloped. Other features include a brachycephalic skull, obtuse mandibular angle, and micrognathia. Patients also have exophthalmia and a parrotlike nose. Pectus excavatum and hypoplastic clavicles may be present, and kyphosis, scoliosis, genu valgum, and bowing of the long bones occur. Pathologic fractures are seen that heal well. Severe anemia and hepatosplenomegaly do not occur. In adults, there is gradual elimination of the marrow spaces in the jaws, resulting in a susceptibility to osteomyelitis in some cases. Ruprecht and colleagues (1988) reviewed some of the common features of sclerotic bone diseases, including pyknodysostosis.

As normal bone develops, precursor elements lay down woven bone that is replaced by lamellar bone. This occurs through a resorption and remodeling process, whereby bone trabeculae are added and aligned to support function, while maintaining spaces for the marrow elements between the trabeculae. In osteopetrosis, the primary spongiosum or initial bone does not remodel because of the defective function of osteoclasts. Some osteoclasts are present; however, they remain inactive. The resulting bone is dense but weak and susceptible to fracture. Healing occurs because osteoblastic function is unimpaired. In addition, bone continues to be laid down because of normal osteoblastic function; ultimately, the marrow spaces are obliterated because of the defective osteoclastic function. Hyperplasia of the extraosseous blood-forming elements develops, resulting in hepatomegaly, splenomegaly, and enlarged lymph nodes. Because of the resulting severe anemia in some patients, infection is a very serious complication in osteopetrosis. Serum calcium, phosphorus, and alkaline phosphatase levels usually are normal.

Shafer and colleagues (1983) described the histologic features of osteopetrosis. There is endosteal production of bone, with a lack of physiologic resorption. Osteoblasts are prominent, and significant numbers of osteoclasts seldom are seen. In endochondral bones, there is persistence of cartilaginous cores of bony trabeculae long after their ossification should have occurred. The arrangement of the trabeculae is disorderly, and the marrow tissue is usually fibrous. In the benign form, the histologic picture is different, with evidence of remodeling resulting from osteoblastic and osteoclastic activity; however, the bone is deficient in collagen matrix. Under polarized light, fibrils rarely cross from one osteotome to another, accounting for the tendency for fracture in these patients.

Clinical Features

Benign Osteopetrosis

Some patients with the benign type have no symptoms, and the diagnosis is made when radiographs are taken for other reasons. Anemia and hepatosplenomegaly are rare. Neurologic disturbances may be present, resulting from narrowing of the cranial nerve exit foramina and pressure on nerve trunks. Some families with the benign pleitropic type show a pattern of bony sclerosis similar to that of the malignant form. Pathologic fractures are a problem in the benign form; however, healing is normal. Infections also are prone to occur; however, the prognosis is better than that of the malignant form because these patients usually are not anemic.

Malignant Osteopetrosis

The clinical features of the malignant form include hepatomegaly, splenomegaly, enlarged lymph nodes, retarded growth, genu valgum, frontal bossing, hypertelorism, mandibular prognathism, and anemia. Complications include pathologic fractures that heal, osteomyelitis that rarely heals, and neurogenic disorders most frequently resulting from optic and facial nerve compression. Death usually results from anemia or infection.

Osteomyelitis in Osteopetrosis

In their review of the literature, Steiner and colleagues (1983) found a generally equal sex distribution, with no racial predilection reported; however, in their review of 57 cases of jaw involvement and osteomyelitis, they found a slight male predilection, with a ratio of 1.4:1. The youngest patient with osteomyelitis was 3 weeks old and the oldest 70 years. Approximately 72% of patients experienced the initial symptoms of osteomyelitis within the first 3 decades of life. Steiner and colleagues (1983) reported that the mandible was involved in 49 of 57 patients (86%), the maxilla in 3 patients (5%), and the mandible and maxilla in 5 patients (9%). They found that severely carious teeth with pathologic conditions of the pulp, postextraction infection, and trauma commonly contributed to the development of osteomyelitis.

Treatment/Prognosis

Teeth

Smith (1966) and Dick and Simpson (1972) investigated the dental changes in osteopetrosis and reported certain anomalies. The crowns are described as poorly formed and possibly poorly calcified; as a result, they are more susceptible to caries. Thus, any preventive measures directed at aborting caries and the subsequent pulpal infections or the need for extraction are recommended because they can be lifesaving for these patients. Endodontic procedures are preferable to extractions and may be lifesaving. Extraction may result in postoperative infection or pathologic fracture, even in relatively simple cases. Surgical procedures, including periodontal treatment, should be avoided if possible, and even the simplest procedures should be performed with antibiotic coverage. In severe cases, osteopetrotic bone contains irregular tracts of necrotic bone devoid of any blood supply, and is similar to osteoradionecrotic bone in some respects.

Osteomyelitis

Steiner and colleagues (1983) reviewed osteomyelitis in association with osteopetrosis in 57 patients. Treatment included incision and drainage, antibiotics, sequestrectomy, extraction of teeth, saucerization, decortication, resection of the jaw, and hyperbaric oxygen, singularly or in combination. Among all of the reviewed cases, the only successful methods of management were total removal of the mandible and hyperbaric oxygen therapy. It must be emphasized that many of these patients had a protracted course and many died with their infections.

Pathologic Fractures

As mentioned previously, pathologic fractures occur rarely in the jaws. Fractures also may be induced iatrogenically during simple exodontic procedures. Although such fractures will heal, a common complication is the development of osteomyelitis. This was the final outcome in the case reported by Smith (1966).

Prognosis of the Benign Form

The benign form is mild and compatible with a normal life span in many patients. Rubin (1964) estimated that 28% of benign cases are diagnosed in patients older than 21 years. In fact, if a patient survives beyond the age of 20 years, he or she almost certainly has the benign type.

Prognosis of the Malignant Form

The malignant form is severe, with affected patients rarely surviving beyond the age of 20 years. The earlier the diagnosis, the poorer is the prognosis. Some cases have been detected in utero, and many such fetuses are born dead. Those with the recessive pleiotropic type rarely survive beyond the age of 2 years.

◆ *RADIOLOGY (Figs. 18–34 to 18–40)*

Osteopetrosis commonly is diagnosed by radiographic examination and interpretation. The disease is characterized by changes in bone density that vary from none to extreme. It is usually generalized, affecting many bones of the skeleton. The characteristic appearance is an amorphous, structureless density involving the entire bone. The least affected bone in the skeleton may be the mandible, with the calvaria and phalanges exhibiting the mildest changes; however, at times these bones also may be affected severely.

Radiologic Features of the Jaws

Location. The manifestations of osteopetrosis in the jaws have been reviewed by Worth (1963). The maxilla and facial bones probably are affected more commonly than the mandible; both the mandible and maxilla may be affected. According to Worth (1963), the mandible does not appear to be involved when there are no changes in the maxilla. When the jaws are involved, the changes are bilateral.

Radiologic Features. Within the jaws, the alveolar bone is the least likely to be affected. In less severe cases, there is an overall increase in density; however, trabeculation still can be seen. The trabeculae become thickened and the marrow spaces diminished. In several cases of minor mandibular involvement, we observed thickening of the inferior cortex of the mandible, with a zone of more densely homogeneous opaque bone adjacent to the inferior cortex, a greater degree of involvement toward the anterior body of the mandible, and diminishing involvement toward the angle. Above this diffusely homogeneous layer is an additional zone characterized by thickened, coarse trabeculae with prominent marrow spaces. There may be thickening of the cortical outlines of the inferior alveolar canal and walls of the antrum. A frequently reported finding is generalized thickening of the lamina dura when the jaws are involved. With more severe involvement, there is homogeneous opacification of both jaws and significant enlargement of the overall dimension. In some instances, the bone is so dense that the root outlines and lamina dura cannot be seen. Sometimes the inferior alveolar canal remains visible, but this structure also may be obliterated by the bone density.

Encroachment upon the mandibular foramen or mandibular canal may cause neurogenic symptoms such as paresthe-

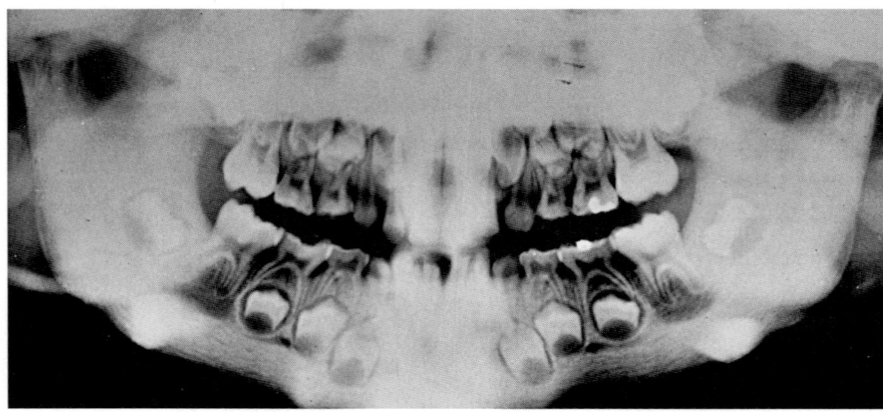

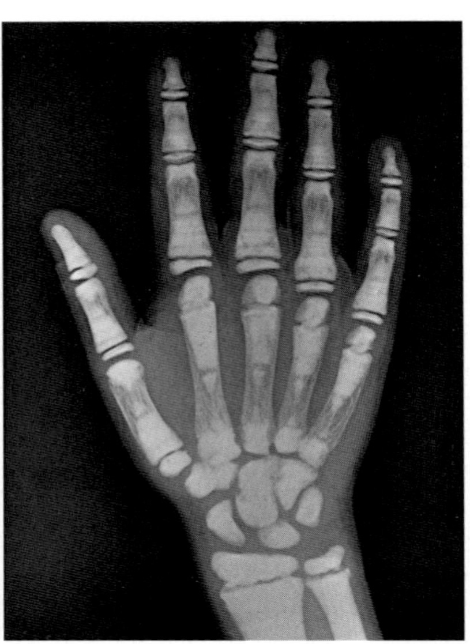

A B

FIGURE 18–34.

Malignant Osteopetrosis: Case in a 6-year-old boy. A, Severe involvement of jaws, including hyoid bone. B. "Bone within a bone" feature in phalanges and metacarpals. Bones of wrist, radius, and ulna also are affected. (Courtesy of L. Alfaro, University of Chile School of Dentistry, Pathology Referral Center, Santiago, Chile.)

sia of the lip, although this is a rare occurrence. In osteopetrosis, the mandibular angle may become much more obtuse. In such cases the mandible appears only mildly curved. Such an appearance could be seen in the cases reported by Steiner and co-workers (1983) and Ruprecht and colleagues (1988). In addition, Ruprecht and colleagues (1988) stated that such changes may be accompanied by the development of an Angle class III malocclusion. Worth (1963) mentioned two important points that must be remembered with jaw involvement: (1) when periapical infection occurs, it is not likely to be identified in the image; and (2) minor infections unlikely to cause major changes in a normal person may cause intractable osteomyelitis in osteopetrosis.

Relationship to Teeth

Changes in the teeth may be seen in osteopetrosis. These have been reviewed by Smith (1966) and Dick and Simpson (1972). According to Dick and Simpson (1972), development of the dentition invariably is affected, with the degree of dental malformation being somewhat proportional to the severity of bone disease. They hypothesized that the pathogenesis of the dental changes relates to the anemia, which may interfere with normal metabolism and differentiation of the relatively avascular metabolically more active dental tissues. They believed that a relative state of malnutrition particularly affects the initial mineralization process, resulting in calcium-deficient tooth tissues. These defects have been reported as enamel hypoplasia and crown defects causing an increased susceptibility to caries, stunted and deformed roots with an irregular covering of cementum, pulp chambers with a diminished size, delayed eruption, early loss of teeth, and missing teeth. In the case reported by Smith (1966), there was significant hypercementosis, which may have been an incidental finding. Dick and Simpson (1972) emphasized that dental changes are seen in the benign and malignant forms.

Radiologic Features of the Skull

In the skull, the base is more likely to be involved than the calvaria. This may be because this part of the skull is preformed by cartilage. The base of the skull appears densely sclerotic, and there may be clubbing and thickening of the posterior clinoid process; the pituitary fossa may appear small. The frontal and nasal bones may be dense and enlarged and the paranasal sinuses obliterated. Worth (1963) stated that leontiasis ossea does not appear in osteopetrosis, but we have seen several cases with this pattern. In the case reported by Steiner and associates (1983), leontiasis ossea was a prominent feature. When the calvaria is affected, the entire cranial vault may appear uniformly thickened, with a loss of the diploic space. The various sutural and vascular markings may be lost, and the cranium may have a homogeneous amorphous density and resemble a "bladder of lard." The cranial foramina may appear diminished in size.

Radiologic Features of the Skeleton

The skeletal changes have been described by Edeiken (1981) and are similar to those previously described. Changes are characterized by a gradual appearance of a single amorphous density. The iliac bones are the earliest to be affected. In the long bones, a lack of modeling causes a flaring of the ends, causing them to have a clubbed or Erlenmeyer flask appearance. The shafts also may be widened. Radiolucent transverse bands or longitudinal streaking may be seen in

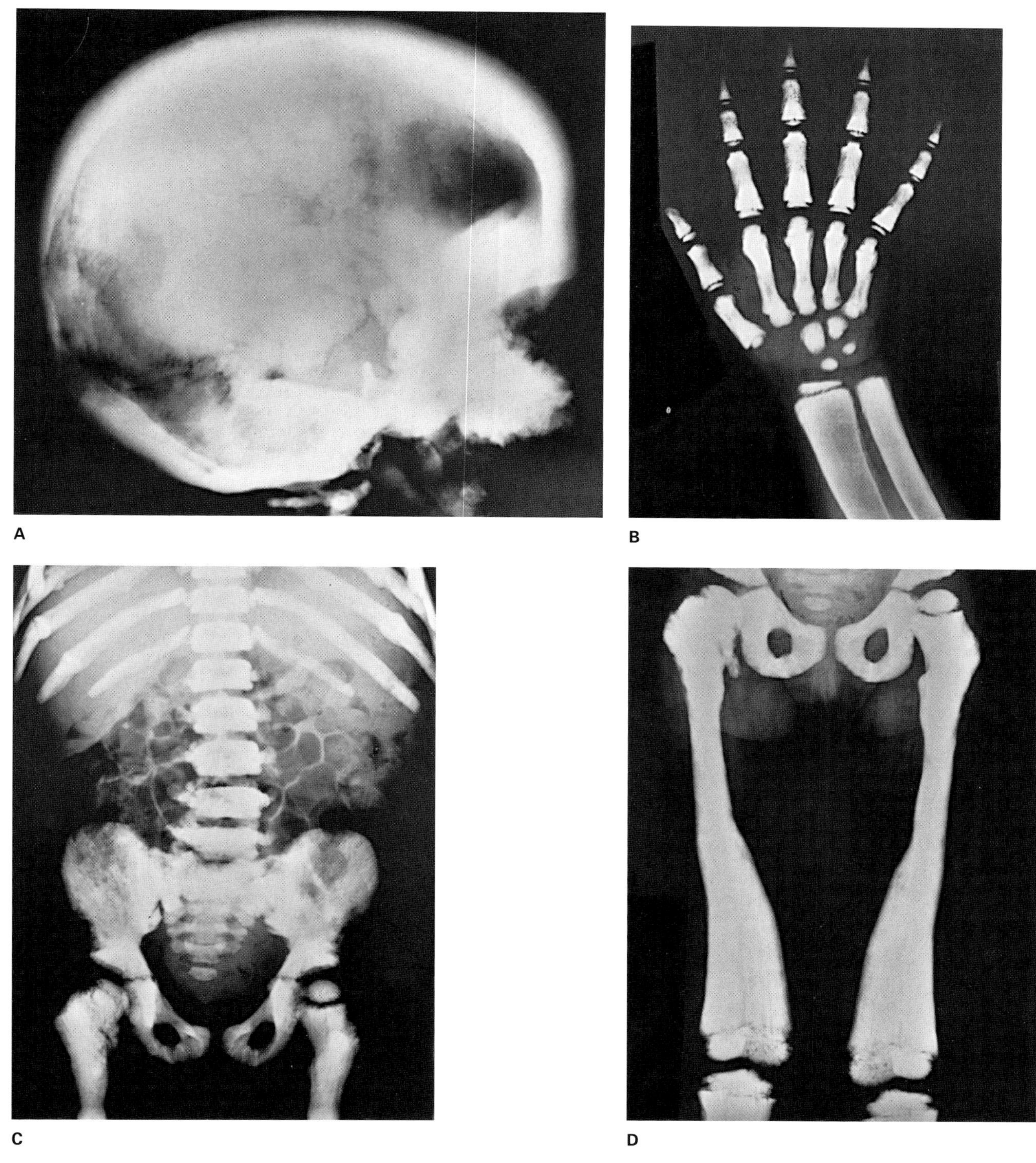

FIGURE 18–35.

Malignant Osteopetrosis: Severe involvement of entire skeleton in a child. A, Skull and facial bones. B, Hand, wrist, radius, and ulna. C, Ribs, spine, and pelvis. D, Femurs with Erlenmeyer flask deformity at distal ends. (Courtesy of R. Cone, San Antonio, TX.)

the metaphases of some bones. Sometimes, the pattern of a bone within a bone may be seen, with a relatively denser area appearing in the central part of the bone. This occurs in the small tubular bones and vertebrae. The vertebrae may have more radiolucent centers with a densely sclerotic radiopaque outline. Pathologic fracture may be observed in any of the bones, especially the tubular ones. A condition known as melorheostosis greatly resembles osteopetrosis; however,

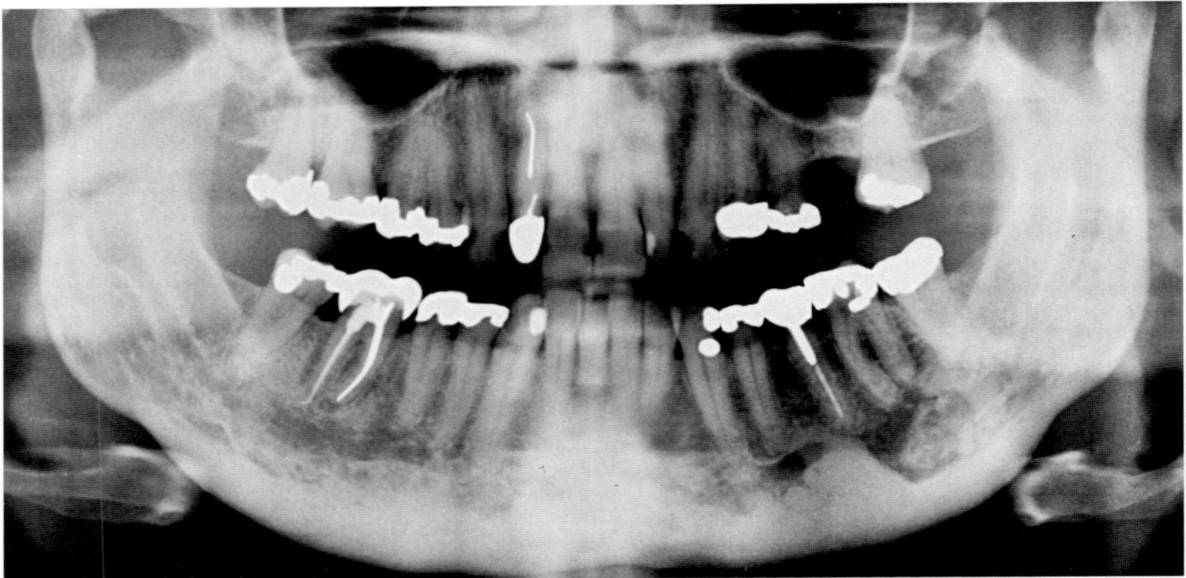

A

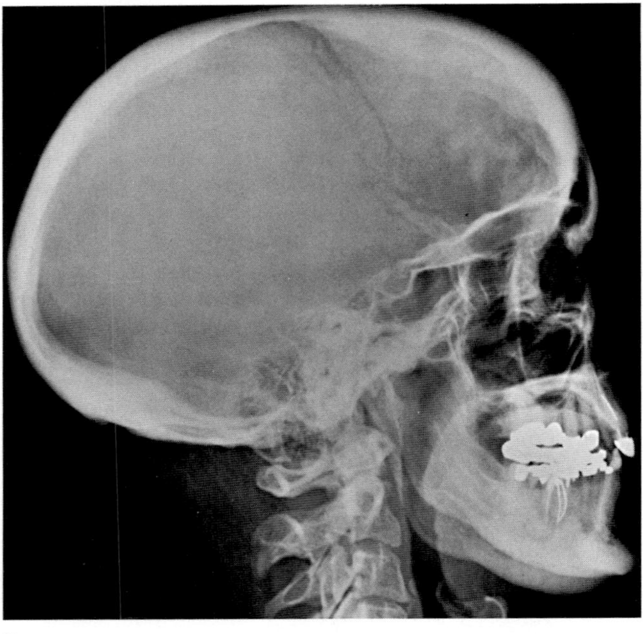

B

FIGURE 18–36.

Benign Osteopetrosis: Case in a 54-year-old woman. A, Hyperostosis of endosteal surface of mandibular cortex, increasing toward midline. There are thickened trabeculations in region, and the wall of the inferior alveolar canal and antrum is increased in thickness. B, Mild involvement of vault with hyperostosis frontalis interna. There is loss of the diploic space because of cortical thickening. Discrete areas of increased density in frontal area resulted from endosteal thickening of inner table. There is no involvement of base of skull or spine.

it is limited to a single extremity only. Sclerosteosis also is similar to osteopetrosis, and its description follows in this chapter.

SCLEROSTEOSIS (Sklerosteose)

Sclerosteosis is one of a group of disorders known as the sclerosing bone dysplasias. The condition first was described by Truswell (1958), who believed that it was a morphologic variant of osteopetrosis. In 1967, Hansen suggested the term "sklerosteose," which has been Anglicized to sclerosteosis. Wood and colleagues (1988) presented a review of this condition and a case report, describing a patient in whom osteopetrosis was diagnosed initially. Beighton and colleagues (1976) presented a review of 25 cases.

Pathologic Characteristics

Sclerosteosis almost uniquely occurs in the White Afrikaner population in South Africa. Several cases have been reported in white and black families in the United States, one case in Switzerland, and one in Japan. No cases have been reported in the Netherlands, where most of the Afrikaner population in South Africa had its origins. Paradoxically, sclerosteosis is very similar to van Buchem's syndrome

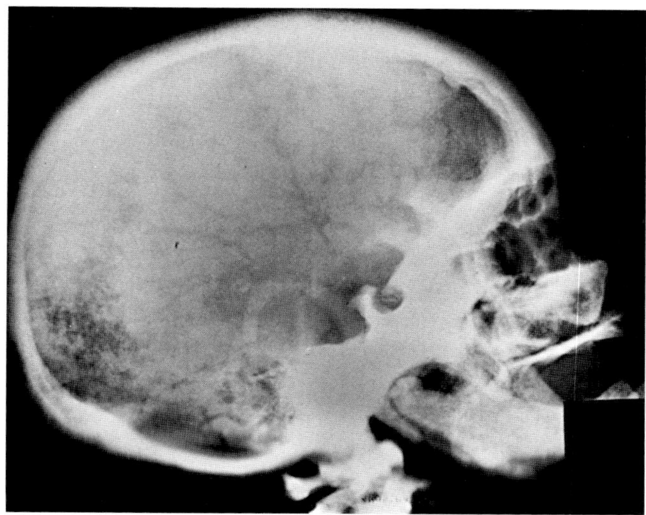

FIGURE 18–37.

Osteopetrosis: Mild involvement of vault, with severe hyperostotic change in cranial base, clubbing of dorsum sellae, and obliteration of the sphenoid, ethmoid, and frontal sinuses.

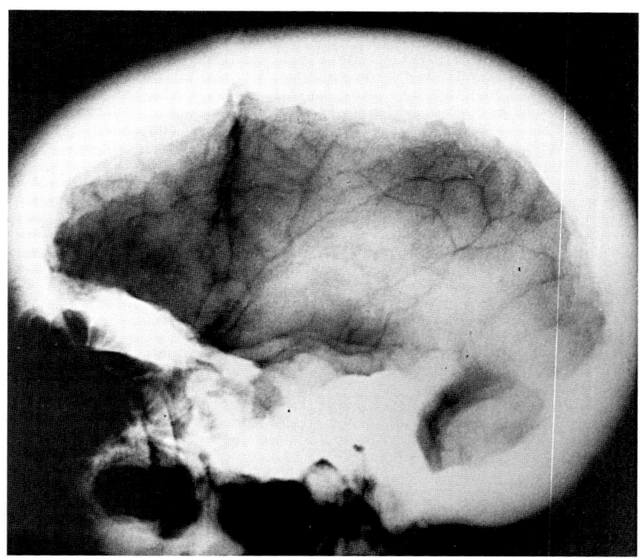

A

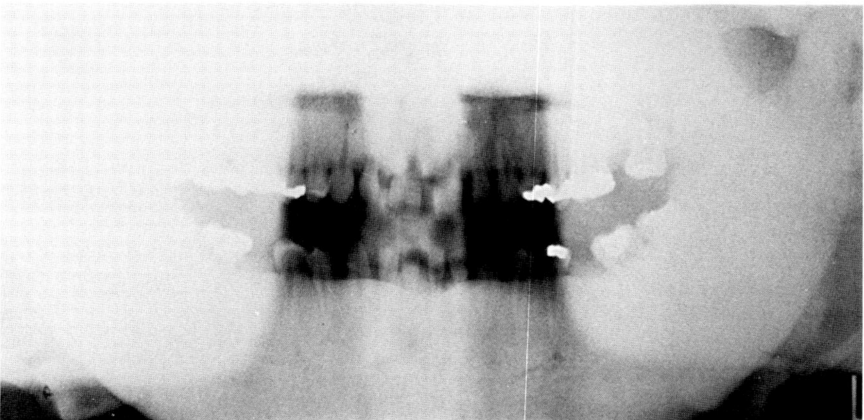

B

FIGURE 18–38.

Osteopetrosis: A, Severe involvement of the vault and base of the skull. B, Lack of penetration resulting from severe osteopetrotic change in jaws. (From Ruprecht A, Wagner H, Engle H: Osteopetrosis: report of a case and discussion of the differential diagnosis. Oral Surg Oral Med Oral Pathol 66:674, 1988.)

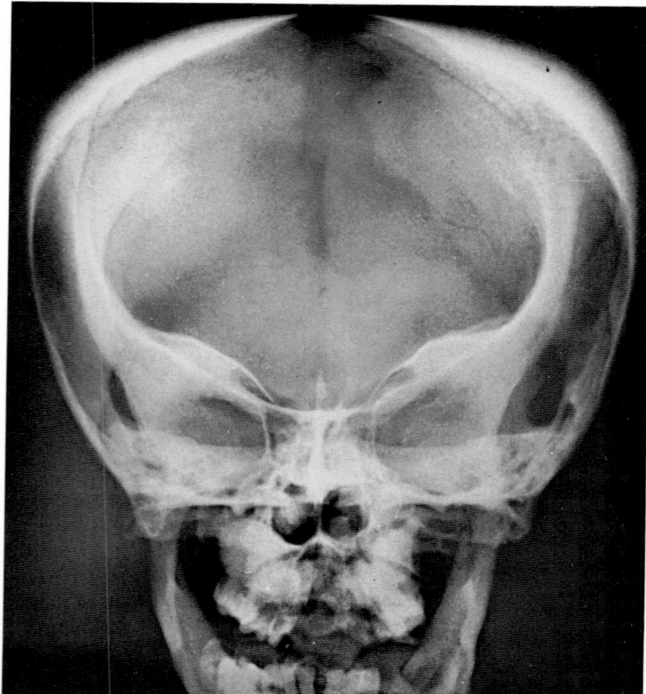

A

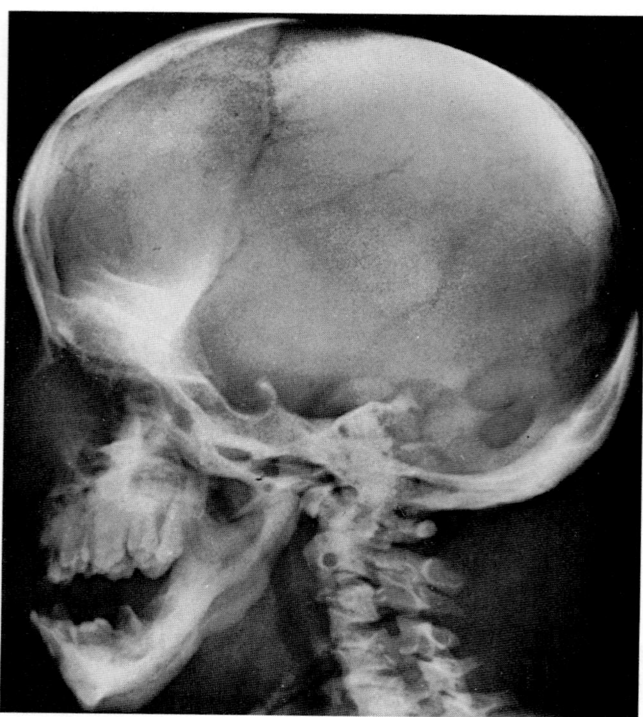

B

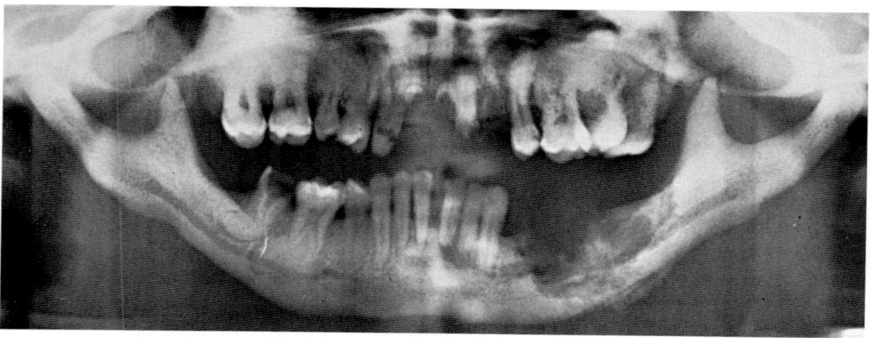

C

FIGURE 18–39.

Osteopetrosis: Case in a 26-year-old woman. A, Open anterior fontanel and frontal suture; mild leontiasis ossea in orbital regions. B, Open posterior fontanel and lambdoid sutures in occipital region; mild involvement of base of skull, with clubbing of the dorsum sellae; and acute angle of mandible. C, Acute angle of mandible, with coronoid processes pointing upward; osteomyelitis in left mandible, with an associated periosteal reaction.

(generalized cortical hyperostosis), which first was described by van Buchem (1955) in a group of Dutch patients living in Holland. Both conditions are inherited in an autosomal recessive manner, and the clinical and radiologic manifestations are similar.

Clinical Features

The clinical features of sclerosteosis include severely distorted facies, caused by mandibular enlargement with class III malocclusion, mandibular prognathism, relative midface hypoplasia. There is transient facial nerve palsy with permanent bilateral facial nerve paralysis in adults, resulting from a narrowing of the cranial nerve exit foramina; and progressive diminution of cranial capacity, producing elevated intracranial pressure and associated headaches. Patients are tall; some authors describe their stature as gigantism. Hand changes often may be present, especially cutaneous or bony syndactyle of the fingers and radial deviation of the second and third fingers, sometimes with dystrophic nails on the affected fingers. The serum calcium phosphorus and alkaline phosphatase levels are normal.

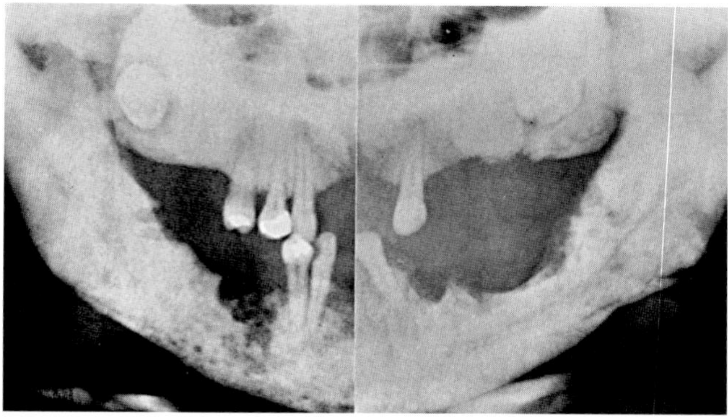

FIGURE 18–40.

Osteopetrosis: Bilateral osteomyelitis in mandible, with motheaten and permeative changes. Gonial angles are obtuse, and maxillary third molars are unerupted. (From Steiner M, Gould AR, Means WR: Osteomyelitis of the mandible associated with osteopetrosis. J Oral Maxillofac Surg 41:395, 1983.)

Treatment/Prognosis

The most severe complication is sudden death in adults with a history of chronic headache. Increased intracranial pressure may result in impaction of the medulla oblongata in the foramen magnum, resulting in sudden death. Cranial decompression by prophylactic craniotomy and cerebrospinal shunt therapy are lifesaving in such patients. Because of this complication, it is important to distinguish sclerosteosis from osteopetrosis and generalized cortical hyperostosis. Such differences have been discussed by Wood and colleagues (1988). From a treatment point of view, patients with sclerosteosis do not have anemia develop, are not susceptible to osteomyelitis, and do not manifest pathologic fractures. Extractions are difficult, however, because of the dense and unyielding nature of the alveolar bone.

◆ *RADIOLOGY (Fig. 18–41)*

The major radiologic features may be listed as follows: (1) hyperostosis of the calvaria, base of the skull, and mandible; (2) lack of normal diaphyseal constriction in the tubular bones; and (3) hyperostosis and thickening of the cortex in the tubular bones.

Beighton (1980) classified sclerosteosis as a type of craniotubular hyperostosis, with all types resembling each other to some degree. The radiographs are helpful in distinguishing them: (1) endosteal hyperostosis (van Buchem disease), (2) sclerosteosis, (3) diaphyseal dysplasia (Camurati-Englemann syndrome), (4) infantile cortical hyperostosis (ICH) (Caffey's disease), (5) osteoclasia with hyperphosphatemia, and (6) osteitis deformans (Paget's disease).

Radiologic Features of the Jaws

The mandible becomes densely sclerotic and massive, and mandibular involvement is a characteristic feature of the condition. In the case reported by Wood and colleagues (1988), the patient, a 24-year-old Afrikaner, complained that his chin and lower jaw had become so enlarged that the chin strap on his motorcycle helmet no longer fit. The mandible was increased in its vertical dimension, and the alveolar process of the maxilla was widened bilaterally. The occlusion was normal. The alveolar bone appeared to be denser in the posterior mandible and maxilla, such that it was progressively difficult to see the root and even coronal outlines of the molars, with progressive worsening toward the posterior. The inferior alveolar canal was obliterated in some areas. Severe rounding or increased obtuseness of the mandibular angle is seen in some cases but may be absent in others. The obtuseness of the angle may increase with the severity of mandibular involvement. It is said that mandibular involvement is more severe in sclerosteosis than in van Buchem's disease.

Radiologic Features of the Skull

The calvarium is widened and densely sclerotic. Some of the widening occurs at the expense of the cranial cavity. The cranial markings were still present in the case of Wood and colleagues (1988). The base of the skull becomes significantly hyperostotic, especially toward the sphenoid and occipital regions. Cranial nerve foramina are diminished in size or even obliterated. The sinuses remain patent, and the sella turcica may appear hyperostotic. Large, punched-out radiolucent areas measuring 1 to 3 inches in diameter may be seen in the frontal or other regions of the cranium. These represent an absence of bone, resulting from craniotomy procedures to decompress the cranial contents.

Radiologic Features of the Skeleton

The small tubular bones of the hands lack diaphyseal constriction, a sign of a remodeling disorder. The bones become opacified because of cortical thickening. Although the medullary spaces may be difficult to see, they do remain, and occasionally they are detected on careful examination. The phalanges are curved in a radial direction. It is said that the remodeling defect in the tubular bones of the hands is more severe than that in van Buchem's disease. When present, syndactyly distinguishes this disease from all others it may resemble.

The long bones characteristically appear hyperostotic because of cortical thickening. A marrow space usually is found on close scrutiny. Diaphyseal constriction is absent because of a remodeling defect. The cortical outline may be irregular. Hyperostotic changes also can be seen in the spine, chest, and pelvis.

ENDOSTEAL HYPEROSTOSIS (van Buchem's disease, hyperostosis corticalis generalisata familiaris, generalized cortical hyperostosis, hyperostosis corticalis generalisata congenita)

Endosteal hyperostosis is a hereditary systemic disease of the skeleton characterized by hyperostosis in the skull, mandible, and long bones. Endosteal hyperostosis first was described by van Buchem and co-authors in 1955. Van Buchem has been associated with multiple subsequent reports, thus

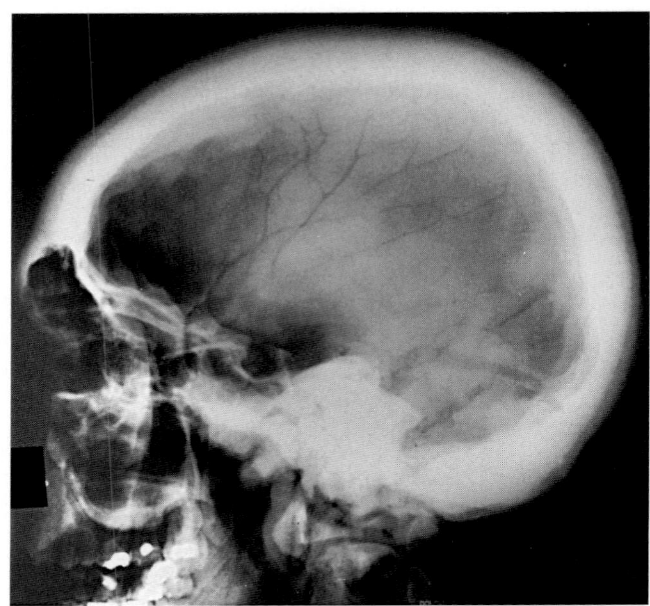

A

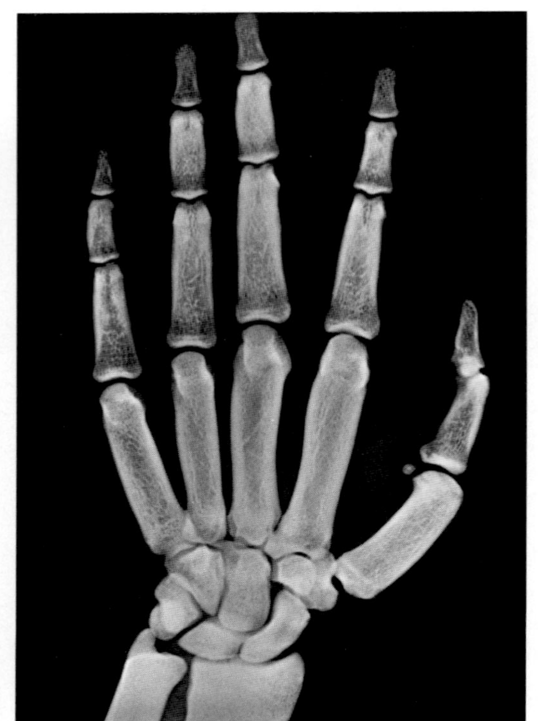

B

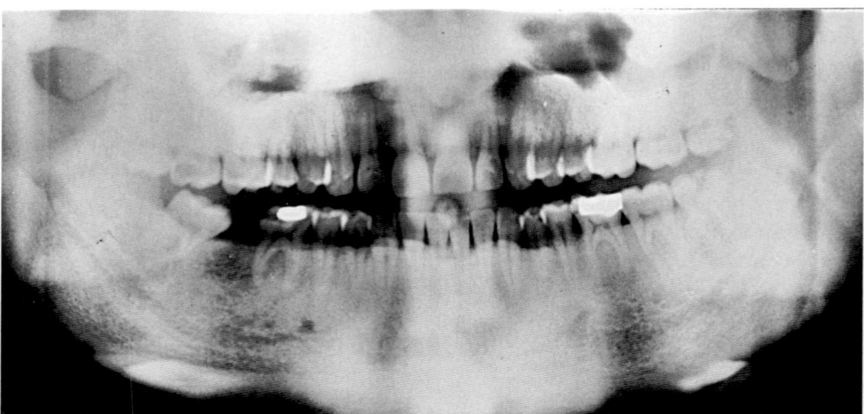

C

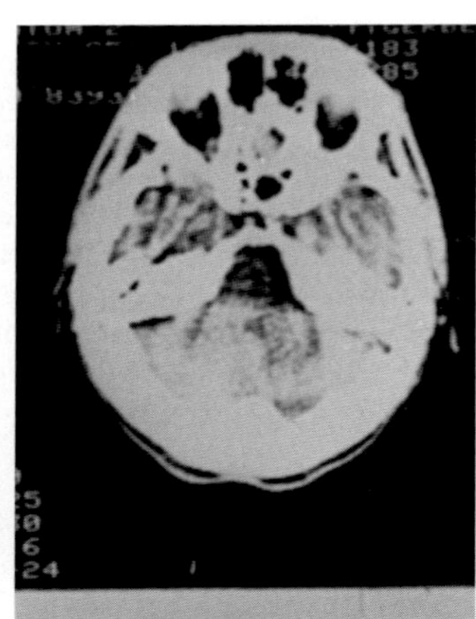
TOM 2
TYGERBE
183
85
8393
25
6
24

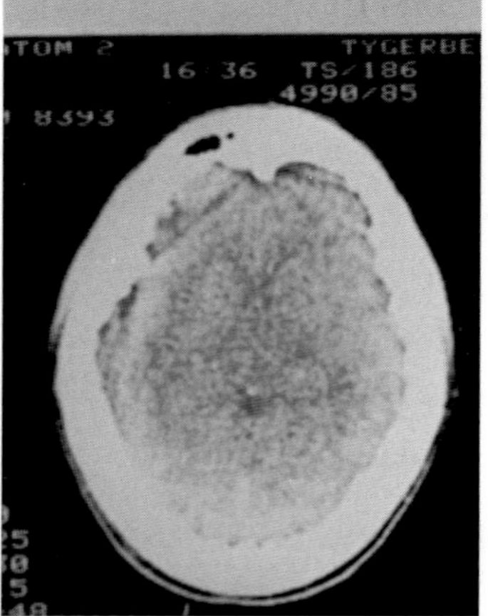
TOM 2
TYGERBE
16 36 TS/186
4990/85
8393

D

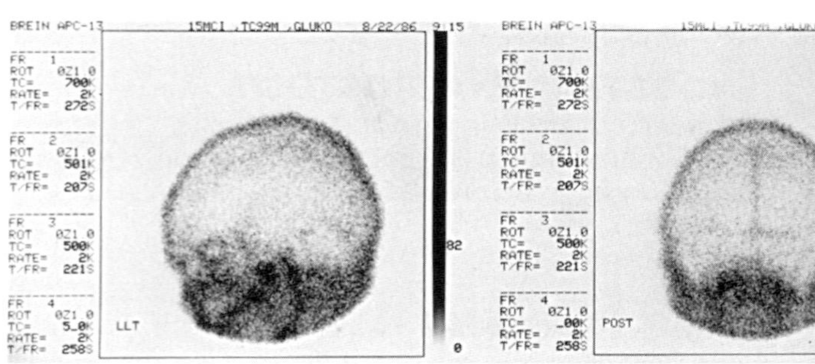
BREIN APC-13
15MCI ,TC99M ,GLUKO
8/22/86
FR 1
ROT 0Z1.0
TC= 700K
RATE= 2K
T/FR= 272S
FR 2
ROT 0Z1.0
TC= 501K
RATE= 2K
T/FR= 207S
FR 3
ROT 0Z1.0
TC= 500K
RATE= 2K
T/FR= 221S
FR 4
ROT 0Z1.0
RATE= 2K
T/FR= 258S
LLT
82
0
BREIN APC-13
FR 1
ROT 0Z1.0
TC= 700K
RATE= 2K
T/FR= 272S
FR 2
ROT 0Z1.0
TC= 501K
RATE= 2K
T/FR= 207S
FR 3
ROT 0Z1.0
TC= 500K
RATE= 2K
T/FR= 221S
FR 4
ROT 0Z1.0
RATE= 2K
T/FR= 258S
POST

E

the eponym van Buchem's disease is widely accepted. The disease subsequently was divided into two major subtypes: (1) the more severe autosomal recessive van Buchem type, and (2) the mild autosomal dominant Worth type.

Pathologic Characteristics

Endosteal hyperostosis has been categorized by Beighton (1978) as one type of craniotubular hyperostosis. All of these types are characterized by overgrowth of bone, and the predominant radiologic feature is an increase in the density of the skeleton. The types of craniotubular hyperostosis are as follows: (1) endosteal hyperostosis, (2) sclerosteosis, (3) diaphyseal dysplasia, (4) osteoclasia with hyperphosphatemia, (5) infantile cortical hyperostosis, and (6) osteitis deformans.

Endosteal hyperostosis is associated with increased bone deposition in selected sites. This is associated with elevated levels of serum alkaline phosphatase of bone origin in children and adults. According to van Buchem and co-workers (1976), the elevated alkaline phosphatase level varies in any given patient from normal to elevated values ranging from 50 to 250% above normal. The latter finding occurs during periods of increased bone deposition. Bone resorption appears to be normal, and the levels of hormones controlling bone resorption—calcitonin and parathyroid hormone—are within normal limits. Serum calcium and phosphorus levels also are normal. Van Buchem and colleagues (1976) found that high doses of calcitonin administered to healthy rats and rabbits caused widening of the cortex of the long bones, which were otherwise normal in structure. They reviewed some investigations and concluded that, although calcitonin inhibits bone resorption by acting on parathyroid hormone, calcitonin also may stimulate osteoblastic activity and that such a mechanism may be partially responsible for cortical thickening in this disease.

Microscopically, the thickened bone appears normal in structure, and occasional osteoblasts and osteoclasts can be seen. Microradiographic studies show that although there is thickening of affected bones, the degree of mineralization is within normal limits. Even though the thickening of the cortex is on the endosteal surface, normal healthy marrow is present in sufficient quantities.

Clinical Features

The autosomal recessive van Buchem form may have been identified in less than 30 patients, with most residing in Holland and aggregation in an inbred community on the island of Urk. In this form, there is severe sclerosis and hyperostosis of the calvarium, base of the skull, and mandible, along with diaphyseal thickening of the long bones. The mandible is grossly enlarged and asymmetric; the brow also is enlarged because of hyperostosis of the calvarium. The clinical signs and symptoms are almost entirely neurologic in nature, including facial nerve paralysis, deafness, and impaired vision. Dixon and colleagues (1982) hypothesized that conductive deafness resulted from sclerosis affecting the bony ossicles, and nerve deafness was caused by encroachment on the acoustic nerve within the auditory meatus. Dixon and coauthors (1982) stated that headaches and mental impairment also have been reported. In their 2 cases, intracranial pressure was diagnosed, for which craniotomies were performed. The 2 patients subsequently lived more than 50 years without development of mental deficit. Although craniotomy is performed rarely in patients with van Buchem's disease, Dixon and associates (1982) emphasized the importance of this procedure in relieving increased intracranial pressure and in preventing later mental deficits.

The autosomal dominant Worth form was reported first by Worth and Wollin in 1966. In 1971, Maroteaux and colleagues discussed its autosomal dominant inheritance. This variant has been reviewed by Beighton (1978) and Horan and Beighton (1982), who stated that cases have been reported in a variety of locations, including the United Kingdom, France, the United States, and Canada. Although the radiologic features are very similar to those of the van Buchem type, the extent of involvement is less severe, the clinical course is milder, and cranial nerve involvement is seen very rarely. Thus, patients with the Worth type have less overgrowth of the jaws and usually have no symptoms.

Treatment/Prognosis

Most patients with endosteal hyperostosis of either type lead relatively normal lives without complaints. In late life, serious cerebral complications may occur, such as cerebellar compression resulting from encroachment on the posterior cranial fossa or paralysis caused by compression of the spinal cord. Other complications include blindness, deafness, and epilepsy.

◆ *RADIOLOGY (Fig. 18–42)*

The salient radiologic features include the following: hyperostosis of the calvaria and base of the skull, gross enlargement and hyperostosis of the mandible, and endosteal thickening of the diaphyses of the tubular bones.

FIGURE 18–41.

Sclerosteosis: Case in a 24-year-old man is described in text. A. Skull, with hyperostosis of vault and cranial base. B, Hand, with lack of diaphyseal constriction and increased density of bones. C, Hyperostosis of jaws and rounded angle of mandible. D, Hyperostosis of all facial bones and thickening of vault at the expense of the cranial cavity. E, Bone scan showing mild increased uptake in outer cortex of vault, mandibular cortex, coronoid process or pterygoid plate area, maxillary midline, nasal area, and the base of the skull. (From Wood RE, Kleyn G, Nortjé C, Grotepass F: Jaw involvement in sclerosteosis: a case report. Dentomaxillofac Radiol 17:145, 1988.)

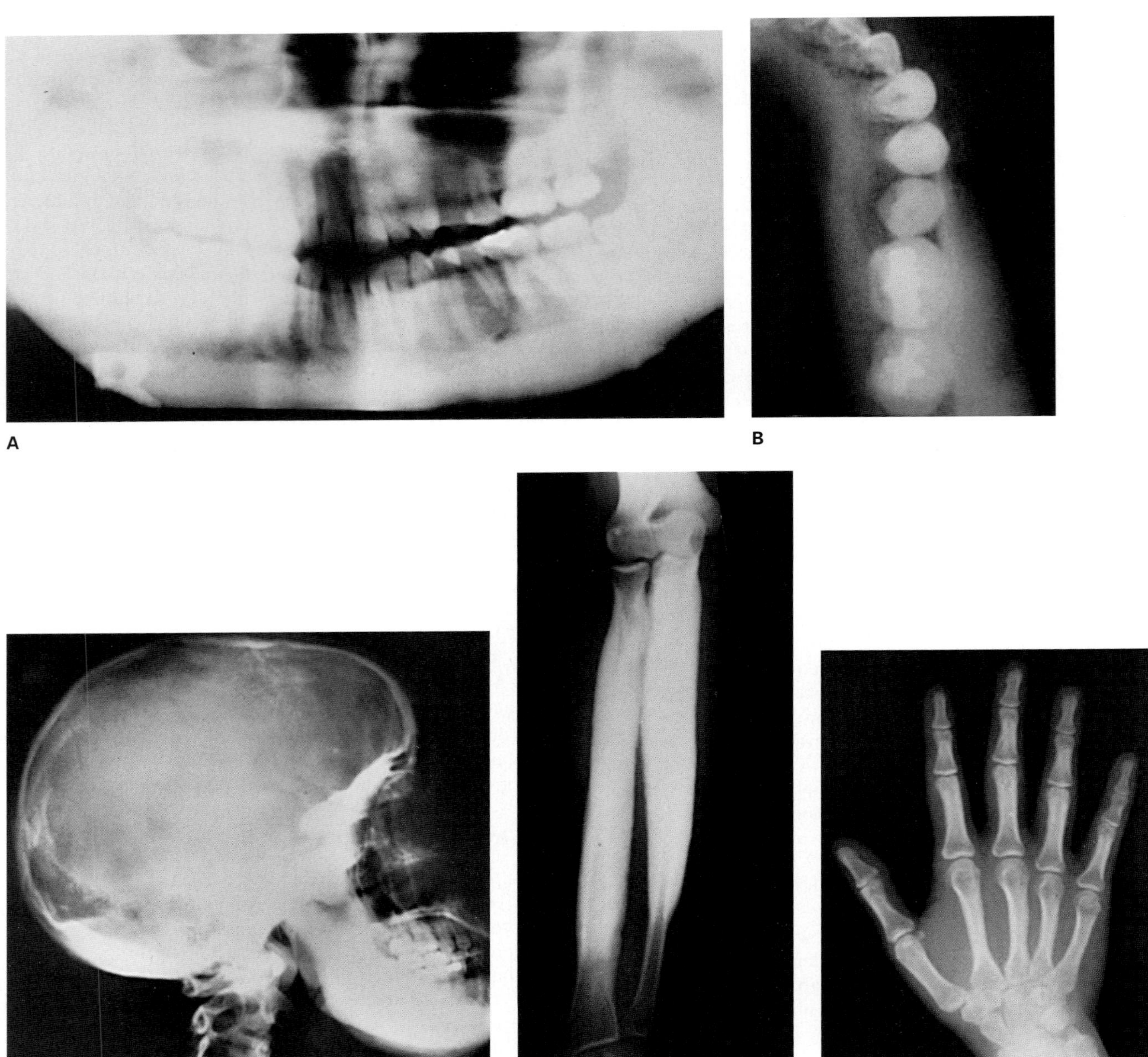

FIGURE 18–42.

Endosteal Hyperostosis: Autosomal dominant Worth type in a 21-year-old white American woman of unknown ethnic origin. A and B, In the jaws, there is a lack of penetration because of thickened cortex. Occlusal view shows endosteal thickening of cortex. C, In the skull, there is hyperostosis in the occipital area, base of skull, and mandible. The angle of the mandible is obtuse. D, The long bones show enlargement and increased density resulting from proliferation of cortex. The marrow space is narrowed but not obliterated. E, In the hands, there is endosteal thickening of the cortex in proximal phalanges and metacarpals.

Radiologic Features of the Jaws

The maxilla is affected rarely, and development of the paranasal sinuses usually is normal, even with severe involvement of the base of the skull. The mandible appears densely sclerotic in the lateral view, with a flattened, obtuse mandibular angle. The mandible appears widened in a superior-inferior and bucco-lingual direction. In the panoramic radiograph, the inferior cortex is grossly thickened. The entire ramus may appear densely sclerotic, with a homogeneous texture. This is increased because of prominent ghosting and superimposition of the contralateral rami. The alveolar bone may be seen along with the root outlines. The outlines of the maxillary and mandibular posterior teeth may be obscured by the superimposition of prominent ghost images of the contralateral mandible. In the occlusal views, the buccal and lingual cortices are grossly thickened. Small bony excrescences may be seen projecting on the periosteal surfaces of the mandible. These may have smooth and rounded external surfaces, or they may be more pointed and spiculelike in shape. The occlusion may be normal. There is no tendency for pathologic fracture or the development of osteomyelitis.

Radiologic Features of the Skull

The base of the skull and calvaria are involved. The calvaria is thickened, and the diploic space appears obliterated. Nodular areas of increased density may be observed occasionally in the lateral view. These are round, with sharp, well-defined, smooth margins and no tendency to coalesce. Their diameters may range from several millimeters to several centimeters. These represent nodular excrescences on the outer surface of the skull. Evidence of craniotomy, usually in the parietal area, was shown in the case of Dixon and colleagues (1982). The base of the skull appears densely sclerotic; however, the pituitary fossa is usually normal in size. The paranasal sinuses usually are present and well developed.

Radiologic Features of the Skeleton

The tubular bones show diaphyseal thickening on the endosteal surface. This causes widening of the cortex, without increasing the diameter of the bone. Such thickening is seen in the long bones, metacarpals, and phalanges. When this occurs, the bones appear more tubular in shape, lacking diaphyseal constriction. In this case, the problem does not result from abnormal remodeling, but rather from selective deposition of excess cortical bone. Bony excrescences also may be seen in the long bones on the periosteal surface. Other involved bones include the clavicles and ribs. The vertebral column may be affected, particularly the spinous processes, which appear hyperostotic. Pathologic fracture is not a problem.

INFANTILE CORTICAL HYPEROSTOSIS
(Caffey's disease, Caffey-Silverman syndrome)

Infantile cortical hyperostosis (ICH) is an idiopathic disorder of infants characterized by sudden painful soft tissue swelling in the mandible and extremities, followed by transient cortical hyperostosis in the underlying bone and spontaneous resolution. The condition first was described in 1930 by Roske, who recognized that common infections were not the cause. In 1945, Caffey and Silverman published the definitive report of four cases and coined the term ''infantile cortical hyperostosis.'' As stated by Snook and King (1989), similar changes have been described occasionally in pigs, dogs, and monkeys.

Pathologic Characteristics

Although the condition still is thought to be idiopathic, genetic theories are the most prevalent. Paradoxically, the acute inflammatory nature of the disorder differentiates it from a genetic disease. Caffey's disease is divided into two subtypes: (1) familial ICH, which is thought to be autosomal dominant with variable expressivity; and (2) sporadic ICH, which is considered to result from environmentally induced phenocopies.

Clinical Features

Familial ICH is believed by many, including Saul and colleagues (1982), to occur more commonly since 1960. This disorder often is congenital, with 24% of cases present at birth according to these authors. Invariably, it is diagnosed within the first 3 months of life, with rare cases recognized in utero or in children as old as 4 years of age. The onset is sudden. During the first or acute phase, the infant usually becomes irritable, and hard, extremely tender, soft tissue swellings are found in the deep muscles. Other common features include fever and an elevated erythrocyte sedimentation rate. Some less common findings are leukocytosis, monocytosis, and elevated alkaline phosphatase levels. In familial ICH, the soft tissue swellings are more likely to be found over the extremities than in the mandible, but the lower jaw is involved in many cases. Initially, there is no radiologic evidence of hyperostosis in the bones contiguous with the soft tissue swellings. Once present, the radiologic changes persist long after resolution of the soft tissue swelling. Pleurisy may be present when the overlying ribs are involved.

It is believed that sporadic ICH occurred much more commonly before 1960. It exhibits the same characteristics as familial ICH, but with the following differences: (1) sporadic ICH is rarely present at birth; and (2) the mandible almost invariably is involved.

Most reports stated that sporadic and familial ICH occur with no sex predilection, although Worth (1963) asserted that male patients are affected more commonly than female patients. Snook and King (1989) reviewed the pathogenesis and stated that, although the disease is characterized by subperiosteal new bone formation, the presence of periosteal inflammation is disputed. Some authors, such as Potter and Craig (1976), reported acute periostitis, whereas Aegerter and Kirkpatrick (1975) described subacute or no inflammation. Most believe that periostitis leads to an osteoblastic and fibrous tissue reaction, resulting in deposition of radically oriented fine spicules of new bone on the subperiosteal surface of the pre-existing cortical bone. The marrow spaces of the new bone are filled with loose fibrous connective tissue. Ultimately, the bone appears thickened and hyperostotic.

Treatment/Prognosis

Milder forms of the disease may resolve rapidly within weeks or months. Although antibiotics are not helpful in this disease, corticosteroids may be useful in arresting the process or stimulating resolution. Occasionally, the disease may persist for years or recur intermittently. Roske's (1930) original case involving the mandible persisted for 7 years. In such instances, the condition is referred to as chronic ICH; however, cases usually heal, even chronic cases with little evidence of disease.

◆ *RADIOLOGY (Fig. 18–43)*

The radiologic changes consist of perifocal soft tissue swelling and new bone formation.

Location

The mandible is one of the most common locations, but long bone involvement may precede jaw changes. According to Worth (1963), the maxilla is not involved. Edeiken (1981) stated that the following bones are affected most commonly (in order of frequency): (1) mandible, (2) clavicle, and (3) ulna. This author stated, however, that every bone has been affected, except the phalanges and vertebral bodies.

Radiologic Features of the Jaws

Worth (1963) presented the most extensive radiologic description of the mandibular changes. Involvement of the mandible usually is bilateral, although one side may be more involved than the other. Unilateral involvement may occur in rare instances. According to Caffey (1961), the mandible is involved before a child is 6 months of age. It appears larger because of the deposition of subperiosteal new bone. Occasionally, the original outline of the mandible can be seen through the new bone, but at other times this may not be possible because of the density of the new bone. The surface of the new bone in the mandible tends to be smooth, although it may be slightly irregular in some cases. At the peak of bone deposition, the new bone appears very homogeneous and granular. The mandible seems grossly enlarged, and although it maintains its contours, the minor elevations and depressions on the surface are eliminated. During resolution, onion skin-like laminations of bone may be seen. The appearance usually returns to normal within 1 year.

According to Worth (1963), the teeth, lamina dura, and cortices of developing tooth follicles remain unaffected, although they may become difficult to see during maximum hyperostosis. With appropriate exposure values, swelling of the soft tissues adjacent to the jaws may be observed, with or without contiguous mandibular involvement.

Radiologic Features of the Skeleton

In the long bones, hyperostosis affects the diaphyses and spares the epiphyses. An outline of the original bone often is seen within the hyperostotic new bone. Although the outline of the new bone may be smooth, it is often irregular. At times, the hyperostotic bone can be seen to consist of multiple, densely compacted, thin striae of new bone projecting at right angles to the original bone. The bones may be grossly thickened and sclerotic. In severe, grossly involved cases, there may be bridging between the commonly involved ulna to the adjacent radius. According to Edeiken (1981), there is no periosteal layering, except during healing. Caffey (1961) asserted that scapular involvement is usually unilateral and most often occurs before a child is 6 months of age. Resolution is usually uneventful, although Pajewski and Vure (1967) reported bowing of the long bones, enlarged marrow cavities, and thin cortices with streaks of incom-

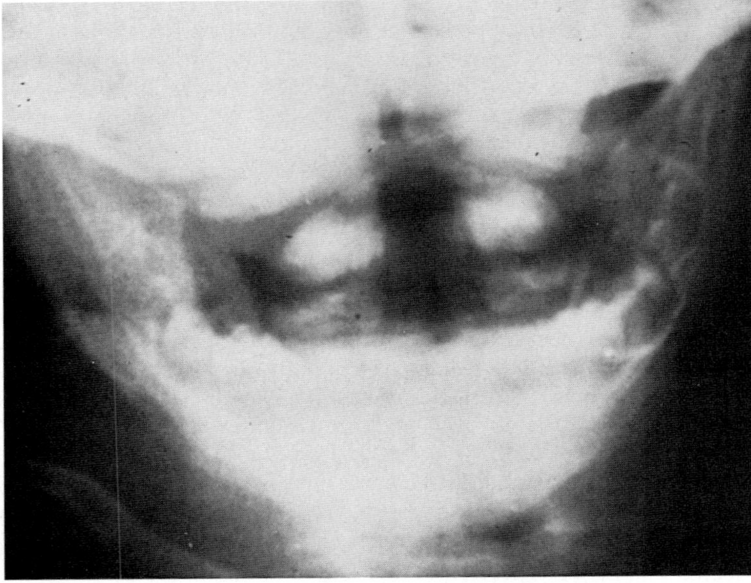

A

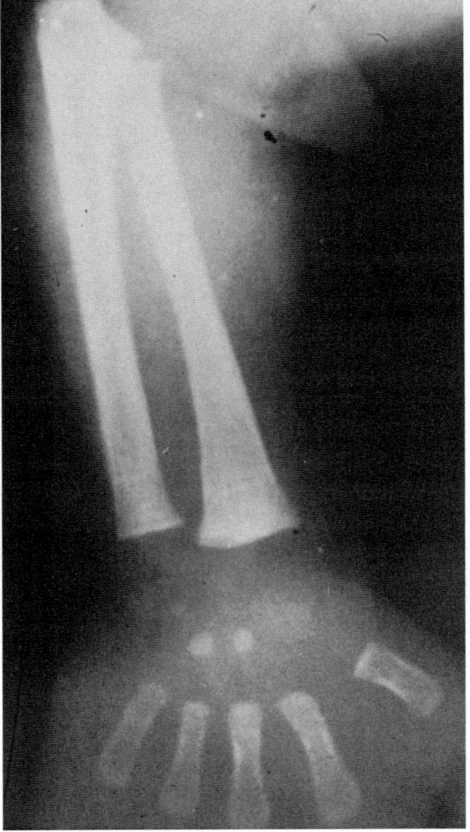

B

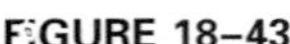

FIGURE 18–43.

Infantile Cortical Hyperostosis: A, Affecting mandible of an infant. B, Affecting radius and ulna of forearm in another child. (Courtesy of R. Cone, San Antonio, TX.)

pletely resorbed cortical bone as rare residual signs in some adults.

DOMINANT CRANIOMETAPHYSEAL DYSPLASIA

In 1969, Gorlin and colleagues critically analyzed the literature for conditions that could be grouped as craniotubular bone dysplasias. Their classic report separated craniometaphyseal dysplasia (CMD) as a distinct entity and further classified CMD into dominant and recessive forms.

Gorlin and colleagues (1969) included the following conditions among the craniotubular bone dysplasias: (1) Pyle's disease, (2) dominant CMD, (3) recessive CMD, (4) craniodiaphyseal dysplasia, (4) frontometaphyseal dysplasia, (6) dysosteosclerosis, (7) Schwartz-Lelek syndrome, and (8) occulodentodigital dysplasia.

Pathologic Characteristics

The autosomal dominant transmission of CMD proposed by Gorlin and co-workers (1969) has been supported in reports by Spiro and associates (1975) and Beighton and colleagues (1970); however, in these cases, affected family members had varying degrees of expression of the signs and symptoms associated with dominant CMD. For example, the father exhibited a prominent asymmetric jaw and right facial palsy, but no frontal bossing. His three children each had prominent paranasal sinus obliteration and frontal bossing. It is uncertain whether these variations are age related or representative of minor degrees of phenotypic expression.

The precise mechanism of pathogenesis in dominant CMD is unknown. It has been suggested that disturbances in calcium metabolism or vascularity may be implicated. Jackson and colleagues (1954) and Rubin (1964) suggested that decreased osteoclastic activity in the endosteal and periosteal layers results in failure to resorb and remodel the secondary spongiosum in long bones; Mori and Holt (1956) proposed that failure of normal periosteal resorption could contribute to hyperostosis in cranial bones.

Clinical Features

Bricker and colleagues (1983) reviewed the literature and described the following clinical characteristics of the dominant form of CMD: (1) ocular hypertelorism; (2) broadening of the base of the nose; (3) an open mouth resulting from narrowing of the nasal lumen; (4) deafness, usually before puberty; and (5) rarely, facial paralysis or defective vision. The radiographic findings include the following: (1) frontal and occipital hyperostosis, (2) long bones with a club-shaped metaphyseal flare milder than in Pyle's disease, and (3) short tubular bones exhibiting similar changes.

Treatment/Prognosis

Keitzer and Paparella (1969) classified the hearing loss associated with dominant CMD as sensorineural and, less often, conductive. The sensorineural loss results from constriction of the cranial foramina. The hyperostosis of the skull affects the middle ear chamber and ossicles, and, hence, sound conduction. Successful surgical repair of this conductive disorder has been reported by Shea and colleagues (1981).

If orthodontic treatment of malocclusion is contemplated, the alveolar bone should be evaluated for involvement, and this should be a consideration when determining the prognosis of the treatment plan.

◆ *RADIOLOGY (Fig. 18–44)*

The radiologic changes may be summarized as follows: (1) frontal and occipital hyperostosis; (2) a mild, club-shaped metaphyseal flare in the long bones and short tubular bones; and (3) sclerotic changes in the jaw bones and abnormalities of the dentition.

Radiologic Features of the Jaws

The jaws appear densely sclerotic. The sclerosis seems to be limited primarily to the alveolar bone and is more severe in the anterior regions. We have observed that sclerosis of the alveolar bone appears to begin locally around the developing dental papilla at the apical region of the tooth. The sclerotic area is immediately adjacent to the apical dental papilla, with no normal bone in between. The focal areas enlarge and coalesce to involve all of the alveolar bone diffusely. The areas of increased density appear homogeneous, and the trabeculae look granular, resembling an orange peel. This is especially true in the maxilla. In such affected areas, the lamina dura appears absent, but it actually is obscured by the densely sclerotic adjacent granular bone apical to the affected alveolar bone. There may be a zone of normal bone between this region and the inferior cortex of the mandible. In the maxilla, the granular bone may extend to the antral and nasal regions, with a lack of development of the maxillary sinus. The mandible appears normally developed, including a normal gonial angle. Mandibular prognathism may be present. Maxillary sclerosis could be more severe than in the mandible. Eruption of most of the permanent teeth may be delayed. We observed incompletely erupted mandibular second molars and second premolars and impacted maxillary second premolars and molars in a 15-year-old boy; the maxilla had more severe sclerotic changes than the mandible. In addition, prominent diastemata were between many teeth, especially the maxillary anterior teeth. This may have resulted partially from the net additive nature of the disease and more severe involvement of the maxilla, especially in the anterior region. We also observed retained root tips of the mandibular primary second molars in association with the erupting second premolars.

Radiologic Features of the Skull

In the skull, one may see hyperostosis of the base of the skull and a lack of pneumatization of the paranasal sinuses and mastoid air spaces. The cranium appears more radiodense. Hyperostosis frontalis interna and hyperostosis occipitalis interna may be found. The soft tissue outline in the lateral view may show the typical open mouth caused by mouth breathing, resulting from a flattened nasal bridge and obstructed airway.

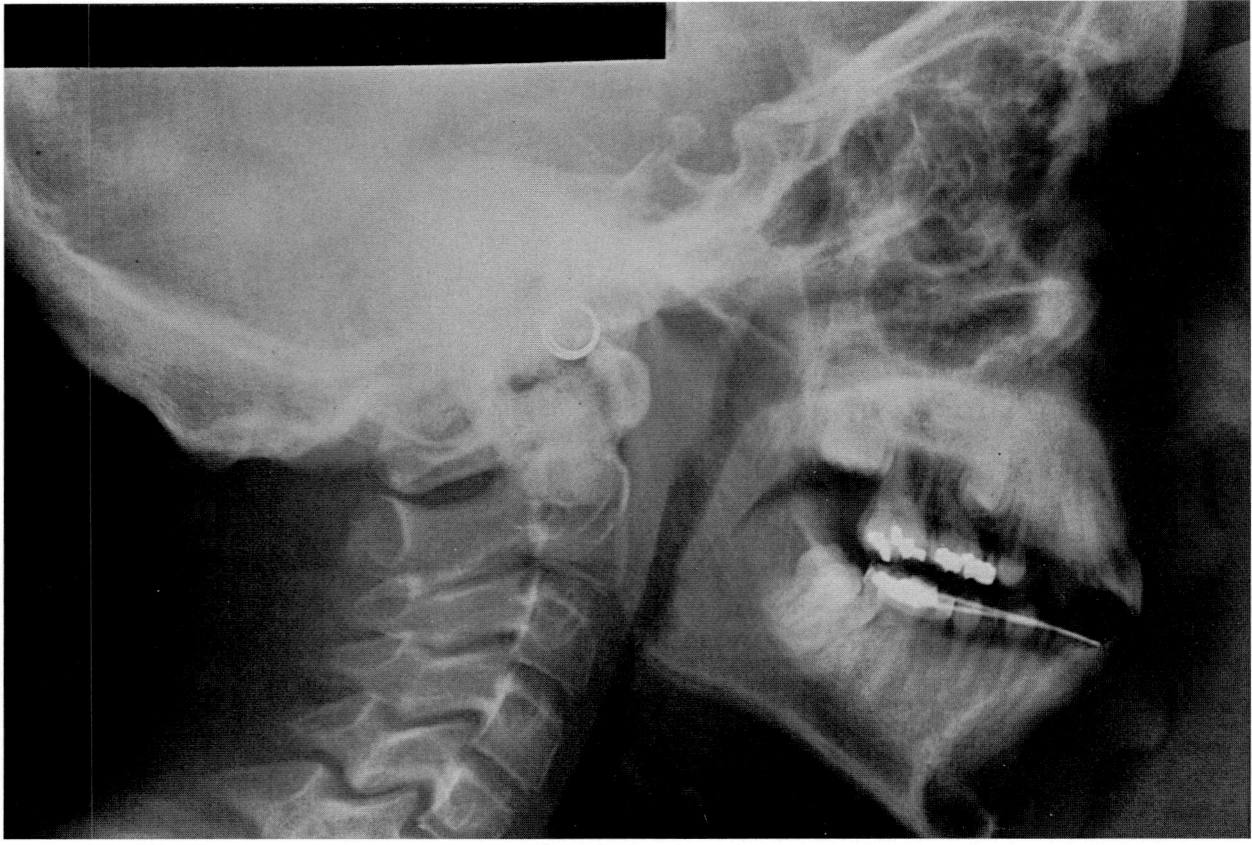

A

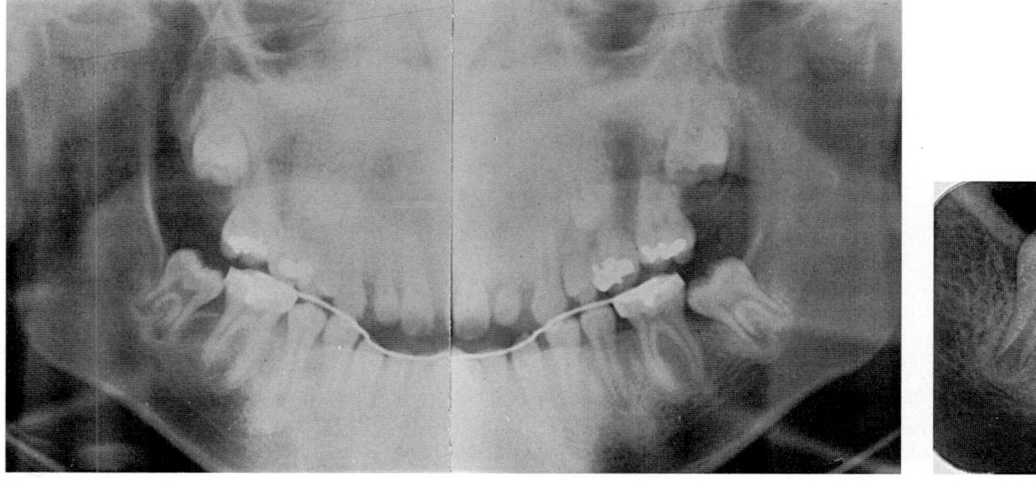

B

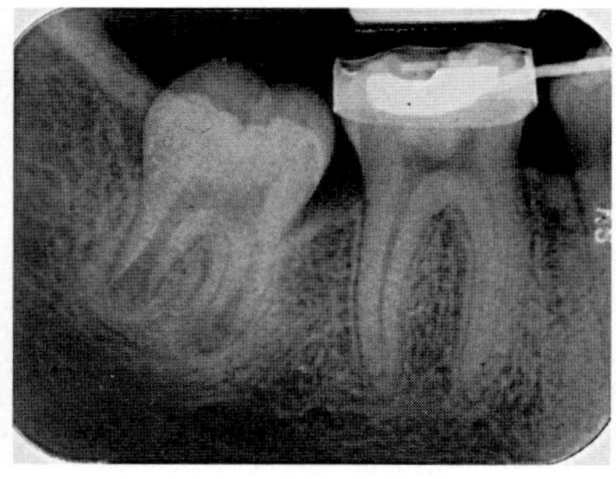

C

FIGURE 18–44.

Dominant Craniometaphyseal Dysplasia: Case in a 15-year-old boy. A, Hyperostosis of the base of the skull, including sella turcica and hyperostosis occipitalis interna, and hyperostosis of maxillary and mandibular alveolar bone. B, Hyperostosis in alveolar bone producing ground glass appearance; lamina dura is absent in affected areas. C, Alveolar hyperostosis appearing to originate in lamina dura of developing teeth.

(*continued*)

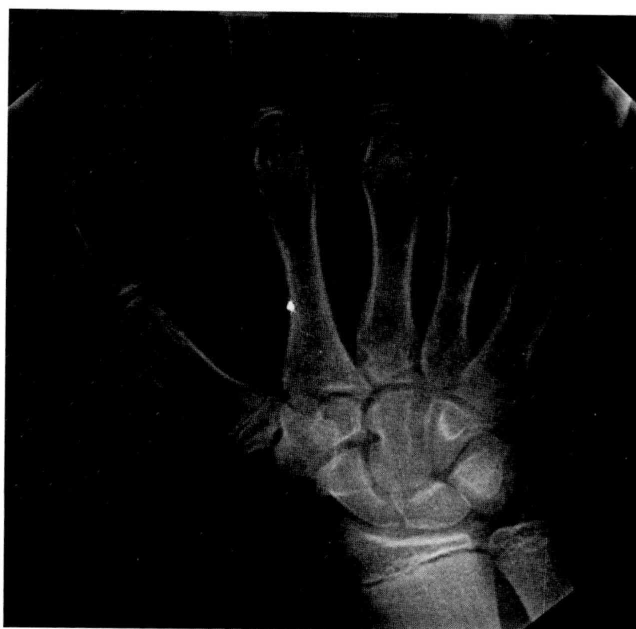

D

FIGURE 18–44. *(continued)*

D. Brachydactyly of fourth metacarpal and tubular defect in fifth metacarpal.

Radiologic Features of the Skeleton

The metaphyseal flare of the long bones produces an Erlenmeyer flask appearance, causing the genu valgum or knock-knee clinical sign. The tubular defect in the small bones of the hands causes a lack of diaphyseal narrowing, thus demonstrating the remodeling defect. The cortices have a normal thickness.

References

Gardner's Syndrome

Bochetto JF, Raycroft JF, DeInnocentes LW: Multiple polyposis, exostosis and soft tissue tumors. Surg Gynecol Obstet 117:489, 1963.

Chang CHJ, Piatt ED, Thomas KE, Watne AL: Bone abnormalities in Gardner's syndrome. Am J Roentgenol Radium Ther Nucl Med 103:6645, 1968.

Devic A, Bussy H: Un cas de polypose adénomateuse généralisée a tout pintestin. Arch Mal Appar Diag 6:278, 1912.

Fader M, Kline S, Spatz S, Zubrow HJ: Gardner's syndrome and a new dental discovery. Oral Surg Oral Med Oral Pathol 15:153, 1962.

Fitzgerald GM: Multiple composite odontoma: coincidental with other tumorous conditions: report of a case. J Am Dent Assoc 30:1408, 1943.

Gardner EJ, Plenk HP: Hereditary pattern for multiple osteomas in a family group. Am J Hum Genet 4:31, 1952.

Gardner EJ, Richards RC: Multiple cutaneous and subcutaneous lesions occurring simultaneously with hereditary polyposis and osteomatosis. Am J Hum Genet 5:139, 1953.

Gardner EJ, Stephens FE: Cancer and the lower digestive tract in one family group. Am J Hum Genet 2:41, 1950.

Ida M, Nakamura T, Utsumorniya J: Osteomatous changes and tooth abnormalities found in the jaws of patients with adenomatosis coli. Oral Surg Oral Med Oral Pathol 52:2, 1981.

Jones EL, Cornell WP: Gardner's syndrome. Arch Surg 92:287, 1966.

Komatsu I: A clinical genetic study on multiple intestinal polyposis and allied conditions. Jinrui Idengaku Zasshi 12:246, 1968.

Marshall KA, et al: Excision of multiple epidermal facial cysts in Gardner's syndrome. Am J Surg 150:615, 1985.

O'Brien SP, Wels P: Synchronous occurrence of benign fibrous tissue neoplasia, in hereditary adenosis of colon and rectum. NY J Med 55:1877, 1955.

Offerhaus GJA, et al: Gastroenterology 93:490, 1987.

Reed TE, Neel JV: A genetic study of multiple polyposis of the colon. Am J Hum Genet 7:236, 1955.

Robbins S: Textbook of Pathology. Philadelphia:WB Saunders, 1957, p. 795.

Small IA, Shandler H, Husain M, David H: Gardner's syndrome with an unusual fibro-osseous lesion of the mandible. Oral Surg Oral Med Oral Pathol 49:477, 1980.

Whitson WE, Orcutt JC, Walkinshaw MD: Orbital osteoma in Gardner's syndrome. Am J Ophthalmol 101:236, 1986.

Florid Cemento-osseous Dysplasia

Agazzi C, Belloni L: Gli odontomi duri dei mascellari: contributo clinicoromtgeriologico e anatomo-microscopico con particolare reguardo alle for me ad ampia estensione e alla comparsa familiare. Arch Ital Otal 64(suppl 16):3, 1953.

Bhaskar SN, Cutright DE: Multiple enostosis: report of 16 cases. J Oral Surg 26:321, 1968.

Friedman N, Goldman RC: Cementoma of the long bones. Clin Orthop 67: 243, 1969.

Goldstein BH, Byrne JE, Miller AS: Chronic sclerosing osteomyelitis. J Oral Surg 37:101, 1979.

Kaugars GE, Cale AD: Traumatic bone cyst. Oral Surg Oral Med Oral Pathol 63:318, 1987.

Melrose RJ, Abrams AM, Mills BG: Florid osseous dysplasia: a clinical pathologic study of 34 cases. Oral Surg Oral Med Oral Pathol 41:62, 1976.

Mincer HH, McGinnis JP, Wyatt JR: Ultrastructure of sclerotic cemental masses. Oral Surg Oral Med Oral Pathol 43:70, 1977.

Mirra JM, et al: Cementum-like bone production in solitary bone cysts (so-called "cementoma of the long bones"): report of 3 cases. Clin Orthop 135, 1978.

Sedano A, Kuba R, Gorlin RI: Autosomal dominant cemental dysplasia. Oral Surg Oral Med Oral Pathol 54:642, 1982.

Shafer WG: Chronic sclerosing osteomyelitis. J Oral Surg 15:138, 1957.

Waldron CA, Giangantì JS, Browand BC: Sclerotic cemental masses of the jaws (so-called chronic sclerosing osteomyelitis, sclerosing osteitis, multiple enostosis, and gigantiform cementoma). Oral Surg Oral Med Oral Pathol 39:590, 1975.

Waldron CA: Fibro-osseous lesions of the jaws. J Oral Maxillofac Surg 43:249, 1985.

Diffuse Sclerosing Osteomyelitis

Hardmeier T, Uehlinger E, Mugglie A: Primar chronische sklerosierende osteomyelitis. Verh Dtsch Ges Pathol 58:474, 1974.

Jacobsson S: Diffuse sclerosing osteomyelitis of the mandible. Int J Oral Surg 13:363, 1984.

Jacobsson S, Heyden G: Chronic sclerosing osteomyelitis of the mandible: histologic and histochemical findings. Oral Surg Oral Med Oral Pathol 43:357, 1977.

Jacobsson S, Hollender L: Treatment and prognosis of diffuse sclerosing osteomyelitis (DSO) of the mandible. Oral Surg Oral Med Oral Pathol 49:7, 1980.

Shafer WG, Hine M, Levy BM: A Textbook of Oral Pathology. 4th Ed. Philadelphia:WB Saunders, 1983, p. 502.

van Merkesteyn JPR, Groot RH, Bras J, Bakker DJ: Diffuse sclerosing osteomyelitis of the mandible: clinical, radiographic, and histologic findings in twenty seven patients. J Oral Maxillofac Surg 46:825, 1988.

van Merkesteyn JPR, et al: Diffuse sclerosing osteomyelitis of the mandible: a new concept of its etiology. Oral Surg Oral Med Oral Pathol 70:414, 1990.

Fibrous Dysplasia

Albright F, Butler AM, Hampton AO, Smith P: Syndrome characterized by osteitis fibrosa disseminata, areas of pigmentation and endocrine dysfunction with precocious puberty in females: report of five cases. N Engl J Med 216:727, 1937.

Dahlin DC: Bone Tumors. 3rd Ed. Springfield, IL:Charles C Thomas, 1978, p. 362.
Daves ML, Yardley JH: Fibrous dysplasia of bone. Am J Med Sci 234: 590, 1957.
Daramola JO, et al: Fibrous dysplasia in the jaws of Nigerians. Oral Surg Oral Med Oral Pathol 42:290, 1976.
Edeiken J: Roentgen Diagnosis of Diseases of Bone. 3rd Ed. Baltimore: Williams & Wilkins, 1981, p. 994.
El Deeb M, Sedano HD, Waite DE: Aneurysmal bone cyst of the jaws: report of a case associated with fibrous dysplasia and review of the literature. Int J Oral Surg 9:301, 1980.
El Deeb M, Waite DE, Jaspers MT: Fibrous dysplasia of the jaws: report of 5 cases. Oral Surg Oral Med Oral Pathol 48:312, 1979.
Eversole LR, Sabes WR, Rovin S: Fibrous dysplasia: a nosologic problem in the diagnosis of fibro-osseous lesions of the jaws. J Oral Pathol 1: 189, 1972.
Farman AG, Nortjé CJ, Grotepass FW: Pathological conditions of the mandible: their effect on the radiographic appearance of the inferior dental (mandibular) canal. Br J Oral Surg 15:64, 1977.
Giunta JL, Heffez L, Doku HC: Superior and buccal displacement of the mandibular canal in fibrous dysplasia. J Oral Maxillofac Surg 43:460, 1985.
Goldberg MH, Sperling A: Gross displacement of the mandibular canal: a radiographic sign of benign fibro-osseous bone disease. Oral Surg Oral Med Oral Pathol 51:225, 1981.
Harris WH, Dudley HR Jr, Barry RJ: The natural history of fibrous dysplasia. J Bone Joint Surg (Am) 44:207, 1962.
Lichtenstein L, Jaffe HL: Fibrous dysplasia of bone. Arch Pathol 33:777, 1942.
Lichtenstein L: Polyostotic fibrous dysplasia. Arch Surg 36:874, 1938.
McCune DJ, Burch H: Osteodystrophia fibrosa. Am J Dis Child 54:806, 1937.
Mirra JM, Picci P, Gold RH: Bone Tumors: Clinical Radiologic and Pathologic Correlations. Philadelphia:Lea & Febiger, 1989, p. 191.
Obisesan AA, et al: The radiologic features of fibrous dysplasia of the craniofacial bones. Oral Surg Oral Med Oral Pathol 44:949, 1977.
Schlumberger HG: Monostotic fibrous dysplasia. Milit Surg 99:504, 1946.
Schwartz DT, Alpert M: The malignant transformation of fibrous dysplasia. Am J Med Sci 247:1, 1964.
Shafer WG, Hine MK, Levy BM: A Textbook of Oral Pathology. 4th Ed. Philadelphia:WB Saunders, 1983, p. 694.
Slow IN, Stern D, Friedman FW: Osteogenic sarcoma arising in preexisting fibrous dysplasia. J Oral Surg 29:126, 1971.
Stafne EC, Gibilisco JA: Oral Roentgenographic Diagnosis. 4th Ed. Philadelphia:WB Saunders, 1975, p. 222.
von Recklinghausen F: Die fibrose oder deformiende osteite. Festschrift R. Virchow zu Seinem 71 Geburtstage. Berlin, 1891.
Waldron CA, Giansanti JS: Benign fibro-osseous lesions of the jaws. Part 1: fibrous dysplasia of the jaws. Oral Surg Oral Med Oral Pathol 35: 190, 1973.
Waldron CA: Fibro-osseous lesions of the jaws. J Oral Maxillofac Surg 43:249, 1985.
Wannfors K, Lindskog S, Olander KJ, Hammarstrom L: Fibrous dysplasia of bone concomitant with dysplastic changes in the dentin. Oral Surg Oral Med Oral Pathol 59:394, 1985.
Worth HM: Principles and Practice of Oral Radiologic Interpretation. Chicago:Year Book Medical Publishers, 1963, p. 606.
Zimmerman DC, Dahlin DC, Stafne EC: Fibrous dysplasia of the maxilla and the mandible. Oral Surg Oral Med Oral Pathol 11:55, 1958.

Paget's Disease

Brooke RI: Giant cell tumor in patients with Paget's disease. Oral Surg Oral Med Oral Pathol 30:230, 1970.
Burket LW: Oral Medicine: Diagnosis and Treatment. Philadelphia:JB Lippincott, 1971, p. 360.
Dickson DD, Camp JD, Ghormley RA: Osteitis deformans Paget's disease of bone. Radiology 44:449, 1945.
Goldstein BH, Laskin BM: Giant cell tumor of the maxilla complicating Paget's disease of bone. J Oral Surg 32:209, 1974.
Greenspan A, Norman A, Sterling AP: Precocious onset of Paget's disease: a report of three cases and review of the literature. J Can Assoc Radiol 28:69, 1977.
Guyer PB, Clough PWC: Paget's disease of bone: some observations on the relation of the skeletal distribution to pathogenesis. Clin Radiol 29: 421, 1978.
Hamdy R: The signs and treatment of Paget's disease. Geriatrics 32:89, 1977.
Hutter RVP, Foote FW, Frazell EL, Francis KC: Giant cell tumors complicating Paget's disease of bone. Cancer 16:1044, 1963.
Jaffe HL: Metabolic Degenerative and Inflammatory Diseases of Bones and joints. Philadelphia:Lea & Febiger, p. 355, 1972.
Krane SM: Paget's disease of bone. Clin Orthop 127:24, 1977.
Maldague B, Malghem A: Dynamic radiologic patterns of Paget's disease of bone. Clin Orthop 217:126, 1987.
Marks JM, Dunkelberger FB: Paget's disease. J Am Dent Assoc 101:49, 1980.
Meunier PJ, et al: Skeletal distribution of biochemical parameters of Paget's disease. Clin Orthop 217:37, 1987.
Mirra J, Bauer F, Grant T: Giant cell tumor with viral-like intranuclear inclusions associated with Paget's disease. Clin Orthop 158:243, 1981.
Mirra JM, Picci P, Gold RH: Bone Tumors: Clinical Radiologic and Pathologic Correlations. Philadelphia:Lea & Febiger, 1989, p. 893.
Paget J: On a form of chronic inflammation of bones (osteitis deformans). Med Chir Tr 60:37, 1877.
Poretta CA, Dahlin DC, Jarres JM: Sarcoma in Paget's disease of bone. J Bone Joint Surg (Am) 39:1314, 1957.
Sofaer JA: Dental extractions in Paget's disease of bone. Int J Oral Surg 13:79, 1984.
Schmorl G: Ulser osteitis deformans Paget. Virchows Arch [A] 282:694, 1932.
Schuller A: Dysostosis hypophoria. Br J Radiol 31:156, 1926.
Singer FR, Schiller AL, Pyle EB, Krane SM: Paget's disease of bone. In: Avioli LV, Krane SM, eds. Metabolic Bone Disease. 2nd Ed. New York:Academic Press, p. 481, 1978.
Smith BJ, Eveson JW: Paget's disease of bone with particular reference to density. J Oral Pathol 10:233, 1981.
Sosman MC: Radiology as an aid in the diagnosis of skull and intracranial lesions. Radiology 9:396, 1927.
Stafne EC, Austin LT: Study of dental roentgenograms in cases of Paget's disease (osteitis deformans) osteitis fibrosis cystica and osteoma. J Am Dent Assoc 25:1202, 1938.
Standish SM, Gorlin RJ: Bone disorders affecting jaws. In: Gorlin RJ, Goodman HM, eds. Thoma's Oral Pathology. 6th Ed. St. Louis:CV Mosby, p. 546, 1970.
Sutton D: Textbook of Radiology. 2nd Ed. Edinburgh:Churchill Livingstone, 1975, p. 78.
Tillman HH: Paget's disease of bone: a clinical, radiographic and histopathologic study of 24 cases involving the jaws. Oral Surg Oral Med Oral Pathol 15:1125, 1962.
Vacher-Lavenu M, et al: Inclusion tubulofilamenteuses intranucléaires dans les cellules multinuclées des tumeures à cellules géantes des os: étude ultrastructurale d'une série de 31 tumeures. CR Acad Sci 293:639, 1981.
Welfare RD: Paget's disease. Br Dent J 158:90, 1985.
Worth HM: Principles and Practice of Radiologic Interpretation. Chicago: Year Book Medical Publishers, 1963, p. 638.

Osteopetrosis

Albers-Schönberg HE: Röentgenbilder einer seltenen Knochenerkrankung. Munch Med Wochenschr 51:365, 1904.
Dick HM, Simpson WJ: Dental changes in osteopetrosis. Oral Surg Oral Med Oral Pathol 34:408, 1972.
Edeiken J: Roentgen Diagnosis of Diseases of Bone. 3rd Ed. Baltimore: Williams & Wilkins, 1981, p. 1347.
Hanhart E: Uber de genetik der eintoch-rezessiven formen der armorknachenkrankheit and zwei ents prechande stammbaume aus der schweiz. Helv Paediatr Acta 3:113, 1948.
Karshner RG: Osteopetrosis. AJR 16:405, 1926.
Rubin P: Dynamic Classification of Bone Dysplasias. Chicago:Yearbook Medical Publishers, 1964, p. 267.
Ruprecht A, Wagner H, Engle H: Osteopetrosis: report of a case and discussion of the differential diagnosis. Oral Surg Oral Med Oral Pathol 66: 674, 1988.
Schulze F: Das Wesen des Krankenheitsbildes der Marmorknochen (Albers-Schönberg). Arch Klin Chir 118:411, 1921.

Shafer WG, Hine MK, Levy BM: A Textbook of Oral Pathology. 3rd Ed. Philadelphia:WB Saunders, 1983, p. 684.

Sly WS, et al: Carbonic anhydrase II deficiency in 12 families with autosomal recessive syndrome of osteopetrosis with renal tubular acidosis and cerebral calcifications. N Engl 5 Med 3132:139, 1985.

Smith NHH: Albers-Schonberg disease (osteopetrosis): report of a case and review of the literature. Oral Surg Oral Med Oral Pathol 22:699, 1966.

Steiner M, Gould AR, Means WR: Osteomyelitis of the mandible associated with osteopetrosis. J Oral Maxillofac Surg 41:395, 1983.

Worth HM: Principles and Practice of Oral Radiologic Interpretation. Chicago:Yearbook Medical Publishers, 1963, p. 128.

Zachariades N, Koundouris I: Maxillofacial symptoms in two patients with pyknodysostosis. J Oral Maxillofac Surg 42:819, 1984.

Sclerosteosis

Beighton P, Cremin BJ: Sclerosing Bone Dysplasias. Berlin:Springer-Verlag, 1980, p. 19.

Beighton P, Davidson J, Durr L, Hamersma H: The clinical features of sclerosteosis: a review of manifestations in 25 affected individuals. Ann Intern Med 84:393, 1976.

Hansen HG: Sklerosteose. In: Opitz H, Schmidt F, eds. Handbach der Kinderheilkunde. Vol 6. Berlin:Springer, 1967, p. 351.

Truswell AS: Osteopetrosis with syndactyle: a morphological variant of Albers-Schonberg disease. J Bone Joint Surg (Br) 40:208, 1958.

van Buchem FSP, Hadders HN, Ubbens R: An uncommon familial systemic disease of the skeleton: hyperostosis corticalis generalisata familiaris. Acta Radiol 44:109, 1955.

Wood RE, Kleyn G, Nortjé CJ, Grotepass F: Jaw involvement in sclerosteosis: a case report. Dentomaxillofac Radiol 17:145, 1988.

Endosteal Hyperostosis

Beighton P: Inherited Disorders of the Skeleton. Edinburgh:Churchill Livingstone, 1978, p. 119.

Dixon JM, Cull RE, Gamble P: Two cases of van Buchem's disease. J Neurol Neurosurg Psychiatry 45:913, 1982.

Horan F, Beighton P: Orthopaedic Problems in Inherited Disorders. Berlin: Springer-Verlag, 1982, p. 71.

Maroteaux P, Fontaine G, Scharfman W, Farriaux JP: L'hyperostose corticale generalisee, a transmission dominante. Arch Fr Pediatr 28:685, 1971.

van Buchem FSP, Hadders HN, Ubbens R: An uncommon familial systemic disease of the skeleton: hyperostosis corticalis generalisata familiaris. Acta Radiol 44:109, 1955.

van Buchem FSP, Prick JJG, Jaspar HHJ: Hyperostosis Corticalis Generalisata Familiaris (van Buchem's Disease). Amsterdam:Exerpta Medica, 1976, p. 3.

Worth HM, Wollin DG: Hyperostosis corticalis generalisata congenita. J Can Assoc Radiol 17:67, 1966.

Infantile Cortical Hyperostosis

Aegerter E, Kirkpatrick JA Jr: Infantile cortical hyperostosis. In: Aegerter E, Kirkpatrick JA Jr, eds. Orthopedic Diseases. Philadelphia:WB Saunders, 1975, p. 70.

Caffey J, Silverman WA: Infantile cortical hyperostosis: preliminary report of a new syndrome. AJR 54:1, 1945.

Caffey J: Pediatric X-ray Diagnosis. Chicago:Year Book Medical Publishers, 1961, p. 240.

Edeiken J: Roentgen Diagnosis of Diseases of Bone. 3rd Ed. Baltimore: Williams & Wilkins, 1981, p. 817.

Pajewski M, Vure E: Late manifestations of infantile cortical hyperostosis (Caffey's disease). Br J Radiol 40:90, 1967.

Potter LE, Craig MM: Pathology of the Fetus and Infant. 3rd Ed. Chicago: Year Book Medical Publishers, 1976, p. 568.

Roske G: Eine eigenartige knochenerkrankung im sauglingsalter. Monatsschr Kinderheilkd 47:385, 1930.

Saul RA, Lee WH, Stevenson RE: Caffey's disease revisited. Am J Dis Child 136:56, 1982.

Snook SS, King NW: Familial infantile cortical hyperostosis (Caffey's disease) in rhesus Monkeys (macaca mulatta). Vet Pathol 26:274, 1989.

Worth HM: Principles and Practice of Oral Radiologic Interpretation. Chicago:Year Book Medical Publishers, 1963, p. 603.

Dominant Craniometaphyseal Dysplasia

Beighton P, Hamersma H, Horan F: Craniometaphyseal dysplasia: variability of expression within a large family. Clin Genet 15:252, 1970.

Bricker SL, Langlais RP, Van Dis ML: Dominant craniometaphyseal dysplasia: literature review and case report. Dentomaxillofac Radiol 12: 95, 1983.

Gorlin RJ, Springer J, Koszalka MF: Genetic craniotubular bone dysplasias and hyperostosis: a critical analysis. Birth Defects 4:79, 1969.

Jackson WPU, et al: Metaphyseal dysplasia, epiphyseal dysplasia, diaphyseal dysplasia and related conditions. Arch Intern Med 94:871, 1954.

Keitzer G, Paparella MM: Otolaryngological disorders in craniometaphyseal dysplasia. Laryngoscope 79:921, 1969.

Mori PA, Holt JF: Cranial manifestations of familial metaphyseal dysplasia. Radiology 66:335, 1956.

Rubin P: Dynamic Classification of Bone Dysplasias. Chicago:Year Book Medical Publishers, 1964, p. 89.

Shea J, Gerbe R, Ayani N: Craniometaphyseal dysplasia: the first successful surgical treatment for associated hearing loss. Laryngoscope 91:1369, 1981.

Spiro PC, Hamersma H, Beighton P: Radiology of the autosomal dominant form of craniometaphyseal dysplasia. S Afr Med J 49:839, 1975.

Chapter 19

Soft Tissue Radiopacities

FOREIGN BODIES

A foreign body, which is a mass or particle of material normally not located in a certain place, may be found within the jaws or surrounding soft tissues. According to Gibilisco (1980), more foreign bodies are discovered in the region of the face than any other part of the body. The most common foreign bodies within the jaws are amalgam, gutta percha, cements, whole or parts of teeth, elastic impression materials such as rubber base, and dental instruments such as broaches, curette tips, elevator tips, and burs. In the soft tissues, the following may be found: hypodermic needles, pins, needles, birdshot, bullets, and metal and glass fragments often resulting from accidents. Wood fragments, toothbrush bristles, fish bones, and popcorn husks may become impacted in soft tissue and not be visible on radiographs. According to Alattan and colleagues (1980), 0.3 to 2.8% of all pathologic lesions consist of foreign bodies.

Clinical Features

The most common foreign body in the jaws is amalgam. In most cases, it is found in edentulous areas, having fallen into the socket during an extraction. Because it does not interfere with healing, it is not detected immediately. In other instances, the alloy becomes embedded beneath the periosteum or within the marginal gingiva during a crown preparation with a diamond bur. In this latter instance, small fragments of the amalgam buildup are embedded into the gingiva by contact with the bur. These areas clinically appear bluish purple and are seen most often within the gingiva of the edentulous ridge or the marginal gingiva around a full crown. Amalgam fragments also may be found in the buccal mucosa, floor of the mouth, and palate. Some radiopaque foreign bodies are introduced deliberately for diagnostic, therapeutic, cosmetic, or functional reasons and include contrast medium, radon particles, and metal plates and screws to reduce fractures and surgical margins. Various implants commonly are seen. Most foreign bodies cause no symptoms, but the patient may have longstanding symptoms such as paresthesia if there is pressure on a nerve.

If a patient swallows or aspirates a foreign body, it must be determined immediately whether the object has entered the alimentary canal or respiratory tract. Laryngeal foreign bodies may produce stupor, hoarseness, coughing, and gagging. According to Wintrobe and colleagues (1970), the rapidity of the laryngeal reflex usually prevents the foreign body from slipping into the lungs. When a foreign body enters the esophagus, coughing, gagging, neck pain, and difficulty in swallowing may result and the patient may complain of something stuck in the throat. In such instances, there are no signs of respiratory distress. According to Edwards (1948), the patient should be referred to a radiologist, who can ascertain the location and nature of the foreign object.

◆ *RADIOLOGY (Figs. 19–1 to 19–4)*

Metal objects usually are more radiopaque than enamel, which helps the radiologist to distinguish these from tooth fragments. The nature of the object often may be ascertained by its shape and density. Thus, broken dental burs and instruments, BB shot, shotgun pellets, and bullets usually are identified easily. Stanhope (1955) reported a case in which the beaks of broken forceps were left within the jaws. Tooth fragments show a root canal space and pulp chamber, as well as differing densities of enamel and dentin. These fragments often may be found within the maxillary sinus, usually resulting from extraction or accidental trauma; they also may be detected within the soft tissues, including the tongue, floor of the mouth, and lips, and usually are caused by trauma. The foreign body usually is well tolerated by the host bone, but it should be removed if there is evidence of inflammatory or reactive changes.

ELONGATED STYLOID PROCESS

The styloid process is connected to the temporal bone anterior to the stylomastoid foramen by cartilaginous tissue. Worth (1963) reported that the styloid process varies in length in different people and often on two sides of the same person. Eagle (1948) stated that the normal length of the styloid process is 25 mm. Worth (1963) asserted that an elongated styloid process is common and almost always results from ossification in the stylohyoid or stylomandibular ligaments. The ossification usually arises in the upper end of the ligament and is in continuity with the styloid process, but it sometimes starts at the lower end of the stylohyoid ligament at the lesser cornu of the hyoid bone and less commonly in the midportion, usually in older people. Mineralization or calcification of the stylohyoid complex is relatively common. The reported incidence varies between 1.4%, as found by Grossman and Tarsitano (1977), and 28%, as stated by Kaufman and associates (1970); Correll and associates (1979) discovered an incidence of 18% on panoramic radiographs in a review of 1771 cases. Most authors agreed that few of these elongated processes produce symptoms. Kauf-

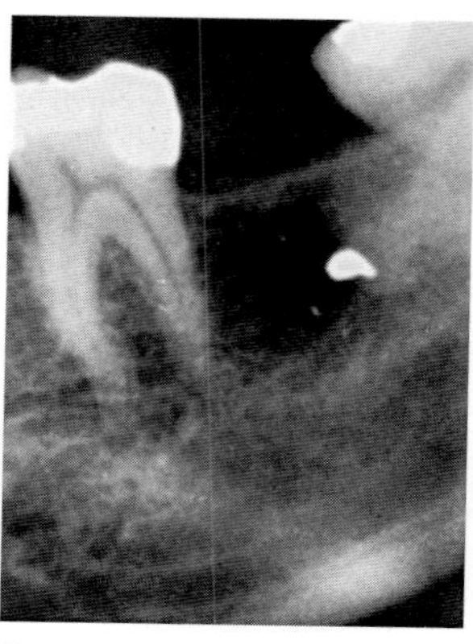

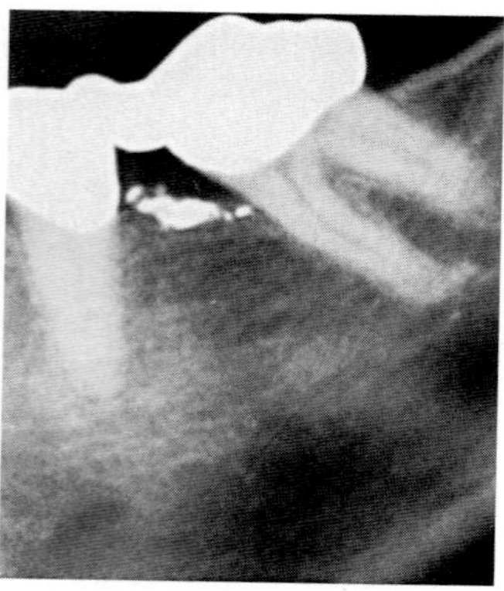

A B

FIGURE 19–1.

Foreign Body: Amalgam fragments. A, Within healed socket. B, At crest of ridge. Amalgam tattoo is visible clinically.

man and associates (1970) examined 68 patients with elongated processes and found 7 (10%) definite and 12 questionable (total of 28%) positive responses regarding the existence of clinical symptoms; Correll and co-authors (1979) established that 8 of 103 (8%) patients with elongated styloid processes showed related clinical symptoms.

Anatomic Considerations

The styloid process projects downward, forward, and slightly medially. Of pathogenic importance is the spatial position of the tip of this process. It is positioned between the internal and external carotid arteries and lies posterior to the tonsillar fossa and lateral to the pharyngeal wall. Muscular and ligamentous structures are attached at various locations on the process. The attached muscles are the stylopharyngeus (arising from the base), stylohyoid (attached to the middle portion), and styloglossus muscles (originating from the extremity of the process); the innervations of these three muscles are through the glossopharyngeal, facial, and hypoglossal nerves, respectively. At the apex of the process, two ligaments are inserted: the stylohyoid ligament, attached at its far end to the lesser cornu of the hyoid bone, and the stylomandibular ligament, which attaches at the angle of the mandible. The stylohyoid chain consists of the styloid process and the lesser cornu or horn of the hyoid bone and its connecting ligament, usually the stylohyoid ligament. Its embryologic derivation is from the second branchial or hyoid arch, also known as Reichert's cartilage.

Clinical Features

Dwight (1907) concluded from radiographic observations that the most striking cases of stylohyoid chain ossification occurred in people younger than 31 years of age; however, Grossman and Tarsitano (1977), Balasubramian (1964), Kaufman and colleagues (1970), and Barclay (1970) reported that the few patients who do have symptoms usually are older than 40 years of age. The sex incidence seems to be equal. Keur and associates (1986) reported on a sample of 1135 edentulous patients and found an abnormality in the styloid-stylohyoid complex in 33% of the women and 28% of the men. When symptoms are present, the condition is known as Eagle's syndrome, elongated styloid process syndrome, styloid process-carotid artery syndrome, stylohyoid syndrome, or styloid process neuralgia.

Eagle first presented two cases of symptomatic elongated calcified stylohyoid processes in 1937. In the first case, symptoms began immediately after tonsillectomy and were believed to be caused by a fibrous scar, which, when associated with the subjacent elongated styloid process, produced stimulation of the sensory nerve endings of cranial nerve V, VII, IX, or X or all of these nerves. The symptoms included subjective complaints of throat pain, which the patient attributed to improper postsurgical healing; a sensation of a foreign body, such as a fish bone stuck in the throat; pain on swallowing; and, frequently, referred pain to the ear on the affected side. A clinical finding of "tenting" or a firm bulge in the tonsillar fossa sometimes is present. When the tonsillar

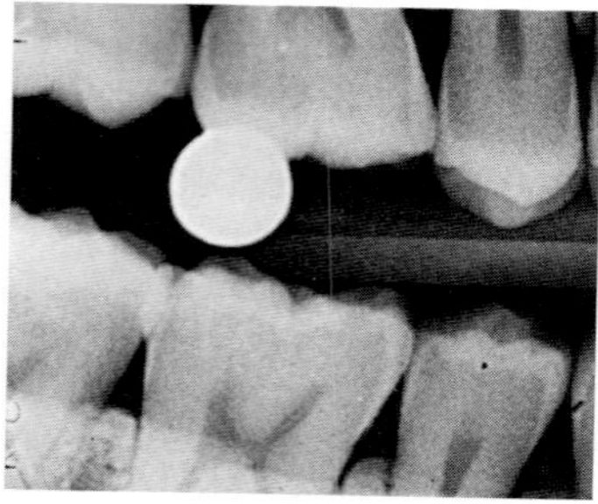

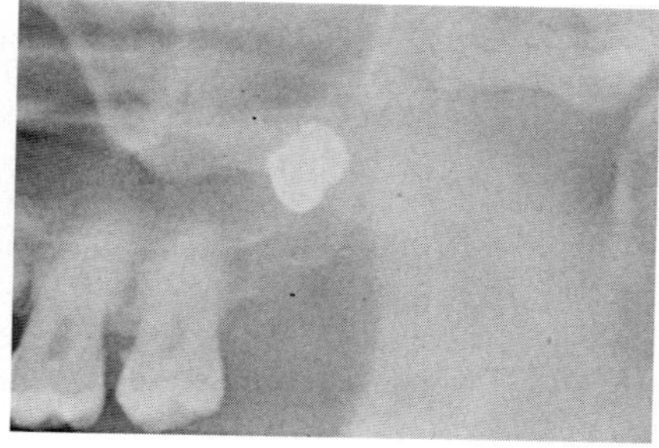

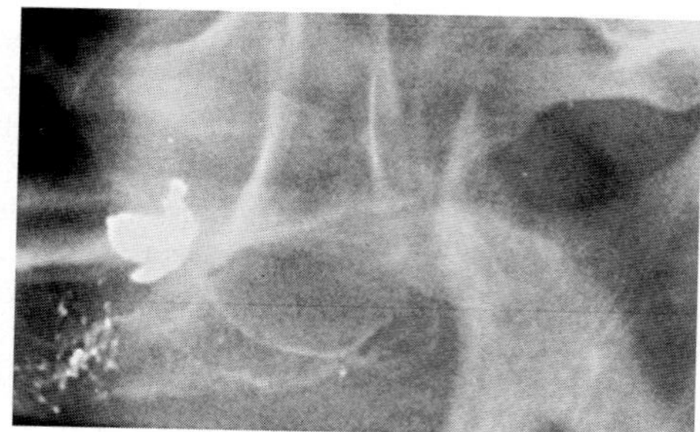

A B C

FIGURE 19–2.

Foreign Body: Missiles. A, BB shot in buccal mucosa. B, Pellet in cheek. C, Bullet in maxilla lodged near root of zygoma.

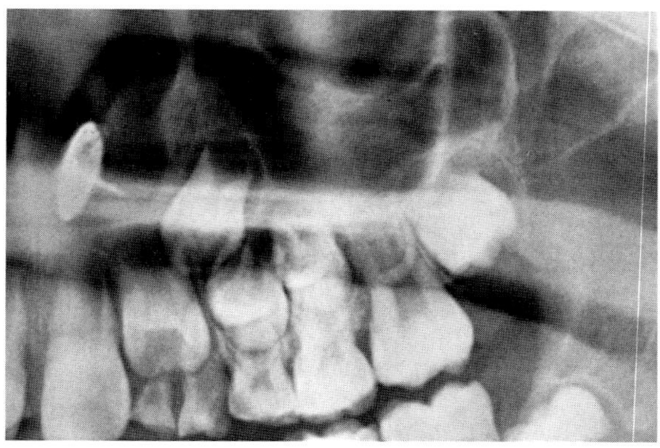
A

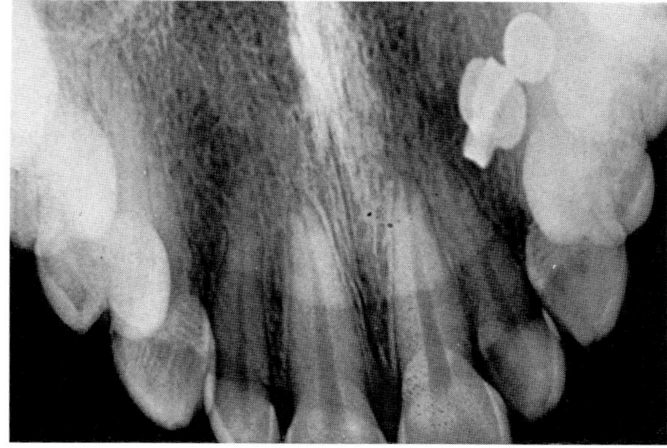
B

FIGURE 19-3.

Foreign Body: Objects in nose. A, Thumb tack. B, Jewelry.

fossa is palpated, firm resistance is met and symptoms usually are elicited. In the second case, as originally cited by Eagle (1937), the elongated styloid process produced impingement or compression of the internal or external carotid artery. The symptoms were attributed mainly to irritation of the rich sympathetic nerve supply to the walls of the carotid arteries, producing referred pain in the areas supplied by these vessels. Additionally, when the external carotid artery is involved, regional carotidynia, tinnitus, pain in the anterior cervical triangle, or pain on turning the head may occur. When the internal carotid artery is affected, the patient may have headaches in the orbital area and other sites supplied by this vessel. Although the condition is usually bilateral, paradoxically, the symptoms are typically unilateral. Other symptoms include transitory dizziness or lightheadedness, especially on turning the head; cervical pain; a sensation of a frequent need to swallow; and other painful symptoms.

After a detailed review of the literature regarding the association of cervicopharyngeal pain and stylohyoid ossification, Camarda and associates (1989) concluded that three syndromes are involved: Eagle's syndrome, stylohyoid syndrome, and pseudohyoid syndrome. Eagle's syndrome should be applied to patients with symptoms, according to the following criteria: patient may be of any age and there is a recent history of neck trauma or surgery (e.g., tonsillectomy), radiographic evidence of an elongated styloid process or stylohyoid chain ossification, clinical palpation of such elongation or ossification, and no pretraumatic clinical or radiographic evidence of styloid process elongation or stylohyoid chain ossification. The stylohyoid syndrome applies to patients of any age, but they usually are older than 40 years. There is no history of previous neck trauma, but the patient has radiographic evidence of stylohyoid chain ossification (in part or whole) at a young age. It is possible that such ossification may be palpated clinically. Most patients with symptoms with true stylohyoid chain ossification are 40 years of age and older. The pseudostylohyoid syndrome is reserved for patients 40 years of age and older with no history of trauma, radiographic evidence of stylohyoid chain ossification (in part or whole), or clinical palpation of such ossification. These are older patients who have symptoms identical to those of stylohyoid syndrome but have no radiographic findings, clinical findings (on palpation), or evidence of stylohyoid ossification. These people probably have tendinitis at the junction of the stylohyoid ligament and the lesser horn of the hyoid bone.

The differential diagnosis, depending on the symptoms, includes glossopharyngeal neuralgia, sphenopalatine neuralgia or Sluder's syndrome, histamine cephalalgia or cluster headaches, migraine headaches, carotidynia, myofascial pain-dysfunction or temporomandibular joint syndrome, impacted third molars, and other conditions associated with dysphagia, otalgia, or tinnitus.

Treatment

Camarda and associates (1989) stated that, in Eagle's syndrome, surgery is the initial treatment of choice because of the severity of the rapidly occurring ossification and symptoms, to which the patient has no time to adapt. In stylohyoid syndrome, however, the initial treatment should be more reversible. Camarda and associates (1989) proposed a two-phase treatment for these patients. The first phase involves

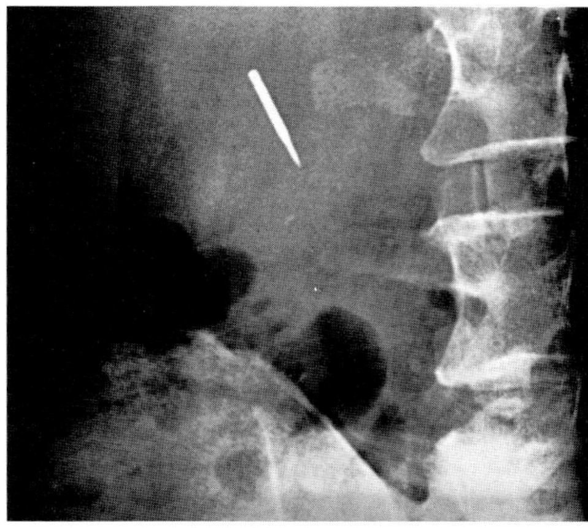

FIGURE 19-4.

Foreign Body: Swallowed foreign body: finishing bur in colon. (Courtesy of Dr. A. Del Balso, SUNY School of Medicine, Buffalo, NY.)

reassurance and injection of long-acting local anesthetics and steroidal solutions regionally to confirm the diagnosis and provide relief. Depending on the response to this initial treatment, surgery may then be considered. In pseudostylohyoid syndrome, this treatment is all that is necessary. In patients with stylohyoid syndrome, who are refractive to such initial treatments and cannot adapt to their developing symptoms, surgical treatment may be required. This usually consists of excision of the excessive mineralized portion of the stylohyoid complex, most often by a transpharyngeal or lateral neck approach. If the styloid process is excessive or radical amounts must be removed, the extraoral approach is a direct, anatomically concise approach to the styloid process; furthermore, if major vessel hemorrhage is encountered, it can be managed in a well-visualized and controlled manner.

◆ RADIOLOGY (Figs. 19–5 to 19–9)

Classification

Langlais and associates (1986) proposed a radiographic classification of the elongated and mineralized stylohyoid ligament complex. It included three types of radiographic appearances and four patterns of calcification or mineralization.

Morphologic Characteristics. Three types of radiographic appearances are proposed.

Type I: Elongated. The radiographic appearance of this type of mineralized complex is characterized by uninterrupted integrity of the styloid image. Langlais and associates (1986) accepted the normal length of the styloid process to be 25 mm for most radiographic projections; however, if panoramic radiographs are studies, measurements as long as 28 mm may be considered within the normal range because of the inherent magnification in most panoramic projections.

Type II: Pseudoarticulated. The styloid process apparently is joined to the mineralized stylomandicular or stylohyoid ligament by a single pseudoarticulation, which usually is located superior to a level tangential to the inferior border of the mandible. This gives an overall picture of an apparently articulated elongated styloid process. Langlais and associates (1986) believed that this type of mineralized complex is seen regularly, although much less frequently than Type I.

Type III: Segmented. Type III consists of short or long noncontinuous portions of the styloid process or interrupted segments of mineralized ligament. In either instance, two or more segments are seen, with interruptions above or below the inferior border of the mandible, or both. The overall appearance is of a segmented mineralized stylohyoid complex. In the study by Grossman and Tarsitano (1977), there was an approximately 27% incidence of segmented versions of the stylohyoid complex. Frommer (1974) described fibrous or cartilaginous unions between mineralized segments in his dissections.

Pattern of Calcification. Four patterns are proposed.

Calcified Outline. This pattern describes a thin radiopaque border with a central radiolucency that constitutes

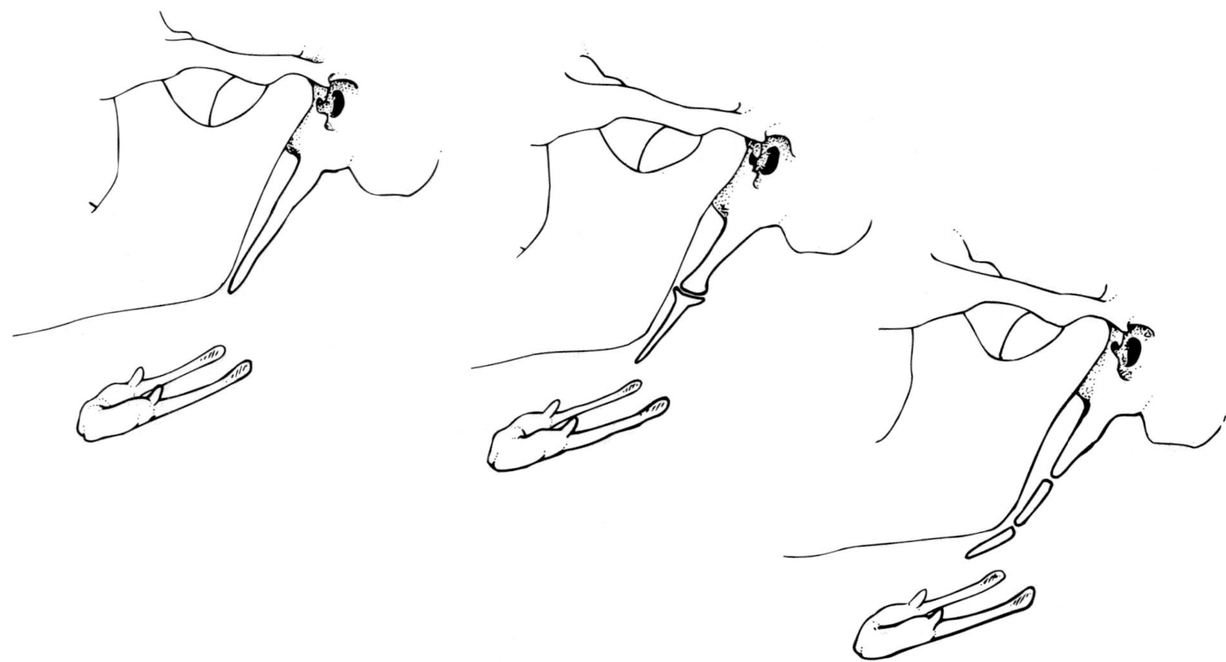

FIGURE 19–5.

Elongated Styloid Process: Classification from left to right: type 1, elongated; type 2, pseudoarticulated; type 3, segmented.

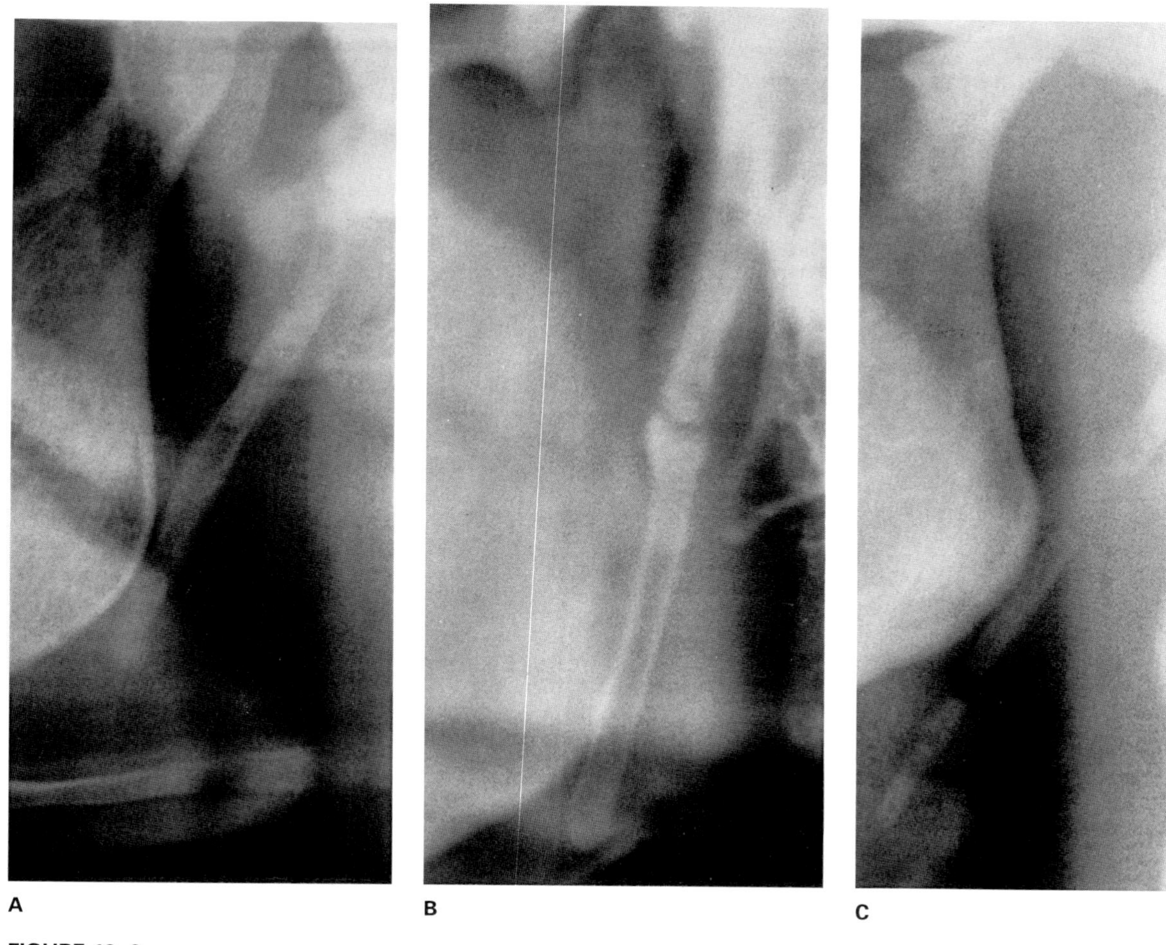

FIGURE 19–6.

Elongated Styloid Process: A, Type 1, elongated. B, Type 2, pseudoarticulated. C, Type 3, segmented.

most of the process. This pattern is reminiscent of the radiographic appearance of a long bone.

Partially Calcified. This pattern shows a process that has a thicker radiopaque outline, with almost complete opacification but a small, sometimes discontinuous, radiolucent core.

Nodular Complex. This pattern has a knobby or scalloped outline. It may be partially or completely calcified, with varying degrees of central radiolucency.

Completely Calcified. This pattern is totally radiopaque, with no evidence of a radiolucent interior.

Radiologic Features

Elongation and mineralization of the stylohyoid ligament complex are observed readily on panoramic radiographs. Kaufman and associates (1970), Correll and colleagues (1979), and Keur and co-workers (1986) considered any styloid process or mineralized stylohyoid ligament complex abnormal if it was 30 mm or longer on the radiograph. The mineralized stylohyoid ligament may be distinguished more definitively when it extends below the inferior border of the mandible or its attachment to the inferior cornu of the hyoid bone is seen. No radiographic features can be used to identify or distinguish symptomatic from asymptomatic elongated styloid processes. The Eagle's syndrome subtype cannot be determined on the basis of the radiographic appearance alone; however, the posteroanterior radiographs may show medial deviation of the process. In the presence of symptoms, this finding may be suggestive of the carotid artery subtype of Eagle's syndrome.

ERUPTION SEQUESTRUM

The eruption sequestrum, an anomaly associated with the eruption of teeth in children, first was described by Starkey and Shafer (1963). It is a tiny fragment of nonviable bone overlying an erupting permanent molar that is visible clinically and radiographically. As the molars erupt through the alveolar bone, the eruption sequestrum separates and isolates a central area of bone over the occlusal surface of the tooth.

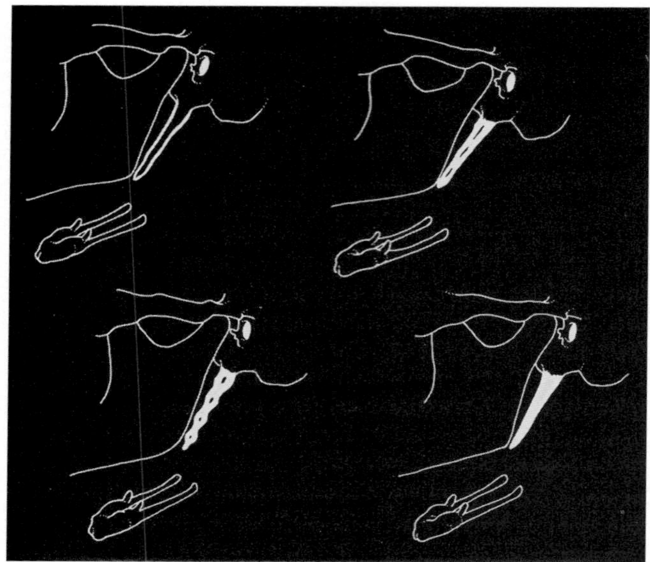

FIGURE 19–7.

Elongated Styloid Process: Patterns of mineralization from left to right, top to bottom: mineralized outline, partially mineralized, nodular, homogeneous.

Clinical Features

Normally, an erupting molar breaks into soft tissue and the intervening bone resorbs. When an eruption sequestrum occurs, it may cause mild discomfort, probably produced by compression of the soft tissue over the spicule during mastication. For a few days, the bone fragment may be seen lying on the crest of the ridge in a tiny depression. At this point, it can be removed easily. The condition is temporary and self-limiting. No treatment is necessary.

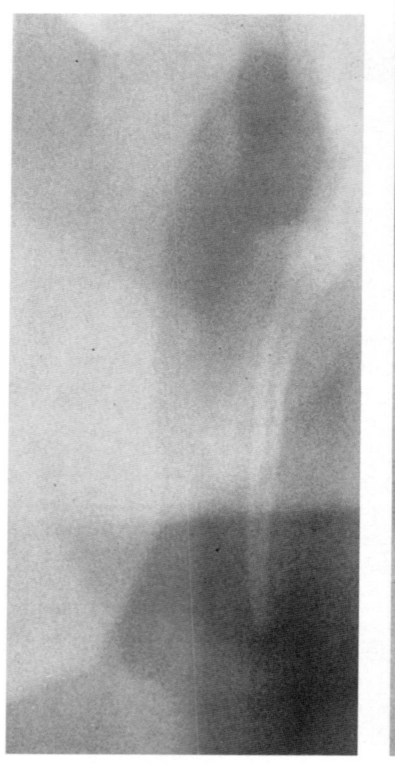

A

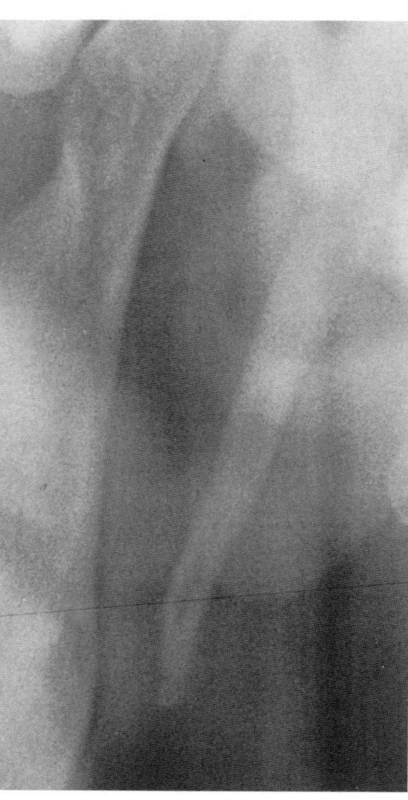

B

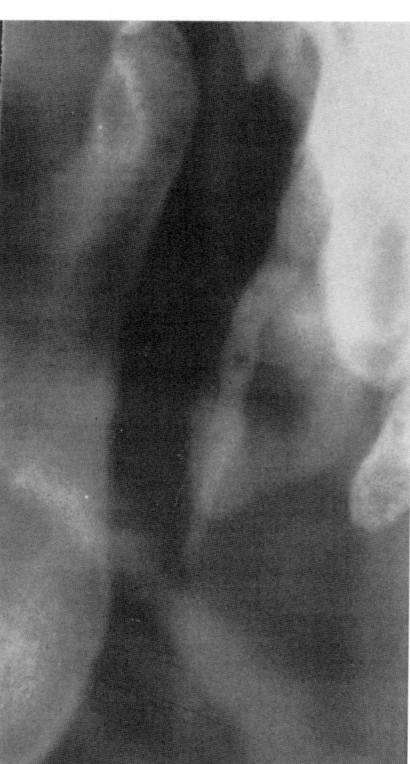

C

FIGURE 19–8.

Elongated Styloid Process: Patterns of mineralization. A, Mineralized outline. B, Partially mineralized. C, Nodular.

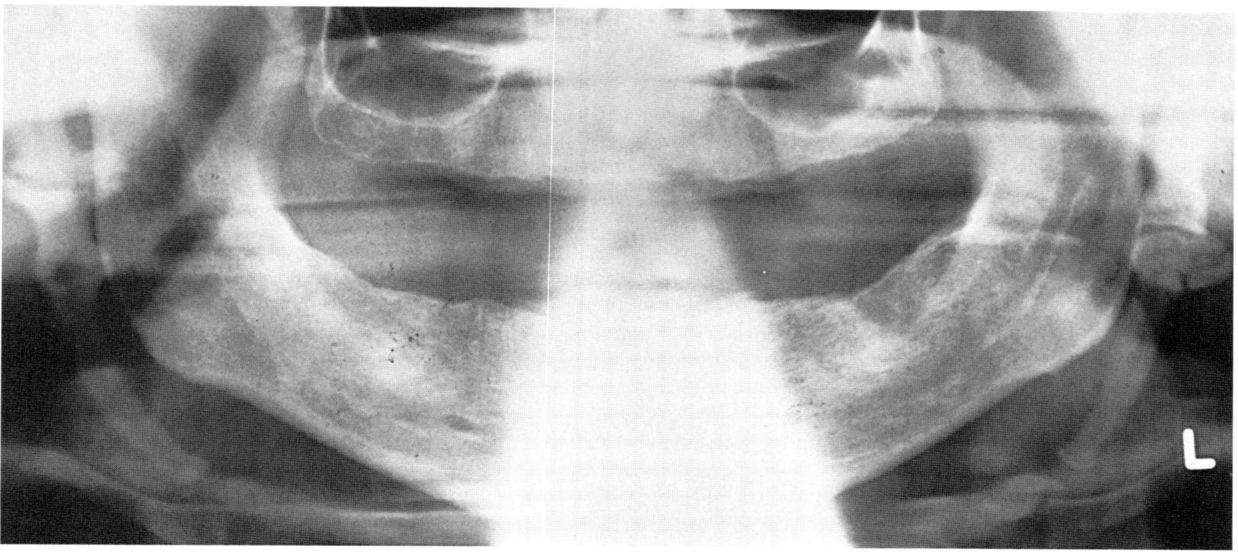

FIGURE 19–9.

Eagle's Syndrome: A 54-year-old man had a history of lightheadedness when turning his head to one side only. Bilateral pseudoarticulated, partially mineralized; only left side had symptoms. (Courtesy of Drs. D. Miles and M. Van Dis, Indiana University, Indianapolis, IN.)

◆ *RADIOLOGY (Figs. 19–10)*

The bony spicule (eruption sequestrum) appears to float in the soft-tissue overlying the crown of the erupting tooth. It is seen most frequently as a narrow radiopaque band that may be pencil thin, crescent shaped, figure-eight shaped, round, or ovoid. The sequestrum has the same density as the adjacent alveolar bone. If the overlying soft tissue can be seen, the sequestrum may be entirely within the soft tissue, partially within it, or in close approximation to the oral surface of the soft tissue. In the latter two instances, the sequestrum is visible clinically and, therefore, easy to locate if it is to be removed; in the first instance, the small bone fragment is not visible clinically.

SIALOLITH

Sialoliths are calcareous deposits in the ducts of major or minor salivary glands or within the glands themselves. The major salivary glands are the submandibular, parotid, and sublingual; minor salivary glands are located in the labial mucosa, cheeks, soft palate, and tongue. Among diseases of the salivary glands, sialolithiasis is second in frequency only to mumps, and it is probably the most frequent disease of the salivary glands in people older than 20 years of age.

Pathologic Characteristics

It is believed that sialoliths form by the deposition of calcium salts around a central nidus that may consist of desquamated epithelial cells, foreign bodies, bacteria, abnormal mucoid material, or bacterial debris. Salivary gland calculi have a laminated structure; calcium phosphate and carbonate are the major inorganic substances. Alternate layers of white calcareous mineral and organic, brownish yellow, resinous material are superimposed on the nucleus. Although the cause and pathogenesis of salivary calculi are not known, several theories have been proposed. Gorlin and Goldman (1970), Levy and associates (1962), and Baurmash and Mandel (1959) generally believe that the process of stone formation is enhanced by the stasis of salivary flow within the duct of the gland. Rabinov and Weber (1985) stated that the pathogenesis of salivary gland calculi appears to be related to the greater alkalinity of the submandibular gland as opposed to the more acidic product of the parotid gland; this difference in pH may explain the greater incidence of stone formation in the submandibular gland. Jensen and colleagues (1979) and Eversole and Sabes (1971) stated that the locali-

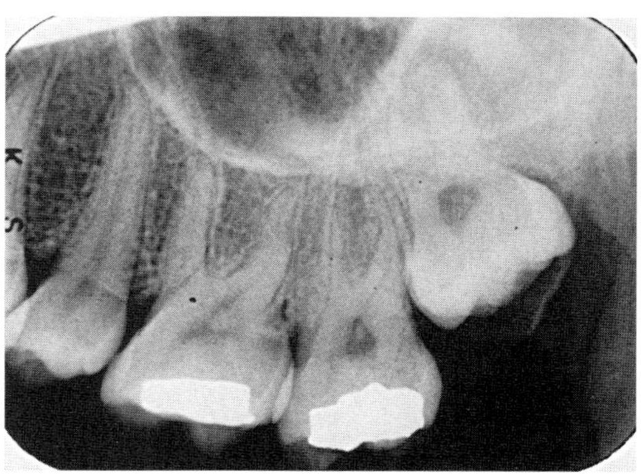

FIGURE 19–10.

Eruption Sequestrum: Clinically small fragment of bone can be teased from soft tissue.

zation of major salivary calculi primarily to the submandibular gland and the minor salivary gland calculi to the buccal mucosa suggests that local factors, such as trauma and duct morphologic characteristics, may be involved. Wharton's duct of the submandibular gland is much more irregular and longer than Stenson's duct of the parotid; Wharton's duct follows an uphill course that encourages stagnation of saliva, and stagnation leads to calculus formation. The lengths of the ducts of the labial and buccal mucosal salivary glands are longer than in the glands of the palatal mucosa. Certain other factors may facilitate stone formation. The mucus content of the submandibular gland may become more viscous, thus promoting stone formation.

When sialoliths reach a critical size or position, they effect a partial or complete obstruction of the duct. If the duct (usually Wharton's duct) becomes occluded, acute sialadenitis occurs when secondary pathogenic bacteria ascend the duct from the mouth, reaching the saliva stagnating in the dilated ducts proximal to the calculus. Inflammation resulting from bacterial infection will cause edema in the duct, and the duct will close around the calculus, resulting in obstructive symptoms of pain and swelling. If the acute sialadenitis is not treated properly, a chronic process eventually may lead to fibrosis and atrophy of the gland. Rabinov and Weber (1985) suggested that submandibular calculi form rapidly and infection follows as a consequence of obstruction, whereas parotid calculi form secondarily as result of infection. Of patients with recurrent chronic sialadenitis, 65% have had sialolithiasis.

Clinical Features

Rauch (1959) stated that stones form in patients ranging from the first decade of life to old age, with the peak incidence between 30 and 50 years; the author also reported that sialolithiasis occurs twice as often in men as women. Sometimes the stone presents no symptoms, and it is detected by bimanual palpation of Wharton's or Stenson's duct or incidentally on a radiograph. Many patients with sialolithiasis complain of a painful swelling of the gland that is most pronounced just before, during, and immediately after meals or during other times, such as brushing the teeth, drinking coffee or tea, or eating bitter or sour foods such as a lemon or candy. The involved gland may be tender and painful. The severity of symptoms depends on the degree of obstruction related to the size and location of the calculus. Stones within the gland tend to cause less severe symptoms and may lead to formation of a tender, inflammatory mass. Complete ductal obstruction may result in a continuously swollen gland, with severe pain, swelling in the floor of the mouth or cheek, and pus emanating from the duct orifice. In some cases, the swelling is diffuse and simulates cellulitis. Parotid stones generally are diagnosed 1 to 2 months after the onset of symptoms as opposed to approximately 1.5 years for submandibular stones.

In the minor salivary glands, stones may cause very little discomfort and may be expressed spontaneously. They appear as solitary, asymptomatic, small submucosal nodules that are hard or firm in consistency and freely movable in the surrounding tissue. In studies of sialolithiasis of minor salivary glands, Jensen and colleagues (1979), Anneroth and associates (1975), and Anneroth and Hansen (1983) observed that these calculi have a striking predilection for the upper lip and buccal mucosa of adults in their sixth, seventh, and eighth decades of life. Jensen and colleagues (1979) found a slight female predilection, whereas Anneroth and associates (1975) reported a male preponderance, which is in accordance with the findings of Bahn and Tabachnick (1971) and Pullon and Miller (1972).

The differential diagnosis of a sialolith should include a calcified lymph node, an avulsed or embedded tooth, a foreign body, a phlebolith (calcified thrombus), calcification in the facial artery, myositis ossificans, and the hyoid bone.

Treatment

The stones are removed surgically. Removal of calculi near the duct orifice sometimes may be accomplished by a small surgical nick at the duct orifice. If secondary infection is causing complications, it should be eliminated before the stone is removed surgically. A sialogram may have questionable value before surgery, especially in the anterior ductal stone, because injection of the contrast media may dislodge the calculus and carry it to the posterior part of the duct; preoperative sialography is indicated in cases of posterior ductal or intraglandular stones. If the sialolith is present near or in the substance of the gland itself, surgical extirpation of the gland may be necessary. Before removal of the gland, patients should know that the major glands contribute approximately 50% of the volume of saliva and the minor glands contribute the remainder.

◆ *RADIOLOGY (Figs. 19–11 to 19–15)*

Radiographic studies of patients with suspected salivary gland calculi consist of conventional plain radiographs, followed by sialography. For investigation of the parotid calculi, anteroposterior puffed-cheek, true lateral, lateral oblique, or panoramic views are obtained. The occlusal, true lateral, lateral oblique, basal views, and panoramic views are indicated for examination of the submandibular gland. The intraoral occlusal view should encompass the entire floor of the oral cavity posteriorly to the molar region. This projection usually shows the entire Wharton's duct, including the right-angle bend near the hilum of the gland. Most duct calculi occupy a position near the anterior end of Wharton's duct so that they are free of any overlying bone in the intraoral occlusal projection. Soft tissue radiographs may be useful in supporting a clinical diagnosis of minor salivary gland calculi. For instance, Jensen and co-workers (1979), Barnett (1971), DeGregori and Pippen (1970), and Alexander and Andrews (1965) found small radiopacities in soft tissue radiographs. Failure to detect a radiopacity in a lesion suspected of being a minor salivary gland calculus does not rule out that possibility because there is a wide variability in the degree of mineralization of these calculi. Sialoliths were not apparent on soft tissue radiographs as reported by Holst (1968) and Moskow and associates (1964).

It is not unusual for the image of salivary calculi to appear on a periapical radiograph incidental to routine dental radio-

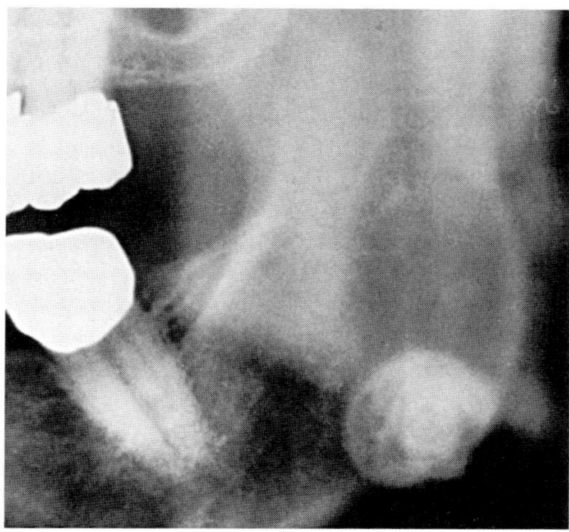
A

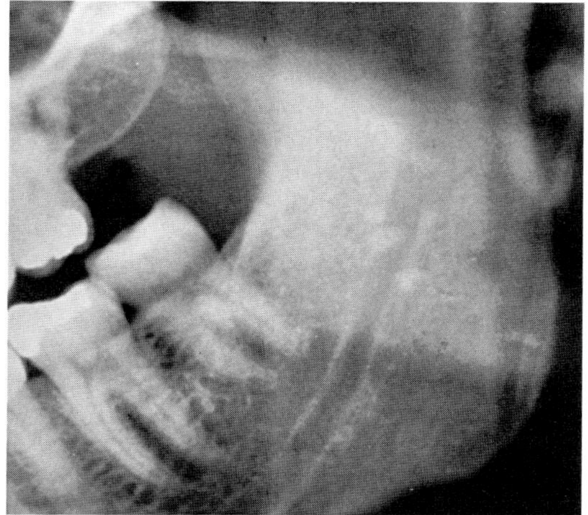
B

FIGURE 19–11.

Sialolith: A, Submandibular gland. B, Parotid gland; multiple calculi in midramus.

graphic examination. Those that occur in Wharton's duct are disclosed most often, particularly when radiographs are taken of the edentulous mandible, because there is a tendency to place the films deeper in the vestibule and thereby include the floor of the mouth and its contents. When superimposed on the mandible, the image may be interpreted as sclerotic bone or enostosis within the bone.

Location

Gorlin and Goldman (1970) reported that 92% of salivary calculi occur in the submandibular gland, 6% in the parotid gland, and 2% in both the sublingual and minor salivary glands. In a study of 180 cases of salivary calculi, Levy and associates (1962) found that 80% occurred in Wharton's duct, 18% in Stenson's duct, and 2% within the sublingual and minor salivary glands. Multiple calculi do occur in the same gland. Noehren (1923) stated that, in approximately 20% of patients with salivary calculi, the submandibular gland contains two calculi, and 5% of patients have more than two stones; multiple calculi occur frequently in the parotid gland. Rauch (1959) determined the following locations of submandibular stones: near the ostium (30%), middle third of the duct (20%), right-angle bend of Wharton's duct (35%), and proximal to the right-angle bend and hilum of the submandibular gland (15%). It is usual for duct calculi to be solitary, but frequently there are two and very rarely even more. Stones of the parotid gland frequently are located in Stenson's duct and usually are smaller than submandibular stones. Rauch (1959) reported the ratio of intraglandular versus extraglandular parotid stones as 1:35.

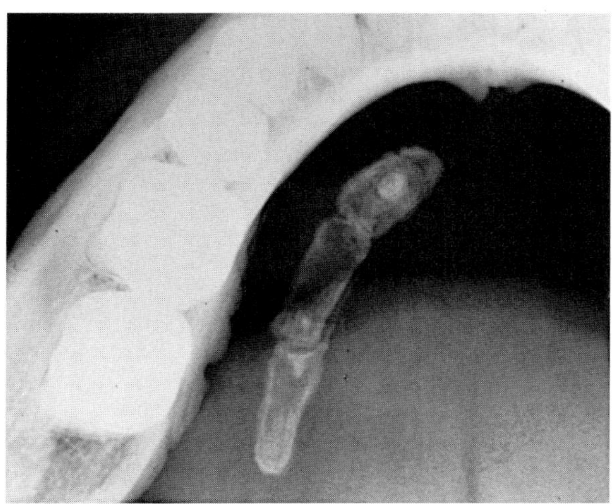
A

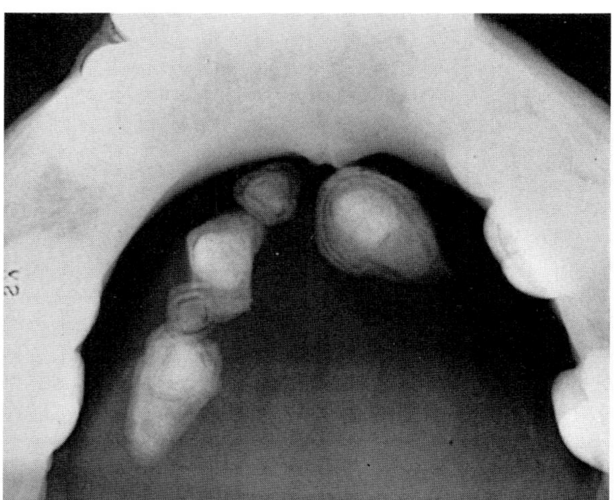
B

FIGURE 19–12.

Sialolith: Multiple salivary calculi. A, Unilateral. B, Bilateral. (Courtesy of Professor L. Alfaro, University of Chile School of Dentistry, Santiago, Chile.)

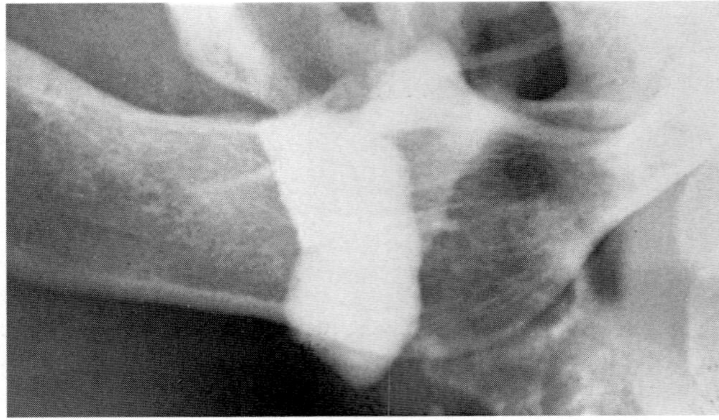

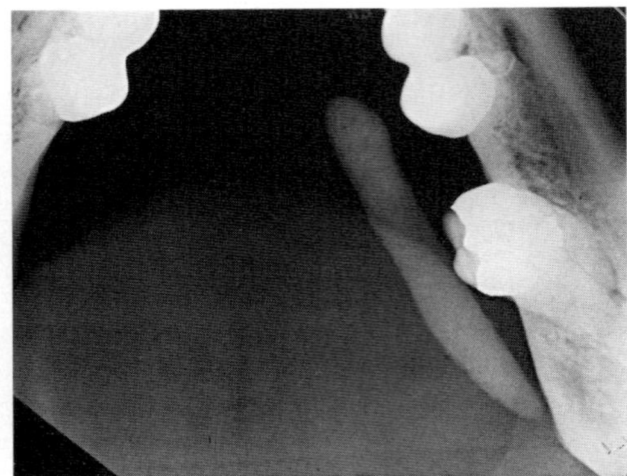

A B

FIGURE 19–13.

Sialolith: Gigantiform salivary calculi. A, Lateral ramus view. B, Occlusal view. (From Isacsson G, Persson NE: The gigantiform salivary calculus. Int J Oral Surg 11:135, 1982.)

Radiologic Features

Rubin and Holt (1957) stated that 20% of the stones of the submandibular gland are radiolucent, whereas 40% of those in the parotid gland are radiolucent. Thus, without sialography, parotid calculi are diagnosed less frequently. Most stones are round to oval or elliptic. In some cases the shape of the single calculus simulates a whole tooth or root. A cluster of calculi sometimes is present. The surface is smooth or slightly irregular and rough. The roughness is caused by short, sharp projections from the surface. Rauch (1959) pointed out that stones of the parotid gland often are irregular in size and shape, with pointed projections that may cause considerable pain. The size of the stones varies from small grains in smaller ducts to large stones in the main duct, especially Wharton's duct. Anneroth and co-workers (1975) reported that the average size is approximately 18 mm long with a girth of 3 mm. Isacsson and Persson (1982) described a 3.6 cm-long gigantiform salivary calculus located in Wharton's duct.

Radiographically, salivary calculus appears as a white or gray opacity in the region of the glandular apparatus. The radiographic density reflects the mineral composition of calculus. The degree of the radiopacity varies. Long-standing stones that have reached an appreciable size may have a greater radiographic density than normal bone and are shown readily. Those in which the organic content may be relatively high are not seen clearly, and, in some instances, the calculi may not be seen without sialography.

Sialography

Sialography with water-soluble contrast media material usually is the only means of ruling out salivary calculi. According to Levy and co-workers (1962), these calculi are radiolucent in 20% of cases, and Rubin and Holt (1957) reported that radiolucent stones are found in 20% of submandibular gland cases and 40% of parotid gland cases.

Sialography can be used to detect radiolucent calculi. Any delay in evacuation of the contrast media from within the

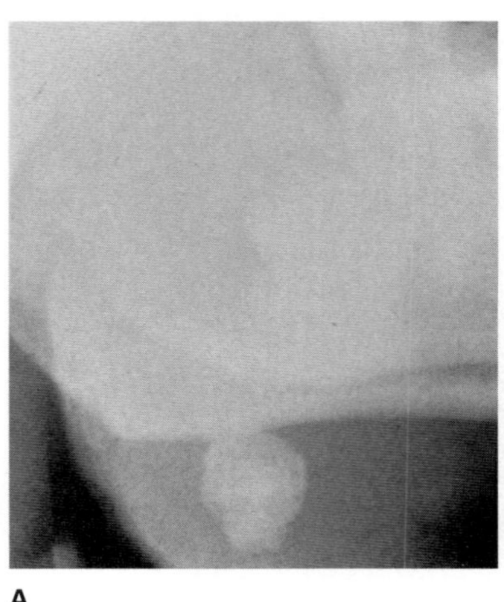

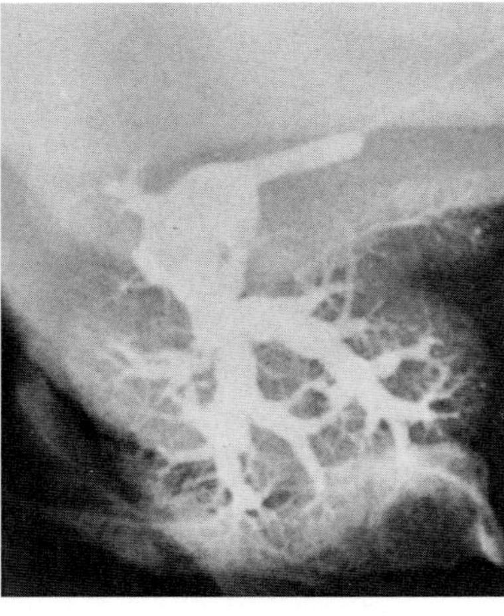

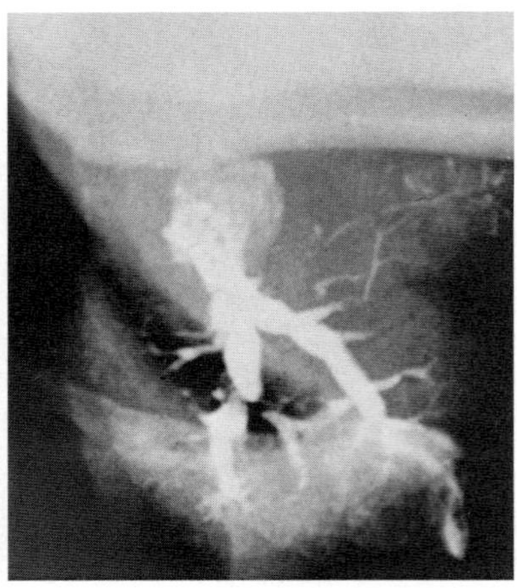

A B C

FIGURE 19–14.

Sialolith: Sialogram. A, Scout film. B, Terminal opacification. C, Ten-minute emptying; calculus is within ductal system. (Courtesy of Dr. M. Van Dis, Indiana University, Indianapolis, IN.)

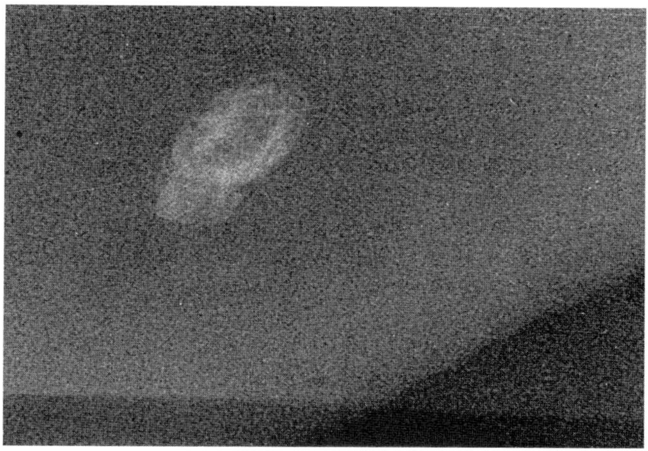

FIGURE 19–15.

Sialolith: Accessory salivary gland calculus in upper lip. (From van der Waal I: Sialoliths of minor salivary glands: how rare? J Oral Surg 29:815, 1971.)

main duct or branches may indicate obstruction by a radiolucent stone. Large radiopaque stones may obstruct the main duct completely. The interface between the stone and contrast medium is characterized by a crescent-shaped defect. In most instances, the contrast material will bypass the stone, which causes a filling defect of varying shape and size. Variable degrees of dilation of the main duct or intraglandular branches proximal to the stone also may be seen. Smaller stones may be obscured completely by the contrast medium during the filling phase, although fluoroscopic examination may show a temporary delay in the flow of the contrast material at the location of the stone. Rarely, salivary stones perforate the duct system and form a fistula into the oral cavity or skin.

CALCIFIED LYMPH NODES

In the head and neck area, submandibular, cervical, and digastric nodes usually are enlarged during inflammatory processes. After being involved by infection, the nodes become fibrous, and foci of dystrophic calcification subsequently develop. Tuberculous lymphadenitis (scrofula) is probably the most prevalent disease process in which calcification develops. Actinomycosis, histoplasmosis, cat-scratch fever, and other chronic inflammatory diseases also may become dormant (burned-out) eventually, with dystrophic calcification of sclerotic nodes.

Clinical Features

A calcified submandibular lymph node is sometimes difficult to differentiate from a sialolith within the submandibular salivary gland system. Wood and Goaz (1980) stated that the relative incidence favors the sialolith; also, if painful swelling accompanies a calcified mass in the submandibular space, this strongly indicates a sialolith. A calcified lymph node represents an old burned-out asymptomatic lesion.

A sialogram is useful in distinguishing between these two entities. When a history of tuberculous lymphadenitis (scrofula) or other diseases associated with chronic lymphadenitis is given, calcified lymph nodes should be considered, particularly when the radiopacities are located in an area where lymph nodes are known to occur. In the differential diagnosis of calcified lymph nodes, sialoliths, phleboliths, or foreign bodies should be included. Usually there is no treatment for calcified lymph nodes.

◆ *RADIOLOGY (Fig. 19–16)*

On the radiograph, the calcifications appear as mottled areas of calcific density, which are often multiple, and are distributed along the course of the cervical, submandibular, and digastric node chains. Radiographically, a single ovoid calcification or clustered calcifications may be seen in regions where groups of lymph nodes typically are found. Multiple calcifications may be in a chainlike arrangement as subsequent nodes calcify within the same chain. Calcified lymph nodes may be smooth in contour, or they often may be irregular, with a cauliflowerlike appearance. Within the affected node, radiolucent areas may be observed, and, rarely, lamellations of differing density as seen in some sialoliths. Calcified lymph nodes will not be within the ductal system of a salivary gland on sialograms; however, they may cause ductal compression, which may be associated with intermittent symptoms of ductal obstruction or even chronic sialadenitis.

The localized single mass is most likely to be mistaken for a submandibular salivary calculus. If doubt remains and findings on palpation do not determine the diagnosis, it is reasonable to take a sialogram; however, this usually is not necessary.

TONSILLOLITH

Tonsillar calculi are oropharyngeal concretions stemming from a reactive foreign nidus. Most cases occur in people with prior chronic tonsillitis and little access to physician's care or antibiotics early in the course of the disease. Samant and Gupta (1975) described two cases of lithiasis in the peritonsillar region after spontaneous rupture of peritonsillar abscesses. Cooper and associates (1983) stated that tonsil calculi entail the standard pathophysiologic process of calcium stone formation. They removed a tonsillolith from an elderly woman with acceptable renal function and normal serum calcium levels. The patient's stone had equal parts of calcium and phosphorous. Cooper and co-workers (1983) stated that any infectious agent related to actinomyces, fungi, or bacteria causing tonsillitis can initiate a tonsillolith. Actinomyces is a common resident of an abnormal tonsil and appears as large, gritty "sulfurous granules." Clarke and Long (1954) asserted that tuberculous foci may act as starting points for these masses.

A

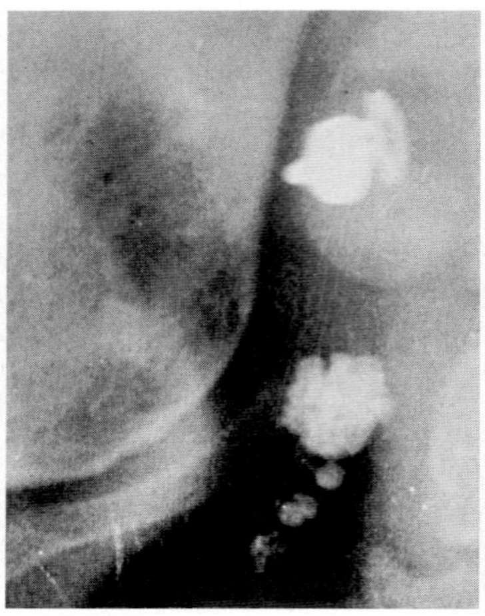

B

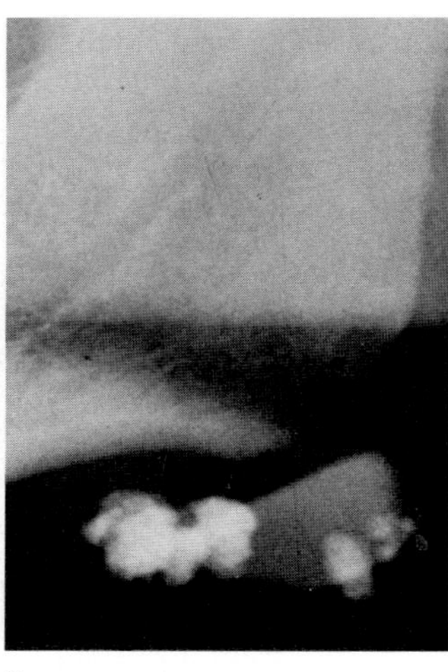

C

FIGURE 19–16.

Calcified Lymph Node: A, Parotid in 30-year-old man with chronic parotitis. (Courtesy of Drs. A. and G. Castro Delgado, Universidad Javeriana, Santa Fé de Bogotá, Colombia.) B, Cervical lymph node that is cauliflower shaped and chainlike. C, Submandibular lymph nodes.

Clinical Features

In review of 23 cases of tonsilloliths by Cooper and associates (1983), the average patient age at medical intervention was 46 years (42 years for male and 51 for female patients). There was no sex predilection. The tonsillolith was located in the right tonsillar fossa in 13 patients, the left in 6 patients, the palatine in 3 patients, and the right supratonsillar area in 1 patient. The average size of the tonsilloliths was 5.5 mm, with a range from 0.5 to 14.5 mm. Of the 17 patients with symptoms, 13 complained of pain or soreness, including 3 with dysphagia; 4 had a mass, swelling, or stone; 3 had infection; 1 had ''heaviness''; 2 had halitosis; and 1 had calculus that was found incidentally on a radiograph. The differential diagnosis of a tonsillolith should include a foreign body, elongated styloid process, calcified lymph nodes, or sialolith. Larger calculi, with a preponderance of patients having pain, infection, and swallowing abnormalities (similar to a Zenker's diverticulum syndrome), require removal. Also, if there is a potential for additional oral and pulmonary complications because of the tonsillolith, the mass should be explored to determine its origin and it should be evaluated for removal.

◆ *RADIOLOGY (Fig. 19–17)*

Katz and colleagues (1989) reported on a localization radiographic technique called ''the known object view,'' a variation of the buccal object rule. This is used to identify the location of soft tissue calcifications in the third molar ramus region of the mandible. It is a valuable technique in determining the position of tonsilloliths. This is diagnostically important because tonsilloliths and parotid calculi resemble each other and are seen in a similar location; however, parotid calculi are buccal to the ramus and tonsilloliths are lingual to the ramus. As reported by Hoffman (1978) and Shrimali and Bhatin (1972), tonsilloliths may be misinterpreted as abnormalities of the mandibular rami.

Tonsilloliths are radiopacities of various sizes and shapes seen in the peritonsillar or midramus region. They may be round, ovoid, irregular, ragged, or smooth and are often multiple and clustered. A tonsillar soft tissue enlargement sometimes may be seen. A lateral skull radiograph of a patient presented by Samant and Gupta (1975) showed a large elliptic radiopacity superimposed over the mandibular third molar region.

ANTROLITH

Antrolith first was reported by Wright in 1927. He described a patient who, after nasal antrostomy for chronic sinusitis,

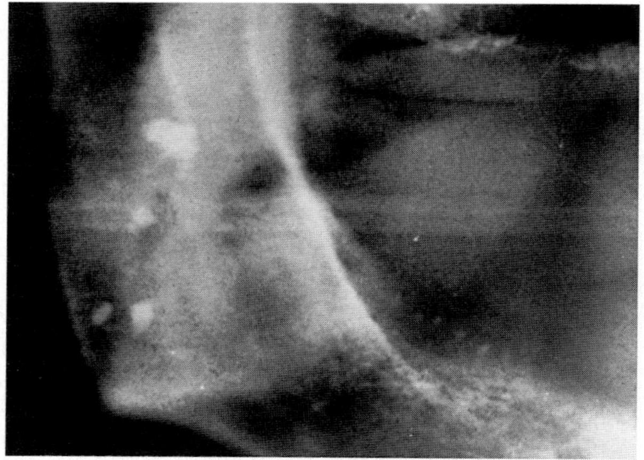

FIGURE 19–17.

Tonsillith: Palatine tonsil on right side only; ghost locates calculi toward the lingual side.

spontaneously dislodged an antrolith 6 weeks after surgery. The stone had a nucleus of a tooth root that had been dislodged into the antrum years previously. In 1944, Lord reviewed the world literature and found an additional five instances of antroliths. He described a patient from whom an antrolith with a paper nucleus was removed after surgery after 12 months of chronic sinusitis. In 1975, Evans reported on 17 cases of calculi within or partially within the antrum, reported in the English literature. Antroliths of the maxillary sinus were referred to by Bowerman (1969) as resulting from complete or partial encrustation of an antral foreign body usually of endogenous origin and occasionally of exogenous origin. They are hard calcareous structures with a rough irregular surface consisting of a central nidus upon which mineral salts, especially calcium phosphate and carbonate, and magnesium are deposited gradually. The nidus is usually endogenous and may be a blood clot, bone fragment, tooth, or tooth fragment or inspissated pus or mucus. The enveloping salts probably are derived from antral secretions or inflammatory exudates. The foreign body with complete or partial encrustation may have been in situ for many years before actual diagnosis and associated with long-term chronic infection.

Clinical Features

The occurrence of calculi in the maxillary antrum or a stone lying partially in the nasal cavity and the antrum is rare. The maxillary antrolith may occur in patients at any age and of either sex. In a review of several case reports of antroliths by Karges and associates (1971), the age range was 23 to 66 years, with a mean age of 39 years. Usually there are no symptoms, but larger stones may cause pain, sinusitis, nasal obstruction, or a foul discharge and epistaxis. A purulent discharge may have been present for a long time. Cunningham and associates (1945) reported a case that lasted 30 years. Of the 17 cases of maxillary antroliths reported by Evans (1975), 14 were associated with maxillary sinusitis; 5 of the 17 cases had associated oroantral fistulas. Also, according to Blaschke and Brady (1979), many antroliths are discovered during radiographic examination in which an opaque shadow is evident in the sinus. Patients with antroliths should be referred to an oral and maxillofacial surgeon or otolaryngologist for evaluation and management. Generally, the antrolith is removed surgically by the Caldwell-Luc approach. Because it is essential to evaluate the mass histopathologically, removal of the mass is justified even in patients with no symptoms.

◆ *RADIOLOGY (Fig. 19–18)*

In viewing antroliths, the panoramic radiograph is not always the best because of the normal superimpositions of the inferior conchae and zygomatic processes over the sinuses. The panoramic radiograph should be supplemented by the Waters projection and other paranasal sinus projections.

The exact location within the maxillary sinus usually can be determined by conventional or tomographic radiography. The antrolith must be separate from the nasal fossa and alveolar process; this is the key feature that differentiates the antrolith from a rhinolith or an odontogenic tumor such as a complex odontoma. Blaschke and Brady (1979) showed the value of tomography in establishing the size, structure, and position of the antrolith in the case they reported. The periapical radiograph may be useful in determining the position of the floor of the sinus in relation to an impacted tooth or retained tooth fragment.

Radiologic Features

Antroliths are radiopaque masses of calcific density situated in the antrum. They may be round to ovoid and irregular, ragged, or smooth in outline. Antroliths may appear as a dense homogeneous radiopacity or show concentric rings of radiopaque and radiolucent material. The size of the antrolith varies from a few millimeters to the dimensions of a hazelnut; despite its texture, the mass can be broken up with strong

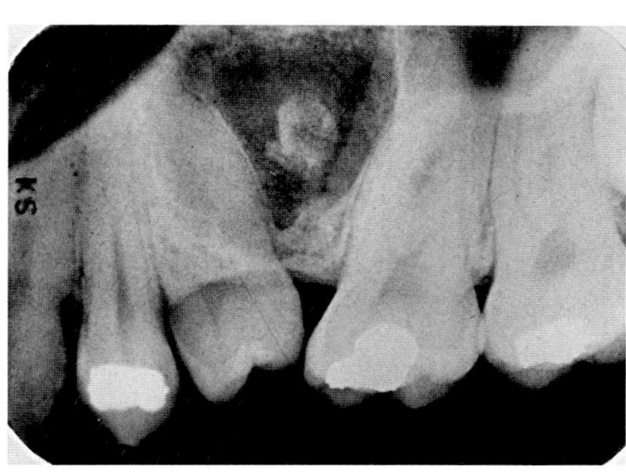

A

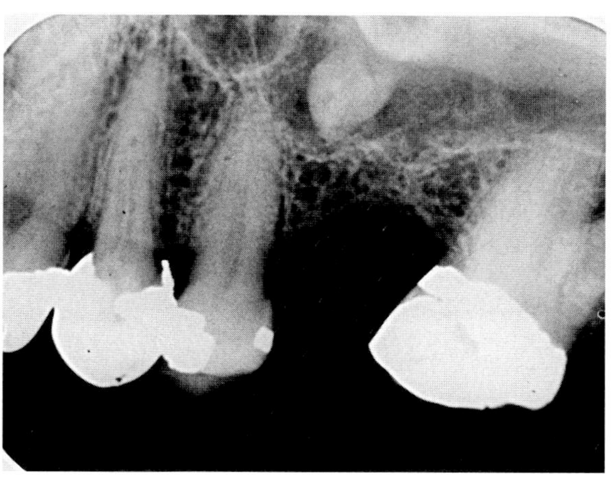

B

FIGURE 19–18.

Antrolith: A, Possibly endogenous origin. B, Nidus is a root tip.

forceps. In some cases, minute radiolucent areas are distributed haphazardly throughout the radiopaque mass. The antrolith may be much more radiopaque than a comparable-sized soft tissue mass, such as a mucous retention cyst.

Most antroliths are associated with the typical radiographic sign of sinusitis consisting of mucoperiosteal thickening, polyps, and air-fluid levels in one or both maxillary sinuses.

RHINOLITH

Rhinoliths were described in the early sixteenth century. According to Polson (1943), nasal concretions or rhinoliths were reported by Bartholin in 1654. Approximately 550 cases have been reported since then, mostly in dental and otorhinolaryngology literature. Terrafranca and Zellis (1952) believed that rhinoliths previously used to occur more frequently than they do now. Eliachar and Schalit (1970) stated that the number of reported cases is declining, presumably because of more frequent medical examinations by schools, armed services, industry, and insurance companies. Rhinoliths are sclerotic masses that result from lime salt deposition around a foreign body in the nasal cavity. A rhinolith occurs when a foreign body remains in a nasal cavity for a considerable length of time. Chemically, rhinoliths consist chiefly of calcium phosphate, magnesium phosphate, calcium carbonate, organic matter, and water. The nuclei of these nasal concretions are classified as exogenous (false) and endogenous (true) types. Those of endogenous origin include displaced teeth, bone fragments, blood clots, desquamated epithelium, clumps of bacteria, or inspissated (dried) mucus. The most common exogenous foreign bodies include fruit seeds, buttons, and paper fragments or other substances.

Clinical Features

Rhinoliths vary in size, from that of a small pebble to one reported by Merideth and Grossman (1952) that weighed 115 g and was the size of a hen's egg. They may be bilateral or multiple, but they are usually unilateral. Bicknell (1970) and Brown and Allen (1957) asserted that rhinoliths may expand to erode surrounding structures.

Dodd and Jing (1977) stated that rhinoliths are more common in adults than in children and are found more frequently in female than male patients. Clinically, there may be no symptoms for years, but sooner or later a unilateral nasal obstruction occurs, with foul-smelling discharge. Pain and recurrent hemorrhage (epistaxis) ensue if the object is rough and causes pressure with resultant swelling or ulceration. Rhinorrhea develops first, and purulent rhinitis follows. This reaction, known as rhinolithic rhinitis, is usually unilateral and is caused by a rhinolith. Harrison and Lamming (1969) stated that the differential diagnosis should include calcified polyps, granulomas, opaque foreign bodies, osteomas, and sequestration after local osteomyelitis. Ballenger (1969) reported that removal of the rhinolith cures the unilateral fetid discharge or obstruction. Blechman and colleagues (1974) and Marano and associates (1970) reported that a rhinolith may be removed if it is pushed into the nasopharynx and removed through the oropharynx.

◆ *RADIOLOGY (Fig. 19–19)*

Allen and Liston (1979) related that panoramic radiographs have drawbacks when used to identify the position of radiopaque lesions, such as a rhinolith, in the nasal cavity. In their case, the rhinolith within the nasal cavity appeared superimposed on the right maxillary sinus. They stated that the position of the rhinolith in panoramic radiographs must be con-

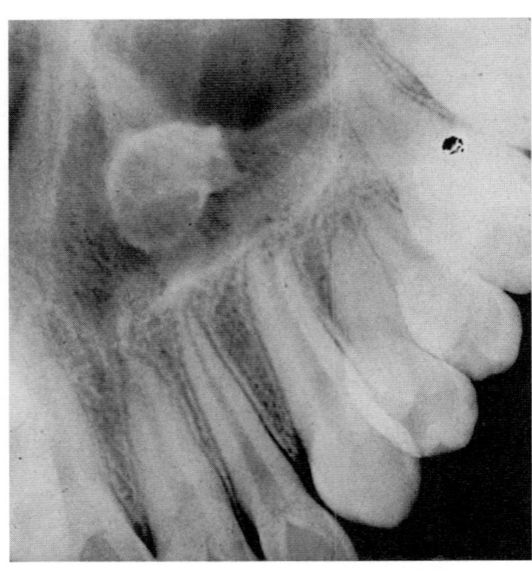

A

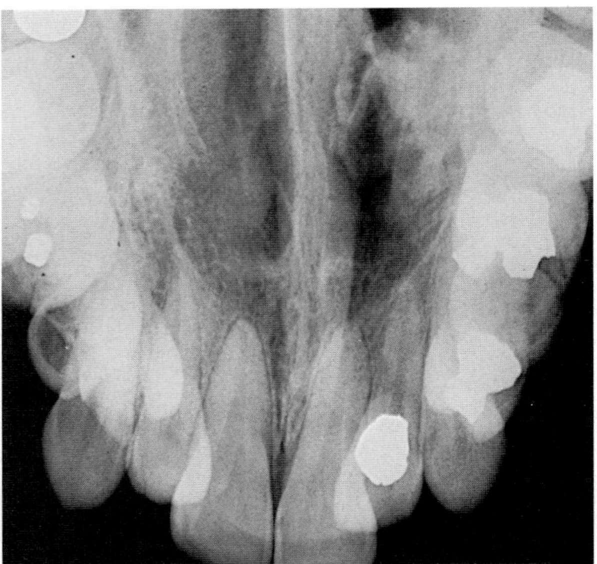

B

FIGURE 19–19.

Rhinolith: A, Case in a 14-year-old boy. B, Case in an 18-year-old boy.

firmed by other radiographic studies, such as the Waters and lateral skull views of the nasal cavity. The panoramic image of the nasal cavity and maxillary sinus can be improved by taking a second view with the patient positioned approximately 1 to 2 cm forward of the normal position.

Location

The most common locations for rhinoliths are the inferior meatus and the space between the inferior turbinate and septum. They usually are unilateral, although bilateral occurrences have been reported.

Radiologic Features

Radiographically, a rhinolith is seen as a dense, irregular, calcified mass lying within the nasal passage, with no demonstrable osseous connection or origin. Dodd and Jing (1977) listed the following radiologic features of rhinoliths:

1. Calcified mass in the nasal fossa. Such masses may vary in size and shape but usually conform to the available space. A coral-like appearance may be seen occasionally.
2. Displacement and perforation of the nasal septum. This may result from swelling and pressure of the rhinolith.
3. Thinning and expansion of the lateral wall of the nasal cavity with large radiopaque masses.
4. Destruction of the nasal wall. This change is uncommon and usually results from superimposed osteomyelitis.

Terrafranca and Zellis (1952) reported a 75-year-old patient with a unilateral nasal discharge. The patient had constant frontal headaches and pain in the left maxillary sinus. The radiographs of the nasal cavity showed a dense, irregular, calcific mass, which was nonhomogeneous and coral-like in appearance, occupying almost the entire left nasal space. Examination of the material removed from the nose indicated that the rhinolith consisted of several fragments of a fruit stone, possibly that of a plum.

CALCIFIED SCAR

Scars are new formations of connective tissue that replace substance lost in the corium or deeper parts as a result of injury or disease; this occurs as part of the normal reparative and healing process. A form of dystrophic calcification that may be seen in dental radiographs may occur on the face in degenerated tissue and hypertrophic scarring from lesions of acne, smallpox, trauma, syphilis, and lupus erythematous.

Clinical Features

Scars with certain characteristics are typical of a particular injury or disease of the skin so they have a diagnostic value. Scars of lupus erythematosus are shiny, rigid, telangiectatic, and minutely pitted, corresponding to glandular orifices. Burn scars are a mixture of thin, depressed, atrophic, and hypertrophic raised or fibrous lesions with a keloid tendency. Smallpox scars are innumerable small, white, rounded, pit-like depressions usually on the face. Atrophic acne, a variety of acne vulgaris, is characterized by tiny residual atrophic pits and scars. Keloidal scars are seen not only in black people, but also less often in white people, and frequently appear in the beard region.

◆ *RADIOLOGY (Fig. 19–20)*

Dystrophic calcifications of scarred tissue from acne vulgaris, smallpox, trauma, syphilis, and lupus erythematosus may go unnoticed on routine dental radiographs, particularly if they are sparse and small; however, if an occlusal or periapical film is placed in the vestibule in the mouth between the teeth and cheek and the exposure reduced considerably, the calcifications may be seen clearly. Ennis demonstrated this technique in 1964 and reported the radiographic features of calcified acne lesions.

Radiologic Features

Ennis (1964) stated that because areas of scarring vary greatly in shape, size, and density, the appearance of dys-

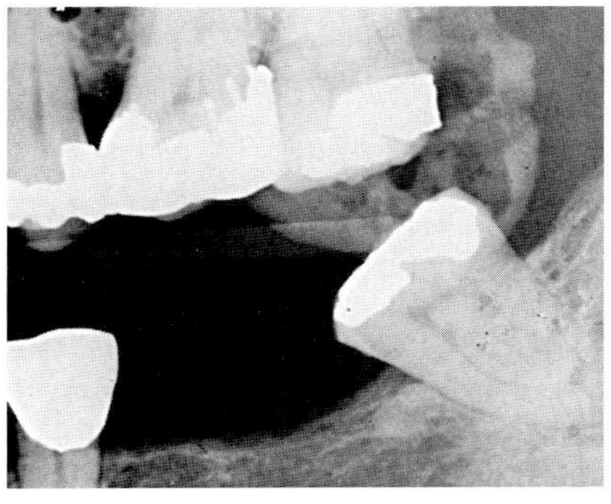

A

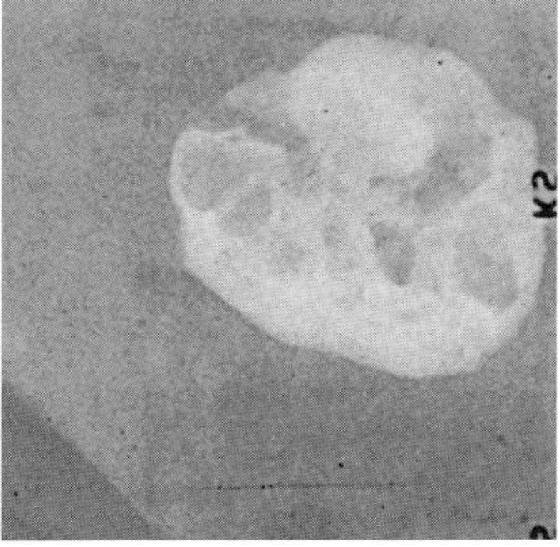

B

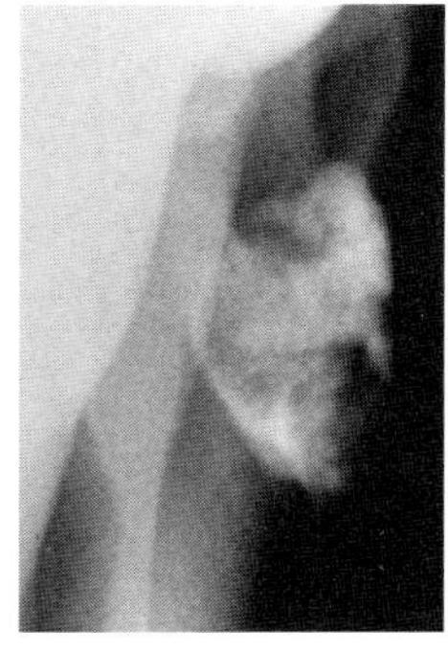

C

FIGURE 19–20.

Calcified Scar: Case in a 46-year-old woman with Baraquer's syndrome, characterized by diminished adipose tissue in the head and neck. A full-thickness skin graft was placed 25 years previously. A, Bitewing. B, Buccal mucosa. C, Anteroposterior view.

trophic calcific scarring will differ accordingly on the radiographs. He stated that these radiographic appearances resembled snowflakes. One of the most important aspects of the radiologic appearance of scars is that they do not resemble any of the other specific conditions, such as miliary osteomas or phleboliths, and they correlate well with the changes observed on the face.

CYSTICERCOSIS CUTIS

The natural intermediate host of the pork tapeworm, taenia solium, is the pig, but under some circumstances humans act in this role. The larval stage of the pork tapeworm, taenia solium, is cysticercus cellulosae. Cysticercosis is more prevalent in countries where pigs feed on human feces. Normally, the pig is the intermediate host of cysticercus cellulosae, and human infestation occurs when humans ingest food contaminated with eggs (e.g, by eating uncooked pork) or by reverse peristalsis of eggs or proglottides, which are segments of tapeworm, from the intestine to the stomach. Here, the eggs hatch, freeing the oncospheres, the larva of the tapeworm. They enter the general circulation and form cysts in various parts of the body, such as striated muscle and the brain, eye, heart, and lung. Humans infected in this manner act as the intermediate host. Thus, the disease develops in a person who ingests ova or water or food contaminated with human fecal material of a person who carries the intestinal parasite, or, in some instances, by autoinfection.

Clinical Features

In the subcutaneous tissues, the lesions are usually painless nodules that contain cysticerci. When the larvae are alive, there is no radiographic evidence of their presence; however, after the larvae die, the cystic spaces are filled with fibrous tissue that in turn may undergo calcific degeneration. The nodules are more or less stationary, usually numerous, and often calcified, so they can be seen on the radiograph. A positive diagnosis is established solely by incision and examination of the interior of the calcified mass, where the parasite will be found. Levin and colleagues (1986) summarized the use of praziquantel (Biltricide, Miles Pharmaceuticals, New Haven, CT) in the treatment of cysticercosis cutis. The drug is given in doses as low as 10 mg per kg body weight as a 1-day treatment and is said to cure almost every patient with tapeworm (taenia solium). Five times the dose is required if the central nervous system is involved.

◆ *RADIOLOGY (Fig. 19–21)*

The encysted parasites may become calcified sufficiently to be seen radiographically as small or slightly elongated masses of 1 mm to several millimeters in diameter or length. Those situated in muscle or subcutaneous tissue that have undergone calcification are seen most often as elliptic or ovoid radiopaque objects. They often resemble grains of rice. The small size of the calcifications and their wide dissemination, particularly in the brain, meninges, and muscles, are highly suggestive of the diagnosis.

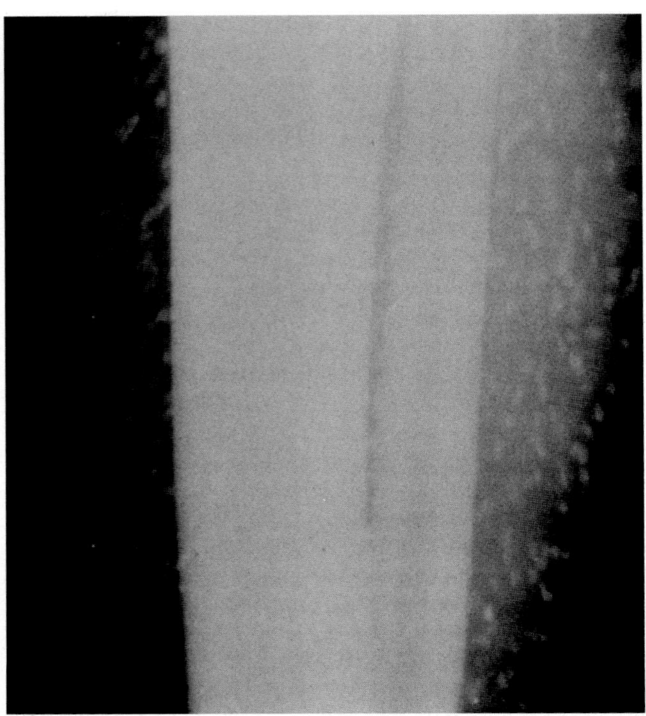

FIGURE 19–21.

Cysticercosis: Leg of a patient who was residing in South America.

Differential Diagnosis

These other conditions in which opacities occur in soft tissues should be in the differential diagnosis of cysticercosis cutis: calcifications in cavernous hemangiomas, phleboliths, sialoliths, and calcified lymph nodes. In Ehlers-Danlos syndrome (cutis hyperelastica), rounded opacities sometimes occur in the soft tissues, but they have a different shape and size compared with those in cysticercosis cutis. The encysted embryos of Trichinella spiralis are said to undergo calcification very frequently, but the parasite is so small that it cannot be seen readily on radiographs, so trichinosis usually cannot be diagnosed from radiographic examination.

MYOSITIS OSSIFICANS

Calcification with subsequent ossification of a muscle often follows a single acute traumatic episode or a series of minor traumatic episodes to the deep tissues of the extremities and is called traumatic myositis ossificans. So-called calcified hematomas involving the muscles of the thigh are observed frequently in athletes, particularly football players, but they may follow any local injury sufficient to cause bruising of the muscle or a frank hemorrhage within it; an injury of this nature that is severe enough to cause a deep muscle bruise often traumatizes the periosteum as well, and there may be hemorrhage beneath it that frequently undergoes calcification. The muscles commonly involved in this condition are those of the thigh and arm; Eversole (1984) has reported that the masseter, temporal, pterygoid, and geniohyoid muscles have been involved.

Traumatic myositis ossificans should not be confused with the disease known as progressive myositis ossificans. This is a rare disorder of unknown cause and appears to represent a congenital dysplasia. The disease progresses slowly from childhood, but eventually there is widespread ossification of muscles. The patient's body becomes immobile and death ensues.

Clinical Features

Abdin and Prabhu (1984) reviewed the literature involving traumatic myositis ossificans of the muscles of the face. They found that 14 of 16 cases involved the masseter muscles, 1 affected the medial pterygoid muscle, and 1 involved the suprahyoid musculature. Their case affected the lateral pterygoid muscle. Goodsell (1962) and Plezia and associates (1977) reviewed the literature for traumatic myositis of the masseter muscles and found that, in most reported cases, a painless swelling of the calcified lesion was rapid, a maximum size was obtained, and then the lesion remained static or even became smaller. It usually developed into a progressive severe trismus. Chronic cases of myositis ossificans are usually asymptomatic and may be discovered accidentally; such cases develop after a single acute traumatic injury that produces a firm, painless mass within 1 to 4 weeks. Cases have been reported in which osteogenic sarcoma has developed in an area of traumatic myositis ossificans, but these appear to be rare.

Treatment

There are different philosophies regarding treatment; however, Palumbo and associates (1964) suggested that early surgical removal has had the most favorable results, with no recurrence or abnormal function. Mulherin and Schow (1980) and Ramesh and Dixon (1974) indicated that there is a tendency for the condition to recur. The recurrence rate is greater if the surgery is performed during the active osteoblastic stage, thus Ramesh and Dixon (1974) recommended a period of watchful waiting before surgical removal of the affected muscle. The prognosis is good because the lesion is localized and inflammatory.

◆ *RADIOLOGY*

Flynn and Graham (1964) and Vernale (1968) reported that a hematoma after trauma to a muscle seems to be the precursor in traumatic myositis ossificans. The hematoma undergoes calcification and may become visible as an image of increased density within a few weeks after the initiating trauma.

The first finding is that of a soft tissue swelling. Calcification subsequently develops in a centrifugal pattern that is flocculent at first, becomes more dense, and finally shows the appearance of bone. Usually after a period of time, the mineralization gradually decreases in size and some of the smaller masses may disappear completely.

Radiographically, traumatic myositis ossificans may appear as a mass with a laminated character caused by hemorrhage dissecting along the muscle and fascial planes or as a solitary irregular calcified mass occurring in a single hematoma.

The lesion must be differentiated from a malignant one such as juxtacortical osteosarcoma. Radiographic signs favoring a benign lesion include a lucent zone between the lesion and adjacent bone, intact underlying cortex, dense calcification at the periphery, and loss of volume or a decrease in size with time. In addition, the most dense calcification is peripheral in this lesion, as opposed to the dense central calcification in most tumors.

CALCINOSIS CUTIS

This condition is marked by deposits of calcium salts in the skin in the form of nodules or plaques. There are several varieties of calcium deposition in the skin, and calcium may be combined with elements of damaged or altered tissue. Such dystrophic calcification may occur in small localized areas (calcinosis circumscripta) or large widespread areas (calcinosis universalis).

Calcinosis Circumscripta

This is a localized type of calcinosis. The deposits of calcium salts consisting of calcium phosphate apatite appear in the skin in the form of nodules, plaques, and tumors, and the sizes range from 2 to 30 mm. They occur chiefly in the upper extremities, particularly on the fingers or wrists, with a tendency to be situated over or along the course of the flexor tendons of the hands and the extensor tendons of the elbows and knees (i.e., in locations subject to frequent trauma and frequent motion).

As the lesions enlarge and the overlying skin becomes adherent and inflamed, it eventually breaks down. Creamy material containing small gritty particles of calcium slowly is exuded. Calcinosis cutis circumscripta is seen in scleroderma associated with CREST syndrome (an acronym for calcinosis cutis, Raynaud's phenomenon, esophageal dysmobility, scleroderma, and telangiectasia). Magalini (1971) stated that calcinosis circumscripta occurs more commonly in women. Wang and colleagues (1988) reported a remarkable treatment response to aluminum hydroxide, 15 to 20 ml four times a day for 1 year, in a patient with dermatomyositis and disfiguring calcinosis cutis.

◆ *RADIOLOGY (Fig. 19–22)*

The calcification may be in the form of a few tiny rounded subcutaneous nodules or may occur as larger masses. These are found commonly in the terminal phalanges or along margins of joints. Other radiographic signs of scleroderma are often present:

1. Diminution in the amount of soft tissue in the tips of the fingers so that these digits show a tapered or almost pointed appearance.

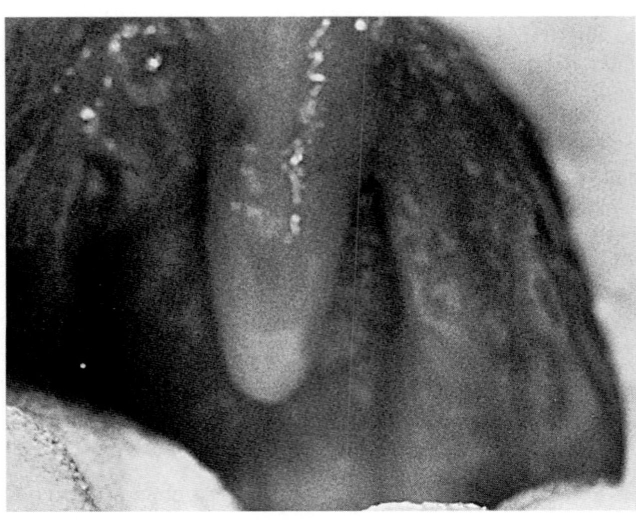

A

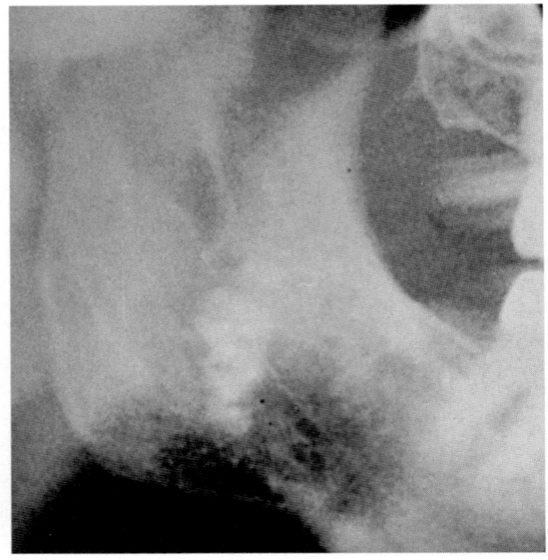

B

FIGURE 19–22.

Calcinosis Circumscripta: Uvula in a 56-year-old man with a history of snoring. A, Elongated, enlarged, and firm uvula. B, Image superimposed on angle area. (Courtesy of Dr. J. Katz, University of Missouri at Kansas City, Kansas City, MO.)

2. Uniform density of the subcutaneous tissues, with loss of normal soft tissue architecture.
3. Absorption of bone.

Calcinosis Universalis

This type of diffuse calcification of the skin usually affects the deeper subcutaneous tissues and the dermis and often involves the proximal parts of the extremities and pelvic girdle. The cause is unknown. It may be a mucopolysaccharide or collagen disorder. Approximately one third of the cases are secondary to scleroderma or dermatomyositis; cases also may be associated with the CREST syndrome. The muscles and tendons may be involved, and the joints can become swollen and immobile. According to Worth (1963), calcinosis universalis does not affect the face, but it does occur in the neck. It is found more frequently in female patients, and its onset is in the first 2 decades life. Symptoms include fatigue, difficulty in locomotion, muscular pain, low-grade fever, palpable calcific plaques in subcutaneous or deeper tissues, and high levels of gamma-carboxyglutamic acid in involved tissues and the urine. At first, skin plaques are painless and the overlying skin is movable and normal. Later, pain and tenderness develop and, finally, necrosis and ulceration of the skin, with discharge of a chalklike material. The sinus tracts are difficult to heal because of superimposed infections. The calcium deposits may disappear spontaneously and return in years. This condition usually takes a chronic course. Septicemia frequently develops when ulcerations occur.

◆ *RADIOLOGY*

On the radiograph, calcific deposits of various sizes and shapes are seen that are mostly long bands of symmetric subcutaneous calcifications with progressive spread to deeper connective tissues such as tendons, ligaments, and nerve sheaths. There is an extraskeletal uptake of ^{99}technetium MDP. In scleroderma and dermatomyositis, the calcification occurs in the form of thin plaques. With scleroderma, they are limited to the skin and immediate subcutaneous tissues, whereas in dermatomyositis, calcifications also occur in the muscles. In addition to plaque, there is a general loss of soft tissue differentiation, with the subcutaneous fat layer becoming very scanty or disappearing altogether.

MILIARY OSTEOMA (Osteoma cutis)

Miliary osteomas are a type of osteoma cutis, which consists of a lesion histologically identical to the bony osteoma but located within the dermis of the skin or oral epithelium. Arnold and co-workers (1990) stated that osteoma cutis may be **primary** in cases in which there is no preceding lesion or **metastatic** when ossification occurs in a pre-existing lesion or inflammatory process. The primary type is rare, whereas the metastatic type is common. Primary osteoma cutis is seen in Albright's syndrome; other types of primary osteoma cutis include widespread or single plaque-like osteomas present at birth or early life, single osteomas occurring in later life, and miliary osteomas of the face. Metastatic osteoma cutis consists of bone deposits in the skin that arise from metaplasia; these occur most frequently in pilomatricoma, a tumor from hair matrix cells usually of the face, neck, and arms, or other lesions in which bone formation may occur, such as basal cell epithelioma, intradermal nevi, mixed tumor of the skin, scars, scleroderma, dermatomyositis, and inflammatory diseases of many types. Miliary osteoma of the skin is a relatively rare condition. This condition first was mentioned by Virchow in 1864.

Clinical Features

The following are theories regarding the possible cause of multiple miliary osteomas of the skin: (1) metaplastic ossification secondary to a chronic inflammatory process, (2) neoplastic ossification, and (3) embryonal cell rests of osteoblastic elements. Miliary osteomas range in size from 0.5 to 2.0 mm in diameter. Cases involving the skin of the face, forehead, and chin have been reported by Carney and Radcliffe (1951), Costello (1947), and Gasner (1954). They are round or oval and surrounded by a capsule of fibrous tissue. Hopkins (1928) and Leider (1948) reported that miliary osteoma cutis does not cause visible changes in the skin. Stafne and Gibilisco (1975) observed 11 patients radiographically. In all of these patients, multiple miliary osteomas occurred bilaterally; only 1 had blemishes on the surface of the skin, and these were nodules of previous acne. Domonkos and co-workers (1982) reported three cases of miliary osteomas of the skin occurring in middle-aged men with seborrheic dermatitis. The differential diagnosis mainly concerns calcinosis cutis, in which the mineralized substance is soft and crumbly, whereas the osteoma cutis is hard and does not disintegrate on pressure. The small osteomas of the skin are incised and then removed easily with a small spoon curette.

◆ *RADIOLOGY (Figs. 19–23 and 19–24)*

Radiographically, the occlusal view of the blown-out cheek of the patient is useful in detecting multiple miliary osteomas of the cheek. The occlusal film is positioned posterior to and at right angles to the surface of the cheek of the patient. The central beam is directed through the cheek, perpendicular to the film, and the 60-kV exposure is made with the patient blowing the cheek outward. Another method involves placing the film in the vestibule between the teeth and cheek, with a similar low kilovolt exposure. Miliary osteomas vary in density from one lesion to another within the same case and from patient to patient, depending on the degree of mineralization present and the radiation exposure factors used.

The images of multiple miliary osteomas of the skin conform to the architecture of the osteoma. Typically, each miliary osteoma appears as a small doughnut-shaped image with a radiolucent center representing the central marrow cavity. In other instances, tiny but solid round or ovoid flecks are seen. In more mature lesions, the central radiolucent area becomes invisible and the osteomas appear as small radiopaque areas.

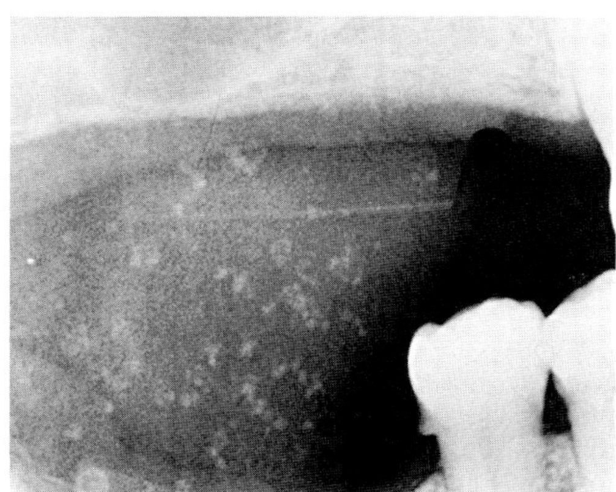

FIGURE 19–23.

Miliary Osteoma: Typical minute radiopacities forming ovoid and circular structures.

INTRAORAL OSSEOUS CHORISTOMA
(Soft tissue osteoma)

True osteomas have been defined by Lucas (1976) as "growths that consist of cancellous or compact bone and increase in size by continuous formation of compact bone." Most solitary osteomas are associated with the skeletal structures of the face and skull and may occur in a central or a peripheral location. These have been described in the chapter titled Focal Radiopacities. In addition to osteomas associated with skeletal structures, lesions consistent with the definition of true osteoma have been found in soft tissues not associated with bone. Krolls and associates (1971) suggested that the term "osseous choristoma" be reserved for extraosseous benign bone-forming lesions, and the term osteoma designates lesions occurring in association with the skeletal structure. Choristoma refers to a tumorlike growth that has developed from primordial cells in a site remote from the original tissue or organ; thus, the choristoma is histologically normal tissue in an abnormal site. Reviews have been reported by Mesa and co-workers (1982) and Tohill and colleagues, who found 72 cases of osseous choristoma in the literature in 1987. The first case of intraoral osseous choristoma was reported by Monserrat in 1913; his case was located in the patient's tongue. According to Krolls and colleagues (1971), osseous choristomas in the buccal mucosa are rare, with only seven reported cases.

Pathologic Characteristics

The cause of osseous choristomas is unknown. There are two main theories on the histogenesis of the lesion: (1) metaplasia of pluripotential-mesenchymal cells, or (2) proliferation of "hematopoietic" embryonic rests. Tohill and associates (1987), Herd (1976), and Sookasam and Philipsen (1986) believed that lesions of the buccal mucosa and anterior aspect of the tongue are post-traumatic centers of ossification and those of the posterior tongue are developmental abnormalities. On histologic examination, normal, well-circumscribed, lamellar bone with dense or loose trabecular bone is found. Haversian canals and osteocytes are present.

Clinical Features

Most osseous choristomas are found in the submucosa on the dorsal surface of the tongue in the area of the circumvallate papilla or the foramen cecum and rarely in the buccal mucosa and buccal submucosa. In a study of 25 cases of osseous choristoma of the intraoral soft tissues, which was conducted by Krolls and colleagues (1971), the patients' ages ranged from 9 to 73 years and there was a female-to-

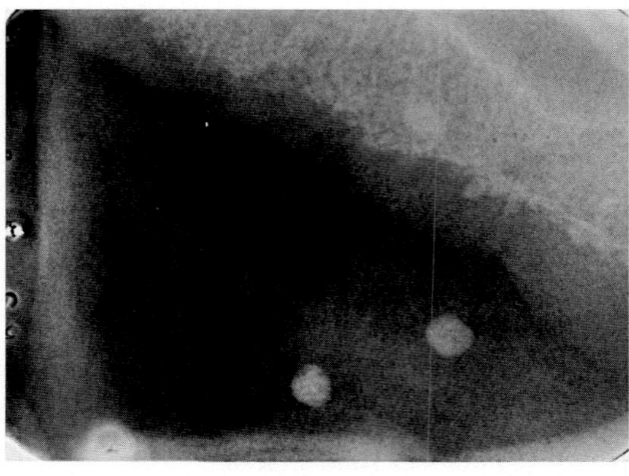
A

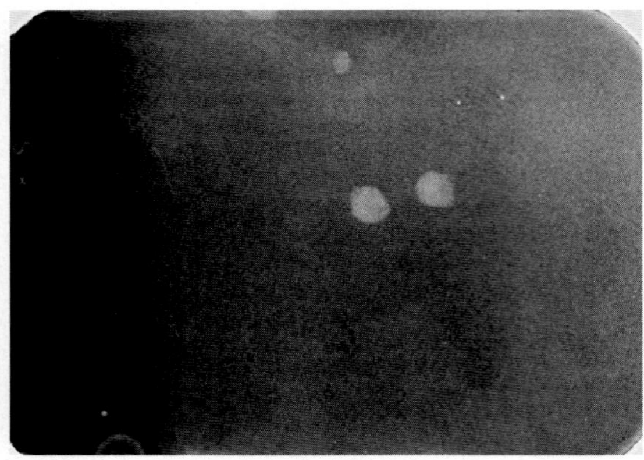
B

FIGURE 19–24.

Miliary Osteoma: A, Film placed palatal to edentulous ridge. B, Film placed buccal to ridge.

male ratio of 3:1. The duration of the lesions ranged from 2.5 months to several years. The mean age of the 7 patients with reported cases of buccal osseous choristoma was 48 years (range, 33 to 75 years), and the sex distribution was almost equal. The lesions were found predominantly in white patients and generally were present for 1 to 2 years.

Lesions vary in size from 0.5 to 2 cm in diameter. When symptoms were stated, 11 of the 25 patients with tongue lesions had a sensation of gagging or a similar complaint; 8 had no symptoms.

The lesions invariably were reported as soft, with the clinical appearance of a fibroma, papilloma, or hyperplastic papilla. Radiologically, the differential diagnosis should include myositis ossificans, calcinosis cutis, osteoma cutis, and soft tissue chondroma.

Treatment

The nodules usually are excised, and healing is uneventful. As reported by Krolls and colleagues (1971), Davis (1980), and Shafer and co-workers (1983), osseous choristomas do not recur; however, Long and Koutnik (1991) reported a case of an intraoral osseous choristoma of the buccal mucosa that recurred. The original and second lesions were located in the same site, were unattached to the underlying bone and easily removed from the surrounding soft tissue, and were diagnosed histologically as osteomas.

◆ *RADIOLOGY (Figs. 19–25 to 19–27)*

Location

Most intraoral osseous choristomas are in the tongue, usually the dorsum, and in rare instances in the buccal mucosa. Posterior lesions in the tongue and buccal mucosa may be superimposed on bone and appear as a focal radiopacity within or on the surface. In such instances, another view, such as an occlusal radiograph of the tongue or buccal mucosa, is necessary. If the lesion is posterior in the tongue, it is possible that bilateral images will be seen in the panoramic radiograph.

Radiologic Features

The radiograph usually shows a well-circumscribed radiopaque nodule, which may be round or ovoid, with a smooth or bosselated outline. The lesion may appear as a solid radiopaque nodule, or one may see a more radiolucent center marginated by condensed bone. Occasionally there is no condensed bone at the periphery, and a prominent trabecular pattern can be seen throughout.

SOFT TISSUE CHONDROMA

The chondroma is a benign tumor usually arising in bone and composed of mature cartilage. It is uncommon in the maxilla and mandible; Chaudhry and co-workers (1961) found only 18 cases affecting the jaws in the English literature published between 1912 and 1959. Occasionally, intraoral soft tissue chondromas have been found, such as in the soft palate, as described by Gardner and Paterson (1968), or the more common chondroma or osteochondroma of the tongue. The relationship of these intraoral soft tissue chondromas, especially those of the tongue, to the well-recognized chondroma of soft parts as reviewed by Chung and Enzinger (1978) is not clearly established.

Pathologic Characteristics

Cartilage normally is not found in the tongue, and the exact histogenesis of lingual chondroma is unknown; however, there are two possible explanations—the embryonal and cellular metaplasia theories. Cellular metaplasia involves differentiation of pluripotential mesenchymal cells into chondrocytes or cartilaginous metaplasia of the connective tissue. This metaplasia presumably is stimulated by some type of trauma or chronic inflammation. The embryonal theory postulates that the tumor results from proliferation of heterotopic (occurring in an abnormal place) fetal cartilage remnants in the tongue. Yasuoka and associates (1984) believed that the metaplastic transformation theory best explains the histogenesis of lesions at the lateral borders of the tongue, whereas the embryonal theory best describes the histogene-

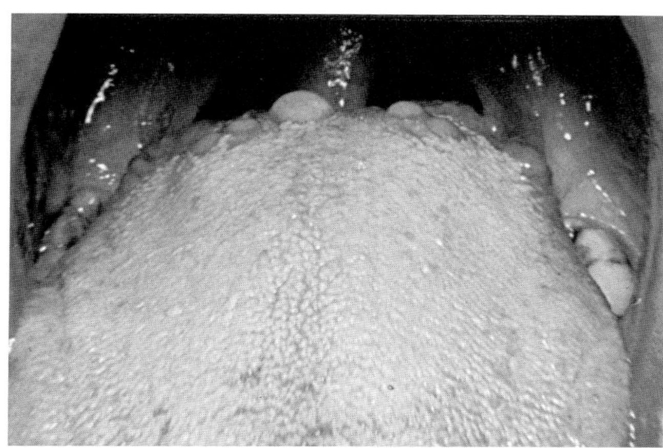

A

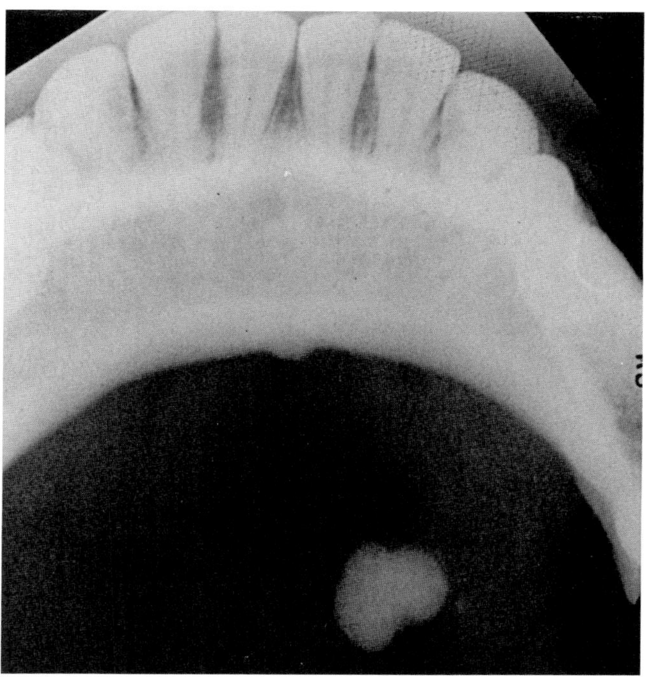

B

FIGURE 19–25.

Soft Tissue Osteoma: A, Slight swelling on left side of tongue. B, Osseous choristoma within same patient. (Courtesy of Dr. B. Alexander, University of Mississippi School of Dentistry, Jackson, MS.)

sis of the chondroma on the dorsum of the tongue. Del Rio (1978) and, later, Ling (1986) summarized the cases of chondroma of the tongue reported in the English language literature until 1982. Of the total of 16 cases, 9 were pure chondromas and 7 were histologic variants, such as fibrochondroma (1 case), osteochondroma (4 cases), and chondromas with osteoid tissue (2 cases).

Clinical Features

The average age of the 16 patients reviewed by Ling (1986) was 31 years, with ages ranging from 10 to 50 years. The male-to-female ratio was 1:1. The average duration of the lesions before diagnosis was 8 years. The lesions were in the region of the lateral margin in six patients, on the dorsum of the tongue in eight patients, and on the ventral surface in one case. The diameters ranged from 0.3 to 0.5 cm. Tongue lesions consist of a nontender protrusion much like a nipple that is usually mobile, hard when palpated, and covered with mucosa-colored smooth epithelium that is free of ulceration. There is no associated lymph node enlargement. Plessier and Leroux-Robert (1932) and Ramachandran and Viswanathan (1968) discussed cases in which multiple chondromas of the tongue were associated with intraoral anomalies, such as cleft palate, in very young patients.

Treatment/Prognosis

When treatment was mentioned for cases, it was surgical. No recurrences were reported for cases with available follow-up data. Vassar (1958) and Forman (1967) reported cases of primary chondrosarcoma of the tongue. Vassar's case showed no evidence that lesions arose from a benign tumor. In Forman's case, the tumor showed areas of apparently benign cartilaginous structure and peripheral areas strongly indicative of malignant transformation. Stout and Verner (1953), however, concluded from seven cases of chondrosarcoma of soft tissues that the tumor usually arises de novo rather than in a pre-existing chondroma.

◆ *RADIOLOGY*

Typical chondroid calcification may be found within soft tissue masses of the tongue on the radiograph. In some lesions, there may be no calcification of the chondroid tissue. When chondroid calcification is present, it is characterized as multiple, tiny, punctate flecks, referred to as calcific foci. These begin as tiny pinpoint structures of rather faint density, somewhat less than that of bone, and ultimately become more radiopaque as calcification progresses. Calcific foci typically are arranged in clusters, sometimes resembling a snowflake. In older lesions calcific foci become larger, in which case they are referred to as flocculent, but the tendency to form clusters may persist. At times, larger clumps of calcified cartilage may be present. Generally, calcific foci, flocculi, and clumps tend to be rounded, and even if the margins are irregular, they are smooth and spiculation generally is absent. If osseous tissue is present as in osteochondroma, then trabeculation and more irregularly shaped osseous foci with pointed spicules at the margins also may be seen admixed with the cartilaginous calcification.

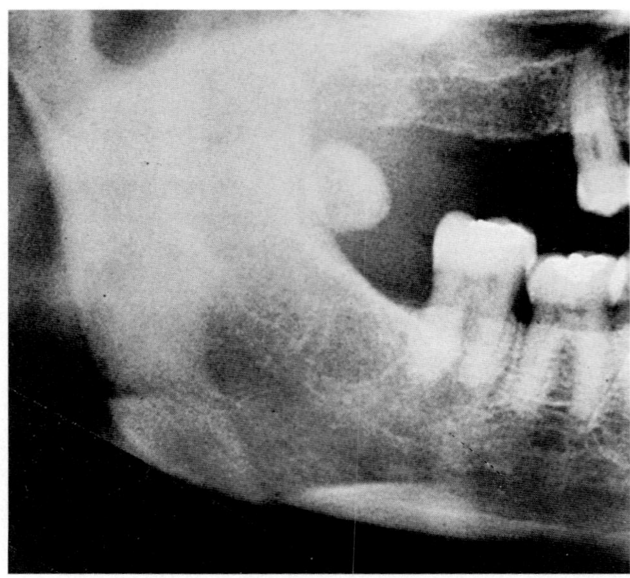

A

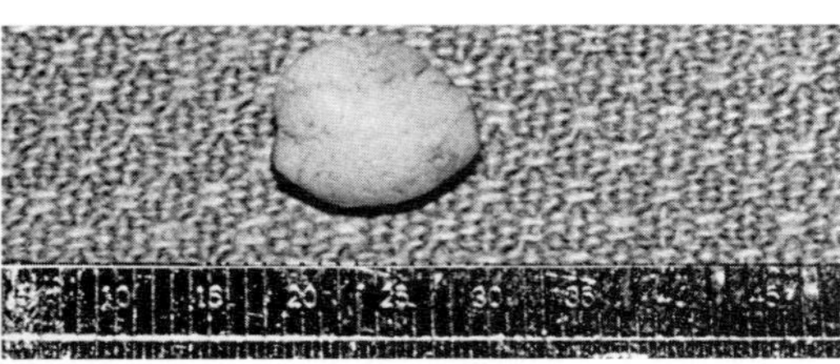

B

FIGURE 19–26.

Soft Tissue Osteoma: A, Recurrent lesion in buccal mucosa. B, Surgical specimen. (From Long DE, Koutnik AW: Recurrent intraosseous choristoma. Oral Surg Oral Med Oral Pathol 72: 337, 1991.)

ARTERIAL CALCIFICATION

Calcification frequently is found in the walls of the larger arteries of the abdomen and extremities in radiographs of middle-aged and older patients. The observation of arterial calcifications by radiologists is used to determine the severity and prognosis of several diseases. Parfitt (1969), Peterson (1978), Meema and associates (1976), Rifkin and co-workers (1979), and Ferrier (1964) reported on calcifications in diseases such as primary and secondary hyperparathyroidism, coronary heart disease, and diabetes. Bagdade (1975) reported that the incidence of accelerated atherosclerosis in patients on hemodialysis was many times that of normal or hypertensive populations. Facial artery calcification first was observed in two cases reported by Ennis and Burket (1942). Stafne and Gibilisco (1975), Hays and co-authors (1966), and Wood and Goaz (1980) have reported similar facial arterial calcifications on intraoral and panoramic radiographs. Friedlander and Lande (1981) showed carotid arterial plaques on panoramic radiographs.

Clinical Features

Miles and Craig (1983) examined 2422 panoramic radiographs in 1980 to 1981 and found 7 cases of calcified facial arteries. The age range for the 7 patients was 54 to 68 years; the median age was 61 years. All involvement was bilateral. Six of the 7 patients were men, an expected finding because the patients were seen at a Veterans Administration Hospital, which has a predominately male population. Five of the 7 patients had chronic renal failure, and 4 of these were receiving hemodialysis therapy. Of the 3 patients who were diabetic, 2 also had chronic renal failure. In 1 patient, only atherosclerotic vascular disease was diagnosed.

There are three major types of pathologic calcification of arteries. One of the three types, diffuse arteriolar sclerosis, is not included in this discussion because the small size of the involved vessels precludes radiographic examination, even when dense calcification is present. The other two types, Monckeberg's medial arteriosclerosis and intimal arteriosclerosis (atherosclerosis), have certain radiologic characteristics by which they often can be identified.

Monckeberg's Medial Arteriosclerosis

Monckeberg's medial arteriosclerosis, named after Johann Georg Monckeberg (1877 to 1925), a German pathologist at Bonn University, is characterized by the deposition of calcium in the medial layer of an artery. These calcium deposits do not narrow the vessel lumen or interfere with flow. Monckeberg's arteriosclerosis is an almost constant finding in elderly people, and it is seen frequently in people 35 to 50 years of age, particularly in diabetic patients. This type of calcification often is seen in people with no evidence of

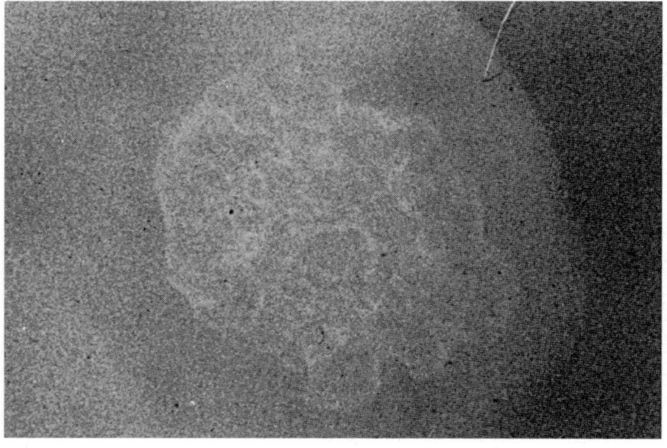

FIGURE 19–27.

Soft Tissue Osteoma: Case in buccal mucosa. (From Mesa ML, Schneider LC, Northington L: Osteoma of the buccal mucosa. J Oral Maxillofac Surg 40:684, 1982.)

occlusive arterial disease. The femoral, popliteal, and radial arteries are affected most often.

Intimal Arteriosclerosis (Atherosclerosis)

Intimal arteriosclerosis is characterized by the formation of atheromatous plaques in the thickened intima of arteries. Because the intima is the innermost layer of the vessel wall, the lumen of the vessel is narrowed and thrombosis may result in complete occlusion. This is the type of arteriosclerosis that leads to symptomatic arterial insufficiency. Fairbairn and colleagues (1972) reported that calcification in the intima of the arteries is a prominent feature in arteriosclerosis obliterans, which is primarily an intimal degenerative process that causes obliteration of the lumen.

Mixed Types (Combined Medial and Intimal Arteriosclerosis)

Combined medial and intimal arteriosclerosis is common, and when advanced medial calcification is present, the intimal plaques may be hidden. In the feet, it usually is difficult to determine the type of disease that may be present. The small vessels are often heavily calcified, and combined forms are frequent. Calcified plaques are seen frequently in the abdominal aorta and iliac vessels. The most frequent type of aortic arteriosclerosis, however, is a form of medial arteriosclerosis that weakens the vessel wall and predisposes the patient to aneurysm formation. There may be enough calcification in the medial wall of an abdominal aortic aneurysm to make it visible. Ultrasonography is indicated when the aneurysm is uncalcified.

◆ *RADIOLOGY (Figs. 19–28 and 19–29)*

Monckeberg's Medial Arteriosclerosis

In Monckeberg's medial arteriosclerosis, the following radiographic features are seen:

1. The calcification occurs in the form of closely spaced, fine concentric rings. These may be complete or incomplete, but the process is diffuse, involving long segments of multiple vessels. In 1950, Lindbom first described the radiographic changes in medial arteriosclerosis as ringlike calcifications with a "pipe-stem" appearance.
2. Calcification that accentuates the lateral margins of the artery to produce a tubular configuration almost always indicates that the deposition of calcium has taken place in the medial layer of the vessel. Hays and co-authors (1966) suggested that this type of calcification often is seen in the elderly and occasionally in middle-aged people with no evidence of occlusive arterial disease.
3. The characteristic changes are seen to best advantage in the femoral, popliteal, and tibial arteries, but often can be identified in other moderate-sized arteries, such as the radial and dorsalis pedis.

Calcifications sometimes may be seen in the facial, internal carotid, external carotid, and maxillary arteries. When a considerable length of the artery is involved, the serpentine outline and a faint radiopacity of the facial artery can be seen on the dental radiograph. Carotid plaques are observed in the lower part of the panoramic radiograph. They may be bilateral and generally appear diffuse and well calcified. A separate discussion follows on this condition.

Intimal Arteriosclerosis

The atheromatous plaques in intimal arteriosclerosis may be calcified. When they are calcified, they are seen as irregular plaques of various sizes, from small flecks to larger areas that are 1 cm or longer. They may be elongated or somewhat triangular, with a considerable variation in shape. They seldom occlude the lumen of the artery completely and are distributed irregularly along the course without any specific arrangement. The amount of visible calcification bears no relationship to the severity of the vascular occlusion, and complete obstruction may exist with no visible calcification. Allen and colleagues (1962) reported that calcified plaques of various sizes and shapes are found in patients with arteriosclerosis obliterans. The term arteriosclerosis obliterans usually refers to atherosclerosis within the arteries of the extremities, and the condition frequently progresses to produce

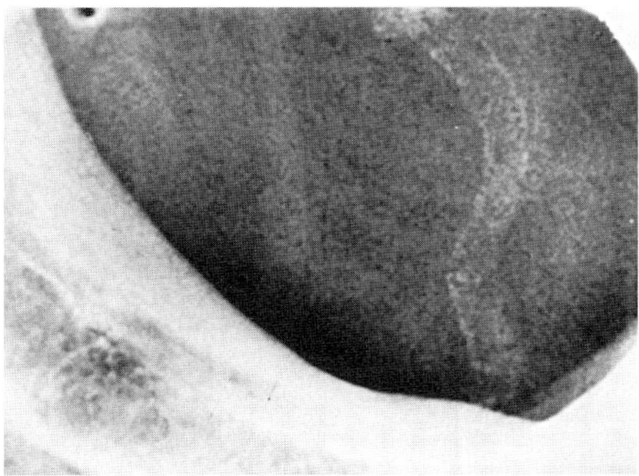

A

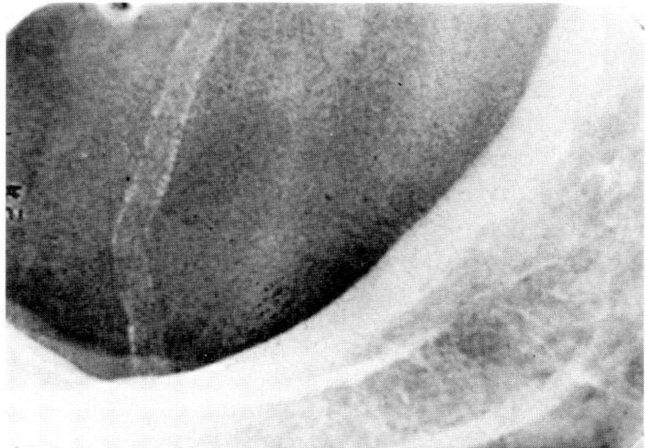

B

FIGURE 19–28.

Calcified Facial Artery: A and B, Bilateral case in an 83-year-old man.

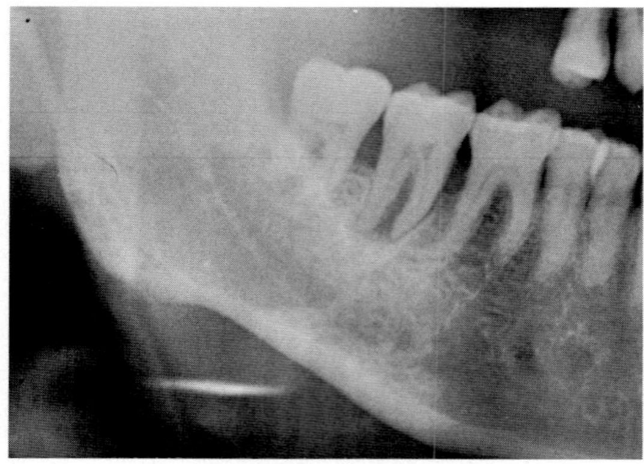
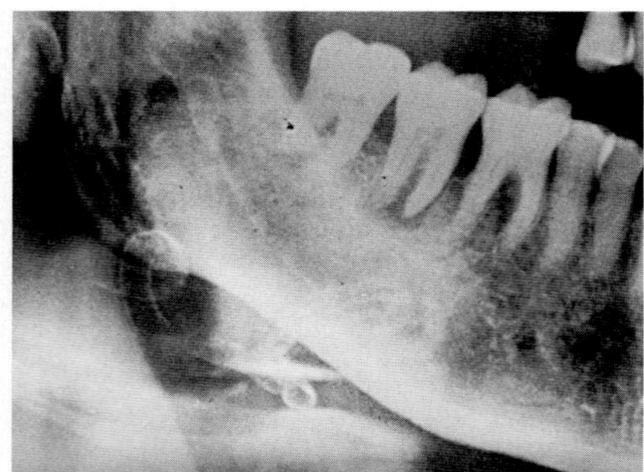

A B

FIGURE 19–29.

Calcified Facial Artery: A, Case in 55-year-old diabetic man. B, Same patient 10 months later, after onset of renal complications; calcification of facial artery at angle of mandible.

stenosis or occlusion of the arterial lumen. The abdominal aorta and iliac, femoral, and popliteal arteries are involved most often.

CAROTID ARTERIAL PLAQUES

In 1875, Gowers was the first to link a stroke with extracranial vascular disease when he described a patient with right hemiplegia and blindness in the left eye and attributed this syndrome to occlusion of the left carotid artery. In 1914, Hunt postulated that obstructed carotid arteries represented a prodrome to vascular lesions of the brain. The most common location for an atherosclerotic plaque lesion is at the carotid bifurcation; thus, this lesion may be visible on panoramic radiographs.

Pathologic Characteristics

Arterial plaque is a form of intimal arteriosclerosis and may be referred to as atherosclerotic plaque, the primary pathologic entity involved in extracranial vascular disease. This consists of focal deposits of fat, primarily cholesterol, in the arterial intima. It is associated with an inflammatory response resulting from fibroblastic proliferation and calcium salt encrustations. These calcium deposits may be seen on radiographs. The common carotid arteries ascend within the neck to approximately the midcervical region; in this area, opposite the upper border of the thyroid cartilage, they bifurcate into the external and internal carotid arteries. When such plaques are seen in the panoramic radiograph, care should be exercised in palpating the neck so that a portion of the plaque is not dislodged.

Clinical Features

Carotid arterial plaques may result in a cerebrovascular accident. Matsumoto and co-workers (1973) found that the annual incidence of new strokes in the United States is 160 per 100,000 people between the ages of 55 and 64 years and 632 per 100,000 people between 65 and 74 years of age; they also showed that the rate is 1.5 times greater in men than women of the same age. Symptoms associated with cerebrovascular disease may be mild or severe, depending on the degree of vascular involvement. A transient ischemic attack may last only a few minutes, and the patient may recover without a residual neurologic deficit. The most common form of transient ischemic attack from carotid artery occlusive plaque yields symptoms of transient monocular blindness or motor dysfunction, usually hemiparesis; a secondary malfunction, such as hemidysesthesia, also may be seen. The symptoms of a complete stroke resulting from carotid artery occlusion involve an element of persistent neurologic deficit that may vary from subtle degrees of weakness to hemiplegia and aphasia.

Treatment/Prognosis

In 1954, Eastcott and associates described the first successful surgical procedure on the extracranial portion of the carotid artery. They removed an atherosclerotic lesion at the carotid bifurcation by resecting the diseased vessel; then they reestablished vessel continuity by anastomosing the remaining portion of the vessel proximally and distally. Extracerebral occlusion in the carotid artery can be managed successfully with endarterectomy or bypass grafting. Little can be done when the lesion is intracerebral.

◆ *RADIOLOGY*

In 1937, Moniz and colleagues reported that arteriography could be used to diagnose carotid artery occlusion. Atherosclerotic calcifications at the origin of the internal carotid artery can be seen on panoramic radiographs. The presence of carotid calcifications may indicate the probable point of occlusion. Friedlander and Lande (1981) evaluated panoramic radiographs of 1000 men between the ages of 50 and 75 years. Soft tissue calcification in the region of the carotid artery was identified on 2% of the radiographs. Approximately 88% of the soft tissue calcifications were interpreted as calcifications in the region of the carotid bifurcation, and 12% represented salivary calculi, phleboliths, or calcified lymph nodes.

PHLEBOLITH

Vascular calcifications are usually associated with the walls of arteries, as previously described. Venous calcifications are rarely seen in radiographs, although calcification in a thrombosed vein is common, especially in the leg. These calcifications are known as phleboliths and, by definition, are calcified thrombi. In the head and neck, phleboliths most frequently occur in association with vascular lesions. In reports such as those of Keathley and associates (1983), phleboliths have been documented in association with hemangiomas and arteriovenous malformations, usually within the soft tissues of the face or neck.

◆ *RADIOLOGY (Fig. 19–30)*

Phleboliths usually occur within soft tissue; thus, they may overlie the osseous structures within which their images are seen radiographically, or they may also be seen within the soft tissues beyond the confines of an adjacent bone. Phleboliths are round or ovoid and vary in diameter from several millimeters to 1 cm. They are rarely solitary and may number from several to dozens within the affected area. Each phlebolith consists of concentric lamellae of calcified material separated by radiolucent bands of uncalcified layers of the thrombus. The outer layer as seen in the radiograph is always calcified, whereas the central part is most often radiolucent, although this area may also be radiopaque. Whereas the most typical appearance resembles calcified onion rings, some lesions merely consist of a calcified outer shell, a radiolucent layer beneath this shell, and a radiopaque central core.

STURGE-WEBER SYNDROME
(Encephalotrigeminal angiomatosis)

Sturge-Weber syndrome is the concurrence of a port-wine stain or nevus flammeus, a form of capillary hemangioma, within the distribution of the the trigeminal nerve, especially the ophthalmic division, and associated with ipsilateral leptomeningeal vascular anomalies. In a review of port-wine stains by Enjoiras and co-authors (1985), they found that 90 of 106 patients had only cutaneous vascular abnormalities, without a leptomeningeal component. Thus, most patients with port-wine stains do not have Sturge-Weber syndrome. Incomplete forms of Sturge-Weber syndrome have been discussed by Bergstrand and associates (1936), and many cases have been called Sturge-Weber syndrome without proof of cerebral angiomatosis. Brain involvement consists of an angioma of the leptomeninges that consist of the pia-arachnoid membranes over the posterior parietal or occipital lobes. The angiomatosis consists of thin-walled venous vessels with convolutional, gyriform calcification that develops after the second year. These calcifications are discernible in cranial radiographs.

Clinical Features

Although port-wine hemangiomas may be widespread and involve as much as half of the body, they often are located on the face and neck. They are present at birth and range from small red macules to large red patches, which are partially or completely blanched by diascopic pressure. The

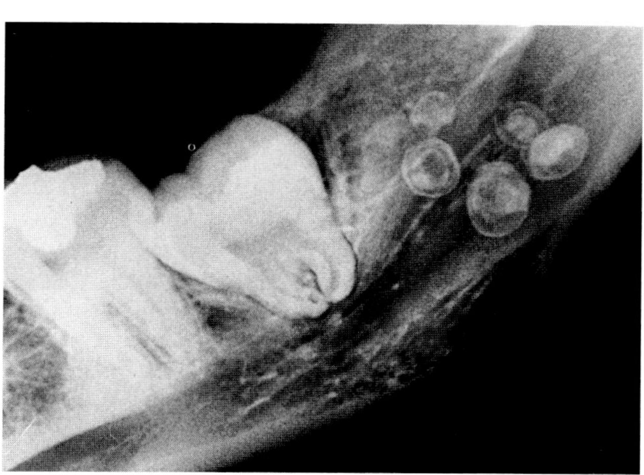

A

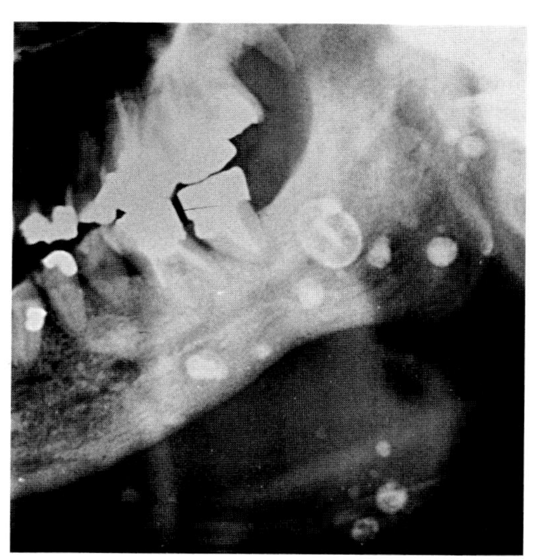

B

FIGURE 19–30.

Phleboliths: A and B, Facial hemangioma was present. (A, Courtesy of Dr. D. Barnet, Portland, OR; B, Courtesy of Dr. L. Alfaro, University of Chile School of Dentistry, Pathology Referral Center, Santiago, Chile.)

most common appearance is a unilateral distribution on the face, especially along the ophthalmic and other divisions of the trigeminal nerve. Port-wine hemangiomas do not tend to cross the midline, but they may. They vary in color from pink to dark or bluish red. The mucous membrane of the mouth may be involved when the distribution of the lesions is over the maxillary or mandibular divisions of the trigeminal nerve. A diagnosis of Sturge-Weber syndrome requires concurrence of port-wine stain within the ophthalmic division of the trigeminal nerve, intracranial calcifications associated with cerebral angiomatosis, and the onset of the characteristic symptoms.

The following symptoms may occur: glaucoma, contralateral jacksonian epilepsy, paralysis, mental retardation, and retinal detachment. Peterman and colleagues (1958) reported that epilepsy is common, occurring in 89% of patients with this syndrome at the Mayo Clinic. The seizures are often the jacksonian type and are contralateral to the angiomatosis in the motor cortex. The classic ophthalmic lesion is a choroidal (posterior vascular coat of eyeball) angioma. Buphthalmos (enlargement and distention of fibrous coats of eye) and glaucoma frequently are found. In the survey by Alexander and Norman (1960), buphthalmos was seen in 48 and glaucoma in 25 of the 257 cases analyzed. Peterman and colleagues (1958) reported that at least one third of children with Sturge-Weber syndrome are mentally retarded. These manifestations result directly from the leptomeningeal angiomas and calcifications. The most frequent oral sign is a port-wine stain lesion in the oral mucosa. Vascular lesions may be seen on the lips, buccal mucosa, gingiva, hard and soft palate, tongue, and floor of the mouth; they may be more bluish red than the surrounding normal mucosa.

Treatment/Prognosis

Because severe brain damage sometimes is seen in patients with Sturge-Weber syndrome, it is important to diagnose the leptomeningeal angiomatosis as soon as possible. Cerebral lobectomy must be considered while the patient is an infant, before epilepsy occurs. In cases that already have resulted in hemiparesis, hemispherectomy has yielded promising results. The epilepsy sometimes can be controlled by anticonvulsant medications. Mental retardation and hemiparesis eventually develop if surgery does not prevent them. Treatment of nevus flammeus is difficult; tattooing with skin-colored pigments has been performed for years, but it has been difficult to match the varied natural skin colors and impossible to match the changing color of normal skin. Laser therapy has been used, with increasing satisfactory results; the best results have been achieved with the dark purplish lesions in older patients.

◆ *RADIOLOGY (Fig. 19–31)*

The characteristic calcification seen in the leptomeninges consists of double-contoured "tram-lines," following the convolutions of the cerebral cortex. Brushfield and Wyatt (1928) stated that this tram-line calcification is pathognomonic of the syndrome. These are seen best in the lateral skull view, with the affected side closest to the film, and the basilar or anteroposterior view may show the distribution from superficial to deeper parts of the leptomeninges. Because the vascular anomalies tend to be convoluted and the vessel walls calcified, anastomosing interconnections of the vascular network are seen easily on radiographs, especially in more severe lesions. According to Alexander and Norman (1960), the calcification remains rather stationary after the second decade of life; the severity of brain-associated symptoms increases with greater distribution of the intracerebral lesions. Horing (1960) described asymmetry of the skull in patients with Sturge-Weber syndrome.

PERIPHERAL ODONTOGENIC TUMORS WITH CALCIFICATION (Extraosseous odontogenic tumors, soft tissue odontogenic tumors)

Buchner and Sciubba (1987) defined peripheral odontogenic tumors as showing the histologic characteristics of their intraosseous counterparts, but occurring solely in the soft tissue covering the tooth-bearing portion of the mandible and maxilla. Odontogenic tumors that have been described as originating in gingiva include the ameloblastoma, adenomatoid odontogenic tumor (AOT), calcifying epithelial odontogenic tumor (CEOT), squamous odontogenic tumor (SOT), and odontogenic fibroma (World Health Organization [WHO] type). The calcifying odontogenic cyst also can originate in gingiva and is not as rare as the odontogenic tumors. In reviews of gingival lesions, Freedman and associates (1975) found that 22% of their cases and Fejerskov and Krogh (1972) reported 30% of their cases were calcifying odontogenic cysts. Odontogenic tumors are uncommon lesions in the oral cavity; Regezi and co-workers (1978) found that odontogenic tumors represented only 1.3% of 55,000 biopsy specimens processed within the Michigan Dental School biopsy service. In a literature review by Buchner and Sciubba (1987) in 1987, only 48 well-documented cases of peripheral epithelial odontogenic tumor were reported.

Peripheral Ameloblastoma

The peripheral ameloblastoma (PA) has all the histologic characteristics of its intraosseous counterpart but occurs in the gingival soft tissues overlying the tooth-bearing areas of the maxilla and mandible. Gardner (1977), Waldron (1972), and Simpson (1974) believed that basal cell carcinoma arising in the gingiva and PA are essentially the same lesion. In 1987, Buchner and Sciubba (1987), in a review of the English language literature for peripheral epithelial odontogenic tumors, found 26 well-documented cases of PA. Buchner and Sciubba (1987) combined the 26 cases of PA of the tooth-bearing areas and the 6 cases reported as basal cell carcinoma of the gingiva. The mean patient age at diagnosis was 52 years. The highest incidence was in the fifth and sixth decades of life, with 44% of the patients in these age groups. The male-to-female ratio was 1.7:1. Most of the PA lesions occurred as painless sessile epulislike growths described as firm and exophytic. The color of the lesion was usually normal or pink, and in some cases it was described

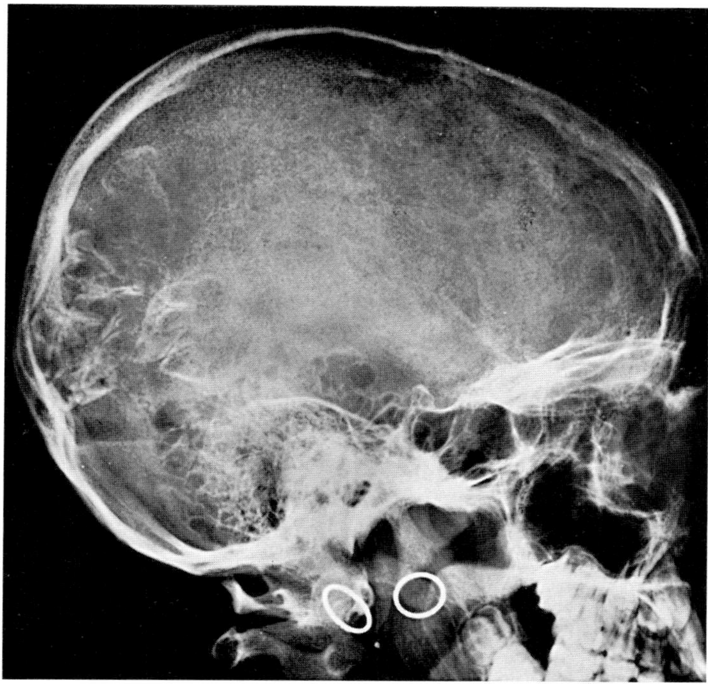

A

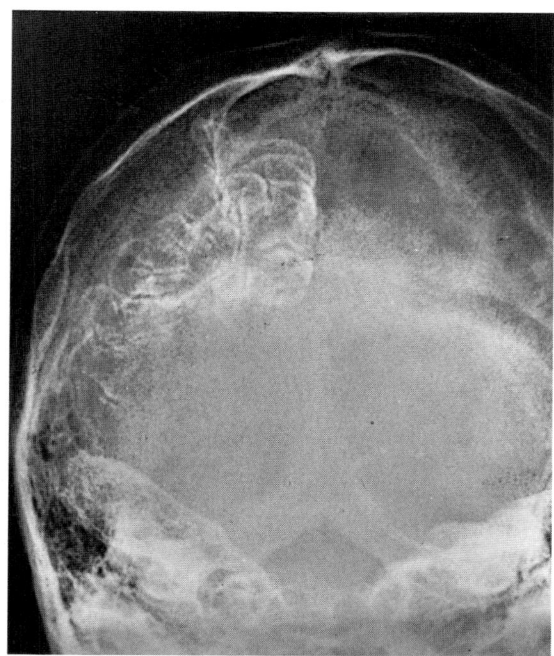

B

FIGURE 19–31.

Sturge-Weber Syndrome: A and B, "Tram line" pattern of calcification within intracranial vascular lesion.

as red or dark red. The size of the lesion ranged from 0.3 to 2.0 cm at the greatest diameter. Although the intraosseous ameloblastoma is a locally aggressive neoplasm capable of invasion and destruction of bone, the PA does not manifest such behavior. As the treatment of choice, Gardner (1977) and Guralnick and associates (1983) recommended conservative excision of the growth with adequate margins, which is usually curative. Also, because experience is limited with this lesion, long-term follow-up is necessary.

◆ *RADIOLOGY*

The mandible was the most common site for PA (59%), and most mandibular lesions occurred in the canine-premolar region; the most common location in the maxilla was the soft tissue of the tuberosity area. In 29 of the 32 cases of PA reviewed by Buchner and Sciubba (1987), there was no radiologic evidence of bone involvement. In 2 cases, superficial saucerization of the alveolar bone was seen. In 5 cases, including the 2 cases with radiographic evidence of superficial saucerization of bone, a shallow bony depression of the underlying bone was observed at surgery.

Peripheral Adenomatoid Odontogenic Tumor

A review of the literature by Giansanti and associates in 1970 revealed more than 100 cases of intraosseous AOT, and a second review by Courtney and Kerr in 1975 increased the number to almost 150 cases. AOT rarely occurs within soft tissues. Buchner and Sciubba (1987) found only 6 acceptable well-documented cases of peripheral AOT; the histomorphologic features of peripheral AOT are similar to those observed in the intraosseous lesions. Abrams and coworkers (1968) suggested that their 3 cases of peripheral AOT were associated with an unerupted tooth and postulated that when normal eruption of the tooth progressed, the tumor was pushed to one side and those portions not destroyed by the erupting tooth remained as a peripheral AOT. Yazdi and Nowparast (1974), however, suggested that the basal layer of the surface epithelium is the source of origin of the peripheral AOT. The patients' ages ranged from 9 to 16 years, with a mean age of 14 years. According to Courtney and Kerr's (1975) review of patients with intraosseous AOT, the age range was 5 to 53 years, with a mean age of 18 years. Of the 6 patients with peripheral AOT, 5 were female and 1 was male. The gender distribution for intraosseous AOT also showed a predilection for female patients (64%). All the peripheral AOTs were evident clinically as painless gingival swellings. All peripheral AOTs were treated by surgical excision. Follow-up histories were available in 3 cases; no recurrences were reported and none should be expected because there is no evidence that the intraosseous AOT recurs.

◆ *RADIOLOGY*

Peripheral AOTs occurred primarily in the maxillary arch (83%). No lesions were found distal to the canine region. The intraosseous AOT has a predilection for the incisor and canine regions of the maxillary arch. In one case, the radiologic appearance suggested a shallow erosion of the underlying bone. In another case, a bony depression was observed immediately beneath the lesion. Although not mentioned, the characteristic mineralization within the lesion would be expected, especially in the occlusal view. One should recognize grouping of flecks into patterns in an even generalized distribution and the capsule space.

Peripheral Calcifying Epithelial Odontogenic Tumor

A review by Franklin and Pindborg in 1976 reported that 108 intraosseous CEOTs have been described since Pindborg's original article in 1955. The lesion rarely occurs in soft tissues; Buchner and Sciubba (1987) found only 9 acceptable, well-documented cases in the literature. Histomorphologically, the peripheral CEOT lesions are identical to their intraosseous counterparts. Krolls and Pindborg (1974) considered the intraosseous CEOT to be locally invasive, but it does not extend into the intratrabecular spaces as readily as the ameloblastoma. The location of the peripheral CEOT suggests that it may arise from rests of Serres of the dental lamina, which are located in the gingiva, or from the basal cells of the surface epithelium. In Buchner and Sciubba's 1987 review, the age range of the 9 patients with peripheral CEOTs was 12 to 60 years; the mean patient age at the initial diagnosis was 32 years. According to the review by Franklin and Pindborg (1976), the age range for the patients with intraosseous lesions was 8 to 92 years, with a mean age of 40 years. Of the 9 peripheral cases in Buchner and Sciubba's 1987 review, 6 occurred in female patients and 3 in male patients. Franklin and Pindborg (1976) reported a nearly equal distribution of intraosseous CEOTs between male and female patients.

Clinically, the peripheral CEOT appears most commonly as a painless, firm gingival mass. In most cases, they were pink. Five of the nine peripheral CEOTs were treated by simple excision, and in one case the lesion was excised with electrocautery and the underlying bone was cauterized. In another case, Takeda and co-workers (1983) excised the underlying bone, and Ai-ru and co-workers (1982) performed a ''partial mandibular resection'' in an additional case. To our knowledge, no recurrences of these lesions have been recorded. For intraosseous CEOT, Franklin and Pindborg (1976) reported a recurrence rate of 14%.

◆ *RADIOLOGY*

Among the nine peripheral lesions, most were in the mandibular arch (67%) and the incisor and canine-premolar regions. Intraosseous CEOTs are found primarily in the mandible and located mainly in the molar region. To our knowledge, no one has mentioned the appearance of calcifications within peripheral CEOTs. If present, they would be expected more toward one part of the lesion, perhaps the deeper aspect, closest to the underlying gingival tissue. The mineralized amyloid histologically resembles a droplet; thus, even larger clumps would be expected to have rounded outlines. We are not certain whether the ''driven snow'' pattern can occur without an associated impacted tooth. As the coronal aspect of the impacted tooth is pushed toward the periphery of the lesion, it leaves behind linear streaks of calcified amyloid that originate at the occlusal or incisal surface and continue to form until additional displacement of the associated tooth is impeded by the outer cortex of the jaw. If tooth movement occurs before mineralization of the amyloid, clumps of calcified amyloid are seen in close association with the occlusal or incisal surface, without streaking.

Peripheral Squamous Odontogenic Tumor

Pullon and associates first described the SOT in 1975. Buchner and Sciubba (1987) stated that 22 cases of intraosseous SOT have been reported through the end of 1985. A single case of peripheral SOT was reported in 1985 by Hietanen and co-workers. The lesion occurred in an 11-year-old girl as a nodule in the palatal mucosa in the region of the right maxillary canine and first premolar. It was excised and recurred 13 years later in the same location. The histologic features of the recurrent lesion were similar to those of the primary tumor, and it was diagnosed as a recurrent peripheral SOT.

◆ *RADIOLOGY*

Radiographic examination did not show bony involvement, and at surgery the lesion appeared entirely extraosseous.

Peripheral Odontogenic Fibroma (WHO Type) (Fig. 19–32)

At one time, the terms peripheral ossifying fibroma and peripheral odontogenic fibroma were used interchangeably; however, the WHO, in its classification of odontogenic tumors, used the term peripheral odontogenic fibroma as a specific entity, quite separate from peripheral ossifying fibroma. In the past, the peripheral odontogenic fibroma has been termed an odontogenic gingiva epithelial hamartoma by Baden and co-workers (1968) and a peripheral ameloblastic fibrodentinoma by McKelvy and Cherrick (1976). The peripheral odontogenic fibroma (WHO type) is a rare lesion. The largest series of cases was reported by Farman (1975), who found only 5 cases in an extensive review of the English literature and added 10 new cases. It is a fibroblastic neoplasm containing varying amounts of odontogenic epithelium; sometimes the proliferation of odontogenic epithelium is so significant that it may be difficult to distinguish the lesion from a PA. Mineralized tissue may be present in the peripheral odontogenic fibroma. When observed, it may resemble trabeculae of bone or osteoid, dentin or osteodentin, or cementum-like material. The ages of the 15 reported patients ranged from 5 to 65 years, spaced throughout the various decades. There was no sex predilection. The lesions were described as slow-growing, solid, firmly attached gingival masses, sometimes arising between teeth and sometimes displacing teeth. Treatment is surgical excision. In the

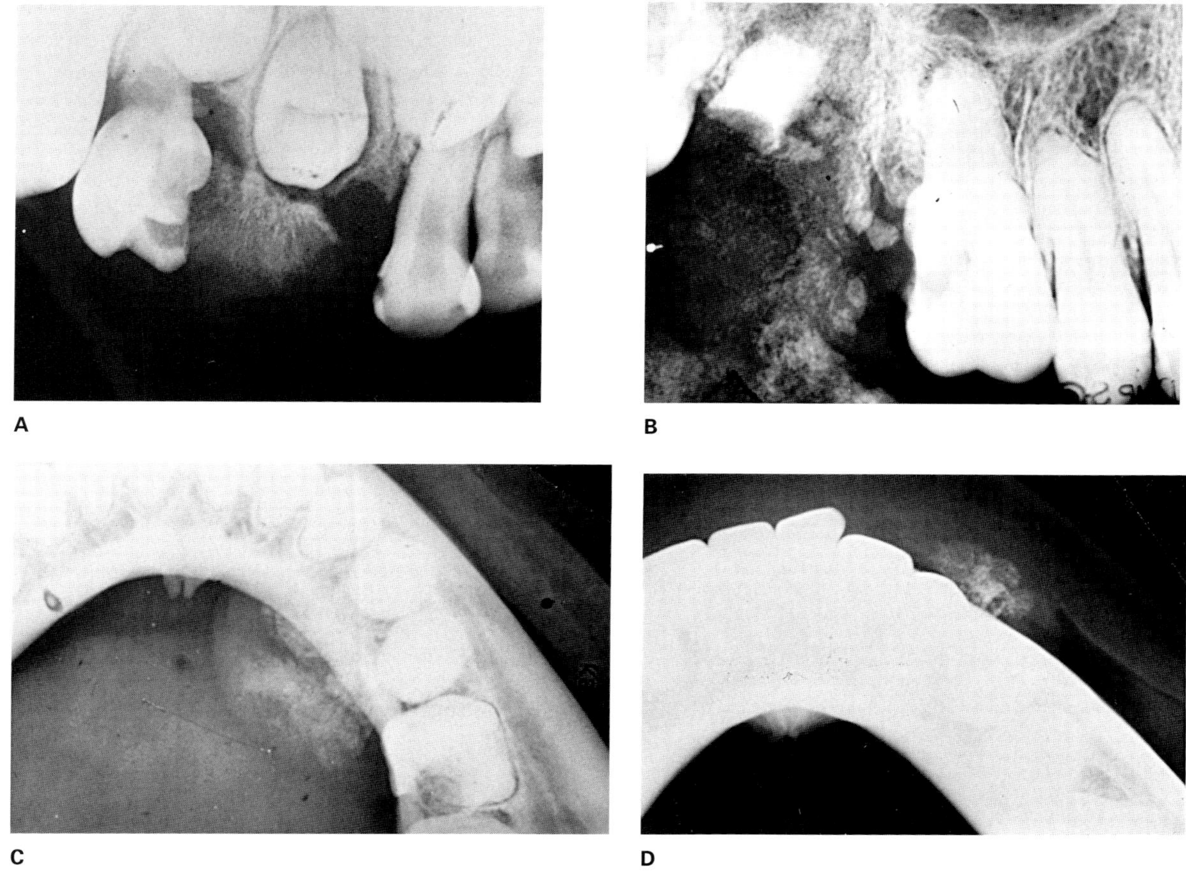

FIGURE 19–32.

Peripheral Fibroma with Calcifications: A to D, Various patterns of mineralization within lesion. (A and B, Courtesy of Dr. L. Alfaro, University of Chile School of Dentistry, Pathology Referral Center, Santiago, Chile; C, Courtesy of Dr. P. Dhiravarangkura, Chulalonghorn University, Bangkok, Thailand; D, Courtesy of Drs. M. Araki and K. Hashimoto, Nihon University, Tokyo, Japan.)

series reported by Farman (1975), no lesion was known to recur.

◆ RADIOLOGY

Eleven of the 15 cases were in the mandible and 4 in the maxilla. Some lesions of peripheral odontogenic fibroma contain a calcified stalk at surgery, and this, or other islands of calcified material, may be seen as radiopaque flecks on the radiograph. On careful examination of the radiograph, bony tissue should show trabeculation or flecks with pointed spicules at the margins. If the material is dentinlike, an appearance similar to that of odontoma should be expected; in well-organized lesions, a sunray appearance or dentinal tubulelike structures might be observed. When the mineralized component consists of cementum, the presence of calcific spherules with a density somewhat less than that of bone and forming circular structures with a radiolucent center and evidence of coalescence to form a central massule or mass are noted. These observations can be made on the basis of the illustrations provided in this chapter; however, we have no histologic correlations in any of our cases.

References

Foreign Bodies

Alattan MM, Baughman RA, Collett WK: A survey of panoramic radiographs for evaluation of normal and pathologic findings. Oral Surg Oral Med Oral Pathol 50:472, 1980.

Edwards RW: Accidents of dental origin: foreign bodies in the bronchi and stomach. J Oral Surg 6:75, 1948.

Gibilisco JA: Stafne's Oral Radiographic Diagnosis. 5th Ed. Philadelphia: WB Saunders, 1980, p. 371.

Stanhope EO: A case of retained forceps blade. Br Dent J 99:434, 1955.

Wintrobe MM, et al: Harrison's Principles of Internal Medicine. 6th Ed. New York:McGraw-Hill, 1970, pp. 1333, 1336, 1337, 1442, 1467.

Elongated Styloid Process

Balasubramian S: The ossification of the stylohyoid ligament and its relation to facial pain. Br Dent J 116:108, 1964.

Barclay JK: Panoramic radiology of the edentulous jaw, a survey of 100 patients. NZ Dent J 66:53, 1970.

Camarda AJ, Deschamps C, Forest D: Stylohyoid chain ossification: a discussion of etiology. Oral Surg Oral Med Oral Pathol 67:515, 1989.

Correll RW, Jensen JL, Taylor JB, Rhyne RR: Mineralization of the stylohyoid-stylomandibular ligament complex. Oral Surg Oral Med Oral Pathol 48:286, 1979.

Dwight T: Stylo-hyoid ossification. Ann Surg 46:721, 1907.

Eagle WW: Elongated styloid process. Arch Otolaryngol 25:584, 1937.
Frommer J: Anatomic variations in the stylohyoid chain and their possible clinical significance. Oral Surg Oral Med Oral Pathol 38:659, 1974.
Grossman JR Jr, Tarsitano JJ: The styloid-stylohyoid syndrome. J Oral Surg 35:555, 1977.
Kaufman SM, Elzay RP, Irish EF: Styloid process variation. Arch Otolaryngol 191:463, 1970.
Keur JJ, Campbell JPS, McCarthy JF, Ralph WJ: The clinical significance of the elongated styloid process. Oral Surg Oral Med Oral Pathol 61: 399, 1986.
Langlais RP, Miles DA, Van Dis ML: Elongated and mineralized stylohyoid ligament complex: a proposed classification and report of a case of Eagle's syndrome. Oral Surg Oral Med Oral Pathol 61:527, 1986.
Worth HM: Principles and Practice of Oral Radiologic Interpretation. Chicago:Year Book Medical Publishers, 1963, p. 327.

Eruption Sequestrum

Starkey PE, Shafer WG: Eruption sequestration in children. J Dent Child 30:84, 1963.

Sialolith

Alexander WN, Andrews JL: Minor salivary gland sialolithiasis: report of a case. J Oral Surg 23:461, 1965.
Anneroth G, Hansen LS: Minor salivary gland calculi: a clinical and histopathological study of 49 cases. Int J Oral Surg 12:80, 1983.
Anneroth G, Everoth C-M, Isacsson G: Morphology of salivary calculus. J Oral Pathol 4:257, 1975.
Bahn SL, Tabachnick TT: Sialolithiasis of minor salivary glands. Oral Surg Oral Med Oral Pathol 32:371, 1971.
Barnett ML: Sialolithiasis of labial gland. Oral Surg Oral Med Oral Pathol 32:22, 1971.
Baurmach H, Mandel L: Surgical excision of miniature sialoliths in Wharton's duct. Oral Surg Oral Med Oral Pathol 12:165, 1959.
DeGregori G, Pippen R: Sialolithiasis with sialadenitis of a minor salivary gland: report of a case. Oral Surg Oral Med Oral Pathol 30:320, 1970.
Eversole LR, Sabes WR: Minor salivary duct changes due to obstruction. Arch Otolaryngol 94:19, 1971.
Gorlin RJ, Goldman HM: Thoma's Oral Pathology. 6th Ed. St. Louis:CV Mosby, 1970, p. 997.
Holst E: Sialolithiasis of the minor salivary glands: report of three cases. J Oral Surg 26:354, 1968.
Isacsson G, Persson NE: The gigantiform salivary calculus. Int J Oral Surg 11:135, 1982.
Jensen JL, Howell FU, Rick GM, Correll RW: Minor salivary gland calculi. Oral Surg Oral Med Oral Pathol 47:44, 1979.
Levy DM, ReMine WH, Devine KD: Salivary gland calculi. JAMA 181: 1115, 1962.
Moskow R, Moskow BS, Robinson HL: Minor salivary gland sialolithiasis. Oral Surg Oral Med Oral Pathol 17:225, 1964.
Noehren HH: Multiple calculi in Stensen's duct. JAMA 80:25, 1923.
Pullon PA, Miller AS: Sialolithiasis of accessory salivary glands: review of 55 cases. J Oral Surg 39:832, 1972.
Rabinov K, Weber AC: Radiology of the salivary glands. Boston:CK Hull Med Publishers, 1985, p. 154.
Rauch S: Sperchelsteine (Sialolithiasis) In Die Speicheldrusen des Menchen. Stuttgart:Georg Thieme Verlag, 1959, p. 434.
Rubin P, Holt JF: Secretory sialography in diseases of the major salivary glands. AJR Am J Roentgenol 77:575, 1957.

Calcified Lymph Nodes

Wood NK, Goaz PW: Periapical Radiopacities in Differential Diagnosis of Oral Lesions. St. Louis:CV Mosby, 1980, p. 557.

Tonsillolith

Bhaskar SN: Synopsis of Oral Pathology. St. Louis:CV Mosby, 1961, p. 401.
Clarke PRR, Long MB: Tonsilar calculi. Lancet 266:1112, 1954.
Cooper MM, Steinberg JJ, Lastra M, Antopol S: Tonsillar calculi: report of a case and review of literature. Oral Surg Oral Med Oral Pathol 55: 239, 1983.
Hoffman H: Tonsillolith. Practitioner 188:93, 1978.
Katz JO, Langlais RP, Underhill TE, Kimura K: Localization of paraoral soft tissue calcifications: the known object rule. Oral Surg Oral Med Oral Pathol 67:459, 1989.
Samant HC, Gupta OP: Oral Surg Oral Med Oral Pathol 40:56, 1975.
Shrimali R, Bhatin PL: A giant radiopaque tonsillolith. J Indian Med Assoc 58:174, 1972.

Antrolith

Blaschke DD, Brady FA: The maxillary antrolith. Oral Surg Oral Med Oral Pathol 48:187, 1979.
Bowerman JE: The maxillary antrolith. J Laryngol Otol 83:873, 1969.
Cunningham AT, Lord OC, Manley CH, Polson CJ: Rhinoliths: the report of an antral and three nasal stones. J Laryngol 60:253, 1945.
Evans J: Maxillary antrolith: a case report. Br J Oral Surg 13:73, 1975.
Karges MA, Eversole LR, Poindexter BJ Jr: Antrolith: report of case and review of literature. J Oral Surg 29:812, 1971.
Lord OC: Antral rhinoliths. J Laryngol 59:218, 1944.
Wright AJ: A case of chronic and antral sinusitis due to a rhinolith. J Laryngol 42:192, 1927.

Rhinolith

Allen GA, Liston SL: Rhinolith: unusual appearance on panoramic radiograph. J Oral Surg 37:54, 1979.
Ballenger JJ: Diseases of the Nose, Throat and Ear. 11th Ed. Philadelphia: Lea & Febiger, 1969, p. 80.
Bicknell PG: Rhinolith perforating the hard palate. J Laryngol Otol 84: 1161, 1970.
Blechman M, Bonakdarpoui A, Ronis M: Rhinolithiasis: a report of 2 cases. Diagn Radiol 113:615, 1974.
Brown CJ Jr, Allen RE: Antral rhinolith: report of a case. J Oral Surg 15: 153, 1957.
Dodd GD, Jing BS: Radiology of the Nose, Paranasal Sinuses and Nasopharynx. Baltimore:Williams & Wilkins, 1977, p. 33.
Eliachar I, Schalit M: Rhinolithiasis: report of eight cases. Arch Otolaryngol 91:88, 1970.
Harrison BB, Lamming RL: Exogenous nasal rhinolith. Br J Radiol 42: 838, 1969.
Marano PD, Smart EA, Kolodny SC: Rhinolith simulating osseous lesion: a report of a case. J Oral Surg 28:615, 1970.
Merideth HW, Grossman JW: Rhinolith. Arch Otolaryngol 55:475, 1952.
Polson CJ: On rhinoliths. J Laryngol Otol 58:79, Mar 1943.
Terrafranca RJ, Zellis A: Rhinolith. Radiology 58:405, 1952.

Calcified Scar

Ennis LM: Roentgenographic appearance of calcified acne lesions. J Am Dent Assoc 68:351, Mar 1964.

Cysticercosis Cutis

Levin JA, et al: Praziquantel in the treatment of cysticercosis [letter]. JAMA 256:349, 1986.

Myositis Ossificans

Abdin HA, Prabhu SR: Traumatic myositis ossificans of lateral pterygoid muscle. J Oral Med 39:54, 1984.
Eversole L: Clinical Outline of Oral Pathology. 2nd Ed. Philadelphia:Lea & Febiger, 1984, p. 292.
Flynn JE, Graham JH: Myositis ossificans. Surg Gynecol Obstet 118:1101, 1964.
Goodsell JO: Traumatic myositis ossificans of the masseter muscle: review of literature and report of a case. J Oral Surg 20:116, 1962.
Mulherin D, Schow CE Jr: Traumatic myositis ossificans after genioplasty. J Oral Surg 38:786, 1980.
Palumbo VD, Sills AH, Hinds EC: Limited mandibular motion associated with bone pathosis: report of cases. J Oral Surg 11:531, 1964.
Plezia RA, Mintz SM, Calligaro P: Myositis ossificans traumatism of the masseter muscle: report of a case. J Oral Surg 44:351, 1977.
Ramesh N, Dixon RA Jr: Myositis ossificans: medial pterygoid muscle: a case report. Br J Oral Surg 12:229, 1974.
Vernale CA: Traumatic myositis ossificans of the masseter muscle: report of 2 cases. Oral Surg Oral Med Oral Pathol 16:8, 1968.

Calcinosis Cutis

Magalini S: Dictionary of Medical Syndromes. Philadelphia:JB Lippincott, 1971, p. 86.

Wang WJ, et al: Calcinosis cutis in juvenile dermatomyositis: remarkable response to aluminum hydroxide therapy. Arch Dermatol 124:1721, 1988.

Worth HM: Principles and Practice of Oral Radiologic Interpretation. Chicago:Year Book Medical Publishers, 1963, p. 648.

Miliary Osteoma

Arnold HL, Odom RB, James WP: Andrews' Diseases of the Skin. Philadelphia:WB Saunders, 1990, p. 636.

Carney RG, Radcliffe CE: Multiple miliary osteomas of the skin. Arch Dermatol Syph 64:483, 1951.

Costello MJ: Metaplasia of bone: report of a case. Arch Dermatol Syph 56:536, 1947.

Domonkos AN, Arnold HL, Odom RB: Andrews' Diseases of the Skin. 7th Ed. Philadelphia:WB Saunders, 1982, p. 776.

Gasner WG: Primary osteoma cutis: report of case. Arch Dermatol Syph 69:101, 1954.

Hopkins JG: Multiple miliary osteomas of the skin: report of a case. Arch Dermatol Syph 18:706, 1928.

Leider M: Osteoma cutis: report of a case. Arch Dermatol Syph 58:168, 1948.

Monserrat M: Ostéome de la langue. Bull Soc Anat 88:282, 1913.

Stafne EC, Gibilisco JA: Oral Roentgenographic Diagnosis. 4th Ed. Philadelphia:WB Saunders, 1975, p. 146.

Virchow R: Die Krankhaften Geschwulste. Vol 2. Berlin:A. Hirschwold, 1864, p. 103.

Intraoral Osseous Choristoma

Davis GB: Intraoral osseous choristoma: report of case. J Oral Surg 38: 144, 1980.

Herd JR: Extra-osseous osteoma. Aust Dent J 21:469, 1976.

Lucas RB: Pathology of Tumors of the Oral Tissues. 2nd Ed. Baltimore: Williams & Wilkins, 1972, p. 182.

Krolls SO, Jacoway JR, Alexander WN: Osseous choristomas (osteomas) of intraoral soft tissues. Oral Surg Oral Med Oral Pathol 32:588, 1971.

Long DE, Koutnik AW: Recurrent intraosseous choristoma. Oral Surg Oral Med Oral Pathol 72:337, 1991.

Mesa ML, Schneider LC, Northington L: Osteoma of the buccal mucosa. J Oral Maxillofac Surg 40:684, 1982.

Shafer WG, Hine MK, Levy BM: A Textbook of Oral Pathology. 4th Ed. Philadelphia:WB Saunders, 1983, p. 163.

Sookasam M, Philipsen HP: The intra-oral soft tissue osteoma: report of two cases. J Dent Assoc Thai 36:229, 1986.

Tohill MJ, Green JG, Cohen DM: Intraoral osseous and cartilaginous choristomas: report of three cases and review of the literature. Oral Surg Oral Med Oral Pathol 63:506, 1987.

Soft Tissue Chondroma

Chaudhry AP, Robinovitch MR, Mitchell DF: Chondrogenic tumors of the jaws. Am J Surg 102:403, 1961.

Chung EB, Enzinger FM: Chondroma of soft parts. Cancer 41:1414, 1978.

del Rio C: Chondroma of the tongue: review of the literature and case report. J Oral Med 33:54, 1978.

Forman G: Chondrosarcoma of the tongue. Br J Oral Surg 4:218, 1967.

Gardner DG, Paterson JC: Chondroma or metaplastic chondroma of soft palate. Oral Surg Oral Med Oral Pathol 26:601, 1968.

Ling KC: Chondroma of the tongue. J Oral Maxillofac Surg 44:156, 1986.

Plessier P, Leroux-Robert J: Dysembryoplasies linguales multiples a conteau carhlaneux. Ann Anat Pathol 9:430, 1932.

Ramachandran KR, Viswanathan R: Chondroma of the tongue. Oral Surg Oral Med Oral Pathol 25:487, 1968.

Stout AP, Verner EW: Chondrosarcoma of the extra-skeletal soft tissues. Cancer 6:581, 1953.

Vassar PS: Chondrosarcoma of the tongue. Arch Pathol 65:261, 1958.

Yasuoka T, Handa Y, Watanabe F, Oka N: Chondroma of the tongue. J Maxillofac Surg 12:189, 1984.

Arterial Calcification

Allen EV, Barker NW, Hinds EA Jr: Peripheral Vascular Diseases. 4th Ed. Philadelphia:WB Saunders, 1962, pp. 261, 312.

Bagdade JD: Atherosclerosis in patients undergoing maintenance hemodialysis. Kidney Int 7:S-370, 1975.

Ennis LM, Burket LW: Calcified vessels of the cheeks: demonstration by means of dental roentgenograms. Ann Dent 1:111, 1942.

Fairbairn JF II, Juergens JC, Spittell JA Jr: Peripheral Vascular Diseases. 4th Ed. Philadelphia:WB Saunders, 1972, p. 179.

Ferrier TM: Radiologically demonstrable arterial calcification in diabetes mellitus. Aust Ann Med 13:222, 1964.

Friedlander AH, Lande A: Panoramic radiographic identification of carotid arterial plaques. Oral Surg Oral Med Oral Pathol 52:102, 1981.

Hays JB, Gibilisco JA, Juergens JL: Calcification of vessels in cheek of patient with medial arteriosclerosis. Oral Surg Oral Med Oral Pathol 21:299, 1966.

Lindbom A: Arteriosclerosis and arterial thrombosis in the lower limb: a roentgenological study. Acta Radiol 80(suppl):1, 1950.

Meema HE, Oreopoulous DG, de Veber GA: Arterial calcification in severe chronic renal disease and their relationship to dialysis treatment, renal transplant, and parathyroidectomy. Radiology 121:315, 1976.

Miles DA, Craig RM: The calcified facial artery. Oral Surg Oral Med Oral Pathol 55:214, 1983.

Parfitt MA: Soft tissue calcification in uremia. Arch Intern Med 124:544, 1969.

Peterson R: Small vessel calcification and its relationship to secondary hyperparathyroidism in the renal homotransplant patient. Radiology 126:627, 1978.

Rifkin RD, Parisi AF, Folland E: Coronary calcification in the diagnosis of coronary artery disease. Am J Cardiol 44:141, 1979.

Stafne EC, Gibilisco JA: Oral Roentgenographic Diagnosis. 4th Ed. Philadelphia:WB Saunders, 1975, p. 140.

Wood NK, Goaz P: Differential Diagnosis of Oral Lesions. 2nd Ed. St. Louis:CV Mosby, 1980, p. 559.

Carotid Arterial Plaques

Eastcott HHG, Pickering GW, Rob CG: Reconstruction of internal carotid artery in a patient with intermittent attacks of hemiplegia. Lancet 2: 994, 1954.

Friedlander AH, Lande A: Panoramic radiographic identification of carotid arterial plaques. Oral Surg Oral Med Oral Pathol 52:102, 1981.

Gowers WR: In a case of simultaneous embolism of central retinal and middle cerebral arteries. Lancet 2:794, 1875.

Hunt JR: The role of the carotid arteries in the causation of vascular lesions of the brain: with remarks on certain special features of the symptomology. Am J Med Sci 147:704, 1914.

Matsumoto N, Whisnant JP, Karland LT, Okuzaki H: Natural history of stroke in Rochester, Minnesota, 1955 through 1969: an extension of a previous study, 1945 through 1954. Stroke 4:20 1973.

Moniz E, Lima A, De Lacerda R: Hémiplégie par thrombose de la carotide interne. Presse Med 45:977, 1937.

Phlebolith

Keathley CJ, Campbell RL, Isbell JW: Arteriovenous malformation and associated phleboliths: report of a case. Oral Surg Oral Med Oral Pathol 56:132, 1983.

Sturge-Weber Syndrome

Bergstrand H, Olivecrona H, Tonnis W: Gefassmissbildungen und Gefassgeschwulste des Gehirns. Stuttgart:Georg Thieme Verlag, 1936.

Brushfield T, Wyatt W: Sturge-Weber disease. Br J Child Dis 24:98, 209, 1927; 25:96, 1928.

Enjoiras O, et al: Facial port-wine stains and Sturge-Weber syndrome. Pediatrics 76:48, 1985.

Horing H: Zin Lokalisation mesenchymalev Dysplasien ber Sturge-Weber Krankhert. Arch Klin Exp Derm 209:615, 1960.

Peterman AF, et al: Encephalotrigeminal angiomatosis (Sturge-Weber disease): clinical study of 35 cases. JAMA 167:2169, 1958.

Peripheral Odontogenic Tumors with Calcification

Abrams AM, Melrose RJ, Howell FV: Adenoameloblastoma: a clinical pathologic study of the ten new cases. Cancer 22:175, 1968.

Ai-ru L, Zhen L, Jian S: Calcifying epithelial odontogenic tumors: a clinicopathologic study of nine cases. J Oral Pathol 11:399, 1982.

Baden E, Moskow BS, Moscow R: Odontogenic gingival epithelial hamartoma. J Oral Surg 26:702, 1968.
Buchner A, Sciubba JJ: Peripheral odontogenic tumors: a review. Oral Surg Oral Med Oral Pathol 63:688, 1987.
Courtney RM, Kerr DA: The odontogenic adenomatoid tumor: a comprehensive study of twenty new cases. Oral Surg Oral Med Oral Pathol 39:424, 1975.
Farman AG: The peripheral odontogenic fibroma. Oral Surg Oral Med Oral Pathol 40:82, 1975.
Fejerskov O, Krogh J: The calcifying ghost cell odontogenic tumor—or the calcifying odontogenic cyst. J Oral Pathol 1:273, 1972.
Franklin CD, Pindborg JJ: The calcifying epithelial odontogenic tumor: a review and analysis of 113 cases. Oral Surg Oral Med Oral Pathol 42: 753, 1976.
Freedman PD, Lumerman H, Gee JK: Calcifying odontogenic cyst: a review and analysis of seventy cases. Oral Surg Oral Med Oral Pathol 40:93, 1975.
Gardner DG: Peripheral ameloblastoma: a study of 21 cases, including 5 reported as basal cell carcinoma of the gingiva. Cancer 39:1625, 1977.
Giansanti JS, Someren A, Waldron CA: Odontogenic adenomatoid tumor (adenoameloblastoma). Oral Surg Oral Med Oral Pathol 30:69, 1970.
Guralnick W, Chuong R, Goodman M: Peripheral ameloblastoma of the gingiva. J Oral Maxillofac Surg 41:536, 1983.
Hietanen J, et al: Peripheral squamous odontogenic tumor. Br J Oral Maxillofac Surg 23:362, 1985.
Krolls SO, Pindborg JJ: Calcifying epithelial odontogenic tumor. Arch Pathol 98:206, 1974.
McKelvy BD, Cherrick HM: Peripheral ameloblastic fibrodentinoma. J Oral Surg 34:826, 1976.
Pindborg JJ: Calcifying epithelial odontogenic tumor. Acta Pathol Microbiol Scand 111(suppl):71, 1955.
Pullon PA, et al: Squamous odontogenic tumor. Oral Surg Oral Med Oral Pathol 40:616, 1975.
Regezi JA, Kerr DA, Courtney RM: Odontogenic tumors: analysis of 706 cases. J Oral Surg 36:771, 1978.
Simpson HE: Basal cell carcinoma and peripheral ameloblastoma. Oral Surg Oral Med Oral Pathol 38:233, 1974.
Takeda Y, Suzuki A, Sekiyama S: Peripheral calcifying epithelial odontogenic tumor. Oral Surg Oral Med Oral Pathol 56:71, 1983.
Waldron, CA: Comment on basal cell carcinoma of the oral cavity. J Oral Surg 30:66, 1972.
Yazdi I, Nowparast B: Extraosseous adenomatoid odontogenic tumor with special reference to the probability of the basal cell layer of the oral epithelium as a potential source of origin. Oral Surg Oral Med Oral Pathol 37:249, 1974.

Index